The GALE ENCYCLOPEDIA of CHILDREN'S HEALTH

INFANCY THROUGH ADOLESCENCE

SECOND EDITION

The GALE ENCYCLOPEDIA *of* CHILDREN'S HEALTH

INFANCY THROUGH ADOLESCENCE

SECOND EDITION

VOLUME

2

D–K

JACQUELINE L. LONGE, EDITOR

GALE
CENGAGE Learning™

Detroit • New York • San Francisco • New Haven, Conn • Waterville, Maine • London

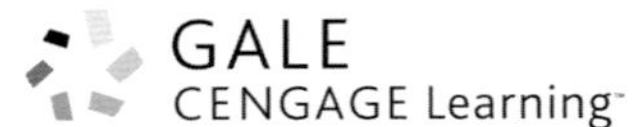

Gale Encyclopedia of Children's Health: Infancy through Adolescence, Second Edition

Project Editor: Jacqueline L. Longe

Editorial: Donna Batten, Laurie Fundukian, Kristin Key, Kristin Mallegg, Brigham Narins, Alejandro Valtierra, Jeffrey Wilson

Product Manager: Kate Hanley

Editorial Support Services: Andrea Lopeman

Indexing Services: Factiva, a Dow Jones Company

Rights Acquisition and Management: Tracie Richardson and Robyn V. Young

Composition: Evi Abou-El-Seoud

Manufacturing: Wendy Blurton

Imaging: John Watkins

Product Design: Kristine Julien

LIBRARY OF CONGRESS CATALOGING-IN-PUBLICATION DATA

Gale encyclopedia of children's health: infancy through adolescence / project editor, Jacqueline L. Longe. -- 2nd ed.
p. cm.
Includes bibliographical references and index.
ISBN 978-1-4144-8641-3 (set : alk. paper) -- ISBN 978-1-4144-8642-0 (volume 1 : alk. paper) -- ISBN 978-1-4144-8643-7 (volume 2 : alk. paper) -- ISBN 978-1-4144-8644-4 (volume 3 : alk. paper) -- ISBN 978-1-4144-8645-1 (volume 4 : alk. paper)
1. Children–Health and hygiene–Encyclopedias. 2. Children–Diseases–Encyclopedias. 3. Pediatrics–Encyclopedias. I. Longe, Jacqueline L. II. Title: Encyclopedia of children's health.
RJ26.G35 2011
618.920003–dc22

2011002635

Gale
27500 Drake Rd.
Farmington Hills, MI, 48331-3535

ISBN13: 978-1-4144-8641-3 (set) ISBN10: 1-4144-8641-3 (set)
ISBN13: 978-1-4144-8642-0 (vol. 1) ISBN10: 1-4144-8642-1 (vol. 1)
ISBN13: 978-1-4144-8643-7 (vol. 2) ISBN10: 1-4144-8643-X (vol. 2)
ISBN13: 978-1-4144-8644-4 (vol. 3) ISBN10: 1-4144-8644-8 (vol. 3)
ISBN13: 978-1-4144-8645-1 (vol. 4) ISBN10: 1-4144-8645-6 (vol. 4)

This title is also available as an e-book.
ISBN-13: 978-1-4144-8692-5 ISBN-10: 1-4144-8692-8
Contact your Gale, a part of Cengage Learning sales representative for ordering information.

Printed in China
1 2 3 4 5 6 7 15 14 13 12 11

CONTENTS

LIST OF ENTRIES

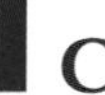

C

D

E

F

G

H

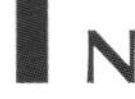

N

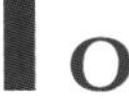

O

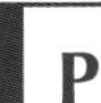

P

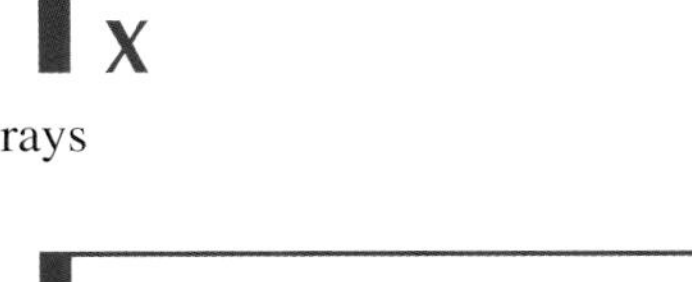

PLEASE READ—IMPORTANT INFORMATION

The *Gale Encyclopedia of Children's Health: Infancy through Adolescence* is a health reference product designed to inform and educate readers about a wide variety of topics related to children's health. Cengage Learning believes the product to be comprehensive, but not necessarily definitive. It is intended to supplement, not replace, consultation with a physician or other healthcare practitioners. While Cengage Learning has made substantial efforts to provide information that is accurate, comprehensive, and up-to-date, Cengage Learning makes no representations or warranties of any kind, including without limitation, warranties of merchantability or fitness for a particular purpose, nor does it guarantee the accuracy, comprehensiveness, or timeliness of the information contained in this product. Readers should be aware that the universe of medical knowledge is constantly growing and changing, and that differences of opinion exist among authorities. Readers are also advised to seek professional diagnosis and treatment for any medical condition, and to discuss information obtained from this book with their healthcare provider.

INTRODUCTION

The *Gale Encyclopedia of Children's Health: Infancy through Adolescence* is a one-stop source for medical information that covers common and rare diseases and medical conditions, immunizations and drugs, procedures, and developmental issues. It particularly addresses parents' concerns about their children's health from before birth through age 18. The book avoids medical jargon, making it easier for the layperson to use. The *Gale Encyclopedia of Children's Health* presents authoritative, balanced information and is more comprehensive than single-volume family medical guides.

SCOPE

Approximately 800 full-length articles are included in The *Gale Encyclopedia of Children's Health*. Articles follow a standardized format that provides information at a glance. Rubrics include:

Disease

- Definition
- Description
- Demographics
- Causes and symptoms
- Diagnosis
- Treatment
- Prognosis
- Prevention
- Clinical trials
- Parental concerns
- Resources
- Key terms

Procedures

- Definition
- Purpose
- Description
- Risks
- Results
- Parental concerns
- Resources
- Key terms

Drugs/Immunizations

- Definition
- Purpose
- Description
- Recommended dosage
- Precautions
- Side effects
- Interactions
- Parental concerns
- Resources
- Key Terms

Development

- Definition
- Description
- Common problems
- Interactions
- Parental concerns
- Resources
- Key Terms

INCLUSION CRITERIA

A preliminary list of topics was compiled from a wide variety of sources, including professional medical guides and textbooks, as well as consumer guides and encyclopedias. The advisory board, made up of medical doctors and nurses, evaluated the topics and made suggestions for inclusion. Final selection of topics to include was made by the advisory board in conjunction with the editor.

ABOUT THE CONTRIBUTORS

The essays were compiled by experienced medical writers, including physicians, pharmacists, nurses, and other health care professionals. The advisors reviewed the completed essays to ensure that they are appropriate, up-to-date, and medically accurate.

HOW TO USE THIS BOOK

The *Gale Encyclopedia of Children's Health* has been designed with ready reference in mind.

- Straight **alphabetical arrangement** of topics allows users to locate information quickly.
- **Bold-faced terms** within entries direct the reader to related articles.
- **Cross-references** placed throughout the encyclopedia direct readers from alternate names and related topics to entries.
- A list of **key terms** is provided where appropriate to define unfamiliar terms or concepts. A full glossary is available as an appendix.
- The **Resources** section for entries directs readers to additional sources of medical information on a topic.
- An appendix of updated growth charts from the U.S. Centers for Disease Control for children from birth through age 20 is included.
- A comprehensive **general index** guides readers to all topics mentioned in the text.

GRAPHICS

The *Gale Encyclopedia of Children's Health* is also enhanced by over 350 color photographs, illustrations, and tables.

ADVISORS

A number of experts in the medical community provided invaluable assistance in the formulation of this encyclopedia. Our advisory board performed a myriad of duties, from defining the scope of coverage to reviewing individual entries for accuracy and accessibility. The editor would like to express her appreciation to them.

Rosalyn Carson-DeWitt, MD
Medical Editor and Writer
Durham, North Carolina

Paul Checchia, MD, FAAP
Director, Pediatric Cardiac Intensive Care Program
St. Louis Children's Hospital
Assistant Professor of Pediatric
Critical Care and Cardiology
Washington University School of Medicine
St. Louis, Missouri

Melinda Granger Oberleitner, RN, DNS
Acting Department Head and Associate Professor
Department of Nursing
University of Louisiana at Lafayette
Lafayette, Louisiana

Brenda Wilmoth Lerner, RN
Medical Editor and Writer

Chitra Venkatasubramanian, MD
Clinical Assistant Professor, Neurology and Neurological Sciences
Stanford University School of Medicine
Palo Alto, California

CONTRIBUTORS

Margaret Alic, Ph.D.
Science Writer
Eastsound, Washington

Kim Saltel Allan, RD, BHEcol
Clinical Dietitian
Winnipeg, Manitoba, Canada

Linda K. Bennington, C.N.S., M. S.N.
Clinical Nurse Specialist
Department of Nursing
Old Dominion University
Norfolk, Virginia

Mark A. Best, MD, MBA, MPH
Pathologist
Eastview, Kentucky

Rosalyn Carson-DeWitt, MD
Durham, North Carolina

Paul Checchia, MD, FAAP
Director, Pediatric Cardiac Intensive Care Program
St. Louis Children's Hospital
Assistant Professor of Pediatric
Critical Care and Cardiology
Washington University School of Medicine
St. Louis, Missouri

Lata Cherath, PhD
Science Writer
Franklin Park, New York

Angela Costello
Medical Editor
Cleveland, Ohio

L. Lee Culvert
Medical Writer
Alna, Maine

Tish Davidson, AM
Medical Writer
Fremont, California

L. Fleming Fallon Jr., MD, DrPH
Professor of Public Health
Bowling Green University
Bowling Green, Ohio

Paula Ford-Martin
Medical Writer
Warwick, Rhode Island

Janie Franz
Medical Writer
Grand Forks, North Dakota

Rebecca J. Frey, PhD
Research and Administrative Associate
East Rock Institute
New Haven, Connecticut

Melinda Granger Oberleitner, RN, DNS
Acting Department Head and Associate Professor
Department of Nursing
University of Louisiana at Lafayette
Lafayette, Louisiana

Maureen Haggerty
Medical Writer
Ambler, Pennsylvania

Clare Hanrahan
Medical Writer
Asheville, North Carolina

Crystal H. Kaczkowski, MSc
Medical Writer
Chicago, Illinois

Christine Kuehn Kelly
Medical Writer
Havertown, Pennsylvania

Monique Laberge, PhD
Research Associate
Department of Biochemistry and Biophysics
McGill University
Montreal, Quebec Canada

Brenda Wilmoth Lerner, RN
Medical Editor and Writer

Aliene S. Linwood, BSN, DPA, FACHE
Medical and Science Writer
Athens, Ohio

Mark A. Mitchell, MD
Medical Writer
Seattle, Washington

Deborah L. Nurmi, MS
Medical Writer, Public Health Researcher
Atlanta, Georgia

Teresa G. Odle
Medical Writer
Albuquerque, New Mexico

Martha Reilly, OD
Clinical Optometrist
Madison, Wisconsin

Joan Schonbeck, RN
Medical Writer
Nursing
Massachusetts Department of Mental Health
Marlborough, Massachusetts

Stephanie Dionne Sherk
Medical Writer
Ann Arbor, Michigan

Judith Sims, MS
Science Writer
Logan, Utah

Jennifer E. Sisk, MA
Medical Writer
Philadelphia, Pennsylvania

Genevieve Slomski, PhD
Medical Writer
New Britain, Connecticut

Deanna M. Swartout-Corbeil, RN
Medical Writer
Thompsons Station, Tennessee

Samuel Uretsky, PharmD
Medical Writer
Wantagh, New York

Chitra Venkatasubramanian, MD
Clinical Assistant Professor, Neurology and Neurological Sciences
Stanford University School of Medicine
Palo Alto, California

James E. Waun, MD, MA, RPh
Adjunct Assistant Professor of Clinical Pharmacy
Ferris State University
East Lansing, Michigan

Ken R. Wells
Freelance Writer
Laguna Hills, California

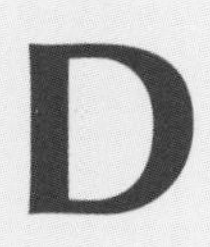

Dandruff *see* **Seborrheic dermatitis**

Day care

Definition

Day care is supervision for infants, **preschool**, and school-aged children in institutional facilities or private (**family**) homes.

Demographics

According to the National Center for Education Statistics, about three-quarters of all American children ages three to five years and not yet enrolled in kindergarten were cared for at least once a week on a regular basis by someone other than a parent. Of these children in child care, 57% were primarily in center-based care, about 23% were cared for by a member of their extended family (most often a grandparent), and 12% were cared for in a home setting by someone who was not a related to them. Some children were cared for in multiple

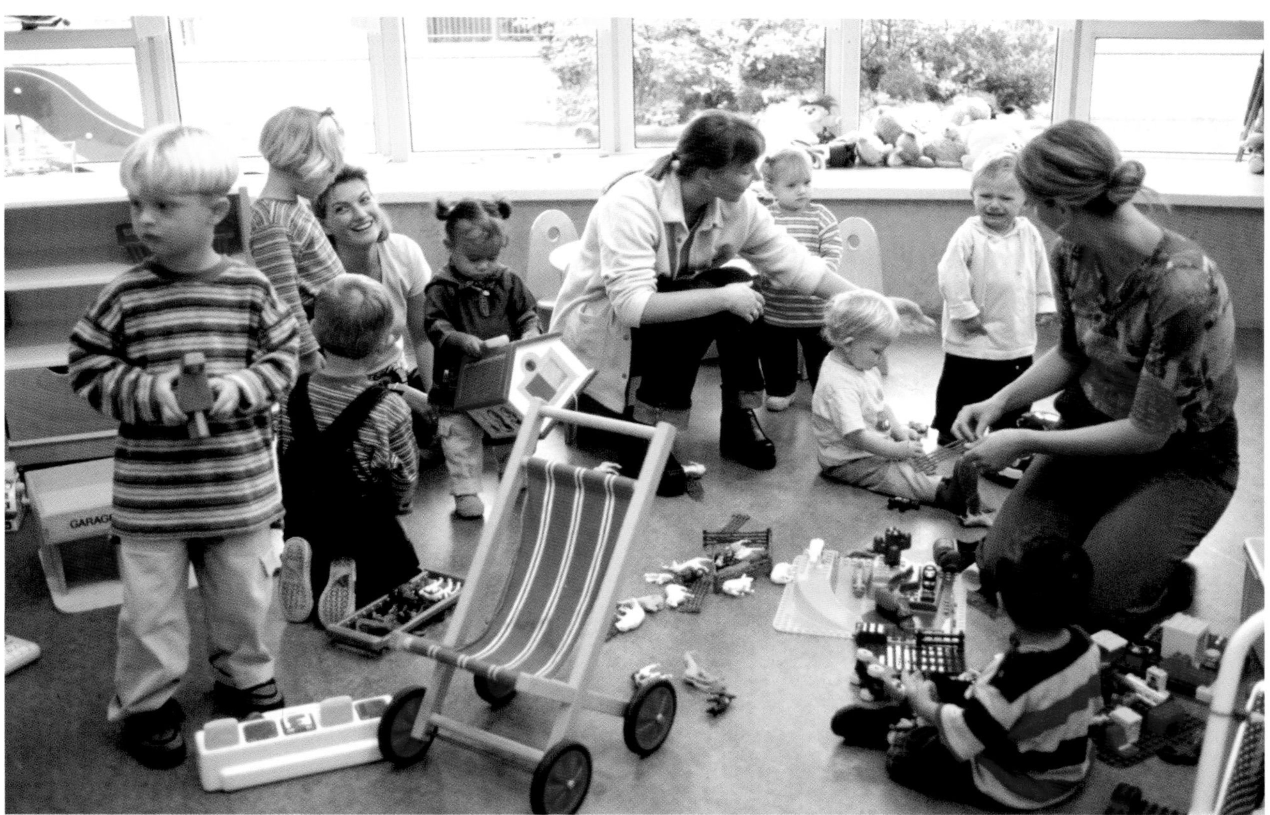

Children during playtime at a daycare center. *(© Picture Partners/Alamy.)*

settings (e.g., half a day at a child care center and half with a relative). Children from **birth** through age five or being cared for by a nonrelative in a home setting spent an average of 26.7 hours per week in nonparental care. Those being cared for by relatives spent an average of 24.3 hours per week in nonparental care, while those attending child care centers spent an average of 24.8 in center-based care.

Description

Day care centers have emerged as an important option for care of infants, preschool, and school-age children. There are two main types of day care facilities: the day care center, which is located in a public facility and equipped with a staff, and the family day care center, which is run in a home setting by a private **caregiver**. It is difficult to generalize about day care centers of either type, because structure, focus, and quality of care vary greatly. To help families in selecting day care, most states have regulations for licensing day care centers. A license is not a guarantee of quality care, but it does signify that the day care center meets certain standards of **safety**, group size, ratio of adults to children, and staff qualifications. In 2005, the number of children ages 3–6 in day care centers was almost double the number in family day care.

Effects of day care on child development

Much research has studied the effects of day care on emotional and **cognitive development**. When family factors, parents' personality traits, the child's **temperament**, and the number of different child care arrangements the child has experienced are all taken into account, most researchers conclude that day care has little or no effect on the child's emotional and cognitive development. In other words, it is difficult both to evaluate the effects of day care objectively because of the wide variation in day care experiences and to separate the effects of day care from the complex interaction of other factors such as the child's temperament and other family factors.

Day care centers

Each state sets its own regulation of day care centers. However, the National Association for the Education of Young Children (NAEYC), a professional membership organization dedicated to the healthy development of young children, issues recommendations relating to the structure and organization of day care centers, particularly those that accept infants and toddlers. These recommendations are considered to be the minimum standards a day care center should observe; a lower ratio of children to caregivers is always encouraged.

- A maximum of four infants (birth to 12 months) per caregiver, and a maximum of eight infants and two caregivers per group.
- A maximum of four young toddlers (12–24 months) per caregiver, and a maximum of 12 young toddlers and three caregivers per group.
- A maximum of six older toddlers (24–36 months) per caregiver, and a maximum of 12 older toddlers and two caregivers per group.

Benefits

Day care centers offer parents reliable, consistent care from early morning to early evening. Parents employed in weekend or evening shift positions are largely unable to secure institutional day care. Employers, such as hospitals, that rely on around-the-clock employee shifts, are increasingly being pressured to offer child care on their premises for employees. Day care centers provide young children with experience in social interaction through structured activities. Most day care centers are staffed with full-time and part-time workers, all or some of whom may have received training in child development, **first aid**, and safety procedures. Many communities require staff training as part of the day care center licensing procedure.

Precautions

Disadvantages of day care centers may include overlooking the child as an individual due to over-enrollment, inflexible center hours, and the possibility that the center management will bypass or fail to meet licensing regulations. In addition, while some day care center staff have specialized training in early childhood education and first aid, some do not. Staffing challenges are amplified by high turnover rates due to generally low wages and poor (or no) employee benefits such as medical insurance, paid vacations, and sick leave.

Family day care

Family day care centers, where children are cared for by a caregiver in her home, are often registered or licensed by their communities. Licensing requirements vary depending on the age and number of children being cared for. Many informal family day care situations where there are only a few and/or part time children on the premises are not required to be licensed in many states. Advantages of family day care include the home-like setting, offering comfort to both parents and child, potential for greater scheduling flexibility; and lower overall number of children being cared for.

The National Association for Family Child Care (NAFCC), a professional membership organization, offers these minimum standards for family day care settings:

- No more than six children per family day care provider, including the provider's own children.
- No more than two of the children in a family day care group should be under age two.
- The family day care provider should be at least 18 years old.
- The family day care provider should have completed basic training in first aid, safety, and child development.

Benefits

An individual caregiver may develop a stronger, more nurturing bond with the children she (or less often, he) cares for, and may be able to accommodate a family's need for care outside the normal business day.

Precautions

One of the key differences between day care centers and family day care is the consistency and reliability of care. Individual caretakers and relatives are less able to provide for a substitute caretaker in the event of an emergency, illness, or schedule conflict.

The decision to use day care—whether in a facility or home setting—is highly individualized. Parents should observe the activities at more than one center before making their day care choice. State and community agencies can provide guidance in identifying nearby centers to consider. Ultimately, the parents must evaluate what factors are important to them, and which staff seems to reflect the parent's own temperament, child-rearing style, and values.

Resources

BOOKS

Powers, Julie, and Yvonne Pearson. *Not Just A Babysitter: Making Child Care Work for You.* St. Paul, MN: Redleaf Press, 2005.

OTHER

Child Care. MedlinePlus. June 29, 2010 [accessed July 8, 2010], http://www.nlm.nih.gov/medlineplus/childcare.html.

National Association of Child Care Resource and Referral Agencies. [accessed July 8, 2010], http://www.naccrra.org.

ORGANIZATIONS

National Association for the Education of Young Children, 1313 L Street, NW, Suite 500, Washington DC, 20005, (202)232-8777, (800) 424-2460 or (866) NAEYC-4U, (202) 328-1846, http://www.naeyc.org.

National Association for Family Child Care (NAFCC), 1743 W. Alexander Street, Salt Lake City UT, (801) 866-2322, (800) 359-3817, (801) 866-2325, nafcc@nafcc.org, http://www.nafcc.org.

Tish Davidson, AM

Death and mourning

Definition

Mourning is a person's understanding and adjusting to death and loss at various stages of life.

Description

Almost every child or adolescent faces the death of someone close—a relative, friend, or even a pet—at some point in his or her life. In fact, it is estimated that about five percent of children under age 15, or about 1 in

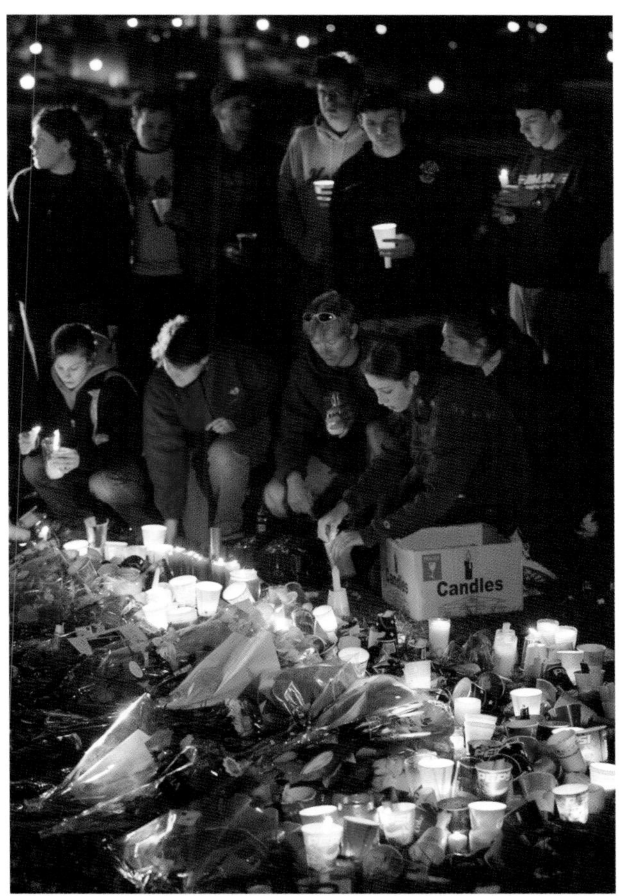

Students gather around a memorial on a college campus in remembrance of classmates killed in a school shooting. *(Scott Olson/Getty Images News/Getty Images.)*

20, will lose one or both parents. The loss of a parent before age 18 has been shown to have lasting effects on the child's later development, including his or her sense of identity. With regard to the loss of a pet, parents should keep in mind that for many children, the death of a beloved cat, dog, or other pet is usually their first encounter with death. They should let the child know that pets are also members of the **family** and that it is normal and natural to grieve for them when they die; they should never say things like, "Well, it was just an animal, it's no big deal." Many doctors think that it is helpful to allow the child to care for the pet in its last illness and to say good-bye to it before it dies.

Causes and symptoms

Parents, caregivers, and teachers can provide support and minimize **fear** by answering a child's questions about death, whether of humans or animals, honestly. Encouraging communication will help the child through the essential grieving period. At one time, well-meaning adults felt that it was in the child's best interests to avoid discussing death. Research has shown, however, that children cope more successfully with a loss or death if they feel included in the group that has experienced the loss, and share in grieving and mourning.

When listening to a child's observations about death, adults must keep an open mind. A child may respond to the death of a grandmother who used to make cupcakes for her by observing that there will be no more cupcakes for dessert. This response could be interpreted as selfish, but it is in fact an expression of the child's loss in her own very personal terms. When a child learns of the accidental death of a playmate, he may ask to go out to play. This too may be an expression of the loss, as the child might want to remember his friend by engaging in the activity the two of them shared. The child's response to loss can be misunderstood by adults, especially by those who are also grieving. By passing judgment on the child's reactions ("I can't believe you said that! Don't you feel sad that Grandma died?"), adults undermine the child's feelings and make the loss even more difficult for the child to handle.

In the days, weeks, and months that follow a death or loss, adults should refrain from criticizing or reacting negatively to the child's feelings. When the child seems to repeat the same questions over and over, the same answers, as open and honest as possible, must be repeated patiently. Young children may express concern, either directly or through behavior, about being abandoned or neglected, or fears that they may have in some way caused the death. Changes in appetite, complaints of feeling sick, and changes in activity patterns can be indications that the child is worried or anxious. Adults can help a child deal with these fears by acknowledging them and by reassuring the child that he will still be cared for, and that no one can cause a death by thoughts and feelings.

When the death or loss is unanticipated, as in the case of accidents, violence, or sudden heart attack or **stroke**, children may grieve longer and more intensely. Sad feelings may resurface over the years when the child experiences the loss anew, such as on holidays or other occasions. In addition, every death that the child experiences in later life will tend to reopen memories of the first loss. When a parent is deeply affected by the death of a loved person, the child may need the steady support of another adult. Books about illness and death can also be helpful. Adults should review the books in advance or ask a librarian, teacher, spiritual leader, or counselor for advice. Issues of concern include age-appropriateness, situation-appropriateness, and religious point of view.

Preschool and school-age years

By the time a child is about two and a half or three, he will be able to acknowledge that a death has occurred, but he will not really understand the reality of death. Research indicates that by ages five to seven, children begin to understand that death is permanent. They also begin to acknowledge the universality of death—that it happens to everyone. Around this age, children are often ready to be part of rituals of death, such as visits with the deceased's family, wakes, funerals, or memorial services. Prior to participating in a visit or funeral, it is helpful to prepare the child for the experience, and to explain the purpose of the visit—to grieve and help the family. If a child expresses reluctance to participate in any aspect of the rituals of death, adults should accept his feelings and not exert pressure.

School-aged children can understand what death means, but they may be so overwhelmed that they act as if nothing has happened. Unexpressed feelings may surface in the form of such physical symptoms as **stomachache**, **headache**, and feeling unusually tired. Behavior may also change, demonstrated by reluctance to go to school, daydreaming in class, or a decline in academic performance. On the other hand, children do not have long and sustained periods of sadness like adults. They will sometimes want to play or have fun even while they are working through their grief. Parents should not shame them or accuse them of disrespect or of not loving the person who died.

Children will both grieve alone and share their grief with others. Families can take a number of actions to support emotional healing, such as openly acknowledging the death, letting children participate in the rituals, and maintaining such familiar routines as school and bedtime activities. Parents should also let children see them grieve. Rather than avoid any mention of the deceased, it may help to display a photograph in a prominent place as a way of letting family members maintain memories. The visual reminder provides a way to help the child understand that it is okay to talk about the person who died. In many cases children benefit from attending a support group of other recently bereaved children.

Adolescence

Teenagers have an adult understanding of death, but may find it even more difficult than younger children to deal with their sorrow. Behavior problems, dropping out of school, physical complaints such as headache or chest **pain**, sexual promiscuity, and even **suicide** attempts may result from their feelings of pain and loss. Oftentimes, teenagers are reluctant to talk to adults who may help them through their grief.

The death of a peer—even someone they hardly knew—affects adolescents differently than the death of an older person. They must cope not only with the shock of life's unpredictability but also their own mortality. Adolescents may also have a similar reaction to the death of a celebrity or entertainer with whom they identified, particularly if the famous person committed suicide. It is not unusual for a celebrity's suicide to trigger a wave of copycat suicides among vulnerable adolescents.

Special circumstances

There are some situations in which children's grief will resolve more slowly because of the circumstances of the loved one's death:

- When the death occurs in the emergency department (ED) of a hospital. In most cases these are sudden and unexpected deaths, in many cases they are traumatic, and in many EDs, staff have not been trained to offer grief support even though they are usually the persons who must notify the family.
- When the death is a suicide. If it is difficult to explain death to young children, it is doubly difficult to explain why the loved one took his or her own life. While parents should not hesitate to ask a spiritual leader or grief counselor to help them explain suicide to the child, they should never lie to the child about the fact of suicide. The American Association of Suicidology maintains that "secrecy about the suicide in the hopes of protecting children may cause further complications."
- When the death results from a natural or transportation disaster. Children very often develop a form of post-traumatic stress disorder when a loved one is killed in a plane crash, avalanche, tsunami, or similar disaster. If the child was also involved in the disaster but survived, he or she may develop a form of survivor's guilt for living when the loved one died. In addition, grieving families often have their privacy violated by news media after major disasters. It is a good idea to have a trustworthy friend of the family or a grief counselor available to deal with the media and answer questions for reporters to minimize stress on the family.
- When a parent dies in military service. In addition to suffering a sudden loss, the child may not have seen the deployed parent for some time. In this situation also, there is the problem of media attention, sometimes compounded by outsiders who want to exploit military funerals as occasions for political protest.

Parental concerns

Most bereaved people begin to feel at least somewhat better within a few months after the loved one's death and to slowly return to normal activities and interests. In some cases, however, the person does not seem to be adjusting to the loss and beginning to look to the future, but is preoccupied with thoughts of the dead person, seeks him or her constantly, and is excessively lonely. Children who are having problems with complicated grief may show one or more of the following:

- a long period of depression marked by lack of interest in daily activities
- sleep disorders and/or loss of appetite
- excessive fear of being alone
- frequently dressing like or imitating the dead person
- talking repeatedly about wanting to join the dead person
- avoiding friends
- school refusal or sharp drop in academic performance

If these signs persist, the parents may want to consult a therapist who can help the child with the grieving process.

Resources

BOOKS

Barton Ross, Cheri. *Pet Loss and Human Emotion: A Guide to Recovery.* New York: Routledge, 2006.

Buckingham, R. W. *Care of the Dying Child: A Practical Guide for Those Who Help Others.* New York: Continuum, 1989.

Fiorini, Jodi J., and Jody Ann Mullen. *Counseling Children and Adolescents through Grief and Loss.* Champaign, IL: Research Press, 2006.

Harris, Maxine, Ph.D. *The Loss That Is Forever: The Lifelong Impact of the Early Death of a Mother or Father.* New York: Dutton, 1995.

O'Connor, Joey. *Children and Grief: Helping Your Child Understand Death.* Grand Rapids, MI: Revell, 2004.

Rubel, Barbara. *But I Didn't Say Goodbye: For Parents and Professionals Helping Child Suicide Survivors*. Kendall Park, NJ: Griefwork Center, 1999.

Webb, N. B., ed. *Helping Bereaved Children: A Handbook for Practitioners*. New York: Guilford Press, 1993.

PERIODICALS

Brant, Martha. "No Child Left Behind: More Than 1,200 U.S. Kids Have Lost a Parent in Iraq or Afghanistan. How the Pentagon Is Helping Them Cope." *Newsweek* April 24, 2006: 32.

Isaacs, Eric, MD, and Peter D'Souza, MD. "Grief Support in the ED." *eMedicine*, topic 694, March 16, 2006. Available online at http://www.emedicine.com/emerg/topic694.htm.

Knapp, Jane, MD, and Deborah Mulligan-Smith, MD. "Death of a Child in the Emergency Department." *Pediatrics* 115 (May 2005): 1432-1437.

Smith, Karen, and Karen Boardman. "Comforting a Child When Someone Close Dies." *Nursing* 25 (October 1995): 58-60.

Veciana-Suarez, Ana, and Julie Bourland. "A Death in the Family." *Parenting* 9 (October 1995): 80-85.

Westmoreland, Paula. "Coping with Death: Helping Students Grieve." *Childhood Education* 72 (Spring 1996): 157-160.

OTHER

American Academy of Child and Adolescent Psychiatry (AACAP). Facts for Families #78. *When a Pet Dies* Washington, DC: AACAP, 2000.

American Academy of Child and Adolescent Psychiatry (AACAP). Facts for Families #8. *Children and Grief* Washington, DC: AACAP, 2004.

American Association of Suicidology (AAS) Fact Sheet. *Survivors of Suicide* Washington, DC: AAS, 2006.

Dolan, Paul R. *Public Grief and the News Media* Miami, FL: Hospice Foundation of America, 2003. Available online at http://www.hospicefoundation.org/teleconference/2003/dolan.asp.

Fassler, David MD. *Talking to Children about the Death of a Public Figure* Washington, DC: American Academy of Child and Adolescent Psychiatry (AACAP), 2006. Available online at http://www.aacap.org.

Hospice Foundation of America (HFA). *Eight Myths about Children and Loss* Miami, FL: HFA, 2006. Available online at http://www.hospicefoundation.org/griefAndLoss/myths_children.asp.

ORGANIZATIONS

American Academy of Child and Adolescent Psychiatry (AACAP), 3615 Wisconsin Avenue NW, Washington DC, 20016-3007, (800) 333-7636 (202) 966-7300, http://www.aacap.org.

American Association of Suicidology, 5221 Wisconsin Avenue, NW, Washington DC, 20015, (202) 237-2280, (800) 273-TALK, http://www.suicidology.org.

Hospice Foundation of America (HFA), 12000 Biscayne Boulevard #505, Miami FL, 33181, (800) 854-3402, http://www.hospicefoundation.org.

Decongestants

Definition

Decongestants are medicines used to relieve nasal congestion (stuffy nose).

Purpose

A congested or stuffy nose is a common symptom of colds and **allergies**. This congestion results when membranes lining the nose become swollen. Decongestants relieve the swelling by narrowing the blood vessels that supply the nose. This reduces the blood supply to the swollen membranes, causing the membranes to shrink.

These medicines do not cure colds or reverse the effects of histamines—chemicals released as part of the allergic reaction. They will not relieve all of the symptoms associated with colds and allergies, only the stuffiness.

When considering whether to use a decongestant for cold symptoms, keep in mind that most colds go away with or without treatment and that taking medicine is not the only way to relieve a stuffy nose. Drinking hot tea or broth or eating chicken soup may help. There are also adhesive strips that can be placed on the nose to help widen the nasal passages, making breathing through the nasal passages a bit easier when congestion is present.

Precautions

Over the counter medications pose a significant potential risk to children's (under the age of 18) health and well being. Approximately 7,000 children under the age of 13 are treated in emergency rooms annually for adverse reactions from these medicines. A majority of them are under the age of five.

Children may also be more sensitive to the effects of decongestants. Before giving any decongestant to a child, check the package label carefully. Some of these medicines are too strong for use in children. Serious side effects are possible if they are given large amounts of these drugs or if they swallow nose drops, nasal spray or eye drops. If this happens, call a physician or poison center immediately.

General use

A congested or stuffy nose is a common symptom of colds and allergies. This congestion results when membranes lining the nose become swollen. Decongestants relieve the swelling by narrowing the blood vessels that supply the nose. This narrowing reduces the blood supply to the swollen membranes, causing them to shrink.

These medicines do not cure colds or reverse the effects of histamines, chemicals released as part of the allergic reaction. They will not relieve all of the symptoms associated with colds and allergies, only the stuffiness.

Nasal decongestants may be used in many forms, including tablets, nose drops, and nasal sprays.

Side effects

DECONGESTANT NASAL SPRAYS AND NOSE DROPS The most common side effects from decongestant nasal sprays and nose drops are sneezing and temporary burning, stinging, or dryness. These effects are usually temporary and do not need medical attention. If any of the following side effects occur after using a decongestant nasal spray or nose drops, stop using the medicine immediately and call the physician:

- increased blood pressure
- headache
- fast, slow, or fluttery heartbeat
- nervousness
- dizziness
- nausea
- sleep problems

DECONGESTANTS TAKEN BY MOUTH The most common side effects of decongestants taken by mouth are nervousness, restlessness, excitability, **dizziness**, drowsiness, **headache**, nausea, weakness, and **sleep** problems. Anyone who has these symptoms while taking decongestants should stop taking them immediately.

Patients who have these symptoms while taking decongestants should call the physician immediately:

- increased blood pressure
- fast, irregular, or fluttery heartbeat
- severe headache
- tightness or discomfort in the chest
- breathing problems
- fear or anxiety
- hallucinations
- trembling or shaking
- convulsions (seizures)
- pale skin
- painful or difficult urination

Other side effects may occur. Anyone who has unusual symptoms after taking a decongestant should get in touch with his or her physician.

KEY TERMS

Fetus—A developing baby inside the womb.

Hallucination—A false or distorted perception of objects, sounds, or events that seems real. Hallucinations usually result from drugs or mental disorders.

Interactions with other medicines

Decongestants do not have any interactions with drugs that would be taken by a generally healthy child. Even so, people using decongestants should review their drug therapy with a physician or pharmacist before starting treatment.

Although decongestants have the potential for serious side effects and adverse effects, they are very safe when used properly. However, nasal decongestants should only be used for three days at a time to avoid significant rebound effect. The most severe adverse effects can be avoided by using nose drops and nasal sprays in place of tablets or capsules.

Description

Decongestants are sold in many forms, including tablets, capsules, caplets, gelcaps, liqui-caps, liquids, nasal sprays, and nose drops. These drugs are sometimes combined with other medicines in cold and allergy products designed to relieve several symptoms. Some decongestant products require a physician's prescription, but there are also many nonprescription (over-the-counter) products. Ask a physician or pharmacist about choosing an appropriate decongestant.

The recommended dosage depends on the drug. Check with the physician who prescribed the drug or the pharmacist who filled the prescription for the correct dosage, and always take the medicine exactly as directed. If using nonprescription (over-the-counter) types, follow the directions on the package label or ask a pharmacist for assistance. Never give children larger or more frequent doses, and do not give the drug for longer than directed.

Risks

There are several reasons that children are more likely to have problems with drugs that can be purchased without a prescription:

- Children are more likely than adults to experience drowsiness or excitement from the antihistamines and alcohol in adult cough medicines.
- Dosing errors are more likely to occur if household devices, like teaspoons, are used to measure and administer medications instead of the droppers provided with medication packages.
- Many products, like cough and cold medicines and sleep aids, contain the same drugs, like acetaminophen, ibuprophen or antihistamines, making overdosing more likely.
- Over the counter drugs were developed for adults, and then used in children.
- Except for ibuprophen and acetaminophen, used to treat fever or discomfort, over the counter medicines have not been thoroughly tested for safety or effectiveness in children.

Parental concerns

Parents administering these drugs to their children should use nose drops or nasal spray and avoid tablets or capsules, which are more likely to cause adverse effects. They should also review the proper administration of nose drops and nasal spray with a physician or nurse.

Decongestants are subject to abuse. Parents should observe the behavior of adolescents and teens who may be purposely overdosing on these drugs.

In the event of severe adverse effects, parents should get medical care immediately for their child.

What parents should keep in mind when giving over the counter medicines to children.

- To avoid drug duplication and possible overdose, know what drug(s) are in every over the counter product you give children.
- Give medications only according to package directions using the delivery device provided.
- Over the counter medicines do not treat the underlying causes of the symptoms of a cold or flu and have no effect on how long they last.
- Your pharmacist is a valuable resource for information and advice on over the counter medications.
- Non-drug treatments for the discomforts of coughs and colds include sucking on hard candy or lozenges and drinking extra cold beverages.

Resources

PERIODICALS

Henderson, Charles W. "Voluntary Withdrawal of Cold and Allergy Products Announced." *Medical Letter on the CDC and FDA*, November 26, 2000.

"An Ingredient Under Fire: Drugmakers are Jittery Afteran FDA Panel Ruling." *Newsweek* October 30, 2000: 59.

OTHER

"Giving Medication to Children: Q & A with Dianne Murphy, MD." FDA Consumer Health Information, http://www.fda.gov/consumer (accessed December 15, 2010).

Medline Plus Health Information. U.S. National Library of Medicine. http://www.nlm.nih.gov/medlineplus.

James Waun, MD, RPh, MA
Deanna M. Swartout-Corbeil, RN

Deductive reasoning

Definition

Deductive reasoning is reasoning that constructs or tests the validity of deductive arguments. Deductive arguments in turn attempt to show that a conclusion must follow necessarily from a set of premises. A deductive argument moves from the general to the particular, in contrast to inductive reasoning, which moves from the particular to the general.

Purpose

Deductive reasoning is used in a wide variety of fields, most often mathematics, philosophy, and computer science, although it also has many applications in law and detective work. Many of the famous Sherlock Holmes stories contain examples of the master sleuth's skill at deductive reasoning. In a short story titled "A Scandal in Bohemia," Holmes astounds his friend Dr. Watson by deducing from the appearance of the doctor's boots that he had recently gotten soaked in the rain and that he had a clumsy and careless servant. "[My method] is simplicity itself.... My eyes tell me that on the inside of your left shoe, just where the firelight strikes it, the leather is scored by six almost parallel cuts. Obviously they have been caused by someone who has very carelessly scraped round the edges of the sole in order to remove crusted mud from it. Hence, you see, my double deduction that you had been out in vile weather, and that you had a particularly malignant boot-slitting specimen of the London [servant girl]."

The Holmes example shows that people often use deductive reasoning in everyday life even when they are not aware of the formal structure of the process. An example might be a scientist packing for a field trip to the American Southwest in the summer. She knows on the basis of general information that people should dress comfortably in the summer but also protect themselves against sun exposure. She also knows that summer in the Southwest is characterized by high heat and few clouds to block the sun. She therefore packs a hat and plenty of sunscreen in her suitcase as well as easy-care shirts and shorts.

Description

The most common example of deductive reasoning is the syllogism, which goes back at least as far as the Greek philosopher Aristotle (384–322 BC). Aristotle defined a syllogism as a type of logical argument in which one proposition—the conclusion—is deduced from two propositions known as premises. The first premise is called the major premise and the second one is called the minor premise. An example of a syllogism is as follows: All cats are animals. Blackie is a cat. Therefore Blackie is an animal.

The deductive reasoning used by the traveling scientist could also be put in the form of a syllogism: People should dress appropriately for hot weather and high sun. It is hot in the American Southwest in the summer and the sunlight is intense. Therefore, I should take appropriate clothing and sun protection when I travel to the Southwest in summertime.

Stages in learning deductive reasoning

Deductive reasoning is a skill that humans develop in stages, beginning in middle childhood. The best-known researcher in the field of children's **cognitive development** is Jean Piaget (1896–1980), a Swiss psychologist. Piaget became interested in the development of children's reasoning abilities when he began working with Alfred Binet (1857–1911), a French psychologist who developed the first widely used **intelligence** test. Piaget noticed as he was scoring children's answers to Binet's tests that younger children made types of mistakes that older children and adults did not. He came to think that children's cognitive development, including the ability to reason, unfolds in stages, and that these stages are age-related. The stages that are most important for understanding children's development of deductive reasoning are as follows:

- The preoperational stage (ages two to seven years). In this stage, children have not yet learned to perform purely mental operations. For example, if a child in this stage wishes to add three blocks in a line to two blocks, he or she will have to move the blocks physically to perform the addition. Children in this stage also make errors in deductive logic. For example, if a child is shown a picture of six cats and three dogs and asked whether there are more cats than dogs in the picture, he or she will usually give the correct answer. But when asked whether there are more cats than animals in the picture, the child will usually state again that there are more cats.
- The concrete operational stage (ages seven to 11 years). In this stage the child begins to use deductive reasoning correctly. One example is transitivity: if the child knows that object A is taller than B and that B is taller than C, he or she will state that A is taller than C. In this stage, however, children are still not capable of working with abstract concepts; they can solve only problems that involve concrete objects or specific events. In the example of concrete operational thinking, a little boy is told that a glass hit with a hammer will break. He is then asked what happens when an imaginary child named Don hits a glass with a hammer. The boy answers immediately that the glass will break.
- The formal operational phase (age 11 to adulthood). In this stage, people are able to move beyond concrete objects; they begin to think abstractly, reason logically, and draw conclusions from the information available. They can also apply these reasoning processes to hypothetical situations. Adolescents are able to devise plans for solving problems and testing possible solutions, using a form of deductive reasoning to eliminate the unsatisfactory approaches. Many begin to apply their new skills at the high school level in such subjects as mathematics (particularly plane geometry) and the laboratory sciences. At the college level, students who are interested can take courses in formal logic in either the philosophy or mathematics department; they may also be encouraged to apply deductive reasoning in such fields as history or psychology. Adults can use deductive reasoning in many occupations; for example, a doctor who is working on a differential diagnosis is carrying out a systematic process of considering various possible causes of the patient's symptoms and eliminating those that do not fit the laboratory test results or the patient's history.

Common problems

Deductive reasoning depends on the accuracy of the facts used in the deduction to yield reliable results. It is possible for a syllogism to be valid without being sound. A syllogism is valid when its conclusion follows logically from its premises, even though the premises may be false. An example: All cats are rats. All rats are

KEY TERMS

Cognitive—Pertaining to such mental processes as thinking, knowing, remembering, analyzing, and other forms of information processing.

Logic—The branch of philosophy that deals with correct reasoning and the analysis of arguments.

Premise—An assertion or proposition used in deductive reasoning to arrive at a conclusion.

Sound—Referring to a syllogism that is both valid and based on true premises.

Syllogism—A form of argument in which two premises are stated and a conclusion is drawn from them.

Valid—Referring to a syllogism whose conclusion follows logically from its premises even though the premises may be false.

dogs. Therefore all cats are dogs. Both premises are false but the conclusion is still valid.

In contrast, a sound syllogism is one in which the conclusion follows logically from premises that are true. Older children, adolescents, and adults wishing to improve their skills in deductive reasoning should make sure that they are working with known or verifiable facts.

Parental concerns

As with other cognitive skills, children do not develop the ability to identify and use deductive reasoning at the same rate. Parents who are concerned that their child is having difficulty with logical reasoning should consult the child's teacher. In many cases tutoring can help, particularly if the child's difficulty is showing up in a mathematics class. There are puzzles, games of logic, and other strategies that teachers can use with older children or teenagers to help them learn deductive reasoning.

Resources

BOOKS

Inhelder, Barbel, and Jean Piaget. *The Growth of Logical Thinking from Childhood to Adolescence; An Essay on the Construction of Formal Operational Structures*, translated by Anne Parsons and Stanley Milgram. New York: Basic Books, 1958.

Ross, Debra Ann. *Master Math: Geometry: Including Everything from Triangles, Polygons, Proofs, and Deductive Reasoning to Circles, Solids, Similarity, and Coordinate Geometry*. Clifton Park, NY: Thomson/ Delmar Learning, 2005.

Salmon, Merrilee H. *Introduction to Logic and Critical Thinking*. 5th ed. Belmont, CA: Thomson Wadsworth, 2007.

PERIODICALS

McFeeters, P. Janelle, and Ralph T. Mason. "Learning Deductive Reasoning through Games of Logic." *Mathematics Teacher* 103 (November 2009): 284.

Pillow, B.H., et al. "Children's and Adults' Judgments of the Certainty of Deductive Inferences, Inductive Inferences, and Guesses." *Journal of Genetic Psychology* 171 (July-September 2010): 203–17.

Wanko, Jeffrey J. "Deductive Puzzling." *Mathematics Teaching in the Middle School* 15 (May 2010): 524.

ORGANIZATIONS

American Psychological Association (APA), 750 First Street NE, Washington DC, 20002, (202) 336-5500, (800) 374–2721, http://www.apa.org.

Jean Piaget Society (JPS), c/o Geoffrey Saxe, 4315 Tolman Hall, University of California, Berkeley, Berkeley CA United States, 94704, (510) 643–6627, saxe@socrates.berkeley.edu, http://www.piaget.org.

Society for Research in Child Development (SRCD), 2950 S. State Street, Suite 401, Ann Arbor MI, 48104, (734) 926-0600, (734) 926-0601, info@srcd.org, http://www.srcd.org.

National Council of Teachers of Mathematics (NCTM), 1906 Association Drive, Reston VA, 20191, (703) 620-9840, (800) 235-7566, (703) 476-2970, nctm@nctm.org, http://www.nctm.org.

Rebecca J. Frey, PhD

Defense mechanisms

Definition

Defense mechanisms are unconscious strategies used by humans for avoiding or reducing such threatening feelings as **fear** and **anxiety**; to cope with upsetting events in the real world; and to repair damage to or maintain one's self-image. They should not be confused with coping strategies.

Purpose

Defense mechanisms serve several purposes: to ease the transitions from childhood to **adolescence** and mature adulthood; to protect a person's ego or sense of self from anxiety; to provide a person with a temporary respite from a frightening or traumatic situation until they can better cope with it; and to allow a mature person to integrate conflicting thoughts and feelings in an effective fashion.

Demographics

Defense mechanisms are ubiquitous in human beings; some, in fact, are part of the normal process of human intellectual and psychological maturation. People vary, however, in their ability to replace relatively immature defense mechanisms with more mature forms as they grow older, and they vary in their ability to use defense mechanisms flexibly and appropriately.

Description

The concept of the defense mechanism originated with Sigmund Freud (1856–1939), the inventor of psychoanalysis, and was later elaborated by other psychodynamically oriented theorists, notably his daughter Anna Freud (1895–1982). According to Freudian theory, defense mechanisms allow negative feelings to be lessened without an alteration of the situation that is producing them, often by distorting the reality of that situation in some way. In more recent years, however, psychiatrists have moved away from Freud's understanding of defense mechanisms as related to drives to interpreting them as devices to maintain the individual's **self-esteem**.

While defense mechanisms can help in coping with environmental or interpersonal stress, they pose a danger because the reduction of stress can be so appealing that the defenses are maintained and become habitual. They can also be harmful if they become a person's primary mode of responding to problems. In children, excessive dependence on defense mechanisms may produce social isolation and distortion of reality and hamper the ability to engage in and learn from new experiences.

While there is no list or classification of defense mechanisms that is universally accepted, the four-tier categorization introduced by George Vaillant (1934–), an American psychiatrist, in 1977 is widely used. Vaillant classified defense mechanisms according to the level of psychological development that they represent. His four levels are I, pathological; II, immature; III, neurotic; and IV, mature. The *Diagnostic and Statistical Manual of Mental Disorders-IV, Text Revision* (also known as the DSM-IV-TR), which is the standard manual used by psychiatrists in the United States, uses a modified version of Vaillant's classification.

Level I defense mechanisms

Level I defense mechanisms are considered pathological because they involve reconstructing external phenomena or events in order to eliminate the need to deal with the real world. These defenses are typically found in patients diagnosed with **schizophrenia** and other psychoses, but may also occur in young children.

- Delusional projection. This defense involves imposing gross delusions on the external world; the delusions often involve feelings of persecution. An example would be a person who interprets a routine traffic stop as proof that he is being investigated by the FBI or that the police officer is a secret agent of a foreign power.
- Denial. In denial, an unpleasant reality is ignored, and a realistic interpretation of potentially threatening events is replaced by a benign but inaccurate one. Denial is a common defense mechanism in alcoholics and drug addicts in that they will typically deny that they have a problem with substance abuse or that it is affecting their employment and family life. In very young children, however, a degree of denial is normal. One way of coping with the relative powerlessness of childhood is for young children to sometimes act as if they can change reality by refusing to acknowledge it, thereby ascribing magical powers to their thoughts and wishes. For example, a child who is told that her parents are divorcing may deny that it is happening or deny that she is upset about the divorce. Denial has been shown to be effective in reducing the arousal caused by a threatening situation. In a criminal attack, plane crash or severe auto accident, or other extreme situations, denial can temporarily be useful in helping people cope with the immediate impact of the event, but in the long term painful feelings and events must be acknowledged in order to avoid further psychological and emotional problems.
- Distortion. Distortion represents an exaggerated and irrational reshaping of a real-world situation to meet the person's emotional needs. An example would be that of an abusive parent who interprets a baby's crying as a failure or refusal on the child's part to take care of the parent. Another common example of distortion is accusing someone who accidentally makes a mess (spilling food, splashing mud on a pedestrian while driving along a rain-soaked street, a baby soiling its diaper) of having done so deliberately.
- Splitting. Sometimes called all-or-nothing thinking, splitting is a primitive defense mechanism in which a person sees others as all good or all bad; they are unable to understand others as mixtures of different qualities. Splitting is commonly observed in persons with borderline or narcissistic personality disorder.
- Extreme projection. In projection, undesirable feelings are attributed to another person or persons. An angry person believes others are angry at her; a person who is critical of others believes they are critical of him. Very young children are especially prone to projection because of their egocentric orientation, which blurs the

boundary between themselves and others, making it easier to also blur the distinction between their feelings and those of others.

Level II defense mechanisms

Vaillant classifies level II defense mechanisms as immature. They are normal in adolescents, but used excessively in adults, they lead to difficulties in coping, unpopularity with other people, and finding oneself in potentially dangerous situations:

- Acting out. Acting out refers to carrying out a behavior—usually an antisocial act—rather than managing or controlling the underlying feelings or the impulse to perform the act. Taking drugs, sexual promiscuity, shoplifting, or throwing a temper tantrum are common forms of acting out.
- Fantasy. Fantasy as a defense mechanism involves living in a dream world. A classic literary example is the short story by James Thurber titled "The Secret Life of Walter Mitty." In this story the central character variously imagines himself as a heroic Navy pilot, a brilliant surgeon, a participant in a courtroom drama, a World War I air ace, and a condemned man facing a firing squad.
- Idealization. Idealization refers to the unconscious perception of another person or situation as better or more desirable than is really the case. For example, a person may consider a job offer to be "perfect" and overlook the downside of the job requirements, company location, etc.
- Passive aggression. Passive aggression refers to an unconscious resistance to following through on commitments or fulfilling the expectations of others. It includes such behaviors as procrastination, "forgetting" a request or assignment, stubbornness, a generally sullen attitude while obeying an order, or repeated failure to complete assigned tasks.
- Projective identification. Projective identification is a process of interaction characterized by a self-fulfilling prophecy; the affected person has a false belief about the other and acts toward the other in accordance with that false belief. Eventually the other person responds by altering their behavior to make the belief come true. An example would be that of someone who is convinced another person dislikes him, so he acts in a hostile or irritable fashion toward the other. Sooner or later the other will usually come to dislike and reject him in actuality.
- Somatization. Somatization is a defense mechanism in which the person's unconscious feelings are turned against the body and emerge in the form of physical symptoms. An example would be that of someone who is afraid to tell an abusive relative what they think of them in words, but feel nauseated and vomit when they have to spend a long period of time visiting the abusive person. Somatization can also take the form of chronic headaches, skin rashes, diarrhea, and fatigue.

Level III defense mechanisms

Level III defense mechanisms are characterized as neurotic; that is, they reflect emotional distress but do not involve delusions, hallucinations, or behaviors that fall outside social norms. Neurotic defense mechanisms are commonplace in adults; they can be useful in short-term coping but can cause long-term damage to relationships and employment.

- Displacement. Displacement is a defense in which an impulse perceived as dangerous is displaced, either through redirection toward a different object or replacement by another impulse. In the first type, known as object displacement, anger or another emotion is initially felt toward a person against whom it is unsafe to express it (in children, for example, toward a parent). Displacement functions as a means by which the impulse can still be expressed, allowing release of the original emotion, but toward a safer target, such as a sibling, peer, or even a toy. In the second type of displacement, known as drive displacement, the object of the emotion remains the same but the emotion itself is replaced by a less threatening one.
- Dissociation. Dissociation refers to a compartmentalization or sealing-off of strong emotions in order to avoid being overwhelmed by them at the time of a traumatic event. Dissociation may include amnesia (loss of memory) of the event, psychological numbing, depersonalization (a feeling that the self is unreal), or derealization (a feeling that the environment is unreal or dreamlike). Dissociation is a characteristic feature of post-traumatic stress disorder (PTSD).
- Hypochondriasis. Hypochondriasis refers to excessive worry about having a serious illness.
- Intellectualization. Intellectualization is a defense mechanism in which a person uses reasoning or intellectual analysis of a situation as a way of distancing themselves from strong emotions aroused by the situation. An example might be someone who deals with fears of a relationship breaking up by making a list of reasons why the other person is sure to stay in the relationship.
- Isolation. Isolation is a rather complicated defense. It involves compartmentalizing one's experience so that an event becomes separated from the feelings that accompanied it, allowing it to be consciously available without the threat of painful feelings. For example, a witness of a murder might describe the murder in graphic detail without any emotional response or reaction.

- Rationalization. Rationalization represents an attempt to deny one's true motives to oneself or others by using a reason (or rationale) that is more logical or socially acceptable than one's own impulses. Typical rationalizations include such statements as "I don't care that I wasn't chosen for the team; I didn't really want to play soccer anyway" and "I couldn't get my homework done because I had too many other things to do." Adolescents, caught between their own unruly impulses and adult expectations that seem unreasonable, are especially prone to rationalizing their behavior. Their advanced cognitive development makes many adolescents adept at this strategy.
- Repression. Repression is a defense mechanism in which painful feelings are conscious initially and then forgotten. However, they are stored in the unconscious, from which they can be retrieved under certain circumstances—a phenomenon Freud called "the return of the repressed." Repression can range from momentary memory lapses to forgetting the details of a catastrophic event, such as a murder or an earthquake. Complete amnesia can even occur in cases where a person has experienced something very painful. Other situations may also occasion the repression of hostile feelings toward a loved one, especially a parent. Possibly the most extreme is child abuse, the memory of which may remain repressed long into adulthood, sometimes being deliberately retrieved in therapy through hypnosis and other techniques.
- Reaction formation. Reaction formation involves behavior that is diametrically opposed to the impulses or feelings that one is repressing. For example, a parent who is repressing feelings of resentment or rejection toward a child may overcompensate by appearing to be lavishly generous and solicitous of the child's welfare. In this type of situation, the child generally senses the true hostility underlying the parent's behavior. A child who is being toilet trained may show an exaggerated sense of fastidiousness to counter conflicts over controlling elimination. The Freudian stage of sexual latency in middle childhood is yet another example of reaction formation: in order to repress their sexual feelings, children at this age evince a strong sense of indifference or even hostility toward the opposite sex. In adults, reaction formation is often noticeable by its exaggerated and inflexible nature. For example, a person in whom cleanliness is a reaction formation against a desire to soil or defile their surroundings will clean their room (or themselves) several times a day and become extremely upset about a minor speck of dirt on the floor or their clothing.
- Undoing. Undoing refers to managing an unhealthy, destructive, or otherwise threatening thought by performing a contrary behavior. An example would be being overly nice to someone after feeling a desire to hurt them in some way.

Level IV defense mechanisms

Level IV defense mechanisms represent mature ways to integrate conflicting thoughts and emotions and enhance the person's satisfaction in life. Mature defenses may originate during earlier stages of personal development but are used effectively in adult life to increase the chances of success in work and relationships. They include:

- Altruism. Altruism represents constructive forms of service to others (including animals or the environment) that lead to personal satisfaction. Altruism includes such actions as volunteering one's time to help others, giving up one's seat on a bus to an elderly or disabled person, or donating money to a charity.
- Humor. Humor is a defense that includes the ability to see the absurd or funny features of an otherwise distressing event and to express these features in a way that relieves tension and may help others to laugh as well. Humor is, however, often relative to a specific culture or setting and may need to be interpreted within that context. A real-life example concerns an American ballerina who was performing on a European stage that slanted toward the audience rather than being completely level. She lost her balance, fell, and slid forward for some distance. Her partner mimicked the arm gestures of a baseball umpire and yelled "Safe!" Those who understood baseball (including the ballerina) could laugh about the incident rather than getting upset and disrupting the entire ballet.
- Anticipation. Anticipation is a defense mechanism that allows a person to make realistic plans about a future problem or unpleasant event, such as putting aside money for retirement or having one's car checked and serviced before a cross-country trip.
- Thought suppression. Thought suppression involves a conscious effort to manage unpleasant feelings through a decision not to think about them. Suppression differs from repression and denial in that the undesirable feelings are available but deliberately ignored—unlike repression and denial, in which the person is completely unaware of these feelings. Suppression generally works by replacing unpleasant thoughts with others that do not produce stress. Thought suppression may be done instinctively, or it may be done deliberately in a therapeutic context. Cognitive behavior therapy makes use of this technique to help people combat negative thought patterns that produce maladaptive emotions and behavior. For example, a child may be instructed to block feelings of

fear by thinking about a pleasant experience, such as a party, an academic achievement, or a victory in a sporting event. Suppression is considered one of the more mature and healthy defense mechanisms.

- Identification. In identification, a person unconsciously models their own character and behavior on that of someone they admire. Identification is basic to human development and an essential part of the learning process, but it can also serve as a defense mechanism. It can be negative as well as positive. Taking on the characteristics of someone else can enable a person to engage in impulses or behavior that she sees as forbidden to her but acceptable for the person with whom she is identifying. Still another motive for identification is a fear of losing the person with whom one identifies. One particularly well-known variety of identification is identification with the aggressor, in which someone who is victimized in some way takes on the traits of the victimizer to combat feelings of powerlessness. This type of projection occurs when a child who is abused by his parents abuses others in turn.
- Introjection. Introjection refers to identifying with or internalizing an idea or object so deeply that it becomes a part of that person. It is less inclusive than identification; in introjection, only a particular aspect of someone else's personality or character is internalized.
- Sublimation. Sublimation is considered one of the healthiest defense mechanisms. It involves rechanneling the energy connected with an unacceptable impulse into one that is more socially acceptable. In this way, inappropriate sexual or aggressive impulses can be released in sports, art or dance, writing and other creative pursuits, religious worship, or other worthwhile activities. Undesired feelings can also be sublimated into altruistic impulses, from which one may derive the vicarious pleasure of helping others.

Common problems

Common problems with defense mechanisms range from the lack of an agreed-upon classification or interpretation of them to the difficulty of identifying or dealing with them in one's own **family** or workplace context. The average person (that is, one who is not a trained psychoanalyst or psychotherapist) may find themselves having recurrent problems with a family member or colleague at work without being able to pinpoint the source of the problems or how to cope with them. In many cases, the person who is using immature, neurotic, or pathological defense mechanisms is just as puzzled by their occupational setbacks or interpersonal rejections. In addition, the very nature of defense mechanisms makes it difficult for the affected person to accept a health care professional's identification of their problem, as their self-esteem is at stake.

One measure that can be used with adolescents and adults in assessing problematic defense mechanisms is a self-report questionnaire known as the Defense Style Questionnaire-40 or the DSQ-40, first published in 1993. The DSQ-40 is a set of 40 questions intended to identify the test-taker's characteristic defense mechanisms. The person is instructed to rate each of the 40 items on a scale from 1 (strongly disagree) to 9 (strongly agree). There are two items for each of 20 defense mechanisms, grouped into three broad defensive styles: mature, which consists of four mechanisms (humor, suppression, sublimation, and anticipation); neurotic, which consists of four mechanisms (reaction formation, idealization, pseudo-altruism, and undoing); and immature, which includes 12 mechanisms (rationalization, autistic fantasy, displacement, isolation, dissociation, devaluation, splitting, denial, passive aggression, somatization, **acting out**, and projection). It will be noted that the DSQ-40 categorization overlaps with Vaillant's, although it identifies some of his neurotic defense mechanisms as immature.

Most adults and older adolescents who are having difficulties in life from the use of immature or neurotic defense mechanisms can benefit from some form of insight-oriented therapy, although it is critical that those abusing drugs or alcohol receive treatment for their **substance abuse** and stop using prior to psychiatric treatment. Cognitive **behavioral therapy** (CBT) is the most widely used form of insight-oriented therapy in treating emotional disorders involving defense mechanisms; however, people whose defense mechanisms originated in childhood as a way to cope with disturbed parents may also benefit from psychodynamic psychotherapy, which is an approach to treatment that includes exploration of childhood history.

Parental concerns

Parental concerns about defense mechanisms are largely related to age-appropriateness in younger children and the possibility of a personality disorder in older adolescents. Some defense mechanisms considered immature in adults are regarded as part of normal psychological and **emotional development** in children and younger adolescents. Parents concerned about their child's use of defense mechanisms—particularly if they involve gross delusions rather than fantasies, or severe splitting—should consult a specialist in child and adolescent psychiatry.

KEY TERMS

Delusion—A fixed belief that is either false or illusory and that is maintained by the individual in spite of contrary evidence.

Insight-oriented therapy—An approach to psychotherapy based on helping the client understand the existence of previously unconscious conflicts and the origin of maladaptive behavior in order to change it.

Latency phase—In Freudian theory, the phase in a child's development in which sexual issues are largely quiet (latent) and the child develops its sense of self and acquires culturally approved skills and values. It is usually identified as the period between the child's starting school between the ages of 3 and 7, and the beginning of puberty.

Psychosis—A severe mental disorder characterized by loss of contact with reality, as evidenced by delusions and hallucinations.

Self-report questionnaire—A type of psychological test in which a person answers a set of questions without the help of the person administering the test. It is also called a self-report inventory.

Resources

BOOKS

American Psychiatric Association. *Diagnostic and Statistical Manual of Mental Disorders*. 4th ed., Text rev. Washington, D.C.: American Psychiatric Association, 2000.

Cramer, Phebe. *Protecting the Self: Defense Mechanisms in Action*. New York: Guilford Press, 2006.

Freud, Sigmund. *An Outline of Psychoanalysis*. New York: Norton, 1987.

Hentschel, Uwe, et al., eds. *Defense Mechanisms: Theoretical, Research and Clinical Perspectives*. Boston, MA: Elsevier, 2004.

Subbotsky, Eugene. *Magic and the Mind: Mechanisms, Functions, and Development of Magical Thinking and Behavior*. New York: Oxford University Press, 2010.

Vaillant, George E. *Adaptation to Life*. Boston, MA: Little, Brown, 1977.

PERIODICALS

Bowins, B. "Personality Disorders: A Dimensional Defense Mechanism Approach." *American Journal of Psychotherapy* 64 (February 2010): 153–69.

Brown, S., and E. Locker. "Defensive Responses to an Emotive Anti-alcohol Message." *Psychology and Health* 24 (June 2009): 517–28.

Klimstra, T.A., et al. "Identity Formation in Adolescence: Change or Stability?" *Journal of Youth and Adolescence* 39 (February 2010): 150–62.

Levitt, H.M., and D.C. Williams. "Facilitating Client Change: Principles Based upon the Experience of Eminent Psychotherapists." *Psychotherapy Research* 20 (May 2010): 337–52.

Presniak, M.D., et al. "The Role of Defense Mechanisms in Borderline and Antisocial Personalities." *Journal of Personality Assessment* 92 (March 2010): 137–45.

Tull, M.T., et al. "Emotion Suppression: A Preliminary Experimental Investigation of Its Immediate Effects and Role in Subsequent Reactivity to Novel Stimuli." *Cognitive Behaviour Therapy* 39 (June 2010): 114–25.

Yu, Y., et al. "Personality and Defense Mechanisms in Late Adulthood." *Journal of Aging and Health* 20 (August 2008): 526–44.

OTHER

American Academy of Child and Adolescent Psychiatry (AACAP). *Facts for Families: When to Seek Help for Your Child*, http://www.aacap.org/cs/root/facts_for_families/when_to_seek_help_for_your_child.

KidsHealth for Parents. *Taking Your Child to a Therapist*, http://kidshealth.org/parent/positive/family/finding_therapist.html.

Mayo Clinic Adult Health. *Denial: Learn to Cope with Painful Situations*. Includes advice about helping loved ones move past denial, http://www.mayoclinic.com/health/denial/SR00043.

Thurber, James. "The Secret Life of Walter Mitty." http://www.all-story.com/issues.cgi?action=show_story&story_id=100.

Ziegler-Hill, V., and D.W. Pratt. "Defense Styles and the Interpersonal Circumplex: The Interpersonal Nature of Psychological Defense." *Journal of Psychiatry, Psychology and Mental Health* 1 (Winter 2007): 1–15, http://www.scientificjournals.org/journals2007/articles/1183.pdf.

ORGANIZATIONS

American Academy of Child and Adolescent Psychiatry (AACAP), 3615 Wisconsin Avenue, N.W., Washington DC, 20016-3007, 202-966-7300, 202-966-2891, http://www.aacap.org/.

American Psychiatric Association, 1000 Wilson Boulevard, Suite 1825, Arlington VA, 22209-3901, 703-907-7300, apa@psych.org, http://www.psych.org/.

American Psychoanalytic Association (APsaA), 309 East 49th Street, New York NY, 10017, 212-752-0450, 212-593-0571, info@apsa.org, http://www.apsa.org/.

American Psychological Association (APA), 750 First Street NE, Washington DC, 20002, 202-336-5500, 800-374-2721, http://www.apa.org/index.aspx.

International Psychoanalytic Association (IPA), Broomhills, Woodside Lane, London United Kingdom, N12 8UD, +44 20 8446 8324, +44 20 8445 4729, ipa@ipa.og.uk, http://www.ipa.org.uk/Public/.

National Institute of Mental Health (NIMH), 6001 Executive Boulevard, Room 8184, MSC 9663, Bethesda MD, 20892-9663, 301-443-4513, 866-615-6464, 301-443-4279 nimhinfo@nih.gov, http://www.nimh.nih.gov/index.shtml.

Rebecca J. Frey, PhD

Dehydration

Definition

Dehydration is a condition in which the body loses too much water usually as a result of excess sweating, **vomiting**, and/or **diarrhea**. Hydration describes a condition of fluid balance (water homeostasis) when adequate fluid levels are maintained. When fluid balance is not maintained, the individual is said to be dehydrated.

Demographics

The very young and the very old are most likely to become dehydrated. Young children are at greater risk because they are more likely to get diseases that cause vomiting, diarrhea, and **fever**. Worldwide, dehydration is the leading cause of **death** in children. In the United States, 400–500 children under the age of five die every year of dehydration. The elderly are at risk because they are less likely to drink when they become dehydrated. The thirst mechanism often becomes less sensitive as people age. Also, their kidneys lose the ability to make highly concentrated urine. Older individuals who are confined to wheelchairs or bed and cannot get water for themselves (e.g. nursing home and hospital patients) are at risk of developing chronic dehydration.

Description

Dehydration occurs when more fluid is lost from the body than is taken in. Water is essential to life. Transporting nutrients throughout the body, removing wastes, regulating body temperature, lubrication of joints and membranes, and chemical reactions that occur during cellular metabolism all require water.

Water is distributed throughout three compartments in the body: inside the cells (intracellular), in the tissue (interstitial), and in the bloodstream (intravascular). Each compartment contains differing amounts of electrolytes that must remain in balance in order for body organs and systems to function correctly. Dehydration upsets this delicate balance. Total body water also varies in relation to age, gender, and amount of body fat. Adult males have approximately 60% water content, adult females have 50%, infants have an estimated 77%, and the elderly have 46% to 52%. An increase in body fat causes a decrease in the percent fluid content because fat does not contain significant amounts of water.

The amount of water a person needs to prevent dehydration varies widely depending on the individual's age, weight, level of physical activity, and the environmental temperature. The individual's health and the medications they take may also affect the amount of water a person needs. Most dehydration results from an acute, or sudden, loss of fluid. Slow-developing chronic dehydration can occur, however, most often in the frail elderly and infants and young children who must rely on others to supply them with liquids. Infants are also more likely to develop dehydration than adults because they have a higher metabolic rate and their immature kidneys have difficulty concentrating urine. Children who do not wet their diapers for three hours or more are dehydrated.

Healthy people lose water through urination, elimination of solid wastes, sweating, and breathing out water vapor. This water must be replaced through the diet. The United States Institute of Medicine (IOM) recommended in 2004 that relatively inactive adult men take in about 3.7 L (about 15 cups) of fluids daily and that women take in about of 2.7 L (about 10 cups) to replace lost water. These recommendations are for total fluid intake from both beverages and food. Highly active adults and those living in very warm climates need more fluid.

About 80% of the water the average person needs is replaced by drinking liquids. The other 20% is found in food. Below are listed some foods and the percentage of water that they contain:

- iceberg lettuce 96%
- squash, cooked 90%
- cantaloupe, raw, 90%
- 2% milk 89%
- apple, raw 86%
- cottage cheese 76%
- potato, baked 75%
- macaroni, cooked 66%
- turkey, roasted 62%
- steak, cooked 50%
- cheese, cheddar 37%
- bread, white 36%
- peanuts, dry roasted 2%

Dehydration involves more than just water deficiency. Electrolytes are ions that form when salts dissolve in water or body fluids. In order for cells to function adequately, the various electrolytes, such as sodium (Na+) and potassium (K+), must remain within a very narrow range of concentrations. Often electrolytes are lost along with water. For example, sodium is lost in sweat. To prevent the effects of dehydration, both water and electrolytes must be replaced in the correct proportions.

Risk factors

Risk factors for dehydration in the general population include:

- Geographical location. People lose more water from the body in dry climates and at high altitudes.
- Environmental conditions. Heat waves and natural disasters affecting sanitation can lead to dehydration.
- Occupations requiring outdoor work in warm weather.
- Diseases and disorders that affect the body's water balance. These include diabetes, kidney disease, diseases of the adrenal gland, eating disorders, intestinal parasites, and alcoholism.
- Travel to countries where cholera, dengue, and other diarrheal diseases are endemic.
- Methamphetamine abuse.
- Malnutrition.

Risk factors for dehydration in seniors include:

- Age over age 85.
- Living alone and not drinking enough or having access to fluids.
- Heavy alcohol consumption.
- Taking such medications as diuretics, laxatives, and sedatives.
- Having acute or chronic illnesses that affect normal eating and drinking habits.
- Are confused or have mental problems or communication problems.
- Having difficulty swallowing.

Causes and symptoms

There are three basic types of dehydration, defined by the sodium/water balance in body fluids. Doctors who are treating patients with dehydration must determine the type of water loss to ensure appropriate treatment. In addition, water and sodium levels in the body are closely related; if one is abnormal, the other often is too.

Isotonic dehydration is an equal loss of water and sodium. Isotonic means that the number of particles contained on one side of a permeable membrane is the same as on the other side, thus there is no fluid shift in either direction. The amount of intracellular and extracellular water remains in balance. Isotonic dehydration can be caused by a complete fast, vomiting, and diarrhea.

Hypertonic dehydration occurs when water loss is greater than sodium loss. Blood sodium levels may be >145 mmol/l (normal range=135 to 145 mmol/l). Higher blood sodium levels combined with decreased water in the intravascular space increases the osmotic pressure in the bloodstream, which, in turn, pulls more fluid out of the cells. This type of dehydration is usually caused by extended fever with limited oral rehydration. Mortality is more likely to occur from hypertonic than from isotonic dehydration.

Hypotonic dehydration occurs when sodium loss is greater than water loss. Blood sodium levels may be less than 135 mmol/l; and the osmotic pressure is greater inside the cells, which pulls more fluid out of the intravascular space into the intracellular space. This type of dehydration occurs with overuse of diuretics, which causes excessive sodium and potassium loss. Potassium depletion affects respiration, increases nausea, and, if severe enough, may cause respiratory arrest or central nervous system (CNS) seizures. Potassium depletion may also cause arrhythmias (irregular heartbeat). As a result, patients are told to take diuretics with orange juice or to eat a banana, both of which are high in potassium.

Causes

Diarrhea, often accompanied by vomiting, is the leading cause of dehydration. Both water and electrolytes are lost in large quantities. Diarrhea is often caused by bacteria, viruses, or parasites. Fever that often accompanies disease accelerates the amount of water that is lost through the skin. The smaller the child, the greater the risk of dehydration. Worldwide, acute diarrhea accounts for the death of about 4 million children each year. In the United States, about 220,000 children are hospitalized for dehydration caused by diarrhea annually.

Heavy sweating also causes dehydration and loss of electrolytes. Athletes, especially endurance athletes and individuals with active outdoor professions as roofers and road crew workers are at high risk of becoming dehydrated. Children who play **sports** outdoors can also be vulnerable to dehydration.

Certain chronic illnesses that disrupt fluid balance can cause dehydration. Kidney disease and hormonal disorders, such as diabetes, adrenal gland, or pituitary gland disorders, can cause fluid and electrolyte loss through excessive urination. Such disorders as **cystic fibrosis** or other **genetic disorders** resulting in inadequate absorption of nutrients from the intestines can cause chronic diarrhea that leads to dehydration. Individuals with **eating disorders** who abuse **laxatives**, diuretics, and enemas, or regularly cause themselves to vomit are vulnerable to severe electrolyte imbalances and dehydration. The same is true of people with **alcoholism**. People who have severe **burns** over a large part of their body also are likely to become dehydrated because they no longer have unbroken skin to act as a barrier to evaporation.

Symptoms

Dehydration can be mild, moderate or severe. Mild dehydration occurs when fluid losses equal 3–5%. At this point, the thirst sensation is felt, and is often accompanied by dry mouth and thick saliva.

Moderate dehydration occurs when fluid losses equal 6–9% of their body weight. This condition can occur rapidly in young children who are vomiting and/or have diarrhea. In an infant, a loss of as little as 2–3 cups of liquids can result in moderate dehydration. Signs of moderate dehydration include intense thirst, severely reduced urine production, sunken eyes, **headache**, **dizziness**, irritability, and decreased activity.

Severe dehydration occurs when fluid losses are 10% or more of their body weight. Severe dehydration is a medical emergency for individuals of any age. A loss of fluids equaling 15–20% of a person's body weight is fatal. Signs of severe dehydration include all those of moderate dehydration as well as lack of sweating, little or no urine production, dry skin that has little elasticity, low blood pressure, rapid heartbeat, fever, delirium, or coma.

KEY TERMS

Antiemetic—A type of drug given to stop vomiting.

Diuretic—A drug designed to encourage excretion of urine in people who accumulate excess fluid such as individuals with high blood pressure or heart conditions.

Electrolytes—Substances in the body that are able to conduct electricity. Electrolytes are essential in the normal functioning of body cells and organs.

Endemic—Referring to a disease that is prevalent in a particular location.

Hydration—Taking in water or fluid to replace loss of fluid.

Incontinence—Loss of ability to control urination or to control bowel movements (fecal incontinence).

Postural hypotension (orthostatic hypotension)—A sudden drop in blood pressure when rising from a sitting or lying down position.

Rupture—A tear or break in body tissue of an organ.

Water homeostasis—A condition of adequate fluid level in the body in which fluid loss and fluid intake are equally matched and sodium levels are within normal range.

Diagnosis

Mild dehydration can often be treated at home. However, a doctor should be consulted whenever:

- A child less than three months old develops a fever higher than 100 °F (37.8 °C).
- A child more than three months old develops a fever higher than 102 °F (38.9 °C).
- Symptoms of dehydration in an older child or adult worsen.
- An individual urinates very sparingly, passes dark-colored urine, or does not urinate at all during a six-hour period.
- Dizziness, listlessness, or excessive thirst occur.
- A person who is dieting and using diuretics loses more than 3 lb (1.3 kg) in a day or more than 5 lb (2.3 kg) a week.

A doctor's diagnosis of dehydration includes taking a recent health history, especially checking for the presence of specific illnesses, vomiting, diarrhea, **constipation**, fever, or such other noticeable symptoms as less frequent urination or lack of thirst. The doctor will also want to know about chronic illnesses and current medications.

Examination

In addition to taking the patient's history, dehydration is diagnosed by a physical examination. A healthcare professional or observant adult can usually tell by looking at someone that they are moderately or severely dehydrated. Visual signs are often enough to begin treatment.

Tests

Laboratory tests are important indicators of dehydration; blood tests include complete blood count (CBC), blood chemistries such as electrolytes (i.e., sodium, potassium, chloride), blood urea nitrogen (BUN), and creatinine, among others. Examination of urine and measurement of a 24-hour urine sample may be done to determine if output is normal or decreased. Heart rate and blood pressure will be measured and an electrocardiogram may be taken to see if heart rhythm is altered. In hospitalized patients with possible dehydration, fluid intake and output may be measured to determine if **kidney function** is impaired.

Other laboratory tests may be ordered to determine if an underlying condition (e.g., diabetes or an adrenal gland disorder) is the cause of the dehydration.

Treatment

Traditional

The goal of treatment is to restore fluid and electrolyte balance. For individuals with mild dehydration, this can be done in infants and children by giving them oral rehydration solutions such as Pedialyte, Infalyte, Naturalyte, Oralyte, or Rehydralyte. These are available in supermarkets and pharmacies without a prescription. These solutions have the proper balance of salts and sugars to restore the electrolyte balance. Water, apple juice, chicken broth, sodas, and similar fluids are effective in treating mild dehydration. Oral rehydration fluids can be given young children in small sips as soon as vomiting and diarrhea start. They may continue to vomit and have diarrhea, but some of the fluid will be absorbed.

A child who is vomiting should sip one or two teaspoons of liquid every 10 minutes. A child who is less than a year old and who is not vomiting should be given one tablespoon of liquid every 20 minutes. A child who is more than one year old and who is not vomiting should take two tablespoons of liquid every 30 minutes. A baby who is being breastfed should be given clear liquids for two consecutive feedings before **breastfeeding** is resumed. A bottle-fed baby should be given formula diluted with water to half the formula strength for the first 24 hours after symptoms of dehydration are identified.

To calculate fluid loss accurately, weight changes should be charted every day and a record kept of how many times a patient vomits or has diarrhea. A record of fluid output (including sputum or vomit) and of fluid intake or replacement should be kept for at least 24 to 48 hours to see if balance is being accomplished. Parents should note how many times a baby's diaper must be changed. If dehydration continues, emergency department treatment or hospitalization to receive intravenous fluids and electrolytes may be necessary.

Older children who are dehydrated can be given oral rehydration solutions or sports drinks such as Gatorade for moderate and severe dehydration, otherwise general fluids are fine. Athletes who are dehydrated should be given sports drinks. According to the American College of Sports Medicine, sports drinks are effective in supplying energy for muscles, maintaining blood sugar levels, preventing dehydration, and replacing electrolytes lost in sweat. Adults who are mildly or moderately dehydrated usually improve by drinking water and avoiding coffee, tea, and soft drinks that do not contain **caffeine**.

Individuals of all ages who are seriously dehydrated need to be treated by a medical professional. In the case of severe dehydration, the individual may be hospitalized and fluids given intravenously (IV; directly into the vein). Hospital care will include not only immediate replacement of fluids but may also involve treating an underlying chronic illness such as diabetes, kidney disease, or heart disease, which has resulted in fluid loss and dehydration.

Drugs

Treatment of dehydration may involve changing medications that have caused excessive fluid loss. In some cases patients may be given antiemetics or antidiarrheal drugs to stop the vomiting or diarrhea that may be causing the dehydration.

Home remedies

People can keep rehydration products in the home in case they are needed. Fluid replacement products that contain essential body chemicals and nutrients are available at pharmacies and some supermarkets; pharmacists can offer advice about the best ones to help correct or prevent dehydration and to restore electrolyte balance.

The World Health Organization (WHO) recommends a homemade solution to help the dehydrated person correct fluid levels and also receive needed sugars and nourishment. To rehydrate the body, the following ingredients can be combined and sipped frequently over several hours:

- 1 quart of water
- three-fourths teaspoon of table salt
- 1 teaspoon of baking powder
- 4 tablespoons of sugar
- 1 cup of orange juice

Prognosis

Mild dehydration rarely results in complications. It can usually be reversed by correcting fluid levels through drinking or receiving fluids intravenously. If the cause is eliminated and lost fluid is replaced, mild dehydration can usually be resolved in 24 to 48 hours.

On the other hand, vomiting and diarrhea that continue for several days without adequate fluid replacement can be fatal since more is lost than water and sodium. Severe potassium loss may lead to cardiac arrhythmias, respiratory distress or arrest, or convulsions (seizures). The risk of life-threatening complications is greater for young children and the elderly. Imbalances in the electrolyte sodium can cause too much water to be absorbed by brain cells, causing them to swell and rupture—a serious complication of dehydration. Underlying chronic diseases can complicate the correction of dehydration, resulting in organ system dysfunction. Severe dehydration can lead to shock and kidney failure, which can be life-threatening.

Prevention

Preventing dehydration is easier than treating it once it occurs. Drinking at least eight glasses of water a day prevents dehydration. More may be needed in hot weather. Beginning each day with a glass of water containing a small amount of lemon or other citrus juice helps restore fluid and blood sugar (glucose) levels that have diminished overnight. Water and other clear liquids (tea, juices, and clear soups) can be consumed slowly throughout the day rather than drinking too much at mealtimes, which will dilute digestive juices. Alcoholic beverages and excessive amounts of caffeine–containing drinks, which dehydrate the body, should be avoided.

Another way to prevent dehydration is to be alert to situations in which it could occur, such as exercising in hot weather or vomiting and diarrhea in infants and young children. Athletes and people who work in hot conditions should drink regularly whether or not they feel thirsty. Rehydration of young children should begin at the first sign of fluid loss. A healthcare provider should be consulted before the situation becomes serious. Caregivers of the mobility-impaired elderly and infants and young children who cannot get water for themselves should be offered fluids on a regular basis.

Nutrition/Dietetic concerns

Besides drinking to restore fluid balance, normal consumption of food is necessary when someone is dehydrated. Because intestinal upsets with either diarrhea or vomiting can result in loss of interest in eating or the temporary inability to keep food down or digest it, foods should be kept simple and as soft or liquid as possible, including weak tea, broth, bouillon, plain soups, and lightly cooked vegetables. Large amounts of fluids should not be consumed all at once as this delays gastric emptying and encourages urination. It is recommended that dehydrated individuals sip fluids in small amounts at frequent intervals (e.g. 100–200 mL every 20 minutes) to achieve effective rehydration. Flavored gelatin is often a good fluid replacement and is easy to digest. Such high-fiber foods as whole fruit, bread, grains, and meat should be avoided until the intestinal tract has had a rest. Milk is not a clear liquid and may not be tolerated; milk is not ideal for fluid replacement. Caffeine–containing drinks and alcohol encourage excess urination and should be avoided.

Caregiver concerns for the elderly

Any older individual who has an illness that causes fever, diarrhea, or vomiting may become dehydrated if fluid is not replaced through drinking water and other clear fluids. In these situations, caretakers must always watch for early signs of dehydration such as dry mouth, dark urine, and fatigue or irritability. Older individuals may not drink enough for various reasons: They may not feel thirsty; it may be difficult to hold a glass containing liquid; or they may have difficulty getting up from a chair or bed and want to avoid trips to the bathroom. Some elderly people take diuretic medications and have a time during the day, usually morning, when they urinate frequently. Some will not drink because they are incontinent and want to reduce the possibility of having accidents. Caregivers must always encourage drinking to replace what is excreted or replace fluid loss during certain illnesses through diarrhea, vomiting, or fever. Caregivers should also understand the symptoms of severe dehydration and know when to call the doctor or an ambulance.

Resources

BOOKS

"Dehydration." *The Merck Manual of Diagnosis and Therapy*, Section 6, edited by R. S. Porter. White House Station, NJ: Merck Research Laboratories, 2007.

Isaac, Jeff. *Outward Bound Wilderness First-Aid Handbook*, revised and updated. Guilford, CT: Falcon Guides, 2008.

Knoop, Kevin J. et al., eds. *Atlas of Emergency Medicine*, 3rd ed. New York: McGraw-Hill Professional, 2009.

Maughn, Ronald J., and Louise M. Burke, eds. *Sports Nutrition*. Malden, MA: Blackwell Science, 2002.

Panel on Dietary Reference Intakes for Electrolytes and Water, Standing Committee on the Scientific Evaluation of Dietary Reference Intakes, Food and Nutrition Board. *DRI, Dietary Reference Intakes for Water, Potassium, Sodium, Chloride, and Sulfate*. Washington, DC: National Academies Press, 2005.

Rich, Brent E., and Mitchell K. Pratte. *Tarascon Sports Medicine Pocketbook*. Sudbury, MA: Jones and Bartlett Publishers, 2010.

PERIODICALS

Gregorio, G. V., et al. "Polymer-based Oral Rehydration Solution for Treating Acute Watery Diarrhoea." *Cochrane Database of Systematic Reviews*, April 15, 2009: CD006519.

Levine, D. A. "Antiemetics for Acute Gastroenteritis in Children." *Current Opinion in Pediatrics* 21 (June 2009): 294–298.

Scherb, C. A., et al. "Outcomes Related to Dehydration in the Pediatric Population." *Journal of Pediatric Nursing* 22 (October 2007): 376–382.

Wakefield, B. J., et al. "Risk Factors and Outcomes Associated with Hospital Admission for Dehydration." *Rehabilitation Nursing* 33 (November-December 2008): 233–241.

Wotton, K., et al. "Prevalence, Risk Factors, and Strategies to Prevent Dehydration in Older Adults." *Contemporary Nurse* 31 (December 2008): 44–56.

OTHER

Centers for Disease Control and Prevention (CDC). *Guidelines for the Management of Acute Diarrhea*, http://emergency.cdc.gov/disasters/hurricanes/pdf/dguidelines.pdf.

Lozner, Alison Wiley. "Pediatrics, Dehydration." *eMedicine*, February 5, 2009, http://emedicine.medscape.com/article/801012-overview.

Mayo Clinic. *Dehydration*, http://www.mayoclinic.com/health/dehydration/DS00561.

Medline Plus. *Dehydration*, http://www.nlm.nih.gov/medlineplus/ency/article/000982.htm#visualContent.

Prakash, Chandra. *Patient Information: Nausea and Vomiting*, http://www.acg.gi.org/patients/gihealth/nausea.asp.

Water UK. *Water Requirements in Adults*, http://www.water.org.uk/home/water-for-health/medical-facts/adults.

ORGANIZATIONS

American College of Gastroenterology, P.O. Box 342260, Bethesda MD, 20827-2260, 301-263-9000, http://www.acg.gi.org/.

American College of Sports Medicine (ACSM), P.O. Box 1440, Indianapolis IN, 46206-1440, 317-637-9200, 317-634-7817, http://www.acsm.org//AM/Template.cfm?Section=Home_Page.

Centers for Disease Control and Prevention (CDC), 1600 Clifton Road, Atlanta GA, 30333, 800-232-4636, cdcinfo@cdc.gov, http://www.cdc.gov.

International Society of Travel Medicine (ISTM), 2386 Clower Street, Suite A-102, Snellvile GA, United States, 30078, +1 770 736 060, +1-770 736 0313, istm@istm.org, https://www.istm.org/.

World Health Organization (WHO), Avenue Appia 20, 1211 Geneva 27 Switzerland, + 41 22 791 21 11, + 41 22 791 31 11, info@who.int, http://www.who.int/en/.

Tish Davidson, AM
L. Lee Culvert
Rebecca J. Frey, PhD

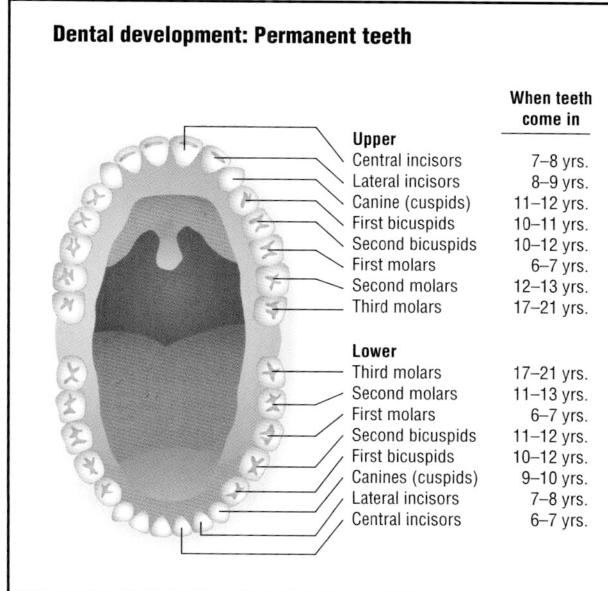

Illustration of the eruption of permanent teeth. *(Illustration by PreMediaGlobal. Reproduced by permission of Gale, a part of Cengage Learning.)*

Dental development: Primary teeth

	When teeth come in	When teeth fall out
Upper		
Central incisors	7–12 mos.	6–8 yrs.
Lateral incisors	9–13 mos.	7–8 yrs.
Canines (cuspids)	16–22 mos.	10–12 yrs.
First molars	13–19 mos.	9–11 yrs.
Second molars	25–33 mos.	10–12 yrs.
Lower		
Second molars	20–31 mos.	10–12 yrs.
First molars	12–18 mos.	9–11 yrs.
Canines (cuspids)	16–23 mos.	9–12 yrs.
Lateral incisors	7–16 mos.	7–8 yrs.
Central incisors	6–10 mos.	6–8 yrs.

Illustration of the eruption of primary, or baby, teeth. *(Illustration by PreMediaGlobal. Reproduced by permission of Gale, a part of Cengage Learning.)*

Dental development

Definition

Dental development or odontogenesis is the process that culminates in the formation of permanent teeth in humans. Dental development begins in the first trimester of prenatal life when the tips or cusps of the primary or deciduous (baby) teeth start to form, and it ends in most individuals when the root ends of the third permanent molars fully calcify and finally close. From start to finish, development and exfoliation (shedding) of the 20 deciduous teeth and the development of the 32 permanent teeth occupy a period of more than two decades.

The 32 permanent teeth in the human adult consist of six molars in each jaw (upper and lower); four premolars in each jaw; two canines (pointed teeth) in each jaw; and four incisors (flat teeth at the front of each dental arch) in each jaw. The molars and premolars are adapted for crushing food, the canines and incisors for tearing and piercing. This combination of shapes in human teeth is thought to be an adaptation to the combination of foods (both meat and fruits or vegetables containing fiber) in the modern human diet. Prehistoric humans are known to have had teeth that were shaped differently from those of humans in historic times.

Demographics

To a large extent, both dental development and tooth size are under genetic control, as shown in twin and sibling comparisons, and there are population differences both in developmental timing and in crown size and shape. Dental development is also affected by such endocrine disorders as hypopituitarism and **hypothyroidism**. Dental development is slightly advanced in obese individuals and slightly retarded in those with chronic **malnutrition**.

The complete lack of teeth in humans is very rare; however, lacking some teeth (called hypodontia) is fairly common in the American population. Between 20% and 23% percent of people lack third molars (the so–called wisdom teeth), while another eight percent lack the second premolars. Hyperdontia, the condition of having one or two extra teeth (most often molars), occurs in one to three percent of Caucasians and five percent of Asian Americans.

Except for the earliest stages of prenatal dental development, and with the possible exception of the third permanent molar (M3), girls are advanced over boys in dental development, by as much as six percent. Girls also have slightly smaller tooth crowns and slightly shorter tooth roots, allowing sex identification of cadavers and skeletal material.

Description

The deciduous teeth start to form in humans between the sixth and eighth weeks of fetal life, with the permanent teeth beginning to develop around the twentieth week. If teeth do not start to develop at or near these times, they will not develop at all.

"Teething," or tooth eruption, the emergence of the deciduous teeth, begins in the middle of the first year of life and ends in the second year with the emergence of the second or deciduous molars (symbolized as "dm2"). Some discomfort is associated with the piercing of the gums, especially so for the large deciduous molars. Eruption of the permanent teeth may also cause some discomfort in the course of emergence through the gums, especially the permanent molars, which have no predecessors to pave the way. Timing of the emergence of baby teeth tends to be hereditary and is quite variable. However, most children have a full set of primary teeth by age two–and–a–half.

There are fewer baby teeth than permanent teeth; in all, humans have only 20 deciduous teeth—two incisors, one canine, and two deciduous molars in each of the four jaw quadrants of the jaw. While the primary teeth are in place, the permanent or adult teeth are forming under the gum. Children begin to lose their baby teeth beginning between ages five and six; the last baby tooth is typically lost around age 12. Most children have all their permanent teeth except the final last set of molars (wisdom teeth) by about age ten. There are typically 32 successional or permanent teeth.

Risk factors

Risk factors for abnormal tooth development in humans include:

- Malnutrition, particularly a lack of vitamins A, C, and D.
- Low birth weight.
- Down syndrome.
- Cystic fibrosis.
- Leukemia.
- Prader–Willi syndrome.
- Fluoride deficiency.
- Chemotherapy for childhood cancer.
- History of severe childhood infections, including HIV infection.
- Crouzon syndrome. Crouzon syndrome is a rare genetic disorder in which a baby's facial and jaw bones fail to develop normally. It is named for the French neurologist who first identified it as a hereditary disorder in the 1930s.
- Obesity. Obesity in children is a risk factor for premature tooth loss as well as caries.

Causes and symptoms

Normal tooth development

Normal tooth development in humans begins with the formation of the tooth bud (sometimes called the tooth germ) in the fetus during the early weeks of pregnancy. The tooth bud forms around the sixth week of pregnancy and has three parts: the enamel organ, the dental papilla, and the dental follicle. The enamel organ eventually gives rise to the enamel—the hard exterior surface of the tooth. The dental papilla gives rise to the pulp in the center of the tooth, and the dental follicle produces the bone around the root of the tooth and the ligaments that hold the tooth in place.

The tooth bud then undergoes several stages of development. In the second stage, called the cap stage, the bud forms a rounded group of cells on its top resembling a cap in shape, and the three parts of the tooth bud (the enamel organ, dental papilla, and dental follicle) begin to differentiate. In the third stage, called the bell stage, the crown of the tooth begins to take shape. It is not known as of 2010 why the various types of teeth in the human mouth have differently shaped crowns. In the maturation stage, the hard tissues of the tooth (the enamel and dentin) begin to form.

Some teeth may fail to form, a condition known as agenesis or hypodontia. The most common missing tooth is the third molar (M3) and—sometimes—the lateral (2nd) incisors, (I2). When M3 and especially I2 are missing, the remaining teeth tend to be reduced in size and late developing as well. Supernumerary (extra) teeth also exist (hyperdontia), although rarely. They usually appear as relatively shapeless pegs, but in some cases there may be a complete extra molar (M4) that is fully formed.

Traditionally, the emergence of the first deciduous or baby tooth was taken as an indication to extend the infant's diet beyond breast milk alone. However, today cereals and other foods are often introduced much earlier then in the past. In turn, completion of the deciduous dentition was taken as a readiness for solid foods, now also introduced far earlier than the end of the second year of life. Traditionally also, emergence of the second permanent molars was considered evidence of the ability to perform "adult," rigorous labor.

Childhood dental disorders

Teething is the first dental problem parents are likely to encounter. It is common for babies who are teething to become fussy, irritable, have trouble sleeping, lose interest in food, or drool more than usual. It is *not* normal, however, for a baby to run a **fever** or develop skin **rashes** or **vomiting** and **diarrhea** from teething alone. If the baby develops these symptoms, parents should call the **pediatrician**.

Other major disorders of dentition during childhood are dental caries (cavities), **malocclusion** (malpositioning of the teeth), and less commonly, accidental injury. The incidence and prevalence of dental caries increased rapidly during the nineteenth century until the middle of the twentieth century, consistent with increased consumption of sugars. Addition of fluorides to the water supply and the use of topical fluorides reversed the incidence of caries in the second half of the twentieth century.

Malocclusions (misalignments of the teeth) are now ubiquitous, with over 90% of children affected to some degree. Although the actual cause of malocclusion is not known, satisfactory dental alignment can be achieved by orthodontic intervention.

Many accidental injuries occur during participation in contact **sports**. Most injuries of this type can be prevented by the use of mouth guards and protective headgear. Another common cause of dental injuries in children is bicycle or car accidents. A third common cause is **child abuse**.

KEY TERMS

Agenesis—Failure to form a body part.

Caries—Tooth cavities.

Deciduous teeth—Also called primary or baby teeth, the first set of teeth in a baby's mouth.

Dental arch—The complete set of teeth in the upper or lower jaw, so named because the 16 teeth in each jaw are arranged in the shape of an arch. The upper dental arch in humans is slightly larger than the lower.

Dentin—A hard substance that forms the largest portion of a tooth's structure and lies underneath the enamel.

Enamel—The hard outer surface of a tooth. It is the hardest and most highly mineralized substance in the human body.

Exfoliation—Shedding of baby teeth.

Hyperdontia—Having one or two extra permanent teeth.

Hypodontia—Having fewer than the normal number of 32 permanent teeth.

Malocclusion—Misalignment of teeth.

Odontogenesis—Formation and development of teeth.

Teething—Eruption of baby teeth in the infant's mouth.

Tooth bud—The collection of cells in the human fetus that eventually gives rise to a complete tooth.

Diagnosis

Examination

The American Dental Association (ADA) recommends that a baby should see the dentist for an initial checkup as soon as the first deciduous tooth erupts, and no later than the first birthday. After the first visit, children should be seen at least once a year and preferably every six months. During the examination, the dentist will evaluate the overall condition of the child's mouth as well as the emergence of teeth, checking for signs of infection, cavities, and malocclusion. The dentist will also give the parents or the child age–appropriate instructions about brushing, flossing, and other aspects of tooth care.

Tests

The dentist may take an x ray of the child's teeth to check for cavities and malocclusion. In older teenagers and young adults, **x rays** can also be used to identify the location of the third molars. Newer machines allow the dentist to view x–ray images of the teeth directly on a computer rather than having to develop film in a darkroom.

Procedures

The dentist may recommend taking an impression of the child's dental arches when malocclusion is suspected. To take an impression, the dentist fills an arch–shaped tray with a soft plastic material and asks the child to bite on it. The tray is removed and the plastic material is allowed to harden. The impression can be used to make a cast of the child's mouth.

Treatment

Traditional

The discomfort of teething can be eased by gently rubbing the baby's gums with a clean gauze pad soaked in cool water or offering the baby a teething ring. The dentist or the baby's pediatrician can recommend a teething ring or a special salve containing a local anesthetic to numb the gums.

The baby's first teeth should be gently brushed with a soft–bristle brush and plain water to prevent cavities. Toothpaste should not be used with children younger than two years. With children older than two, parents can use a pea–sized quantity of fluoride toothpaste when brushing the child's teeth. They should make sure, however, that the child spits out the toothpaste and rinses the mouth thoroughly afterward.

Prognosis

The great majority of children have their baby teeth and permanent teeth emerge on schedule with no major problems. Although malocclusions are common, they can be corrected by an orthodontist. Wisdom teeth often require extraction during late **adolescence** or the early adult years if they are coming in sideways, are only partially erupting, are trapped beneath the gum and bone, are likely to lead to chronic infections, or if there is not enough room in the dental arch for them. According to the American Association of Oral and Maxillofacial Surgeons (AAOMS), about 85% of third molars will eventually need to be removed. Extraction of wisdom teeth is a commonplace oral surgery procedure; patients typically return to the oral surgeon between seven and 10 days after extraction to make sure healing is proceeding normally.

Prevention

The dentist may recommend applying a sealant or fluoride compound to prevent or lower the risk of **tooth decay**.

Common–sense **safety** precautions during contact sports, instruction in **bicycle safety**, and the use of mouth guards can lower the risk of tooth damage or loss from accidental injury.

Resources

BOOKS

Cameron, Angus C., and Richard P. Widmer, editors. *Handbook of Pediatric Dentistry*, 3rd ed. New York: Mosby, 2008.

Sroda, Rebecca. *Nutrition for a Healthy Mouth*, 2nd ed. Philadelphia: Wolters Kluwer Health/Lippincott Williams and Wilkins, 2010.

Taggart, Jose C., editor. *Handbook of Dental Care: Diagnostic, Preventive and Restorative Services*. New York: Nova Biomedical Books, 2009.

PERIODICALS

Atar, M., and E.J. Körperich. "Systemic Disorders and Their Influence on the Development of Dental Hard Tissues: A Literature Review." *Journal of Dentistry* 38 (April 2010): 296–306.

Bei, M. "Molecular Genetics of Tooth Development." *Current Opinion in Genetics and Development* 19 (October 2009): 504–10.

Birnstein, E., and J. Katz. "Obesity in Children: A Challenge That Pediatric Dentistry Should Not Ignore—Review of the Literature." *Journal of Clinical Pediatric Dentistry* 34 (Winter 2009): 103–06.

Fleming, P.S., et al. "Revisiting the Supernumerary: The Epidemiological and Molecular Basis of Extra Teeth." *British Dental Journal* 208 (January 9, 2010): 25–30.

Kugel, G., et al. "Treatment Modalities for Caries Management, Including a New Resin Infiltration System." *Compendium of Continuing Education in Dentistry* 30 (October 2009): 1–10.

McTigue, D.J. "Managing Injuries to the Primary Dentition." *Dental Clinics of North America* 53 (October 2009): 627–38.

O'Connell, S., et al. "Medical, Nutritional, and Dental Considerations in Children with Low Birth Weight." *Pediatric Dentistry* 31 (November–December 2009): 504–12.

OTHER

American Academy of Pediatric Dentistry. "Frequently Asked Questions." http://www.aapd.org/pediatricinformation/faq.asp (accessed September 17, 2010).

American Association of Oral and Maxillofacial Surgeons. "Wisdom Teeth." http://www.aaoms.org/wisdom_teeth.php (accessed September 17, 2010).

American Dental Association. "Teething," http://www.ada.org/3015.aspx?currentTab=1 (accessed September 17, 2010).

American Dental Association. "Tooth Eruption Charts," http://www.ada.org/2930.aspx?currentTab=1 (accessed September 17, 2010).

Mayo Clinic. "Dental Exam for Children," http://www.mayoclinic.com/health/dental–exam–for–children/MY01098 (accessed September 17, 2010).

ORGANIZATIONS

American Academy of Pediatric Dentistry (AAPD), 211 East Chicago Ave., Suite 1700, Chicago IL, 60611, (312) 337-2169, (312) 337-6329, http://www.aapd.org/.

American Association of Oral and Maxillofacial Surgeons (AAOMS), 9700 West Bryn Mawr Ave., Rosemont IL, 60018, (847) 678-6200, (800) 822-6637, (847) 678-6286, http://www.aaoms.org/.

American Dental Association (ADA), 211 East Chicago Ave., Chicago IL, 60611, (312) 440-2500, http://www.ada.org/.

Stanley A. Garn, PhD
Tish Davidson, AM
Rebecca J. Frey, PhD

Dental fillings

Definition

Dental fillings are metal amalgams or composite resins used to fill a cavity.

Purpose

Dentists use dental fillings to restore teeth damaged by dental caries (**tooth decay**). Dental caries are caused by microorganisms that convert sugars in food to acids that erode the enamel of a tooth, creating a hole or cavity. The dentist cleans out the decayed part of the tooth and fills the opening with an artificial material (a filling) to protect the tooth's structure and restore the appearance and utility of the tooth.

Precautions

As in any dental procedure, the dentist and dental assistant will need to use sterile techniques. Gloves and masks are essential as well as the sterilization of equipment and tools. This not only helps prevent the spread of infectious diseases like **AIDS** and hepatitis, but also the **common cold**.

The patient's reaction to anesthesia is the other main concern of the dentist and dental assistant when performing dental fillings. Nitrous oxide should be avoided with pregnant patients, and local anesthetics should be used with caution, though they are considered safe. Local anesthetics like Novocain and lidocaine have been in practical use for decades with few side effects reported. Some patients, however, are allergic to these drugs.

Description

Though dentists are encountering fewer and smaller cavities in their patients, there is still a need for dentists to fill cavities. Old fillings wear out over time and need to be replaced. Recently, patients have begun to request more restorative work on their teeth, sometimes opting for full mouth restorations that involve installing crowns, bleaching teeth or applying veneers, and replacing dark metal fillings with tooth-colored ones that create a monochromatic view in a patient's mouth.

The dentist begins by removing the decayed area of the tooth and preparing the tooth to receive the filling. The dentist has a wide choice of dental filling materials to choose from.

Amalgam fillings

The most common and strongest filling material is amalgam. It is a silver filling that is usually placed on the rear molars, which endure more stress during chewing. Amalgam fillings—used for large, deep cavities—are strong and very resistant to wear. Amalgam has been in use since 1833.

Amalgam is a mixture (which is what the word means) of several metals, including liquid mercury (35% silver, 15% tin or tin and copper, a trace of zinc, and 50% mercury). When it is prepared, it has a malleable consistency that can easily be shaped to fit the prepared tooth. It hardens to a durable metal.

Despite its durability, many dentists and patients avoid amalgam fillings. Dentists have found that amalgam has a tendency to expand with time. As a result, teeth become fractured from the inside, often splitting the tooth. Patients often avoid amalgam for strictly aesthetic reasons. Amalgam fillings darken over time and make teeth look as if they are decayed.

The biggest reason amalgam has lost favor is a health concern due to its 50% mercury content. Although the American Dental Association (ADA) has pronounced amalgam safe in the quantity and composition of amalgam, some patients and dentists are disturbed by various reports of illness in relation to the mercury in amalgam fillings. Mercury is a toxic material. Some states are required to dispose of mercury waste as if it were a hazardous product. There is also an added risk of inhaling mercury particles when old fillings are removed.

Gold fillings

Gold fillings or inlays are created outside of the mouth by a dental technician and then cemented into place. They are also used to fill the back molars. Gold fillings are very durable. Like amalgam, however, they are not as aesthetically pleasing as tooth-colored fillings.

Composite fillings

Composite fillings, often called white fillings, are made of a plastic resin and finely ground glass. They must be applied to the tooth surface in thin layers. Dentists try to match the color of composites with neighboring teeth for a more natural look, making the filling appear invisible. Composite resin fillings often are made smaller than amalgam fillings and require less tooth preparation, thereby saving more natural tooth surface.

Composite fillings are bonded to the tooth so that the tooth becomes stronger than it was before. They are also less sensitive to temperature changes in the mouth that can damage the tooth; therefore there is less chance that the tooth will shatter because of the filling.

These fillings may not be suitable for large cavities in molars. Though composite durability increased in the 1990s, a porcelain inlay or crown may be the best choice for a durable, natural-looking restoration of a molar.

The major drawback of composite resin fillings is cost. They average one-and-a-half to two times more than the price of amalgam fillings. They also can be stained from drinking coffee and tea. Large composite fillings tend to wear out sooner than amalgam fillings.

Composite fillings can last seven to 10 years, which is similar to the lifespan of amalgam fillings.

Resin ionomer

Resin ionomers are new, tooth-colored filling materials that contain a resin and fluoride. They are very suitable for children and for older adults who suffer from root decay that is more likely to occur as a person ages. These fillings seal the tooth and also protect it from future decay because of the fluoride that they release.

Preparation

During a routine checkup, the dentist may find a cavity in a tooth with a metal tooth probe. A new diagnostic tool, the DIAGNOdent, can detect evidence of cavities and pre-cavity conditions on the tooth's surface. A low-powered laser, the DIAGNOdent is able to detect decay so early that a dental cavity can be avoided. These pre-cavity areas can be protected with a sealant, thereby preventing further decay.

If the cavities found are relatively small and not very deep, there may be no need to anesthetize the area where the dental work will be done. High-speed drills often are able to clean out the decay quickly and with little discomfort. If the cavity is not very deep, the drill may not reach the sensitive nerves in the teeth, which usually cause **pain**. Children and some adults may need anesthesia in any case. The dentist and the dental assistant need to be aware of the patient's history and if the patient reacts adversely to local anesthesia.

There are some dentists who use electronic dental anesthesia (EDA), a device that sends electrical charges to the gum through electrodes. Sometimes this is enough anesthesia for the procedure. At other times, EDA numbs the area where the anesthesia is administered, so that the patient does not feel the needle as it goes into the gum. Some dentists also provide soothing music to calm patients during the procedure. Other dentists will use local anesthesia in combination with nitrous oxide-oxygen analgesia to minimize discomfort through the drilling phase of a filling.

Dental lasers that generate a low-powered beam of light are being used to cut away decay, but without the whine of the drill and without using anesthesia. Though a bit slower than the conventional drill, lasers are very efficient at preparing a tooth to receive a filling. Unfortunately, lasers cannot yet remove old fillings or prepare a tooth surface to receive a crown.

Air abrasion is another way to remove decay without using anesthesia. Air abrasion machines produce a spray of air and powder. There is no vibration or heat. Because it has no vibration, it avoids microfractures in the tooth that sometimes occur with drills. Air abrasion removes only a small amount of the tooth's structure. Therefore, it is suitable for small cavities and the repair and replacement of old fillings. It also can repair chipped teeth and clean discolored or stained teeth.

After the cavity is cleaned of decay, the walls of the tooth are shaped and are ready to receive a filling material. If a composite resin filling is used, the tooth next needs to be etched so that the resin will adhere to the tooth. The tooth then is filled, shaped, and polished. The composite filling then must be hardened by shining a special light on it.

KEY TERMS

Amalgam—A mixture of metals, primarily mercury used to make large, durable fillings. Also called silver fillings.

Anesthesia—A condition created by drugs that produces a numb feeling. General anesthesia produces unconsciousness whereas a local anesthesia produces numbness around the site where the drug was introduced.

Composite filling—A resin material that is tooth colored and is used to fill a tooth once decay has been removed. It is used most often in front teeth, but may be used in any tooth for aesthetic reasons.

Crown—An artificial covering prepared by a lab technician to fit over a damaged tooth or one weakened by decay.

Dental caries—Tooth decay caused by microorganisms that convert sugars in food to acids which erode the enamel of a tooth.

Dental laser—A device that generates a low-powered beam of light that is used in place of a dentist's drill to cut away decay from a tooth or remove gum tissue.

Enamel—The hard outer surface of a tooth.

Aftercare

The dentist and dental assistant should advise the patient that the teeth, lips, and tongue may be numb for several hours after the procedure, if a local anesthetic was used. Some patients experience sore gums or a sensitivity to hot and cold in the tooth that has just been filled. Normally, patients are advised to avoid chewing hard foods directly on new amalgam fillings for 24 hours. Composite fillings require no special caution since they set immediately. If patients experience continued pain or an uncomfortable bite, they should call their dentist.

Complications

Some patient's have allergic reactions to local anesthesia. The tooth that received a filling may be sensitive to changes in temperature or may be sore for a short time after the procedure.

Results

Fillings restore a tooth's function and appearance. They permit the patient to continue to eat and chew properly and last for several years. Normal fillings will need to be replaced over a patient's lifetime. Since fewer dental caries had been observed since the last decade of the twentieth century, dentists are initially filling fewer teeth, but are replacing fillings as they fail and sometimes systematically, especially if the patient decides to cosmetically enhance his or her teeth. Since many of the initial cavities are quite small, patients are opting for more aesthetically pleasing filling materials even if they are not as durable.

Health care team roles

When the dentist discovers a cavity, filling options are discussed with the patient. The dental assistant prepares the dentist's workstation and lays out the specific instruments that are needed. The dental assistant prepares the filling material according to the manufacturer's directions and assists the dentist in preparing the tooth for filling and in the filling procedure itself. The dental assistant cleans the patient's mouth and returns the procedure room to order. All of the instruments that have been used are sterilized by the dental assistant.

Resources

BOOKS

Landau, Elaine. *Cavities and Toothaches.* New York: Marshall Cavendish Benchmark, 2008.

Pitts, Nigel, ed. *Detection, Assessment, Diagnosis and Monitoring of Caries.* New York: Krager, 2009.

Sroda, Rebecca. *Nutrition for a Healthy Mouth,* 2nd ed. Philadelphia: Wolters Kluwer Health/Lippincott Williams and Wilkins, 2010.

PERIODICALS

"Improving Patient Awareness: Methods For Optimal Caries Detection." *Practical Procedures and Aesthetic Dentistry.* (September 2008) 20(8): 282–284.

Kolahi, Jafar, Fazilati, Mohamad, and Kadivar, Mahdi. "Towards Tooth Friendly Soft Drinks." *Medical Hypotheses* (October 2009) 73(4): 524–525.

ORGANIZATIONS

American Dental Association, 211 East Chicago Avenue, Chicago IL, 60611-2678, (312) 440-2500, www.ada.org.

American Dental Education Association, 1400 K Street, Suite 1100, Washington DC, 20005, (202) 289-7201, (202) 289-7204, www.adea.org.

American Dental Hygienists' Association, 444 North Michigan Avenue, Suite 3400, Chicago IL, 60611, (312) 440-8900, mail@adha.net, www.adha.org.

Janie F. Franz
Tish Davidson, AM

Dental hygiene ***see* Oral hygiene**

Dental sealants

Definition

A dental sealant is a thin layer of plastic substance that is painted over teeth to discourage the formation of dental caries (cavities).

Demographics

Dental sealants normally are applied to the permanent back teeth (pre-molars and molars) of children soon after these teeth erupt through the gum, most often between the ages of six and 12 years. In a 2005 study, the United States Centers for Disease Control and Prevention (CDC) found that only 32% of children aged 6–19 years had received dental sealants. One of the goals of the United States Department of Health and Human Services Initiative Healthy People 2010 is to increase the percentage of children who receive dental sealants to 50%.

Purpose

The purpose of applying dental sealants is to protect the teeth by sealing out food particles and acids produced by bacteria so that they do not accumulate on the tooth surface and cause decay.

Description

Dental sealants, sometimes called tooth sealants, are plastic material that first appeared in the 1960s. Sealants usually are applied to the chewing teeth—the pre-molars and molars. These are teeth that have what dentists call "pits and fissures" or rough surfaces with deep grooves that a toothbrush has trouble cleaning.

Teeth continuously develop a coating plaque that consists of bacteria and mucin. In order to prevent **tooth decay**, plaque must be removed daily through brushing and flossing. The structure of the pre-molars and molars makes it very difficult to reach all surfaces with a toothbrush. When dental sealant is applied to these teeth, it protects the tooth enamel from plaque. This helps prevent tooth decay and may ultimately save the individual money by eliminating the need for fillings, crowns, or other treatment for tooth decay. Some dental insurance will pay for sealants but may put restrictions on when or to which teeth they may be applied. Individuals should check with their insurance company.

Dental sealants can be applied quickly and painlessly. The procedure is as follows:

- The tooth is cleaned and dried.
- An acid solution is painted on the tooth in order to roughen the surface so that the dental sealant adheres to the tooth better.
- The tooth is rinsed and dried.
- A liquid sealant is applied to the tooth.
- The sealant quickly hardens.

In March 2008, the American Dental Association (ADA) made the following recommendations based on critical evaluation of studies conducted on dental sealants (evidence based medicine):

- Sealants should be placed on pits and fissures of children's and adolescent's permanent teeth when these teeth are at risk for developing dental caries.
- Sealants should be placed on teeth early before cavities develop.
- Resin-based sealants are the preferred type of sealant.

The expert committee appointed by the ADA to investigate sealants suggested that sealants be placed on adult teeth in danger of developing dental caries, However, studies of sealants in adults have not been adequate to make this a firm, evidence-based recommendation. The use of sealants in primary (baby) teeth is left to the discretion of the dentist and the parent.

KEY TERMS

Cavity—A hole or weak spot in the tooth surface caused by decay.

Dental caries—The medical term for tooth decay.

Enamel—The hard, outermost surface of a tooth.

Evidence-based medicine—Recommendations that are based on an evaluation of randomized, controlled trials; non-randomized trials; other experiments; descriptive studies; and reports of expert committees. Each class of evidence is graded (A to D, with A being the most reliable) based on the type and size of study. Recommendations and clinical practice guides can then be made using these grades.

Fluoride—A chemical compound containing fluorine that is used to treat water or applied directly to teeth to prevent decay.

Mucin—A protein in saliva that combines with sugars in the mouth to form plaque.

Plaque—A thin, sticky, colorless film that forms on teeth. Plaque is composed of mucin, sugars from food, and bacteria that live in the plaque.

Benefits

There is clear evidence that sealant applied when secondary pre-molars or molars erupt from the gum will reduce the likelihood of developing dental caries in these teeth. Adults may have sealants applied, but the benefit to adults has not been proven.

Precautions

The tooth must be free of decay before the sealant is applied. If tooth decay has already begun, there exists the possibility that they tooth will continue to decay under the sealant and that this will not be detected until much damage has already been done.

The sealant material may contain small amounts of **bisphenol A** (BPA), a material found in plastics that has been shown to cause **cancer** in animals. As of 2010, the ADA has stated that BPA is rarely used in dental sealants and that the small amount that may be present should not cause health concerns. Some European countries and Canada are considerably more concerned about the health risks of BPA than the United States. They are more likely to regulate the use of this material.

Preparation

The tooth is examined for any sign of decay. If no decay is found, the tooth is cleaned before the sealant is applied. If there is any sign of dental caries, the sealant should not be applied; instead, the decay should be removed and the tooth filled.

Aftercare

Sealants harden very quickly. No aftercare is needed. Sealants last on average five to ten years.

Risks

There are no known risks related to the application of dental sealants except for the concerns mentioned in the Precautions section.

Research and general acceptance

The American Dental Association and most other dental associations in developed countries endorse the use of dental sealants on secondary pre-molars and molars of children. Use of sealants in adults and on primary teeth of children is not specifically endorsed, but is left up to the discretion of the dentist and the patient.

Holistic dentists tend to be less enthusiastic about the use of dental sealants, citing concerns about trapping decay in the tooth and the presence of BPA in the sealant material.

Training and certification

Sealants are applied by a licensed dentist, often with the assistance of a certified dental hygienist.

Resources

BOOKS

Harris, Norman O., Garcia-Godoy, Franklin, and Nathe, Christine Nielsen. *Primary Preventive Dentistry,* 7th ed. Upper Saddle River, NJ: Pearson, 2009.

Hollins, Carole. *Basic Guide to Dental Procedures.* Oxford: Blackwell Publishing, 2008.

Runkle, Richard S. *Taking a Giant Bite Out of Dental Confusion: The Consumer's Guide to 21st Century Dentistry.* Moscow, ID: Luminary Media Group, 2008.

Taggart, Jose C., ed. *Handbook of Dental Care: Diagnostic, Preventive, and Restorative Services.* Hauppauge, NY: Nova Science Publishers, 2009.

PERIODICALS

Hyde, Susan, et al. "Developing an Acceptability Assessment of Preventive Dental Treatments." *Journal of Public Health Dentistry,* (2009) 69(1):18–23.

OTHER

Pit-and-Fissure Sealants. American Dental Association. Undated [accessed January 10, 2010], http://www.ada.org/prof/resources/topics/sealants.asp.

Things to Know About Tooth Sealants. Dental Health Directory Library. Undated [accessed January 10, 2010], http://www.dental–health.com/tooth_sealants.html.

Weil, Andrew. Are Dental Sealants Safe? October.12, 2009, http://www.drweil.com/drw/u/QAA400629/Are-Dental-Sealants-Safe.html.

ORGANIZATIONS

American Dental Association, 211 East Chicago Avenue, Chicago IL, 60611-2678, (312) 440-2500, www.ada.org.

American Dental Education Association, 1400 K Street, Suite 1100, Washington DC, 20005, (202) 289-7201, (202) 289-7204, www.adea.org.

American Dental Hygienists' Association, 444 North Michigan Avenue, Suite 3400, Chicago IL, 60611, (312) 440-8900, mail@adha.net, www.adha.org.

Tish Davidson, AM
Brenda Lerner

Dental trauma

Definition

Dental trauma is injury to the mouth, including teeth, lips, gums, tongue, and jawbones. The most common dental trauma is a broken or lost tooth.

Description

Dental trauma may be inflicted in a number of ways: contact **sports**, motor vehicle accidents, fights, falls, eating hard foods, drinking hot liquids, and other such mishaps. As oral tissues are highly sensitive, injuries to the mouth are typically very painful. Dental trauma should receive prompt treatment from a dentist.

Causes and symptoms

Soft tissue injuries, such as a "fat lip," a burned tongue, or a cut inside the cheek, are characterized by **pain**, redness, and swelling with or without bleeding. A broken tooth often has a sharp edge that may cut the tongue and cheek. Depending on the position of the fracture, the tooth may or may not cause **toothache** pain. When a tooth is knocked out (evulsed), the socket is swollen, painful, and bloody. A jawbone may be broken if the upper and lower teeth no longer fit together properly (**malocclusion**), or if the jaws have pain with limited ability to open and close (mobility), especially around the temporomandibular joint (TMJ).

Diagnosis

Dental trauma is readily apparent upon examination. **Dental x rays** may be taken to determine the extent of the damage to broken teeth. More comprehensive **x rays** are needed to diagnose a broken jaw.

Treatment

Soft tissue injuries may require only cold compresses to reduce swelling. Bleeding may be controlled with direct pressure applied with clean gauze. Deep lacerations and punctures may require stitches. Pain may be managed with aspirin or **acetaminophen** (Tylenol, Aspirin Free Excedrin) or ibuprofen (Motrin, Advil).

Treatment of a broken tooth will vary depending on the severity of the fracture. For immediate **first aid**, the injured tooth and surrounding area should be rinsed gently with warm water to remove dirt, then covered with a cold compress to reduce swelling and ease pain. A dentist should examine the injury as soon as possible. Any pieces from the broken tooth should be saved and brought along.

If a piece of the outer tooth has chipped off, but the inner core (pulp) is undisturbed, the dentist may simply smooth the rough edges or replace the missing section with a small composite filling. In some cases, a fragment of broken tooth may be bonded back into place. If enough tooth is missing to compromise the entire tooth structure, but the pulp is not permanently damaged, the tooth will require a protective coverage with a gold or porcelain crown. If the pulp has been seriously damaged, the tooth will require root canal treatment before it receives a crown. A tooth that is vertically fractured or fractured below the gumline will require root canal treatment and protective restoration. A tooth that no longer has enough remaining structure to retain a crown may have to be extracted (surgically removed).

When a permanent tooth has been knocked out, it may be saved with prompt action. The tooth must be found immediately after it has been lost. It should be picked up by the natural crown (the top part covered by hard enamel). It must not be handled by the root. If the tooth is dirty, it may be gently rinsed under running water. It should never be scrubbed, and it should never be washed with soap, toothpaste, mouthwash, or other chemicals. The tooth should not be dried or wrapped in a tissue or cloth. It must be kept moist at all times.

The tooth may be placed in a clean container of milk, cool water with or without a pinch of salt, or in saliva. If possible, the patient and the tooth should be brought to the dentist within 30 minutes of the tooth loss. Rapid action improves the chances of successful re-implantation; however, it is possible to save a tooth after 30 minutes, if the tooth has been kept moist and handled properly.

The body usually rejects re-implantation of a primary (baby) tooth. In this case, the empty socket is treated as a soft tissue injury and monitored until the permanent tooth erupts.

A broken jaw must be set back into its proper position and stabilized with wires while it heals. Healing may take six weeks or longer, depending on the patient's age and the severity of the fracture.

Alternative treatment

There is no substitute for treatment by a dentist or other medical professional. There are, however, homeopathic remedies and herbs that can be used simultaneously with dental care and throughout the healing process. Homeopathic arnica (*Arnica montana*) should be taken as soon as possible after the injury to help the body deal with the trauma. Repeating a dose several times daily for the duration of healing is also useful. Homeopathic hypericum (*Hypericum perforatum*) can be taken if nerve pain is involved, especially with a **tooth extraction** or root canal. Homeopathic comfrey (officinale) *Symphytum* may be helpful in treating pain due to broken jaw bones, but should only be used after the bones have been reset. Calendula (*Calendula officinalis*) and plantain (*Plantago major*) can be used as a mouth rinse to enhance tissue healing. These herbs should not be used with deep lacerations that need to heal from the inside first.

Prognosis

When dental trauma receives timely attention and proper treatment, the prognosis for healing is good. As with other types of trauma, infection may be a complication, but a course of **antibiotics** is generally effective.

Prevention

Most dental trauma is preventable. Car seat belts should always be worn, and young children should be secured in appropriate car seats. Homes should be monitored for potential tripping and slipping hazards. Child-proofing measures should be taken, especially for toddlers. In addition to placing gates across stairs and padding sharp table edges, electrical cords should be tucked away. Young children may receive severe oral **burns** from gnawing on live power cords.

Everyone who participates in contact sports should wear a mouthguard to avoid dental trauma. Athletes in football, ice hockey, wrestling, and boxing commonly wear mouthguards. The mandatory use of mouthguards in football prevents about 200,000 oral injuries annually. Mouthguards should also be worn along with helmets in noncontact sports such as skateboarding, in-line skating, and bicycling. An athlete who does not wear a mouthguard is 60 times more likely to sustain dental trauma than one who does. Any activity involving speed, an increased chance of falling, and potential contact with a hard piece of equipment has the likelihood of dental trauma that may be prevented or substantially reduced in severity with the use of mouthguards.

KEY TERMS

Crown—The natural part of the tooth covered by enamel. A restorative crown is a protective shell that fits over a tooth.

Eruption—The process of a tooth breaking through the gum tissue to grow into place in the mouth.

Evulsion—The forceful, and usually accidental, removal of a tooth from its socket in the bone.

Extraction—The surgical removal of a tooth from its socket in the bone.

Malocclusion—A problem in the way the upper and lower teeth fit together in biting or chewing.

Pulp—The soft innermost layer of a tooth containing blood vessels and nerves.

Root canal treatment—The process of removing diseased or damaged pulp from a tooth, then filling and sealing the pulp chamber and root canals.

Temporomandibular joint (TMJ)—The jaw joint formed by the mandible (lower jaw bone) moving against the temporal (temple and side) bone of the skull.

ORGANIZATIONS

American Academy of Pediatric Dentistry, 211 East Chicago Ave., Ste. 700, Chicago IL, 60611-2616, (312) 337-2169, http://www.aapd.org.

American Association of Endodontists, 211 East Chicago Ave., Ste. 1100, Chicago IL, 60611-2691, (800) 872-3636, http://www.aae.org.

American Association of Oral and Maxillofacial Surgeons, 9700 West Bryn Mawr Ave., Rosemont IL, 60018-5701, (847) 678-6200, http://www.aaoms.org.

American Dental Association, 211 E. Chicago Ave., Chicago IL, 60611, (312) 440-2500, http://www.ada.org.

Bethany Thivierge

Dental x rays

Definition

Dental **x rays** are pictures taken of the mouth area using high-energy photons with very short wavelengths. They show the teeth and surrounding bone.

Purpose

Dental x rays are effective in discovering **tooth decay**, broken fillings, fractured teeth, tumors, occlusal trauma, or impacted or ectopic teeth that would otherwise be unseen by the eye, in between the teeth and below the gum tissue.

Description

Dental x rays are part of the dental examination for aiding in the diagnostic process. X rays are vital in the diagnosis of root canal treatment on checking the apical of the tooth and the surrounding structures for abscesses or bone loss. Without the aid of dental x rays, 60% of dental decay would be missed. Diagnostic x rays are essential in providing accurate information. The most common x rays taken are:

- bitewing x rays (vertical and horizontal bitewings)
- panoramic x rays
- periapical x rays
- occlusal x rays

Each is used in its own respective degree of diagnosis, with the bitewing x ray being the most common. Bitewings are the most effective in discovering tooth decay in between the teeth and on adjacent teeth. A bitewing shows only the top crown portion of the tooth structure. It is called a bitewing due to the way the patient can bite down and hold the film securely in place. The bitewing is good in diagnosing and evaluating periodontal conditions and bone levels between the teeth. They are also good in detecting tartar buildup.

The panoramic (a type of film used), or Panorex (brand name) is also commonly taken on the initial visit to the dental office. This type of x ray makes a complete circle of the head from one ear to the other, to produce a complete two-dimensional representation of all the teeth. This x ray will also show bone structure beneath the teeth and the temporomandibular joint (TMJ). The panoramic is the most commonly used x ray in the aid of diagnostic decisions regarding third molar extractions (wisdom teeth) for people who are edentulous (the tooth is not there/has not erupted). This special x ray, however, has its advantages and disadvantages.

One advantage of the panoramic is that a broad area is imaged, showing many structures. Furthermore, the exposure level emits low radiation. The panoramic is excellent for evaluation of trauma, tooth development, and certain anomalies. In some cases dental x rays can even reveal non-dental medical conditions. One study at the University of Buffalo School of Dental Medicine demonstrated that calcifications in the carotid arteries, which were exposed on standard panoramic x rays, served as predictors of **death** from cardiovascular disease.

The main disadvantage of panoramic x rays is that the image shown does not provide the fine detail of a bitewing x ray. The procedure for taking a panoramic x ray is also somewhat confining to the patient, as the x-ray machine takes a minute or more to fully encircle the head for the complete picture. These films are not good in aiding the diagnosis of decay, bone level, and certain types of periapical problems.

A periapical x ray is similar to a bitewing. This type of x ray shows the entire tooth area, from crown to root, and the bone surrounding the root from a side view. This type of film will reveal any root anomalies, changes in the bone and surrounding tissue, cysts, bone tumors, and abscesses. The fine detail in the periapical film is necessary in diagnosis and treatment planning, and is commonly taken during root canal treatment and crown restoration procedures.

Occlusal films are least common. These films show the whole bite of the lower or upper jaw. Occlusal x rays, when taken, are mainly taken on children to show the eruption order of the permanent teeth.

X rays pass through hard and soft tissue in the mouth. The x-ray beam is blocked by denser structures, such as teeth, fillings, jaws, and bones. Teeth appear lighter because fewer x rays go through the teeth to reach the film. Cavities and gum disease appear darker (shown by a dark spot in the tooth or loss of bone structure around the tooth) because of more x-ray penetration. On the film, the white images are the dense structures.

Operation

William Roentgen, a German scientist, discovered the x ray in 1895. He found that x rays are energy in the form of waves, similar to visible light. The only difference between light and x rays is that light does not have the ability to penetrate the body as x ray energy does. Light makes pictures of the outside of objects, while x rays have the ability to make pictures of the inside of objects. The roentgen represents the amount of exposure given off by one single energy photon. The amount of absorbed x ray in the body is a unit called a rad. A unit called "rem" accounts for the difference in biological effectiveness of different types of radiation, such as secondary radiation, or cosmic radiation. One rem equals one rad. One rad equals one R and one thousand milliroentgens, more commonly known as mrad; it is equal to one roentgen (R).

Research conducted by the Idaho Radiation Network set a maximum permissible x ray dose for one year at 5R (roentgens). A full mouth set of dental x rays consists of 18 to 20 films (bitewings, periapicals, occlusals, and panoramic x rays). The amount of radiation for receiving the full-mouth set of x rays is 10 to 20 mrads (milliroentgens). The benefits derived from x rays greatly outweigh the radiation concerns. The amount of radiation an average person receives each year from background sources (e.g., outer space, materials in the earth, foods consumed, and naturally radioactive materials in the body) is about 360 mrads.

Secondary radiation consists of the radiation waves left over after the source of radiation is stopped. Most secondary waves can penetrate tissue and are the most damaging waves from radiation. Measures taken to prevent damaging rays are:

- setting radiation exposure to lower settings depending on the patient's age, height, build and structure
- using high-speed films to minimize exposure time
- using lead-filled aprons to shield sensitive body parts, such as thyroid glands and gonads
- x-ray badges worn by dental staff to monitor the amount of radiation exposure in the workplace

Maintenance

Dental x rays are essential in diagnosing and treating oral disease, abnormal tooth development, or trauma. At the initial dental examination, a full-mouth set of x rays may be taken (bitewings and panoramic). Thereafter, it is the dentist who should determine when and how often x rays will be required. Children are usually more cavity prone than adults; x rays may be taken with regard to degree of risk, or at the check-up examination every six months.

An adult presenting a **dental trauma** will need x rays to diagnose what the treatment should be. More x rays may be needed depending on the treatment plan and the extent of the injury.

The American Dental Association (ADA) recommends basic guidelines on taking dental x rays. On average, bitewing x rays should be taken approximately once a year. This is mainly to detect and treat any conditions early in their development. If the overall general health of the mouth is good, x rays can be taken every 18 to 24 months. The ADA also recommends that the type and frequency of dental x rays taken at an examination be based upon clinical judgment after the examination and consideration of the dental health and the general health of the patient.

Health care team roles

A registered dental assistant (RDA) or registered dental hygienist (RDH) commonly takes the x rays during a dental examination. They review the health and dental history, chart, and age of the patient to be x rayed. Adjustments are made to the x-ray unit depending on the size and age of the patient. The RDA then develops and mounts the x rays and presents them to the dentist. The dentist will interpret the x rays and complete the oral examination. A treatment plan will follow.

Training

An RDA and an RDH must have an x-ray certification in order to take and develop x rays. To become certified, full-mouth sets of x rays need to be taken. Knowledge of the x-ray machine unit is needed, as is the number of roentgens emitted from a variety of different x-ray machines. Furthermore, a working knowledge of angles and height of the x-ray unit is needed; this is necessary for taking fine-detailed images. Certification also requires knowledge of the principles of radiation **safety**.

Classes leading to certification as an RDA or RDH are available outside the work setting. Each state has different bylaws regarding x-ray licensing for technicians.

KEY TERMS

Apical—Rounded end of the root of a tooth that is embedded in hard tissue (bone); toward the apex of the root.

Crown—1. The upper part of the tooth, covered by enamel. 2. A dental restoration that is a protective shell fitting over a tooth.

Eruption—The process of a tooth breaking through the gum tissue to grow into place in the mouth.

Pulp—The soft, innermost part of a tooth containing blood and lymph vessels, and nerves.

Root canal treatment—The process of removing diseased or damaged pulp tissue from a tooth, then filling and sealing the pulp chamber and root canals.

The rules of the state in which one is interested in working should be consulted.

Resources

BOOKS

Bunkle, Richard S. *Taking a Giant Bite Out of Dental Confusion: The Consumer's Guide to 21st Century Dentistry.* Moscow, ID: Luminary Media Group, 2008.

Hollins, Carole. *Basic Guide to Dental Procedures.* Oxford: Blackwell Publishing, 2008.

Whaites, Eric. *Radiography and Radiology for Dental Nurses,* 2nd ed. New York: Saunders, 2009.

PERIODICALS

Barge, Katie. "Dental X Rays Accurately Predict Osteoporosis Risk." *Journal of Dental Hygiene* 81, no. 2 (2007): 42.

Robb-Nicholson, Celeste. "By The Way, Doctor. What Kind of Radiation Causes Thyroid Cancer? What About Microwave Ovens and Dental X Rays?" *Harvard Women's Health Watch* 14, no. 6 (February 2007): 8.

ORGANIZATIONS

American Dental Association, 211 East Chicago Avenue, Chicago IL, 60611-2678, (312) 440-2500, www.ada.org.

American Dental Education Association, 1400 K Street, Suite 1100, Washington DC, 20005, (202) 289-7201, (202) 289-7204, www.adea.org.

American Dental Hygienists' Association, 444 North Michigan Avenue, Suite 3400, Chicago IL, 60611, (312) 440-8900, mail@adha.net, www.adha.org.

Cindy F. Ovard, RDA
Tish Davidson, AM
Brenda Lerner

Dependent personality disorder

Definition

Dependent personality disorder is defined as a lack of self-confidence coupled with excessive dependence on others.

Description

Persons affected by dependent personality disorder have a disproportionately low level of confidence in their own **intelligence** and abilities and have difficulty making decisions and undertaking projects on their own.

KEY TERMS

Psychologist—A mental health professional who treats mental and behavioral disorders by support and insight to encourage healthy behavior patterns and personality growth. Psychologists also study the brain, behavior, emotions, and learning.

Psychotherapy—The treatment of mental and behavioral disorders by support and insight to encourage healthy behavior patterns and personality growth.

Causes and symptoms

Dependent personality disorder occurs equally in males and females and begins by early adulthood. It may be linked to either chronic physical illness or separation anxietydisorder earlier in life.

Individuals with this disorder have a pervasive reliance on others, even for minor tasks or decisions, making them exaggeratedly cooperative out of **fear** of alienating those whose help they need. They are reluctant to express disagreement with others and are often willing to go to abnormal lengths to win the approval of those on whom they rely. Another common feature of the disorder is an exaggerated fear of being left to fend for oneself. Adolescents with dependent personality disorder rely on their parents to make even minor decisions for them, such as what they should wear or how they should spend their free time, as well as major ones, such as what college they should attend.

Diagnosis

Individuals believed to have dependent personality disorder should undergo a thorough physical examination and patient history to rule out possible organic causes, or physical reasons for dependency on others. If a psychological cause is suspected, a mental health professional will typically conduct an interview with the patient and administer clinical tests to evaluate psychological status.

Treatment

The primary treatment for dependent personality disorder is psychotherapy, with an emphasis on learning to cope with **anxiety**, developing assertiveness, and improving decision-making skills. Group therapy can also be helpful.

Prognosis

Individuals with this disorder may experience improvement with long term physiological therapy.

Resources

BOOKS

Graham, George. *The Disordered Mind: An Introduction to Philosophy of Mind and Mental Illness.* New York: Routledge, 2010.

Shams, K., MD. *Human Relation and Personified Relational Disorders.* Raleigh, NC: lulu.com, 2009.

ORGANIZATIONS

American Psychiatric Association, 1400 K Street NW, Washington DC, 20005, (888) 357-7924, http://www.psych.org.

American Psychological Association (APA), 750 First St. NE, Washington DC, 20002-4242 (202) 336-5700, http://www.apa.org.

National Alliance for the Mentally Ill (NAMI), Colonial Place Three, 2107 Wilson Blvd., Ste. 300, Arlington VA, 22201-3042 (800) 950-6264, http://www.nami.org.

ORGANIZATIONS

American Psychiatric Association, 1000 Wilson Boulevard, Suite 1825, Arlington VA, 22209, (703) 907-7300, apa@psych.org, http://www.psych.org/.

National Alliance on Mental Illness (NAMI), Colonial Place Three, 2107 Wilson Blvd., Suite 300, Arlington VA, 22201, (703) 524-7600, (800) 950-NAMI (6264), (703) 524-9094, http://www.nami.org/Hometemplate.cfm.

National Institute of Mental Health (NIMH), 6001 Executive Boulevard, Room 8184, MSC 9663, Bethesda MD, 20892, (301) 443-4513, (866) 615-6464, (301) 443-4279, nimhinfo@nih.gov, http://www.nimh.nih.gov/index.shtml.

National Mental Health Association (NMHA), 2000 N. Beauregard Street, 6th Floor, Alexandria VA, 22311, (703) 684-7722, (800) 969-NMHA, (703) 684-5968, http://www1.nmha.org/.

Laura Jean Cataldo, RN, EdD

Depersonalization disorder *see* **Dissociative disorders**

Depression *see* **Depressive disorders**

Depressive disorders

Definition

Depression or depressive disorders (unipolar depression) are mental illnesses characterized by a profound and persistent feeling of sadness or despair and/or a loss of interest in things that once were pleasurable. Disturbance in **sleep**, appetite, and mental processes are a common accompaniment.

Description

Everyone experiences feelings of unhappiness and sadness occasionally. But when these depressed feelings start to dominate everyday life and cause physical and mental deterioration, they become what are known as depressive disorders. There are two main categories of depressive disorders: major depressive disorder and dysthymic disorder. Major depressive disorder is a moderate to severe episode of depression lasting two or more weeks. Individuals experiencing this major depressive episode may have trouble sleeping, lose interest in activities they once took pleasure in, experience a change in weight, have difficulty concentrating, feel worthless and hopeless, or have a preoccupation with **death** or **suicide**. In children, major depression may be characterized by irritability.

In 2006 The National Institutes of Mental Health estimated that about 6.7% of Americans adults are affected by major depressive disorder, and about 1.5% are affected by dyrthmic disorder in a given year. Major depressive disorder has a median age of onset of 32 years, and affects

Percentage of youth ages 12–17 who suffered at least one major depressive episode with severe impairment in the past year, by select demographic characteristics

Age	
12–13	3.1
14–15	6.0
16–17	8.3
Gender	
Male	2.9
Female	9.2
Race/ethnicity	
White[1]	6.5
Black[1]	4.7
American Indian or Alaska Native	6.5
Asian	4.7
Two or more races	10.2
Hispanic	5.1
Total:	**6.0**

[1]Non-Hispanic origin

SOURCE: Substance Abuse and Mental Health Services Administration, Office of Applied Studies, *Results from the 2008 National Survey on Drug Use and Health: National Findings* (2009).

(Table by PreMediaGlobal. Reproduced by permission of Gale, a part of Cengage Learning.)

Depressive disorders

Diagnosis	Symptoms	Treatment
Sadness	Transient, normal depressive response or mood change due to stress.	Emotional support
Bereavement	Sadness related to a major loss that persists for less than two months after the loss. Thoughts of death and morbid preoccupation with worthlessness are also present.	Emotional support, counseling
Sadness problem	Sadness or irritability that begins to resemble major depressive disorder, but lower in severity and more transient.	Support, counseling, medication possible
Adjustment disorder with depressed mood	Symptoms include depressed mood, tearfulness, and hopelessness, and occur within three months of an identifiable stressor. Symptoms resolve in six months.	Psychotherapy, medication
Major depressive disorder	A depressed or irritable mood or diminished pleasure as well as three to seven of the following criteria almost daily for two weeks. The criteria include: recurrent thoughts of death and suicidal ideation, weight loss or gain, fatigue or energy loss, feelings of worthlessness, diminished ability to concentrate, insomnia or hypersomnia, and feeling hyper and jittery or abnormally slow.	Psychotherapy, medication
Dysthymic disorder	Depressed mood for most of the day, for more days than not, for one year, including the presence of two of the following symptoms: poor appetite or overeating, insomnia/hypersomnia, low energy/fatigue, poor concentration, and feelings of hopelessness. Symptoms are less severe than those of a major depressive episode but are more persistent.	Psychotherapy, medication
Bipolar I disorder, most recent episode depressed	Current major depressive episode with a history of one manic or mixed episode. (Manic episode is longer than four days and causes significant impairment in normal functioning.) Moods are not accounted for by another psychiatric disorder.	Psychotherapy, medication
Bipolar II disorder, recurrent major depressive episodes with hypomanic episodes	Presence or history of one major depressive episode and one hypomanic episode (similar to manic episode but shorter and less severe). Symptoms are not accounted for by another psychiatric disorder and cause clinically significant impairment in functioning.	Psychotherapy, medication

SOURCE: Academy of American Family Physicians, http://www.aafp.org.

(Table by PreMediaGlobal. Reproduced by permission of Gale, a part of Cengage Learning.)

women more frequently than men. Dyrthmic disorder has a median age of onset of 31 years. Both disorders may occur in any age group, from children to the elderly.

While major depressive episodes may be acute (intense but short-lived), dysthymic disorder is an ongoing, chronic depression that lasts two or more years (one or more years in children) and has an average duration of 16 years. The mild to moderate depression of dysthymic disorder may rise and fall in intensity, and those afflicted with the disorder may experience some periods of normal, non-depressed mood of up to two months in length. Its onset is gradual, and dysthymic patients may not be able to pinpoint exactly when they started feeling depressed. Individuals with dysthymic disorder may experience a change in sleeping and eating patterns, low **self-esteem**, fatigue, trouble concentrating, and feelings of hopelessness.

Depression also can occur in **bipolar disorder**, an affective mental illness that causes radical emotional changes and mood swings, from manic highs to depressive lows. The majority of bipolar individuals experience alternating episodes of mania and depression.

Causes and symptoms

The causes behind depression are complex and not yet fully understood. While an imbalance of certain neurotransmitters—the chemicals in the brain that transmit messages between nerve cells—is believed to play a key role in depression, external factors such as upbringing and environment (more so in dysthymia than major depression) may be as important. For example, it is speculated that, if an individual is abused and neglected throughout childhood and **adolescence**, a pattern of low self-esteem and negative thinking may emerge. From that, a lifelong pattern of depression may follow. Many different factors have been linked to major depression, including chronic **pain**, severe obesity, and **smoking** (among teenagers).

Heredity seems to play a role in who develops depressive disorders. Individuals with major depression in their immediate family are up to three times more likely to have the disorder themselves. It would seem that biological and genetic factors may make certain individuals predisposed or prone to depressive disorders, but environmental circumstances often may trigger the disorder.

External stressors and significant life changes, such as chronic medical problems, death of a loved one, **divorce** or estrangement, miscarriage, or loss of a job, also can result in a form of depression known as adjustment disorder. Although periods of adjustment disorder usually resolve themselves, occasionally they may evolve into a major depressive disorder.

Major depressive episode

Individuals experiencing a major depressive episode have a depressed mood and/or a diminished interest or pleasure in activities. Children experiencing a major depressive episode may appear or feel irritable rather than depressed. In addition, five or more of the following symptoms will occur on an almost daily basis for a period of at least two weeks:

- Significant change in weight.
- Insomnia or hypersomnia (excessive sleep).
- Psychomotor agitation or retardation.
- Fatigue or loss of energy.
- Feelings of worthlessness or inappropriate guilt.
- Diminished ability to think or to concentrate, or indecisiveness.
- Recurrent thoughts of death or suicide and/or suicide attempts.

Dysthymic disorder

Dysthymia commonly occurs in tandem with other psychiatric and physical conditions. Up to 70% of dysthymic patients have both dysthymic disorder and major depressive disorder, known as double depression. **Substance abuse**, panic disorders, **personality disorders**, social **phobias**, and other psychiatric conditions also are found in many dysthymic patients. Dysthymia and medical conditions often co-occur. The connection between them is unclear, but it may be related to the way the medical condition and/or its pharmacological treatment affects neurotransmitters. Dysthymia is prevalent in patients with multiple sclerosis, **AIDS**, **hypothyroidism**, chronic fatigue syndrome, Parkinson's disease, diabetes, and post-cardiac transplantation. Dysthymic disorder can lengthen or complicate the recovery of patients with these and other medical conditions.

Along with an underlying feeling of depression, people with dysthymic disorder experience two or more of the following symptoms on an almost daily basis for a period for two or more years (many experience them for five or more years), or one year or more for children:

- under or overeating
- insomnia or hypersomnia
- low energy or fatigue
- low self-esteem
- poor concentration or trouble making decisions
- feelings of hopelessness

Diagnosis

In addition to an interview, several clinical inventories or scales may be used to assess a patient's mental status and determine the presence of depressive symptoms. Among these tests are: the Hamilton Depression Scale (HAM-D), Child Depression Inventory (CDI), Geriatric Depression Scale (GDS), Beck Depression Inventory (BDI), and the Zung Self-Rating Scale for Depression. These tests may be administered in an outpatient or hospital setting by a general practitioner, social worker, psychiatrist, or psychologist.

Treatment

Major depressive and dysthymic disorders are typically treated with a combination of antidepressants and psychosocial therapy. Psychosocial therapy focuses on the personal and interpersonal issues behind depression, while antidepressant medication is prescribed to provide more immediate relief for the symptoms of the disorder. When used together correctly, therapy and antidepressants are a powerful treatment plan for the depressed patient.

Antidepressants

Selective serotonin reuptake inhibitors (SSRIs) such as fluoxetine (Prozac) and sertraline (Zoloft) reduce depression by increasing levels of serotonin, a neurotransmitter. Some clinicians prefer SSRIs for treatment of dysthymic disorder. **Anxiety**, **diarrhea**, drowsiness, **headache**, sweating, nausea, poor sexual functioning, and insomnia all are possible side effects of SSRIs. In early 2004, the U.S. Food and Drug Administration (FDA) issued warnings to physicians and parents about increased risk of suicide among children and adolescents taking SSRIs.

Tricyclic antidepressants (TCAs) are less expensive than SSRIs, but have more severe side-effects, which may include persistent dry mouth, sedation, **dizziness**, and cardiac arrhythmias. Because of these side effects, caution is taken when prescribing TCAs to elderly patients. TCAs include amitriptyline (Elavil), imipramine (Tofranil), and nortriptyline (Aventyl, Pamelor). A 10-day supply of TCAs can be lethal if ingested all at once, so these drugs may not be a preferred treatment option for patients at risk for suicide.

Monoamine oxidase inhibitors (MAOIs) such as tranylcypromine (Parnate) and phenelzine (Nardil) block the action of monoamine oxidase (MAO), an enzyme in the central nervous system. Patients taking MAOIs must cut foods high in tyramine (found in aged cheeses and meats) out of their diet to avoid potentially serious hypertensive side effects.

Heterocyclics include bupropion (Wellbutrin) and trazodone (Desyrel). Bupropion should not be prescribed to patients with a **seizure disorder**. Side effects of the drug may include agitation, anxiety, confusion, tremor, dry mouth, fast or irregular heartbeat, headache, low blood pressure, and insomnia. Because trazodone has a sedative effect, it is useful in treating depressed patients with insomnia. Other possible side effects of trazodone include dry mouth, gastrointestinal distress, dizziness, and headache.

Psychosocial therapy

Psychotherapy explores an individual's life to bring to light possible contributing causes of the present depression. During treatment, the therapist helps the patient to become self-aware of his or her thinking patterns and how they came to be. There are several different subtypes of psychotherapy, but all have the common goal of helping the patient develop healthy problem solving and coping skills.

Cognitive-behavioral therapy assumes that the patient's problematic thinking is causing the current depression and focuses on changing the depressed patient's thought patterns and perceptions. The therapist helps the patient identify negative or distorted thought patterns and the emotions and the behaviors that accompany them, and then retrains the depressed individual to recognize the thinking and react differently to it.

Electroconvulsant therapy

ECT, or electroconvulsive therapy, usually is employed after all psychosocial therapy and pharmaceutical treatment options have been explored. However, it is sometimes used early in treatment when severe depression is present and the patient refuses oral medication, or when the patient is becoming dehydrated, extremely suicidal, or psychotic.

The treatment consists of a series of electrical pulses that move into the brain through electrodes on the patient's head. ECT is given under general anesthesia and patients are administered a muscle relaxant to prevent convulsions. Although the exact mechanisms behind the success of ECT therapy are not known, it is believed that the electrical current modifies the electrochemical processes of the brain, consequently relieving depression. Headaches, muscle soreness, nausea, and confusion are possible side effects immediately following an ECT procedure. Memory loss, typically transient, also has been reported in ECT patients.

Alternative treatment

St. John's wort (*Hypericum perforatum*) is used throughout Europe to treat depressive symptoms. Unlike traditional prescription antidepressants, this herbal antidepressant has few reported side effects. Despite uncertainty concerning its effectiveness, it is accepted by many practitioners of alternative medicine. Although St. John's wort appears to be a safe alternative to conventional antidepressants, care should be taken, as the herb can interfere with the actions of some pharmaceuticals, and because herbal supplements are not regulated by the FDA in the same way as conventional medications.

Homeopathic treatment also can be therapeutic in treating depression. Good **nutrition**, proper sleep, **exercise**, and full engagement in life are very important to a healthy mental state.

In several small studies, S-adenosyl-methionine (SAM, SAMe) was shown to be more effective than placebo and equally effective as tricyclic antidepressants in treating depression. The usual dosage is 200 mg to 400 mg twice daily. It may, however, cause some side effects, and an individual should discuss the possible risks and benefits with a doctor.

Prognosis

Untreated or improperly treated depression is the number one cause of suicide in the United States. Proper treatment relieves symptoms in 80–90% of depressed patients. After each major depressive episode, the risk of recurrence climbs significantly—50% after one episode, 70% after two episodes, and 90% after three episodes. For this reason, patients need to be aware of the symptoms of recurring depression and may require long-term maintenance treatment of antidepressants and/or therapy.

Research has found that depression may lead to other problems as well. Increased risk of heart disease has been linked to depression, particularly in postmenopausal women. And while chronic pain may cause depression, some studies indicate that depression may also cause chronic pain.

KEY TERMS

Hypersomnia—The need to sleep excessively; a symptom of dysthymic and major depressive disorder.

Neurotransmitter—A chemical in the brain that transmits messages between neurons, or nerve cells. Changes in the levels of certain neurotransmitters, such as serotonin, norepinephrine, and dopamine, are thought to be related to depressive disorders.

Psychomotor agitation—Disturbed physical and mental processes (e.g., fidgeting, wringing of hands, racing thoughts); a symptom of major depressive disorder.

Psychomotor retardation—Slowed physical and mental processes (e.g., slowed thinking, walking, and talking); a symptom of major depressive disorder.

Prevention

Patient education in the form of therapy or self-help groups is crucial for training patients with depressive disorders to recognize symptoms of depression and to take an active part in their treatment program. Extended maintenance treatment with antidepressants may be required in some patients to prevent relapse. Early intervention for children with depression is usually effective in arresting development of more severe problems.

Resources

BOOKS

Henri, Maurice J., ed. *Trends in Depression Research.* New York: Nova Science Publishers, 2007.

PERIODICALS

"Depression Can Lead to Back Pain." *Biotech Week* March 24, 2004: 576.

"Depression May Be a Risk Factor for Heart Disease, Death in Older Women." *Women's Health Weekly* March 4, 2004: 90.

"FDA Panel Urges Stronger Warnings of Child Suicide." *SCRIP World Pharmaceutical News* February 6, 2004: 24.

"National Study Indicates Obesity Is Linked to Major Depression." *Drug Week* February 13, 2004: 338.

"Researchers See Link Between Depression, Smoking." *Mental Health Weekly* March 1, 2004: 8.

ORGANIZATIONS

American Psychiatric Association, 1400 K Street NW, Washington DC, 20005, (888) 357-7924, http://www.psych.org.

American Psychological Association (APA), 750 First St. NE, Washington DC, 20002-4242 (202) 336-5700, http://www.apa.org.

National Alliance for the Mentally Ill (NAMI), Colonial Place Three, 2107 Wilson Blvd., Ste. 300, Arlington VA, 22201-3042 (800) 950-6264, http://www.nami.org.

National Depressive and Manic-Depressive Association (NDMDA) 730 N. Franklin St., Suite 501, Chicago IL, 60610 (800) 826-3632 http://www.ndmda.org.

National Institute of Mental Health (NIMH), 6001 Executive Boulevard, Room 8184, MSC 9663, Bethesda MD, 20892-9663, (301) 443-4513, (866) 615-6464 nimhinfo@nih.gov, http://www.nimh.nih.gov.

Paula Anne Ford-Martin

Teresa G. Odle

Dermatitis

Definition

Dermatitis is a general term used to describe inflammation of the skin.

Description

Most types of dermatitis are characterized by an itchy pink or red rash.

Contact dermatitis is an allergic reaction to something that irritates the skin and is manifested by one or more lines of red, swollen, blistered skin that may itch or seep. It usually appears within 48 hours after

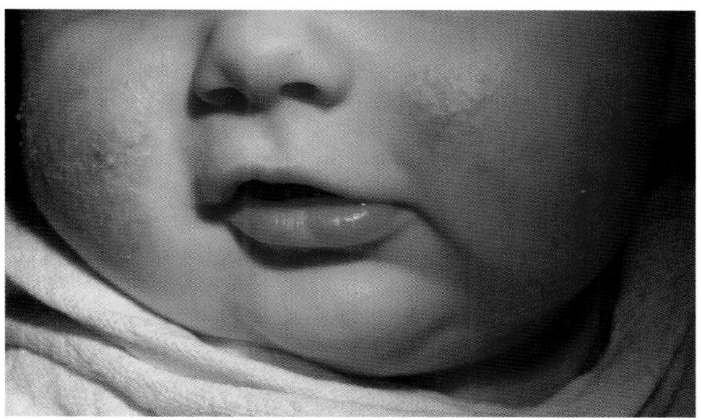

Dry skin on the cheeks of an infant suffering from atopic dermatitis. *(PHANIE/Photo Researchers, Inc.)*

touching or brushing against a substance to which the skin is sensitive. The condition is more common in adults than in children.

Contact dermatitis can occur on any part of the body, but it usually affects the hands, feet, and groin. Contact dermatitis usually does not spread from one person to another, nor does it spread beyond the area exposed to the irritant unless affected skin comes into contact with another part of the body. However, in the case of some irritants, such as **poison ivy**, contact dermatitis can be passed to another person or to another part of the body.

Stasis dermatitis is characterized by scaly, greasy looking skin on the lower legs and around the ankles. Stasis dermatitis is most apt to affect the inner side of the calf.

Nummular dermatitis, which is also called nummular eczematous dermatitis or nummular **eczema**, generally affects the hands, arms, legs, and buttocks of men and women older than 55 years of age. This stubborn inflamed rash forms circular, sometimes itchy, patches and is characterized by flares and periods of inactivity.

Atopic dermatitis is characterized by **itching**, scaling, swelling, and sometimes blistering. In early childhood it is called infantile eczema and is characterized by redness, oozing, and crusting. It is usually found on the face, inside the elbows, and behind the knees.

Seborrheic dermatitis may be dry or moist and is characterized by greasy scales and yellowish crusts on the scalp, eyelids, face, external surfaces of the ears, underarms, breasts, and groin. In infants it is called "cradle cap."

Causes and symptoms

Allergic reactions are genetically determined, and different substances cause contact dermatitis to develop in different people. A reaction to resin produced by poison ivy, **poison oak**, or poison sumac is the most common source of symptoms. It is, in fact, the most common allergy in this country, affecting one of every two people in the United States.

Flowers, herbs, and vegetables can also affect the skin of some people. **Burns** and **sunburn** increase the risk of dermatitis developing, and chemical irritants that can cause the condition include:

- chlorine
- cleansers
- detergents and soaps
- fabric softeners
- glues used on artificial nails
- perfumes
- topical medications

Contact dermatitis can develop when the first contact occurs or after years of use or exposure.

Stasis dermatitis, a consequence of poor circulation, occurs when leg veins can no longer return blood to the heart as efficiently as they once did. When that happens, fluid collects in the lower legs and causes them to swell. Stasis dermatitis can also result in a rash that can break down into sores known as stasis ulcers.

The cause of nummular dermatitis is not known, but it usually occurs in cold weather and is most common in people who have dry skin. Hot weather and stress can aggravate this condition, as can the following:

- allergies
- fabric softeners
- soaps and detergents
- wool clothing
- bathing more than once a day

Atopic dermatitis can be caused by **allergies**, **asthma**, or stress, and there seems to be a genetic predisposition for atopic conditions. It is sometimes caused by an allergy to nickel in jewelry.

Seborrheic dermatitis (for which there may also be a genetic predisposition) is usually caused by overproduction of the oil glands. In adults it can be associated with **diabetes mellitus** or gold allergy. In infants and adults it may be caused by a biotin deficiency.

Diagnosis

The diagnosis of dermatitis is made on the basis of how the rash looks and its location. The doctor may scrape off a small piece of affected skin for microscopic examination or direct the patient to discontinue use of any potential irritant that has recently come into contact with the affected area. Two weeks after the rash disappears, the patient may resume use of the substances, one at a time, until the condition recurs. Eliminating the substance most recently added should eliminate the irritation.

If the origin of the irritation has still not been identified, a dermatologist may perform one or more patch tests. This involves dabbing a small amount of a suspected irritant onto skin on the patient's back. If no irritation develops within a few days, another patch test is performed. The process continues until the patient experiences an allergic reaction at the spot where the irritant was applied.

Treatment

Treating contact dermatitis begins with eliminating or avoiding the source of irritation. Prescription or over-the-counter corticosteroid creams can lessen inflammation and relieve irritation. Creams, lotions, or ointments not specifically formulated for dermatitis can intensify the irritation. Oral **antihistamines** are sometimes recommended to alleviate itching, and **antibiotics** are prescribed if the rash becomes infected. Medications taken by mouth to relieve symptoms of dermatitis can make skin red and scaly and cause hair loss.

Patients who have a history of dermatitis should remove their rings before washing their hands. They should use bath oils or glycerine-based soaps and bathe in lukewarm saltwater.

Patting rather than rubbing the skin after bathing and thoroughly massaging lubricating lotion or nonprescription cortisone creams into still-damp skin can soothe red, irritated nummular dermatitis. Highly concentrated cortisone preparations should not be applied to the face, armpits, groin, or rectal area. Periodic medical monitoring is necessary to detect side effects in patients who use such preparations on **rashes** covering large areas of the body.

Coal-tar salves can help relieve symptoms of nummular dermatitis that have not responded to other treatments, but these ointments have an unpleasant odor and stain clothing.

Patients who have stasis dermatitis should elevate their legs as often as possible and **sleep** with a pillow between the lower legs.

Tar or zinc paste may also be used to treat stasis dermatitis. Because these compounds must remain in contact with the rash for as long as two weeks, the paste and bandages must be applied by a nurse or a doctor.

Coal-tar shampoos may be used for seborrheic dermatitis that occurs on the scalp. Sun exposure after the use of these shampoos should be avoided because the risk of sunburn of the scalp is increased.

Alternative treatment

Some herbal therapies can be useful for skin conditions. Among the herbs most often recommended are:

- Burdock root (*Arctium lappa*)
- Calendula (*Calendula officinalis*) ointment
- Chamomile (*Matricaria recutita*) ointment
- Cleavers (*Galium* ssp.)
- Evening primrose oil (*Oenothera biennis*)
- Nettles (*Urtica dioica*)

Contact dermatitis can be treated botanically and homeopathically. Grindelia (*Grindelia* spp.) and sassafras (*Sassafras albidum*) can help when applied topically.

KEY TERMS

Allergic reaction—An inappropriate or exaggerated genetically determined reaction to a chemical that occurs only on the second or subsequent exposures to the offending agent, after the first contact has sensitized the body.

Corticosteriod—A group of synthetic hormones that are used to prevent or reduce inflammation. Toxic effects may result from rapid withdrawal after prolonged use or from continued use of large doses.

Patch test—A skin test that is done to identify allergens. A suspected substance is applied to the skin. After 24–48 hours, if the area is red and swollen, the test is positive for that substance. If no reaction occurs, another substance is applied. This is continued until the patient experiences an allergic reaction where the irritant was applied to the skin.

Rash—A spotted, pink or red skin eruption that may be accompanied by itching and is caused by disease, contact with an allergen, food ingestion, or drug reaction.

Ulcer—An open sore on the skin, resulting from tissue destruction, that is usually accompanied by redness, pain, or infection.

Determining the source of the problem and eliminating it is essential. Oatmeal baths are very helpful in relieving the itch. Bentonite clay packs or any mud pack draws the fluid out and helps dry up the lesions. Cortisone creams are not recommended.

Stasis dermatitis should be treated by a trained practitioner. This condition responds well to topical herbal therapies, however, the cause must also be addressed. Selenium-based shampoos, topical applications of flax oil and/or olive oil, and biotin supplementation are among the therapies recommended for seborrheic dermatitis.

Prognosis

Dermatitis is often chronic, but symptoms can generally be controlled.

Prevention

Contact dermatitis can be prevented by avoiding the source of irritation. If the irritant cannot be avoided completely, the patient should wear gloves and other protective clothing whenever exposure is likely to occur.

Immediately washing the exposed area with soap and water can stem allergic reactions to poison ivy, poison oak, or poison sumac, but because soaps can dry the skin, patients susceptible to dermatitis should use them only on the face, feet, genitals, and underarms.

Clothing should be loose fitting and 100% cotton. New clothing should be washed in dye-free, unscented detergent before being worn.

Injury to the lower leg can cause stasis dermatitis to ulcerate (form open sores). If stasis ulcers develop, a doctor should be notified immediately.

Yoga and other relaxation techniques may help prevent atopic dermatitis caused by stress.

Avoidance of sweating may aid in preventing seborrheic dermatitis.

A patient who has dermatitis should also notify a doctor if any of the following occurs:

- fever develops
- skin oozes or other signs of infection appear
- symptoms do not begin to subside after seven days' treatment
- he/she comes into contact with someone who has a wart, cold sore, or other viral skin infection

Resources

OTHER

"Allergic Contact Dermatitis." *The Skin Site.* April 10, 1998 (accessed January 11, 2006), http://www.skinsite.com/info_allergic.htm.

Maureen Haggerty

Dermatomyositis

Definition

Dermatomyositis (DM) is a rare inflammatory muscle disease that leads to destruction of muscle tissue usually accompanied by **pain** and weakness.

Description

Dermatomyositis is one of a group of three related diseases called inflammatory **myopathies**. The other two are polymyositis and inclusion-body myositis. These diseases are rare; only about 20,000 people in the United States have dermatomyositis. Another estimates suggest that DM occurs in about 5.5 individuals out of every one million. The disease is of unknown origin and can develop in children and adults. Most often individuals either develop DM either between the ages of five and 14 or they do not develop it until they are over age 45. In all age groups, females are twice as likely to develop the disease than males. Although DM causes pain and weakness, it is not necessarily life threatening. However, adults, but not children, who develop DM have an increased risk of developing **cancer** and should be screened for malignancies regularly.

Causes and symptoms

The exact cause of dermatomyositis is unknown. It is an autoimmune disease. In a healthy body, cells of **immune system** attack only foreign or defective cells in the body to protect it from disease. In an autoimmune disease, the immune system attacks normal body cells. In the case of DM, immune system cells attack healthy cells of small blood vessels in the muscle and skin. Over time, this causes muscle fiber to shrink and sometimes cuts off blood supply to the muscle. DM tends to develop in muscles closest to the center of the body.

As yet, there is no clear explanation of what causes an individual to develop DM. It is thought that the disease may be triggered by a virus or exposure to certain drugs or vaccines. According to the **Muscular Dystrophy** Association, recent research suggests developing DM may be related to the mixing of blood cells that sometimes occurs between the mother and fetus during pregnancy. The disease is not directly inherited, although there may be some genetic sensitivity toward whatever triggers it.

Often the first sign of DM is the development of a patchy, scaly, violet to dark red skin rash on the face, neck, shoulders, upper chest, knees, or back. Often the rash appears before any signs of illness or muscle weakness. About 40% of children and teens develop hard, painful bumps under the skin that are deposits of calcium, a mineral used in bone formation. This condition, called calcinosis, is much less common in adults.

Muscle weakness, especially in the upper arms, hips, thighs, and neck, becomes apparent in activities such as climbing stairs or reaching up over the head. This weakness develops after the rash appears. Some people have difficulty swallowing and chewing when the muscles of the face and esophagus are affected. Individuals may also feel tried, weak, have a low-grade **fever**, weight loss, and joint stiffness. Some individuals have the rash for years before they progress to these symptoms, while in others the onset of symptoms is rapid. In children the development of symptoms is almost always gradual, making diagnosis especially difficult.

Diagnosis

DM can be difficult to diagnose, and often the first doctor an individual sees is a dermatologist for treatment of the rash and then is referred to a rheumatologist, specialist in internal medicine or neurologist when DM is suspected. Many tests may be done to rule out other diseases before a firm diagnosis is made. A blood test is done to measure the level of creatine kinase. Creatine kinase is an enzyme found in muscle tissue. When muscle is damaged, this enzyme leaks out into the blood. An increased level of creatine kinase in the blood suggests DM as a possible diagnosis. Another blood test may be done to test for specific immune system antibodies. Antibodies are proteins made in response to material the body thinks is foreign.

An electromyogram (EMG) is a test that measures electrical activity in muscles as they contract. Individuals with inflammatory myopathies usually have distinct patterns of electrical activity in the affected muscles. However, up to 15% of people with DM have normal electromyogram readings, so this test is not definitive. The definitive test is a muscle biopsy. The doctor takes a small sample of muscle tissue and examines it under a microscope. From this sample, the doctor can differentiate DM from other inflammatory myopathies and other muscle wasting diseases.

Treatment

The goal of treatment is to improve muscle strength and allow the individual to participate in normal daily activities. Individuals are given steroid drugs (prednisone, corticosteroids) that suppress the immune system. Over time, these drugs often produce undesirable side effects, so treatment is usually begun with a large dose, then tapered to the minimum dose needed for maintenance. People who do not respond well to steroid treatment may be treated with other immunosuppressive drugs or intravenous immunoglobulin. Individuals with DM are advised to avoid exposure to the sun, as sunlight worsens the skin rash. Physical therapy is often helpful in keeping joints from stiffening and freezing. Moderate **exercise** is also recommended.

Alternative treatment

A healthy diet high is recommended for all individuals with supplemental protein for those with severe muscle damage.

KEY TERMS

Immunoglobulin—Material containing specific antibodies to fight disease that can be injected into an individual to fight infection.

Inflammation—An infection or irritation of a tissue.

Myopathy—Relating to muscle tissue.

Prognosis

The course of DM is highly variable. In about 20% of people, the disease spontaneously goes into remission and individuals are able to lead symptom-free lives for long periods. On the other hand, in about 5% of individuals the disease progresses to **death** because of heart and lung involvement. The majority of people continue to have some symptoms and require long-term treatment, but their degree of daily activity varies greatly.

Serious complications from DM include involvement of the muscles of the heart and lungs, difficulty eating and swallowing, and a tendency to develop cancer. This association is seen only in adults and not in children. Individuals over age 60 are more likely to have serious complications than younger individuals.

Prevention

There is no known way to prevent this disease.

Resources

PERIODICALS

Koler, Ric A. and Andrew Montemarano. "Dermatomyositis." *American Family Physician* 24, no. 9 (November 1, 2001) 1565-1574 [cited 16 February 2005], http://www.aafp.org/afp/20011101/1565.html.

OTHER

Callen, Jeffrey P. *Dermatomyositis*. December 5, 2002 [cited February 16, 2005], http://www.emedicine.com/derm/topic98.htm.

Hashmat, Aamir and Zaineb Daud. *Dermatomyositis/Polymyositis*. January 16, 2004 [cited February 16, 2005], http://www.emedicine.com/neuro/topic85.htm.

ORGANIZATIONS

American Autoimmune Related Diseases Association, Inc., 22100 Gratiot Avenue E., Detroit MI, 48021, (586) 776-3900, (586) 776-3903 (800) 598-4668, http://www.aarda.org.

Muscular Dystrophy Association, 3300 East Sunrise Dr., Tucson AZ, 85718, (520) 529-2000, (800) 572-1717, http://www.mdausa.org.

Myositis Association, 1233 20th Street, NW, Washington DC, 20036, (800) 821-7356, http://www.myositis.org.

National Organization for Rare Disorders (NORD) 55 Kenosia Avenue, P. O. Box 1968Danbury CT, 06813-1968 (203) 744-0100, (800) 999-6673, http://www.rarediseases.org.

Tish Davidson, AM

Development assessment

Definition

Developmental **assessment** involves the measure of a child's attainment of physical or cognitive skills that allow continued maturation, learning, and function in society.

Purpose

Developmental assessment is used to observe functional ability in children and to identify any deviations from the norm. It is used to recognize whether or not a disability may exist and if so, where the specific problem areas lie. Developmental tests provide information regarding the milestones a child has attained, and can help in determining the course of intervention to attain further milestones. Results of developmental tests may also be used to indicate the level of progress achieved after intervention, and are often used by both clinicians and researchers.

Description

In addition to the use of a test with established reliability and validity, a developmental assessment should include data collection in the form of an interview, history, and clinical observation. The interview should take place with the parents/caregivers and, if age-appropriate, the child, in an informal and friendly setting. The concerns and goals of the parents and child are important to note, and information regarding the child's developmental and medical history may be obtained at this time. In addition to the parent report, it is important to look at medical records if they are available. Information regarding the mother's pregnancy, labor, and delivery, and the child's medical/surgical history, health status, medications, precautions, and other items of relevance is helpful in providing a background for the assessment.

Clinical observation of the child is useful in determining factors that may contribute to developmental difficulties. In addition, it is helpful to watch a child moving under his or her own volition, instead of under a therapist's directions. Observation may include, but is not limited to: the manner in which the infant or child is held by the parent (e.g., posture, support required); preferred means of mobility (e.g., wheelchair, ambulation [walking], **crawling**, scooting, rolling); antigravity posture and movements; equilibrium and righting reactions; balance, including base of support; compensations; and assistance required for stability or mobility.

There are a number of assessment tools available that measure gross motor development.

Screening tests

Screening tests are the most basic form of developmental assessment tool, and are used to determine whether or not a concern exists. The Alberta Infant Motor Scale (AIMS) is used during the first year of life to identify motor delay and to evaluate maturation over time. Fifty-eight items related to posture, movement, and weight bearing in prone, supine, sitting, and standing positions take 10 to 20 minutes to observe. Researchers have found predictive validity, interrater (the consistency of the rating between different people performing the test), and test-retest reliability of the AIMS to be good. In addition, there is high concurrent validity with the Peabody Developmental Motor Scales' gross motor portion.

The Miller First Step Screening Test for Evaluating Preschoolers assesses cognitive and physical function in children 35 to 74 months of age. It uses 18 games that are age-appropriate and takes approximately 20 minutes. The Denver II is a comprehensive screening test encompassing 125 items in the personal-social, fine motor-adaptive, language, and gross motor domains. The test is norm-referenced from **birth** to six years; however, it has been criticized for poor specificity.

Motor assessments

The Test of Infant Motor Performance (TIMP) consists of observation of 28 items and elicitation of 31 items in infants up to four months of age. It is found to be highly sensitive to small changes in development and valid in measuring behaviors of functional relevance. Test-retest reliability has been found to be high; more research needs to be done on predictive validity. Administration takes 25 to 45 minutes.

The Movement Assessment of Infants (MAI) is a criterion-referenced test for infants in the first year of life. Sixty-five items related to muscle strength/tone, primitive reflexes, automatic reactions, and volitional movement, including quality of movement, are assessed. Researchers report that interrater and test-retest reliability is good; however, the MAI has been found to over-identify infants with motor delay (i.e. produce a high rate of false positives).

The Peabody Developmental Motor Scales (PDMS) is a norm- and criterion-referenced test that examines gross and fine motor function in children from birth to 83 months (the second edition includes up to 71 months). The gross motor scale includes reflexes, balance, nonlocomotor, locomotor, and receipt and propulsion of objects. The fine motor scale includes grasp, hand functions, eye-hand coordination, and manual dexterity. High reliability and validity have been reported; however, criticisms of the test prompted the creation of a second edition, the PDMS-2. This edition is updated with new normative data representative of the current U.S. population. Reliability and validity were studied for gender, race, and other subgroups of the normative sample. In addition, more specific scoring criteria and illustrations were added.

The Bruininks-Oseretsky Test of Motor Proficiency (BOTMP) is a norm-referenced test that examines gross and fine motor function in children aged four-and-a-half to fourteen-and-a-half years. The gross motor subtests assess speed and agility, balance, bilateral coordination, and strength. The fine motor subtests assess upper-limb coordination, speed and dexterity, response speed, and visuomotor control. Administration takes 45 to 60 minutes, and reliability (interrater and test-retest) is high. Critics of the test have pointed out, however, that some of the items, for example "tapping feet alternately while making circles with fingers," do not measure skills relevant to everyday function. In addition, it is important to note that failure of items may result as much from cognitive and perceptual difficulties as from motor difficulties.

The Gross Motor Function Measure (GMFM) is designed to evaluate change in motor performance over time in children with **cerebral palsy**. The test contains 88 items in five groups: lying and rolling; sitting; crawling and kneeling; standing; and walking, running, and jumping. Interrater and test-retest reliability have been demonstrated as high.

Comprehensive assessments

The Bayley II consists of a norm-referenced test of motor performance (manipulation, coordination of large muscle groups, dynamic movement, postural imitation, stereognosis [the ability to recognize solid objects by touch]), and mental ability (object permanence, memory, problem solving, complex language) in children from birth to 42 months. It also contains a criterion-referenced behavior scale that looks at affect, interests, activity, and fearfulness. Test-retest and interrater reliability have been found to be higher for older ages than for younger ages with this test. This test takes approximately 45 to 60 minutes to administer.

KEY TERMS

Concurrent validity—Relationship between performance on a given test and another well-established test which is purported to measure the same skills.

Content validity—The likelihood that the test measures what it says it is to measure.

Interrater reliability—Relationship of an individual's score on first administration of a test to the score on second administration.

Predictive validity—The likelihood that a child's performance on the test predicts an actual behavior.

Specificity—Ability of a test to identify those who do not have a disorder.

Test-retest reliability—Index of agreement between two different testers for the same test.

The Early Intervention Developmental Profile (EIDP) consists of six scales in the following areas: perceptual/fine motor; cognition, language, social/emotional; self-care; and gross motor development. It is designed to be administered wholly by any member of a multidisciplinary team to children from birth to 36 months. Content validity, in addition to interrater and test-retest reliability, have been found to be good.

Assessments of functional capabilities are not necessarily developmental milestone-based; however, their use is important in determining whether or not specific disabilities exist. These disabilities may be related to mobility, transfer, self-care or social function. Examples of functional assessments include the Pediatric Evaluation of Disability Inventory (PEDI) and the Functional Independence Measure for Children (WeeFIM).

Results

In a norm-referenced test, the child's score is compared to the average of a group of children. This average is obtained by collecting scores from a large population. In a criterion-referenced test, the scores are interpreted based on absolute criteria such as the number of items performed correctly. Raw scores on tests often can be converted to age equivalent scores, standard scores, motor quotients and percentile rankings.

Once scores are obtained, they must be analyzed along with the information gathered during the interview, history, and observation. Although the normative populations used for the tests are representative of the U.S. population, cultural differences in motor development need to be considered as well. All of this information may be used to guide intervention and/or identify areas of progress or concern. Once specific areas of dysfunction are noted, goals and objectives may be formulated to treat these areas.

Health care team roles

Physical and occupational therapists usually perform developmental motor assessments; however, the more comprehensive scales are often designed for administration by any or all members of the health care team. This team may include any or all of the following: physician, nurse, physical therapist, occupational therapist, speech and language pathologist, special educator, psychologist, and social worker. It is important that whoever administers the test takes care to learn the test and procedure for administration.

Resources

BOOKS

Campbell, Suzann K., Darl W. Vander Linden, and Robert J. Palisano. *Physical Therapy for Children, 2nd ed.* Philadelphia: W. B. Saunders Company, 2000.

Folio, M. Rhonda, and Rebecca R. Fewell. *Peabody Developmental Motor Scales, 2nd Edition: Examiner's Manual.* Austin, TX: PRO-ED, Inc., 2000.

PERIODICALS

Campbell, Suzann K., and Thubi H. A. Kolobe. "Concurrent Validity of the Test of Infant Motor Performance with the Alberta Infant Motor Scale." *Pediatric Physical Therapy* 12, no. 1 (Spring 2000): 2-9.

Fetters, Linda, and Edward Z. Tronick. "Discriminate Power of the Alberta Infant Motor Scale and the Movement Assessment of Infants for Prediction of Peabody Gross Motor Scale Scores of Infants Exposed In Utero to Cocaine." *Pediatric Physical Therapy* 12, no. 1 (Spring 2000): 16-23.

Ketelaar, Marjolijn, and Adri Vermeer. "Functional Motor Abilities of Children with Cerebral Palsy: A Systematic Literature Review of Assessment Measures." *Clinical Rehabilitation* 12 (1998): 369-80.

Koseck, Karen. "Review and Evaluation of Psychometric Properties of the Revised Bayley Scales of Infant Development." *Pediatric Physical Therapy* 11, no. 4 (Winter 1999): 198-204.

OTHER

Levine, Kristin J. "The Bruininks-Oseretsky Test of Motor Proficiency: Usefulness for Assessing Writing Disorders." *OT-Peds website.* 1995, http://www.dartmouth.edu/~kjlevine/ot-peds.

Peggy Campbell Torpey, MPT

Developmental delay

Definition

Developmental delay refers to any delay in a child's physical, cognitive, behavioral, emotional, or social development, due to any number of reasons. The Centers for Disease Control and Prevention (CDC) defines a developmental delay as follows: "A delay occurs when a child reaches a milestone at an age later than the average developmental rate."

Developmental delays are assessed in five areas of human development: cognitive (thinking-related) development; social and **emotional development**; speech and **language development**; fine motor skill development; and gross motor skill development. The last two areas are sometimes grouped together under the heading of physical development or motor skills.

Demographics

Developmental delays and disabilities are common in the general population in North America. According to the U.S. Administration on Developmental Disabilities (ADD), there are about 4.5 million children and adults in the United States with developmental disorders of some type as of 2010. The CDC states that 17% of children in the United States "experience some form of behavioral or developmental disability." Some statistics for specific disorders are as follows:

- Autism: 560,000 persons between the ages of 1 and 21 years.
- Cerebral palsy: 800,000 children and adults.
- Hearing loss: 72,000 children between the ages of 6 and 21.
- Mental retardation: 2 million children and adults between the ages of 6 and 64.

Description

Developmental delay refers to any significant retardation in a child's physical, cognitive, behavioral, emotional, or social development. The two most frequent reasons for classing a child as having developmental delay involve those psychological systems for which there are good norms. This is especially true for motor development and language development. Because it is known that all children begin to crawl by eight months of age and walk by the middle of the second year, any child who was more than five or six months delayed in attaining those two milestones would probably be classified as developmentally delayed and the parents should consult the **pediatrician**.

Most children begin to speak their first words before they are eighteen months old and by three years of age the vast majority are speaking short sentences. Therefore, any child who is not speaking words or sentences by the third birthday would be considered developmentally delayed and, as in motor development delay, the parent should consult the pediatrician.

The other developmental problems that children show are more often called disabilities rather than delays. Thus children with **autism** do not show normal social development; however, these children are usually called disabled or autistic rather than developmentally delayed. Similarly, most children are able to read single words by the second grade of elementary school. Children who cannot do that are normally labeled dyslexic or learning disabled, or in some cases academically delayed, rather than developmentally delayed.

Physical development is assessed by progress in both fine and **gross motor skills**. Possible problems are indicated by muscles that are either too limp or too tight. Jerky or uncertain movements are another cause for concern, as are abnormalities in reflexes. Delays in motor development may indicate the presence of a neurological condition such as mild **cerebral palsy** or Tourette's syndrome. Neurological problems may also be present when a child's head circumference is increasing either too fast or too slowly. Although physical and cognitive delays may occur together, one is not necessarily a sign of the other.

Important cognitive attainments that physicians look for in infants in the first 18 months include object permanence, an awareness of causality, and different reactions to strangers and **family** members. Cognitive delays can signal a wide variety of problems, including **fetal alcohol syndrome** and brain dysfunction. Developmental milestones achieved and then lost should also be investigated, as the loss of function could be a sign of a degenerative neurological condition.

Delays in social and emotional development can be among the most difficult for parents, who feel rejected by a child's failure to respond to them on an emotional level. They expect such responses to social cues as smiling, vocalization, and cuddling, and may feel angry or frustrated when their children do not respond. However, a delay in social responses can be caused by a number of factors, including prenatal stress or deprivation, **prematurity**, **birth** difficulties, including oxygen deprivation, or a hypersensitivity of the nervous system (which creates an aversion to stimuli that are normally tolerated or welcomed). One study, the Millennium Cohort Study, examined the impact **breastfeeding** had on infants and their developmental milestones. From their results, the researchers felt confident stating that breastfeeding does have a positive impact on a child and the attainment of these important developmental markers.

Risk factors

Risk factors for developmental delays fall into two categories, genetic and environmental. Genetic factors include such chromosomal disorders as **Down syndrome**, **Turner syndrome**, **Klinefelter syndrome**, and others caused by defects in the child's chromosomes.

Environmental risk factors for developmental delays include such problems as:

- Exposure to lead or other toxic substances.
- Mother's use of drugs or alcohol during pregnancy.
- Mother's infection with rubella (German measles) or a sexually transmitted disease during pregnancy.
- Malnutrition.
- Premature birth.
- Early surgery for congenital heart defects.
- Lack of care.
- Severe poverty.
- Depression or other psychiatric disturbance in the mother.

Risk factors have a cumulative impact on a child's development; the greater the number of risk factors, the greater the likelihood that the child's development will be delayed in one or more areas, and the greater the likelihood that the delays will eventually result in long-term disabilities.

Causes and symptoms

The causes of developmental delay may range from inherited genetic defects to social and environmental factors. Symptoms depend on the area of development affected. For example, symptoms of an eye disorder may include closing one eye to look at distant objects, tilting the head at an unnatural angle in order to look at objects, or rubbing the eyes frequently. Behavioral warning signs include such behaviors as extreme aggressiveness on the one hand or avoidance of interactions with others on the other hand; avoiding eye contact with others; and inability to concentrate on an activity as long as other children of the same age.

Diagnosis

There are two levels of evaluation for developmental delays, screening and a more intensive developmental examination. Many physicians routinely include developmental screening in physical examinations. The doctor or nurse may talk to the child, play with him or her, or talk with the parents about the child's development.

KEY TERMS

Chronic—Long-term.

Cognitive—Referring to such mental functions as thinking, reasoning, and memory.

Congenital—Present at birth.

Degenerative disorder—A type of disorder in which a child gradually loses certain abilities that he or she had acquired at an earlier age.

Developmental delay—The term used to describe a child's reaching a developmental milestone later than the average age for that specific attainment.

Fine motor skills—Skills that involve the use of the small muscles in the hands and arms for such tasks as writing, using scissors, typing on a keyboard, etc.

Gross motor skills—Skills that involve the larger muscles of the body for such tasks as running, lifting objects, sitting up, etc.

Intervention—In medicine, any action that is intended to produce an effect or interrupt a disease (or disability) process.

Milestone—A physical development or accomplishment that most children reach within a specific age range.

Some doctors will ask the parents to fill out a brief written screening instrument during the office visit.

Some of the physical characteristics or abilities that doctors look for in evaluating a child's development during the **preschool** years are as follows:

- Three months: baby smiles when smiled at, grasps rattle, turns head toward lights or voices.
- Six months: baby can sit in a high chair, imitate parent's hand movements, laugh, and make sing-song noises.
- 12 months: baby can eat finger food, crawl, walk holding parent's hand, respond to music, say first word.
- 18 months: toddler can walk without help, identify an object in a picture book, say 8–10 different words, ask for something by pointing.
- Two years: child can open boxes, drink from a straw, have a vocabulary of several hundred words, hum or try to sing, play with other children.
- Four years: child can eat or drink without spilling; draw simple objects; undress without help; use the toilet alone; tell the difference between the real world and imaginary worlds; speak in complete sentences with good grammar.
- Five years: child can count to 10; has an understanding of time; can hop, climb, skip, and turn somersaults.

Examination

If the doctor's office screening or concerns raised by the parents indicate that the child may have a developmental problem, the child will be referred to a specialist for further evaluation. The specialist may be either a developmental pediatrician or a child psychologist. After an intensive evaluation of the child's physical, cognitive, behavioral, emotional, and social development, the specialist will recommend either early intervention or a treatment plan.

Tests

As of 2010, there are no laboratory or imaging tests that can diagnose developmental delays after birth. The diagnosis is based on a combination of the parents' and clinicians' observations. Although a technique known as chromosomal microarray (CMA) is presently available and used for **genetic testing** of individuals with unexplained developmental delay/intellectual disability (DD/ID), autism spectrum disorders (ASD), or multiple congenital anomalies (MCA), the technique is too expensive as of 2010 to be used for general screening of all children with developmental delays (as distinct from evident disabilities).

Treatment

There are two major forms of treatment for developmental delays, early intervention and individualized education programs or IEPs. Early intervention programs for children under the age of three are administered by Early Start and other early intervention agencies at the local or state level; the local public school system administers these programs for children over the age of three. Early intervention services cover a number of developmental needs, ranging from **nutrition**, hearing services, and speech/language therapy to physical therapy, **occupational therapy**, and psychological counseling.

Individualized education programs (IEPs) are written documents, ordered by federal law, that define a given child's disabilities, state current levels of academic performance, describe the child's educational needs, and specify annual goals and objectives. Setting up an IEP is a lengthy process that begins with a consultation between the child's parents and his or her teacher and doctor. The next step is a meeting with the local **special education** office or school district, followed by an evaluation of the child and drawing up the IEP, if the child is considered eligible for one.

A more elaborate plan is known as an individualized family service plan or ISFP. This type of plan coordinates all the services for the child's family that may be needed as well as early intervention or other services for the child. Federal requirements for both IEPs and ISFPs are complex and detailed.

Prognosis

Children rarely outgrow developmental delays, which is the major reason why screening or intensive evaluation should be carried out as soon as the parents or pediatrician suspect that the child's development is abnormally slow. Another reason for catching any developmental issues early is that a delay in one area can often slow a child's development in others; for example, children with speech problems may avoid other children at school and begin to fall back in their social and behavioral development. The specific prognosis depends on the cause(s) of the developmental delay and the types of interventions that are needed and available.

Prevention

Not all developmental delays can be prevented. Some measures that people can take, to lower their risk of having a child with developmental problems include:

- Genetic screening for both parents, particularly if either father or mother comes from a family with a history of genetic disorders.
- Proper nutrition and health care for the mother during pregnancy.
- Avoidance of drinking, smoking, and drug use during pregnancy.
- Vaccination against rubella before pregnancy if the mother has not been exposed to it.

Resources

BOOKS

Mountstephen, Mary. *How to Detect Developmental Delay and What to Do Next: A Holistic Approach to Intervention.* Philadelphia: Jessica Kingsley Publishers, 2010.

Stroh, Katrin, Thelma Robinson, and Alan Proctor. *Every Child Can Learn: Using Learning Tools and Play to Help Children with Developmental Delay.* Los Angeles, CA: SAGE, 2008.

Taulbee, Jack. *Understanding Children of Special Needs: What Every Parent Needs to Know.* Monrovia, CA: Wayne Publishing, 2005.

PERIODICALS

Bruce, B.B., et al. "Neurologic and Ophthalmic Manifestations of Fetal Alcohol Syndrome." *Reviews in Neurological Diseases* 6 (Winter 2009): 13–20.

Cappiello, M.M., and S. Gahagan. "Early Child Development and Developmental Delay in Indigenous Communities." *Pediatric Clinics of North America* 56 (December 2009): 1501–17.

de Campos, A.C., et al. "Reaching and Grasping Movements in Infants at Risk: A Review." *Research in Developmental Disabilities* 30 (September-October 2009): 819–26.

Miller, D.T., et al. "Consensus Statement: Chromosomal Microarray Is a First-tier Clinical Diagnostic Test for Individuals with Developmental Disabilities or Congenital Anomalies." *American Journal of Human Genetics* 86 (May 14, 2010): 749–64.

Snookes, S.H., et al. "A Systematic Review of Motor and Cognitive Outcomes after Early Surgery for Congenital Heart Disease." *Pediatrics* 125 (April 2010): e818–e827.

Toriello, H.V. "Role of the Dysmorphologic Evaluation in the Child with Developmental Delay." *Pediatric Clinics of North America* 55 (October 2008): 1085–98.

OTHER

Administration on Developmental Disabilities (ADD). *Fact Sheet,* http://www.acf.hhs.gov/opa/fact_sheets/add_factsheet.html.

Centers for Disease Control and Prevention (CDC). *Developmental Screening Fact Sheet,* http://www.cdc.gov/ncbddd/actearly/pdf/parents_pdfs/DevelopmentalScreening.pdf.

Centers for Disease Control and Prevention (CDC). *Learn the Signs; Act Early: Developmental Milestones* This page contains an interactive chart for parents to help them identify their child's progress from 3 months through 5 years of age. The page also includes a video titled "Baby Steps" on developmental milestones; it takes 4-1/2 minutes to play, http://www.cdc.gov/ncbddd/actearly/milestones/index.html.

How Kids Develop. "What Is Developmental Delay and What Services Are Available If I Think My Child Might Be Delayed?" http://www.howkidsdevelop.com/develop DevDelay.html.

Moeschler, John B., et al. "Clinical Genetic Evaluation of the Child with Mental Retardation or Developmental Delays." *Pediatrics* 117 (June 2006): 2304–2316, http://pediatrics.aappublications.org/cgi/content/full/117/6/2304.

University of Michigan Health System. *Developmental Delay,* http://www.med.umich.edu/yourchild/topics/devdel.htm.

ORGANIZATIONS

Administration on Developmental Disabilities (ADD), U.S. Department of Health and Human Services (HHS), 370 L'Enfant Promenade, S.W., Washington DC, 20447, (202) 690-6590, (202) 690-6904, http://www.acf.hhs.gov/programs/add/index.html.

American Academy of Pediatrics (AAP), 141 Northwest Point Boulevard, Elk Grove Village IL, 60007, (847) 434-4000, (847) 434-8000, http://www.aap.org/.

Centers for Disease Control and Prevention (CDC), 1600 Clifton Road, Atlanta GA, 30333, (800) 232-4636, cdcinfo@cdc.gov, http://www.cdc.gov.

National Institute of Child Health and Human Development (NICHD)., Bldg 31, Room 2A32, MSC 2425, 31 Center Drive, Bethesda MD, 20892, (800) 370-2943, (866) 760-5947, NICHDInformationResourceCenter@mail.nih.gov, http://www.nichd.nih.gov/.

Rebecca J. Frey, PhD

Developmental psychology

Definition

Developmental psychology is the branch of psychology that studies the ways in which people develop physically, emotionally, intellectually, and socially over the course of their lives. Developmental psychologists are concerned primarily with how the human mind or personality changes from conception and intrauterine development through childhood, **adolescence**, adulthood, and old age. The field covers nearly all aspects of life and seeks to understand the factors that influence personality, **intelligence**, and behavior. In addition to describing and analyzing the changes that take place in humans over the course of the life cycle, developmental psychology also seeks to understand the principles or mechanisms underlying those changes.

Purpose

Some developmental psychologists are interested in research for its own sake; that is, they are concerned with adding to current understandings of humans and how they develop. One ongoing topic of debate among research psychologists is the nature vs. nurture controversy—whether humans are born with certain skills and abilities "hard-wired" into their brains that cannot be fundamentally changed by life experiences, or whether they are primarily molded by interactions with their environment. The position that emphasizes innate capacities is called nativism, and the position that emphasizes the importance of the environment is called empiricism. Another recurrent debate in developmental psychology has to do with whether human development proceeds in discrete and identifiable stages or whether it is a continuous process of growth that cannot be readily subdivided into phases or stages.

Other developmental psychologists are concerned with clinical applications of this branch of psychology. These applications include forensic developmental psychology, or the study of children's memories and their reliability as witnesses in criminal trials; educational psychology, which includes the **assessment** and diagnosis of children with learning disabilities, the development and testing of new methods of classroom instruction, and the study of intellectually gifted children; and child psychopathology, which investigates the development of mental illnesses and **personality disorders** in children as well as new treatment methods for them.

Description

Developmental psychology began its development in the late nineteenth century with the work of Sigmund Freud (1856–1939), a Viennese physician considered the father of psychiatry. Prior to Freud, there was relatively little interest in the cognitive and **emotional development** of children. One of the major exceptions to this long-standing focus on adults was Augustine of Hippo (354–430), a fifth-century Christian bishop whose examination of his childhood memories in his autobiographical *Confessions* (written around 397) is one of the earliest explorations of children's emotional lives and their differences from adults. Augustine traced back his adult difficulties with impulsiveness, moodiness, and selfishness to his childhood and adolescence.

Classical theories of developmental psychology

FREUDIAN PSYCHOLOGY Sigmund Freud was the first major theorist after the rise of scientific medicine in the nineteenth century to link childhood experience with adult behavior. Freud proposed what is perhaps the most widely known but least understood theory of childhood development. He saw personality development as consisting primarily of conflicts between biology and culture—that is, between the genetically programmed needs of the infant or child and the ability or willingness of the parents to satisfy those needs. Freud laid out a blueprint of development consisting of four stages: oral, anal, phallic, and latency. At each stage of development, which Freud believed occurred at varying ages, infants and children have different needs, all biologically determined. What Freud saw as significant was the degree to which those needs were either met or frustrated by the parents; extremes at either end, whether severe frustration or uninhibited gratification, resulted in fixations that stunted development. Freud's ideas were and continue to be highly controversial, mainly because he attributed feelings of sexuality to infants, but also because of his focus on male concepts and imagery to explain his theories.

BEHAVIORISM Freud was followed in the early twentieth century by the behaviorist school of psychology, whose leaders maintained that psychologists should concern themselves only with externally observable and measurable behaviors rather than internal emotional states. The behaviorist who wrote most extensively on child development was John B. Watson (1878–1958), who took a radically empiricist view of human development. In 1930 Watson published a book titled *Behaviorism*, in which he all but denied the significance of inborn characteristics. Watson issued a famous challenge: "Give me a dozen healthy infants, well-formed, and my own specified world to bring them up in and I'll guarantee to take any one at random and train him [sic] to become any type of specialist I might select—doctor, lawyer, artist, merchant-chief and, yes, even beggar-man and thief, regardless of his talents, penchants, tendencies, abilities, vocations, and race of his ancestors."

Watson also wrote several books on child rearing that have been strongly criticized by later psychologists and pediatricians. Accepting Freud's concept of fixation, Watson urged parents to rear children with a businesslike attitude of emotional detachment and objectivity, treating them as young adults, not holding them in their laps, and limiting kissing to a good-night kiss.

DEVELOPMENTAL STAGE THEORY Developmental psychologists who were not behaviorists also expanded on Freud's work, and proposed new schemes of development. One such theorist was the Swiss zoologist and psychologist Jean Piaget (1896–1980), who revolutionized developmental psychology with his theories of intellectual, or cognitive, development. Piaget's first contribution was to define intelligence as a process of volitional, cognitive endeavor a person undertakes to make sense of the world. He theorized that every individual passing through each of these stages struggles to internalize or understand the novelties inherent in each stage. This process has three phases: assimilation, accommodation, and equilibrium. The stages consist of the sensorimotor (0–2 years), the pre-operational (2–7 years), the concrete operational (7–11 years), and the formal operational (11–15 years). Each stage requires the mastery of the skills and understanding of the previous stage, and not every person reaches every stage.

LIFESPAN APPROACH Developmental psychologists focused primarily on childhood development in the early years of the field, believing that with adulthood personality became rather fixed or static. One of the first to question this notion was Erik Erikson (1902–1979). In his landmark 1950 book, *Eight Ages of Man*, Erikson laid out a schema whereby human personality continues to change and evolve throughout the life-cycle. It was chiefly due to Erikson's work that developmental psychology expanded its view, taking on what is referred to within the field as the lifespan approach.

One of Erikson's main tenets was the idea of crisis, defined as a significant moment when a person's present understanding of himself and his place in the world becomes untenable. The identity crisis, a term Erikson coined, is the most widely known such crisis. Erikson's theory of development is also based on his belief that biology or genetics requires that humans pass through these stages. Once pushed into them, however, culture takes over and the social/family environment greatly determines the success of the crisis resolution. Erikson's stages are laid out as a series of conflicts, thus underlining his concept of crisis. These stages, which occur at varying ages, are: basic trust versus mistrust; autonomy versus shame and doubt; initiative versus guilt; industry versus inferiority; identity versus role confusion; intimacy versus isolation; generativity versus stagnation; integrity versus despair.

MORAL DEVELOPMENT Another area within the field of developmental psychology which has gained interest in recent years is **moral development**, as pioneered by Lawrence Kohlberg (1927–1987). In a series of investigations in which children were presented with moral dilemmas, Kohlberg developed what is called **Kohlberg's theory of moral reasoning**. He observed that moral reasoning develops through three distinct levels occurring between the ages of seven and adolescence. As with all the other theories discussed, the ages at which individuals arrive at the stages vary, and, like Piaget's stages, not everyone arrives at the "highest" stage of moral development. Kohlberg's theory has been criticized by Carol Gilligan (1936–), whose 1982 book *In a Different Voice* argued that Kohlberg's stages of moral development are androcentric and overlook the distinctive but equally valid pattern of moral development in girls and women.

Newer approaches to developmental psychology

ECOLOGICAL SYSTEMS THEORY Ecological systems theory is an approach to psychological development associated with Urie Bronfenbrenner (1917–2005), who was one of the co-founders of the Head Start Program. Bronfenbrenner maintained that human development is shaped by the individual's interactions with five nested environmental systems: the microsystem (the person's immediate social environment: home, **family**, school, neighborhood); the mesosystem (the relations among a person's various contexts, such as the relationship between school environment and home or church environment, relationships between the nuclear and extended family, and so on); the exosystem (involves links between a person and external environments on that person's development, such as the influence of the parents' workplaces on a child); the macrosystem (the larger social culture, class system, and economic system); and the chronosystem (the evolution of the first four systems over the individual's lifetime and their ongoing influence on his or her development).

According to Bronfenbrenner, each of the five systems contains roles, norms and rules that can powerfully shape an individual's development, particularly if the different systems come into conflict. An example might be that of a child from a family that does not value education succeeding in school and going on to college.

ATTACHMENT THEORY Attachment theory is an account of psychological development in childhood associated with John Bowlby (1907–1990), a British psychiatrist, and Mary Ainsworth (1913–1999), a Canadian psychologist who studied under Bowlby. The central thesis of attachment theory is that a young child needs to develop a secure attachment to at least one primary **caregiver** (called the attachment figure) in order for psychological development to proceed normally. The growing child uses the attachment figure(s) as a "secure base" from which to explore the larger world and form relationships with others, such as peer relationships, friendships, and later romantic or sexual relationships.

Ainsworth identified four basic patterns of attachment in the children she studied: secure (child freely explores the environment when the mother is present); anxious-resistant insecure attachment (child is fearful of strangers and anxious about exploring the environment; this pattern is often seen in children whose mothers relate to them only on their terms rather than the child's); anxious-avoidant insecure (child shows little attachment to caregiver and will interact with strangers in the same detached way); and disorganized (frequently seen in children whose mothers had become depressed shortly after the child's **birth**). Cindy Hazen and Phillip Shaver extended Ainsworth's four patterns of attachment to adult romantic relationships in the work in the late 1980s.

SOCIAL LEARNING THEORY Social learning theory is associated with the work of Albert Bandura (1925–), a Canadian psychologist best known for his 1961 Bobo doll experiment. The Bobo doll was an inflatable doll that could be hit with a wooden mallet or a person's hand. Some of the children (aged 3 to 6 years) in the experiment placed in a room with an adult who hit the Bobo doll while others were placed in a room with an adult who did not model aggressive behavior but simply played normally with the doll. Bandura found that the children exposed to an adult's aggressive behavior were more likely to act aggressively themselves. The children were particularly likely to imitate the adult's behavior when the adult was of the same sex as their own.

Bandura concluded that learning in humans has a social dimension, that people learn new behaviors through observing others around them. If the behavior has a positive or beneficial outcome, the learner is likely to imitate and adopt the behavior themselves. Social learning theorists identify three requirements for people to learn and model positive behaviors: retention (remembering what they observe); reproduction (having the ability to imitate or copy the behavior); and motivation (having a good reason to want to adopt the behavior).

KEY TERMS

Androcentric—Referring to the practice, whether conscious or unconscious, placing male human beings or the masculine point of view at the center of one's view of the world and its culture.

Attachment theory—A view of human development that holds that persons need to form a secure attachment with at least one primary caregiver in early childhood for later development to proceed normally.

Behaviorism—A school of psychology that focuses on the analysis, prediction, and control of externally observable behavior rather than internal mental states or thoughts.

Cognitive—Pertaining to such mental processes as thinking, knowing, remembering, analyzing, and other forms of information processing.

Empiricism—In psychology, the belief that experience of the environment is the primary determinant of human development.

Fixation—In Freudian theory, a condition in which a person becomes obsessively attached to another person, activity, object, or being.

Nativism—In psychology, the belief that certain skills or abilities are inborn in humans, thus native to them.

Social learning theory—A theory of development that holds that human behavior is influenced by a person's social environment as well as by individual factors, and that people learn new behaviors by observing and imitating those around them.

Parental concerns

The various schools and theories of developmental psychology are largely discussed within academic and research contexts rather than between parents and teachers or parents and their child's doctor. Parents who wish to learn more about a particular approach to human development or one of the theorists who developed that approach may want to consult a basic history of psychology or look into an online or local community college course on child development.

Resources

BOOKS

Miller, Patricia H. *Theories of Developmental Psychology*, 5th ed. New York: Worth, 2011.

Parke, Ross D., and Mary Gauvain. *Child Psychology: A Contemporary Viewpoint*, 7th ed. Boston, MA: McGraw-Hill, 2009.

Roberts, Michael C., ed. *Handbook of Pediatric Psychology*, 4th ed. New York: Guilford Press, 2009.

Shaffer, David, and Katherrine Kipp. *Developmental Psychology: Childhood and Adolescence*, 8th ed. Belmont, CA: Wadsworth Cengage Learning, 2010.

Thomas, R. Murray. *Comparing Theories of Child Development*, 6th ed. Belmont, CA: Wadsworth Publishing Company, 2004.

PERIODICALS

Hackman, D.A., et al. "Socioeconomic Status and the Brain: Mechanistic Insights from Human and Animal Research." *Nature Reviews: Neuroscience* 11 (September 2010): 651–59.

Kagan, J. "In Defense of Qualitative Changes in Development." *Child Development* 79 (November-December 2008): 1606–24.

Karmiloff-Smith, A. "Nativism versus Neuroconstructivism: Rethinking the Study of Developmental Disorders." *Developmental Psychology* 45 (January 2009): 56–63.

Lewin-Bizan, S., et al. "One Good Thing Leads to Another: Cascades of Positive Youth Development among American Adolescents." *Development and Psychopathology* 22 (November 2010): 759–70.

Osborne, J.W. "Commentary on Retirement, Identity, and Erikson's Developmental Stage Model." *Canadian Journal of Aging* 28 (December 2009): 295–301.

Rapoport, J.L. "Personal Reflections on Observational and Experimental Research Approaches to Childhood Psychopathology." *Journal of Child Psychology and Psychiatry, and Allied Disciplines* 50 (January 2009): 36–43.

Sneed, J.R., et al. "Gender Differences in the Age-changing Relationship between Instrumentality and Family Contact in Emerging Adulthood." *Developmental Psychology* 42 (September 2006): 787–97.

van der Horst, F.C., and R. van der Veer. "The Ontogeny of an Idea: John Bowlby and Contemporaries on Mother-Child Separation." *History of Psychology* 13 (February 2010): 25–45.

OTHER

Centers for Disease Control and Prevention. *Child Development* This is a section of the CDC website that contains tips for positive parenting, overviews of general topics in child development, and resources for parents concerned about developmental delays or disorders, http://www.cdc.gov/ncbddd/child/.

Davidson Films. *Mary Ainsworth: Attachment and the Growth of Love.* This is a four-minute video about Mary Ainsworth's work on attachment theory, http://www.youtube.com/watch?v=SHP_NikTkao&feature=related.

Division 7 Home Page. Division 7 is the subgroup of the American Psychological Association that specializes in developmental psychology, http://ecp.fiu.edu/apa/div7/?a.

ORGANIZATIONS

American Academy of Child and Adolescent Psychiatry (AACAP), 3615 Wisconsin Avenue, N.W., Washington DC, 20016-3007, (202) 966-7300, (202) 966-2891, http://www.aacap.org/.

American Psychological Association (APA), 750 First Street NE, Washington DC, 20002, (202) 336-5500, (800) 374-2721, http://www.apa.org/index.aspx.

National Institute of Child Health and Human Development (NICHD), P.O. Box 3006, Rockville MD, 20847, (800) 370-2943, (866) 760-5947, NICHDInformationResourceCenter@mail.nih.gov, http://www.nichd.nih.gov/.

Society for Research in Child Development (SRCD), 2950 S. State Street, Suite 401, Ann Arbor MI, 48104, (734) 926-0600, (734) 926-0601, info@srcd.org, http://www.srcd.org/.

Rebecca J. Frey, PhD

Developmental reading disorder

Definition

Also referred to as reading disability, reading difficulty, and **dyslexia**, developmental reading disorder is the most commonly diagnosed learning disability in the United States. It is defined by the American Psychiatric Association (APA) as "reading achievement . . . that falls substantially below that expected given the individual's chronological age, measured **intelligence**, and age-appropriate education." Developmental reading disorder is distinct from alexia, which is the term for loss of the ability to read caused by brain damage from injury or disease. However, neurological studies of alexia have helped researchers better understand children's reading disabilities.

Demographics

Estimates of the prevalence of developmental reading disorder in North America vary widely, ranging from less than 5 percent to nearly one fifth of elementary school students. The figure given by the APA is that about 5 out of every 100 school-age children in the United States have a reading disorder, with another 5–10 percent having difficulty with reading. The National Center for Learning Disabilities gives a figure of 15% for the U.S. population as a whole. Some researchers think that as many as 20 percent of American adults have some of the symptoms of dyslexia, including slow or inaccurate reading, problems with spelling and writing, or mixing up words that sound similar.

Reading disabilities are diagnosed up to five times more frequently in boys than girls, although some sources claim that this figure is misleading because boys are more likely to be screened and referred for treatment of learning disabilities due to their higher incidence of disruptive behavior, which draws the attention of educators and other professionals. Epidemiological studies indicate that girls are just as likely as boys to have difficulties with reading. Most reading disabilities were formerly grouped together under the term *dyslexia*, which has largely fallen out of favor with educators and psychologists because of confusion over widespread and inconsistent use of the term in both broad and narrower contexts; nonetheless, many organizations formed to help people with reading disorders still use the term in their materials.

Description

Reading disorder was first identified as a distinctive condition in 1881 by Oswald Berkhan, a German physician. The term *dyslexia* itself was coined by a German ophthalmologist named Rudolf Berlin in 1887. In England, the condition was called pure word blindness, after the title of an 1896 article in the *British Medical Journal* published by W. Pringle Morgan. Later, reading disorders were called developmental alexia. Starting in the 1960s the use of the term dyslexia became widespread in American medicine and education. The word *dyslexia* is derived from two Greek words, *dys*, meaning poor or inadequate, and *lexis* meaning words or language.

Types of reading disorder

Reading disabilities have been classified as either dyseidetic, dysphonetic, or mixed. Children with the dyseidetic type are able to sound out individual letters phonetically but have trouble identifying patterns of letters when they are grouped together. Their spelling tends to be phonetic even when incorrect ("laf" for "laugh"). By comparison, dysphonic readers have difficulty relating letters to sounds, so their spelling is chaotic. They are able to recognize words they have memorized but cannot sound out new ones. They may be able to read near the appropriate grade level but are poor spellers. Children with mixed reading disabilities have both the dyseidetic and dysphonic types of reading disorder.

Risk factors

Risk factors for reading disorders include a concurrent diagnosis of attention-deficit/hyperactivity disorder (**ADHD**); a family history of reading disorders; and delayed early **language development**.

As far as is known as of 2010, race or ethnicity is not a risk factor for a reading disorder.

Causes and symptoms

Causes

The causes of reading disorder are not completely understood as of 2010 but are thought to be related to differences in the structure and functioning of the brain, particularly areas of the brain known as the left perisylvian region, the left temporo-occipital region, and the right fronto-parietal cortex. Children with reading difficulties appear to process information in different parts of the brain from those without reading disorders. The reader should note that **learning to read** is a complex task. It requires coordination of the muscles of the eye to follow a line of print, spatial orientation to interpret letters and words, visual memory to retain the meaning of letters and sight words, sequencing ability, a grasp of sentence structure and grammar, and the ability to categorize and analyze. In addition, the brain must integrate visual cues with memory and associate them with specific sounds. The sounds, or phonemes, must then be associated with specific meanings, and for comprehension, the meanings must be retained while a sentence or passage is read. Reading disorder occurs when any of these processes are disrupted. For that reason, the roots of reading disorder have proved difficult to isolate, and may be different in different individuals.

Although reading disorder has not yet been conclusively traced to specific genes, it is known to run in families. In 2005, a region on chromosome 6 was identified as possibly related to dyslexia, but this finding has not yet been verified.

One surprising finding, reported by a team of researchers at Hong Kong University in 2008, is that the part of the brain affected by dyslexia appears to differ according to the child's primary language. The researchers used **magnetic resonance imaging** (MRI) to compare a group of children whose first language is English with a second group raised to speak Chinese. The scientists found that the English speakers use a different part of the brain when reading from that used by the Chinese students. The difference is apparently related to the fact that English is an alphabetic language whereas Chinese uses symbols to represent words.

Symptoms

Reading disorder can cause severe problems in reading, and consequently in academic work, even in people with normal intelligence, educational opportunity, motivation to learn to read, and emotional self-control. Reading disorder is different from learning slowness or **mental retardation**, because with reading disorder, there is a gap between the expected level of performance and achievement. Difficulties in reading can occur on many levels, and reading disorder may have multiple causes that manifest in different ways. Common problems in people with reading disorder include:

- slow reading speed
- poor comprehension when reading material either aloud or silently
- omission of words while reading
- reversal of words or letters while reading
- difficulty decoding syllables or single words and associating them with specific sounds (phonics)
- limited sight word vocabulary

In addition to having trouble associating letters with sounds and forming memories for words, children with a reading disorder may have some of the following problems with learning:

- learning to speak.
- organizing thoughts and ideas into clear written and spoken language.
- memorizing number facts, such as the multiplication tables.
- reading quickly enough to understand what is being read. Some children with dyslexia read so slowly that they cannot remember the beginning of a sentence by the time they reach the end of it, particularly if it is a long and complicated sentence.
- making their way through longer reading assignments.
- spelling words correctly.
- trouble with making rhymes.
- learning foreign languages, which involves a basic understanding of grammar and the parts of speech.
- performing mathematical calculations correctly.

Diagnosis

Reading disorder is rarely diagnosed in children before age five or six because formal instruction in reading does not begin before kindergarten or first grade in most American schools. Even at the **preschool** stage, however, there are certain problems, such as trouble sounding out words and difficulty memorizing sequence information such as the days of the week, that may foreshadow a reading disability.

Examination

Evaluation of a child's reading ability must be done individually to make a diagnosis of reading disorder and distinguish it from slow learning or low intelligence. The diagnostic process takes several steps. The first step is an office examination by the child's doctor to rule out any disorders of vision or hearing that could interfere with learning. The child may also be referred to a neurologist (a specialist in disorders of the nervous system) for further evaluation to make sure that the child does not have a brain tumor or other physical disease of the brain.

The next step is usually intelligence testing and an evaluation of the child's reading and speaking skills by a qualified expert. This type of evaluation involves testing the child's short-term memory or asking the child to read nonsense words as a test of their ability to link letters and sounds. In addition, the child may be evaluated psychologically to see whether depression, **anxiety**, or social problems are causing the learning difficulty. The examiner must take into account the child's age, intelligence, educational opportunities, and such cultural factors as whether the language spoken at home is different from the language used in school instruction.

Reading disorder is diagnosed when reading achievement is substantially below what would be expected after taking into account the above factors. In addition, to meet the APA's diagnostic criteria for reading disorder, the child's reading problems must substantially interfere with

KEY TERMS

Alexia—A condition in which damage to the brain causes a person to lose the ability to read.

Decoding—In education, the ability to associate letters of the alphabet with sounds.

Dyslexia—A word that is often used as a synonym for reading disorder. Dyslexia, however, usually includes difficulties with spelling and writing as well as reading.

Neurologist—A doctor who specializes in diagnosing and treating disorders of the nervous system.

Phoneme—The smallest detectable sound of a word or language.

Phonics—A method of teaching speakers of English to read and write by learning to connect the sounds of spoken English with letters or groups of letters.

his or her schoolwork or daily life. If a physical condition is present (for example, mental retardation or hearing loss), the reading deficit must be in excess of what one would normally associate with the physical handicap.

Treatment

Traditional

There is no medical or surgical cure for a reading disorder as of 2010; however, dyslexic individuals can learn to read and write with appropriate education or treatment. Treatment for a reading disorder is highly individualized. After the child's specific difficulties in reading and understanding language have been analyzed by an expert, a treatment program is drawn up tailored to his or her needs. Under the provisions of the Individuals with Disabilities Education Act (IDEA) of 2004, any child with a diagnosed learning disability, including reading disorder or dyslexia, should be eligible for an Individual Education Program (IEP) that provides customized instruction at school designed to address his or her disability.

Classroom approaches to remedial reading

Reading disabilities are diagnosed on the basis of individualized testing. Schools are required by law to provide specialized instruction for children with learning disabilities, including developmental reading disorder. The child may receive special help from his or her teacher within the regular classroom setting. Preferably, however, she will work with a reading specialist, either privately or in a small group that meets in a special classroom, generally called a resource room, reading center, or reading lab. (Reading specialists are certified in many states.) A variety of teaching methods are used; in many cases the teacher or specialist will try a variety of techniques with a child to see which ones are most effective for that child.

Children with a severe reading disorder may require tutoring on a one-to-one basis or in small group sessions several times a week. Whereas a child with normal language skills may need 60 to 90 hours to master a specific set of tasks involving reading, children with a reading disorder may need between 80 and 100 hours to make the same progress. In general, the earlier a child is diagnosed and **special education** programs are started, the greater the likelihood that he or she will learn to read well enough to succeed in school. Some children with severe reading disorders, however, may never learn to read or write well and are usually helped by training for occupations or career paths that do not require strong language skills.

The synthetic phonics method, which was once the mainstay of reading instruction nationwide, is often used for remedial reading instruction. Children start by learning basic consonant and vowels sounds, first separately and then in combination (usually starting with consonants and short vowels and progressing from there to three-letter words), and vocabulary words are introduced only when all the letter sounds have already been studied. Students are taught to sound out unfamiliar words one letter or letter-group at a time based on their sounds. With the opposite approach—the whole-word or analytic method—students first acquire a basic vocabulary of words they know by sight and then study the relationships of letters and sounds by analyzing how they operate within these words. Initially a few phonetic units are taught, beginning with consonants and short vowel sounds, and the sounds are combined in a particular sequence, with tracing, writing, and spelling used as supplementary activities.

Another remedial reading technique is the kinesthetic approach (also known as the Orton-Gillingham method), in which new words are taught using a procedure nicknamed VAKT for the four senses that are involved: visual, auditory, kinesthetic, tactual. It is basically a phonetic approach that teaches individual letter sounds and then blends them into words. What is unique is the multisensory component, which involves writing each new letter, sound, or word on an oversize card and having the child trace it with her finger while pronouncing it. This activity is followed by several other steps over a period of weeks, including visualization and memorization.

In contrast to the Orton-Gillingham method—which is most helpful for children with a dyseidetic reading disorder, who learn letter sounds more easily than whole words—the Fernald method uses a kinesthetic approach but emphasizes whole words. In addition to tracing, writing, and saying selected words, the child uses them in sentences and stories, keeping a collection of new words in a special file box.

The language experience, or whole-language approach, which aroused controversy when it was adopted in the regular reading curriculums of many schools in the 1970s and 1980s and has been deemphasized in many curriculums since that time, is also used for remedial reading. A whole-word approach whose main emphasis is on motivation and **creativity**, it attempts to get the child involved in reading by introducing words through colorful, imaginative stories. Other approaches to remedial reading include the color-coding method (which associates letters with specific colors that are then blended to create sounds) and the neuropsychological approach, which utilizes the findings of advanced brain research to devise activities targeting certain types of neurological functioning.

Assistive devices

As of 2010, a new assistive device known as the Intel Reader is being field-tested by the International Dyslexia Association (IDA) for students with reading disorders. The handheld device takes a photograph of printed material with a camera on its bottom edge and then reads the text aloud to the student, who can follow the printed material as the device reads the text aloud. The reader can be used by people with impaired vision as well as by those with reading disorders.

Psychotherapy

Children with reading disorders often need and benefit from psychotherapy because of their struggles with low **self-esteem**. Many come to feel that they are stupid or less capable than they really are; they are likely to drop out of school if they are not diagnosed and treated early.

Prognosis

The prognosis of dyslexia is difficult to predict because an individual child's outcome depends on a number of factors: the severity of the child's language difficulties; the stage at which the dyslexia is diagnosed; the supportiveness of the child's family; the presence of other health problems; and the quality of supplemental teaching and tutoring that the child receives. In general, people who are identified as having a reading disorder before grade three and who receive intensive reading education can do well. Reading disorders can persist into adult life; however, many people with reading disorders do achieve personal and professional success. Some go on to complete advanced degrees while others do well in such fields as business and the performing arts.

Prevention

There is no known way to prevent developmental reading disorder as of 2010. Early intervention is key to successfully preventing the associated symptoms of low self esteem, lack of interest in school, and poor behavior that can accompany low academic achievement.

Resources

BOOKS

American Psychiatric Association. *Diagnostic and Statistical Manual of Mental Disorders.* 4th ed. text revision. Washington D.C.: American Psychiatric Association, 2000.

Hulme, Charles, and Margaret J. Snowling. *Developmental Disorders of Language Learning and Cognition.* Malden, MA: Wiley-Blackwell, 2009.

Moats, Louisa Cook, and Karen E. Dakin. *Basic Facts about Dyslexia and Other Reading Problems.* Baltimore, MD: International Dyslexia Association, 2008.

Thompson, Diane, and Lidia E. Bushnell. *Reading: Learning, Writing, and Disorders.* Hauppauge, NY: Nova Science Publishers, 2009.

PERIODICALS

Dhar, M., et al. "Information Processing Differences and Similarities in Adults with Dyslexia and Adults with Attention Deficit Hyperactivity Disorder during a Continuous Performance Test: A Study of Cortical Potentials." *Neuropsychologia* 48 (August 2010): 3045–3056.

Germano, E., et al. "Comorbidity of ADHD and Dyslexia." *Developmental Neuropsychology* 35 (September 2010): 475–93.

Heim, S., et al. "Interaction of Phonological Awareness and 'Magnocellular' Processing during Normal and Dyslexic Reading: Behavioural and fMRI Investigations." *Dyslexia* 16 (August 2010): 258–82.

Hensler, B.S., et al. "Behavioral Genetic Approach to the Study of Dyslexia." *Journal of Developmental and Behavioral Pediatrics* 31 (September 2010): 525–32.

Thomson, J.M., and T.P. Hogan. "Introduction: Advances in Early Detection of Reading Risk." *Journal of Learning Disabilities* 43 (July-August 2010): 291–93.

Waldie, K.E., and M. Hausmann. "Right Fronto-parietal Dysfunction in Children with ADHD and Developmental Dyslexia as Determined by Line Bisection Judgements." *Neuropsychologia* 48 (October 2010): 3650–3656.

Willcutt, E.G., et al. "Understanding the Complex Etiologies of Developmental Disorders: Behavioral and Molecular Genetic Approaches." *Journal of Developmental and Behavioral Pediatrics* 31 (September 2010): 533–44.

OTHER

Learning Disabilities Association of America (LDA). *Dyslexia,* http://www.ldaamerica.org/aboutld/teachers/understanding/dyslexia.asp.

Mayo Clinic. *Dyslexia,* http://www.mayoclinic.com/health/dyslexia/DS00224.

National Center for Learning Disabilities. *Dyslexia,* http://www.ncld.org/ld-basics/ld-aamp-language/reading/dyslexia.

National Institute of Neurological Disorders and Stroke (NINDS). *Dyslexia Information Page,* http://www.ninds.nih.gov/disorders/dyslexia/dyslexia.htm.

Tynan, W. Douglas. "Learning Disorder, Reading." *eMedicine,* February 25, 2008, http://emedicine.medscape.com/article/1835801-overview.

ORGANIZATIONS

Learning Disabilities Association of America (LDA), 4156 Library Road, Pittsburgh PA, 15234, (412) 341-1515, (412) 344-0224, http://www.ldaamerica.org/index.cfm.

National Center for Learning Disabilities, 381 Park Avenue South, Suite 1401, New York NY, 10016, (212) 545-7510, 888-575-7373, (212) 545-9665, http://www.ncld.org/.

National Institute of Neurological Disorders and Stroke (NINDS), P.O. Box 5801, Bethesda MD, 20824, (800) 352-9424 (301) 496-5751 http://www.ninds.nih.gov/index.htm.

International Dyslexia Association (IDA), 40 York Rd., 4th Floor, Towson MD 21286, (410) 296-0232, (410) 321-5069, http://www.interdys.org/index.htm.

Rebecca J. Frey, PhD

Dextromethorphan *see* **Cough suppressants**

Diabetes mellitus

Definition

Diabetes mellitus is a condition in which the pancreas no longer produces enough insulin or cells stop responding to the insulin that is produced, so that glucose in the blood cannot be absorbed into the cells of the body. Symptoms include frequent urination, lethargy, weight loss, excessive thirst, and hunger. Treatment includes changes in diet, oral medications, and in some cases, daily injections of insulin or other hormone–like medications designed to boost insulin or lower blood sugar.

Demographics

Approximately 23 million Americans have diabetes, according to the American Diabetes Association. Unfortunately, as many as one–;half are unaware they have it. The World Health Organization (WHO) estimates that as of 2010, 230 million people worldwide have diabetes, including 20 million in China, 31 million in India, 8.4 million in Indonesia, 33 million in Europe, 11 million in Africa, and two million in Mexico. WHO estimates that without large–scale, strategic intervention, the number of people with diabetes worldwide could double by 2030.

Description

Diabetes mellitus is a chronic disease that causes serious health complications including renal (kidney) failure, heart disease, **stroke**, limb amputation, and blindness. Every cell in the human body needs energy in order to function. The body's primary energy source is glucose, a simple sugar resulting from the digestion of foods containing carbohydrates (sugars and starches). Glucose from digested food circulates in the blood as a ready energy source for cells. Insulin is a hormone or chemical produced by cells in the pancreas, an organ located behind the stomach. Insulin bonds to a receptor site on the outside of cell and acts like a key to open a doorway into the cell, through which glucose can enter. Some of the glucose can be converted to concentrated energy sources like glycogen or fatty acids and saved for later use. When there is not enough insulin produced or when the doorway no longer recognizes the insulin key, glucose stays in the blood rather entering the cells.

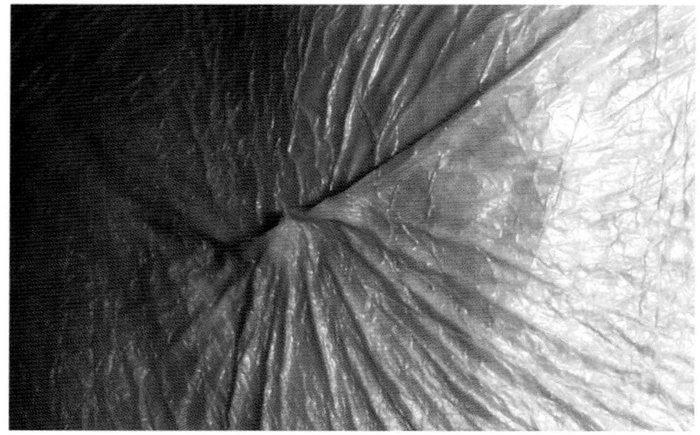

Wrinkled, dehydrated skin of a person in a diabetic coma. Untreated diabetes mellitus results in elevated blood glucose levels, causing a variety of symptoms that can culminate in a diabetic coma. *(Dr. P. Marazzi/SPL/Photo Researchers, Inc.)*

The body will attempt to dilute the high level of glucose in the blood, a condition called **hyperglycemia**, by drawing water out of cells and into the bloodstream in an effort to dilute the sugar and excrete it in the urine. It is not unusual for people with undiagnosed diabetes to be constantly thirsty, drink large quantities of water, and to urinate frequently as their bodies try to get rid of the extra glucose. This creates high levels of glucose in the urine.

At the same time that the body is trying to get rid of glucose from the blood, cells are starving for glucose and sending signals to the body to eat more food, thus making patients extremely hungry. To provide energy for the starving cells, the body also tries to convert fats and proteins to glucose. The breakdown of fats and proteins for energy causes acid compounds called ketones to form in the blood. Ketones also will be excreted in the urine. As ketones build up in the blood, a condition called ketoacidosis can occur. This condition can be life–threatening if left untreated, leading to coma and **death**.

Types of diabetes mellitus

Type I diabetes, earlier called juvenile diabetes, begins most commonly in childhood, **adolescence**, or early adulthood. In this form of diabetes, the body produces little or no insulin. The disease is characterized by a sudden onset and occurs more frequently in populations descended from Northern European countries (Finland, Scotland, Scandinavia) than in those from Southern European countries, the Middle East, or Asia. In the United States, approximately three people in 1,000 develop Type I diabetes. This form is also called insulin–dependent diabetes because people who develop this type require daily injections of insulin.

Brittle diabetics are a subgroup of Type I in which patients have frequent and rapid swings of blood sugar levels between hyperglycemia (a condition where there is too much glucose or sugar in the blood) and **hypoglycemia** (a condition where there are abnormally low levels of glucose or sugar in the blood). These diabetics require several injections of different types of insulin during the day to keep the blood sugar level within a fairly normal range.

The more common form of diabetes, Type II diabetes, occurs in approximately three to five percent of Americans under 50 years of age, and increases to 10–15% in those over 50. More than 90% of the diabetics in the United States are Type II diabetics. Sometimes called adult–onset diabetes, this form of diabetes occurs most often in people who are overweight and who do not **exercise** enough. It is also more common in people of Native American, Hispanic, and African–American descent. People who have migrated to Western cultures from East India, Japan, and Australian Aboriginal cultures also are more likely to develop Type II diabetes than those who remain in their original countries.

Type II is considered a milder form of diabetes because of its slow onset (sometimes developing over the course of several years) and because it frequently can be controlled with diet and oral medication. The consequences of uncontrolled and untreated Type II diabetes, however, are the just as serious as those for Type I. This form is also called non–insulin–dependent diabetes, a term that is somewhat misleading. Many people with Type II diabetes can control the condition with diet and oral medications, however, insulin injections are sometimes necessary if treatment with diet and oral medication is inadequate to maintain normal blood glucose levels

Another form of diabetes called gestational diabetes can develop during pregnancy and generally resolves after the baby is delivered. This diabetic condition develops during the second or third trimester of pregnancy in about two percent of pregnancies. In 2004, the incidence of gestational diabetes was reported to have increased 35% in 10 years. Children of women with gestational diabetes are more likely to be born prematurely, have hypoglycemia, have an excess of body fat, or have severe **jaundice** at **birth**. The condition usually is treated by diet; however, insulin injections may be required. Women who have diabetes during pregnancy are at higher risk for developing Type II diabetes within 5–10 years.

Diabetes also can develop as a result of pancreatic disease, **alcoholism**, **malnutrition**, or other severe illnesses that stress the body.

Causes and symptoms

Causes

The causes of diabetes mellitus are unclear, however, there seem to be both hereditary (genetic factors passed on in families) and environmental factors involved. Research has shown that some people who develop diabetes have common genetic markers. In Type I diabetes, the **immune system**, the body's defense system against infection, is assumed to be triggered by a virus or another microorganism that destroys cells in the pancreas that produce insulin. In Type II diabetes, age, obesity, and family history of diabetes play a role.

In Type II diabetes, the pancreas may produce enough insulin. However, cells have become resistant to the insulin produced and it may not work as effectively. Symptoms of Type II diabetes can begin so gradually that a person may not know that he or she has it. Early signs are lethargy, extreme thirst, and frequent urination. Other symptoms may include sudden weight loss, slow wound healing, urinary tract infections, gum disease, or blurred vision. It is not unusual for Type II diabetes to be detected while a patient is seeing a doctor about another health concern that is actually being caused by the yet undiagnosed diabetes.

Individuals who are at high risk of developing Type II diabetes mellitus include people who:

- are obese (more than 20% above their ideal body weight)
- have a relative with diabetes mellitus
- belong to a high–risk ethnic population (African–American, Native American, Hispanic, or Native Hawaiian)
- have been diagnosed with gestational diabetes or have delivered a baby weighing more than 9 lb (4 kg)
- have high blood pressure (140/90 mmHg or above)
- have a high–density lipoprotein cholesterol level less than or equal to 35 mg/dL and/or a triglyceride level greater than or equal to 250 mg/dL
- have had impaired glucose tolerance or impaired fasting glucose on previous testing

Several common medications can impair the body's use of insulin, causing a condition known as secondary diabetes. These medications include treatments for high blood pressure (furosemide, clonidine, and thiazide diuretics), drugs with hormonal activity (**oral contraceptives**, thyroid hormone, progestins, and glucocorticorids), and the anti–inflammation drug indomethacin. Several drugs that are used to treat **mood disorders** (such as **anxiety** and depression) also can impair glucose absorption. These drugs include haloperidol, lithium carbonate, Zyprexa (olanzapine), Seroquel (quetiapine), phenothiazines, **tricyclic antidepressants**, and adrenergic agonists. Other medications that can cause diabetes symptoms include isoniazid, nicotinic acid, cimetidine, protease inhibitors used to treat HIV, and heparin. A 2004 study found that low levels of the essential mineral chromium in the body may be linked to increased risk for diseases associated with insulin resistance. Vitamin D deficiencies have also been linked with impaired glucose tolerance, and vitamin D deficient diabetics tend to have more difficulty in controlling their blood glucose levels.

Symptoms

Symptoms of diabetes can develop suddenly (over days or weeks) in previously healthy children or adolescents, or can develop gradually (over several years) in overweight adults over the age of 40. The classic symptoms include feeling tired and sick, frequent urination, excessive thirst, excessive hunger, and weight loss.

Ketoacidosis, a condition due to starvation or uncontrolled diabetes, is common in Type I diabetes. Ketones are acid compounds that form in the blood when the body breaks down fats and proteins. Symptoms include abdominal **pain**, **vomiting**, rapid breathing, weight loss, extreme lethargy, and drowsiness. Patients with ketoacidosis also have a sweet breath odor. Left untreated, this condition can lead to coma and death.

With Type II diabetes, the condition may not become evident until the patient presents for medical treatment for some other condition. A patient may have heart disease, chronic infections of the gums and urinary tract, blurred vision, **numbness** in the feet and legs, or slow–healing **wounds**. Women may experience genital **itching**.

Diagnosis

Diabetes is suspected based on symptoms. Urine tests can confirm a diagnosis of diabetes based on the amount of glucose found. Urine tests can also detect ketones and protein in the urine that may help diagnose diabetes and assess how well the kidneys are functioning. These tests also can be used to monitor the disease once the patient is on a standardized diet, oral medications, or insulin.

KEY TERMS

Cataract—A condition in which the lens of the eye becomes cloudy.

Diabetic peripheral neuropathy—A condition in which the sensitivity of nerves to pain, temperature, and pressure is dulled, particularly in the legs and feet.

Diabetic retinopathy—A condition in which the tiny blood vessels to the retina, the tissues that sense light at the back of the eye, are damaged, leading to blurred vision, sudden blindness, or black spots, lines, or flashing lights in the field of vision.

Glaucoma—A condition in which pressure within the eye causes damage to the optic nerve, which sends visual images to the brain.

Hyperglycemia—A condition in which there is too much glucose or sugar in the blood.

Hypoglycemia—A condition in which there is too little glucose or sugar in the blood.

Insulin—A hormone or chemical produced by the pancreas that is needed by cells of the body in order to use glucose (sugar), the body's main source of energy.

Ketoacidosis—A condition due to starvation or uncontrolled Type I diabetes. Ketones are acid compounds that form in the blood when the body breaks down fats and proteins. Symptoms include abdominal pain, vomiting, rapid breathing, extreme tiredness, and drowsiness.

Kidney dialysis—A process during which blood is filtered through a dialysis machine to remove waste products that would normally be removed by the kidneys. The filtered blood is then circulated back into the patient. This process also is called renal dialysis.

Pancreas—A gland located behind the stomach that produces insulin.

Urine tests

Clinistix and Diastix are paper strips or dipsticks that change color when dipped in urine. The test strip is compared to a chart that shows the amount of glucose in the urine based on the change in color. The level of glucose in the urine lags behind the level of glucose in the blood. Testing the urine with a test stick, paper strip, or tablet that changes color when sugar is present is not as accurate as blood testing. However, it can give a fast and simple reading. It is no longer considered appropriate for use by diabetics as a means to assess glucose control.

Ketones in the urine can be detected using similar types of dipstick tests (Acetest or Ketostix). Ketoacidosis can be a life–threatening situation in Type I diabetics, so having a quick and simple test to detect ketones can assist in establishing a diagnosis sooner.

Another dipstick test can determine the presence of protein or albumin in the urine. Protein in the urine can indicate problems with **kidney function** and can be used to track the development of renal failure. A more sensitive test for urine protein uses radioactively tagged chemicals to detect microalbuminuria, small amounts of protein in the urine, that may not show up on dipstick tests.

Blood tests

FASTING GLUCOSE TEST Blood is drawn from a vein in the patient's arm after a period at least eight hours after the patient has last eaten, usually in the morning before breakfast. Red blood cells are separated from the sample and the amount of glucose is measured in the remaining plasma. A plasma level of 7 mmol/L (126 mg/L) or greater can indicate diabetes. The fasting glucose test is usually repeated on another day to confirm the results.

GLYCATED HEMOGLOBIN (A1C) TEST This blood test indicates the average blood glucose level for the previous 60–90 days. Blood is drawn from a vein after the patient has fasted for at least eight hours. An A1C level that equals or exceeds 6.5% or more on two separate test dates indicates diabetes. In 2009, the International Diabetes Federation recommended the A1C test as the preferred method for diagnosing diabetes and monitoring the effectiveness of treatment.

ORAL GLUCOSE TOLERANCE TEST Blood samples are taken from a vein before and after a patient drinks a thick, sweet syrup of glucose. In a non–diabetic, the level of glucose in the blood goes up immediately after the drink and then decreases gradually as insulin is used by the body to metabolize, or absorb, the sugar. In a diabetic, the glucose in the blood goes up and stays high after drinking the sweetened liquid. A plasma glucose level of 11.1 mmol/L (200 mg/dL) or higher at two hours after drinking the syrup confirms the diagnosis of diabetes.

A diagnosis of diabetes is confirmed if there are symptoms of diabetes and a plasma glucose level of at least 11.1 mmol/L, a fasting plasma glucose level of at least seven mmol/L; or a two–hour plasma glucose level of at least 11.1 mmol/L during an oral glucose tolerance test.

Home blood glucose monitoring kits are available so patients with diabetes can monitor their own levels. A small needle or lancet is used to prick the finger and a drop of blood is collected and analyzed by a monitoring device. Some patients may test their blood glucose levels several times during a day and use this information to adjust their doses of insulin.

Treatment

A successful pancreas transplant currently offers the only cure for Type 1 diabetes. Diabetes is usually managed with medication and lifestyle changes so that patients can live a relatively normal life. Treatment of diabetes focuses on two goals: keeping blood glucose within normal range and preventing the development of long–term complications. Careful monitoring of diet, exercise, and blood glucose levels are as important as the use of insulin or oral medications in preventing complications of diabetes.

Dietary changes

Diet and moderate exercise are the first treatments implemented in diabetes. For many Type II diabetics, weight loss may be an important goal in helping them to control their diabetes. A well–balanced, nutritious diet provides approximately 50–;60% of calories from carbohydrates, approximately 10–20% of calories from protein, and less than 30% of calories from fat. The number of calories required by an individual depends on age, weight, and activity level. The calorie intake also needs to be distributed over the course of the entire day, so surges of glucose entering the blood system are kept to a minimum. Carbohydrates such as grains, vegetables, legumes, and fruits are healthier than carbohydrates provided by sweets and snack–type foods.

Keeping track of the number of calories and carbohydrates provided by different foods can become complicated, so patients usually are advised to consult a nutritionist or dietitian. An individualized, easy to manage diet plan can be set up for each patient. Both the American Diabetes Association and the American Dietetic Association recommend diets based on the use of food exchange lists. Each food exchange contains a known amount of calories in the form of protein, fat, or carbohydrate. A patient's diet plan will consist of a certain number of exchanges from each food category (meat or protein, fruits, breads and starches, vegetables, and fats) to be eaten at meal times and as snacks. Patients have flexibility in choosing which foods they eat as long as they stick with the number of exchanges prescribed.

For many Type II diabetics, weight loss is an important factor in controlling their condition. The food exchange system, along with a plan of moderate exercise, can help them lose excess weight and improve their overall health.

Oral medications

Oral medications are available to lower blood glucose in Type II diabetics. In 1990, 23.4 million outpatient prescriptions for oral antidiabetic agents were dispensed.

By 2005, the number had increased to more than 100 million prescriptions. Oral antidiabetic agents accounted for more than $8 billion dollars in worldwide retail sales in 2005 and were the fastest–growing segment of diabetes drugs. There are five distinct classes of hypoglycemic agents available, each class displaying unique pharmacologic properties. These classes are the sulfonylureas, meglitinides, biguanides, thiazolidinediones and alpha–glucosidase inhibitors. In patients for whom diet and exercise do not provide adequate glucose control, therapy with a single oral agent can be tried. The drugs first prescribed for Type II diabetes are in a class of compounds called sulfonylureas and include tolbutamide, tolazamide, acetohexamide, and chlorpropamide. Other drugs in the same class include glyburide, glimeperide, and glipizide. How these drugs work is not well understood. However, they seem to stimulate cells of the pancreas to produce more insulin. Newer medications that are available to treat diabetes include Glucophage (metformin), Precose (acarbose), Glycet (miglitol), Actos (pioglitazone), and Avandia (rosiglitazone). The choice of medication depends in part on the individual patient profile. All drugs have side effects that may make them inappropriate for particular patients. Some for example, may stimulate weight gain or cause stomach irritation, so they may not be the best treatment for someone who is already overweight or who has stomach ulcers. Others, like metformin, have been shown to have positive effects such as reduced cardiovascular mortality. While these medications are an important aspect of treatment for Type II diabetes, they are not a substitute for a well–planned diet and moderate exercise. Oral medications have not been shown effective for Type I diabetes, in which the patient produces little or no insulin.

Constant advances are being made in development of new oral medications for persons with diabetes. One drug called Metaglip combining glipizide and metformin was approved in a single tablet. Along with diet and exercise, the drug is used as initial therapy for Type II diabetes. Another drug approved by the U.S. Food and Drug Administration (FDA) combines metformin and rosiglitazone (Avandia), a medication that increases muscle cells' sensitivity to insulin. It is marketed under the name Avandamet. Other combination drugs include Avandaryl (rosiglitazone and glimepiride), and Duetact (pioglitazone and glimepiride). As of 2010, more combination drugs were under development. So many new drugs are in the pipeline, a record 235 as of mid–2010, with many nearing FDA approval, that it is best to stay in touch with a physician for the latest information. Physicians can find the best drug, diet and exercise program to fit an individual patient's need. In 2007, a study in the *New England Journal of Medicine* suggested the use of Avandia (rosiglitazone) increased the risk of a heart attack and death from heart failure. Other studies regarding Avandia and its effect on heart health were underway as of mid–2010, including a pending review by the FDA. An FDA ruling also required that Avandia, Actos, Avandaryl, and Duetact carry stronger warnings on their labels.

Byetta (exenatide) and Victoza (liraglutide) are the first compunds in a class of injectable medicines called incretin mimetics to improve blood sugar levels in Type II diabetes. Byetta usually requires two injections daily compared to one with Victoza. However, long–term studies are under way to access a possible relationship between Victoza and an increased incidence of pancreatitis and thyroid tumors.

Insulin

Persons with Type I diabetes need daily injections of insulin to help their bodies use glucose. The amount and type of insulin required depends on the height, weight, age, food intake, and activity level of the individual diabetic patient. Some patients with Type II diabetes may need to use insulin injections if their diabetes cannot be controlled with diet, exercise, and oral medication. Injections are given subcutaneously, that is, just under the skin, using a small needle and syringe, using an injection pen, or an insulin pump. Injection sites can be anywhere on the body where there is looser skin, including the upper arm, abdomen, or upper thigh.

Purified human insulin is most commonly used. Insulin from animal sources is no longer used. Insulin may be given as an injection of a single dose of one type of insulin once a day. Different types of insulin can be mixed and given in one dose or split into two or more doses during a day. Patients who require multiple injections over the course of a day may be able to use an insulin pump that administers small doses of insulin on demand. The small battery–operated pump is worn outside the body and is connected to a needle that is inserted into the abdomen. Pumps can be programmed to inject small doses of insulin at various times during the day, or the patient may be able to adjust the insulin doses to coincide with meals and exercise.

Regular insulin is fast–acting and starts to work within 15–30 minutes, with its peak glucose–lowering effect about two hours after it is injected. Its effects last for about four to six hours. NPH (neutral protamine Hagedorn) and Lente insulin are intermediate–acting, starting to work within one to three hours and lasting up to 18–26 hours. Ultra–lente is a long–acting form of insulin that starts to work within four to eight hours and lasts up to 24 hours.

Hypoglycemia, or low blood sugar, can be caused by too much insulin, too little food (or eating too late to coincide with the action of the insulin), alcohol consumption, or increased exercise. A patient with symptoms of hypoglycemia may be hungry, cranky, confused, and tired. The patient may become sweaty and shaky. Left untreated, the patient can lose consciousness or have a seizure. This condition is sometimes called an insulin reaction and should be treated by giving the patient something sweet to eat or drink like a candy, sugar cubes, fruit juice, or another high sugar snack.

Surgery

Transplantation of a healthy pancreas into a diabetic patient is a successful treatment, however, this transplant is usually done only if a kidney transplant is performed at the same time. Although a pancreas transplant is possible, it is often not clear if the potential benefits outweigh the risks of the surgery and drug therapy needed.

Alternative treatment

Since diabetes can be a life–threatening condition if not properly managed, persons should not attempt to treat this condition without medical supervision. A variety of alternative therapies can be helpful in managing the symptoms of diabetes and supporting patients with the disease. Acupuncture can help relieve the pain associated with diabetic neuropathy by stimulation of certain points. A qualified practitioner should be consulted. Herbal remedies also may be helpful in managing diabetes. Although there is no herbal substitute for insulin, some herbs may help adjust blood sugar levels or manage other diabetic symptoms. Some options include:

- fenugreek (*Trigonella foenum–graecum*) has been shown in some studies to reduce blood insulin and glucose levels while also lowering cholesterol
- bilberry (*Vaccinium myrtillus*) may lower blood glucose levels, as well as helping to maintain healthy blood vessels
- garlic (*Allium sativum*) may lower blood sugar and cholesterol levels
- onions (*Allium cepa*) may help lower blood glucose levels by freeing insulin to metabolize them
- cayenne pepper (*Capsicum frutescens*) can help relieve pain in the peripheral nerves (a type of diabetic neuropathy)
- gingko (*Gingko biloba*) may maintain blood flow to the retina, helping to prevent diabetic retinopathy

Other alternative medicine therapies for controlling blood sugar include chromium picolinate, alpha lipoic acid, cinnamon, evening primrose oil, and pygenol (pine bark extract). Any therapy that lowers stress levels also can be useful in treating diabetes by helping to reduce insulin requirements. Among the alternative treatments that aim to lower stress are hypnotherapy, biofeedback, and meditation.

Prognosis

Uncontrolled diabetes is a leading cause of blindness, end–stage renal disease, and limb amputations. It also doubles the risks of heart disease and increases the risk of stroke. Eye problems including cataracts, glaucoma, and diabetic retinopathy also are more common in diabetics.

Diabetic peripheral neuropathy is a condition where nerve endings, particularly in the legs and feet, become less sensitive. Diabetic foot ulcers are a particular problem since the patient does not feel the pain of a blister, callous, or other minor injury. Poor blood circulation in the legs and feet contribute to delayed wound healing. The inability to sense pain along with the complications of delayed wound healing can result in minor injuries, blisters, or calluses becoming infected and difficult to treat. In cases of severe infection, the infected tissue begins to break down and rot away. The most serious consequence of this condition is the need for amputation of toes, feet, or legs due to severe infection.

Heart disease and kidney disease are common complications of diabetes. Long–term complications may include the need for kidney dialysis or a kidney transplant due to kidney failure.

Babies born to diabetic mothers have an increased risk of **birth defects** and distress at birth.

Prevention

Research continues on diabetes prevention and improved detection of those at risk for developing diabetes. As of 2010, research was being conducted in a number of countries, including the United States, China, and Finland. While the onset of Type I diabetes is unpredictable, the risk of developing Type II diabetes can be reduced by maintaining ideal weight and exercising regularly. The physical and emotional stress of surgery, illness, pregnancy, and alcoholism can increase the risks of diabetes, so maintaining a healthy lifestyle is critical to preventing the onset of Type II diabetes and preventing further complications of the disease.

Parental concerns

Parents of children with diabetes must work with their child's teachers and school administrators to ensure that their child is able to test her blood sugars regularly, take insulin as needed, and have access to food or drink to treat a low. Someone at school should also be trained in how to administer a glucagon injection, an emergency treatment for a hypoglycemic episode when a child loses consciousness.

Section 504 of the Rehabilitation Act of 1973 enables parents to develop both a Section 504 plan (which describes a child's medical needs) and an individualized education plan (IEP) (which describes what special accommodations a child requires to address those needs). An IEP should cover such issues as blood glucose monitoring, dietary plans, and treating highs and lows. If school staff has little to no experience with diabetes, bringing in a certified diabetes educator (CDE) to offer basic training may be useful.

Children with diabetes can lead an active life and enjoy most of the activities and foods their peers do, with a few precautions to avoid blood sugar highs or lows. A certified diabetes educator that has experience working with children can help them understand the importance of regular testing as well as methods for minimizing discomfort. Diabetes summer camps, where children can learn about diabetes care in the company of peers and counselors who also live with the disease, may be useful from both a health and a social standpoint. In addition, peer support groups can sometimes help children come to terms with their diabetes.

Hypoglycemia, or low blood sugar, can be caused by too much insulin, too little food (or eating too late to coincide with the action of the insulin), alcohol consumption, or increased exercise. A child with symptoms of hypoglycemia may be hungry, cranky, confused, and tired. The patient may become sweaty and shaky. Left untreated, a child can lose consciousness or have a seizure. This condition is sometimes called an insulin reaction and should be treated by giving the patient something sweet to eat or drink like candy, juice, glucose gel, or another high sugar snack. A child who loses consciousness due to a low should never be given food or drink due to the risk of choking. In these cases, a glucagon injection should be administered and the child should be taken to the nearest emergency care facility.

While exercise can lower blood glucose levels, children with diabetes can and do excel in sports. Proper hydration, frequent testing, and a before-game or practice snack can prevent hypoglycemia. Coaches or another onsite adult should be aware of a child's medical condition and be prepared to treat a hypoglycemic attack if necessary.

The other potential danger to a child with diabetes—diabetic ketoacidosis is uncommon—and most likely to occur prior to a diagnosis. It may also happen if insulin is discontinued or if the body is under stress due to illness or injury. Ketones in the urine can be detected using dipstick tests (e.g., Ketostix), or detected using a home ketone blood monitor. Early detection facilitates early treatment and can prevent full-blown DKA.

Because the symptoms of DKA can mimic the flu, and the flu can increase blood sugar levels, a child who comes down with a flu-like illness should be monitored closely and tested regularly. An increase in insulin may also be necessary; parents of children with diabetes should talk with their pediatrician about a sick day plan for their child before they need it.

Resources

BOOKS

American Diabetes Association. *American Diabetes Association Complete Guide to Diabetes*. New York: Bantam, 2006.

Bernstein, Richard K. *Dr. Bernstein's Diabetes Solution: The Complete Guide to Achieving Normal Blood Sugars*. New York: Little, Brown and Co., 2007.

Remedios, David M. *The Great Physician's Rx for Diabetes* Nashville, TN: Thomas Nelson, 2006.

PERIODICALS

Babbington, Gabrielle. "Metformin Tops Diabetes Trial." *Australian Doctor* (July 27, 2007): 3.

Buchanan, Thomas A., et al. "What is Gestational Diabetes?" *Diabetes Care* (July 2007): S105–S111.

Carmichael, Mary. "Diabetes: A 'Disease of Poverty'?" *Newsweek* (July 2, 2007): 57.

James–Enger, Kelly. "The Dangerous Diabetes–Obesity Connection: How to Reduce Your Risk Now." *Vibrant Life* (July–August 2007): 6–11.

"Study Estimates 15,000 Children and Adolescents Diagnosed With Type 1 Diabetes Annually; Among Youth in U.S., Whites Have Highest Incidence of Diabetes." *Ascribe Higher Education News Service* (June 26, 2007).

OTHER

National Library of Medicine. "Diabetes–Introduction." MedlinePlus, http://www.nlm.nih.gov/medlineplus/tutorials/diabetesintroduction/ht m/index.htm (accessed September 9, 2010).

World Health Organization. "WHO Diabetes Programme." http://www.who.int/diabete s/en/index.html (accessed September 9, 2010).

ORGANIZATIONS

American Diabetes Association, 1701 North Beauregard St., Alexandria VA, 22311, (800) 342–2383, AskADA@diabetes.org, http://www.diabetes.org.

American Dietetic Association, 120 South Riverside Plaza, Suite 2000, Chicago IL, 60606–6995, (312) 899–0040, (800) 877–1600, knowledge@eatright.org, http://www.eatright.org.

Canadian Diabetes Association, National Life Building, 1400–522 University Ave., Toronto ON Canada, M5G

2R5, (800) 226–8464, info@diabetes.ca, http://www.diabetes.ca.

Juvenile Diabetes Research Foundation International, 26 Broadway, 14th Floor, New York NY, 10004, (800) 533–2873, info@jdrf.org, http://www.jdrf.org.

Altha Roberts Edgren
Ken R. Wells

Diagnostic reading tests—DORA and others

Definition

Diagnostic reading tests are **assessment** tests that, in addition to measuring student achievement in reading, also attempt to identify specific reading difficulties. The most widely used diagnostic reading tests include the:

- Diagnostic Online Reading Assessment (DORA), for kindergarten through twelfth grade
- Durrell Analysis of Reading Difficulty (DARD), for grades one through six
- Gates-McKillop-Horowitz Reading Diagnostic Tests, for grades one through six

Purpose

Diagnostic reading tests are used both to assess and track student progress in reading and to identify specific reading deficits that are impeding student progress. The federal mandates in the No Child Left Behind (NCLB) Act, passed during the administration of President George W. Bush, and the subsequent adoption of the National Assessment of Educational Progress (NAEP) to track student achievement nationwide, have led to the replacement of some diagnostic reading tests. However these tests continue to be used by individual teachers, schools, and districts, as well as by home-schooling parents and cooperatives.

Diagnostic reading tests assess the reading level of each individual student, as well as mastery of specific skills that are necessary for reading improvement, so that instruction can be individually tailored. The relatively new Diagnostic Online Reading Assessment (DORA) is being widely adopted for this purpose, at least by schools that possess the required technology. Older paper-and-pencil tests, such as the Durrell Analysis of Reading Difficulty (DARD) and the Gates-McKillop-Horowitz Reading Diagnostic Tests, remain in use.

DORA is a web-based comprehensive diagnostic tool for students from kindergarten through grade 12, in both English and Spanish. DORA:

- assesses student reading ability, using research-based predictors of reading success
- provides the rationales underlying each student's scores
- provides parents, teachers, and administrators with real-time results that can be used to immediately address student needs and implement instructional planning
- makes specific instructional recommendations, based on each student's scores and an integration of the core curriculum with supplemental reading instruction
- helps group students according to their specific needs, including special supplemental reading programs
- connects to various supplemental programs, including Title I and after-school and special education programs
- aids in the development of individualized education programs (IEPs) for special-education students
- is aligned to the most stringent current state standards for language arts content and to the requirements of NCLB
- provides data storage and analysis for long-term monitoring of and intervention for individual students
- provides a means of comparing first-language Spanish students' reading abilities in Spanish and English and utilizing Spanish reading skills to develop English reading skills

The DARD and the Gates-McKillop-Horowitz Reading Diagnostic Tests are older diagnostic reading tests that continue to be used for determining each student's grade level in reading and to identify individual reading strengths and weaknesses. Both tests are also used for instructional program planning. The DARD is designed specifically to screen students for reading difficulties.

The Gates-McKillop-Horowitz tests are used to place students in appropriate instructional groups within classrooms and to screen for reading difficulties in older children. The auditory discrimination and auditory blending subtests of the Gates-McKillop-Horowitz tests can also be used to detect hearing problems that make it difficult for children to discriminate and manipulate certain English language sound units or phonemes. For example, children who suffered from multiple ear infections during key language-acquisition stages sometimes have a degree of hearing loss that interferes with beginning reading skills.

There are various other reading tests, such as the **Gates-MacGinitie Reading Tests (GMRT)**, that purport to be diagnostic. The **GMRTs** are primarily achievement tests, with each test assessing at only a single grade level.

Description

DORA

DORA is an award-winning series that is a component of the Let's Go Learn web-based reading and math assessments and instructional materials. Let's Go Learn was founded in 2000 with a grant from the U.S. Department of Education and has been used for hundreds of thousands of assessments nationwide. DORA was developed by Richard McCallum at the University of California, Berkeley, with new components introduced as recently as 2008 and 2010.

The DORA K–12 series is unique in that it provides individual reading assessments that adapt up and down in difficulty, based on the student's responses. This decreases overall testing time. The initial DORA assessment is based on the student's **birth** date. Each subtest begins with a sample question that is used to adjust the assessment to the student's level. Assessments take about one hour, but vary in length according to the student's skills. DORA utilizes multimedia technology to keep students engaged. DORA use can begin as early as pre-kindergarten.

DORA assesses eight reading sub-skills:

- phonemic awareness—knowledge of and the ability to manipulate the phonemes or individual sounds of spoken English or Spanish
- phonics—connecting phonemes to letters
- word recognition
- high-frequency words
- oral vocabulary
- spelling
- reading comprehension
- fluency in the English-language version

The DORA Phonemic Awareness for grades K–2plus is a complete supplemental assessment of phonemic awareness for readers, struggling readers, and non-readers. It assesses students' phonemic skills—their ability to hear and manipulate the individual sounds of spoken language, including phoneme:

- addition
- deletion
- substitution
- identification
- categorization
- blending
- segmenting
- isolating
- rhyming

DORA links directly to an online intervention system that includes ongoing assessments and self-paced targeted instructional programs—the Unique Reader and Unique Reader Secondary—based on the assessments. The Unique Reader for pre-K–fifth grade includes:

- four instructional tracks based on DORA assessments and ongoing progress
- more than 1,000 tutorials and activities that address critical skills, including phonics, sight words, vocabulary development, and comprehension
- an instructional approach that includes tutorials, reinforcement, and graded review lessons

The Unique Reader Secondary for grades six through 12 focuses on comprehension. It includes:

- supplemental reading lessons for middle and high school students
- explicit instruction in vocabulary, comprehension strategies, and critical thinking
- music, videos, and games to maintain student interest
- engaging, easer-to-read content and random items that focus on repetition and skill mastery

DARD

The DARD was first developed by Donald DeWitt Durrell in the 1930s. The complete DARD was first published in 1937. The third and most recent edition was published in 1980. The DARD is appropriate for non-readers through a sixth-grade reading level. It consists of three parallel subtests for grades one through six:

- listening comprehension
- oral reading
- silent reading

The DARD presents a series of situations and tests that enable the examiner to make detailed observations of different aspects of an individual child's reading. It can identify weaknesses and poor habits that may be addressed with remedial instruction.

Gates-McKillop-Horowitz Reading Diagnostic Tests

The Gates-McKillop-Horowitz Reading Diagnostic Tests were developed by Arthur I. Gates, Anne S. McKillop, and Elizabeth Cliff Horowitz. The second and most recent edition was published in 1981. These are individually administered assessments of reading skills for children in grades one through six, designed to identify strengths and weaknesses in reading and related skills. Although the tests are not timed, they generally take about one hour to complete.

Students do not necessarily take all 11 parts of the Gates-McKillop-Horowitz tests, which include:

- naming letters
- letter sounds
- identifying vowel sounds
- knowledge of phonemes
- recognition and blending of common word parts or phonemes
- auditory discrimination
- auditory blending
- recognition of isolated words
- reading words
- oral reading
- writing ability, assessed with an informal writing sample

The auditory discrimination and auditory blending subtests of the Gates-McKillop-Horowitz are often administered separately to assess phonemic awareness and auditory comprehension. This is because reading difficulties often arise when a child is unable to distinguish sounds or individual phonemes or is unable to combine them into words. The auditory discrimination and blending tests can quickly identify students who have such difficulties, so they can be given remedial instruction. The tests have no time restrictions. The **auditory discrimination test** is often explained to students by being showing them a pen and a pencil and asking whether they are the same or different. The child is then turned away from the teacher. The teacher reads two words and the student responds with whether they are the same or different. Only one trial is allowed. For the auditory blending test, the teacher pronounces the phonemes of each word separately and the student joins them together into the word. Students are allowed a second attempt if their first response on the auditory blending test is incorrect.

Results

DORA is a criterion-referenced test, meaning that it scores on mastery of specific skill areas, rather than comparison of test results to a representative population. It is a research-based program that is considered to have high validity.

KEY TERMS

Criterion-referenced—Test performance measurements based on a defined, independent standard, rather than relative to the performance of a population.

Fluency—The ability to speak, read, and write smoothly, easily, and rapidly.

National Assessment of Educational Progress; NAEP—The largest representative, ongoing national assessment of student progress in various subject areas.

No Child Left Behind; NCLB—Federal legislation first passed in 2001 that mandates standards-based education reform.

Phoneme—A basic unit of sound in a language.

Phonemic awareness—Knowledge of and the ability to manipulate the phonemes or individual sounds of a spoken language.

Phonics—Connecting phonemes or basic sounds to graphemes or letters or symbols.

Screening—A brief test to identify children who may need more intensive assessment.

Title I—Federal aid to school districts for extra educational services for children who are falling behind; available funds are based on the numbers of low-income families in each district.

Validity—The extent to which a test measures the trait that it is designed to assess.

DORA provides detailed student diagnostic profiles, using multiple measures of reading skills. The profiles include specific detailed instructional recommendations, linkage to appropriate instructional programs, and tracking of progress against state standards. Class reports recommend groupings of students with different instructional requirements and track performance of the groups. Parent reports are detailed and graphic and make recommendations for parental participation in student learning.

DARD results are in the form of grade equivalents (GE) for the first through sixth grades. The GE is the grade level of an average student who earned the same score.

The Gates-McKillop-Horowitz Reading Diagnostic Tests report results as raw scores, which are compared to average scores on each specific test. For example, on the auditory discrimination test, the raw score is the number of correct answers. For the auditory blending test, the teacher writes down the student's exact response. The raw score is derived by assigning one point for a correct response on the first trial and a half point for the correct response on the second try.

Resources

BOOKS

Durrell, Donald DeWitt, and J. H. Catterson. *Durrell Analysis of Reading Difficulty.* 3rd ed. New York: Harcourt Brace Jovanovich, 1980.

Durrell, Donald DeWitt. *Durrell Analysis of Reading Difficulty: Reading Paragraphs.* Yonkers-on-Hudson, NY: World Book Co., 1933.

Durrell, Donald DeWitt. *Durrell Analysis of Reading Difficulty.* Yonkers, NY: World Book Co., 1937.

Gates, Arthur I., Anne S. McKillop, and Elizabeth Cliff Horowitz. *Gates-McKillop-Horowitz Reading Diagnostic Tests.* 2nd ed. New York: Teachers College, Columbia University, 1981.

OTHER

"DORA—Diagnostic Online Reading Assessment." Curriculum Associates, http://www.curriculumassociates.com/products/detail.asp?title=DORA (accessed October 3, 2010).

"DORA Phonemic Awareness." Curriculum Associates, http://www.curriculumassociates.com/products/detail.asp?Title=DORA-phonemic (accessed October 4, 2010).

Moradi, Parisa, and Jessica Powell. "Dora: Diagnostic Online Reading Assessment: A Virtual Reading Specialist for Your Classroom!" National Tech Center. 2008, http://www.nationaltechcenter.org/documents/conf08/presentations/techExpo_LetsGoLearn.pdf (accessed October 3, 2010).

"Online Reading Assessment, Math Assessment and Supplemental Instruction." Let's Go Learn, http://www.letsgo-learn.com (accessed October 3, 2010).

"Success for All." Child Trends. July 22, 2010, http://www.childtrends.org/lifecourse/programs/success.htm (accessed October 3, 2010).

ORGANIZATIONS

Child Trends, 4301 Connecticut Ave., NW, Suite 350, Washington DC, 20008, (202) 572-6000, (202) 362-8420, http://www.childtrends.org.

National Institute of Child Health and Human Development Information Resource Center, PO Box 3006, Rockville MD, 20847, (800) 370-2943, (866) 760-5947, NICHDInformationResourceCenter@mail.nih.gov, http://www.nichd.nih.gov.

Reading Rockets, WETA Public Television, 2775 S. Quincy St., Arlington VA, 22206, (703) 998-2001, (703) 998-2060, readingrockets@weta.org, http://www.readingrockets.org.

SkyLearn, 8120 Penn Ave. South, Suite 151 Q, Bloomington MN, 55431, (952) 368-4604, (952) 368-4605, http://skylearn.org/.

Margaret Alic, PhD

Diaper rash

Definition

Dermatitis of the buttocks, genitals, lower abdomen, or thigh folds of an infant or toddler is commonly referred to as diaper rash.

Demographics

Diaper rash is believed to occur with the same frequency in infants who wear cloth or disposable diapers. It occurs most frequently in infants between eight and ten months of age, although it can occur in any child who wears diapers, generally from **birth** through about age three. It is estimated that about 10% of children will experience some significant diaper rash, although many more children will experience mild diaper rash at some time.

Description

Diaper rash is a term that covers a broad variety of skin conditions that occur on the same area of the body. Some babies are more prone to diaper rash than others.

Frequently a flat, red rash is caused by simple chafing of the diaper against tender skin, initiating a friction rash. This type of rash is not seen in the skin folds. It may be more

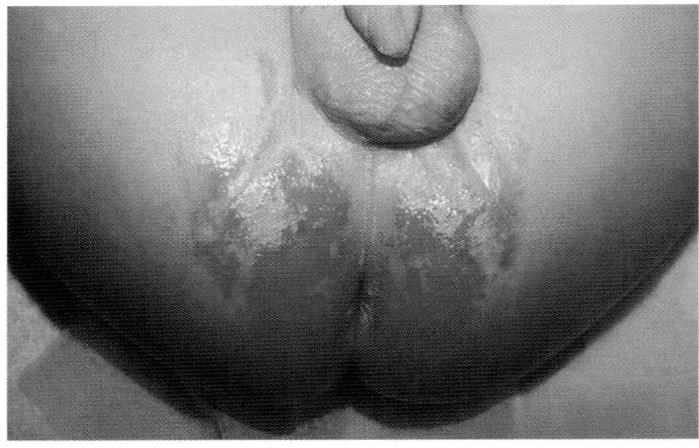

Baby with severe diaper rash. *(Custom Medical Stock Photo, Inc. Reproduced by permission.)*

pronounced around the edges of the diaper, at the waist and leg bands. The baby generally does not appear to experience much discomfort. Sometimes the chemicals or detergents in the diaper are contributing factors and may result in **contact dermatitis**. These **rashes** should clear up easily with proper attention. Ignoring the condition may lead to a secondary infection that is more difficult to resolve.

Friction of skin against itself can cause a rash in the baby's skin folds, called intertrigo. This rash appears as reddened areas that may ooze and is often uncomfortable when the diaper is wet. Intertrigo can also be found on other areas of the body where there are deep skin folds that tend to trap moisture.

Seborrheic dermatitis is the diaper area equivalent of cradle cap. It is scaly and greasy in appearance and may be worse in the folds of the skin.

Yeast, or candidal dermatitis, is the most common infectious cause of diaper rash. The affected areas are raised and quite red with distinct borders, and satellite lesions may occur around the edges. Yeast is part of the normal skin flora, and is often an opportunistic invader when simple diaper rash is left untreated. It is particularly common after treatment with **antibiotics**, which kill the good bacteria that normally keep the yeast population in check. Usual treatments for diaper rash often are not sufficient to treat this rash. Repeated or difficult to resolve episodes of yeast infection may warrant further medical attention, since this is sometimes associated with diabetes or **immune system** problems.

Another infectious cause of diaper rash is **impetigo**. This bacterial infection is characterized by blisters that ooze and crust.

Causes and symptoms

The outside layer of skin normally forms a protective barrier that prevents infection. One of the primary causes of dermatitis in the diaper area is prolonged skin contact with wetness. Under these circumstances, natural oils are stripped away, the outer layer of skin is damaged, and there is increased susceptibility to infection by bacteria or yeast.

Diagnosis

The presence of red, blotchy skin or skin lesions in the diaper area means that the baby has diaper rash. However, there are several types of rash that may require specific treatment in order to heal. It is useful to be able to distinguish them by appearance as described above.

A baby with a rash that does not clear up within two to three days with home treatment or a rash with pustules, blisters, or bleeding should be seen by a healthcare professional for further evaluation. A rash accompanied by other symptoms such as a **fever**, rash on other areas of the body, or **vomiting** should also be seen quickly by the baby's doctor.

Treatment

Traditional

Antibiotics are generally prescribed for rashes caused by bacteria, particularly impetigo. This may be a topical or oral formulation, depending on the size of the area involved and the severity of the infection.

Over–the–counter antifungal creams, such as Lotrimin, are often recommended to treat a rash resulting from yeast. If topical treatment is not effective, an oral antifungal may be prescribed.

Mild steroid creams, such as 0.5–1% hydrocortisone, can be used for seborrheic dermatitis and sometimes intertrigo. Prescription strength creams may be needed for short–term treatment of more stubborn cases.

Alternative

In the event of suspected yeast, a tablespoon of cider vinegar can be added to a cup of warm water and used as a cleansing solution. This is dilute enough that it should not burn, but acidifies the skin pH enough to hamper yeast growth.

What the baby eats can make a difference in stool frequency and acidity. When adding a new food to the diet, the baby should be observed closely to see whether rashes are produced around the baby's mouth or anus. If this occurs, the new food should be discontinued.

Babies who are taking antibiotics are more likely to get rashes due to yeast. To help bring the good bacterial counts back to normal, *Lactobacillus bifidus* can be added to the diet. It is available in powder form from most health food stores.

Some herbal preparations can be useful for diaper rash. Calendula reduces inflammation, tightens tissues, and disinfects. It has been recommended for seborrheic dermatitis as well as for general inflammation of the skin. The ointment should be applied at each diaper change. Chickweed ointment can also be soothing for irritated skin and may be applied once or twice daily.

Home remedies

Good diaper hygiene will prevent or clear up many simple cases of diaper rash. Diapers should be checked very frequently and changed as soon as they are wet or

KEY TERMS

Dermatitis—Inflammation of the skin.

Pustule—A small raised pimple or blister-like swelling of the skin that contains pus.

soiled. Good air circulation is also important for healthy skin. Babies should have some time without wearing a diaper; a waterproof pad can be used to protect the bed or other surface. Rubber pants or other occlusive fabrics should not be used over the diaper area. There is no clear evidence that either cloth or disposable diapers are better at preventing diaper rash. It may be necessary for parents to experiment with diaper types to see if the baby's skin reacts better to cloth or disposable ones or if a particular brand works especially well. If the baby is wearing cloth diapers, they should be washed in a mild detergent and double rinsed. Using a larger size of diaper than normal until the rash heals can help speed healing and increase the baby's comfort.

The diaper area should be cleaned with something mild, even plain water. Some wipes contain alcohol or chemicals that can be irritating for some babies. Plain water may be the best cleansing substance when there is a rash. Using warm water in a spray bottle (or giving a quick bath) and then lightly patting the skin dry can produce less skin trauma than using wipes.

Barrier ointments can be valuable to treat rashes. Those that contain zinc oxide are especially effective. These creams and ointments protect already irritated skin from the additional insult of urine and stool, particularly if the baby has **diarrhea**. It is generally not recommended to use a talcum powder when changing the diaper, as inhaling the powder has been found to cause damage to infant's lungs.

Prognosis

Treated appropriately, diaper rash resolves fairly quickly if there is no underlying health problem or skin disease.

Prevention

Frequent diaper changes are important to keep the skin dry and healthy. Application of powders and ointments is not necessary when there is no rash. Finding the best combination of cleansing and diapering products for the individual baby will also help to prevent diaper rash.

Resources

BOOKS

Bremner, Gavin. J. and Theodore D. Wachs, editors. *The Wiley–Blackwell Handbook of Infant Development,* 2nd ed. Hoboken, NJ: Wiley–Blackwell, 2010.

Shelov, Steven P., and Tanya R. Altman, editors. *American Academy of Pediatrics, Caring for Your Baby and Young Child: Birth to Age 5,* 5th ed. New York: Bantam Books, 2009.

PERIODICALS

Adam, Ralf. "Skin Care of the Diaper Area." *Pediatric Dermatology* 25(4) (July–August 2008): 427–33.

Nield, Linda S., and Deepak Kamat. "Prevention, Diagnosis, and Management of Diaper Dermatitis." *Clinical Pediatrics.* 46(6) (July 2007): 480–486.

ORGANIZATIONS

American Academy of Dermatology (AAD), PO Box 4014, Schaumburg IL, 60168–4014, (847) 330–0230, (866) 503–SKIN (7546), (847) 240–1859, MRC@aad.org, http://www.aad.org.

American Academy of Family Physicians (AAFP), PO Box 11210, Shawnee Mission KS, 66207, (913) 906–6000, (800) 274–2237, (913) 906–6075, http://familydoctor.org.

American Academy of Pediatrics (AAP), 141 Northwest Point Blvd., Elk Grove Village IL, 60007–1098, (847) 434–4000, (847) 434–8000, http://www.aap.org.

Judith Turner
Tish Davidson, AM

Diarrhea

Definition

To most individuals, diarrhea means an increased frequency or decreased consistency of bowel movements; however, the medical definition is more exact than this. In many developed countries, the average number of bowel movements is three per day. However, researchers have found that diarrhea best correlates with an increase in stool weight; stool weights above 10 oz (300 g) per day generally indicates diarrhea. This is mainly due to excess water, which normally makes up 60–85% of fecal matter. In this way, true diarrhea is distinguished from diseases that cause only an increase in the number of bowel movements (hyperdefecation) or incontinence (involuntary loss of bowel contents).

Diarrhea is also classified by physicians into acute, which lasts one or two weeks, and chronic, which continues for longer than 2 or 3 weeks. Viral and bacterial infections are the most common causes of acute diarrhea.

Description

In many cases, acute infectious diarrhea is a mild, limited annoyance. However, worldwide acute infectious diarrhea has a huge impact, causing over five million deaths per year. While most deaths are among children under five years of age in developing nations, the impact, even in developed countries, is considerable. For example, over 250,000 individuals are admitted to hospitals in the United States each year because of one of these episodes. Rapid diagnosis and proper treatment can prevent much of the suffering associated with these devastating illnesses.

Chronic diarrhea also has a considerable effect on health, as well as on social and economic well being. Patients with **celiac disease**, inflammatory bowel disease, and other prolonged diarrheal illnesses develop nutritional deficiencies that diminish growth and immunity. They affect social interaction and result in the loss of many working hours.

Causes and symptoms

Diarrhea occurs because more fluid passes through the large intestine (colon) than that organ can absorb. As a rule, the colon can absorb several times more fluid than is required on a daily basis. However, when this reserve capacity is overwhelmed, diarrhea occurs.

Diarrhea is caused by infections or illnesses that either lead to excess production of fluids or prevent absorption of fluids. Also, certain substances in the colon, such as fats and bile acids, can interfere with water absorption and cause diarrhea. In addition, rapid passage of material through the colon can also do the same.

Symptoms related to any diarrheal illness are often those associated with any injury to the gastrointestinal tract, such as **fever**, nausea, **vomiting**, and abdominal **pain**. All or none of these may be present depending on the disease causing the diarrhea. The number of bowel movements can vary—up to 20 or more per day. In some patients, blood or pus is present in the stool. Bowel movements may be difficult to flush (float) or contain undigested food material.

The most common causes of acute diarrhea are infections (the cause of traveler's diarrhea), **food poisoning**, and medications. Medications are a frequent and often over-looked cause, especially **antibiotics** and antacids. Less often, various sugar free foods, which sometimes contain poorly absorbable materials, cause diarrhea.

Chronic diarrhea is frequently due to many of the same things that cause the shorter episodes (infections, medications, etc.); symptoms just last longer. Some infections can become chronic. This occurs mainly with parasitic infections (such as *Giardia*) or when patients have altered immunity (**AIDS**).

The following are the more usual causes of chronic diarrhea:

- AIDS
- colon cancer and other bowel tumors
- endocrine or hormonal abnormalities (thyroid, diabetes mellitus, etc.)
- food allergy
- inflammatory bowel disease (Crohn's disease and ulcerative colitis)
- lactose intolerance
- malabsorption syndromes (celiac and Whipple's disease)
- other (alcohol, microscopic colitis, radiation, surgery)

Complications

The major effects of diarrhea are **dehydration**, **malnutrition**, and weight loss. Signs of dehydration can be hard to notice, but increasing thirst, dry mouth, weakness or lightheadedness (particularly if worsening on standing), or a darkening/decrease in urination are suggestive. Severe dehydration leads to changes in the body's chemistry and could become life-threatening. Dehydration from diarrhea can result in kidney failure, neurological symptoms, arthritis, and skin problems.

Diagnosis

Most cases of acute diarrhea never need diagnosis or treatment, as many are mild and produce few problems. But patients with fever over 102 °F (38.9 °C), signs of dehydration, bloody bowel movements, severe abdominal pain, known immune disease, or prior use of antibiotics need prompt medical evaluation.

When diagnostic studies are needed, the most useful are stool culture and examination for parasites; however these are often negative and a cause cannot be found in a large number of patients. The earlier cultures are performed, the greater the chance of obtaining a positive result. For those with a history of antibiotic use in the preceding two months, stool samples need to be examined for the toxins that cause antibiotic-associated colitis. Tests are also available to check stool samples for microscopic amounts of blood and for cells that indicate severe inflammation of the colon. Examination with an endoscope is sometimes helpful in determining severity and extent of inflammation. Tests to check changes in blood chemistry (potassium, magnesium, etc.) and a complete blood count (CBC) are also often performed.

Chronic diarrhea is quite different, and most patients with this condition will receive some degree of testing. Many exams are the same as for an acute episode, as some infections and parasites cause both types of diarrhea. A careful history to evaluate medication use, dietary changes, family history of illnesses, and other symptoms is necessary. Key points in determining the seriousness of symptoms are weight loss of over 10 lb (4.5 kg), blood in the stool, and nocturnal diarrhea (symptoms that awaken the patient from **sleep**).

Both prescription and over-the-counter medications can contain additives, such as lactose and sorbitol, that will produce diarrhea in sensitive individuals. Review of **allergies** or skin changes may also point to a cause. Social history may indicate if stress is playing a role or identify activities which can be associated with diarrhea (for example, diarrhea that occurs in runners).

A combination of stool, blood, and urine tests may be needed in the evaluation of chronic diarrhea; in addition a number of endoscopic and x-ray studies are frequently required.

Treatment

Treatment is ideally directed toward correcting the cause; however, the first aim should be to prevent or treat dehydration and nutritional deficiencies. The type of fluid and nutrient replacement will depend on whether oral feedings can be taken and the severity of fluid losses. Oral rehydration solution (ORS) or intravenous fluids are the choices; ORS is preferred if possible.

A physician should be notified if the patient is dehydrated, and if oral replacement is suggested then commercial (Pedialyte and others) or homemade preparations can be used. The World Health Organization (WHO) has provided this easy recipe for home preparation, which can be taken in small frequent sips:

- table salt—3/4 tsp
- baking powder—1 tsp
- orange juice—1 c
- water—1 qt (1L)

When feasible, food intake should be continued even in those with acute diarrhea. A physician should be consulted as to what type and how much food is permitted.

Anti-motility agents (loperamide, diphenoxylate) are useful for those with chronic symptoms; their use is limited or even contraindicated in most individuals with acute diarrhea, especially in those with high fever or bloody bowel movements. They should not be taken without the advice of a physician.

Other treatments are available, depending on the cause of symptoms. For example, the bulk agent psyllium helps some patients by absorbing excess fluid and solidifying stools; cholestyramine, which binds bile acids, is effective in treating bile salt induced diarrhea. Low fat diets or more easily digestible fat is useful in some patients. New antidiarrheal drugs that decrease excessive secretion of fluid by the intestinal tract is another approach for some diseases. Avoidance of medications or other products that are known to cause diarrhea (such as lactose) is curative in some, but should be discussed with a physician.

Alternative treatment

It is especially important to find the cause of diarrhea, since stopping diarrhea when it is the body's way of eliminating something foreign is not helpful and can be harmful in the long run.

One effective alternative approach to preventing and treating diarrhea involves oral supplementation of aspects of the normal flora in the colon with the yeasts *Lactobacillus acidophilus*, *L. bifidus*, or *Saccharomyces boulardii.* In clinical settings, these "biotherapeutic" agents have repeatedly been helpful in the resolution of diarrhea, especially antibiotic-associated diarrhea. Their effectiveness is also supported by the results of a research study published in the *Journal of the American Medical Association*.

Nutrient replacement also plays a role in preventing and treating episodes of diarrhea. Zinc especially appears to have an effect on the **immune system**, and deficiency of this mineral can lead to chronic diarrhea. Also, zinc replacement improves growth in young patients. Plenty of fluids, especially water, should be taken by individuals suffering from diarrhea to prevent dehydration. The BRAT diet also can be useful in helping to resolve diarrhea. This diet limits food intake to bananas, rice, applesauce, and toast. These foods provide soluble and insoluble fiber without irritation. If the toast is slightly burnt, the charcoal can help sequester toxins and pull them from the body.

Acute homeopathic remedies can be very effective for treating diarrhea especially in infants and young children.

Prognosis

Prognosis is related to the cause of the diarrhea; for most individuals in developed countries, a bout of acute, infectious diarrhea is at best uncomfortable. However, in both industrialized and developing areas, serious complications and **death** can occur.

KEY TERMS

Anti-motiltiy medications—Medications such as loperamide (Imodium), diphenoxylate (Lomotil), or medications containing codeine or narcotics that decrease the ability of the intestine to contract. These can worsen the condition of a patient with dysentery or colitis.

Colitis—Inflammation of the colon.

Endoscope—An endoscope, as used in the field of gastroenterology, is a thin flexible tube that uses a lens or miniature camera to view various areas of the gastrointestinal tract. Both diagnosis, through biopsies or other means, and therapeutic procedures can be done with this instrument.

Endoscopy—The performance of an exam using an endoscope is known generally as endoscopy.

Lactose intolerance—An inability to properly digest milk and dairy products.

Oral rehydration solution (ORS)—A liquid preparation developed by the World Health Organization that can decrease fluid loss in persons with diarrhea. Originally developed to be prepared with materials available in the home, commercial preparations have recently come into use.

Steatorrhea—Excessive amounts of fat in the feces.

For those with chronic symptoms, an extensive number of tests are usually necessary to make a proper diagnosis and begin treatment; a specific diagnosis is found in 90% of patients. In some, however, no specific cause is found and only treatment with bulk agents or anti-motility agents is indicated.

Prevention

Proper hygiene and food handling techniques will prevent many cases. Traveler's diarrhea can be avoided by use of Pepto-Bismol and/or antibiotics, if necessary. The most important action is to prevent the complications of dehydration.

Resources

OTHER

"Directory of Digestive Diseases Organizations for Patients." *National Institute of Diabetes and Digestive and Kidney Disease,* http://www.niddk.nih.gov.

"A Neglected Modality for the Treatment and Prevention of Selected Intestinal and Vaginal Infections." *JAMA,* http://pubs.ama-assn.org.

Selected publications and documents on diarrhoeal diseases (including cholera). *World Health Organization (WHO),* http://www.who.ch/chd/pub/cdd/cddpub.htm.

ORGANIZATIONS

World Health Organization, Division of Emerging and Other Communicable Diseases Surveillance and Control, Avenue Appia 20, 1211 Geneva 27 Switzerland (+00 41 22) 791 21 11, http://www.who.int.

David Kaminstein, MD

DiGeorge syndrome

Definition

DiGeorge syndrome (also called 22q11 deletion syndrome, congenital thymic hypoplasia, or third and fourth pharyngeal pouch syndrome) is a **birth** defect that is caused by an abnormality in chromosome 22 and affects the baby's **immune system**. The disorder is marked by absence or underdevelopment of the thymus and parathyroid glands. It is named for Angelo DiGeorge, the **pediatrician** who first described it in 1965. Some researchers prefer to call it DiGeorge anomaly, or DGA, rather than DiGeorge syndrome, on the grounds that the defects associated with the disorder represent the failure of a part of the human embryo to develop normally rather than a collection of symptoms caused by a single disease.

Description

The prevalence of DiGeorge syndrome is debated; the estimates range from 1:4,000 to 1:6,395. Because the symptoms caused by the chromosomal abnormality vary somewhat from patient to patient, the syndrome probably occurs much more often than was previously thought. DiGeorge syndrome is sometimes described as one of the "CATCH 22" disorders, so named because of their characteristics—cardiac defects, abnormal facial features, thymus underdevelopment, **cleft palate**, and hypocalcemia—caused by a deletion of several genes in chromosome 22. The specific facial features associated with DiGeorge syndrome include low-set ears, wide-set eyes, a small jaw, and a short groove in the upper lip. The male/female ratio is 1:1. The syndrome appears to be equally common in all racial and ethnic groups.

Causes and symptoms

DiGeorge syndrome is caused either by inheritance of a defective chromosome 22 or by a new defect in chromosome 22 in the fetus. The type of defect that is involved is called deletion. A deletion occurs when the genetic material in the chromosomes does not recombine properly during the formation of sperm or egg cells. The deletion means that several genes from chromosome 22 are missing in DiGeorge syndrome patients. Although efforts have been made in the early 2000s to identify individual candidate genes for DGA, it appears that a combination of several genes in the deleted area is responsible for the disorder. Detailed genetic mapping of chromosome 22 has, however, identified a so-called DiGeorge critical region (DGCR), which has been completely sequenced.

According to a 1999 study, 6% of children with DiGeorge syndrome inherited the deletion from a parent, while 94% had a new deletion. Other conditions that are associated with DiGeorge syndrome are diabetes (a condition where the pancreas no longer produces enough insulin) in the mother and **fetal alcohol syndrome** (a pattern of **birth defects**, and learning and behavioral problems affecting individuals whose mothers consumed alcohol during pregnancy). Other chromosomal abnormalities that have been found in patients diagnosed with DGA include deletions on chromosomes 10p13, 17p13, and 18q21.

The loss of the genes in the deleted material means that the baby's third and fourth pharyngeal pouches fail to develop normally during the twelfth week of pregnancy. This developmental failure results in a completely or partially absent thymus gland and parathyroid glands. In addition, 74% of fetuses with DiGeorge syndrome have severe heart defects. The child is born with a defective immune system and an abnormally low level of calcium in the blood. Some children with DGA are also born with malformations of the genitals or urinary tract.

These defects usually become apparent within 48 hours of birth. The infant's heart defects may lead to heart failure, or there may be seizures and other evidence of a low level of calcium in the blood (hypocalcemia).

DiGeorge syndrome is also associated with an increased risk of **autoimmune disorders**. Cases have been reported of DGA in association with Graves' disease, immune thrombocytopenic purpura, juvenile rheumatoid arthritis, and severe **eczema**.

Diagnosis

Diagnosis of DiGeorge syndrome can be made by ultrasound examination around the eighteenth week of pregnancy, when abnormalities in the development of the heart or the palate can be detected. Another technique that is used to diagnose the syndrome before birth is called fluorescence in situ hybridization, or FISH. This technique uses DNA probes from the DiGeorge region on chromosome 22. FISH can be performed on cell samples obtained by **amniocentesis** as early as the fourteenth week of pregnancy. It confirms about 95% of cases of DiGeorge syndrome.

If the mother has not had prenatal testing, the diagnosis of DiGeorge syndrome is sometimes suggested by the child's facial features at birth. In other cases, the doctor makes the diagnosis during heart surgery when he or she notices the absence or abnormal location of the thymus gland. The diagnosis can be confirmed by blood tests for calcium, phosphorus, and parathyroid hormone levels, and by the sheep cell test for immune function.

Treatment

Hypocalcemia

Hypocalcemia in DiGeorge patients is unusually difficult to treat. Infants are usually given calcium and vitamin D by mouth. Severe cases have been treated by transplantation of fetal thymus tissue or bone marrow.

Heart defects

Infants with life-threatening heart defects are treated surgically.

Defective immune function

Children with DiGeorge syndrome should be kept on low-phosphorus diets and kept away from crowds or other sources of infection. They should not be immunized with vaccines made from live viruses or given corticosteroids.

Prognosis

The prognosis is variable; many infants with DiGeorge syndrome die from overwhelming infection, seizures, or heart failure within the first year. One study of a series of 558 patients reported 8% mortality within six months of birth, with heart defects accounting for all but one of the deaths. Infections resulting from severe immune deficiency are the second most common cause of **death** in patients with DGA. Advances in heart surgery indicate that the prognosis is most closely linked to the severity of the heart defects and the partial presence of the thymus gland. In most children who survive, the number of T cells, a type of white blood cell, in the blood rises spontaneously as they mature. Survivors are likely to be mentally retarded, however, and to have other

KEY TERMS

Deletion—A genetic abnormality in which a segment of a chromosome is lost. DiGeorge syndrome is caused by a deletion on human chromosome 22.

Fetal alcohol syndrome—A cluster of birth defects that includes abnormal facial features and mental retardation, caused by the mother's consumption of alcoholic beverages during pregnancy.

Fluorescence in situ hybridization (FISH)—A technique for diagnosing DiGeorge syndrome before birth by analyzing cells obtained by amniocentesis with DNA probes. FISH is about 95% accurate.

Hypocalcemia—An abnormally low level of calcium in the blood.

Hypoplasia—A deficiency or underdevelopment of a tissue or body structure.

T cells—A type of white blood cell produced in the thymus gland. T cells are an important part of the immune system. Infants born with an underdeveloped or absent thymus do not have a normal level of T cells in their blood.

developmental difficulties, including seizures or other psychiatric and neurological problems in later life.

Prevention

Genetic counseling is recommended for parents of children with DiGeorge syndrome because the disorder can be detected prior to birth. Although most children with DiGeorge syndrome did not inherit the chromosome deletion from their parents, they have a 50% chance of passing the deletion on to their own children.

Because of the association between DiGeorge syndrome and fetal alcohol syndrome, pregnant women should avoid drinking alcoholic beverages.

Resources

BOOKS

Beers, Mark H., MD, and Robert Berkow, MD, editors. "Immunodeficiency Diseases." In *The Merck Manual of Diagnosis and Therapy*. 18th ed., Whitehouse Station, NJ: Merck Research Laboratories, 2006.

McDonald-McGinn, Donna M., et al. *22q11 Deletion Syndrome*. Philadelphia: The Children's Hospital of Philadelphia, 1999.

PERIODICALS

Guduri, Sridhar, MD, and Iftikhar Hussain, MD. "DiGeorge Syndrome." *eMedicine* May 28, 2002, http://www.emedicine.com/med/topic567.htm.

Verri, A., P. Maraschio, K. Devriendt, et al. "Chromosome 10p Deletion in a Patient with Hypoparathyroidism, Severe Mental Retardation, Autism and Basal Ganglia Calcifications." *Annales de génétique* 47 (July-September 2004): 281–287.

Yatsenko, S. A., A. N. Yatsenko, K. Szigeti, et al. "Interstitial Deletion of 10p and Atrial Septal Defect in DiGeorge 2 Syndrome." *Clinical Genetics* 66 (August 2004): 128–136.

ORGANIZATIONS

Canadian 22q Group, 320 Cote Street Antoine, West Montreal Quebec H3Y 2J4 Canada

Chromosome Deletion Outreach, Inc., PO Box 724, Boca Raton FL, 33429-0724, (888) 236-6680

International DiGeorge/VCF Support Network, c/o Family Voices of New York, 46 1/2 Clinton Avenue, Cortland NY, 13045, (607) 753-1250

National Organization for Rare Disorders (NORD), 55 Kenosia Avenue, P. O. Box 1968Danbury CT, 06813-1968 (203) 744-0100, (800) 999-6673, http://www.rarediseases.org.

Rebecca J. Frey, PhD

Diphenhydramine *see* **Antihistamines**

Diphtheria

Definition

Diphtheria is a potentially fatal, contagious disease that usually involves the nose, throat, and air passages, but may also infect the skin. Its most striking feature is the formation of a grayish membrane covering the tonsils and upper part of the throat.

Demographics

Before 1920 when the diphtheria toxiod was introduced, diphtheria was a major childhood killer, with 200,000 cases reported annually in the United States. In the twenty first century, diphtheria is rare and sporadic in the developed world because of widespread immunization. In countries that do not have routine immunization against this infection, periodic outbreaks occur. The largest recent outbreak occurred in the countries comprising the former Soviet Union and the Baltic States. From 1990–1995, 157,000 cases and 5,000 deaths were reported in this region, accounting for more than 80% of all diphtheria cases reported during those years. Other, smaller outbreaks have been reported in sub–Saharan Africa, India, and France. Like many other upper respiratory diseases, diphtheria is most likely to occur during the cold months. Individuals who have not been immunized may get diphtheria at any age; mortality rates are highest in those under five years or over 40 years of age.

Description

Diphtheria is spread most often by droplets from the coughing or sneezing of an infected person or carrier. The incubation period is two to seven days, with an average of three days. It is vital to seek medical help at once when diphtheria is suspected, because treatment requires emergency measures for adults as well as children.

Risk factors for developing diphtheria include:

- failure to immunize or incomplete immunization
- living in crowded, unhygienic conditions
- having a compromised immune system
- traveling to developing regions of the world where diphtheria is more common

Causes and symptoms

The symptoms of diphtheria are caused by toxins produced by the diphtheria bacillus, *Corynebacterium diphtheriae* (from the Greek for "rubber membrane"). In fact, toxin production is related to infections of the bacillus itself with a particular bacterial virus called a phage (from bacteriophage; a virus that infects bacteria). The infection destroys healthy tissue in the upper area of the throat around the tonsils, or in open **wounds** in the skin. Fluid from dying cells then coagulates to form the telltale gray or grayish–green membrane. Inside the membrane, the bacteria produce an exotoxin, which is a poisonous secretion that causes the life–threatening symptoms of diphtheria. The exotoxin is carried throughout the body in the bloodstream, destroying healthy tissue in other parts of the body.

The most serious complications caused by the exotoxin are inflammations of the heart muscle (myocarditis) and damage to the nervous system. The risk of serious complications is increased as the time between onset of symptoms and the administration of antitoxin increases and as the size of the membrane formed increases. Myocarditis may cause disturbances in the heart rhythm (arrhythmias) and may result in heart failure. Symptoms of nervous system involvement can include seeing double vision (diplopia), painful or difficult swallowing (dysphagia), and slurred speech or loss of voice, which are all indications of the exotoxin's effect on nerve functions. The exotoxin may also cause severe swelling in the neck ("bull neck").

The signs and symptoms of diphtheria vary according to the location of the infection.

Nasal

Nasal diphtheria produces few symptoms other than a watery or bloody discharge. On examination, there may be a small visible membrane in the nasal passages. Nasal infection rarely causes complications by itself, but it is a public health problem because it spreads the disease more rapidly than other forms of diphtheria.

Pharyngeal

Pharyngeal diphtheria gets its name from the pharynx, which is the part of the upper throat that connects the mouth and nasal passages with the voice box (larynx). This is the most common form of diphtheria, causing the characteristic grayish throat membrane. The membrane often bleeds if it is scraped or cut. It is important not to try to remove the membrane because the trauma may increase the body's absorption of the exotoxin. Other signs and symptoms of pharyngeal diphtheria include mild **sore throat**, **fever** of 101–102 °F (38.3–38.9 °C), a rapid pulse, and general body weakness.

Laryngeal

Laryngeal diphtheria, which involves the voice box or larynx, is the form most likely to produce serious complications. The fever is usually higher in this form of diphtheria (103–104 °F or 39.4–40 °C) and the patient is very weak. Patients may have a severe **cough**, have difficulty breathing, or lose their voice completely. The development of a "bull neck" indicates a high level of exotoxin in the bloodstream. Obstruction of the airway may result in difficulty breathing, respiratory compromise, and **death**.

Skin

This form of diphtheria, which is sometimes called cutaneous diphtheria, accounts for about 33% of diphtheria cases. It is found chiefly among people with poor hygiene, and is more common in tropical climates. Any break in the skin can become infected with diphtheria. The infected tissue develops an ulcerated area and a diphtheria membrane may form over the wound but is not always

KEY TERMS

Antitoxin—An antibody against an exotoxin, usually derived from horse serum.

Bacillus—A rod-shaped bacterium, such as the diphtheria bacterium.

Carrier—A person who may harbor an organism without symptoms and may transmit it to others.

Cutaneous—Located in the skin.

Diphtheria–tetanus–pertussis (DTP)—The standard preparation used to immunize children against diphtheria, tetanus, and whooping cough. A so-called "acellular pertussis" vaccine (aP) is usually used since its release in the mid-1990s in a combined vaccine known as DTaP.

Exotoxin—A poisonous secretion produced by bacilli which is carried in the bloodstream to other parts of the body.

Gram's stain—A dye staining technique used in laboratory tests to determine the presence and type of bacteria.

Loeffler's medium—A special substance used to grow diphtheria bacilli to confirm a diagnosis.

Myocarditis—Inflammation of the heart tissue.

Toxoid—A preparation made from inactivated exotoxin, used in immunization.

present. The wound or ulcer is slow to heal and may be numb or insensitive when touched.

Diagnosis

Because diphtheria must be treated as quickly as possible, doctors usually make the diagnosis on the basis of the visible symptoms without waiting for test results.

Examination

In making the diagnosis, the doctor examines the patient's eyes, ears, nose, and throat in order to rule out other diseases that may cause fever and sore throat, such as **infectious mononucleosis**, a sinus infection, or **strep throat**. The most important single symptom that suggests diphtheria is the membrane. When a patient develops skin infections during an outbreak of diphtheria, the doctor will consider the possibility of cutaneous diphtheria and take a smear to confirm the diagnosis.

Tests

The diagnosis of diphtheria can be confirmed by the results of a culture obtained from the infected area. Material from the swab is put on a microscope slide and stained using a procedure called Gram's stain. The diphtheria bacillus is called Gram-positive because it holds the dye after the slide is rinsed with alcohol. Under the microscope, diphtheria bacilli look like beaded rod-shaped cells, grouped in patterns that resemble Chinese characters. Another laboratory test involves growing the diphtheria bacillus on a special material called Loeffler's medium.

Treatment

Diphtheria is a serious disease requiring hospital treatment in an intensive care unit if the patient has developed respiratory symptoms. Treatment includes a combination of medications and supportive care:

Antitoxin

The most important step is prompt administration of diphtheria antitoxin, without waiting for laboratory results. The antitoxin is made from horse serum and works by neutralizing any circulating exotoxin. The doctor must first test the patient for sensitivity to animal serum. Patients who are sensitive (about 10%) must be desensitized with diluted antitoxin, since the antitoxin is the only specific substance that will counteract diphtheria exotoxin. No other type if antitoxin is available for the treatment of diphtheria.

The dose of antitoxin ranges from 20,000–100,000 units, depending on the severity and length of time of symptoms occurring before treatment. Diphtheria antitoxin is usually given intravenously. It must be obtained from the United States Centers for Disease Control and Prevention (CDC) and may not be available in some parts of the world.

Antibiotics

Antibiotics are given to kill the bacteria, to prevent the spread of the disease, and to protect the patient from developing **pneumonia**. They are not a substitute for treatment with antitoxin. Both adults and children may be given penicillin, ampicillin, or erythromycin. Erythromycin appears to be more effective than penicillin in treating people who are carriers because of better penetration into the infected area.

Cutaneous diphtheria is usually treated by cleansing the wound thoroughly with soap and water, and giving the patient antibiotics for 10 days.

Supportive care

Diphtheria patients need bed rest with intensive nursing care, including extra fluids, oxygenation, and monitoring for possible heart problems, airway blockage, or involvement of the nervous system. Patients with laryngeal diphtheria are kept in a **croup** tent or high–humidity environment; they may also need throat suctioning or emergency surgery if their airway is blocked.

Patients recovering from diphtheria should rest at home for a minimum of two to three weeks, especially if they have heart complications. In addition, patients should be immunized against diphtheria after recovery, because having the disease does not always induce antitoxin formation and protect them from re–infection.

Prevention of complications

Diphtheria patients who develop myocarditis may be treated with oxygen and with medications to prevent irregular heart rhythms. An artificial pacemaker may be needed. Patients with difficulty swallowing can be fed through a tube inserted into the stomach through the nose. Patients who cannot breathe are usually put on mechanical respirators.

Prognosis

The prognosis depends on the size and location of the membrane and on early treatment with antitoxin; the longer the delay, the higher the death rate. The most vulnerable patients are children under age five and those who develop pneumonia or myocarditis. Death rates generally range from 5–10% and may reach as high as 20% in young children and older adults. Nasal and cutaneous diphtheria are rarely fatal.

Prevention

Prevention of diphtheria has four aspects:

Immunization

Universal immunization is the most effective means of preventing diphtheria. The standard course of immunization for healthy children is three doses of DTaP (diphtheria–tetanus–acellular **pertussis**) preparation given between two months and six months of age, with booster doses given at 18 months and again between the ages of four and six years. At 12 years a booster shot of is given. Adults should be immunized at 10–year intervals with Td (tetanus–diphtheria) toxoid. A toxoid is a bacterial toxin that is treated to make it harmless but still can induce immunity to the disease.

Isolation of patients

Diphtheria patients must be isolated for one to seven days or until two successive cultures show that they are no longer contagious (up to six weeks). Children placed in isolation are usually assigned a primary nurse for emotional support.

Identification and treatment of contacts

Because diphtheria is highly contagious and has a short incubation period, family members and other contacts of diphtheria patients must be watched for symptoms and tested to see if they are carriers. They are usually given antibiotics for seven days and a booster shot of diphtheria/tetanus toxoid.

Reporting cases to public health authorities

Reporting is necessary to track potential epidemics, to help doctors identify the specific strain of diphtheria, and to see if resistance to penicillin or erythromycin has developed.

Resources

BOOKS

Guilfoile, Patrick. *Diphtheria.* New York: Chelsea House, 2009.

Sears, Robert. *The Vaccine Book: Making The Right Decision for Your Child.* New York: Little, Brown, 2007.

OTHER

"Diphtheria." Mayo Foundation for Education and Research. (April 7, 2009), http://www.mayoclinic.com/health/diphtheria/DS00495 (accessed September 17, 2010).

"Diphtheria." MedlinePlus. (March 27, 2010), http://www.nlm.nih.gov/medlineplus/diphtheria.html (accessed September 17, 2010).

"Diphtheria." World Health Organization. (2010), http://www.who.int/topics/diphtheria/en (accessed September 17, 2010).

"Vaccines." United States Centers for Disease Control and Prevention (CDC). (March 30, 2010), http://www.cdc.gov/vaccines (accessed September 17, 2010).

ORGANIZATIONS

Centers for Disease Control and Prevention (CDC), 1600 Clifton Rd., Atlanta GA, 30333, (404) 639–3534, (800) CDC–INFO (800–232–4636). TTY: (888) 232–6348, inquiry@cdc.gov, http://www.cdc.gov.

World Health Organization (WHO), Avenue Appia 20, 1211 Geneva 27 Switzerland, +22 41 791 21 11, +22 41 791 31 11, info@who.int, http://www.who.int.

Rebecca J. Frey, PhD
Tish Davidson, AM

Diphtheria, tetanus, pertussis vaccine ***see*** **DTP vaccine**

Discipline

Definition

Discipline consists of actions or methods used to achieve controlled behavior.

Description

Discipline used as a noun means orderly, controlled behavior. The verb "to discipline" means different things to different people. Most definitions of "to discipline" fall into two general camps: 1) to control, punish, and correct; or 2) to teach, guide, and influence. The majority of studies today show that the second definition is more effective in producing the desired behavior.

The word discipline often is used as a synonym for punishment, but this is incorrect. Discipline is a system of actions or interactions intended to create orderly behavior. There are a variety of disciplinary systems that show varying degrees of success. Some disciplinary systems use punishment as a tool; others shun punishment, believing it is at best ineffective, at worst destructive or counterproductive.

Punitive systems have been the norm in the West for centuries. Judaeo-Christian religion has traditionally been seen to promote authoritarian parenting: "Spare the rod, spoil the child." is an oft-quoted pseudo-Biblical injunction (the only actual words similar to this in the Bible are "He who spares the rod hates his son, but he who loves him is diligent to discipline him" [Proverbs 13:24, Revised Standard Version]). Some conservative Christians and Jews continue to hold to this style of discipline in the belief that punishment is the only way to teach children proper submission and obedience to parents, other adults, and ultimately God.

Other systems of discipline reject harsh, physical violence. Practices of "logical consequences" and "time-outs" are two well-known examples. Both are **behavior modification** techniques that are used to train a child to behave in socially or parentally acceptable ways. Rewards and punishments are used to control a child's actions. This can be effective in modifying external behaviors, but some see it as doing little to change underlying motivations or attitudes. Some attempts to control a child can actually prevent any lasting influence from occurring. Children instead simply rebel against the imposed limitations, resist authority, and resort to lying, evasion, or manipulation to get their needs and desires met.

KEY TERMS

Authoritarian parenting—Parenting using authority based on force.

Authoritative parenting—Parenting using authority based on experience and expertise.

Nuclear family—The family group made up of parents and their children, as opposed to a multigenerational family unit that also includes grandparents, and other extended family members.

Harshly punitive measures of discipline have been shown to create **anxiety**, **fear**, anger, hatred, apathy, depression, obsessiveness, paranoia, sadomasochism, domestic violence, aggression, crime, and apocalyptic religious views, none of which promotes stable, orderly, socially creative behavior. When children are punished harshly, they remember only the **pain** and humiliation of the punishment, not the reason for the discipline. They lose trust in their parent(s) and become less likely to accept their authority in the future. Physically violent discipline can promote further violence by teaching a child that force is a means to gain control and that violence is acceptable in social and familial relationships. Perhaps the biggest problem with punitive systems of discipline, whether violent or nonviolent, is that eventually the parent runs out of means of control. As the child grows, physical force is less and less effective, and the child continually learns new ways to evade other forms of punishment. At some point, the child becomes largely immune to discipline.

Despite this reality, however, American culture remains wedded to punitive discipline in the vast majority. Many adults approve of spanking and think that it is a necessary part of child rearing. Spanking is a controversial issue however. The **American Academy of Pediatrics** and a variety of other bodies recommend against it. In 1979 Sweden became the first country in the world to outlaw spanking entirely. Since 1979 an additional 23 countries have outlawed it. The trend continues to pick up speed, with seven more countries outlawing corporal punishment by parents against children 2007.

Although spanking is still common in the United States as of 2010, it is less common than it once was. In the 1980s and 1990s a shift began away from punitive discipline toward a more relational style based on attachment, mutual trust and respect, and equality. This occurred for a number of socio-cultural reasons. First, the increasing frequency of self-destructive and socially destructive behaviors on the part of increasingly younger children were believed to be evidence that common forms of discipline then in use were not working. The rise in crime, drug and alcohol abuse, school drop-out rates, and **suicide** were seen as showing a dangerous lack of discipline among children. Punitive measures, such as the "war on drugs," or "getting tough on crime," were seen as ineffective, if not counterproductive. In response, therefore, a number of adults have began to explore alternative systems of discipline that do not rely on control or punishment.

Stages of moral development

Childhood is often divided into 5 approximate stages of moral development:

- Stage 1: Infancy. The child's only sense of right and wrong is what feels good or bad.
- Stage 2: Toddler Years. The child learns "right" and "wrong" from what she or he is told by others.
- Stage 3: Preschool Years. The child begins to internalize family values as his or her own, and begins to perceive the consequences of his or her behavior.
- Stage 4: Ages 7–10 Years. The child begins to question the infallibility of parents, teachers, and other adults, and develops a strong sense of "should" and "should no.t"
- Stage 5: Preteen and Teenage Years. Peers, rather than adults, become of ultimate importance to the child, who begins to try on different values systems to see which fits best; teens also become more aware of and concerned with the larger society, and begin to reason-more abstractly about "right" and "wrong."

Another factor in the shift away from punitive discipline is the historical movement in favor of greater democracy throughout Western culture that has led different subgroups to seek social equality. Today, children and youth are striving for equality as well, refusing to be treated as inferior to adults. Many of today's parents grew up in this atmosphere of increased equality for children and now view their own children as equals.

The cultural trend toward smaller, isolated nuclear **family** units rather than multigenerational extended families that has been underway since World War II (1939–1945) has also created a significant change in the dynamics of childrearing. Today's children are raised by only one or two parents in relative isolation. Long-standing cultural traditions and behaviors are lost as the cultural community disappears. Demands on parents' time and energy may cause them to leave their children with non-family caregivers who may not share their cultural background. Children are further exposed to a much wider range of traditions, values, beliefs, and attitudes today through the media as well. All this makes them less inclined to accept without question what their parents tell them. Children are coming to question their parents', and others', authority at a younger and younger age. Reduced supervision has also given children more freedoms.

A basic tenet of successful democracy is that with freedom comes responsibility. Equality-based disciplinary systems are not permissive; rather, parents seek to guide children to responsible choices. Parenting is authoritative (authority based on experience and expertise) rather than authoritarian (authority based on force). Children cannot be taught to take responsibility unless responsibility is given to them. Therefore, appropriate amounts of freedom to choose, and to experience the consequences of those choices, are granted to children according to their developmental level.

These stages determine the type of guidance given to a child by the adult **caregiver**, and the amount of self-determination the child is allowed. Ideally, the parent or other adult caregiver develops an intimate knowledge of the child, a connection based on close awareness and attachment, so that the adult can provide the guidance needed by that particular child.

No two children are exactly alike, so no one method of discipline can be applied to all children with equal success. Neither will the same form of discipline work with the same child in every situation at every age. Good discipline, therefore, is contingent upon the right relationship between adult and child, not the right techniques. It is also imperative that adults be self-disciplined teachers. Children learn from modeling, so parents must model disciplined behavior. Self-discipline involves **self-esteem**, self-acceptance, and self-respect. A parent's relationship with her or himself, therefore, is as important to good discipline as is the parent's relationship with the child.

Clearly, nonpunitive discipline is a complex endeavor that requires a good deal of maturity and knowledge on the part of the parent. Many books and videos are available to help parents develop the skills necessary to provide their children with effective discipline.

Resources

BOOKS

Lane, Kathleen Lynne, et al. *Managing Challenging Behaviors in Schools: Research-Based Strategies that Work.* New York: Guilford Press, 2011.

Perry, Nancy J., and Debby M. Fields. *Constructive Guidance and Discipline: Preschool and Primary Education,* 5th ed. Boston: Merrill/Pearson, 2010.

Rosemond, John. *The Well-Behaved Child: Discipline That Really Works!* Nashville: Thomas Nelson, 2009.

PERIODICALS

Bodovski, Katerina, and Min-Jong Youn. "Love, Discipline, and Elementary School Achievement: The Role of Family

Emotional Climate." *Social Science Research* 39, no. 4 (July 2010): 585–595.

Taylor, Catherine A., et al. "Mothers' Spanking of 3-Year-Old Children and Subsequent Risk of Children's Aggressive Behavior." *Pediatrics* 125, no. 5 (May 2010): 1049–1050.

ORGANIZATIONS

American Academy of Child and Adolescent Psychiatry, 3615 Wisconsin Avenue, NW, Washington DC, 20016-3007, (202) 966-7300, (202) 966-2891, http://www.aacap.org.

American Academy of Family Physicians, P. O. Box 11210, Shawnee Mission KS, 66207, (913) 906-6000, (800) 274-2237, (913) 906-6075, http://familydoctor.org.

American Academy of Pediatrics, 141 Northwest Point Boulevard, Elk Grove Village IL, 60007-1098, (847) 434-4000, (847) 434-8000, http://www.aap.org.

Dianne K. Daeg de Mott
Tish Davidson, AM

Dissociative disorders

Definition

The dissociative disorders are a group of mental disorders that affect consciousness defined as causing significant interference with the patient's general functioning, including social relationships and employment.

Description

In order to have a clear picture of these disorders, dissociation should first be understood. Dissociation is a mechanism that allows the mind to separate or compartmentalize certain memories or thoughts from normal consciousness. These split-off mental contents are not erased. They may resurface spontaneously or be triggered by objects or events in the person's environment.

Dissociation is a process that occurs along a spectrum of severity. It does not necessarily mean that a person has a dissociative disorder or other mental illness. A mild degree of dissociation occurs with some physical stressors; people who have gone without **sleep** for a long period of time, have had "laughing gas" for dental surgery, or have been in a minor accident often have brief dissociative experiences. Another commonplace example of dissociation is a person becoming involved in a book or movie so completely that the surroundings or the passage of time are not noticed. Another example might be driving on the highway and taking several exits without noticing or remembering. Dissociation is related to hypnosis in that hypnotic trance also involves a temporarily altered state of consciousness. Most patients with dissociative disorders are highly hypnotizable.

People in other cultures sometimes have dissociative experiences in the course of religious (in certain trance states) or other group activities. These occurrences should not be judged in terms of what is considered "normal" in the United States.

Moderate or severe forms of dissociation are caused by such traumatic experiences as childhood abuse, combat, criminal attacks, brainwashing in hostage situations, or involvement in a natural or transportation disaster. Patients with acute stress disorder, post-traumatic stress disorder (PTSD), or conversion disorder and somatization disorder may develop dissociative symptoms. Recent studies of trauma indicate that the human brain stores traumatic memories in a different way than normal memories. Traumatic memories are not processed or integrated into a person's ongoing life in the same fashion as normal memories. Instead they are dissociated, or "split off," and may erupt into consciousness from time to time without warning. The affected person cannot control or "edit" these memories. Over a period of time, these two sets of memories, the normal and the traumatic, may coexist as parallel sets without being combined or blended. In extreme cases, different sets of dissociated memories may alter subpersonalities of patients with dissociative identity disorder (multiple personality disorder).

The dissociative disorders vary in their severity and the suddenness of onset. It is difficult to give statistics for their frequency in the United States because they are a relatively new category and are often misdiagnosed. Criteria for diagnosis require significant impairment in social or vocational functioning.

Dissociative amnesia

Dissociative amnesia is a disorder in which the distinctive feature is the patient's inability to remember important personal information to a degree that cannot be explained by normal forgetfulness. In many cases, it is a reaction to a traumatic accident or witnessing a violent crime. Patients with dissociative amnesia may develop depersonalization or trance states as part of the disorder, but they do not experience a change in identity.

Dissociative fugue

Dissociative fugue is a disorder in which a person temporarily loses his or her sense of personal identity and travels to another location where he or she may assume a new identity. Again, this condition usually follows a major stressor or trauma. Apart from inability to recall their past or personal information, patients with dissociative fugue do not behave strangely or appear disturbed to others. Cases of dissociative fugue are more common in wartime or in communities disrupted by a natural disaster.

Depersonalization disorder

Depersonalization disorder is a disturbance in which the patient's primary symptom is a sense of detachment from the self. Depersonalization as a symptom (not as a disorder) is quite common in college-age populations. It is often associated with sleep deprivation or "recreational" drug use. It may be accompanied by "derealization" (where objects in an environment appear altered). Patients sometimes describe depersonalization as feeling like a robot or watching themselves from the outside. Depersonalization disorder may also involve feelings of numbness or loss of emotional "aliveness."

Dissociative identity disorder (DID)

Dissociative identity disorder (DID) is the newer name for multiple personality disorder (MPD). DID is considered the most severe dissociative disorder and involves all of the major dissociative symptoms.

Dissociative disorder not otherwise specified (DDNOS)

DDNOS is a diagnostic category ascribed to patients with dissociative symptoms that do not meet the full criteria for a specific dissociative disorder.

Causes and symptoms

The moderate to severe dissociation that occurs in patients with dissociative disorders is understood to result from a set of causes:

- an innate ability to dissociate easily
- repeated episodes of severe physical or sexual abuse in childhood
- the lack of a supportive or comforting person to counteract abusive relative(s)
- the influence of other relatives with dissociative symptoms or disorders

The relationship of dissociative disorders to childhood abuse has led to intense controversy and lawsuits concerning the accuracy of childhood memories. The brain's storage, retrieval, and interpretation of memories are still not fully understood. Controversy also exists regarding how much individuals presenting dissociative disorders have been influenced by books and movies to describe a certain set of symptoms (scripting).

The major dissociative symptoms are:

Amnesia

Amnesia in a dissociative disorder is marked by gaps in a patient's memory for long periods of time or for traumatic events. Doctors can distinguish this type of amnesia from loss of memory caused by head injuries or drug intoxication, because the amnesia is "spotty" and related to highly charged events and feelings.

Depersonalization

Depersonalization is a dissociative symptom in which the patient feels that his or her body is unreal, is changing, or is dissolving. Some patients experience depersonalization as being outside their bodies or watching a movie of themselves.

Derealization

Derealization is a dissociative symptom in which the external environment is perceived as unreal. The patient may see walls, buildings, or other objects as changing in shape, size, or color. In some cases, the patient may feel that other persons are machines or robots, though the patient is able to acknowledge the unreality of this feeling.

Identity disturbances

Patients with dissociative fugue, DDNOS, or DID often experience confusion about their identities or even assume new identities. Identity disturbances result from the patient having split off entire personality traits or characteristics as well as memories. When a stressful or traumatic experience triggers the reemergence of these dissociated parts, the patient may act differently, answer to a different name, or appear confused by his or her surroundings.

Diagnosis

When a doctor is evaluating a patient with dissociative symptoms, he or she will first rule out physical conditions that sometimes produce amnesia, depersonalization, or derealization. These physical conditions include **epilepsy**, head injuries, brain disease, side effects of medications, **substance abuse**, intoxication, **AIDS**, dementia complex, or recent periods of extreme physical stress and sleeplessness. In some cases, the doctor may give the patient an electroencephalogram (EEG) to exclude epilepsy or other seizure disorders.

If the patient appears to be physically normal, the doctor will rule out psychotic disturbances, including

KEY TERMS

Amnesia—A general medical term for loss of memory that is not due to ordinary forgetfulness. Amnesia can be caused by head injuries, brain disease, or epilepsy, as well as by dissociation.

Depersonalization—A dissociative symptom in which the patient feels that his or her body is unreal, is changing, or is dissolving.

Derealization—A dissociative symptom in which the external environment is perceived as unreal.

Dissociation—A psychological mechanism that allows the mind to split off traumatic memories or disturbing ideas from conscious awareness.

Fugue—A dissociative experience during which a person travels away from home, has amnesia for their past, and may be confused about their identity but otherwise appear normal.

Hypnosis—The means by which a state of extreme relaxation and suggestibility is induced: used to treat amnesia and identity disturbances that occur in dissociative disorders.

Multiple personality disorder (MPD)—An older term for dissociative identity disorder (DID).

Trauma—A disastrous or life-threatening event that can cause severe emotional distress, including dissociative symptoms and disorders.

schizophrenia. In addition, doctors can use some **psychological tests** to narrow the diagnosis. One is a screener, the Dissociative Experiences Scale (DES). If the patient has a high score on this test, he or she can be evaluated further with the Dissociative Disorders Interview Schedule (DDIS) or the Structured Clinical Interview for *DSM-IV* Dissociative Disorders (SCID-D). It is also possible for doctors to measure a patient's hypnotizability as part of a diagnostic evaluation.

Treatment

Treatment of the dissociative disorders often combines several methods.

Psychotherapy

Patients with dissociative disorders often require treatment by a therapist with some specialized understanding of dissociation. This background is particularly important if the patient's symptoms include identity problems. Many patients with dissociative disorders are helped by group as well as individual treatment.

Medications

Some doctors will prescribe tranquilizers or antidepressants for the **anxiety** and/or depression that often accompany dissociative disorders. Patients with dissociative disorders are, however, at risk for abusing or becoming dependent on medications. There is no drug that can reliably counteract dissociation itself.

Hypnosis

Hypnosis is frequently recommended as a method of treatment for dissociative disorders, partly because hypnosis is related to the process of dissociation. Hypnosis may help patients recover repressed ideas and memories. Therapists treating patients with DID sometimes use hypnosis in the process of "fusing" the patient's alternate personalities.

Prognosis

Prognoses for dissociative disorders vary. Recovery from dissociative fugue is usually rapid. Dissociative amnesia may resolve quickly, but can become a chronic disorder in some patients. Depersonalization disorder, DDNOS, and DID are usually chronic conditions. DID usually requires five or more years of treatment for recovery.

Prevention

Since the primary cause of dissociative disorders is thought to involve extended periods of humanly inflicted trauma, prevention depends on the elimination of **child abuse** and psychological abuse of adult prisoners or hostages.

Resources

BOOKS

Eisendrath, Stuart J. "Psychiatric Disorders." In *Current Medical Diagnosis and Treatment, 1998*, edited by Stephen McPhee, et al., 37th ed. Stamford: Appleton & Lange, 1997.

Rebecca J. Frey, PhD

Divorce

Definition

The legal dissolution of a marriage.

Description

The increase in the United States divorce rate over the past 30 years has had significant consequences for the nation's children, over a million of whom are affected by divorce every year. In spite of the frequently-heard statistic that "half of all American marriages end in divorce," the actual rate is somewhat lower, particularly among the more highly educated. According to the United States Centers for Disease Control and Prevention (CDC), in 2008 there were 7.1 new marriages per 1,000 people in the United States, and 3.5 divorces per 1,000, a ratio which has stayed approximately steady for many years since the 1960s. Longer-term studies indicate that the American divorce rate rose slightly every year from 1890 until the Great Depression of the 1930s, when it underwent a small decline. It rose sharply after World War II and rose sharply again following the introduction of no-fault divorce laws in the 1960s. The divorce rate for all marriages peaked at 41% in the 1980s and has declined since then, standing at about 31% in 2006. The majority of all marriages that end in divorce do so in the first ten years, and more than 80% do so within the first 20 years. One significant change since the 1980s is a divergence in the divorce rate according to level of education. Prior to the 1980s, there was little difference among socioeconomic groups in the divorce rate. Since the 1980s, however, the divorce rate among college graduates has dropped to 20%, roughly half that of less educated couples.

Demographics

Divorce statistics in the United States indicate that women are less satisfied with and more likely to take steps to end their marriages than men. Most divorces at all levels of educational attainment are initiated by women, and have been since 1870. After the introduction of no-fault divorce in the 1960s, 70% of divorce cases were filed by women. As of 2010, this number had remained roughly stable since that time. The most common reason given for seeking a divorce is still infidelity on the husband's part.

Effects

Common childhood and adolescent reactions to parental divorce include a continuing desire for the parents to reunite; fears of desertion; feelings of guilt over having been responsible for the divorce; developmental regression; **sleep disorders**; and physical complaints. While researchers have found that some children recover from the trauma of divorce within one to three years, recent long-term studies have documented persistent negative effects that can follow a child into **adolescence** and beyond, especially with regard to the formation of intimate relationships later in life. The effects of parental divorce have been linked to phenomena as diverse as emotional and behavioral problems, school dropout rates, crime rates, physical and **sexual abuse**, and physical health and well-being in adult life. In addition, some studies have found that children from divorced families are more likely to become divorced themselves as adults than those who grew up in intact families. Mental health professionals, however, continue to debate whether divorce is more damaging for children than the continuation of a troubled marriage.

One reason why the debate over the long-term effects of divorce on children continues is methodological, namely, establishing an adequate baseline for comparison. By definition, almost all children of divorce come from unhappy families; however, children whose parents never divorced represent a range of happy and unhappy families, because some couples choose to stay married in spite of deep dissatisfaction with their marriage. Comparisons of life outcomes or well-being that categorize children as either products of broken or of intact families almost always show poorer outcomes for the group composed entirely of children from broken families. The real question, however, is whether it is better or worse to be the offspring of unhappy parents who divorce, or to be the child of unhappy parents who do not divorce. Researchers would have to identify with reasonable certainty a group of still-married parents who are nonetheless deeply unhappy with each other, which has not been done on a large scale as of 2010.

Infancy and toddlerhood

During these stages of development, children's reactions to divorce stem from interference with the satisfaction of their basic needs. The removal of the noncustodial parent or increased work hours for the custodial parent can cause **separation anxiety**, while the parents' emotional distress tends to be transmitted to children at these ages, upsetting their own emotional equilibrium. The inability of infants and toddlers to understand the concept of divorce on an intellectual level makes the changes in their situation seem frighteningly unpredictable and confusing. The child may temporarily revert to an earlier development stage in such areas as eating, sleeping, **toilet training**, motor activity, language, and emotional independence. Other signs of distress include anger, fearfulness, and withdrawal.

Preschool

At this stage, the child's continued egocentric focus, coupled with a more advanced level of **cognitive development**, leads to feelings of guilt as he becomes convinced that he is the reason for his parents' divorce. Children at this age are also prone to powerful fantasies, which in the case of divorce may include imagined scenarios involving **abandonment** or punishment. The disruption that follows divorce, particularly in the relationship with the father, also becomes an important factor for children at this stage of development. Developmental regression may take the form of insisting on sleeping in the same room or bed as the parent; refusing to eat all but a few types of food; **stuttering** or reverting to baby talk; disruptions in toilet training; and developing an excessive emotional dependence on a parent.

School-age children

By the early elementary grades, children are better able to handle separation from the noncustodial parent. Their greater awareness of the divorce situation, however, may lead to elaborate and frightening fantasies of abandonment or of being replaced in the affections of the noncustodial parent. Typical reactions at this stage include sadness, depression, anger, and generalized **anxiety**. Disruption of basic developmental progress in such areas as eating, sleeping, and elimination is possible but less frequent than in younger children. Many children this age suffer a sharp decline in academic performance that often lasts throughout the entire school year in which the divorce takes place. One effective means of helping early elementary children cope with their feelings is communication by displacement, in which a doll or story character acts out feelings and fantasies the child is reluctant to claim as his or her own.

Children in the upper elementary grades are capable of understanding the divorce process on a relatively sophisticated level. At this stage, the simple fears and fantasies of the younger child are replaced by more complex internal conflicts, such as the struggle to preserve one's allegiance to both parents. Older children become adept at erecting **defense mechanisms** to protect themselves against the pain they feel over a divorce. Such defenses include denial, intellectualization, displacement of feelings, and such physical complaints as fatigue, headaches, and nausea or **vomiting**. Children in the upper elementary grades are most likely to become intensely angry at their parents for divorcing. Other common emotions at this stage of development include loneliness, grief, anxiety, and a sense of powerlessness.

Adolescence

For teenagers, parental divorce is difficult because it is yet another source of upheaval in their lives. Teenage behavior is affected not only by recent divorces but also by those that occurred when the child was much younger. One especially painful effect of divorce on adolescents is the negative attitude it can produce toward one or both parents, whom they need as role models but are often blamed for disappointing them.

Adolescents are also prone to internal conflicts over their parents' divorce. They are torn between love for and anger toward their parents and between conflicting loyalties to both parents. Positive feelings toward their parents' new partners come into conflict with anxiety over the intimacy of these relationships, and the teenager's close affiliation with the custodial parent clashes with his or her need for increased social and emotional independence. Although children at all ages are distressed by parental divorce, by adolescence it can result in potentially dangerous behavior, including drug and alcohol abuse, precocious and/or promiscuous sexual activity, violence, and delinquency.

Helping children cope with divorce

Psychologist Judith S. Wallerstein, an internationally recognized authority on the effects of divorce on children, has proposed that children whose parents divorce face special psychological tasks in addition to the normal developmental tasks all children must accomplish. She outlines the following sequence of seven steps: 1) attaining a realistic understanding of the divorce; 2) achieving enough distance from the situation to continue with their lives; 3) absorbing the loss of the original **family** unit and of the noncustodial parent; 4) handling their anger; 5) dealing with guilt feelings; 6) facing the fact that the divorce is permanent; and 7) remaining optimistic about their own chances for healthy relationships in the future.

Experts agree that it is important for parents who are divorcing to avoid involving their children in their disputes or forcing them to choose sides, and are often advised to avoid criticizing their former mates in front of their children. In order for children to heal from the emotional pain of parental divorce, they need an outlet for open expression of their feelings, whether it be a sibling, friend, adult mentor or counselor, or a divorce support group. Extended families can be a significant source of support for children, providing them with stability and with the reassurance that others care about them. Although parental divorce is undeniably difficult for children of all ages, loving, patient, and enlightened parental support can make a crucial difference in helping children cope with the experience both immediately and over the long term.

Unfortunately, many divorcing and divorced parents do not follow this advice. Mental health and law enforcement professionals are frequently confronted with destructive and hurtful behavior on the part of parents. One disturbingly common tactic is child abduction, which affects about 230,000 children each year in the United States. In these cases one parent refuses to return the child to the other parent at the end of a visit or flees with the child to prevent a visit, usually to gain leverage over the other spouse during divorce proceedings or to act out anger against the other spouse for initiating the divorce. Most cases of child abduction take place within the same state, but about 25 percent involve flight across state lines or even international borders. Twenty-one percent of abducted children are gone for a month or longer. Many states have made interstate child abduction a criminal offense. Fathers and mothers are about equally as likely to abduct their child or children.

Another increasingly frequent occurrence following divorce is parent alienation syndrome, or PAS, first identified by a psychiatrist named Richard Gardner in the 1980s. The syndrome is characterized not only by the alienating parent's attempts to turn the child against the target parent by denigrating him or her but also by the child's active contributions to the process. It is thus not the same as straightforward abuse or neglect. In essence, children are used in PAS to attack the targeted parent as a means of revenge and psychological violence. The alienating parent refuses to comply with court orders, tells the children they do not have to either, and to ignore the authority of the targeted parent. The goal of the alienating parent is to destroy the targeted parent by using the children as weapons or pawns. Dr. Gardner maintains that the gender ratio has shifted from the 1980s, when most of the alienating parents he encountered were women, to a nearly 50/50 male/female ratio. Although PAS has not been officially recognized by any medical or psychiatric professional body, it has been recognized in case law in child **custody** disputes.

Resources

BOOKS

Colson, Mary. *Coping With Absent Parents.* Chicago: Heinemann Library, 2011.

Darnall, Douglas. *Beyond Divorce Casualties: Reunifying the Alienated Family.* Lanham, MD: Taylor Trade Pub., 2010.

Green, Janice. *Divorce After 50: Your Guide to the Unique Legal & Financial Challenges.* Berkeley, CA: Nolo, 2010.

Nowinski, Joseph. *The Divorced Child: Strengthening Your Family Through the First Three Years of Separation.* New York: Palgrave Macmillan, 2010.

Pedro-Carroll, JoAnne. *Putting Children First: Proven Parenting Strategies for Helping Children Thrive Through Divorce.* New York: Avery, 2010.

PERIODICALS

Inoue, Ken. "The Correlation of the Suicide Rates with the Rates of Unemployment and Divorce in the United States During Seventeen Years." *American Journal of Forensic Medicine & Pathology,* 30, no. 3 (September 2009): 311–2.

Wolchik, Sharlene, et al. "Promoting Resilience in Youth From Divorced Families: Lessons Learned from Experimental Trials of the New Beginnings Program." *Journal of Personality,* 77, no. 6 (December 2009): 1833–68.

Yongmin, Sun, & Yuanzhang Li. "Parental Divorce, Sibship Size, Family Resources, and Children's Academic Performance." *Social Science Research,* 38, no. 3 (September 2009): 622–34.

ORGANIZATIONS

The American Academy of Child and Adolescent Psychiatry, 3615 Wisconsin Avenue, N.W., Washington DC, 20016, (202) 966-7300, (202) 966-2891, www.aacap.org.

Child Welfare League of America., 2345 Crystal Drive, Suite 250, Arlington VA, 22202, (703) 412-2400, (703) 412-2401, http://www.cwla.org.

Tish Davidson, AM

Dizziness

Definition

As a disorder, dizziness is classified into three categories–vertigo, syncope, and nonsyncope nonvertigo. Each category has a characteristic set of symptoms, all related to the sense of balance. In general, syncope is defined by a brief loss of consciousness (fainting) or by dimmed vision and feeling uncoordinated, confused, and lightheaded. Many people experience a sensation like syncope when they stand up too fast. Vertigo is the feeling that either the individual or the surroundings are spinning. This sensation is like being on a spinning amusement park ride. Individuals with nonsyncope nonvertigo dizziness feel as though they cannot keep their balance. This feeling may become worse with movement.

Description

The brain coordinates information from the eyes, the inner ear, and the body's senses to maintain balance. If any of these information sources is disrupted, the brain may not be able to compensate. For example, people sometimes experience **motion sickness** because the information from their body tells the brain that they are sitting still, but information from the eyes indicates that they are moving. The messages do not correspond and dizziness results.

Vision and the body's senses are the most important systems for maintaining balance, but problems in the inner ear are the most frequent cause of dizziness. The inner ear, also called the vestibular system, contains fluid that helps fine tune the information the brain receives from the eyes and the body. When fluid volume or pressure in one inner ear changes, information about balance is altered. The discrepancy gives conflicting messages to the brain about balance and induces dizziness.

Certain medical conditions can cause dizziness, because they affect the systems that maintain balance.

For example, the inner ear is very sensitive to changes in blood flow. Because medical conditions such as high blood pressure or low blood sugar can affect blood flow, these conditions are frequently accompanied by dizziness. Circulation disorders are the most common causes of dizziness. Other causes are **head injury**, ear infection, **allergies**, and nervous system disorders.

Dizziness often disappears without treatment or with treatment of the underlying problem, but it can be long term or chronic. According to the National Institutes of Health, 42% of Americans will seek medical help for dizziness at some point in their lives. The costs may exceed a billion dollars and account for five million doctor visits annually. Episodes of dizziness increase with age. Among people aged 75 or older, dizziness is the most frequent reason for seeing a doctor.

Causes and symptoms

Careful attention to symptoms can help determine the underlying cause of the dizziness. Underlying problems may be benign and easily treated or they may be dangerous and in need of intensive therapy. Not all cases of dizziness can be linked to a specific cause. More than one type of dizziness can be experienced at the same time and symptoms may be mixed. Episodes of dizziness may last for a few seconds or for days. The length of an episode is related to the underlying cause.

The symptoms of syncope include dimmed vision, loss of coordination, confusion, lightheadedness, and sweating. These symptoms can lead to a brief loss of consciousness or fainting. They are related to a reduced flow of blood to the brain; they often occur when a person is standing up and can be relieved by sitting or lying down. Vertigo is characterized by a sensation of spinning or turning, accompanied by nausea, **vomiting**, ringing in the ears, **headache**, or fatigue. An individual may have trouble walking, remaining coordinated, or keeping balance. Nonsyncope nonvertigo dizziness is characterized by a feeling of being off balance that becomes worse if the individual tries moving or performing detail-intense tasks.

A person may experience dizziness for many reasons. Syncope is associated with low blood pressure, heart problems, and disorders in the autonomic nervous system, the system of involuntary functions such as breathing. Syncope may also arise from emotional distress, **pain**, and other reactions to outside stressors. Nonsyncope nonvertigo dizziness may be caused by rapid breathing, low blood sugar, or migraine headache, as well as by more serious medical conditions.

Vertigo is often associated with inner ear problems called vestibular disorders. A particularly intense vestibular disorder, Méniére's disease, interferes with the volume of fluid in the inner ear. This disease, which affects approximately one in every 1,000 people, causes intermittent vertigo over the course of weeks, months, or years. Méniére's disease is often accompanied by ringing or buzzing in the ear, hearing loss, and a feeling that the ear is blocked. Damage to the nerve that leads from the ear to the brain can also cause vertigo. Such damage can result from head injury or a tumor. An acoustic neuroma, for example, is a benign tumor that wraps around the nerve. Vertigo can also be caused by disorders of the central nervous system and the cirulatory system, such as hardening of the arteries (arteriosclerosis), **stroke**, or multiple sclerosis.

Some medications cause changes in blood pressure or blood flow. These medications can cause dizziness in some people. Prescription medications carry warnings of such side effects, but common drugs, such as **caffeine** or nicotine, can also cause dizziness. Certain **antibiotics** can damage the inner ear and cause hearing loss and dizziness.

Diet may cause dizziness. The role of diet may be direct, as through alcohol intake. It may be also be indirect, as through arteriosclerosis caused by a high-fat diet. Some people experience a slight dip in blood sugar and mild dizziness if they miss a meal, but this condition is rarely dangerous unless the person is diabetic. Food sensitivities or allergies can also be a cause of dizziness. Chronic conditions, such as heart disease, and serious acute problems, such as seizures and strokes, can cause dizziness. However, such conditions usually exhibit other characteristic symptoms.

Diagnosis

During the initial medical examination, an individual with dizziness should provide a detailed description of the type of dizziness experienced, when it occurs, and how often each episode lasts. A diary of symptoms may help track this information. Report any symptoms that accompany the dizziness, such as a ringing in the ear or nausea, any recent injury or infection, and any medication taken.

Blood pressure, pulse, respiration, and body temperature are checked, and the ear, nose, and throat are scrutinized. The sense of balance is assessed by moving the individual's head to various positions or by tilt-table testing. In tilt-table testing, the person lies on a table that can be shifted into different positions and reports any dizziness that occurs.

Further tests may be indicated by the initial examination. Hearing tests help assess ear damage. **X rays**, computed tomography scan (CT scan), and **magnetic resonance imaging** (MRI) can pinpoint evidence of nerve damage, tumor, or other structural problems. If a vestibular disorder is suspected, a technique called electronystagmography (ENG) may be used. ENG measures the electrical impulses generated by eye movements. Blood tests can determine diabetes, high **cholesterol**, and other diseases. In some cases, a heart evaluation may be useful. Despite thorough testing, an underlying cause cannot always be determined.

Treatment

Treatment is determined by the underlying cause. If an individual has a cold or **influenza**, a few days of bed rest is usually adequate to resolve dizziness. Other causes of dizziness, such as mild vestibular system damage, may resolve without medical treatment.

If dizziness continues, drug therapy may prove helpful. Because circulatory problems often cause dizziness, medication may be prescribed to control blood pressure or to treat arteriosclerosis. Sedatives may be useful to relieve the tension that can trigger or aggravate dizziness. Low blood sugar associated with diabetes sometimes causes dizziness and is treated by controlling blood sugar levels. An individual may be asked to avoid caffeine, nicotine, alcohol, and any substances that cause allergic reactions. A low-salt diet may also help some people.

When other measures have failed, surgery may be suggested to relieve pressure on the inner ear. If the dizziness is not treatable by drugs, surgery, or other means, physical therapy may be used and the patient may be taught coping mechanisms for the problem.

Alternative treatment

Because dizziness may arise from serious conditions, it is advisable to seek medical treatment. Alternative treatments can often be used alongside conventional medicine without conflict. Relaxation techniques, such as **yoga** and **massage therapy** that focus on relieving tension, are popularly recommended methods for reducing stress. Aromatherapists recommend a warm bath scented with essential oils of lavender, geranium, and sandalwood.

Homeopathic therapies can work very effectively for dizziness, and are especially applicable when no organic cause can be identified. An osteopath or chiropractor may suggest adjustments of the head, jaw, neck, and lower back to relieve pressure on the inner ear. Acupuncturists also offer some treatment options for acute and chronic cases of dizziness. Nutritionists may be able to offer advice and guidance in choosing dietary supplements, identifying foods to avoid, and balancing nutritional needs.

KEY TERMS

Acoustic neuroma—A benign tumor that grows on the nerve leading from the inner ear to the brain. As the tumor grows, it exerts pressure on the inner ear and causes severe vertigo.

Arteriosclerosis—Hardening of the arteries caused by high blood cholesterol and high blood pressure.

Autonomic nervous system—The part of the nervous system that controls involuntary functions such as breathing and heart beat.

Computed tomography (CT)—An imaging technique in which cross-sectional x rays of the body are compiled to create a three-dimensional image of the body's internal structures.

Electronystagmography—A method for measuring the electricity generated by eye movements. Electrodes are placed on the skin around the eye and the individual is subjected to a variety of stimuli so that the quality of eye movements can be assessed.

Magnetic resonance imaging (MRI)—An imaging technique that uses a large circular magnet and radio waves to generate signals from atoms in the body. These signals are used to construct images of internal structures.

Vestibular system—The area of the inner ear that helps maintain balance.

Prognosis

Outcome depends on the cause of dizziness. Controlling or curing the underlying factors usually relieves dizziness. In some cases, dizziness disappears without treatment. In a few cases, dizziness can become a permanent disabling condition and a person's options are limited.

Prevention

Most people learn through experience that certain activities will make them dizzy and they learn to avoid them. For example, if reading in a car produces motion sickness, an individual leaves reading materials for after the trip. Changes to the diet can also cut down on episodes of dizziness in susceptible people. Relaxation techniques can help ward off tension and **anxiety** that can cause dizziness.

These techniques can help minimize or even prevent dizziness for people with chronic diseases. For example, persons with Méniére's disease may avoid episodes of vertigo by leaving salt, alcohol, and caffeine out of their diets. Reducing blood cholesterol can help diminish arteriosclerosis and indirectly treat dizziness.

Some cases of dizziness cannot be prevented. Acoustic neuromas, for example, are not predictable or preventable. When the underlying cause of dizziness cannot be discovered, it may be difficult to recommend preventive measures. Alternative approaches designed to rebalance the body's energy flow, such as acupuncture and constitutional homeopathy, may be helpful in cases where the cause of dizziness cannot be pinpointed.

ORGANIZATIONS

Méniére's Network, 1817 Patterson St., Nashville TN, 37203, (800) 545-4327, http://www.earfoundation.org.

Vestibular Disorders Association, PO Box 4467, Portland OR, 97208-4467 (503) 229-7705, http://www.teleport.com/~veda.

Julia Barrett

Down syndrome

Definition

Down syndrome is the most common chromosome disorder and genetic cause of intellectual disability. It occurs because of the presence of an extra copy of chromosome 21. For this reason, it is also called trisomy 21.

Demographics

As of 2009, the Centers for Disease Control (CDC) estimate that each year about 3,357 babies in the United States are born with Down syndrome. In other words, about 13 of every 10,000 babies born in the United States each year is born with Down syndrome. It affects an equal number of male and female babies. The majority of cases of Down syndrome occur due to an extra chromosome 21 within the egg cell supplied by the mother (nondisjunction).

Down syndrome occurs with equal frequency across all ethnic groups and subpopulations.

Description

Named after John Langdon Down, the first physician to identify the syndrome, Down syndrome is the result of genetic variations. When the reproductive cells, the sperm and ovum, combine at fertilization, the fertilized egg that results contains 23 chromosome pairs. A normal fertilized egg that will develop into a female contains chromosome pairs 1 through 22, and the XX pair. A normal fertilized egg that will develop into a male contains chromosome pairs 1 through 22, and the XY pair. When the fertilized egg contains extra material from chromosome number 21, this results in Down syndrome. This event is called nondisjunction and it occurs in 95% of Down syndrome cases. The baby, therefore, receives an extra chromosome at conception. Because of this extra chromosome 21, individuals affected with Down syndrome have 47 instead of 46 chromosomes. This additional genetic material disrupts the normal course of development, causing the characteristic features of Down syndrome.

Risk factors

Parents who have already have a baby with Down syndrome or who have abnormalities in their own chromosome 21 are at higher risk for having a baby with Down syndrome. The chance of having a baby with Down syndrome also increases as a woman gets older. As a woman's age (maternal age) increases, the risk of having a Down syndrome baby increases significantly. By the time the woman is age 35, the risk increases to one in 400; by age 40 the risk increases to one in 110; and, by age 45, the risk becomes one in 35. There is no increased risk of either mosaicism or translocation with increased maternal age.

Causes and symptoms

Down syndrome is a chromosomal disorder caused by an error in cell division that results in the presence of an additional third chromosome 21. In approximately one to two percent of Down syndrome cases, the original egg and sperm cells contain the correct number of chromosomes, 23 each.. The problem occurs sometime shortly after fertilization—during the phase when cells are dividing rapidly. One cell divides abnormally, creating a line of cells with an extra copy of chromosome 21. This form of genetic disorder is called mosaicism. The individual with this type of Down syndrome has two types of cells: those with 46 chromosomes (the normal number), and those with 47 chromosomes (as occurs in Down syndrome). Individuals affected with this mosaic form of Down syndrome generally have less severe signs and symptoms of the disorder.

Another relatively rare genetic accident that causes Down syndrome is called translocation. During cell division, chromosome 21 somehow breaks. The broken off piece of this chromosome then becomes attached to another chromosome. Each cell still has 46 chromosomes,

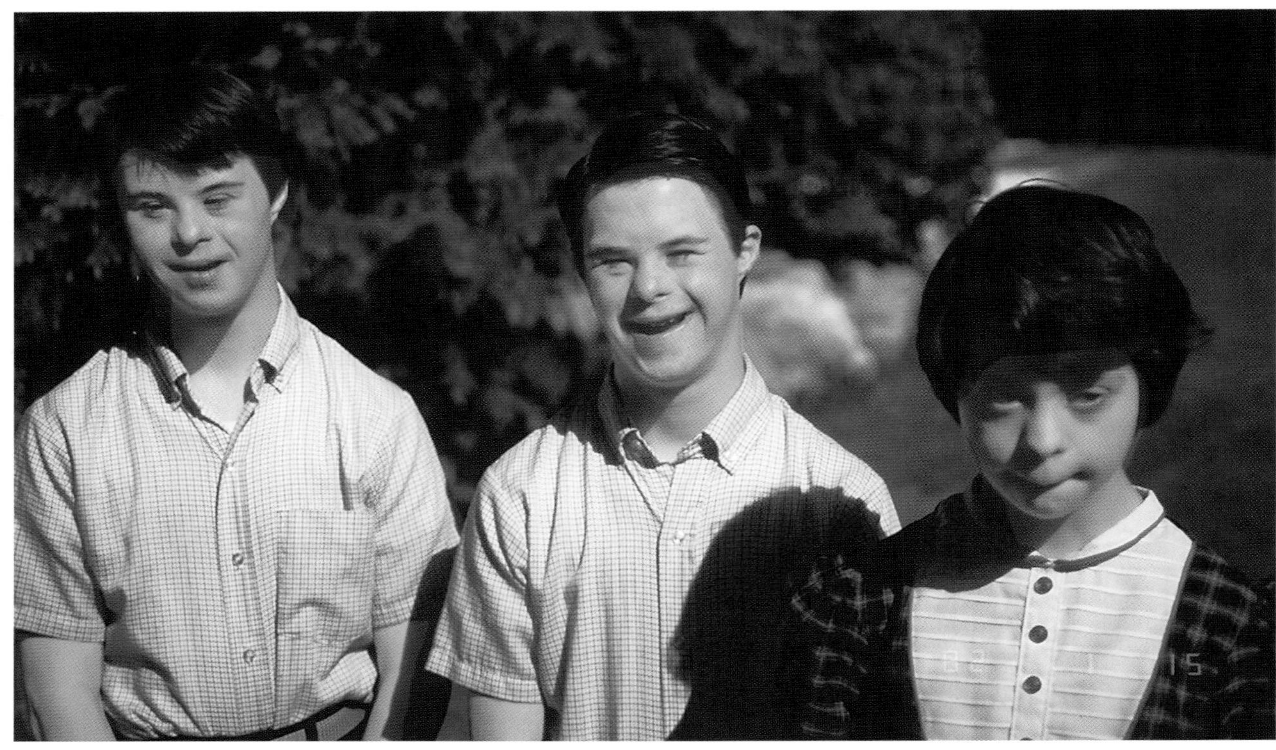

Children with Down syndrome. The disease is caused by trisomy 21, meaning their bodies' cells have an extra chromosome 21. *(© Lester V. Bergman/Corbis.)*

but the extra piece of chromosome 21 results in the signs and symptoms of Down syndrome. Translocations occur in about 3–4% of cases of Down syndrome.

While Down syndrome is a chromosomal disorder, a baby is usually identified at **birth** through observation of a set of common physical characteristics. Not all affected babies will exhibit all of the symptoms discussed. There is a large variability in the number and severity of these characteristics from one affected individual to the next. Babies with Down syndrome tend to be overly quiet, less responsive to stimuli, and have weak, floppy muscles. A number of physical signs may also be present. These include: a flat appearing face; a small head; a flat bridge of the nose; a smaller than normal, low–set nose; small mouth, which causes the tongue to stick out and to appear overly large; upward slanting eyes; bright speckles on the iris of the eye (Brushfield spots); extra folds of skin located at the inside corner of each eye near the nose (epicanthal folds); rounded cheeks; small, misshapen ears; small, wide hands; an unusual deep crease across the center of the palm (simian crease); an inwardly curved little finger; a wide space between the great and the second toes; unusual creases on the soles of the feet; overly flexible joints (sometimes referred to as being double–jointed); and shorter–than–normal stature.

Other types of defects often accompany Down syndrome. Approximately 30–50% of all children with Down syndrome are found to have heart defects. A number of different heart defects are common in Down syndrome. All of these result in abnormal patterns of blood flow within the heart. Abnormal blood flow within the heart often means that less oxygen is sent into circulation throughout the body, which can cause fatigue, a lack of energy, and poor muscle tone.

Malformations of the gastrointestinal tract are present in about 5–7% of children with Down syndrome. The most common malformation is a narrowed, obstructed duodenum (the part of the intestine into which the stomach empties). This disorder, called duodenal atresia, interferes with the baby's milk or formula leaving the stomach and entering the intestine for digestion. The baby often vomits forcibly after feeding, and cannot gain weight appropriately until the defect is repaired.

Another malformation of the gastrointestinal tract that is seen in patients with Down syndrome is an abnormal connection between the windpipe (trachea) and the digestive tube of the throat (esophagus) called a tracheo–esophageal fistula (T–E fistula). This connection interferes with eating and/or breathing because it allows air to enter the digestive system and/or food to enter the airway.

KEY TERMS

Chromosome—A microscopic thread–like structure found within each cell of the body and consists of a complex of proteins and DNA. Humans have 46 chromosomes arranged into 23 pairs. Changes in either the total number of chromosomes or their shape and size (structure) may lead to physical or mental abnormalities.

Karyotype—A standard arrangement of photographic or computer–generated images of chromosome pairs from a cell in ascending numerical order, from largest to smallest.

Mental retardation—Significant impairment in intellectual function and adaptation in society. Usually associated an intelligence quotient (IQ) below 70.

Mosaic—A term referring to a genetic situation in which an individual's cells do not have the exact same composition of chromosomes. In Down syndrome, this may mean that some of the individual's cells have a normal 46 chromosomes, while other cells have an abnormal 47 chromosomes.

Nondisjunction—Non–separation of a chromosome pair, during either meiosis or mitosis.

Translocation—The transfer of one part of a chromosome to another chromosome during cell division. A balanced translocation occurs when pieces from two different chromosomes exchange places without loss or gain of any chromosome material. An unbalanced translocation involves the unequal loss or gain of genetic information between two chromosomes.

Trisomy—The condition of having three identical chromosomes, instead of the normal two, in a cell.

Other medical conditions occurring in patients with Down syndrome include an increased chance of developing infections, especially ear infections and **pneumonia**; certain kidney disorders; thyroid disease (especially low or hypothyroid); hearing loss; vision impairment requiring glasses (corrective lenses); and a 20 times greater chance than the population as a whole of developing leukemia.

Development in a baby and child affected with Down syndrome occurs at a much slower than normal rate. Because of weak, floppy muscles (**hypotonia**), babies learn to sit up, crawl, and walk much later than their unaffected peers. Talking is also quite delayed. The level of **mental retardation** is considered to be mild–to–moderate in Down syndrome. The degree of mental retardation varies a great deal from one child to the next. While it is impossible to predict the severity of Down syndrome at birth, with proper education, children who have Down syndrome are capable of learning. Most children affected with Down syndrome can read and write and are placed in **special education** classes in school. The majority of individuals with Down syndrome become semi–independent adults, meaning that they can take care of their own needs with some assistance.

As people with Down syndrome age, they face an increased chance of developing the brain disease called Alzheimer's (sometimes referred to as dementia or senility). Most people have a 12% chance of developing Alzheimer's, but almost all people with Down syndrome will have either Alzheimer disease or a similar type of dementia by the age of 50. Alzheimer disease causes the brain to shrink and to break down. The number of brain cells decreases, and abnormal deposits and structural arrangements occur. This process results in a loss of brain functioning. People with Alzheimer's have strikingly faulty memories. Over time, people with Alzheimer's disease will lapse into an increasingly unresponsive state.

As people with Down syndrome age, they also have an increased chance of developing a number of other illnesses, including cataracts, thyroid problems, diabetes, and seizure disorders.

Diagnosis

Examination

Diagnosis is usually suspected at birth, when the characteristic physical signs of Down syndrome are observed.

Tests

Once Down syndrome is suspected, **genetic testing** (chromosome analysis) can be undertaken in order to verify the presence of the disorder. This testing is usually done on a blood sample, although chromosome analysis can also be done on other types of tissue, including the skin. The cells to be studied are prepared in a laboratory. Chemical stain is added to make the characteristics of the cells and the chromosomes stand out. Chemicals are added to prompt the cells to go through normal development, up to the point where the chromosomes are most visible, prior to cell division. At this point, they are examined under a microscope and photographed. The photograph is used to sort the different sizes and shapes of chromosomes into pairs. In most cases of Down syndrome, one extra chromosome 21 will be revealed. The final result of such testing, with the photographed chromosomes paired and organized by shape and size, is called the individual's karyotype. An individual with Down syndrome will have a 47 XX+21 karyotype if they are female and a 47 XY+21 karyotype if they are male.

Women who become pregnant after the age of 35 are offered prenatal tests to determine whether or not their developing baby is affected with Down syndrome. A genetic counselor meets with these families to inform them of the risks and to discuss the types of tests available to make a diagnosis prior to delivery. Because there is a slight risk of miscarriage following some prenatal tests, all testing is optional, and couples need to decide whether or not they desire to take this risk in order to learn the status of their unborn baby.

Screening tests are used to estimate the chance that an individual woman will have a baby with Down syndrome. A test called the maternal serum alpha–fetoprotein test (MSAFP) is offered to all pregnant women under the age of 35. If the mother decides to have this test, it is performed between 15 and 22 weeks of pregnancy. The MSAFP screen measures a protein and two hormones that are normally found in maternal blood during pregnancy. A specific pattern of these hormones and protein can indicate an increased risk for having a baby born with Down syndrome. However, this is only a risk and MSAFP cannot diagnose Down syndrome directly. Women found to have an increased risk of their babies being affected with Down syndrome are offered **amniocentesis**. The MSAFP test can detect up to 60% of all babies who will be born with Down syndrome.

Ultrasound screening for Down syndrome is also available. This is generally performed in the mid–trimester of pregnancy. Abnormal growth patterns characteristic of Down syndrome such as growth retardation, heart defects, duodenal atresia, T–E fistula, shorter than normal long–bone lengths, and extra folds of skin along the back of the neck of the developing fetus may all be observed via ultrasonic imaging.

The only way to definitively establish (with about 99% accuracy) the presence or absence of Down syndrome in a developing baby is to test tissue during the pregnancy itself. This is usually done either by amniocentesis, or chorionic villus sampling (CVS). All women under the age of 35 who show a high risk for having a baby affected with Down syndrome via an MSAFP screen and all mothers over the age of 35 are offered either CVS or amniocentesis. In CVS, a tiny tube is inserted into the opening of the uterus to retrieve a small sample of the placenta (the organ that attaches the growing baby to the mother via the umbilical cord, and provides oxygen and nutrition). In amniocentesis, a small amount of the fluid in which the baby is floating is withdrawn with a long, thin needle. CVS may be performed as early as 10 to 12 weeks into a pregnancy. Amniocentesis is generally not performed until at least the fifteenth week. Both CVS and amniocentesis carry small risks of miscarriage. Approximately 1% of women miscarry after undergoing CVS testing, while approximately one–half of one percent miscarry after undergoing amniocentesis. Both amniocentesis and CVS allow the baby's own karyotype to be determined.

Approximately 75% of all babies diagnosed prenatally as affected with Down syndrome do not survive to term and spontaneously miscarry. In addition, these prenatal tests can only diagnose Down syndrome, not the severity of the symptoms that the unborn child will experience. For this reason, a couple might use this information to begin to prepare for the arrival of a baby with Down syndrome, to terminate the pregnancy, or in the case of miscarriage or termination, decide whether to consider **adoption** as an alternative.

Treatment

Traditional

No treatment is available to cure Down syndrome. Treatment is directed at addressing the individual concerns of a particular patient. For example, heart defects may require surgical repair, as will duodenal atresia and T–E fistula. Many Down syndrome patients will need to wear glasses to correct vision. Patients with hearing impairment benefit from hearing aids.

While some decades ago all children with Down syndrome were quickly placed into institutions for lifelong care, research shows very clearly that the best outlook for children with Down syndrome is a normal **family** life in their own home. This requires careful support and education of the parents and the siblings. It is a life–changing event to learn that a new baby has a permanent condition that will affect essentially all aspects of his or her development. Some community groups help families deal with the emotional effects of raising a child with Down syndrome. Schools are required to provide services to children with Down syndrome, sometimes in separate special education classrooms, and sometimes in regular classrooms (this is called mainstreaming or inclusion).

As of May 2000, the genetic sequence for chromosome 21 was fully determined, which opens the door to new approaches to the treatment of Down syndrome through the development of gene–specific therapies.

Alternative

Clinical trials for the treatment of Down syndrome are currently sponsored by the National Institutes of

Health (NIH) and other agencies. In 2009, NIH reported 20 on–going or recently completed studies.

A few examples include:

- The evaluation of a new prenatal blood test for Down syndrome. (NCT00877292)
- The evaluation of the efficacy on language and cognitive function in Down syndrome patients who take Rivastigmine. (NCT00748007)
- The evaluation of the efficacy and tolerability of Continuous Positive Pressure in case of SAOS by Down Syndrome patients. (NCT00394290)
- A study to assess whether memantine is effective and safe in preventing age related cognitive deterioration in people with Down's syndrome (DS) age 40 and over. (NCT00240760)

Clinical trial information is constantly updated by NIH and the most recent information on Down syndrome trials can be found at: http://clinicaltrials.gov/.

Prognosis

The prognosis for an individual with Down syndrome is quite variable, depending on the types of complications (heart defects, susceptibility to infections, development of leukemia, etc.). The severity of the retardation can also vary significantly. Without the presence of heart defects, about 90% of children with Down syndrome live into their teens. People with Down syndrome appear to go through the normal physical changes of aging more rapidly, however. The average age of **death** for an individual with Down syndrome is about 50 to 55 years.

Still, the prognosis for a baby born with Down syndrome is better than ever before. Because of modern medical treatments, including **antibiotics** to treat infections, and surgery to treat heart defects and duodenal atresia, life expectancy has greatly increased. Community and family support allows people with Down syndrome to have rich, meaningful relationships. Because of educational programs, some people with Down syndrome are able to hold jobs.

Prevention

There is no known way to prevent the Down syndrome. Women expecting to give birth, can take steps before and during pregnancy to have a healthy pregnancy. Steps include taking a daily multivitamin with **folic acid** (400 mg), not **smoking**, and not drinking alcohol during pregnancy. Once a couple has had one baby with Down syndrome, they are often concerned about the likelihood of future offspring also being born with the disorder.

When a baby with Down syndrome has the type that results from a translocation, it is possible that one of the two parents is a carrier of a balanced translocation. A carrier has rearranged chromosomal information and can pass it on, but he or she does not have an extra chromosome and therefore is not affected with the disorder. When one parent is a carrier of a translocation, the chance of future offspring having Down syndrome is greatly increased. The specific risk will have to be assessed by a genetic counsellor. Approximately 60% of women with Down syndrome are fully capable of having children. The risk of a woman with trisomy 21 having a child affected with Down syndrome is 50%.

Resources

BOOKS

Groneberg, Jennifer Graf. *Road Map to Holland: How I Found My Way Through My Son's First Two Years With Down Syndrome.* New York, NY: New American Library (Penguin), 2008.

Kumin, Libby. *Helping Children with Down Syndrome Communicate Better: Speech and Language Skills for Ages 6–14.* Bethesda, MD: Woodbine House, 2008.

McGuire, Dennis, and Brian Chicoine. *Mental Wellness in Adults with Down Syndrome: A Guide to Emotional and Behavioral Strengths and Challenges.* Bethesda, MD: Woodbine House, 2006.

Moore–Mallinos, Jennifer. *My Friend Has Down Syndrome.* Hauppauge, NY: Barron's Educational Series, 2008.

Selikowitz, Mark. *Down Syndrome.* New York, NY: Oxford University Press, 2008.

Skallerup, Susan J., editor. *Babies with Down Syndrome: A New Parents' Guide.* Bethesda, MD: Woodbine House, 2008.

PERIODICALS

Creavin, A. L., and R. D. Brown. "Ophthalmic abnormalities in children with Down syndrome." *Journal of Pediatric Ophthalmology and Strabismus* 46, no. 2 (March–April 2009): 76–82.

Hartway, S. "A parent's guide to the genetics of Down syndrome." *Advances in Neonatal Care* 9, no. 1 (February 2009): 27–30.

Kusters, M. A., et al. "Intrinsic defect of the immune system in children with Down syndrome: a review." *Clinical and Experimental Immunology* 156, no. 2 (May 2009): 189–193.

Mégarbané, A., et al. "The 50th anniversary of the discovery of trisomy 21: the past, present, and future of research and treatment of Down syndrome." *Genetics in Medicine* 11, no. 9 (September 2009): 611–616.

Park, J., et al. "Function and regulation of Dyrk1A: towards understanding Down syndrome." *Cellular and Molecular Life Sciences* 66, no. 20 (October 2009): 3235–3240.

Patterson, D. "Molecular genetic analysis of Down syndrome." *Human Genetics* 126, no. 1 (July 2009): 195–214.

Ranweiler, R. "Assessment and care of the newborn with Down syndrome." *Advances in Neonatal Care* 9, no. 1 (February 2009): 17–24.

Wiseman, F. K., et al. "Down syndrome—recent progress and future prospects." *Human Molecular Genetics* 18, no. R1 (April 2009): R75–R83.

OTHER

"Chromosome 21." *Genetics Home Reference* Information Page, http://ghr.nlm.nih.gov/chromosome=21 (accessed December 14, 2009).

"Down Syndrome." *CDC* Information Page, http://www.cdc.gov/ncbddd/birthdefects/DownSyndrome.htm (accessed December 14, 2009).

"Down Syndrome." *Genetics Home Reference* Information Page, http://ghr.nlm.nih.gov/condition=downsyndrome (accessed December 14, 2009).

"Down Syndrome." *March of Dimes* Information Page, http://www.marchofdimes.com/professionals/14332_1214.asp (accessed December 14, 2009).

"Down Syndrome." *Medline Plus* Health Topics, http://www.nlm.nih.gov/medlineplus/downsyndrome.html (accessed December 14, 2009).

"Down Syndrome." *NICHD* Information Page, http://www.nichd.nih.gov/health/topics/Down_Syndrome.cfm (accessed December 14, 2009).

ORGANIZATIONS

March of Dimes Foundation, 1275 Mamaroneck Avenue, White Plains NY, 10605, (914) 428-7100, (888) MOD-IMES, (914) 428-8203, askus@marchofdimes.com, http://www.marchofdimes.com.

National Association for Down Syndrome (NADS), PO Box 206, Wilmette IL, 60091, (630) 325-9112, info@nads.org, http://www.nads.org.

National Center on Birth Defects and Developmental Disabilities, Centers for Disease Control and Prevention, 1600 Clifton Rd., Atlanta GA, 75231, (800) 232-4636, http://www.cdc.gov/ncbddd/index.html.

National Down Syndrome Society, 666 Broadway, 8th Floor, New York NY, 10012, (800) 221-4602, (212) 979-2873, info@ndss.org, http://www.ndss.org.

National Institute of Child Health and Human Development (NICHD), 31 Center Drive, Rm. 2A32, MSC 2425, Bethesda MD, 20892-2425, (301) 496-5133, (301) 496-7101, http://www.nichd.nih.gov.

Paul A. Johnson
Monique Laberge, PhD

Doxycycline **see Tetracyclines**

Draw-A-Person test

Used to measure nonverbal **intelligence** or to screen for emotional or behavioral disorders.

Based on children's **drawings** of human figures, this test can be used with two different scoring systems for different purposes. One measures nonverbal intelligence while the other screens for emotional or behavioral disorders. Drawings obtained from a child during a single administration may be used with both systems. During the testing session, which can be completed in 15 minutes, the child is asked to draw three figures—a man, a woman, and him- or herself. Draw a Person:QSS (Quantitative Scoring System) assesses intellectual ability by analyzing 14 different aspects of the drawings, such as specific body parts and clothing, for various criteria, including presence or absence, detail, and proportion. In all, there are 64 scoring items for each drawing. A separate standard score is recorded for each one, and a total score for all three. The use of a nonverbal, nonthreatening task to evaluate intelligence is intended to eliminate possible sources of bias by reducing variables like primary language, verbal skills, communication disabilities, and sensitivity to working under pressure. However, test results can be influenced by previous drawing experience, a factor that may account for the tendency of middle-class children to score higher on this test than lower-class children, who often have fewer opportunities to draw. Draw a Person: SPED (Screening Procedure for Emotional Disturbance) uses the test's figure drawings as a means of identifying emotional problems. The scoring system is composed of two types of criteria. For the first type, eight dimensions of each drawing are evaluated against norms for the child's age group. For the second type, 47 different items are considered for each drawing.

Resources

BOOKS

Chandler, Louis A., and Virginia J. Johnson. *Using Projective Techniques with Children: A Guide to Clinical Assessment.* Springfield, IL: C.C. Thomas, 1991.

Mortensen, Karen Vibeke. *Form and Content in Children's Human Figure Drawings: Development, Sex Differences, and Body Experience.* New York: New York University Press, 1991.

Wortham, Sue Clark. *Tests and Measurement in Early Childhood Education.* Columbus: Merrill Publishing Co., 1990.

Drawings

Definition

Humans have expressed themselves with symbols throughout history. Drawing, or making two-dimensional representations of objects or abstract ideas, is one of the oldest forms of self-expression.

Purpose

People draw for both enjoyment and as a means of individual expression. When used by a trained art therapist, drawing can reveal emotions and help in healing.

Description

Instruction in the technique and interpretation of drawing is a component of the curriculum in many schools. In addition, classroom teachers can employ drawing as one component of activities designed to allow students to develop skills of reflection and expression. Narrative drawings can be incorporated into writing lessons, or used independently to strengthen skills of observation and description. Drawings are also effective tools of communication for students with limited verbal and written communication. Art instruction also helps develop **fine motor skills**.

Drawings can help a psychologist determine a child's personality characteristics. A number of tests, such as **Draw-A-Person Test**, and **Goodenough-Harris Drawing Test**, are based on the notion that the ability to accurately draw human figures is one nonverbal measure of **intelligence**.

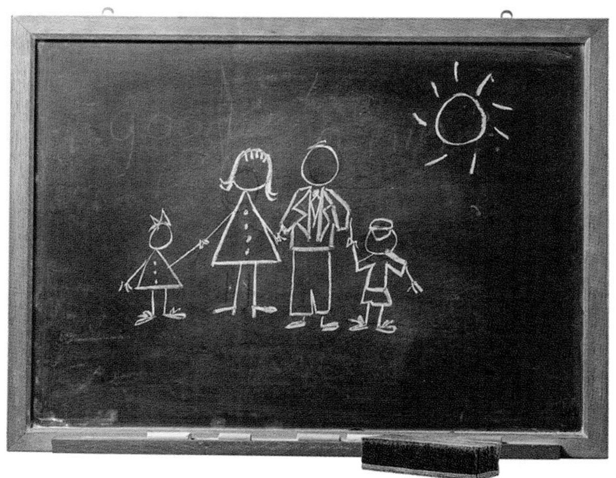

Drawing by a young child depicting a family. *(© Lawrence Manning/Corbis.)*

KEY TERMS

Art therapy—A type of psychotherapy that encourages people to express and understand emotions through artistic expression and through the creative process.

Art therapy

For individuals with behavior or **personality disorders**, art therapy is one of the tools available to explore and treat the symptoms and causes of the disorder. Margaret Naumburg was a follower of both Freud and Jung, and incorporated art into psychotherapy as a means for her clients to visualize and recognize the unconscious. She founded the Walden School in 1915, where she used students' artworks in psychological counseling. She published extensively on the subject and taught seminars on the technique at New York University in the 1950s. She is considered the founder of art therapy in the United States.

Art therapy is based on the assumption that visual symbols and images are the most accessible and natural form of communication to the human experience. Clients are encouraged to visualize, and then create, the thoughts and emotions that they cannot talk about. The resulting artwork is then reviewed and its meaning interpreted by the client. Ideally, art therapy provides the client-artist with critical insight into emotions, thoughts, and feelings.

Art therapy often is one aspect of a psychiatric inpatient or outpatient treatment program and can take place in individual or group therapy sessions. It frequently is employed in the treatment of **eating disorders**, in coping with chronic illness or long-term hospitalization and in the education of autistic children. Group art therapy sessions often take place in hospital, clinic, shelter, and community program settings. These group therapy sessions can have the added benefits of positive social interaction, empathy, and support from peers. The client-artist can learn that others have similar concerns and issues.

Resources

BOOKS

Buchalter, Susan I. *Art Therapy Techniques and Applications.* Philadelphia: Jessica Kingsley, 2009.

Rubin, Judith A. *Introduction to Art Therapy: Sources and Resources.* New York: Brunner-Routledge, 2009.

Wadeson, Harriet. *Art Psychotherapy,* 2nd ed. Hoboken, NJ: John Wiley and Sons, 2010.

PERIODICALS

Dyer, Geraldine, and Hunter, Ernest. "Creative Recovery: Art for Mental Health's Sake." *Australasian Psychiatry,* 17S, no. 1 (August 2009): S146–50.

Kropf, Aleisha. "The Transforming Power of Art." *American Journal of Public Health* 99, no. 5 (May 2009): 778.

ORGANIZATIONS

American Art Therapy Association, 225 North Fairfax Street, Alexandra VA, 22314, (703) 548-5860, (888) 290-0878, (703) 783-8468, www.arttherapy.org.

Art Therapy Credentials Board, 3 Terrace Way, Greensboro NC, 27403, (336) 482-2856, (877) 213-2822, (336) 482-2852, atcb@nbcc.org, www.atcb.org.

Tish Davidson, AM

Drowning **see Near-drowning**

Drug abuse **see Substance abuse and dependence**

KEY TERMS

Booster immunization—An additional dose of a vaccine to maintain immunity to the disease.

Encephalopathy—Any abnormality in the structure or function of brain tissues.

Larynx—Also known as the voice box, the larynx is the part of the airway that lies between the pharynx and the trachea. It is composed of cartilage that contains the apparatus for voice production—the vocal cords and the muscles and ligaments that move the cords.

Toxin—A poisonous substance usually produced by a microorganism or plant.

DTaP vaccine

Definition

DTaP vaccine confers immunity to **diphtheria**, **tetanus**, and **pertussis**. DTaP replaced an earlier vaccine known as DTP (also called DPT or DTwP) in the United States in 1991. DTaP contains multiple diphtheria and tetanus toxoids combined with acellular pertussis. The original vaccine, which is still used in some parts of the world, contains whole cells of *Bordatella pertussis*, the organism that causes pertussis, better known as **whooping cough**. Both vaccines are equally effective in stimulating immunity, but DTaP has reduced side effects by as much as 90%.

Purpose

Diphtheria and tetanus toxoids and acellular pertussis, taken together, provides immunity against diphtheria, tetanus, and whooping **cough**. The vaccine is normally given to children somewhere between the ages of two months and seven years of age (prior to their seventh birthday). Because these diseases can pose a severe problem in early childhood, the shots should be given as early in life as possible.

Description

DTaP vaccine conveys immunity to three different infectious diseases:

- Diphtheria is a potentially fatal disease that usually involves the nose, throat, and air passages, but may also infect the skin. It can result in heart and nervous system complications. The most striking feature of diphtheria is the formation of a grayish membrane covering the tonsils and upper part of the throat. It is caused by the bacterium *Corynebacterium diphtheriae*. Routine vaccination has almost eradicated diphtheria from the United States, but it is still seen in many parts of the world.
- Tetanus, sometimes called lockjaw, is a disease caused by the toxin of *Clostridium tetani*. The disease affects the central nervous system and causes painful muscle contractions. Food is not given by mouth to those with muscle spasm but may be given via nasogastric tube or intravenously. Tetanus is often fatal.
- Pertussis, also called whooping cough, is a respiratory disease caused by *Bordatella pertussis*. The name comes from a typical cough which starts with a deep inhalation, followed by a series of quick, short coughs that continues until the air is expelled from the lungs, and ends with a long shrill, whooping inhalation. Pertussis is very contagious and usually affects young children.

Recommended dosage

DTaP is given in a series of five doses. Usually, the doses are given at two, four, and six months of age, at 15–18 months of age and at four to six years. The vaccine is not approved for people over age seven years. Individuals ages 11–64 years should receive one booster shot of another vaccine Tdap, which is similar to DTaP. After that, every 10 years, adults should receive a Td **vaccination** that protects against tetanus and diphtheria. They should not receive additional injections of DTaP or Tdap. Children and adults who have missed the early childhood DTaP injections should consult their physician about a special catch–up immunization schedule.

Pre–term infants should be vaccinated according to their chronological age from **birth**. Interruption of the recommended schedule with a delay between doses should not interfere with the final immunity achieved. There is no need to start the series over again, regardless of the time between doses.

Precautions

DTaP vaccine should not be given to children seven years of age or older. Moreover, children who are allergic to any component of the vaccine should not receive the drug. Because there are several different brands on the market, some children may be allergic to one brand and not to another. Because some of the bacterial cultures are grown in beef broth, the injections may be inadvisable for children who are allergic to beef. Children who have an allergic reaction after the first shot should be referred to an allergist before continuing with the DTaP injections. Children who within a week after vaccination develop encephalopathy that cannot be traced to any other cause should not receive further injections. These children may be treated with DT (diphtheria–tetanus) vaccine. Also, DTaP vaccine should be used with caution in patients who are receiving anticoagulant therapy. If a patient with a history of fevers and febrile convulsions is to be given DTaP, the patient should receive **acetaminophen** at the time of the injection and for the following 24 hours. Children with only minor illness (e.g., a cold but no **fever**) can be vaccinated. Children who are more seriously ill or have a fever should wait until they are well to be vaccinated.

Side effects

Older DTP vaccine has been associated with severe allergic reactions, seizures, and encephalopathy at the rate of about one per 140,000 children. These reactions are still possible with DTaP, but are extremely rare and are estimated to occur in less than one per 1,000,000 children. The most serious risk of DTaP vaccine is a severe allergic reaction. Unpleasant side effects are more likely to occur as the series of shots progresses, with a greater likelihood of adverse effects after the fourth or fifth shot. Giving a child dose of acetaminophen (Tylenol) before the injection may help reduce common side effects. Mild side effects include:

- irritability (about 66% of children)
- redness, irritation, and itching at injection site (about 25% of children)
- fever (about 25% of children)
- loss of appetite about 10% of children)
- vomiting (about 2% of children)

Interactions

Because DTaP vaccine is injected deep into the muscle, it should be given with care to patients receiving anticoagulant therapy. Also, immunosuppressant drugs, including **steroids** and **cancer** drugs, may reduce the ability of the body to produce antibodies in response to DTaP vaccine.

Resources

BOOKS

Sears, Robert. *The Vaccine Book: Making The Right Decision for Your Child.* New York: Little, Brown, 2007.

OTHER

"Diphtheria, Tetanus & Pertussis Vaccines: What You Need to Know." United States Centers for Disease Control and Protection (CDC). (May 17, 2007) http://www.cdc.gov/vaccines/pubs/vis/downloads/vis-dtap.pdf (accessed September 17, 2010).

"DTaP Immunization (Vaccine)." MedlinePlus. (June 17, 2008) http://www.nlm.nih.gov/medlineplus/ency/article/002021.htm (accessed September 17, 2010).

"Vaccines." United States Centers for Disease Control and Prevention (CDC). (March 30, 2010) http://www.cdc.gov/vaccines (accessed September 17, 2010).

ORGANIZATIONS

American Academy of Family Physicians (AAFP), PO Box 11210, Shawnee Mission KS, 66207, (913) 906–6000, (800) 274–2237, (913) 906–6075, http://familydoctor.org

American Academy of Pediatrics (AAP), 141 Northwest Point Blvd., Elk Grove Village IL, 60007–1098, (847) 434–4000, (847) 434–8000, http://www.aap.org

Centers for Disease Control and Prevention (CDC), 1600 Clifton Rd., Atlanta GA, 30333, (404) 639–3534, (800) CDC–INFO (800–232–4636). TTY: (888) 232–6348, inquiry@cdc.gov http://www.cdc.gov

World Health Organization (WHO), Avenue Appia 20, 1211 Geneva 27 Switzerland, +22 41 791 21 11, +22 41 791 31 11, info@who.int, http://www.who.int

Samuel Uretsky, PharmD
Tish Davidson, AM

Duodenal obstruction

Definition

Duodenal obstruction is a failure of food to pass out of the stomach either from a complete or partial obstruction.

Description

The duodenum is the first part of the intestine, into which the stomach, the gall bladder, and the pancreas empty their contents. The pylorus connects the duodenum with the stomach and contains the valve that regulates stomach emptying. Obstruction usually occurs right at this outlet, so that the gall bladder and pancreas are unable to drain their secretions without hindrance.

Causes and symptoms

Obstruction of the duodenum occurs in adults and infants, each for a different set of reasons. In adults, the usual cause is a peptic ulcer of such antiquity that repeated cycles of injury and scarring have narrowed the passageway. Medical treatment of ulcers has progressed to the point where such obstinate ulcer disease is rarely seen any more. In infants, the conditions are congenital—either the channel is underdeveloped or the pylorus is overdeveloped. The first type is called duodenal hypoplasia and the second is termed hypertrophic pyloric stenosis. In rare cases, the channel may be missing altogether, a condition called duodenal atresia. To say that these anomalies are congenital is not to say their cause is understood. As with most **birth defects**, the specific cause is not known.

Food that cannot exit the stomach in the forward direction will return whence it came. **Vomiting** is the constant symptom of duodenal obstruction. It may be preceded by indigestion and nausea as the stomach attempts to squeeze its contents through an ever narrowing outlet.

Hypertrophic pyloric stenosis appears soon after **birth**. The infant will vomit feedings, lose weight, and be restless and irritable.

Diagnosis

X rays taken with contrast material in the stomach readily demonstrate the site of the blockage and often the ulcer that caused it. Gastroscopy is another way to evaluate the problem. In infants, x rays may not be necessary to detect pyloric stenosis. It is often possible to feel the enlarged pylorus, like an olive, deep under the ribs and see the stomach rippling as it labors to force food through.

KEY TERMS

Atresia—Failure to develop; complete absence.

Contrast agent—A substance that produces shadows on an x ray so that hollow structures can be more easily seen.

Gastroscopy—Looking into the stomach with a flexible viewing instrument called a gastroscope.

Hypoplasia—Incomplete development.

Peptic ulcer—A wound in the lower stomach and duodenum caused by stomach acid and a newly discovered germ called *Helicobacter pylori.*

Treatment

Bowel obstruction requires a surgeon, sometimes immediately. Newer surgical techniques constantly improve the outcome, but obstruction is a mechanical problem that needs a mechanical solution. Most adults who come to surgery for obstruction have suffered for years from peptic ulcer disease. They will usually benefit from ulcer surgery at the same time their obstruction is relieved. The surgeon will therefore select a procedure that combines relief of obstruction with remedy for ulcer disease. There are many choices. In fact, even without obstruction, functional considerations require ulcer surgery to include enhancement of stomach emptying.

To treat an infant with hypertrophic pyloric stenosis, some surgeons have had success with forceful balloon dilation of the pylorus done through a gastroscope, but the standard procedure is to cut across the overdeveloped circular muscle that is constricting the stomach outlet. There are reports of infant hypertrophic pyloric stenosis remitting without surgery following a very careful feeding schedule, but mortality is unacceptably high.

Prognosis

A functioning and unrestricted intestine is a prerequisite for living independent of the most advanced and continuous medical care available. Achieving this desirable goal is the rule with surgery for duodenal obstructions of all types. The bowel is so malleable that there is a rearrangement to suit every occasion. The variety of possible configurations is limited only by the surgeon's imagination.

Prevention

Prompt and effective treatment of peptic ulcers will prevent chronic scarring and narrowing. Drugs developed over the past few decades have all but eliminated the need for ulcer surgery.

Resources

BOOKS

Redel, Carol A., and R. Jeff Zeiwner. "Anatomy and Anomalies of the Stomach and Duodenum." In *Sleisenger & Fordtran's Gastrointestinal and Liver Disease*, edited by Mark Feldman, et al. Philadelphia: W. B. Saunders Co., 1997.

J. Ricker Polsdorfer, MD

Dwarfism

Definition

While dwarfism is sometimes used specifically to describe achondroplasia, a condition characterized by short stature and disproportionately short arms and legs, it is also used more broadly to refer to a variety of conditions resulting in unusually short stature in both children and adults. In some cases, physical development may be disproportionate, as in achondroplasia, but in others the parts of the body develop proportionately. Short stature may be unaccompanied by other symptoms, or it may occur together with other problems, both physical and mental. Adult males under 5 ft (1.5 m) tall and females under 4 ft 8 in (1.4 m) are classified as short-statured. Children are considered unusually short if they fall below the third percentile of height for their age group.

Dwarfism has many causes, and parents of average height can give **birth** to a child who is a dwarf. Some prenatal factors known to contribute to growth retardation include a variety of maternal health problems, including toxemia, kidney and heart disease, infections such as **rubella**, and maternal **malnutrition**. Maternal age is also a factor (adolescent mothers are prone to have undersize babies), as is uterine constraint (which occurs when the uterus is too small for the baby). Possible causes that center on the fetus rather than the mother include chromosomal abnormalities, genetic and other syndromes that impair skeletal growth, and defects of the placenta or umbilical cord. Environmental factors that influence intrauterine growth include maternal use of drugs (including alcohol and tobacco). Some infants who are small at birth (especially **twins**) may attain normal stature within the first year of life, while others remain small throughout their lives.

The four most common causes of dwarfism in children are achondroplasia, **Turner syndrome**, inadequate pituitary function, and lack of emotional or physical nurturance. Achondroplasia (short-limbed dwarfism) is a genetic disorder that impairs embryonic development, resulting in abnormalities in bone growth and cartilage development. It is one of a class of illnesses called chondrodystrophies, all of which involve cartilage abnormalities and result in short stature. In achondroplasia, the long bones fail to develop normally, making the arms and legs disproportionately short and stubby (and sometimes curved). Overly long fibulae (one of two bones in the lower leg) cause the bowlegs that are characteristic of the condition. In addition, the head is disproportionately large and the bridge of the nose is depressed. Persons with achondroplasia are between 3–5 ft

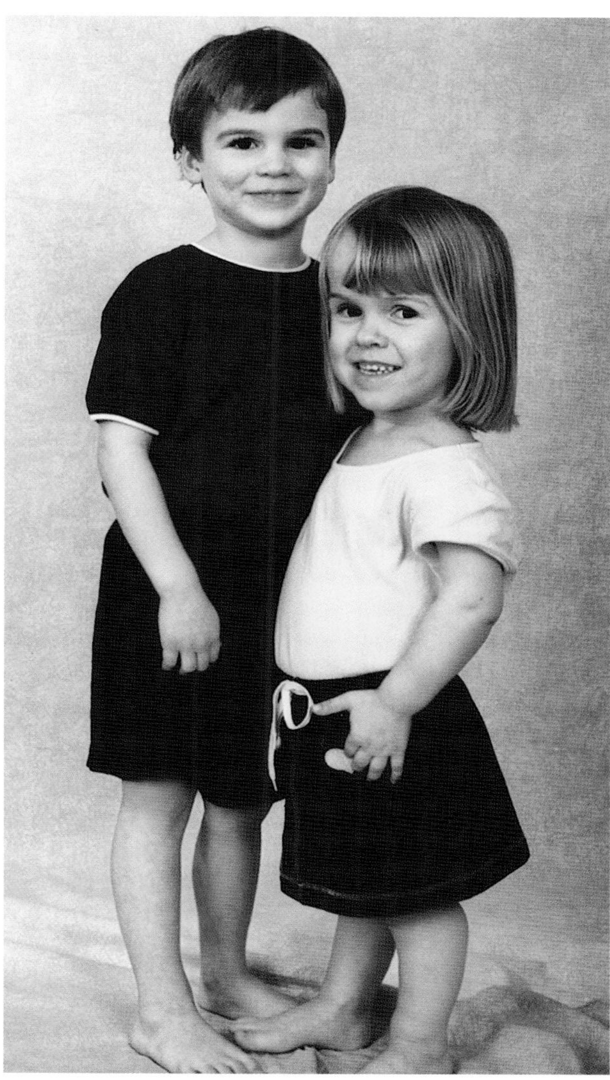

Young female dwarf standing next to a boy of normal stature. *(Courtesy of Dr. Richard Pauli/U. of Wisconsin, Madison, Clinical Genetics Center. Reproduced by permission.)*

(91–152 cm) tall and of normal **intelligence**. Their reproductive development is normal, and they have greater than normal muscular strength. The condition occurs in 1 out of every 10,000 births, and its prevalence increases with the age of the parents, especially the father. Achondroplasia can be detected through prenatal screening. Many infants with the condition are stillborn.

Turner syndrome is a chromosomal abnormality occurring only in females in whom one of the X chromosomes is missing or defective. Girls with Turner syndrome are usually between 4.5–5 ft (137–152 cm) high. Their ovaries are undeveloped, and they do not undergo **puberty**. Besides short stature, other physical characteristics include a stocky build and a webbed neck.

Endocrine and metabolic disorders are another important cause of growth problems. Growth can be impaired by conditions affecting the pituitary, thyroid, parathyroid, and adrenal glands (all part of the endocrine system). Probably the best known of these conditions is growth hormone (GH) deficiency, which is associated with the pituitary and hypothalamus glands. If the deficiency begins before birth, the baby will still be of normal size and weight at birth but will then experience slowed growth. Weight gain still tends to be normal, leading to overweight and a higher than average proportion of body fat. The facial structures of children with this condition are immature, making them look younger than their actual age. Adults in whom growth hormone deficiency has not been treated attain a height of only about 2.5 ft (76 cm). They also have high-pitched voices, high foreheads, and wrinkled skin. Another endocrine disorder that can interfere with growth is **hypothyroidism**, a condition resulting from insufficient activity of the thyroid gland. Hypothyroidism can have a variety of causes, including underdevelopment, absence, or removal of the thyroid gland, lack of an enzyme needed for adequate thyroid function, iodine deficiency, or an underactive pituitary gland. In addition to retarding growth, it can cause **mental retardation** if thyroid hormones are not administered in the first months of an infant's life. If the condition goes untreated, it causes impaired mental development in 50% of affected children by the age of six months.

About 15% of short stature in children is caused by chronic diseases, of which endocrine disorders are only one type. Many of these conditions do not appear until after the fifth year of life. Children with renal disease often experience growth retardation, especially if the condition is congenital. **Congenital heart disease** can cause slow growth, either directly or through secondary problems. Short stature can also result from a variety of conditions related to inadequate **nutrition**, including malabsorption syndromes (in which the body is lacking a substance—often an enzyme—necessary for proper absorption of an important nutrient), chronic inflammatory **bowel disorders**, caloric deficiencies, and zinc deficiency.

A form of severe malnutrition called marasmus retards growth in all parts of the body, including the head and causes mental as well as physical retardation. Marasmus can be caused by being weaned very early and not adequately fed afterwards; if the intake of calories and protein is limited severely enough, the body wastes away. Although the mental and emotional effects of the condition can be reversed with changes in environment, the growth retardation it causes is permanent. On occasion, growth retardation may also be caused solely by emotional deprivation.

Since growth problems are so varied, there is a wide variety of treatments for them, including nutritional changes, medications to treat underlying conditions, and, where appropriate, hormone replacement therapy. Growth hormone for therapeutic purposes was originally derived from the pituitary glands of deceased persons. However, natural growth hormone, aside from being prohibitively expensive, posed health hazards due to contamination. In the 1980s, men who had received growth hormone therapy in childhood were found to have developed Kreuzfeldt-Jakob disease, a fatal neurological disorder. Since then, natural growth hormone has been replaced by a biosynthetic hormone that received FDA approval in 1985.

Resources

BOOKS

Hall, Judith G. *Dwarfism: Medical and Psychosocial Aspects of Profound Short Stature.* Baltimore, MD: Johns Hopkins University Press, 2005.

Jorgensen, Jens Otto Lunde, and Jens Sandahl Christiansen., eds. *Growth Hormone Deficiency in Adults.* New York: Karger, 2005.

OTHER

Kemp, Stephen. "Growth Hormone Deficiency." eMedicine.com, April 19, 2006, http://www.emedicine.com/ped/topic1810.htm.

Park, Joo-Hee Grace and Robert Wallerstein. "Achondroplasia." eMedicine.com, April 4, 2006, http://www.emedicine.com/ped/topic12.htm.

P. M. Medical Health News. *21st Century Complete Medical Guide to Dwarfism, Authoritative Government Documents, Clinical References, and Practical Information for Patients and Physicians (CD-ROM).* Progressive Management, 2004.

Sirotnak, Andrew P. "Child Abuse & Neglect: Psychosocial Dwarfism." eMedicine.com, March 1, 2006, http://www.emedicine.com/ped/topic566.htm.

ORGANIZATIONS

Human Growth Foundation, 7777 Leesburg Pike (PO Box 309), Falls Church VA, 22043, (703) 883-1773, (703) 883-1776 (800) 451-6434, http://www.hgfound.org.

Little People of America, P.O. Box 745, Lubbock TX, 79408, (806) 737-8186, (888) LPA-2001, lpadatabase@juno.com, http://www.lpaonline.org.

Parents of Dwarfed Children, 11524 Colt Terrace, Silver Spring MD, 20902, (301) 649-3275

Short Stature Foundation and Information Center, 17200J Jamboree Rd., Suite J, Irvine CA, 92714-5828, (714) 474-4554, (714) 261-9035

Tish Davidson, AM

Dyslexia

Definition

Dyslexia is a learning disability noted for spatial reversals and shifts. It is characterized by problems in reading, spelling, writing, and sometimes math. In many cases, dyslexia appears to be inherited.

Demographics

Estimates of people with dyslexia range from 2–15% of the United States population. Most research studies give a figure of 5%. Originally it was thought that dyslexia affected more boys than girls (in a ratio of 5:1), but later studies found boys to be only slightly more likely than girls to be dyslexic. Figures for diagnosed child dyslexics are skewed because for various reasons boys tend to be referred more frequently for **special education**. Diagnosis is complicated by the fact that anywhere from 20–55% of dyslexics also suffer from attention deficit/hyperactivity disorder (**ADHD**), a behavioral disorder that may aggravate reading problems.

The owl was a bird.
Teh owl saw a K brid.
The owl was

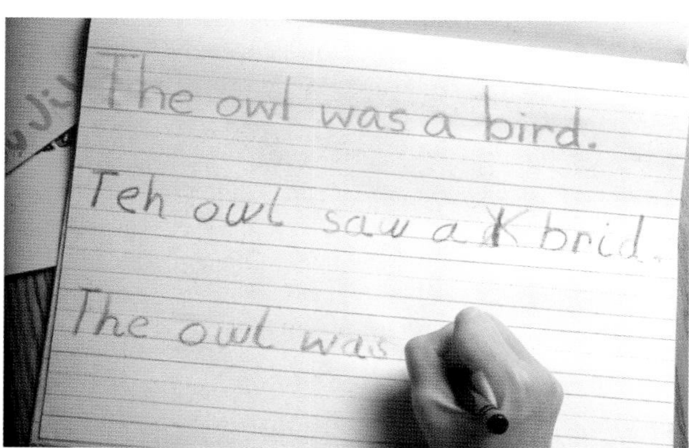

A student with dyslexia has difficulty copying words. *(Will & Deni McIntyre/Science Source/Photo Researchers, Inc.)*

Description

Dyslexia is a specific learning disability characterized by a significant disparity between an individual's general **intelligence** and his or her language skills, usually reflected in school performance. The word dyslexia is derived from the Greek word, *dys* (meaning poor or inadequate) and the word *lexis* (meaning words or language). The term was coined in 1887 by German physician Rudolf Berlin who published a case study of a young boy who had difficulties with reading and writing in spite of having normal intelligence. In 1896, W. Pringle Morgan, a British doctor, published the first English-language case study of dyslexia. It concerned a 14-year-old boy who had not yet learned to read, even though his other intellectual abilities were well within the normal range.

Most individuals with dyslexia have average or above average intelligence, and it is speculated that they have heightened visual-spatial and motor awareness. Many famous inventors, artists, and other creative people have had dyslexia; Thomas Edison, Albert Einstein, Winston Churchill, Michael Faraday, Woodrow Wilson, Guglielmo Marconi, General George Patton, and Auguste Rodin are all thought to have been dyslexic.

Risk factors

Dyslexia is believed to be strongly familial. About 40% of boys and 20% of girls with a dyslexic parent develop the disorder. Dyslexia is believed to occur equally in all races.

Causes and symptoms

There are many different theories about the causes and classifications of different types of dyslexia, but few hard conclusions. It is generally agreed that there is a strong hereditary component of dyslexia. Several genetic studies have found gene linkages on chromosomes 1 and 6 that demonstrate heterogeneous (multiple methods of) transmission. As of 2009, four specific genes linked to dyslexia have been identified, and all four participate in brain development. Positron emission tomography (PET) studies have shown that dyslexics assigned reading tasks show a lower level of activity than children with normal reading skills in a part of the brain known as the left inferior parietal cortex, a region that is necessary for the rapid perception of word forms. Studies using functional **magnetic resonance imaging** (fMRI) pinpointed the left inferior frontal gyrus, the left inferior parietal lobule, and the left middle temporal gyrus as areas of low activation in dyslexic children given word tests to complete. Another indication that specific areas of the brain are involved in dyslexia comes from case studies of children who have suffered **stroke**. In one study reported in 2006, a six-year-old boy had suffered a stroke affecting the left hemisphere of his brain. He was able to read words that he had learned prior to the stroke, but attempts to read unfamiliar words were unsuccessful until he received special training.

The most obvious symptoms of the dyslexic show up in reading and writing; however, listening, speaking, and general organizational skills are also affected. The individual with dyslexia may have trouble transferring information across modalities, for example from verbal to written forms. The dyslexic's characteristic reversal of letters, confusion between such similar letters as "b" and "d," omission of words when reading aloud, trouble sounding out words, and difficulty following written instructions were first thought to be the result of vision and perceptual problems—that is, a failure of taking in the stimulus. Only a small percentage of dyslexics have vision disorders, however, and it is now generally agreed by physicians, researchers, and educators that dyslexia is primarily a **language disorder**. Whereas the non-dyslexic intuitively learns phonic (sound) rules while **learning to read**, the dyslexic needs specific and methodical drills and practice to learn the visual-auditory associations necessary for reading comprehension and written expression.

The most common symptoms of dyslexia include:

- lack of awareness of sounds
- delayed speech
- difficulty understanding spoken words
- difficulty reading single words
- extreme difficulty spelling words
- extreme difficulty with handwriting
- difficulty with locational and time indicators: up/down, right/left, yesterday/tomorrow
- lack of enjoyment in reading
- difficulty transferring information across modalities: writing down thoughts or speech, reading out loud

Diagnosis

Anyone who is suspected to have dyslexia should have a comprehensive evaluation, including hearing, vision, and intelligence testing. The test should include all areas of learning and learning processes, not just reading.

Currently, children and adults are usually referred for testing for dyslexia because of repeated problems in school or work settings. As further research pinpoints the genes responsible for some cases of dyslexia, there is a possibility that earlier testing will be established to allow for early interventions. Earlier interventions could help to prevent the negative educational outcomes that can be associated with dyslexia.

Tests

Children who demonstrate a reading level greater than two SEs below expected level for their age, intelligence, and education are generally diagnosed as dyslexic. Once reading problems are identified, a comprehensive series of tests of neuropsychological function (vision, hearing, and speech), intelligence, and achievement (word and letter recognition) will determine the existence of visual and auditory problems, behavior problems, or subnormal intelligence, all of which may have symptoms similar to dyslexia. Because children of different ages have different levels of normal language skill, the specific tests used will differ by age group.

A child normally develops phonological awareness—the ability to differentiate between speech sounds and recognize their written symbols—while learning to read. The ability to sound out nonsense words (for example, the lines from Lewis Carroll's poem "Jabberwocky": "Twas brillig and the slithy toves/ Did gyre and gimble in the wabe") is a strong indicator of phonological awareness. In cases in which the dyslexic has compensated for the disability by paying special attention to context or simply by rote memorization, a nonsense-word test may reveal the reader's underlying phonological disability despite his academic success.

While teachers and physicians are trained to recognize some language problems, many symptoms of dyslexia will be noticeable to parents. Contrary to popular thought, a child's mirror writing (writing backwards), reversal of letters, and confusion over which hand to use are not definitively signs of dyslexia, and may only indicate lack of development.

Treatment

If caught early, especially before the third grade, dyslexia is highly treatable through special education. Dyslexia is categorized as a learning disability under the national **Education for All Handicapped Children Act** passed in 1975. Dyslexic children are entitled to a comprehensive evaluation by a team of educational specialists, to an individualized education plan (IEP), and to ongoing evaluation under the terms of the federal Individuals with Disabilities Education Act (IDEA), first passed in 1990 and amended in 2004. Parents or caretakers may request the initial evaluation, may participate in all levels of the process, and must give their consent before the treatment plan begins.

Traditional

There are many treatment approaches available to the public, ranging from visual stimulation to diets to enhancement of regular language education. But it is generally agreed that specialized education is the only successful remedy, and the American Academy of Ophthalmology, the **American Academy of Pediatrics**, and the American Association for Pediatric Ophthalmology and **Strabismus** have issued a policy statement warning against visual treatments and recommending a cross-disciplinary educational approach. In fact, the first researcher to identify and study dyslexia, Dr. Samuel Torrey Orton, developed the core principles of such an approach in the 1920s. The work of three of his followers—Bessie Stillman, Anna Gillingham, and Beth Slingerland—underlies many of the programs in wide use today such as project READ, the Wilson Reading System, and programs based on the Herman method. These and other successful programs have three characteristics in common. They are:

- (1) Sound/symbol based. They break words down into their smallest visual components: letters and the sounds associated with them.
- (2) Multisensory. They attempt to form and strengthen mental associations among visual, auditory, and kinesthetic channels of stimulation. The student simultaneously sees, feels, and says the sound-symbol association; for example, a child may trace the letter or letter combination with his finger while pronouncing a word out loud.
- (3) Highly structured. Remediation begins at the level of the single letter-sound, works up to digraphs, then syllables, then into words and sentences in a very systematic fashion. Repetitive drill and practice serve to form necessary sound-symbol associations.

Whatever remediation program is used, the IEP itself should define the student's specific problems and learning objectives, rather than make vague or general recommendations such as "John needs more support in reading comprehension." A good example of a specific learning objective would be "Max will be able to identify the following sound/symbol association in nonsense words: consonants, short and long vowels, and blends." When ADD is co-diagnosed with dyslexia, special care should be taken to identify specific reading problems and to define cognitive as well as behavioral learning objectives.

Drugs

Treatment for dyslexia can sometimes include use of anti-motion drugs, addressing the symptoms of balance and coordination which results from visual perception alterations; stimulant drugs, such as pemoline (Cylert) or **methylphenidate** (Ritalin), to address symptoms of low self esteem, restlessness, and distractibility, and 'nootropics' drugs, a class of drugs believed to improve cognitive function. The stimulant drugs may be more effective for **learning disorders** related to ADHD or ADD than for dyslexia. The drug piracetam (Nootropil), a nootropic, although reported as a possible treatment for dyslexia, is also reported to have legal issues because it has not been approved for use in the United States by the Food and Drug Administration (FDA).

Reported potential side effects of the stimulants include nervousness and insomnia, and are contraindicated with **epilepsy**, **allergies**, blood pressure problems, or with use of monoamine oxidase (MAO) inhibitors. Long-term use of stimulants in children are reported to adversely affect growth, may ironically depress the nervous system or lead to loss of consciousness. By reducing natural levels of stimulants in the brain, they may also cause dependence. The stimulants and nootropics are said to increase the effects of alcohol and amphetamines. Other possible interactions include use of anti-convulsants or anti-epileptics; tricyclic anti-depressants; anti-coagulants, like Coumadin; and "atropine-like drugs" that blocks the neurotransmitter acetylcholine.

Alternative

Ronald D. Davis, writing in *The Gift of Dyslexia* outlines an alternative and complementary treatment consistent with the "moving point of view" model. According to this model, and the reason why letters seem to change shape and float, why lines of print appear to move, and why words appear to be other than they are is that the dyslexic individual sees the world predominantly through his or her "mind's eye," rather than through his or her physiologic eye. In other words, people with dyslexia more than all others, sees what they 'think' they see, rather than what their eyeballs see. To further complicate matters, they do this so quickly that they easily become confused when the multiple facets do not produce a solid view.

The object of treatment proposed by Ronald Davis, a dyslexic individual himself, is to train the mind's eye to return to a learned, anchored, viewpoint when they realize they are seeing with their mind, and not with their eyeballs. This is accomplished with **assessment** testing, followed by one-on-one exercises that retrain mental perception pathways. Using the gifts of the dyslexic individual—their imagination and curiosity—these exercises involve creative physical activities, including the use of modeling clay, "koosh" balls, and movement training. Davis founded the Reading Research Council's Dyslexia Correction Center in 1982, and the Davis Dyslexia Association International, which trains educators and therapists, in 1995.

KEY TERMS

Attention deficit disorder (ADD)—A learning disability characterized by an inability to pay attention. It may be different from dyslexia in that dyslexic individuals are highly aware and able to pay attention, but unable to make sense of their perceptions.

Attention deficit hyperactivity disorder (ADHD)—A learning disability characterized by an inability to sit still or concentrate well. It has been demonstrated to be diagnostically different from dyslexia by speech and vocalization patterns.

Monoamine oxidase (MAO) inhibitors—A group of anti-depressant drugs.

Neurotransmitter—A chemical substance which facilitates the passing of messages along nerve pathways. There are several different neurotransmitters used in the human nervous system, each with distinct effects on mood, movement and perception.

Point of view—In a person with dyslexia, this term is used to describe the angle from which their mind's eye views an object. This point of view may be unanchored and moving about, as if several different people were telling what they see all at the same time.

Prognosis

If left unaddressed, a person with dyslexia may become "functionally illiterate," able to function limited by their ability to read, spell, have their handwriting understood, or do arithmetic. Recognizing that dyslexia is a developed learning disorder affecting people of extraordinary curiosity, imagination and intelligence—people of genius, often—from a productive or functional point of view, dyslexia may contribute significantly, positively or negatively, to performance levels. From an emotional or psychological point of view, dyslexia affects self esteem, and promotes confusion and frustration, that may contribute to under achievement.

Many people with dyslexia becoming very successful. The eventual outcome for an individual with dyslexia depends on a wide variety of factors, including severity of the disorder, age of diagnosis, and achievement level in other non-language areas. Early diagnosis and intervention are important in improving long-term outcomes.

Prevention

There is no known way to prevent dyslexia.

Resources

BOOKS

Berninger, Virginia W., and Beverly Wolf. *Teaching Students with Dyslexia and Dysgraphia: Lessons From Teaching and Science.* Baltimore: Paul H. Brooks Publishing, 2009.

Brunswick, Nicola. *Dyslexia: A Beginner's Guide.* Oxford: Oneworld, 2009.

Pugh, Ken, and Peggy McCardle, eds. *How Children Learn to Read: Current Issues and New Directions in the Integration of Cognition, Neurobiology, and Genetics of Reading and Dyslexia Research and Practice.* New York: Psychology Press, 2009.

Reid, Gavin, ed. *The Routledge Companion to Dyslexia.* New York: Routledge, 2009.

PERIODICALS

American Academy of Pediatrics, Section on Ophthalmology, Council on Children with Disabilities. American Academy of Ophthalmology. American Association for Pediatric Ophthalmology and Strabismus. American Association of Certified Orthoptists "Joint Statement-Learning Disabilities, Dyslexia, and Vision." *Pediatrics,* (August 2009): 837-844.

Gabriele, J.D. "Dyslexia: A New Synergy Between Education and Cognitive Neuroscience." *Science* (July 17, 2009): 325.

ORGANIZATIONS

Council for Learning Disabilities, 11184 Antioch Road, Box 405, Overland Park KS, 66210, (913) 491-1011, (913) 491-1012, http://www.cldinternational.org.

International Dyslexia Association, 40 York Road, 4th Floor, Baltimore MD, 21204, (410) 296-0232, (410) 321-5069, http://www.interdys.org.

Katy Nelson, ND
Tish Davidson, AM

Dysmenorrhea

Definition

Dysmenorrhea is the occurrence of painful cramps during a woman's menstrual period. The English word comes from three Greek words that mean "painful," "month," and "flow." Most women experience some discomfort during their periods; however, dysmenorrhea is diagnosed when the **pain** is so severe as to limit the woman's normal activities or require medical or surgical treatment.

Demographics

Dysmenorrhea is by definition a disorder that affects only females of childbearing age. Some studies indicate that the rate of dysmenorrhea is highest among adolescents and young adults, and declines with age.

Survey results are highly variable, ranging from 29% in one family practice setting to 90% in a group of Swedish adolescents. One group of researchers reported that 67% of teenagers in their sample reported dysmenorrhea, compared to 27% of women in their 30s. Primary dysmenorrhea is the leading cause of recurrent short-term absence from school among adolescent American girls. In the workplace, dysmenorrhea causes 600 million missed work hours in the United States each year and an economic loss of $2 billion.

Secondary dysmenorrhea is more common in older women than in teenagers; in general, women who experience dysmenorrhea for the first time after age 25 have secondary dysmenorrhea.

As far as is known as of 2010, race or ethnicity is not a risk factor for dysmenorrhea.

Description

Women with dysmenorrhea describe the pain in their abdomens as variously shooting, stabbing, burning, sharp, throbbing, or nauseating. Dysmenorrhea may precede the onset of the woman's period by several days, or accompany it. It usually subsides as the woman's flow tapers off.

In some women, dysmenorrhea is accompanied by unusually heavy blood loss—a condition known as menorrhagia.

Risk factors

The likelihood that a woman will have painful cramps increases if she:

- has a family history of painful periods
- leads a stressful life
- smokes
- has never borne a child
- is below 20 years of age
- began puberty before age 11
- has heavy periods
- doesn't get enough exercise
- drinks large quantities of beverages containing caffeine (coffee, tea, cola, energy drinks)
- has attempted to lose weight rapidly
- has pelvic inflammatory disease (PID)
- has a history of sexual abuse

Causes and symptoms

Dysmenorrhea is called "primary" when there is no specific abnormality, and "secondary" when the pain is caused by an underlying gynecological problem. It is believed that primary dysmenorrhea occurs when prostaglandins, hormone-like substances produced by uterine tissue, trigger strong muscle contractions in the uterus during **menstruation**. However, the level of prostaglandins does not seem to correlate with how strong a woman's cramps are. Some women have high levels of prostaglandins and no cramps, whereas other women with low levels have severe cramps. This is why experts assume that cramps must also be related to other causes, such as diets, genetics, stress, and different body types, in addition to prostaglandins. The first year or two

KEY TERMS

Cervix—The neck or lower narrow portion of the uterus that opens into the upper end of the vagina.

Ectopic pregnancy—A pregnancy in which the fertilized egg has implanted outside the uterus, most often in the Fallopian tubes, although in some cases the pregnancy implants in the ovary or in the abdomen. A ruptured ectopic pregnancy is a medical emergency.

Endometrioma—A type of cyst formed when endometrial tissue grows within the ovary.

Endometriosis—The growth of uterine tissue outside the uterus.

Fibroids—Benign (noncancerous) growths that arise from the smooth muscle layer and connective tissue of the uterus. They sometimes cause secondary dysmenorrhea.

Hormone—A chemical messenger secreted by a gland and released into the blood, where it travels to distant cells to exert an effect.

Hysterectomy—Surgical removal of the entire uterus.

Menorrhagia—Unusually heavy or prolonged menstrual period. It may or may not be associated with dysmenorrhea.

Ovary—One of the two almond-shaped glands in the female body that produces the hormones estrogen and progesterone.

Ovulation—The monthly release of an egg from an ovary.

Progesterone—The hormone produced by the ovary after ovulation that prepares the uterine lining for a fertilized egg.

Uterus—The female reproductive organ that contains and nourishes a fetus from implantation of the fertilized egg until birth.

of a girl's periods are not usually very painful. However, once ovulation begins, the blood levels of the prostaglandins rise, leading to stronger contractions.

Secondary dysmenorrhea may be caused by endometriosis, fibroids, ovarian cysts, an ectopic pregnancy, or an infection in the pelvis.

Symptoms of dysmenorrhea include a dull, throbbing cramping in the lower abdomen that may radiate to the lower back and thighs. In addition, some women may experience nausea and **vomiting**; **diarrhea** or **constipation**; hypersensitivity to lights, sounds, or odors; general irritability and fatigue; heavy sweating; or **dizziness**. Cramps usually last for two or three days at the beginning of each menstrual period. Many women often notice their painful periods disappear after they have their first child, probably due to the stretching of the opening of the uterus or because the **birth** improves the uterine blood supply and muscle activity, although other women do not notice a change in their level of menstrual discomfort after **childbirth**.

Diagnosis

A doctor should perform a thorough pelvic exam and take a patient history to rule out any underlying condition that could cause unusually painful cramps. The patient history will include such information as the patient's age at the time of her first period, family history of painful periods, sexual activity (if any), method of **contraception** used (if any), number of children, the regularity of the menstrual cycle, the cycle's length, date of the last menstrual period, and duration and amount of menstrual flow.

Examination

An office examination of the patient's abdomen is usually sufficient in adolescents who have not been sexually active. Women who are sexually active should have a pelvic examination.

Tests

There are no laboratory tests that can be used to diagnose primary dysmenorrhea; however, the doctor may order a blood test to rule out a systemic infection, or take a smear of the cervix to evaluate the patient for a sexually transmitted disease.

If the abdominal and pelvic examinations suggest secondary dysmenorrhea, an ultrasound of the pelvis is the next step in evaluating endometriosis or ovarian cysts as possible causes of the dysmenorrhea. Other imaging studies that can be used include CT scans and MRIs.

Procedures

The doctor may recommend either a hysteroscopy or a laparoscopy to check for such causes of secondary dysmenorrhea as fibroids, ovarian cysts, endometriosis, or an ectopic pregnancy. In a hysteroscopy, the doctor inserts a thin lighted tube called an endoscope into the uterine cavity. The doctor can remove a small sample of uterine tissue for biopsy as well as examining the interior of the uterus visually. In a laparoscopy, the doctor makes small incisions in the skin of the abdomen and inserts an endoscope with a small camera lens. Laparoscopy can also be used for surgical removal of endometriomas, which are a type of cyst formed when endometrial tissue grows inside the ovaries rather than in the uterus. In extreme cases, the doctor may recommend a hysterectomy—surgical removal of the entire uterus.

A qualified physician is required in order to fit a woman with the Mirena (an intrauterine device described below). The woman's cervix must be dilated before insertion; the process is uncomfortable, and some doctors use a local anesthetic to reduce discomfort.

Treatment

Drugs

Several over-the-counter medications can lessen or completely eliminate the pain of primary dysmenorrhea. Most popular are the **nonsteroidal anti-inflammatory drugs** (NSAIDs), which prevent or decrease the formation of prostaglandins. These include aspirin, ibuprofen (Advil), and naproxen (Aleve). For more severe pain, prescription-strength ibuprofen (Motrin) is available. These drugs are usually begun at the first sign of the period and taken for a day or two. Although NSAIDs are effective in providing short-term relief from cramps, some researchers think that long-term use of these medications increases the risk of side effects, particularly diarrhea and peptic ulcer.

If an NSAID is not available, **acetaminophen** (Tylenol) may also help ease the pain. Heat applied to the painful area may bring relief, and a warm bath twice a day also may help.

Hormonal therapy is another approach to dysmenorrhea that works for many women, although it involves prescription medications rather than over-the-counter pain relievers. Birth control pills and Depo-Provera, an injected contraceptive that must be given every three months, work by preventing ovulation. Depo-Provera is also given as a treatment for endometriosis as well as contraception.

Studies of a drug patch containing glyceryl trinitrate to treat dysmenorrhea suggest that it also may help ease pain. This drug has been used in the past to ease preterm contractions in pregnant women. One common side effect of the patch, however, is **headache**.

In 2002, an intrauterine device (IUD) was introduced to help eliminate the pain of menstrual cramps related to endometriosis. The IUD, known as Mirena, is approved for use in the United States as a contraceptive. The device works by releasing small amounts of progestin (a hormone) as well as preventing a fertilized egg from implanting in the lining of the uterus. Mirena cannot, however, be used by women with a history of **pelvic inflammatory disease**, current **gonorrhea** or chlamydia infection, or cervical or breast **cancer**.

There are two drugs that can be given to completely suppress menstrual periods—danazol (Danocrine) and leuprolide acetate (Lupron). These are generally regarded as treatments of last resort for secondary dysmenorrhea that is not helped by other medications. Both Danocrine and Lupron are expensive drugs with severe side effects.

Alternative

There are a variety of alternative therapies for dysmenorrhea. As of 2010, however, most of these have not been well studied.

NUTRITIONAL THERAPY The following dietary changes may help prevent or treat menstrual pain:

- Increased dietary intake of foods such as fiber, calcium, soy foods, fruits and vegetables.
- Decreased consumption of foods that exacerbate PMS. They include caffeine, salt and sugar.
- Quitting smoking. Smoking has been found to worsen cramps.
- Taking daily multi-vitamin and mineral supplements that contain high doses of magnesium and vitamin B_6 (pyridoxine), and flaxseed or fish oil supplements. Recent research suggests that vitamin B supplements, primarily vitamin B_6 in complex, magnesium, calcium, zinc, vitamin E, and fish oil supplements (omega-3 fatty acids) also may help relieve cramps.

HERBAL THERAPY An herbalist may recommend one of the following herbal remedies for menstrual pain:

- Chasteberry (*Vitex agnus-castus*) for women who also experience breast pain, irregular periods, and ovarian cysts.
- Dong quai (*Angelica sinensis*) for women with typical menstrual pain.
- Licorice (*Glycyrrhiza glabra*) for abdominal bloating and cramping.
- Black cohosh (*Cimifuga racemosa*) for relief of menstrual pain as well as mood swing and depression.

PHYSICAL EXERCISE Several **yoga** positions are popular as methods to ease menstrual pain. In the "cat stretch" position, the woman rests on her hands and knees, slowly arching the back. The pelvic tilt is another popular yoga position, in which the woman lies with knees bent, and then lifts the pelvis and buttocks.

Exercise may be a way to reduce the pain of menstrual cramps through the brain's production of endorphins, the body's own painkillers.

OTHER REMEDIES Acupuncture and Chinese herbs are other popular alternative treatments for cramps. There are particular formulas depending on the pattern of imbalance. Aromatherapy and massage may ease pain for some women. Transcutaneous electrical nerve stimulation (TENS) has been touted as a safe and practical way to relieve the pain of dysmenorrhea. It works by using electrodes to stimulate nerve fibers. Some women find relief through visualization, concentrating on the pain as a particular color and gaining control of the sensations. Others find that imagining a white light hovering over the painful area can actually lessen the pain for brief periods. Simply changing the position of the body can help ease cramps. The simplest technique is assuming the fetal position with knee pulled up to the chest while hugging a heating pad or pillow to the abdomen. Also, orgasm can make a woman feel more comfortable by releasing tension in the pelvic muscles.

Prognosis

Dysmenorrhea is a treatable condition with a good-to-excellent prognosis in most women. As noted above, most adolescents with primary dysmenorrhea outgrow their painful cramps as they enter their 20s and 30s. Older women with secondary dysmenorrhea usually do well after surgery to remove fibroids or endometriomas; some of these procedures can be done in outpatient surgical clinics. A complete hysterectomy is usually done as an inpatient procedure, but most women recover without complications.

Prevention

Most of the causes of secondary dysmenorrhea cannot be prevented as of 2010. However, avoidance of **caffeine**, alcohol, and sugar prior to the onset of the period, and NSAIDs taken a day before the period begins may eliminate cramps for some women with primary dysmenorrhea.

Resources

BOOKS

Emans, S. Jean Herriot, Marc R. Laufer, and Donald P. Goldstein. *Pediatric and Adolescent Gynecology*, 5th ed. Philiadelphia: Lippincott Williams and Wilkins, 2005.

Goodwin, T. Murphy, et al., eds. *Management of Common Problems in Obstetrics and Gynecology*, 5th ed. Chichester, West Sussex: Wiley-Blackwell, 2010.

Gordon, Catherine M., et al., eds. *The Menstrual Cycle and Adolescent Health*. Boston, MA: Blackwell, 2008.

PERIODICALS

Cho, S.H., and E.W. Hwang. "Acupuncture for Primary Dysmenorrhoea: A Systematic Review." *BJOG* 117 (April 2010): 509–21.

Guerrera, M.P., et al. "Therapeutic Uses of Magnesium." *American Family Physician* 80 (July 15, 2009): 157–62.

Lloyd, K.B., and L.B. Hornsby. "Complementary and Alternative Medications for Women's Health Issues." *Nutrition in Clinical Practice* 24 (October-November 2009): 589–608.

Morrow, C., and E.H. Naumburg. "Dysmenorrhea." *Primary Care* 36 (March 2009): 19–32.

Quinn, M. "Endometriosis: The Elusive Epiphenomenon." *Journal of Obstetrics and Gynecology* 29 (October 2009): 590–93.

Rose, S., et al. "Mirena (Levonorgestrel Intrauterine System): A Successful Novel Drug Delivery Option in Contraception." *Advanced Drug Delivery Reviews* 61 (August 10, 2009): 808–12.

Zahradnik, H.P., et al. "Nonsteroidal Anti-inflammatory Drugs and Hormonal Contraceptives for Pain Relief from Dysmenorrhea: A Review." *Contraception* 81 (March 2010): 185–96.

OTHER

American Congress of Obstetricians and Gynecologists (ACOG). *Dysmenorrhea*, http://www.acog.org/publications/patient_education/bp046.cfm.

Calis, Karim Anton, et al. "Dysmenorrhea." *eMedicine*, January 28, 2009, http://emedicine.medscape.com/article/253812-overview.

French, Linda. "Dysmenorrhea." *American Family Physician* 71 (January 15, 2005): 285–91, http://www.aafp.org/afp/2005/0115/p285.html.

Mayo Clinic. *Menstrual Cramps*, http://www.mayoclinic.com/health/menstrual-cramps/DS00506.

MedlinePlus Medical Encyclopedia. *Painful Menstrual Periods*, http://www.nlm.nih.gov/medlineplus/ency/article/003150.htm.

ORGANIZATIONS

American Congress of Obstetricians and Gynecologists (ACOG), 409 12th St., S.W., P.O. Box 96920, Washington DC, 20090-6920, (202) 638-5577, resources@acog.org, http://www.acog.org/.

Society for Adolescent Health and Medicine (SAHM), 111 Deer Lake Road, Suite 100, Deerfield IL, 60015, (847) 753-5226, (847) 480-9282, info@adolescenthealth.org, http://www.adolescenthealth.org.

Mai Tran
Teresa G. Odle
Rebecca J. Frey, PhD

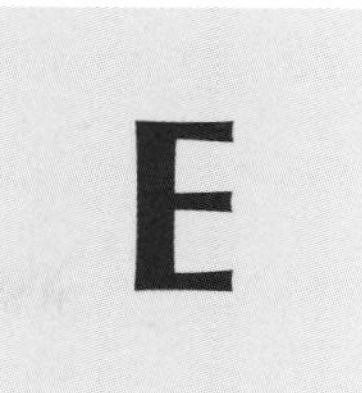

E. coli infection **see Enterobacterial infections**

Ear exam with an otoscope

Definition

An otoscope is a hand-held instrument with a tiny light and a cone-shaped attachment called an ear speculum, which is used to examine the ear canal. An ear examination is a normal part of most physical examinations by a doctor or nurse. It is also done when an ear infection or other type of ear problem is suspected.

Purpose

An otoscope is used to look into the ear canal to see the ear drum. Redness or fluid in the eardrum can indicate an ear infection. Some otoscopes can deliver a small puff of air to the eardrum to see if the eardrum will vibrate (which is normal). This type of ear examination with an otoscope can also detect a build up of wax in the ear canal or a rupture or puncture of the eardrum.

Precautions

No special precautions are required. However, if an ear infection is present, an ear examination may cause some discomfort or **pain**.

Description

An ear examination with an otoscope is usually done by a doctor or a nurse as part of a complete physical examination. The ears may also be examined if an ear infection is suspected due to **fever**, ear pain, or hearing loss. The patient will often be asked to tip the head slightly toward the shoulder so the ear to be examined is pointing up. The doctor or nurse may hold the ear lobe as the speculum is inserted into the ear and may adjust the position of the otoscope to get a better view of the ear canal and eardrum. Both ears are usually examined, even if there seems to be a problem with just one ear.

Preparation

No special preparation is required prior to an ear examination with an otoscope. The ear speculum, which is inserted into the ear, is cleaned and sanitized before it

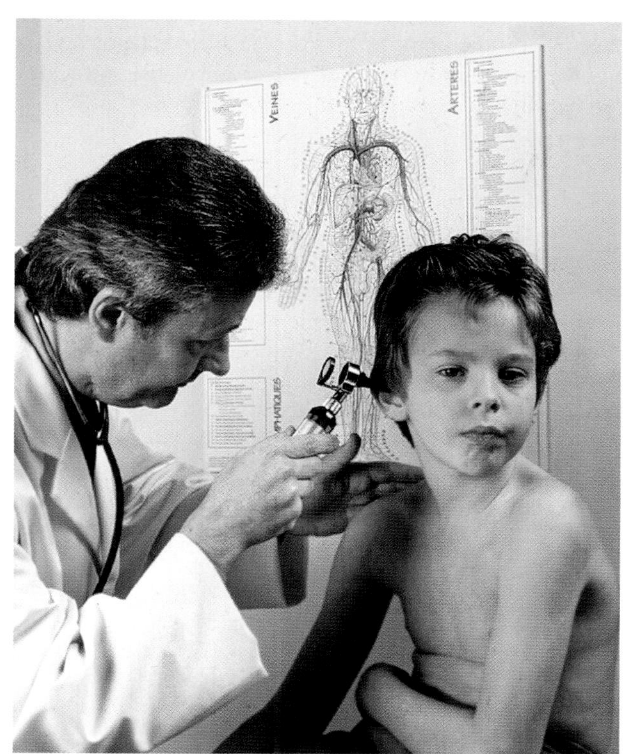

Doctor examining a boy's ear canal with an otoscope, an instrument with a tiny light and cone-shaped attachment called an ear speculum. *(Custom Medical Stock Photo, Inc. Reproduced by permission.)*

is used. The speculums come in various sizes, and the doctor or nurse will select the size that will be most comfortable for the patient's ear.

Aftercare

If an ear infection is diagnosed, the patient may require treatment with **antibiotics**. If there is a buildup of wax in the ear canal, it might be rinsed or scraped out.

Risks

This type of ear examination is simple and generally harmless. Caution should always be used any time an object is inserted into the ear. This process could irritate an infected external ear canal and could rupture an eardrum if performed improperly or if the patient moves.

Normal results

The ear canal is normally skin-colored and is covered with tiny hairs. It is normal for the ear canal to have some yellowish-brown earwax. The eardrum is typically thin, shiny, and pearly-white to light gray in color. The tiny bones in the middle ear can be seen pushing on the eardrum membrane like tent poles. The light from the otoscope will reflect off of the surface of the ear drum.

Abnormal results

An ear infection will cause the eardrum to look red and swollen. In cases where the eardrum has ruptured, there may be fluid draining from the middle ear. A doctor may also see scarring, retraction of the eardrum, or bulging of the eardrum.

Resources

OTHER

"Ear Test." HealthAnswers.com. http://www.healthanswers.com

ORGANIZATIONS

American Academy of Otolaryngology—Head and Neck Surgery, One Prince Street, Alexandria, VA, 22314-3357, (703) 836-4444, http://www.entnet.org.

Ear Foundation, 1817 Patterson St., Nashville TN, 37203, (800) 545-4327, http://www.earfoundation.org.

Altha Roberts Edgren

KEY TERMS

Ear speculum—A cone- or funnel-shaped attachment for an otoscope which is inserted into the ear canal to examine the eardrum.

Otoscope—A hand-held instrument with a tiny light and a funnel-shaped attachment called an ear speculum, which is used to examine the ear canal and eardrum.

Ear infection, middle **see Otitis media**

Ear infection, outer **see Otitis externa**

Ear tubes **see Myringotomy and ear tubes**

Ear wax impaction **see Cerumen impaction**

Eardrum perforation **see Perforated eardrum**

Early childhood development

Definition

Early childhood begins around age 2.5–3 years and extends through age five or until a child enters kindergarten.

Description

Early childhood is a period in which children is actively explore and learn about their environment. Cognitive and language skills expand. Also during this time children become more focused on people other than their primary **caregiver**. Friendships begin to develop and social relationships start to be shaped more strongly by the child's culture.

Fine motor development

Fine motor skills involve deliberate and controlled movements requiring both muscle development and maturation of the central nervous system. During early childhood, the central nervous system and muscle response is still in the process of maturing sufficiently for complex messages from the brain to get to the child's fingers and translate into controlled actions.

By the age of three, many children can control a pencil, although the grip tends to be broad rather than delicate. Three year olds often can draw a circle, although their attempts at drawing people are still very primitive. It is common for four year olds to be able to use scissors, copy geometric shapes and letters, button large buttons, and form clay shapes with two or three sections. Some can print their own names. By age four or five years, children have begun to acquire the fine motor skills needed for daily self-care (e.g., dressing, washing, toileting) They can fasten large, visible buttons (as opposed to those at the back of clothing). By age five or six, most children can manipulate silverware. For example, they can spread jelly or butter on bread with a knife and cut the bread. Most can tie shoelace bows. By age six, they can trace, and cut, paste, and shapes with reasonable proficiency.

Gross motor development

Gross motor skills involve the ability to control the large muscles of the body for walking, running, sitting, **crawling**, and other activities. **Preschool** children are very active. Parents often put a lot of emphasis on gross motor skills, especially walking, toward the end second half of **infancy**, with more emphasis **cognitive development** during early childhood. In addition, during the early childhood years, gross motor activity requires increasing amounts of space, equipment, and adult supervision.

By the age of three, children walk with good posture without watching their feet. They can also walk backwards and run with enough control for stops or changes of direction. They can hop, stand on one foot, and negotiate the rungs of a jungle gym. At the beginning of early childhood, children can walk up stairs alternating feet but usually still walk down putting both feet on each step. Other achievements include riding a tricycle and throwing a ball, although children in this age group have trouble catching balls because they hold their arms out in front of their bodies no matter what direction the ball comes from and their **hand-eye coordination** is still developing.

Four-year-old children typically can balance or hop on one foot, jump forward and backward over objects, and climb and descend stairs alternating feet. They can bounce and catch balls and throw accurately. Some four-year-olds also can skip, as can most five year olds.

Five-year-old children can skip, jump rope, catch a bounced ball, walk on their tiptoes, balance on one foot for over eight seconds, and engage in beginning acrobatics. A few can even ride a small two-wheeler bicycle without training wheels. Children at this age have gained an increased degree of self-consciousness about their motor activities that leads to increased feelings of pride and success when they master a new skill or failure when they fall behind their peers. Although many children begin organized **sports** (T-ball, soccer) by age of five or six, most have a short attention span and still-developing coordination and motor skills that may leave athletically ambitious parents frustrated.

Speech and understanding language

Children's expressive language skills greatly improve during early childhood. Vocabulary expands and sentences become more varied and complex. Reading to children in early childhood is important both for expanding vocabulary and sentence stucture and for developing an interest in the printed word. Pre-reading skills develop during this period. These include letter-sound recognition, the ability to re-tell a story, and to the ability to anticipate what will happen next in a story. Some children are reading by age five.

Cognitive development

The preoperational stage (ages two to six years) characterizes cognitive development during early childhood. This stage involves the manipulation of images and symbols. One object can represent another, as when a broom is turned into a "horsey" that can be ridden around the room. A child's play expands to include "let's pretend" games, spending hours playing hours, pretending to be a fireman and put out fires, or similar activities.

Language acquisition is yet another way of manipulating symbols. Key concepts involved in the logical organization of thoughts, such as causality, time, and perspective, are still absent, as is an awareness that substances retain the same volume even when shifted into containers of different sizes and shapes.

Today it is widely accepted that a child's intellectual ability is determined by a combination of heredity and environment. Thus, although a child's genetic inheritance is unchangeable, there are definite ways that parents can enhance their children's intellectual development through environmental factors. They can provide stimulating learning materials and experiences from an early age, reading to and talking with their children and helping them explore the world around them. As children mature, parents can both challenge and support the child's talents. Although a supportive environment in early childhood provides a clear advantage for a child, it is possible to make up for some early losses in cognitive development if a supportive environment is provided at some later period, in contrast to early disruptions in physical development, which are often irreversible.

Emotional development

Children's capacity to regulate their emotional behavior continues to advance during early childhood. During this time, parents or regular caregivers are the primary socializing force, teaching and modeling appropriate emotional expression in children. Moreover, children learn at about age three that expressions of anger and aggression are to be controlled in the presence of adults. Around peers, however, children are much less likely to suppress negative emotional behavior.

Beginning at about age four, children acquire the ability to alter their emotional expressions, a skill of high value in cultures that require frequent disingenuous social displays. For example, in Western culture, we teach children that they should smile and say thank you when receiving a gift, even if they really do not like the present.

Beginning at about age four or five, children develop a more sophisticated understanding of others' emotional states. Although it has been demonstrated that empathy emerges at quite a young age, with rudimentary displays emerging by age two, increasing cognitive development enables preschoolers to arrive at a more complex understanding of emotions. Pretend play, for example, helps children imagine the world through the eyes of others. Through repeated experiences, children begin to develop their own theories of others' emotional states by referring to causes and consequences of emotions and by observing and being sensitive to behavioral cues that indicate emotional distress.

Social development

Social development is closely linked to **emotional development**. In the early childhood years, socially competent children separate from parents and engage with peers in shared play activities, particularly fantasy play. As these children are just learning to coordinate their social behavior, their interactions are often short and marked by frequent squabbles, and friendships are less stable than at later developmental stages. In addition, physical rough-and-tumble play is common, particularly among boys. During the preschool and early grade school years, children are primarily focused on group acceptance and having companions to spend time with and play with.

Common problems

Children generally are sick less than they were in infancy, although they still get many colds and viral illnesses. By this time parents usually have a developed relationship with a **pediatrician** that they trust. Well-child check ups occur at longer intervals. By the end of early childhood, a large part of the recommended **vaccination** schedule should have been completed

KEY TERMS

Authoritative parenting—Parenting style in which the parents are both responsive and demanding; they are firm, but they discipline with love and affection rather than power, and they are likely to explain rules and expectations to their children instead of simply asserting them.

Authoritarian parenting—A parenting style in which the parents are highly demanding, but strict disciplinarians, frequently relying on physical punishment and the withdrawal of affection to shape their child's behavior.

Disengaged parenting—A parenting style in which parents are neither responsive nor demanding; they may be neglectful or unaware of the child's needs for affection and discipline.

Permissive parenting—A parenting style in which parents are responsive, but not especially demanding; they have few expectations of their children and impose little discipline.

Common problems tend to be related to developmental milestones and behavioral issues. Children who are lagging substantially behind in developmental milestones should be evaluated. Some problems, such as hearing loss, only become apparent when the child does not develop age-appropriate language skills.

Multiple behavior issues can arise during early childhood—everything from refusal to use the toilet to violent, age-inappropriate temper **tantrums** to withdrawal and refusal to play with other children. In early childhood, children often have brief friendships and turbulent relationships with other children, something that is normal for the age. Life situations, such as **divorce**. moving to a new house, or the arrival a new baby can strongly (but usually temporarily) affect behavior. In addition, research has shown that aspects of children's behavior and psychological development are linked to the style of parenting with which they have been raised. Generally, preschoolers with authoritative parents tend to be curious about new situations, focused and skilled at play, self-reliant, self-controlled, and cheerful. Children who are routinely treated in an authoritarian way tend to be moody, unhappy, fearful, withdrawn, lacking in spontaneity, and irritable. Children of permissive parents tend to be low in both social responsibility and independence, but they are usually more cheerful than the conflicted and irritable children of authoritarian parents. Finally, children whose parents are disengaged tend to have a higher proportion of psychological difficulties than other youngsters. A pediatrician can help determine whether specific behavioral issues are normal for the age or whether referral to a family therapist, child psychologist or child psychiatrist are appropriate.

Parental concerns

Many parents are concerned that their child will be prepared for school and do well academically. Some parents put great emphasis on early reading, but reading early is not necessarily a sign that the child is unusually intelligent. Other parents put a great deal of emphasis on sports. Early development of gross motor skills often does correlate to athletic ability. However, there is no correlation between gross motor skills and **intelligence**.

In terms of social and emotional development, parents may rightly be concerned that family turmoil, divorce, domestic abuse, **death** of a family member, and other life-changing events that alter the family dynamic can have a serious impact on a child. Sensitivity to the child's feelings and early professional intervention for the child or the entire family can help the child cope with these issues.

Parents who have a child with disabilities or who suspect they have a child with disabilities may be coming to grips with the limitations of the disability and how it will affect family dynamics. Any parent who feels their child is seriously lagging behind in any area of development should ask for a professional evaluation. Early intervention is the best way to overcome or minimize a **developmental delay**.

Resources

BOOKS

American Academy of Pediatrics. *Caring for Your Baby and Young Child: Birth to Age 5*/5th ed. New York: Bantam, 2009.

Borba, Michele. *The Big Book of Parenting Solutions: 101 Answers to Your Everyday Challenges and Wildest Worries.* San Francisco: Jossey-Bass, 2009.

Trawick-Smith, Jeffrey W. *Early Childhood Development: A Multicultural Perspective*/5th ed. Upper Saddle River, NJ: Pearson Merrill Prentice Hall, 2010.

OTHER

Child Development Chart: Preschool Milestones. Mayo Foundation for Medical Education and Research. July 30, 2010. http://www.mayoclinic.com/health/child-development/MY00136 (accessed September 15, 2010).

Child Development. PBS Parents. Undated, http://www.pbs.org/parents/childdevelopment (accessed September 15, 2010).

Preschoolers (3–5 Years Old). Centers for Disease Control and Prevention. July 26, 2010, http://www.cdc.gov/ncbddd/child/preschoolers.htm (accessed September 15, 2010).

Toddlers (2–3 Years Old). United States Centers for Disease Control and Prevention. July 26, 2010, http://www.cdc.gov/ncbddd/child/toddlers2.htm (accessed September 15, 2010).

ORGANIZATIONS

American Academy of Family Physicians, P. O. Box 11210, Shawnee Mission, KS, 66207, (913)906-6000, (800) 274-2237, (913) 906-6075, http://familydoctor.org.

American Academy of Pediatrics, 141 Northwest Point Boulevard, Elk Grove, Village IL, 60007-1098, (847) 434-4000, (847) 434-8000, http://www.aap.org.

National Association for the Education of Young Children, 1313 L Street, NW, Suite 500, Washington, DC, 20005, (202)232-8777, (800) 424-2460 or (866) NAEYC-4U, (202) 328-1846, http://www.naeyc.org.

National Institute of Child Health and Human Development (NICHD), P.O. Box 3006, Rockville, MD, 20847, (800) 370-2943, (800)320-6942, (866) 760-5947, NICHDInformationResourceCenter@mail.nih.gov, http://www.nichd.nih.gov/publications/pubs/endometriosis.

Tish Davidson, AM

Early childhood education

Definition

Early childhood education (ECE) programs are educational programs for children prior to their entering elementary school.

Description

Any educational program servicing children in the **preschool** years, employing trained adults and administering a program designed to enhance later school performance might be considered an example of early childhood education (ECE). However, the original impetus behind what is now a heterogeneous collection of programs was the desire to provide young children living in poverty—and sometimes their families—with assistance to minimize the risks to their later academic growth and development. Probably the most well-known public early childhood program in the United States is the Head Start Program. Many other U.S. programs fall under the auspices of Title I of the Elementary and Secondary Education Act.

Title I preschool (i.e., prekindergarten) programs operate under a system of federal, state, and local cooperation. Local educational agencies apply to state agencies for program approval, and programs are funded with federal money. Local programs are monitored by state agencies but have the freedom to choose their own educational approaches. **Head Start programs** are funded by the U.S. Department of Health and Human Services, providing grants directly to community organizations. Private centers are tuition-based and may receive assistance from private foundations or hold contracts to serve a certain number of children through Title I or other need-based programs.

There are several models of service delivery. Some programs are child centered, offering educational programs to groups of three- to five-year-olds in schools or other centers. Adjunct social services also may be available. Specialized services (e.g., health, speech-language therapy, **occupational therapy**) may be administered through the local public school or through other providers. Head Start programs, for example, are mandated to provide education, health and social services, and parent services.

Another type of program is one that is more **family** focused. Such programs provide family support services, often through home visits or parent education centers. Their goal is to educate and nurture parents to provide more appropriate stimulation and care for the child at home.

Still other programs attempt to meet both child- and family-centered goals. They may provide center-based care and education for children while parents attend school themselves or obtain job training. A major objective of these programs is to help families move out of poverty, ameliorating some of the risk factors that necessitated early childhood education in the first place.

Benefits

What evidence is there to suggest that ECE offers children a "head start" in their academic careers? Several model programs around the United States—the Abecedarian Project in North Carolina, Houston Parent Child Center, Milwaukee Project, and Syracuse Family Development Research Program, for example—have provided some answers. Studies indicate improvement in **IQ** scores and achievement among children who attend model programs compared to their peers who do not. At least in some projects, gains in IQ persist into **adolescence** when children had been enrolled in programs offering full-day educational childcare. The most uniform effects, however, tend to be in areas of school performance.

Graduates of ECE programs are more likely to progress through their subsequent school years without being retained in grade (i.e., repeating), are less likely to be enrolled in **special education** classes, and are more likely to graduate from high school compared to other children from similar backgrounds who did not attend early childhood programs They also are judged by their elementary school teachers to be better adjusted and seem to show more pride in their achievements compared to their unenrolled peers.

Of course, many of these results are from model programs. Do the benefits extend to programs that are more typical of what is available in most communities? Studies indicate that they do when the community programs meet basic guidelines for quality (e.g., teacher to child ratio, staff training), but the benefits, while still sizable, are somewhat dampened. The most effective programs appear to be those that offer small class size, ongoing support to teachers, ongoing communication with parents or guardians, and curriculum content and methods that are not too different from what the child will encounter in their early school years.

Evidence suggests that experience in elementary school contributes substantially to sustaining the benefits of early childhood education. Even a temporary cognitive boost can enable a child to take full advantage of experiences in the primary grades, prevent placement in lower tracks, avoid grade retention, improve the expectations of teachers, and generally smooth the transition to the early school years. The effects begin to accumulate and may be enhanced by schools that provide supports such as small class size in the early grades, which has been shown to offer advantages to students that persist even when they move into larger classes in later grades.

Changes in the lives of children and families have contributed to the expansion of ECE efforts in recent years. Increasing numbers of single parent families and families in which both parents are employed have prompted the need for more private programs. Children of high-income households are more likely than their low-income peers to be enrolled in a prekindergarten program. Children of parents with at least a Bachelor's degree are about twice as likely to attend an early education program than children of a parent with less than a high school degree.

Children of the wealthy and highly educated, however, are not the ones who will benefit most from their ECE experiences. Wealthy families frequently have resources to provide their children with educational

KEY TERMS

Child-and-Family-Centered Program—An early childhood education program that provides education and services to the young child while simultaneously providing vocational training or additional education to the parents.

Child-Centered Program—An early childhood education program that provides education and other services to three to five year old children.

Family-Centered Program—An early childhood education program that provides education in a more family-centered situation, including home visits and interaction with parents.

advantages in the home, including stimulating **toys**, games, books, computer programs, and access to play spaces, as well as basic **safety**, **nutrition**, and health care. Families who are living in poverty, however, often do not have such resources. In fact, these families frequently face multiple risks stemming from their poverty, including neighborhood violence, **undernutrition**, and poor health care. Therefore, it is not surprising that early childhood education offers the most to children of poverty, who otherwise have the least.

Although there is resistance to providing full funding for federal early childhood initiatives, it is estimated that national cost of failing to offer two years of quality ECE is approximately $100,000 for each child born into poverty, or $400 billion for all impoverished children under the age of five. By comparison, some estimate the cost of full ECE funding at $25 or $30 billion per year, a substantial portion of the annual federal budget, but a fraction of the eventual costs of not offering ECE to each poverty-stricken child who may benefit from it. The demographic trends suggest that early childhood education has become—and will continue to be—an important aspect of achieving an educational standard applicable to all youth.

Resources

BOOKS

Gonzalez-Mena, Janet. *Foundations of Early Childhood Education: Teaching Children in a Diverse Society,* 5th ed. Boston: McGraw Hill, 2011.

Hess, Robert D. and Roberta Meyer Bear. *Early Formal Education: Current Theory, Research, and Practice.* New Brunswick, NJ: AldineTransaction, 2010.

Mawson, W. B. *Collaborative Play in Early Childhood Education.* Hauppauge, NY: Nova Science Publishers, 2010.

PERIODICALS

Al-Momani, Ibrahim, A., et al. "Teaching Reading in the Early Years: Exploring Home and Kindergarten Relationships." *Early Child Development & Care* (July 2010) 180(6): 767-785.

Gillespie, Catherine Wilson, and Kendra R. Glider. "Preschool Teachers' Use of Music to Scaffold Children's Learning and Behaviour." *Early Child Development & Care,* (July 2010) 180(6): 799-808.

ORGANIZATIONS

Association for Childhood Education International, 17904 Georgia Ave, Suite 215, Olney, MD, 20832, (301) 570-2111, (800) 423-3563, (301) 570-2212, headquarters@acei.org, www.acei.org.

The National Association for the Education of Young Children, 1313 L Street, NW, Suite 500, Washington, DC, 20005, (202) 232-8777, (800) 424-2460, (202) 328-1846, www.naeyc.org.

Tish Davidson, A.M.

Early puberty *see* **Precocious puberty**

Eating disorders

Definition

Eating disorders are psychiatric illnesses that result in abnormal eating patterns that have a negative effect on health.

Demographics

In general, more women have eating disorders than men. About 90% of people with **anorexia nervosa** and **bulimia nervosa** are female. Almost as many men as women develop binge-eating disorder. Anorexia athletica, muscle dysmorphic disorder, and orthorexia nervosa tend to be more common in men. Rumination, **pica**, and **Prader-Willi syndrome** affect men and women equally.

Anorexia can occur in people as young as age 7. However, the disorder most often begins during **adolescence**. It is most likely to start at one of two times, either age 14 or 18 and affects mainly white girls. There is a secondary peak of individuals who become anorexic in their 40s.

Bulimia is the most common eating disorder in the United States. Overall, about 3% of people living in the United States are bulimic. Of these 85–90% are female. The rate is highest among adolescents and college women, averaging 5–6%. In men, the disorder is more often diagnosed in homosexuals than in heterosexuals. Bulimia usually develops in women their late teens and early twenties and in men around age 25 or later. It affects all racial, ethnic, and socioeconomic groups.

Estimates of the number of Americans who have binge-eating disorder range from less than 1–4%, with 2% being the most commonly cited figure. Although women with binge-eating disorder outnumber men three to two, **binge eating** is the most common male eating disorder. Binge-eating disorder is a problem of middle age and affects blacks and whites equally.

Prader-Willi syndrome begins in the toddler years. Not enough is known about the other disorders to determine when they are most likely to develop or which races or ethnic groups are most likely to be at risk.

Description

Eating disorders are mental disorders. They develop when a person has an unrealistic attitude toward or abnormal perception of his or her body. This causes behaviors that lead to destructive eating patterns that have negative physical and emotional consequences. Individuals with eating disorders often hide their symptoms and resist seeking treatment. Depression, **anxiety** disorders, and other mental illnesses often are present in people who have eating disorders, although it is not clear whether these cause the eating disorder or are a result of it.

The two best-known eating disorders, anorexia nervosa and bulimia nervosa, have formal diagnostic criteria and are recognized as psychiatric disorders in the *Diagnostic and Statistical Manual for Mental Disorders Fourth Edition (DSM-IV-TR)* published by the American Psychiatric Association (APA). Other eating disorders have recognized sets of symptoms but have not been researched thoroughly enough to be considered separate psychiatric disorders as defined by the APA.

Anorexia nervosa

In the North America and Europe, anorexia nervosa is the most publicized of all eating disorders. It gained widespread public attention with the rise of the ultra-thin fashion model. People who have anorexia nervosa are obsessed with body weight. They constantly monitor their food intake and starve themselves to become thin. No matter how much weight they lose, they continue to restrict their calorie intake in an effort to become ever thinner. Some anorectics **exercise** to the extreme or abuse drugs or herbal remedies that they believe will help them burn calories faster. A few purge their body of the few calories they do eat by abusing **laxatives**, enemas, and diuretics. In time, they reach a point where their health is seriously, and potentially fatally, impaired.

People with anorexia nervosa have an abnormal perception of their body. They genuinely believe that they are fat, even when they clearly are life-threateningly thin. They will deny that they are too thin, or, if they admit they are thin, deny that their behavior will affect their health. People with anorexia will lie to **family**, friends, and healthcare providers about how much they eat. Many vigorously resist treatment and accuse the people trying to cure them of wanting to make them fat. Anorexia nervosa is the most difficult eating disorder to recover from.

Competitive athletes of all races have an increased risk of developing anorexia nervosa, especially in **sports** where weight os tied to performance. Jockeys, wrestlers, figure skaters, cross-country runners, and gymnasts (especially female gymnasts) have higher than average rates of anorexia. People such as actors, models, cheerleaders, and dancers (especially ballet dancers) who are judged mainly on their appearance are also at high risk of developing the disorder. This same group of people is also at higher risk for developing bulimia nervosa.

Bulimia nervosa

Bulimia nervosa is the only other eating disorder with specific diagnostic criteria defined by the *DSM-IV-TR*. People with bulimia often consume unreasonably large amounts of food in a short time. Afterwards, they purge their body of calories. This is done typically by self-induced **vomiting**, often accompanied by laxative abuse. A subset of people with bulimia does not vomit after eating, but fast and exercise obsessively to burn calories. Both behaviors result in impaired health.

People with bulimia feel out of control when they are binge eating. Unlike people with anorexia, they recognize that their behavior is abnormal. Often they are ashamed and feel guilty about their behavior and will go to great lengths to hide their binge/purge cycles from their family and friends. People with bulimia are often of normal weight. Although their behavior results in negative health consequences, because they are less likely to be ultra-thin, these consequences are less likely to be life-threatening.

Binge eating disorder

Binge eating is quite common, but it only rises to the level of a disorder only when binging occurs at least twice a week for three months or more. People with binge-eating disorder may eat thousands of calories in an hour or two. While they are eating, they feel out of control and may continue to eat long after they feel full. Binge eaters do not purge or exercise to get rid of the calories they have eaten. As a result, many, but not all, people with binge-eating disorder are obese, although not all obese people are binge eaters.

Binge eaters are usually ashamed of their behavior and try to hide it by eating in secret and hording food for future binges. After a binge, they usually feel disgusted with themselves and are guilty about their eating behavior. They often promise themselves that they will never binge again, but are unable to keep this promise. Binge-eating disorder often takes the form of an endless cycle—rigorous dieting followed by an eating binge followed by guilt and rigorous dieting, followed by another eating binge. The main health consequences of binge eating are the development of obesity-related diseases, such as type 2 diabetes, sleep apnea, **stroke**, and heart attack.

Lesser-known eating disorders

Quite a few eating problems are called disorders even though they do not have formal diagnostic criteria. They fall under the APA definition of eating disorders not otherwise specified. Many have only recently come to the attention of researchers and have been the subject of only a few small studies. Some have been known to the medical community for years but are rare.

Purge disorder is thought by some experts to be a separate disorder from bulimia. It is distinguished from bulimia by the fact that the individual maintains a normal or near normal weight despite purging by vomiting or laxative, enema, or diuretic abuse.

Anorexia athletica is a disorder of compulsive exercising. The individual places exercise above work, school, or relationships and defines his or her self-worth in terms of athletic performance. People with anorexia athletica also tend to be obsessed less with body weight than with maintaining an abnormally low percentage of body fat. This disorder is common among elite athletes.

Muscle dysmorphic disorder is the opposite of anorexia nervosa. Where the anorectic thinks she is always too fat, the person with muscle dysmorphic disorder believes he is always too small. This believe is maintained even when the person is clearly well muscled. Abnormal eating patterns are less of a problem in people with muscle dysmorphic disorder than damage from compulsive exercising (even when injured) and the abuse of muscle-building drugs such as anabolic **steroids**.

Orthorexia nervosa is a term coined by Steven Bratman, a Colorado physician, to describe "a pathological fixation on eating 'proper,' 'pure,' or 'superior' foods." People with orthorexia allow their fixation with eating the correct amount of properly prepared healthy foods at the correct time of day to take over their lives. This obsession interferes with relationships and daily activities. For example, they may be unwilling to eat at restaurants or friends' homes because the food is "impure" or improperly prepared. The limitations they put on what they will eat can cause serious vitamin and mineral imbalances. Orthorectics are judgmental about what other people eat to the point where it interferes with personal relationships. They justify their fixation by claiming that their way of eating is healthy. Some experts believe orthorexia may be a variation of **obsessive-compulsive disorder**.

Rumination syndrome occurs when an individual, either voluntarily or involuntarily, regurgitates food almost immediately after swallowing it, chews it, and then either swallows it or spits it out. Regurgitation syndrome is the human equivalent of a cow chewing its cud. The behavior often lasts up to two hours after eating. It must continue for at least one month to be considered a disorder. Occasionally the behavior simply stops on its own, but it can last for years.

Pica is eating of non-food substances by people developmentally past the stage where this is normal (usually around age 2). Earth and clay are the most common non-foods eaten, although people have been known to eat hair, feces, lead, laundry starch chalk, burnt matches, cigarette butts, light bulbs, and other equally bizarre non-foods. This disorder has been known to the medical community for years, and in some cultures (mainly tribes living in equatorial Africa) is considered normal. Pica is most common among people with **mental retardation** and developmental delays. It only rises to the level of a disorder when health complications require medical treatment.

Prader-Willi syndrome is a genetic defect that spontaneously arises in chromosome 15. It causes low muscle tone, short stature, incomplete sexual development, mental retardation, and an uncontrollable urge to eat. People with Prader-Willi syndrome never feel full. The only way to stop them from eating themselves to death is to keep them in environments where food is locked up and not available. Prader-Willi syndrome is a rare disease, and although it is caused by a genetic defect, tends not to run in families, but rather is an accident of development. Only 12,000–15,000 people in the United States have Prader-Willi syndrome.

Causes and symptoms

Eating disorders have multiple causes. There appears to be a genetic predisposition in some people toward developing an eating disorder. Biochemistry also seems to play a role. Neurotransmitters in the brain, such as serotonin, play a role in regulating appetite. Abnormalities in the amount of some neurotransmitters are thought to play a role in anorexia, bulimia, and binge-eating disorder. Other disorders have not been studied enough to draw any conclusions. Interestingly, serotonin also helps regulate mood, and low serotonin levels are thought to play a role in causing depression.

Personality type can also put people at risk for developing an eating disorder. Low self-worth is common among all people with eating disorders. Binge eaters and people with bulimia tend to have problems with impulse control and anger management. A tendency toward obsessive-compulsive behavior and black-or-white, all-or-nothing thinking also put people at higher risk.

Social and environmental factors also affect the development and maintenance of eating disorders and may trigger relapses during recovery. Relationship conflict, a disordered, unstructured home life, job or school stress, transition events such as moving or starting a new job all seems to act as triggers for some people to begin disordered eating behaviors. Dieting (nutritional and social stress) is the most common trigger of all. The United States in the early twenty-first century is a culture obsessed with thinness. The media constantly send the message through words and images that being not just thin, but ultra-thin, is fashionable and desirable. Magazines aimed mostly at women devote thousands of words every month to diet and exercise advice that creates a sense of dissatisfaction, unrealistic goals, and a distorted body image.

Signs and symptoms of anorexia and bulimia

Eating disorders have physical and psychological consequences. These include:

- excessive weight loss; loss of muscle
- stunted growth and delayed sexual maturation in preteens
- gastrointestinal complications: liver damage, diarrhea, constipation, bloating, stomach pain
- cardiovascular complications: irregular heartbeat, low pulse rate, cardiac arrest
- urinary system complications: kidney damage, kidney failure, incontinence, urinary tract infections
- skeletal system complications: loss of bone mass, increased risk of fractures, teeth eroded by stomach acid from repeat vomiting
- reproductive system complications (women): irregular menstrual periods, amenorhhea, infertility
- reproductive system complications (men): loss of sex drive, infertility
- fatigue, irritation, headaches, depression, anxiety, impaired judgment and thinking
- fainting, seizures, low blood sugar
- chronically cold hands and feet
- weakened immune system, swollen glands, increased susceptibility to infections
- development of fine hair called lanugos on the shoulders, back, arms, and face, head hair loss, blotchy, dry skin
- potentially life-threatening electrolyte imbalances
- coma
- increased risk of self-mutilation (cutting)
- increased risk of suicide
- death

Signs and symptoms of binge eating

Symptoms of binge eating may be difficult to detect. Binge eating is different from continuously snacking. Binge eaters are often secretive about food and their bingeing is often done in private. Obesity and obesity-related diseases such as **hypertension** (high blood pressure,) type 2 diabetes, and joint **pain** are signs that binge-eating disorder could be present, but not all obese people are binge-eaters. Behaviors such as secretive eating, constant dieting without losing weight, obsessive concern about weight, depression, anxiety, and **substance abuse** are all clues, but none of these signs are definitive. The individual may complain about symptoms related to obesity, such as fatigue and shortness of breath, or mention unsuccessful dieting, but again, these signs are not definitive.

Diagnosis

Diagnosis is based on several factors including a patient history, physical examination, laboratory tests, and a mental status evaluation. A patient history is less helpful in diagnosing eating disorders than in diagnosing many diseases because many people with an eating disorder lie repeatedly about how much they eat, purge, or use laxatives, enemas, and medications. The patient may, however, complain about related symptoms such as fatigue, headaches, **dizziness**, **constipation**, or frequent infections.

Tests

A physical examination begins with weight and blood pressure and moves through all the signs listed above. Based on the physical exam, the physician will order laboratory tests. In general these tests will include a complete blood count (CBC), urinalysis, blood chemistries (to determine electrolyte levels), and **liver function**

KEY TERMS

Body dysmorphic disorder—A psychiatric disorder marked by preoccupation with an imagined physical defect.

Diuretic—a substance that removes water from the body by increasing urine production.

Electrolyte—ions in the body that participate in metabolic reactions. The major human electrolytes are sodium (Na+), potassium (K+), calcium (Ca 2+), magnesium (Mg2+), chloride (Cl-), phosphate (HPO4 2-), bicarbonate (HCO3-), and sulfate (SO4 2-).

Lanugos—A soft, downy body hair that develops on the chest and arms of anorexic women.

Neurotransmitter—One of a group of chemicals secreted by a nerve cell (neuron) to carry a chemical message to another nerve cell, often as a way of transmitting a nerve impulse. Examples of neurotransmitters include acetylcholine, dopamine, serotonin, and norepinephrine.

Purging—The use of vomiting, diuretics, or laxatives to clear the stomach and intestines after a binge.

Serotonin—5-Hydroxytryptamine; a substance that occurs throughout the body with numerous effects including neurotransmission. Inadequate amounts of serotonin are implicated in some forms of depression and obsessive-compulsive disorder.

tests. The physician may also order an electrocardiogram to look for heart abnormalities. Other conditions, including metabolic disorders, brain tumors (especially hypothalamus and pituitary gland lesions), diseases of the digestive tract, and a condition called superior mesenteric artery syndrome, can cause weight loss or vomiting after eating. People with this condition sometimes vomit after meals because the blood supply to the intestine is blocked. The physician may perform tests needed to rule out the presence of these disorders and assess the patient's nutritional status.

The individual may be referred to a psychiatrist for a mental status evaluation. The physician will evaluate things such as whether the person is oriented in time and space, appearance, observable state of emotion (affect), attitude toward food and weight, delusional thinking, and thoughts of self-harm or **suicide**. This evaluation helps to distinguish between an eating disorder and other psychiatric disorders, including depression, **schizophrenia**, social phobia, obsessive-compulsive disorder, and **body dysmorphic disorder**. Two diagnostic tests that are often used are the Eating Attitudes Test (EAT) and the Eating Disorder Inventory (EDI).

Treatment

Treatment depends on the degree to which the individual's health is impaired.

Traditional medical treatment

Hospitalization is recommended for anorectics or bulimics with any of the following characteristics:

- weight of 40% or more below normal; or weight loss over a three-month period of more than 30 pounds
- severely disturbed metabolism
- severe binging and purging
- signs of psychosis
- severe depression or risk of suicide
- family in crisis

Hospital inpatient care is first geared toward correcting problems that present as immediate medical crises, such as severe **malnutrition**, severe electrolyte imbalance, irregular heart beat, pulse below 45 beats per minute, or low body temperature. Patients are hospitalized if they are a high suicide risk, have severe clinical depression, or exhibit signs of an altered mental state. They may also need to be hospitalized to interrupt weight loss, stop the cycle of vomiting, exercising and/or laxative abuse, treat substance disorders, or for additional medical evaluation.

Individuals with eating disorders are treated with a variety of medications to address physical problems brought about by their eating disorder and to treat additional psychiatric problems, such as depression, anxiety, and suicidal thoughts. The medications used will vary depending on the individual; however, depression is common among people with eating disorders and is most often treated with **antidepressant drugs**.

Psychotherapy

The mainstay of treatment is psychotherapy. An appropriate therapy is selected based on the type of eating disorder and the individual's psychological profile. Some of the common therapies used in treating eating disorders include:

- Cognitive behavior therapy (CBT) is designed to confront and then change the individual's thoughts and feelings about his or her body and behaviors toward food, but it does not address why those thoughts or feelings exist. Strategies to maintain self-control may be explored. This therapy is relatively short-term. CBT is often the therapy of choice for people with eating disorders.

- Psychodynamic therapy, also called psychoanalytic therapy, attempts to help the individual gain insight into the cause of the emotions that trigger their dysfunctional behavior. This therapy tends to be more long term than CBT.
- Interpersonal therapy is short-term therapy that helps the individual identify specific issues and problems in relationships. The individual may be asked to look back at his or her family history to try to recognize problem areas or stresses and work toward resolving them.
- Dialectical behavior therapy consists of structured private and group sessions in which the therapist and patient(s) work at reducing behaviors that interfere with quality of life, finding alternate solutions to current problem situations, and learning to regulate emotions.
- Family and couples therapy is helpful in dealing with conflict or disorder that may be a factor in perpetuating the eating disorder. Family therapy is especially useful in helping parents who are anorectics avoid passing on their attitudes and behaviors on to their children.

Nutrition education

A nutrition consultant or dietitian is an essential part of the team needed to successfully treat eating disorders. The first treatment concern is to get the individual medically stable by increasing calorie intake and balancing electrolytes. After that, nutritional therapy is needed to support the long process of recovery and stable weight gain. This is an intensive process involving of nutrition education, meal planning, nutrition monitoring, and helping the anorectic develop a healthy relationship with food. However, nutritional counseling alone will not resolve an eating disorder.

Alternative and complementary treatment

Alternative treatments should complement conventional treatment program. Alternative therapies for anorexia nervosa include diet and nutrition counseling, herbal therapy, hydrotherapy, aromatherapy, Ayurvedic medicine, and mind/body medicine.

The following herbs may help reduce anxiety and depression which are often associated with this disorder:

- chamomile (*Matricaria recutita*)
- lemon balm (*Melissa officinalis*)
- linden (*Tilia* spp.) flowers

Essential oils of herbs such as bergamot, basil, chamomile, sage, and lavender may help stimulate appetite, relax the body, and fight depression. They can be diffused into the air, inhaled, massaged, or put in bath water.

Relaxation techniques such as **yoga**, meditation, and t'ai chi can relax the body and release stress, anxiety, and depression.

Hypnotherapy may help resolve unconscious issues that contribute to anorexic behavior.

Other alternative treatments that may be helpful include hydrotherapy, magnetic field therapy, acupuncture, biofeedback, Ayurvedic medicine, and traditional Chinese medicine.

Prognosis

Recovery from eating disorders can be along, difficult process interrupted by relapses. About half of all anorectics recover. Up to 20% die of complications of the disorder. The recovery rate for people with bulimia is slightly higher. Binge eaters experience many relapses and may have trouble controlling their weight even if they stop bingeing. Not enough is known about the other eating disorders to determine recovery rates. All eating disorders have serious social and emotional consequences. All except rumination disorder have serious health consequences. The sooner a person with an eating disorder gets professional help, the better the chance of recovery.

Prevention

Prevention involves both preventing and relieving stresses and enlisting professional help as soon as abnormal eating patterns develop. Some things that may help prevent an eating disorder from developing are:

- Parents should not obsess about their weight, appearance, and diet in front of their children.
- Parents should not put their child on a diet unless instructed to by a pediatrician.
- Do not tease people about their body shapes or compare them to others.
- Make it clear that family members are loved and accepted as they are.
- Try to eat meals together as a family whenever possible; avoid eating alone.
- Avoid using food for comfort in times of stress.
- Monitoring negative self-talk; practice positive self-talk.
- Spend time doing something enjoyable every day.
- Stay busy, but not overly busy; get enough sleep every night.

- Become aware of the situations that are personal triggers for abnormal eating behaviors and look for ways to avoid or defuse them.
- Do not go on extreme diets.
- Be alert to signs of low self-worth, anxiety, depression, and drug or alcohol abuse and seek help as soon as these signs appear.

Resources

BOOKS

Carleton, Pamela, and Deborah Ashin. *Take Charge of Your Child's Eating Disorder: A Physician's Step-By-Step Guide to Defeating Anorexia and Bulimia.* New York: Marlowe & Co., 2007.

Heaton, Jeanne A., and Claudia J. Strauss. *Talking to Eating Disorders: Simple Ways to Support Someone Who Has Anorexia, Bulimia, Binge Eating or Body Image Issues.* New York, NY: New American Library, 2005.

Liu, Aimee. *Gaining: The Truth About Life After Eating Disorders.* New York, NY: Warner Books, 2007.

Messinger, Lisa, and Merle Goldberg. *My Thin Excuse: Understanding, Recognizing, and Overcoming Eating Disorders.* Garden City Park, NY: Square One Publishers, 2006.

Rubin, Jerome S., ed. *Eating Disorders and Weight Loss Research.* Hauppauge, NY: Nova Science Publishers, 2006.

Walsh, B. Timothy. *If Your Adolescent Has an Eating Disorder: An Essential Resource for Parents.* New York, NY: Oxford University Press, 2005.

OTHER

"Eating Disorders." American Psychological Association. April 2009, http://www.apa.org/topics/topiceating.html (accessed June 23, 2009).

Medline Plus. "Eating Disorders." U.S. National Library of Medicine, May 15, 2009, http://www.nlm.nih.gov/medlineplus/eatingdisorders.html (accessed June 23, 2009).

ORGANIZATIONS

American Psychological Association, 750 First Street, NE, Washington, DC, 20002-4242, (202) 336-5500, TDD/TTY: (202)336-6123, (800) 374-2721, apa@psych.org, http://www.apa.org.

National Association of Anorexia Nervosa and Related Eating Disorders (ANAD), P.O. Box 7, Highland Park, IL, 60035, (847) 831-3438, (847) 433-3996, http://www.anad.org.

National Eating Disorders Association, 603 Stewart Street, Suite 803, Seattle, WA, 98101, (206) 382-3587, Help and Referral Line: (800) 931-2237, (206) 829-8501, info@NationalEatingDisorder.org, http://www.nationaleatingdisorders.org.

Tish Davidson, A.M.

Eczema

Definition

Eczema, also called **atopic dermatitis** (AD), is a non-contagious inflammation of the skin characterized by dry, red, itchy, and oozing lesions that become scaly, crusty, or hardened. Various other types of **dermatitis** are sometimes referred to as eczema or eczematous, although AD is the most common type.

Demographics

Worldwide, 10–20% of people develop atopic dermatitis at some point in their lives. Although eczema can affect anyone at any age, it is most common in children under age five. An estimated 65% of eczema cases begin during the first year of life and 90% develop before the age of five. The incidence of eczema and other allergic diseases appears to have increased in recent decades. As of 2009 it was estimated that almost 1 in 10 babies in the United States develop eczema.

Description

Eczema is sometimes described as "the itch that rashes," because scratching irritated areas sometimes initiates a rash. Eczema can be mild and intermittent or severe and chronic, disappearing as children grow up or lasting a lifetime. Eczema is frequently related to some form of allergy, including **allergies** to foods or inhalants.

The areas of the body affected by eczema tend to vary with age. Infants frequently have eczema on the face and other areas of the head. The stomach and limbs also may be affected. Older children commonly have more severe eczema on flexor surfaces—the inner wrists and elbows, backs of the knees, and tops of the ankles, as well as the hands and feet. The knees, elbows, hands, and feet may continue to be a problem into adulthood. Occasionally eczema becomes widespread throughout the body.

Other types of dermatitis that may be described as eczematous, but which usually affect older children and adults, include:

- contact dermatitis, which results from skin contact with an irritant or allergen
- nummular dermatitis, which usually affects people over the age of 55
- stasis dermatitis, which results from poor circulation in the legs

Risk factors

The major risk factor for eczema appears to be a family history of eczema and/or allergies.

KEY TERMS

Allergic reaction—An immune system reaction to a substance in the environment; symptoms include rash, inflammation, sneezing, itchy watery eyes, runny nose, or skin irritations.

Antigen—A foreign protein or particle that causes the body to produce specific antibodies that bind to the antigen.

Atopy—Allergies, such as eczema, that are probably hereditary, with symptoms that develop upon exposure to specific environmental allergens.

Corticosteroids—A group of hormones produced by the adrenal glands or manufactured synthetically. They are often used to treat inflammation. Examples include cortisone and prednisone.

Dermatitis—Inflammation of the skin.

Patch test—Scratch test; a test to identify allergens, in which the suspected substance is pricked or scratched into the skin and observed for the development of redness and swelling that are indicative of an allergic reaction.

Rash—Spotted, pink or red skin eruptions that may be accompanied by itching.

Causes and symptoms

In many cases the exact cause of eczema is unknown, although it often appears to result from an interaction between an inherited genetic predisposition towards allergies and exposure to specific environmental allergens, especially those that are inhaled or ingested.

The hallmark sign of eczema is a red, itchy rash and skin that is abnormally dry. Chronic or severe cases of eczema can result in thick plaques (patches of slightly raised skin), serous (watery) exudates, or infection.

Diagnosis

Examination

Eczema is diagnosed by the appearance and location of the rash. An individual or family history of allergies, including **food allergies**, hay **fever**, or **asthma**, supports the diagnosis of eczema.

Tests

There are no laboratory tests for diagnosing eczema. Sometimes dermatologists conduct skin tests—scratch or patch tests or intradermal injections—to attempt to identify suspected allergens. A small amount of the suspected allergen is dabbed, scratched, or pricked into the skin, usually on the back. If no irritation develops within a few days, patch tests for other suspected allergens may be performed sequentially. Blood tests can measure the levels of immunoglobulin E (IgE)—the antibodies involved in allergic reactions—and, in some cases, the levels of IgE that are specific for a given antigen.

Procedures

In rare cases a skin biopsy may be required to rule out certain diseases.

Treatment

Traditional

The best treatment for eczema is to identify the cause and eliminate it. Since this is often not possible, medications and home treatments for hydrating the skin are the best options. Since **itching** or scratching eczema can irritate and damage the skin and cause **rashes**, any treatment that reduces the itching is helpful.

Drugs

Drug treatments for eczema include:

- oral antihistamines to decrease itching
- calamine lotion
- mild topical corticosteroids containing at least 1% hydrocortisone
- rarely, oral corticosteroids for severe itching and inflammation
- topical antibiotics to prevent or treat infection
- oral antibiotics for widespread infection
- topical pimecrolimus (Elidel) and tacrolimus (Protopic)—immunomodulators that may be used in adults and children over age two when other treatments have failed

Alternative

Light therapy or phototherapy can effectively treat eczema, either by controlled exposure to natural sunlight or artificial ultraviolet A (UVA) and/or ultraviolet B (UVB) light. However, a dermatologist should be consulted about the benefits and risks of phototherapy.

There are a number of alternative therapies that may prove helpful for treating eczema:

- acupuncture
- autogenic training, meditation, and self-hypnosis
- hypnotherapy—using the power of suggestion to relieve itching

- massage to reduce stress
- reflexology focusing on areas of the body corresponding to the eczema-affected patches, as well the solar plexus, adrenal glands, pituitary gland, liver, kidneys, gastrointestinal tract, and reproductive glands
- aromatherapy with small amounts of essential oils of lavender, bergamot, and geranium to decrease itching and inflammation; however, improper dilutions of essential oils can worsen eczema
- evening primrose (*Oenothera biennis*) oil (EPO) diluted in a carrier oil and massaged into the skin

Herbal therapies that are often recommended for skin conditions such as eczema include:

- calendula (*Calendula officinalis*) ointment, for its anti-inflammatory and antiseptic properties
- chickweed (*Stellaria media*) ointment, to soothe itching
- evening primrose oil—topically to relieve itching and internally as a fatty acid supplement
- German chamomile (*Chamomilla recutita*) ointment, for its anti-inflammatory properties
- nettle (*Urtica dioica*) ointment, to relieve itching
- peppermint (*Menta piperita*) lotion, for its antibacterial and antiseptic properties
- traditional Chinese herbal formulas, both applied topically and taken internally, to moisten the skin, prevent itching, nourish the blood, and encourage healing Individuals vary in their responses to herbal treatments. Chronic, severe, or infected eczema requires the attention of a healthcare professional.

Various nutritional supplements may aid in treating eczema:

- Oral EPO, which contains gamma-linolenic acid, has been shown to significantly reduce itching from eczema at doses of approximately 6 grams (g) daily.
- Fish oil at a dose of about 1.8 g per day has been shown to improve AD.
- Vitamin C can promote both skin healing and the immune system. Doses of 50–75 milligrams per kilogram (mg/kg) of body weight have been shown to relieve symptoms of AD.
- Supplemental copper may be required with high doses of vitamin C.
- Vitamin E may be of use in treating eczema.

Home remedies

Home care for eczema focuses on keeping the skin clean and moist and avoiding irritants and known allergens as much as possible. Frequent long, tepid soaks help hydrate very dry skin; however, soaking in plain water can be painful during severe episodes of eczema:

- Adding one-half cup of table salt to one-half tub of water creates a normal saline solution, similar to that present in the body tissues, and may relieve burning.
- Adding baking soda, a muslin bag filled with milled oats, or the commercial preparation Aveeno to the water can be soothing.
- Research has shown that dilute bleach baths—one-half cup (118 milliliters) of bleach in 40 gallons (151 liters) of warm water—can treat eczema by killing bacteria growing on the skin. The affected areas should be soaked for 5–10 minutes once or twice per week.
- Commercial Domeboro powder may be helpful.
- Bath water should cover as much of the skin as possible. Wet towels may be draped around the shoulders, upper trunk, and arms if they are above the water level.
- The face should be dabbed frequently during bathing to keep it moist.
- The use of soap should be minimized and limited to very mild agents such as Cetaphil.

Drying off should involve two to three minutes of gentle patting, followed by the thick application of a water-barrier ointment, such as Aquaphor, Unibase, or Vaseline. Oil or creams applied to damp skin can seal in moisture. However, moisturizing lotions containing alcohol dry the skin and may burn when applied to eczema. Babies' skin should be kept lubricated with appropriate bath oils, lotions, creams, or ointments.

Soaking wraps are an alternative to bathing. Cotton towels or other cloths are soaked in tepid water, possibly containing table salt or Domeboro powder, and used to cover the bare skin as thoroughly as possible. The patient lies on a bed with a waterproof sheet and is covered by a second waterproof covering, such as vinyl sheeting or plastic wrap, to slow evaporation. The wraps are left in place for as long as possible, but for at least 30 minutes, followed by the application of a water barrier and any topical medications.

Environmental changes can provide relief for many eczema sufferers:

- Pet dander and cigarette smoke should be kept out of the home, or at least out of the room.
- Clothing should be loose fitting to prevent irritation from rubbing.
- Clothing and bedding should be 100% soft cotton.
- Clothing and bedding should be washed before initial use to rid them of potentially irritating residues.
- Laundry soap should by dye- and perfume-free.

- Laundry should be run through a double-rinse cycle to remove any vestiges of detergent.
- Bedding should be washed in hot water to kill dust mites, which can be major irritants to people with eczema.
- Fabric softener or dryer sheets are frequently scented and may be irritating.
- Clothes and bedding should not be dried outdoors where pollen and other potential allergens can cling to them.
- Mattresses and pillowcases can be covered by special casings that are impervious to microscopic dust mites.
- Dust-collecting items, such as curtains, carpeting, and stuffed animals, should be kept to a minimum.
- Vacuuming and dusting should be performed regularly when the patient is out of the room.

Temperature extremes can aggravate eczema, so heating and cooling should be employed appropriately, along with the use of a home humidifier. Eczema can interfere with normal body temperature regulation and can be aggravated by sweating. Central air-conditioning is preferable to evaporative cooling or open windows that can bring allergens into the house. Car air-conditioning is preferable to open windows. Electrostatic filters and vent covers can remove irritants from household air. These should be changed or cleaned frequently. A HEPA filter unit and a vacuum with a built-in HEPA filter can remove a high percentage of the dust and pollen.

It is difficult to keep children from scratching and damaging irritated and itchy skin:

- Fingernails should be kept short, using a nail file for a smoother edge.
- Pajamas and clothing with maximum coverage help to protect the bare skin from fingernails.
- Mittens or socks can be used to prevent scratching at night.
- Infant gowns with hand coverings are useful for very young children.

Prognosis

Although there is no cure for eczema, most children improve with age, often by age five. For others however, eczema is a lifelong problem. Diligent daily skin care and avoidance of known triggers can largely control most cases. However, as many as 75% of children with eczema will develop other allergies, including hay fever, food allergies, or asthma.

Prevention

Breastfeeding an infant may help prevent eczema, particularly if there is a family history of eczema or allergies. It also may help for the breastfeeding mother to avoid foods that are common allergens. These include wheat, eggs, milk products, peanuts, and fish. If breastfeeding is not possible, a hypoallergenic formula should be used if there is family history of allergies.

Avoidance of known triggers and diligent skin care can minimize eczema flare-ups. A twice-daily emollient (moisturizing) routine should be followed even when the eczema appears to be under control. Eczematous skin is more susceptible to infection and patients should try to avoid contact with people infected with **chickenpox**, **cold sores**, and other contagious skin infections.

Resources

BOOKS

Balch, James F., Mark Stengler, and Robin Young-Balch. *Prescription for Drug Alternatives: All-Natural Options for Better Health Without the Side Effects.* Hoboken, NJ: John Wiley & Sons, 2008.

Joneja, Janice M. Vickerstaff. *Dealing with Food Allergies in Babies and Children.* Boulder, CO: Bull Publishing Co., 2007.

Sutton, Amy L. *Allergies Sourcebook.* Detroit: Omnigraphics, 2007.

PERIODICALS

Bieber, T. "Mechanisms of Disease: Atopic Dermatitis." *New England Journal of Medicine* 358 (2008): 1483.

Huang, J. T., et al. "Treatment of *Staphylococcus aureus* Colonization in Atopic Dermatitis Decreases Disease Severity." *Pediatrics* 123 no. 5 (May 1, 2009): e808-814.

Lawton, S. "Assessing and Treating Adult Patients with Eczema." *Nursing Standard* 23 no. 43 (July 1–7, 2009): 49-56.

Shrieves, Linda. "Childhood Eczema is a Growing Problem." *Connecticut Post* (April 20, 2009).

Van Bever, Hugo, Birgit Lane, and John Common. "Gene Defects and Allergy." *British Medical Journal* 339 no. 7712 (July 11, 2009): 58.

Watkins, Jean. "Eczema: Types, Presentation, Causes and Management." *Practice Nurse* 38 no. 4 (September 4, 2009): 11-16.

OTHER

"Atopic Dermatitis." National Institute of Arthritis and Musculoskeletal and Skin Diseases, http://www.niams.nih.gov/Health_Info/Atopic_Dermatitis/atopic_dermatitis_ff.asp

"Eczema." MedlinePlus, http://www.nlm.nih.gov/medlineplus/eczema.html

"Eczema/Atopic Dermatitis." American Academy of Dermatology, http://www.aad.org/public/publications/pamphlets/skin_eczema.html

"Eczema Quick Fact Sheet." National Eczema Association, http://www.nationaleczema.org/living/eczema_quick_fact_sheet.htm

"Evening Primrose Oil." NCCAM Publication No. D341, http://nccam.nih.gov/health/eveningprimrose/

Mayo Clinic Staff. "Atopic Dermatitis (Eczema)." Mayo Clinic Web site, http://www.mayoclinic.com/health/eczema/DS00986

Sampson, Hugh A. "Food Allergy Testing: When, Why, and What Does It Mean?" Food Allergy & Anaphylaxis Network, http://www.foodallergy.org/featuredtopic1.htm

"What is Eczema?" American Academy of Dermatology, http://www.skincarephysicians.com/eczemanet/whatis.html

ORGANIZATIONS

American Academy of Dermatology, PO Box 4014, Schaumburg, IL, 60168, (847) 240-1280, (866) 503-SKIN (503-7546), (847) 240-1859, http://www.aad.org.

American Academy of Family Physicians, 11400 Tomahawk Creek Parkway, Leawood, KS, 66211-2680, (913) 906-6000, (800) 274-6000, (913) 906-6075, http://www.aafp.org/online/en/home.html.

Food Allergy & Anaphylaxis Network, 11781 Lee Jackson Hwy., Suite 160, Fairfax, VA, 22033-3309, (800) 929-4040, (703) 691-2713, faan@foodallergy.org, http://www.foodallergy.org.

National Center for Complementary and Alternative Medicine, National Institutes of Health, 9000 Rockville Pike, Bethesda, MD, 20892, info@nccam.nih.gov, http://nccam.nih.gov.

National Eczema Association, 4460 Redwood Highway, Suite 16D, San Rafael, CA, 94903-1953, (415) 499-3474, (800) 818-7546, info@nationaleczema.org, http://www.nationaleczema.org.

National Institute of Arthritis and Musculoskeletal and Skin Diseases (NIAMS), Information Clearinghouse, National Institutes of Health, 1 AMS Circle, Bethesda, MD, 20892-3675, (301) 495-4484, (877) 22-NIAMS (226-4267), (301) 718-6366, NIAMSinfo@mail.nih.gov, http://www.niams.nih.gov.

Judith Turner
Teresa G. Odle
Margaret Alic, PhD

Education for All Handicapped Children Act

Definition

The Education for All Handicapped Children Act seeks to assure equal opportunity in education for all handicapped children between the ages of 5 and 18, and in most cases for children 3–5 and 18–21 as well. Handicapped children may not be excluded from public school because of their disability and school districts are required to provide special services to meet the needs of handicapped children. The law requires that handicapped children be taught in a setting that resembles the regular school program as closely as possible, while also meeting their special needs. Programs vary according to the individual needs of the special student. Some handicapped children may be placed in a regular classroom, but have special resources available to them; other students may need training at a special school.

Purpose

The law provides for screening so children with special needs are recognized and treated accordingly. The law also requires that an Individualized Education Program (IEP) be developed for each special needs student, with input from the student and student's parents, as well as the student's teachers and therapists. Students must have access to specialized materials and equipment if necessary, such as Braille books for blind students. Handicapped students are also entitled to have specially trained teachers to meet their particular needs. The law provides for ongoing monitoring of the handicapped student's program and an appeals process for both the school and the parents of the handicapped child, so that no child is put in or kept out of **special education** without the consent and agreement of parents and teachers.

Description

The first step in the special education process is to identify children with various educational challenges. States and school districts operate programs to find children with disabilities, and to make their parents aware as soon as possible the resources available to them. Children with a wide range of handicaps are eligible for special education. Blind, deaf, or physically handicapped children are eligible, as are children who may have a mild speech disorder such as a stammer, a learning disability that makes it very difficult for a child to learn to read, or a behavioral or emotional problem that interferes with learning. In some cases, the parents may identify the child as having a problem that needs further evaluation; in others, the teacher may alert the parents.

If parents or school officials note a possible problem in a child, the child is referred for an evaluation. The law requires that parents be notified in writing, in their native language, of the reason for the referral, and be given a description of the evaluation process. The parents'

KEY TERMS

Education for all handicapped children act— Known as Public Law 94-142, a federal law mandating that all handicapped children have available to them free public education suited to their needs.

written consent is required before a child can undergo the evaluation. The parents may also request, in writing, that their child be evaluated.

The next step in the process is evaluation. The law specifies that the evaluation be done by a multidisciplinary team, and not by a single person. Different states have different teams, but they usually include a social worker, a psychologist, and the child's classroom teacher. The parents must be a part of the evaluation team by law. The law recognizes that parents know the child best, and their input is essential. The child will usually be given a variety of standardized tests to determine specific aptitudes and weaknesses. The evaluation team may also observe the child in the classroom, review his or her classroom work, and consult with a guidance counselor, tutor, or other school staff who has worked closely with the child.

If the child is found to need special education, the parents will be asked to meet with a special team to help draw up an Individualized Education Plan (IEP). This team is separate from the evaluation team, though it may include some of the same school district staff. The child may be transferred to a special school or allowed to work with a specialist in the school, depending on what the team decides will help the child most. Parents must give their written consent before the IEP is implemented.

Evaluation and follow-up

The law requires that the IEP be reviewed by the IEP team at least once a year. Also, all students in special education must be reevaluated at least once every three years. If the parents or the school requests it, the reevaluation may be conducted sooner.

Resources

BOOKS

Cutler, Barbara Coyne, ed. *You, Your Child, and Special Education: A Guide to Dealing With the System.* Baltimore, MD: Brookes Publishing, 2010.

Giangreco, Michael F., et al. *Choosing Outcomes and Accommodations for Children (COACH): A Guide to Educational Planning for Students with Disabilities,* 2nd ed. Baltimore, MD: Brookes Publishing, 2010.

Mauro, Terri. *50 Ways to Support Your Child's Special Education: From IEPs to Assorted Therapies, an Empowering Guide to Taking Action, Every Day.* Avon, MA: Adams Media, 2009.

Siegel, Lawrence M. *The Complete IEP Guide: How to Advocate for Your Special Ed Child,* 6th ed. Berkley, CA: NOLO, 2009.

ORGANIZATIONS

National Dissemination Center for Children with Disabilities (NICHCY), 1825 Connecticut Ave NW, Suite 700, Washington, DC, 20009, (800) 695-0285, (202) 884-8441, http://www.nichcy.org/Pages/Home.aspx.

National Information Center for Children and Youth with-Disabilities, P.O. Box 1492, Washington, DC; 20013; 884-8200, (202) 695-0285, http://www.icdri.org/.

Laura Jean Cataldo, RN, Ed.D

Edwards' syndrome

Definition

Edwards' syndrome is caused by an extra copy of chromosome 18. For this reason, it is also called trisomy 18 syndrome. The extra chromosome is lethal for most

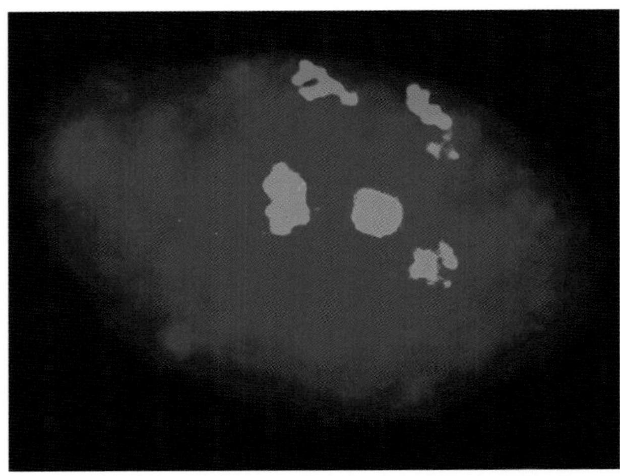

Micrograph showing trisomy 18, three copies of chromosome 18 (green) in cell's nucleus (blue) versus the normal two. The two fuchsia spots are the sex chromosomes, XX, a female. *(Department of Clinical Cytogenetics, Addenbrookes Hospital/Science Photo Library/ Photo Researchers, Inc.)*

babies born with this condition. It causes major physical abnormalities and severe **mental retardation**, and very few children afflicted with this disease survive beyond a year.

Description

Humans normally have 23 pairs of chromosomes. Chromosomes are numbered 1–22, and the 23rd pair is composed of the sex chromosomes, X and Y. A person inherits one set of 23 chromosomes from each parent. Occasionally, a genetic error occurs during egg or sperm cell formation. A child conceived with such an egg or sperm cell may inherit an incorrect number of chromosomes.

In the case of Edwards' syndrome, the child inherits three, rather than two, copies of chromosome 18. Trisomy 18 occurs in approximately one in every 3,000 newborns and affects girls more often than boys. Women older than their early thirties have a greater risk of conceiving a child with trisomy 18, but it can occur in younger women.

Causes and symptoms

A third copy of chromosome 18 causes numerous abnormalities. Most children born with Edwards' syndrome appear weak and fragile, and they are often underweight. The head is unusually small and the back of the head is prominent. The ears are malformed and low-set, and the mouth and jaw are small. The baby may also have a **cleft lip** or **cleft palate**. Frequently, the hands are clenched into fists, and the index finger overlaps the other fingers. The child may have clubfeet and toes may be webbed or fused.

Numerous problems involving the internal organs may be present. Abnormalities often occur in the lungs and diaphragm (the muscle that controls breathing), and heart defects and blood vessel malformations are common. The child may also have malformed kidneys and abnormalities of the urogenital system.

Diagnosis

Physical abnormalities point to Edwards' syndrome, but definitive diagnosis relies on karyotyping. Karyotyping involves drawing the baby's blood or bone marrow for a microscopic examination of the chromosomes. Using special stains and microscopy, individual chromosomes are identified, and the presence of an extra chromosome 18 is revealed.

Trisomy 18 can be detected before **birth**. If a pregnant woman is older than 35, has a family history of genetic abnormalities, has previously conceived a child with a genetic abnormality, or has suffered earlier miscarriages, she may undergo tests to determine whether her child carries genetic abnormalities. Potential tests include maternal serum analysis or screening, ultrasonography, **amniocentesis**, and chorionic villus sampling.

KEY TERMS

Aminocentesis—A procedure in which a needle is inserted through a pregnant woman's abdomen and into her uterus to withdraw a small sample of amniotic fluid. The amniotic fluid can be examined for signs of disease or other problems afflicting the fetus.

Chorionic villus sampling—A medical test that is best done during weeks 10–12 of a pregnancy. The procedure involves inserting a needle into the placenta and withdrawing a small amount of the chorionic membrane for analysis.

Chromosome—A structure composed of deoxyribonucleic acid (DNA) contained within a cell's nucleus (center) where genetic information is stored. Human have 23 pairs of chromosomes, each of which has recognizable characteristics (such as length and staining patterns) that allow individual chromosomes to be identified. Identification is assigned by number (1–22) or letter (X or Y).

Karyotyping—A laboratory test used to study an individual's chromosome make-up. Chromosomes are separated from cells, stained, and arranged in order from largest to smallest so that their number and structure can be studied under a microscope.

Maternal serum analyte screening—A medical procedure in which a pregnant woman's blood is drawn and analyzed for the levels of certain hormones and proteins. These levels can indicate whether there may be an abnormality in the unborn child. This test is not a definitive indicator of a problem and is followed by more specific testing such as amniocentesis or chorionic villus sampling.

Trisomy—A condition in which a third copy of a chromosome is inherited. Normally only two copies should be inherited.

Ultrasound—A medical test that is also called ultrasonography. Sound waves are directed against internal structures in the body. As sound waves bounce off the internal structure, they create an image on a video screen. An ultrasound of a fetus at weeks 16–20 of a pregnancy can be used to determine structural abnormalities.

Treatment

There is no cure for Edwards' syndrome. Since trisomy 18 babies frequently have major physical abnormalities, doctors and parents face difficult choices regarding treatment. Abnormalities can be treated to a certain degree with surgery, but extreme invasive procedures may not be in the best interests of an infant whose lifespan is measured in days or weeks. Medical therapy often consists of supportive care with the goal of making the infant comfortable, rather than prolonging life.

Prognosis

Most children born with trisomy 18 die within their first year of life. The average lifespan is less than two months for 50% of the children, and 90–95% die before their first birthday. The 5–10% of children who survive their first year are severely mentally retarded. They need support to walk, and learning is limited. Verbal communication is also limited, but they can learn to recognize and interact with others.

Prevention

Edwards' syndrome cannot be prevented.

ORGANIZATIONS

Chromosome 18 Registry & Research Society, 6302 Fox Head, San Antonio, TX, 78247, (210) 657-4968, http://www.chromosome18.org.

Support Organization for Trisomy 18, 13, and Related Disorders (SOFT), 2982 South Union St., Rochester, NY, 14624 (800) 716-SOFT, http://www.trisomy.org.

Julia Barrett

EEG ***see*** **Electroencephalography**

Ehlers-Danlos syndrome

Definition

The Ehlers-Danlos syndromes (EDS) refer to a group of inherited disorders that affect collagen structure and function. Genetic abnormalities in the manufacturing of collagen within the body affect connective tissues, causing them to be abnormally weak.

Description

Collagen is a strong, fibrous protein that lends strength and elasticity to connective tissues, such as the skin, tendons, organ walls, cartilage, and blood vessels. Each of these connective tissues requires collagen tailored to meet its specific purposes. The many roles of collagen are reflected in the number of genes dedicated to its production. There are at least 28 genes in humans that encode at least 19 different types of collagen. Mutations in these genes can affect basic construction as well as the fine-tuned processing of the collagen.

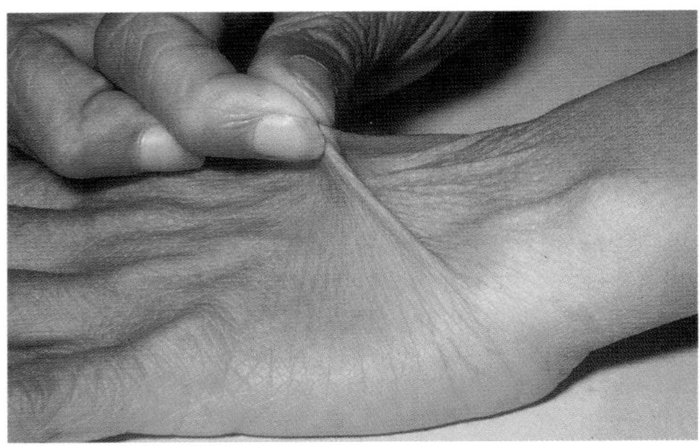

Elasticity of the skin is one characteristic of Ehlers-Danlos syndrome. *(Biophoto Associates/Photo Researchers, Inc.)*

EDS was originally described by Dr. Van Meekeren in 1682. Dr. Ehlers and Dr. Danlos further characterized the disease in 1901 and 1908, respectively. Today, according to the Ehlers-Danlos National Foundation, one in 5,000 to one in 10,000 people are affected by some form of EDS.

EDS is a group of **genetic disorders** that usually affects the skin, ligaments, joints, and blood vessels. Classification of EDS types was revised in 1997. The new classification involves categorizing the different forms of EDS into six major sub-types, including classical, hypermobility, vascular, kyphoscoliosis, arthrochalasia, and dermatosparaxis, and a collection of rare or poorly defined varieties. This new classification is simpler and based more on descriptions of the actual symptoms.

Classical type

Under the old classification system, EDS classical type was divided into two separate types: type I and type II. The major symptoms involved in EDS classical type are the skin and joints. The skin has a smooth, velvety texture and **bruises** easily. Affected individuals typically have extensive scarring, particularly at the knees, elbows, forehead, and chin. The joints are hyperextensible, giving a tendency towards dislocation of the hip, shoulder, elbow, knee, or clavicle. Due to decreased muscle tone, affected infants may experience a delay in reaching motor milestones. Children may have a tendency to develop hernias or other organ shifts within the abdomen. **Sprains** and partial or complete joint dilocations are also common. Symptoms can range from mild to severe. EDS classical type is inherited in an autosomal dominant manner.

There are three major clinical diagnostic criteria for EDS classical type. These include skin hyperextensibility, unusually wide scars, and joint hypermobility. At this time there is no definitive test for the diagnosis of classical EDS. Both DNA and biochemical studies have been used to help identify affected individuals. In some cases, a skin biopsy has been found to be useful in confirming a diagnosis. Unfortunately, these tests are not sensitive enough to identify all individuals with classical EDS. If there are multiple affected individuals in a family, it may be possible to perform prenatal diagnosis using a DNA information technique known as a linkage study.

Hypermobility type

Excessively loose joints are the hallmark of this EDS type, formerly known as EDS type III. Both large joints, such as the elbows and knees, and small joints, such as toes and fingers, are affected. Partial and total joint dislocations are common, and particularly involve the jaw, knee, and shoulder. Many individuals experience chronic limb and joint **pain**, although **x rays** of these joints appear normal. The skin may also bruise easily. Osteoarthritis is a common occurrence in adults. EDS hypermobility type is inherited in an autosomal dominant manner.

There are two major clinical diagnostic criteria for EDS hypermobility type. These include skin involvement (either hyperextensible skin or smooth and velvety skin) and generalized joint hypermobility. At this time there is no test for this form of EDS.

Vascular type

Formerly called EDS type IV, EDS vascular type is the most severe form. The connective tissue in the intestines, arteries, uterus, and other hollow organs may be unusually weak, leading to organ or blood vessel rupture. Such ruptures are most likely between ages 20 and 40, although they can occur any time and may be life-threatening.

There is a classic facial appearance associated with EDS vascular type. Affected individuals tend to have large eyes, a thin pinched nose, thin lips, and a slim body. The skin is thin and translucent, with veins dramatically visible, particularly across the chest.

The large joints have normal stability, but small joints in the hands and feet are loose, showing hyperextensibility. The skin bruises easily. Other complications may include collapsed lungs, premature aging of the skin on the hands and feet, and ruptured arteries and veins. After surgery there tends to be poor wound healing, a complication that tends to be frequent and severe. Pregnancy also carries the risk complications. During and after pregnancy there is an increased risk of the uterus rupturing and of arterial bleeding. Due to the severe complications associated with EDS type IV, **death** usually occurs before the fifth decade. A study of 419 individuals with EDS vascular type, completed in 2000, found that the median survival rate was 48 years, with a range of 6–73 years. EDS vascular type is inherited in an autosomal dominant manner.

There are four major clinical diagnostic criteria for EDS vascular type. These include thin translucent skin, arterial/intestinal/uterine fragility or rupture, extensive bruising, and characteristic facial appearance. EDS vascular type is caused by a change in the gene COL3A1, which codes for one of the collagen chains used to build Collage type III. Laboratory testing is available for this form of EDS. A skin biopsy may be used to demonstrate the structurally abnormal collagen. This type of biochemical test identifies more than 95% of individuals with EDS vascular type. Laboratory testing is recommended for individuals with two or more of the major criteria.

DNA analysis may also be used to identify the change within the COL3A1 gene. This information may be helpful for genetic counseling purposes. Prenatal testing is available for pregnancies in which an affected parent has been identified and their DNA mutation is known or their biochemical defect has been demonstrated.

Kyphoscoliosis type

The major symptoms of kyphoscoliosis type, formerly called EDS type VI, are general joint looseness. At **birth**, the muscle tone is poor, and motor skill development is subsequently delayed. Also, infants with this type of EDS have an abnormal curvature of the spine (**scoliosis**). The scoliosis becomes progressively worse with age, with affected individuals usually unable to walk by age 20. The eyes and skin are fragile and easily damaged, and blood vessel involvement is a possibility. The bones may also be affected as demonstrated by a decrease in bone mass. Kyphoscoliosis type is inherited in an autosomal recessive manner.

There are four major clinical diagnostic criteria for EDS kyphoscoliosis type. These include generaly loose joints, low muscle tone at birth, scoliosis at birth (which worsens with age), and a fragility of the eyes, which may give the white area of the eye a blue tint or cause the eye to rupture. This form of EDS is caused by a change in the

PLOD gene on chromosome 1, which encodes the enzyme lysyl hydroxylase. A laboratory test is available in which urinary hydroxylysyl pryridinoline is measured. This test, performed on urine is extremely senstive and specific for EDS kyphoscolios type. Laboratory testing is recommended for infants with three or more of the major diagnostic criteria.

Prenatal testing is available if a pregnancy is known to be at risk and an identified affected family member has had positive laboratory testing. An **amniocentesis** may be performed in which fetal cells are removed from the amniotic fluid and enzyme activity is measured.

Arthrochalasia type

Dislocation of the hip joint typically accompanies arthrochalasia type EDS, formerly called EDS type VIIB. Other joints are also unusually loose, leading to recurrent partial and total dislocations. The skin has a high degree of stretchability and bruises easily. Individuals with this type of EDS may also experience mildly diminished bone mass, scoliosis, and poor muscle tone. Arthrochalasia type is inherited in an autosomal dominant manner.

There are two major clinical diagnostic criteria for EDS arthrochalasia type. These include severe generalized joing hypermobility and bilateral hip dislocation present at birth. This form of EDS is caused by a change in either of two components of Collage type I, called proa1(I) type A and proa2(I) type B. A skin biopsy may be preformed to demonstrate an abnormality in either components. Direct DNA testing is also available.

Dermatosparaxis type

Individuals with this type of EDS, once called type VIIC, have extremely fragile skin that bruises easily but does not scar excessively. The skin is soft and may sag, leading to an aged appearance even in young adults. Individuals may also experience hernias. Dermatosparaxis type is inherited in an autosomal recessive manner.

There are two major clinical diagnostic criteria for EDS dematosparaxis type. These include severe skin fragility and sagging or aged appearing skin. This form of EDS is caused by a change in the enzyme called procollagen I N-terminal peptidase. A skin biopsy may be preformed for a definitive diagnosis of Dermatosparaxis type.

Other types

There are several other forms of EDS that have not been as clearly defined as the aforementioned types. Forms of EDS within this category may present with soft, mildly stretchable skin, shortened bones, chronic **diarrhea**, joint hypermobility and dislocation, bladder rupture, or poor wound healing. Inheritance patterns within this group include X-linked recessive, autosomal dominant, and autosomal recessive.

Causes and symptoms

There are numerous types of EDS, all caused by changes in one of several genes. The manner in which EDS is inherited depends on the specific gene involved. There are three patterns of inheritance for EDS: autosomal dominant, autosomal recessive, and X-linked (extremely rare).

Chromosomes are made up of hundreds of small units known as genes, which contain the genetic material necessary for an individual to develop and function. Humans have 46 chromosomes, which are matched into 23 pairs. Because chromosomes are inherited in pairs, each individual receives two copies of each chromosome and likewise two copies of each gene.

Changes or mutations in genes can cause genetic diseases in several different ways, many of which are represented within the spectrum of EDS. In autosomal dominant EDS, only one copy of a specific gene must be changed for a person to have EDS. In autosomal recessive EDS, both copies of a specific gene must be changed for a person to have EDS. If only one copy of an autosomal recessive EDS gene is changed the person is referred to as a carrier, meaning they do not have any of the signs or symptoms of the disease itself, but carry the possibility of passing on the disorder to a future child. In X-linked EDS a specific gene on the X chromosome must be changed. However, this affects males and females differently because males and females have a different number of X chromosomes.

The few X-linked forms of EDS fall under the category of X-linked recessive. As with autosomal recessive, this implies that both copies of a specific gene must be changed for a person to be affected. However, because males only have one X-chromosome, they are affected if an X-linked recessive EDS gene is changed on their single X-chromosome. That is, they are affected even though they have only one changed copy. On the other hand, that same gene must be changed on both of the X-chromosomes in a female for her to be affected.

Although there is much information regarding the changes in genes that cause EDS and their various inheritance patterns, the exact gene mutation for all types of EDS is not known.

Diagnosis

Clinical symptoms, such as extreme joint looseness and unusual skin qualities, along with family history, can lead to a diagnosis of EDS. Specific tests, such as skin biopsies are available for diagnosis of certain types of EDS, including vascular, arthrochalasia, and dermatosparaxis types. A skin biopsy involves removing a small sample of skin and examining its microscopic structure. A urine test is available for the Kyphoscoliosis type.

Management of all types of EDS may include genetic counseling to help the affected individual and their family understand the disorder and its impact on other family members and future children.

If a couple has had a child diagnosed with EDS the chance that they will have another child with the same disorder depends on with what form of EDS the child has been diagnosed and if either parent is affected by the same disease or not.

Individuals diagnosed with an autosomal dominant form of EDS have a 50% chance of passing the same disorder on to a child in each pregnancy. Individuals diagnosed with an autosomal recessive form of EDS have an extremely low risk of having a child with the same disorder.

X-linked recessive EDS is accompanied by a slightly more complicated pattern of inheritance. If a father with an X-linked recessive form of EDS passes a copy of his X chromosome to his children, the sons will be unaffected and the daughters will be carriers. If a mother is a carrier for an X-linked recessive form of EDS, she may have affected or unaffected sons, or carrier or unaffected daughters, depending on the second sex chromosome inherited from the father.

Prenatal diagnosis is available for specific forms of EDS, including kyphosocliosis type and vascular type. However, prenatal testing is only a possibility in these types if the underlying defect has been found in another family member.

Treatment

Medical therapy relies on managing symptoms and trying to prevent further complications. There is no cure for EDS.

Braces may be prescribed to stabilize joints, although surgery is sometimes necessary to repair joint damage caused by repeated dislocations. Physical therapy teaches individuals how to strengthen muscles around joints and may help to prevent or limit damage. Elective surgery is discouraged due to the high possibility of complications.

Alternative treatment

There are anecdotal reports that large daily doses 0.04–0.14 oz (1–4 g) of vitamin C may help decrease bruising and aid in wound healing. Constitutional homeopathic treatment may be helpful in maintaining optimal health in persons with a diagnosis of EDS. An

KEY TERMS

Arthrochalasia—Excessive looseness of the joints.

Blood vessels—General term for arteries, veins, and capillaries that transport blood throughout the body.

Cartilage—Supportive connective tissue that cushions bone at the joints or which connects muscle to bone.

Collagen—The main supportive protein of cartilage, connective tissue, tendon, skin, and bone.

Connective tissue—A group of tissues responsible for support throughout the body; includes cartilage, bone, fat, tissue underlying skin, and tissues that support organs, blood vessels, and nerves throughout the body.

Dermatosparaxis—Skin fragility caused by abnormal collagen.

Hernia—A rupture in the wall of a body cavity, through which an organ may protrude.

Homeopathic—A holistic and natural approach to healthcare.

Hyperextensibility—The ability to extend a joint beyond the normal range.

Hypermobility—Unusual flexibility of the joints, allowing them to be bent or moved beyond their normal range of motion.

Joint dislocation—The displacement of a bone.

Kyphoscoliosis—Abnormal front-to-back and side-to-side curvature of the spine.

Ligament—A type of connective tissue that connects bones or cartilage and provides support and strength to joints.

Osteoarthritis—A degenerative joint disease that causes pain and stiffness.

Scoliosis—An abnormal, side-to-side curvature of the spine.

Tendon—A strong connective tissue that connects muscle to bone.

Uterus—A muscular, hollow organ of the female reproductive tract. The uterus contains and nourishes the embryo and fetus from the time the fertilized egg is implanted until birth.

Vascular—Having to do with blood vessels.

individual with EDS should discuss these types of therapies with their doctor before beginning them on their own. Therapy that does not require medical consultation involves protecting the skin with sunscreen and avoiding activities that place stress on the joints.

Prognosis

The outlook for individuals with EDS depends on the type of EDS with which they have been diagnosed. Symptoms vary in severity, even within one sub-type, and the frequency of complications changes on an individual basis. Some individuals have negligible symptoms while others are severely restricted in their daily life. Extreme joint instability and scoliosis may limit a person's mobility. Most individuals will have a normal lifespan. However, those with blood vessel involvement, particularly those with EDS vascular type, have an increased risk of fatal complications.

EDS is a lifelong condition. Affected individuals may face social obstacles related to their disease on a daily basis. Some people with EDS have reported living with fears of significant and painful skin ruptures, becoming pregnant (especially those with EDS vascular type), their condition worsening, becoming unemployed due to physical and emotional burdens, and social stigmatization in general.

Constant bruises, skin **wounds**, and trips to the hospital take their toll on both affected children and their parents. Prior to diagnosis parents of children with EDS have found themselves under suspicion of **child abuse**.

Some people with EDS are not diagnosed until well into adulthood and, in the case of EDS vascular type, occasionally not until after death due to complications of the disorder. Not only may the diagnosis itself be devastating to the family, but in many cases other family members also find out for the first time they are at risk for being affected.

Although individuals with EDS face significant challenges, it is important to remember that each person is unique, with their own distinguished qualities and potential. Persons with EDS go on to have families, to have careers, and to be accomplished citizens, surmounting the challenges of their disease.

Resources

PERIODICALS

"Clinical and Genetic Features of Ehlers-DanlosSyndrome Type IV, the Vascular Type." *The New England Journal of Medicine* 342 no. 10 (2000).

"Living a Restricted Life with Ehlers-DanlosSyndrome." *International Journal of Nursing Studies* 37 (2000): 111–118.

OTHER

GeneClinics. http://www.geneclinics.org

ORGANIZATIONS

Ehlers-Danlos Support Group, PO Box 335, Farnham, Surrey, UK GU10 1XJ, +441252 690 940, http://www.atv.ndirect.co.uk.

Elhers-Danlos National Foundation, 6399 Wilshire Blvd., Ste 203, Los Angeles, CA, 90048, (323) 651-3038, (323) 651-1366, http://www.ednf.org.

Java O. Solis, MS

Elbow injury **see** **Nursemaid's elbow**

Electric and magnetic fields

Definition

Electric and magnetic fields, referred to as EMF, are the fields of energy surrounding electric power wires and other current-carrying devices.

Description

Electric power lines, household wiring, and appliances all carry electric current. Since the late 1970s, concerns have been raised about the link between electric and magnetic fields (EMFs), the invisible lines of force that surround all electrical devices, and the development of **cancer**. EMFs are a form of non-ionizing radiation and as such, are not as likely to cause tissue damage as forms of ionizing radiation.

Alternating current (AC), the form of electric power used in the United States, produces fields that induce weak electric currents in objects that conduct electricity, including humans. Direct current, the form of current produced by batteries, is unlikely to induce electric current in humans. The currents induced by AC fields have been the focus of most research on how EMFs may affect human health.

Some studies in epidemiology (studies with humans to understand the cause and progression of disease) have suggested a possible link may exist between exposure to power-frequency electric and magnetic fields (EMFs) and certain types of cancer, primarily leukemia and brain cancer.

From 1979 to 1993, 14 studies analyzed the possible association between proximity to power lines and types of childhood cancer. Of these, eight reported correlations between proximity to power lines and some form of cancer. Four of the 14 studies showed a statistically significant association with the development of leukemia.

Since the late 1970s there have been over 100 epidemiological studies conducted to determine the impact of EMF exposure in the home or workplace on the development of cancer and other diseases and conditions. A recent document, focused on extremely low frequency magnetic fields (ELFs), was released by the World Health Organization in 2007 and stated that some questions related to carcinogenicity of ELFs have not been resolved. Therefore, the International Agency for Research on Cancer (IARC) has determined that exposure to 50-60 Hz magnetic fields is potentially carcinogenic to humans and there is some limited evidence to link residential exposure to childhood leukemia. More recent studies conducted in Japan, Canada, Germany, the United States, and the United Kingdom have continued to uncover links between exposure to ELF magnetic fields and childhood and other types of cancer particularly in individuals living closest to electrical lines with the highest levels of magnetic fields for the longest amounts of time.

For the typical homeowner, identifying and measuring sources of EMF exposure is complex: EMF fields change constantly, depending on the power usage in the person's environment, and his or her proximity to the power source. People living close to large power lines tend to have higher overall exposures to electric fields, since fields close to transmission lines are much stronger than those surrounding household appliances. Magnetic fields, on the other hand, are stronger in close proximity to household appliances than directly beneath power lines. These magnetic fields decrease in strength with distance from the source more quickly than do electric fields.

To find out about EMFs from a particular power line, homeowners may contact the utility that operates the power line. Most utilities will conduct EMF measurements for customers at no charge. Other options are to hire an independent technician (often listed in the yellow pages of the telephone directory under "Engineers, environmental"), or to purchase a gaussmeter for self-monitoring of EMF levels.

Prevention

For most people who live in urban communities and for many people living in rural areas, it is virtually impossible to prevent all exposure to EMFs. Strategies for minimizing exposure to EMFs are: increase the distance between yourself and the EMF source (keep appliances and electronics at arm's length); avoid unnecessary proximity to high EMF sources (don't play under power lines or on top of power transformers for underground lines); and reduce the time appliances operate (for example, turn off the computer monitor when not in use).

Resources

PERIODICALS

Comba, P., and L. Fazzo. "Health Effects of Magnetic Fields Generated from Power Lines: New Clues from an Old Puzzle." *Ann 1st Super Sanita* (2009) 45(3): 233–37.

Schuz, J., et al. "Nighttime Exposure to Electromagnetic Fields and Childhood Leukemia: An Extended Pooled Analysis." *American Journal of Epidemiology.* (2007) 166: 263–9.

Wood, A. W. "How Dangerous are Mobile Phones, Transmission Masts and Electricity Pylons?" *Archives of Disease in Childhood* (April 2006) 91(4): 361–66.

OTHER

"Electric and Magnetic Fields." National Institute of Environmental Health Sciences National Institutes of Health. http://www.niehs.nih.gov/health/topics/agents/emf (accessed July 5, 2010).

Melinda Granger Oberleitner, RN, DNS, APRN, CNS

Electric shock injuries

Definition

Electricity is a form of energy generated by the flow of electrons across a potential gradient from high to low concentration through a conductive material. Electrical injuries in humans are caused by contact with an electrical current, either natural lightning or mechanically generated.

Demographics

Electrical injuries were rare in industrialized societies until the 1870s and 1880s, when a series of inventions by Thomas Edison (1847–1931) and George Westinghouse (1846–1914) made it possible to transmit electricity over long-distance wires from one location to another for commercial and scientific purposes. The first fatal industrial accident involving an electric shock occurred in Lyon, France, in 1879.

As of 2010, electrical injuries were responsible for about 1,000 deaths in the United States each year, or about 1% of all accidental deaths. About a quarter of these fatalities are caused by natural lightning. Electric shocks are responsible for 5% of all admissions to specialized burn treatment units in North America.

In the United States, 80% of all electrical injuries occur in adult men, largely because of occupational choices. Among children, the male:female ratio is 3:1. Low-voltage injuries are most common among toddlers; high-voltage injuries primarily affect risk-taking adolescents and adults in high-risk occupations.

According to the U.S. Bureau of Labor Statistics, electric shocks are the second leading cause of **death** in the construction industry in North America. With regard to injuries caused by contact with overhead powerlines, between 27% and 60% of cases resulted in over 31 days lost from work—compared to 18%–20% for all other occupational injury and illness. Injuries caused by electric shocks are also costly to employers; a researcher at the Electric Power Research Institute in Palo Alto, California, estimates that the cost to American employers is approximately $15.75 million *per case* in direct and indirect costs.

Description

Accidental electrical injuries

Electrical injuries are classified according to three factors: power source (lightning or human-generated electricity; voltage (high or low); and type of current (alternating or direct). Each is associated with certain patterns of injury. Most electrical injuries are accidental.

The minimum current that humans can feel is 1 milliampere (abbreviated mA). An ampere, named for the French mathematician and physicist André-Marie Ampère (1775–1836), is a measure of the amount of electric charge passing a given point per unit time. One ampere represents 6.241 x 10^{18} electrons passing a given point in a wire in one second of time. In general, a current of 100 mA will be lethal if it passes through sensitive parts of the human body; a current as low as 60 mA can cause ventricular fibrillation, irregular contraction of the muscles in the two lower chambers of the heart.

Intentional use of electric shocks

Electric shocks have been used in medicine to treat mental illness, particularly depression (electroconvulsive therapy or ECT); to correct irregular heart rhythms (defibrillation and cardioversion); and to relieve **pain** by stimulating opioid receptors in the central nervous system (transcutaneous electrical nerve stimulation or TENS).

Electricity was used as a form of torture or punishment almost as soon as it was known to cause accidental workplace injuries. Since the 1930s, the Nazis and other tyrannical regimes have used cattle prods and similar devices to torture people. The tasers currently used by some police departments are electroshock devices that cause strong involuntary contractions of the muscles controlling movement, thus temporarily incapacitating violent or intoxicated suspects.

Electrocution as a method of capital punishment was introduced in the late 1880s on the recommendation of a committee in New York State seeking a more humane method of execution than hanging. Thomas Edison recommended the use of alternating current to electrocute criminals, maintaining that it would cause instantaneous death. The first use of the electric chair in New York in 1890, however, was a disaster, requiring eight minutes to cause death. George Westinghouse is reported to have said that it would have been more humane to use an axe. As of 2010, only six states still used the electric chair as an option for execution.

Risk factors

Risk factors for electrical injuries include:

- working or playing outside during an electrical storm
- employment in an occupation related to the generation of electricity or servicing of electrical equipment or power lines
- employment in the construction industry, mining, or public transportation
- natural disasters, including hurricanes, tornadoes, earthquakes, and ice storms, which bring down or disrupt high-voltage power lines
- theft of copper and other metals from construction sites and other areas close to high-voltage wires

Causes and symptoms

Causes

Electricity damages the cells in human tissues in two basic ways: heating and blast force. The passage of electrical current through cell membranes causes their temperatures to rise, leading to disruption of the cell membrane itself (at 108°F); denaturation of protein molecules in the cell (at 113°F); and destruction of DNA (at 149°F or higher). In most cases of high-voltage electrical shock, heat damage occurs immediately at contact points but requires 1–3 seconds to injure deeper tissues. The blast force of electric current can cause significant blunt trauma injuries.

The overall severity of electrical injury depends on the current's pressure (voltage), the amount of current (amperage), the type of current (direct vs. alternating), the body's resistance to the current, the current's path through the body, and how long the body remains in contact with the current. The interplay of these factors can produce effects ranging from barely noticeable **tingling** to instant death; every part of the body is vulnerable. Although the severity of injury is determined primarily by the voltage, low voltage can be just as dangerous as high voltage under the right circumstances. People have been killed by shocks of just 50 volts. Electric voltage of 380 volts or less is considered low voltage. The United States national electric code defines high voltage as 600 volts or higher. High voltage is generated at power plants and is transformed down to approximately 120 volts for most wall outlets in homes.

Symptoms

Electric shocks can affect all the major organ systems in the human body. How electric shocks affect the skin is determined by the skin's resistance, which in turn is dependent upon the wetness, thickness, and cleanliness of the skin. Thin or wet skin is much less resistant than thick or dry skin. When skin resistance is low, the current may cause little or no skin damage but severely burn internal organs and tissues. Conversely, high skin resistance can produce severe skin **burns** but prevent the current from entering the body.

The nervous system (the brain, spinal cord, and nerves) is particularly vulnerable to injury. Neurological problems are the most common kind of nonlethal harm suffered by electric shock victims. Some neurological damage is minor and clears up on its own or with medical treatment, but some is severe and permanent. Neurological problems may be apparent immediately after the accident, or gradually develop over a period of up to three years.

Damage to the respiratory and cardiovascular systems is most acute at the moment of injury. Electric shocks can paralyze the respiratory system or disrupt heart action, causing instant death. Also at risk are the smaller veins and arteries, which dissipate heat less easily than the larger blood vessels and can develop blood clots. Damage to the

KEY TERMS

Alternating current (AC)—An electric current in which the flow of the electric charge periodically reverses direction. AC is the form in which electricity is usually delivered to homes. The usual household wall outlet (120 volts) provides a current with 120 reversals of the direction of flow occurring each second and is termed 60-cycle alternating current.

Amperage—A measurement of the amount of electric charge passing a given point per unit time. One ampere represents about 6.241×10^{18} electrons passing a given point in a wire in one second of time.

Antibiotics—Substances used against microorganisms that cause infection.

Arc flash—A type of electrical explosion resulting from electrical breakdown of the gases in air, which normally does not conduct electricity. Arc flashes can occur where there is sufficient voltage in an electrical system and a path to the ground or to lower voltage.

Cataract—Clouding of the lens of the eye or its capsule (surrounding membrane).

Computed tomography scan (CT scan)—A process that uses x rays to create three-dimensional images of structures inside the body.

Direct current (DC)—An electric current in which the electric charge moves in only one direction. It is the type of current produced by batteries and solar cells.

Electrolytes—Substances that conduct electric current within the body and are essential for sustaining life.

Magnetic resonance imaging (MRI)—The use of electromagnetic energy to create images of structures inside the body.

Skin grafting—A technique in which a piece of healthy skin from the patient's body (or a donor's) is used to cover another part of the patient's body that has lost its skin.

Taser—Also called a conducted electrical weapon (CEW), a taser is an electroshock device used by some police departments in various countries to subdue armed or otherwise dangerous suspects without having to use lethal force. Tasers work by interfering with the brain's capacity to control voluntary muscles. The name *taser* is an acronym for *Thomas A. Swift's Electric Rifle*, an adventure novel about a fictional weapon published in 1911.

Voltage—The force necessary to drive an electric current between two specified points. A large voltage exerts a greater force, which moves more electrons through a wire at a given rate of time.

smaller vessels is probably one reason why amputation is often required following high-voltage injuries.

Many other sorts of injuries are possible after an electric shock, including cataracts, kidney failure, and substantial destruction of muscle tissue. The victim may suffer a fall or be hit by debris from exploding equipment. An electric arc flash may set clothing or nearby flammable substances on fire. Arc flashes can produce light intense enough to cause permanent blindness as well as heat intense enough (5000°F to 7000°F) to melt bone and vaporize the surfaces of nearby human beings and other objects. Strong shocks are often accompanied by violent **muscle spasms** that can break and dislocate bones. These spasms can also freeze the victim in place and prevent him or her from breaking away from the source of the current. Alternating current is considered three times as dangerous as direct current for this reason: high-voltage DC tends to cause one strong muscle spasm that throws the victim away from the source, whereas the cyclical flow of electrons in AC of the same voltage causes paralysis of the muscles that holds the victim in contact with the current.

Diagnosis

Diagnosis relies on gathering information about the circumstances of the accident, a thorough physical examination, and monitoring of cardiovascular and kidney activity. When at all possible, witnesses of the accident should be questioned about the circumstances of the event, particularly if the victim has lost consciousness or normal mental status. The victim's neurological condition can fluctuate rapidly and requires close observation. A computed tomography scan (CT scan) or **magnetic resonance imaging** (MRI) may be necessary to check for brain injury. Blood and urine samples may be taken. In some cases, the doctor may make a trial incision into burned muscle to assess the extent of tissue damage. The tissue sample is frozen and examined under a microscope to see whether the muscle tissue is still viable. If an arm or leg damaged by electricity is determined not to be viable, immediate amputation is necessary.

Treatment

Treatment of an electrical injury usually begins at the scene, although first responders will generally take the victim to an emergency department or specialized burn or trauma center as soon as possible. The victim of a severe electrical injury may be examined and treated by a variety of specialists, including emergency physicians, plastic surgeons, neurologists, ophthalmologists, and orthopedic surgeons.

Traditional

When an electric shock accident happens at home or in the workplace, the main power should immediately be shut off and 911 should be called. If that cannot be done, and current is still flowing through the victim, the alternative is to stand on a dry, nonconducting surface such as a folded newspaper, flattened cardboard carton, or plastic or rubber mat and use a nonconducting object such as a wooden broomstick (never a damp or metallic object) to push the victim away from the source of the current. The victim and the source of the current must not be touched while the current is still flowing, for this contact can electrocute the rescuer. Emergency medical help should be summoned as quickly as possible. Trained electricians must use lineman's gloves to separate the victim from the circuit by a specially insulated pole. Looping a polydacron rope around the injured patient is another method of pulling him or her from the electric power source. Ideally, the electrician or first responder should stand on a dry surface during the rescue. People who are trained to perform **cardiopulmonary resuscitation** (CPR) should, if appropriate, begin **first aid** while waiting for emergency medical help to arrive.

Burn victims usually require treatment at a specialized burn center. Fluid replacement therapy is necessary to restore lost fluids and electrolytes. Severely injured tissue is repaired surgically, which can involve skin grafting or amputation. **Antibiotics** and antibacterial creams are used to prevent infection. Victims may also require treatment for kidney failure. Following surgery, physical therapy to facilitate recovery, and psychological counseling to cope with disfigurement, may be necessary.

Prognosis

The mortality rate for electrical injuries in the United States as of 2010 was 3–5%. Many survivors, however, require amputation or are permanently disfigured by their burns. **Anxiety** disorders are common in survivors of high-voltage electrical injuries. About 73% of pregnant women injured by lightning or high-voltage electricity lose the baby. Injuries from household appliances and other low-voltage sources are less likely to produce extreme damage.

Prevention

Prevention of electrical injuries in the home or workplace begins with age-appropriate education about the nature of electricity and the importance of **safety** measures. The National Safety Council in the United States and Hydro-Québec (a power company) in Canada have handouts, videos, quizzes, and fact sheets about electrical safety on their websites (http://www.nsc.org/ and http://www.hydroquebec.com/security/index.html), some of which are listed under Resources at the end of this article. These materials are written for the general public and are intended to help people recognize dangerous situations and take steps to protect themselves and their families before an electrical accident occurs.

People who are employed in workplaces with high-voltage electrical equipment or whose jobs require working with electricity should follow all safety precautions recommended by the National Safety Council:

- Those working near high-voltage lines should wear Class B helmets, which are designed to withstand 20,000 volts of AC for 3 minutes.
- Special insulated gloves should be worn, either Class 2 (provides protection against 20,000 volts) or Class 4 (protection against 40,000 volts), along with tinted eyewear to protect the eyes against arc flashes.
- Only employees with special training and authorization should work on high-voltage lines or equipment; other workers should not try to perform tasks for which they are not qualified or trained.
- Rubber-soled shoes or work boots must be worn on damp or wet surfaces.
- Workers should check that circuits, wiring, insulation, equipment, and cords or extension cords are in good repair.
- Hazards of any kind, including water or spills as well as damaged or defective equipment, should be reported to supervisors at once.

Parents and other adults need to be alert to possible electric dangers in the home. Damaged electric appliances, wiring, cords, and plugs should be repaired or replaced. Electrical repairs should be attempted only by people with the proper training. Hair dryers, radios, and other electric appliances should never be used in the bathroom or anywhere else they might accidentally come in contact with water. Young children need to be kept away from electric appliances and should be taught about the dangers of electricity as soon as they are old enough. Electric outlets require safety covers in homes with young children.

People should be particularly careful when using metal ladders outside, accidental contact with an overhead power line can be fatal.

During thunderstorms, people should go indoors immediately, even if no rain is falling, and boaters should return to shore as rapidly as possible. People who cannot reach indoor shelter should move away from such metallic objects as golf clubs and fishing rods and lie down in low-ground areas. Standing or lying under or next to trees and tall or metallic structures is unsafe. An automobile is appropriate cover, as long as the radio is off. Telephones, computers, hair dryers, and other appliances that can act as conduits for lightning should not be used during thunderstorms.

Resources

BOOKS

Bledsoe, Bryan E., and Randall W. Benner. *Critical Care Paramedic*. Upper Saddle River, NJ: Pearson Prentice Hall, 2006.

Denegar, Craig R., et al. *Therapeutic Modalities for Musculoskeletal Injuries*, 3rd ed. Champaign, IL: Human Kinetics, 2010.

Fish, Raymond M., and Leslie A. Geddes, eds. *Electrical Injuries: Medical and Bioengineering Aspects*, 2nd ed. Tucson, AZ: Lawyers and Judges Publishing, 2009.

PERIODICALS

Chudasama, S., et al. "Does Voltage Predict Return to Work and Neuropsychiatric Sequelae Following Electrical Burn Injury?" *Annals of Plastic Surgery* 64 (May 2010): 522–25.

Curinga, G., et al. "Electrical Injuries Due to Theft of Copper." *Journal of Burn Care and Research* 31 (March-April 2010): 341–46.

Fichet, J. "Left Ventricular Function and High-Voltage Electrical Injury." *Critical Care Medicine* 37 (November 2009): 2995.

Fish, R.M., and L.A. Geddes. "Conduction of Electrical Current to and through the Human Body: A Review." *Eplasty* 9 (October 12, 2009): e44.

Lakosha, H., et al. "High-Voltage Electrical Trauma to the Eye." *Canadian Journal of Ophthalmology* 44 (October 2009): 605–06.

Li, A.L., et al. "Effectiveness of Pain Management Following Electrical Injury." *Journal of Burn Care and Research* 31 (January-February 2010): 73–82.

Murphy, P., et al. "A Shocking Call: Prehospital Assessment and Management of Electrical Injuries and Lightning Strikes." *EMS Magazine* 39 (February 2010): 46–53.

Nagesh, K.R., et al. "Arcing Injuries in a Fatal Electrocution." *American Journal of Forensic Medicine and Pathology* 30 (June 2009): 183–85.

OTHER

Chicago Electrical Trauma Research Institute (CETRI). "Electrical Injury." http://www.cetri.org/electrical_injury.html

Cushing, Tracy A., and Ronald K. Wright. "Electrical Injuries." eMedicine, April 10, 2010, http://emedicine.medscape.com/article/770179-overview

Edlich, Richard F., and David B. Drake. "Burns, Electrical." eMedicine, March 4, 2010, http://emedicine.medscape.com/article/1277496-overview

Hydro-Québec. "Effects of an Electric Current on the body." http://www.hydroquebec.com/security/effet_courant.html

———. “The Four Shock Factors.” http://www.hydroquebec.com/security/pop_4acteurs.html

———. “What to do in Case of Electric Shock.” http://www.hydroquebec.com/security/que_faire_choc.html

National Safety Council (NSC). “Electrical Safety.” http://www.nsc.org/news_resources/Resources/Documents/Electrical_Safety.pdf

ORGANIZATIONS

American Burn Association, 625 N. Michigan Ave., Suite 2550, Chicago, IL, 60611, (312) 642-9260, (312) 642-9130, info@ameriburn.org, http://www.ameriburn.org/.

American College of Emergency Physicians (ACEP), 1125 Executive Circle, Irving, TX, 75038-2522, (972) 550-0911, (800) 798-1822, (972) 580-2816, http://www.acep.org/.

American Society of Plastic Surgeons (ASPS), 444 East Algonquin Road, Arlington Heights, IL, 60005, (847) 228-9900, http://www.plasticsurgery.org/.

Chicago Electrical Trauma Research Institute (CETRI), 4047 West 40th Street, Chicago, IL, 60632, (800) 516-8709, info@cetri.org, http://www.cetri.org/.

National Safety Council (NSC), 1121 Spring Lake Drive, Itasca, IL, 60143, (630) 285-1121, (800) 621-7615, (630) 285-1315, http://www.nsc.org/Pages/Home.aspx.

Howard Baker
Rebecca J. Frey, PhD

Electroencephalography

Definition

Electroencephalography, or EEG, is a neurological test that uses an electronic monitoring device to measure and record electrical activity in the brain.

Purpose

The EEG is a key tool in the diagnosis and management of **epilepsy** and other seizure disorders. It is also used to assist in the diagnosis of brain damage and disease (e.g., **stroke**, tumors, **encephalitis**), **mental retardation**, **sleep disorders**, degenerative diseases like Alzheimer’s disease and Parkinson’s disease, and certain mental disorders (e.g., **alcoholism**, **schizophrenia**, **autism**).

An EEG may also be used to monitor brain activity during surgery and to determine brain **death**.

Precautions

Electroencephalography should be administered and interpreted by a trained medical professional only.

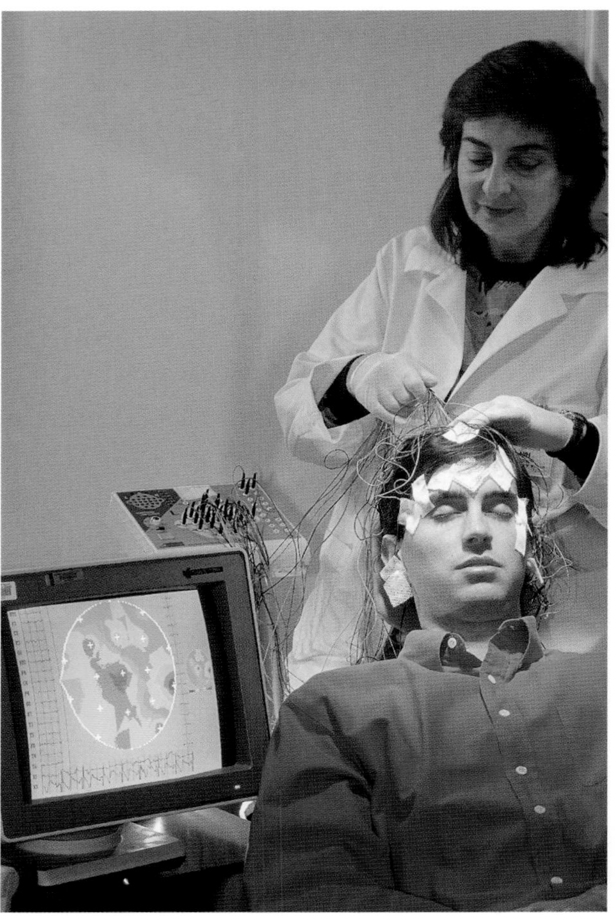

Patient receiving an electroencephalogram, a neurological test to measure and record electrical activity in the brain. *(© Richard T. Nowitz/Corbis.)*

Data from an EEG is only one element of a complete medical and/or psychological patient assessment and should never be used alone as the sole basis for a diagnosis.

Description

Before the EEG begins, a nurse or technician attaches approximately 16–20 electrodes to the patient’s scalp with a conductive, washable paste. Depending on the purpose for the EEG, implantable or invasive electrodes are occasionally used. Implantable electrodes include sphenoidal electrodes, which are fine wires inserted under the zygomatic arch, or cheekbone; and depth electrodes, which are surgically-implanted into the brain. The EEG electrodes are painless, and are used to measure the electrical activity in various regions of the brain.

For the test, the patient lies on a bed, padded table, or comfortable chair and is asked to relax and remain still during the EEG testing period. An EEG usually takes no more than one hour. During the test procedure, the patient may be asked to breathe slowly or quickly; visual stimuli such as flashing lights or a patterned board may be used to stimulate certain types of brain activity. Throughout the procedure, the electroencephalograph machine makes a continuous graphic record of the patient's brain activity, or brainwaves, on a long strip of recording paper or on a computer screen. This graphic record is called an electroencephalogram.

The sleep EEG uses the same equipment and procedures as a regular EEG. Patients undergoing a sleep EEG are encouraged to fall asleep completely rather than just relax. They are typically provided a bed and a quiet room conducive to sleep. A sleep EEG lasts up to three hours.

In an ambulatory EEG, patients are hooked up to a portable cassette recorder. They then go about their normal activities, and take their normal rest and sleep for a period of up to 24 hours. During this period, the patient and patient's family record any symptoms or abnormal behaviors, which can later be correlated with the EEG to see if they represent seizures.

Many insurance plans provide reimbursement for EEG testing. Costs for an EEG range from $100 to more than $500, depending on the purpose and type of test (i.e., asleep or awake, invasive or non-invasive electrodes). Because coverage may be dependent on the disorder or illness the EEG is evaluating, patients should check with their individual insurance plan.

Preparation

Full instructions should be given to EEG patients when they schedule their test. Typically, individuals on medications that affect the central nervous system, such as anticonvulsants, stimulants, or antidepressants, are told to discontinue their prescription for a short time prior to the test (usually one to two days). Patients may be asked to avoid food and beverages that contain **caffeine**, a central nervous system stimulant. However, any such request should be cleared by the treating physician. Patients may also be asked to arrive for the test with clean hair free of spray or other styling products.

Patients undergoing a sleep EEG may be asked to remain awake the night before their test. They may be given a sedative prior to the test to induce sleep.

Aftercare

If the patient has suspended regular medication for the test, the EEG nurse or technician should advise him when he can begin taking it again.

KEY TERMS

Epilepsy—A neurological disorder characterized by recurrent seizures with or without a loss of consciousness.

Ictal EEG—Used to measure brain activity during a seizure. May be useful in learning more about patients who aren't responding to conventional treatments.

Risks

Being off medication for one to two days may trigger seizures. Certain procedures used during EEG may trigger seizures in patients with epilepsy. Those procedures include flashing lights and deep breathing. If the EEG is being used as a diagnostic for epilepsy (i.e., to determine the type of seizures an individual is suffering from), this may be a desired effect, although the patient needs to be monitored closely so that the seizure can be aborted if necessary. This type of test is known as an ictal EEG.

Normal results

In reading and interpreting brainwave patterns, a neurologist or other physician will evaluate the type of brainwaves and the symmetry, location, and consistency of brainwave patterns. He will also look at the brainwave response to certain stimuli presented during the EEG test (such as flashing lights or noise). There are four basic types of brainwaves: alpha, beta, theta, and delta. "Normal" brainwave patterns vary widely, depending on factors of age and activity. For example, awake and relaxed individuals typically register an alpha wave pattern of 8–13 cycles per second. Young children and sleeping adults may have a delta wave pattern of under four cycles per second.

Abnormal results

The EEG readings of patients with epilepsy or other seizure disorders display bursts or spikes of electrical activity. In focal epilepsy, spikes are restricted to one hemisphere of the brain. If spikes are generalized to both hemispheres of the brain, multifocal epilepsy may be present.

The diagnostic brainwave patterns of other disorders varies widely. The appearance of excess theta waves (four to eight cycles per second) may indicate brain injury. Brain wave patterns in patients with brain disease, mental retardation, and brain injury show overall slowing. A trained medical specialist should interpret EEG results in the context of the patient's medical history, and other pertinent medical test results.

Resources

BOOKS

Restak, Richard M. *Brainscapes: An Introduction to What Neuroscience Has Learned About the Structure, Function, and Abilities of the Brain.* NewYork: Hyperion, 1995.

Paula Anne Ford-Martin

Electrolyte disorders

Definition

An electrolyte disorder is an imbalance of certain ionized components (i.e., bicarbonate, calcium, chloride, magnesium, phosphate, potassium, and sodium) in the blood.

Description

Electrolytes are ionized molecules found throughout the blood, tissues, and cells of the body. These molecules, which are either positive (cations) or negative (anions), conduct an electric current and help to balance pH and acid-base levels in the body. Electrolytes also facilitate the passage of fluid between and within cells through a process known as osmosis and play a part in regulating the function of the cardiovascular, neuromuscular, endocrine, and excretory systems.

The serum electrolytes include:

- Sodium (Na). A positively charged electrolyte that helps to balance fluid levels in the body and facilitates neuromuscular functioning.
- Potassium (K). A main component of cellular fluid, this positive electrolyte helps to regulate neuromuscular function and osmotic pressure.
- Calcium (Ca). A cation, or positive electrolyte, that affects neuromuscular performance and contributes to skeletal growth and blood coagulation.
- Magnesium (Mg). Influences muscle contractions and intracellular activity. A cation.
- Chloride (Cl). An anion, or negative electrolyte, that regulates blood pressure.
- Phosphate (HPO_4). Negative electrolyte that impacts metabolism and regulates acid-base balance and calcium levels.
- Bicarbonate (HCO_3). A negatively charged electrolyte that assists in the regulation of blood pH levels. Bicarbonate insufficiencies and elevations cause acid-base disorders (i.e., acidosis, alkalosis).

Risk factors

Medications, chronic diseases, and trauma (for example, **burns**, or **fractures** may cause the concentration of certain electrolytes in the body to become too high (hyper-) or too low (hypo-). When this happens, an electrolyte imbalance, or disorder, results.

Causes and symptoms

Sodium

HYPERNATREMIA Sodium helps the kidneys to regulate the amount of water the body retains or excretes. Consequently, individuals with elevated serum sodium levels experience a loss of fluids, or **dehydration**. Hypernatremia can be caused by inadequate water intake, excessive fluid loss (i.e., diabetes insipidus, kidney disease, severe burns, and prolonged **vomiting** or **diarrhea**), or sodium retention (caused by excessive sodium intake or aldosteronism). In addition, certain drugs, including loop diuretics, corticosteroids, and antihypertensive medications may cause elevated sodium levels.

Symptoms of hypernatremia include:

- thirst
- orthostatic hypotension
- dry mouth and mucous membranes
- dark, concentrated urine
- loss of elasticity in the skin
- irregular heartbeat (tachycardia)
- irritability
- fatigue
- lethargy
- heavy, labored breathing
- muscle twitching and/or seizures

HYPONATREMIA Up to 1% of all hospitalized patients and as many as 18% of nursing home patients develop hyponatremia, making it one of the most common electrolyte disorders. Diuretics, certain psychoactive drugs (i.e., fluoxetine, sertraline, haloperidol), specific antipsychotics (lithium), vasopressin, chlorpropamide, the illicit drug ecstasy, and other pharmaceuticals can cause decreased sodium levels. Low sodium levels may also be triggered by inadequate dietary intake of sodium, excessive perspiration, water intoxication, and impairment of adrenal gland or **kidney function**.

Symptoms of hyponatremia include:

- nausea, abdominal cramping, and/or vomiting
- headache
- edema (swelling)
- muscle weakness and/or tremor
- paralysis
- disorientation
- slowed breathing
- seizures
- coma

Potassium

HYPERKALEMIA Hyperkalemia may be caused by ketoacidosis (diabetic coma), myocardial infarction (heart attack), severe burns, kidney failure, fasting, **bulimia nervosa**, gastrointestinal bleeding, adrenal insufficiency, or Addison's disease. Diuretic drugs, cyclosporin, lithium, heparin, ACE inhibitors, beta blockers, and trimethoprim can increase serum potassium levels, as can heavy **exercise**. The condition may also be secondary to hypernatremia. Symptoms may include:

- weakness
- nausea and/or abdominal pain
- irregular heartbeat (arrhythmia)
- diarrhea
- muscle pain

HYPOKALEMIA Severe dehydration, aldosteronism, Cushing's syndrome, kidney disease, long-term diuretic therapy, certain **penicillins**, laxative abuse, congestive heart failure, and adrenal gland impairments can all cause depletion of potassium levels in the bloodstream. A substance known as glycyrrhetinic acid, which is found in licorice and chewing tobacco, can also deplete potassium serum levels. Symptoms of hypokalemia include:

- weakness
- paralysis
- increased urination
- irregular heartbeat (arrhythmia)
- orthostatic hypotension
- muscle pain
- tetany

Calcium

HYPERCALCEMIA Blood calcium levels may be elevated in cases of thyroid disorder, multiple myeloma, metastatic **cancer**, multiple bone fractures, milk-alkali syndrome, and Paget's disease. Excessive use of calcium-containing supplements and certain over-the-counter medications (i.e., antacids) may also cause hypercalcemia. In infants, lesser known causes may include blue diaper syndrome, **Williams syndrome**, secondary hyperparathyroidism from maternal hypocalcemia, and dietary phosphate deficiency. Symptoms include:

- fatigue
- constipation
- depression
- confusion
- muscle pain
- nausea and vomiting
- dehydration
- increased urination
- irregular heartbeat (arrhythmia)

HYPOCALCEMIA Thyroid disorders, kidney failure, severe burns, sepsis, **vitamin D deficiency**, and medications such as heparin and glucogan can deplete blood calcium levels. Lowered levels cause:

- muscle cramps and spasms
- tetany and/or convulsions
- mood changes (depression, irritability)
- dry skin
- brittle nails
- facial twitching

Magnesium

HYPERMAGNESEMIA Excessive magnesium levels may occur with end-stage renal disease, Addison's disease, or an overdose of magnesium salts. Hypermagnesemia is characterized by:

- lethargy
- hypotension
- decreased heart and respiratory rate
- muscle weakness
- diminished tendon reflexes

HYPOMAGNESEMIA Inadequate dietary intake of magnesium, often caused by chronic **alcoholism** or **malnutrition**, is a common cause of hypomagnesemia. Other causes include malabsorption syndromes, pancreatitis, aldosteronism, burns, hyperparathyroidism, digestive system disorders, and diuretic use. Symptoms of low serum magnesium levels include:

- leg and foot cramps
- weight loss
- vomiting
- muscle spasms, twitching, and tremors
- seizures
- muscle weakness
- arrthymia

Chloride

HYPERCHLOREMIA Severe dehydration, kidney failure, hemodialysis, traumatic brain injury, and aldosteronism can cause hyperchloremia. Drugs such as boric acid and ammonium chloride and the intravenous (IV) infusion of sodium chloride can also boost chloride levels, resulting in hyperchloremic metabolic acidosis. Symptoms include:

- weakness
- headache
- nausea
- cardiac arrest

HYPOCHLOREMIA Hypochloremia usually occurs as a result of sodium and potassium depletion (i.e., hyponatremia, hypokalemia). Severe depletion of serum chloride levels causes metabolic alkalosis. This alkalization of the bloodstream is characterized by:

- mental confusion
- slowed breathing
- paralysis
- muscle tension or spasm

Phosphate

HYPERPHOSPHATEMIA Skeletal fractures or disease, kidney failure, hypoparathyroidism, hemodialysis, diabetic ketoacidosis, **acromegaly**, systemic infection, and intestinal obstruction can all cause phosphate retention and build-up in the blood. The disorder occurs concurrently with hypocalcemia. Individuals with mild hyperphosphatemia are typically asymptomatic, but signs of severe hyperphosphatemia include:

- tingling in hands and fingers
- muscle spasms and cramps
- convulsions
- cardiac arrest

HYPOPHOSPHATEMIA Serum phosphate levels of 2 mg/dL or below may be caused by hypomagnesemia and hypokalemia. Severe burns, alcoholism, diabetic ketoacidosis, kidney disease, hyperparathyroidism, **hypothyroidism**, Cushing's syndrome, malnutrition, hemodialysis, vitamin D deficiency, and prolonged diuretic therapy can also diminish blood phosphate levels. There are typically few physical signs of mild phosphate depletion. Symptoms of severe hypophosphatemia include:

- muscle weakness
- weight loss
- bone deformities (osteomalacia)

KEY TERMS

Acid-base balance—A balance of acidity and alkalinity of fluids in the body that keeps the pH level of blood around 7.35–7.45.

Aldosteronism—A condition defined by high serum levels of aldosterone, a hormone secreted by the adrenal gland that is responsible for increasing sodium reabsorption in the kidneys.

Addison's disease—A disease characterized by a deficiency in adrenocortical hormones due to destruction of the adrenal gland.

Bulimia nervosa—An eating disorder characterized by binging and purging (self-induced vomiting) behaviors.

Milk-alkali syndrome—Elevated blood calcium levels and alkalosis caused by excessive intake of milk and alkalis. Usually occurs in the treatment of peptic ulcer.

Orthostatic hypotension—A drop in blood pressure that causes faintness or dizziness and occurs when one rises to a standing position. Also known as postural hypotension.

Osmotic pressure—Pressure that occurs when two solutions of differing concentrations are separated by a semipermeable membrane, such as a cellular wall, and the lower concentration solute is drawn across the membrane into the higher concentration solute (osmosis).

Tetany—A disorder of the nervous system characterized by muscle cramps, spasms of the arms and legs, and numbness of the extremities.

Diagnosis

Examination

Diagnosis is performed by a physician or other qualified healthcare provider who will take a medical history, discuss symptoms, perform a complete physical examination, and prescribe appropriate laboratory tests. Because electrolyte disorders commonly affect the neuromuscular system, the provider will test reflexes. If a calcium imbalance is suspected, the physician will also check for Chvostek's sign, a reflex test that triggers an involuntary facial twitch, and Trousseau's sign, a muscle spasm that occurs in response to pressure on the upper arm.

Tests

Serum electrolyte imbalances can be detected through blood tests. Blood is drawn from a vein on the back of the hand or inside of the elbow by a medical technician, or phlebotomist, and analyzed at a lab.

Normal levels of electrolytes are:

- Sodium: 135–145 mEq/L (serum)
- Potassium: 3.5–5.5 mEq/L (serum)
- Calcium: 8.8–10.4 mg/dL (total Ca; serum); 4.7–5.2 mg/dL (unbound Ca; serum)
- Magnesium: 1.4–2.1 mEq/L (plasma)
- Chloride: 100–108 mEq/L (serum)
- Phosphate: 2.5–4.5 mg/dL (plasma; adults)

Standard ranges for test results may vary due to differing laboratory standards and physiological variances (gender, age, and other factors). Other blood tests that determine pH levels and acid-base balance may be performed.

Treatment

Treatment of electrolyte disorders depends on the underlying cause of the problem and the type of electrolyte involved. If the disorder is caused by poor diet or improper fluid intake, nutritional changes may be prescribed. If medications, such as diuretics, triggered the imbalance, discontinuing or adjusting the drug therapy may effectively treat the condition. Fluid and electrolyte replacement therapy, either intravenously or by mouth, can reverse electrolyte depletion.

Hemodialysis treatment may be required to reduce serum potassium levels in hyperkalemic patients with impaired kidney function. It may also be recommended for renal patients with severe hypermagnesemia.

Prognosis

A patient's long-term prognosis depends upon the root cause of the electrolyte disorder. When treated quickly and appropriately, electrolyte imbalances in and of themselves are usually effectively reversed.

When they are mild, some electrolyte imbalances have few to no symptoms and may pass unnoticed. For example, transient hyperphosphatemia is usually fairly benign. However, long-term elevations of blood phosphate levels can lead to potentially fatal soft tissue and vascular calcifications and bone disease, and severe serum phosphate deficiencies (hypophosphatemia) can cause encephalopathy, coma, and **death**.

Severe hypernatremia has a mortality rate of 40–60%. Death is commonly due to cerebrovascular damage and hemorrhage resulting from dehydration and shrinkage of the brain cells.

Prevention

Physicians should use caution when prescribing drugs known to affect electrolyte levels and acid-base balance. Individuals with kidney disease, thyroid problems, and other conditions that may place them at risk for developing an electrolyte disorder should be educated on the signs and symptoms.

Resources

PERIODICALS

Ghali, J.K. "Mechanisms, Risks, and New Treatment Optons for Hyponatremia." *Cardiology* 111 no. 3 (April 2008): 147–57.

Lumachi, F., A. Brunello, A. Roma, and U. Basso. "Medical Treatment of Malignancy Associated Hypercalcemia." *Current Medicinal Chemistry* 15 no. 4 (2008): 415–21.

Shingarev, R., and M. Allon. "A Physiologic-Based Approach to the Treatment of Acute Hyperkalemia." *American Journal of Kidney Disease* (June 4, 2010):

Paula Anne Ford-Martin
Teresa G. Odle
Melinda G. Oberleitner, RN, DNS, APRN, CNS

Electrolyte supplements

Definition

Electrolyte supplements are a varied group of prescription and nonprescription preparations used to correct imbalances in the body's electrolyte levels. Electrolytes themselves are substances that dissociate into ions (electrically charged atoms or atom groups) when they melt or are dissolved, thus serving to conduct electricity. In the human body, electrolytes are critical to the proper distribution of water, muscle contraction and expansion, transmission of nerve impulses, delivery of oxygen to body tissues, heart rate and rhythm, acid-base balance, and other important functions or conditions.

The ions that are formed when electrolytes are dissolved in body fluids are either positively or negatively charged. Positively charged ions are called cation and are formed when an atom or atom group loses electrons. The most important cations in the human body are sodium, potassium, magnesium, and calcium ions. Negatively charged ions are called anions and are formed when an atom or atom group gains electrons. The principal anions in the body include bicarbonate, chloride, phosphate, and sulfate ions, as well as ions formed by certain protein compounds or organic acids.

About 60% of an adult human male's total body weight is water. In adult women, the figure is about 55%, and is lower in the elderly and in obese people. Two-thirds of total body water (TBW) lies inside cells and is known as intracellular fluid or ICF. The remaining third of TBW lies outside the cells and is called extracellular fluid or ECF. About 75% of ECF lies in connective tissue or the spaces between tissues outside the blood vessels (interstitial spaces), while the remaining 25% is within the blood vessels. In addition to representing different proportions of TBW, ICF and ECF differ significantly in their electrolyte content. Whereas the major cation in ICF is potassium, the most important cation in ECF is sodium. These differences in electrolyte levels help to regulate the movement of water between ICF and ECF.

Children are more vulnerable than adults to fluid and electrolyte imbalances, in part because they have different ratios of TBW to total body weight, and of ICF to ECF. A newborn baby carried to full term has a TBW ratio between 75 and 80%. The baby's total body water ratio decreases by 4–5% during the first week after **birth** and reaches the adult level of 60% by 12 months of age. Similarly, a newborn has an ICF:ECF ratio of 55:45, which falls to the adult ratio of 70:30 during the first year of life. In addition to these different fluid ratios, children's kidneys are less efficient than adults in regulating water balance; children have smaller organ systems that dissipate body heat less efficiently; and their core body temperature rises faster than that of an adult when they become dehydrated. All these factors help to explain why some electrolyte supplements are formulated specifically for children.

Purpose

The purpose of electrolyte supplements is to restore the proper ratio of total body water to total body weight and the correct proportions of the various electrolytes in body fluids. Electrolyte imbalances may result from excessive intake or inadequate elimination of electrolytes on the one hand or by insufficient intake or excessive elimination on the other hand.

Body regulation of water and electrolytes

Under normal conditions, the water and electrolyte content of the body is regulated by the kidneys, the secretion of antidiuretic hormone, and the sensation of thirst. The average adult needs to take in about 700–800 mL (about 1.5–1.7 pints) of water per day in order to match the water lost through perspiration, breathing, and excretion of waste products (urine and feces). The water taken in by mouth is added to the 200–300 mL (0.42–0.63 pints) of water that are formed in the body each day through tissue breakdown.

The amount of water needed to match fluid losses may be considerably greater than the average during **exercise** or in patients with **fever**, severe **vomiting**, or **diarrhea**. Adults with fever typically lose an additional 0.75–1.0 oz of fluid per day for each degree that their temperature rises above normal. With regard to diarrhea, adults with cholera have been reported to lose as much as a quart of fluid per hour in their stools. The fluid lost in this way contains sodium, potassium, and chloride, resulting in electrolyte imbalances in cholera patients as well as **dehydration**.

Exercise raises the total metabolism of the body to 5–15 times the resting rate. Most of this energy (70–90%) is released as heat, which is partially dissipated by the evaporation of sweat. Depending on weather conditions, the type and weight of clothing being worn, and the intensity of exercise or physical work performed, adults may lose anywhere from 1–2.5 qt of fluid per hour through perspiration. Sweat contains sodium chloride as well as smaller amounts of potassium, calcium, and magnesium. In order to maintain the proper balance of electrolytes in the body as well as fluid, athletes or people employed in outdoor work during warm weather may need to replace the electrolytes lost in sweat by taking capsules or drinking beverages containing supplemental electrolytes.

With regard to the sense of thirst, it is not always an accurate indication of the body's need for water. Researchers have found that many people do not feel thirsty until they have already lost about 2% of their total body weight through fluid losses. As a result, most people do not replace enough fluid during exercise or hot weather simply by drinking water until they no longer feel thirsty. In addition, the aging process, certain mental disorders, or drugs may affect a person's sense of thirst.

At the other extreme of water intake, a person may drink excessive amounts of water due to misunderstandings about their need for extra fluid during exercise. This condition is known as water intoxication or hyperhydration. It leads to abnormally low levels of sodium in the blood, a condition known as hyponatremia. This condition is also known as exercise-associated hyponatremia (EAH). Water intoxication may lead to swelling of the brain, confusion, disorientation, and eventually coma or **death**. Several marathon runners have died from water intoxication, as have teenagers who consumed large amounts of water after taking doses of Ecstasy (MDMA), a so-called "club drug." Other persons at risk for water intoxication include people with **eating disorders** and children with **mental retardation**. Research reported in the *New England Journal of Medicine* revealed that as many as 13% of marathon runners developed hyponatremia during the course of a race as a result of drinking too much water, usually 3 qt or more. Female athletes appear to be at greater risk of water intoxication and hyponatremia than male athletes.

Conditions associated with fluid and electrolyte imbalance

Several common conditions can lead to fluid and electrolyte imbalance:

- Exposure to extended periods of extremely hot weather.
- High levels of athletic activity, military training, or outdoor work in such fields as construction, agriculture, forestry, fishing, and certain types of manufacturing.
- Extreme changes in diet.
- Reduced fluid intake.
- Medication side effects. Certain drugs, particularly diuretics, beta-blockers, and vasodilators, may increase the loss of electrolytes in urine and/or interfere with the body's ability to regulate its temperature during exercise or in hot weather.
- Severe illnesses characterized by high fever, recurrent diarrhea, and/or frequent vomiting. Such illnesses include cholera, viral gastroenteritis (stomach flu), shigellosis, and amebic dysentery.
- Severe burns covering more than 10% of the body.
- Surgical creation of a stoma or urinary diversion. These operations sometimes lead to an increased loss of body fluids while the patient's body is adjusting to the changes in urination and excretion resulting from the surgery. In addition, some forms of weight loss surgery intended to bypass parts of the small intestine in which food absorption occurs have a 70% rate of electrolyte imbalances as a complication of the operation.
- Diseases affecting the kidneys. These include diabetes mellitus, diabetes insipidus, and syndrome of inappropriate antidiuretic hormone secretion (SIADH), as well as cancer or infections of the kidneys.
- In infants, premature birth.

Description

The various electrolyte supplements used in the United States and Canada are intended to prevent or treat electrolyte imbalances in very different situations or groups of patients. They range from sports drinks and other supplements used by amateur or professional athletes to prevent **muscle cramps** and improve athletic performance, to liquids used at home to prevent dehydration in children with diarrhea, to injections administered as part of enteral (feeding through a tube or stoma directly into the small intestine) or parenteral **nutrition** (intravenous feeding that bypasses the digestive tract).

The major categories of electrolyte supplements are:

- Sports drinks. Sports drinks are beverages specially formulated to contain appropriate amounts of electrolytes and carbohydrates as well as water to replace the fluid and sodium lost through sweat during athletic activities. These beverages are popular with athletes at the college level. According to the American College of Sports Medicine as well as dietitians' associations in the United States and Canada sports drinks are effective in supplying food energy for the muscles, maintaining proper levels of blood sugar, maintaining the proper functioning of the thirst mechanism, and lowering the risk of dehydration or hyponatremia. Other researchers have noted that the flavoring added to sports drinks encourages athletes to drink more during periods of exercise and thus maintain proper levels of hydration. Sports drinks can be purchased in supermarkets and health food stores; they include such well-known beverages as Gatorade and Powerade. Some of these supplements come in a semisolid form known as energy gels, which contain caffeine or various herbal compounds as well as carbohydrates and electrolytes.
- Over-the-counter powders and tablets. Some athletes—particularly those who participate in long-distance running or endurance cycling—prefer capsules or concentrated powders to maintain their electrolyte balance during exercise. The powders are mixed with 12 or 16 oz of cold water prior to drinking, while the capsules can be taken before, during, and after exercise. Most contain flavorings to mask the naturally salty or

bitter taste of the electrolytes themselves. Common brand names include eForce, NutriBiotic, and Endurolytes. These products are regarded by the Food and Drug Administration (FDA) as dietary supplements.

- Over-the-counter electrolyte replenishers for children. Infants and young children are more vulnerable to dehydration than adults, particularly from severe gastroenteritis or diarrhea. A child may become dehydrated in less than a day from recurrent vomiting or episodes of diarrhea. Some doctors recommend that parents keep oral rehydration fluids containing mixtures of carbohydrates and electrolytes specially formulated for children in the medicine chest at home in case the child becomes dehydrated from a stomach virus or similar illness. Common brand names for these products, which are regulated by the FDA as medical foods, include Pedialyte, Infalyte, Naturalyte, and Rehydralyte. Most come in a powdered form to be mixed with water as well as liquid forms; Pedialyte is also available as fruit-flavored freezer pops.
- Oral rehydration formulae for children and adults. Oral rehydration salts, also known as ORS, have been a staple of treatment for cholera and other diseases accompanied by severe diarrhea in developing countries since about the 1970s. First researched in the 1940s, oral rehydration salts were adopted by the World Health Organization (WHO) in 1978 in order to reduce the risk of death from dehydration caused by cholera-related diarrhea. Since the introduction of ORS, the number of children around the world who die from acute diarrhea has been reduced from 5 million per year to 1.3 million. Reformulated by WHO in 2002, the ORS salts come in packets to be kept in the home and mixed with water as soon as a child (or adult) falls ill. The formula is a low-glucose and low-sodium mixture. If the WHO packets are unavailable, a comparable form of oral rehydration solution can be made by adding 8 tsp of table sugar, $\frac{1}{2}$ tsp of salt, $\frac{1}{2}$ tsp of baking soda (bicarbonate of soda), and $\frac{1}{3}$ tsp of potassium chloride to 1 L (1.05 qt) of water. In an emergency, a solution prepared from 1 tbsp of sugar and $\frac{1}{2}$ tsp of salt added to 1 L of water can be used to treat diarrhea.
- Multiple electrolyte injections. Various mixtures of electrolytes are available by prescription in injectable form to be added to enteral or parenteral nutrition formulae. These forms of feeding are used in patients who require supplementation or complete replacement of feeding by mouth, including patients with various intestinal disorders, AIDS, or severe burns. Basic solutions for total parenteral nutrition, or TPN, contain the electrolytes sodium, potassium, chloride, phosphate, and magnesium, although the exact proportion of electrolytes can be tailored to an individual patient's needs. Some injectable formulae contain dextrose, a sugar, and acetate or lactate as well as the five major electrolytes. Common brand names include TPN Electrolytes, Lypholyte, Nutrilyte, Plasma-Lyte 148, and others. Some patients are taught to use these injectable formulae at home.

Recommended dosage

Recommended dosages for electrolyte supplements are:

- Sports drinks. Since sports drinks and energy gels are not medications in the strict sense, the amount consumed will vary not only from person to person but also in a given individual from day to day depending on weather conditions, level of athletic conditioning, length of activity, and other factors. To lower the risk of dehydration in adults in hot weather, the American College of Sports Medicine recommends drinking approximately 2 to 3 mL/lb of body weight of water or sports drink four hours before exercising. Overhydration during this time period should be avoided. During exercise, enough fluid should be consumed to prevent a water deficit greater than 2% of body weight. Recommended beverages are those that contain electrolytes and carbohydrates. If the exercise event lasts longer than an hour, consumption of carbohydrate beverages that contain 6–8% carbohydrate is recommended. After exercise, rapid and complete recovery from exercise-induced dehydration can be accomplished by drinking at least 16–24 oz (450–675 mL) of fluid for every pound of weight lost during exercise. To replace fluids and electrolytes lost during endurance events lasting longer than two hours, the current recommendation is consumption of sports drinks that contain 0.5–0.7 g/L of sodium and 0.8–2.0 g/L of potassium and that also contain carbohydrate.
- Over-the-counter powders and tablets. The usual recommended dose of powdered electrolytes is one scoopful (or prepackaged envelope) of powder dissolved in 12–16 oz of water before exercising. Capsules may be taken as follows: 1–3 capsules 30–60 minutes before exercising; 1–6 capsules per hour during the workout; and 1–3 capsules after exercising.
- Over-the-counter electrolyte replenishers for children. Dosages for Pedialyte and similar oral rehydration solutions for children are usually based on the child's age and weight. The child's doctor should determine the quantity to be given if the child is younger than 12 months of age. Children between the ages of one and

KEY TERMS

Anion—An ion carrying a negative charge owing to a surplus of electrons. Anions in the body include bicarbonate, chloride, phosphate, sulfate, certain organic acids, and certain protein compounds.

Cation—An ion carrying a positive charge due to a loss of electrons. Cations in the body include sodium, potassium, magnesium, and calcium ions.

Cholera—A severe bacterial infection of the small intestine characterized by profuse diarrhea and eventual dehydration. Cholera is still a frequent cause of death among children in developing countries.

Electron—An elementary particle carrying a negative charge. Electrons may exist either independently or as components of an atom outside its nucleus.

Enteral nutrition—Nourishment given through a tube or stoma directly into the small intestine, thus bypassing the upper digestive tract.

Hyponatremia—Insufficient sodium in the blood.

Interstitial spaces—Spaces within body tissues that are outside the blood vessels. Also known as interstitial compartments.

Ion—An atom or group of atoms that acquires an electrical charge by the gain or loss of electrons.

Metabolism—The sum of an organism's physical and chemical processes that produce and maintain living tissue, and make energy available to the organism. Insulin resistance is a disorder of metabolism.

Parenteral nutrition—Nutrition supplied intravenously, thus bypassing the patient's digestive tract entirely.

Stoma—A surgical opening made in the abdominal wall to allow waste products to pass directly to the outside.

Water intoxication—A potentially life-threatening condition caused by drinking too much water, which leads to hyponatremia and may result in seizures, coma, and death.

two years are usually given 34 mL of electrolyte solution per pound of body weight during the first eight hours of treatment and 75 mL per pound of body weight during the next 16 hours, although the doctor may adjust the dose if the child is very thirsty. Children between the ages of 2 and 10 are given 23 mL of electrolyte solution per pound of body weight for the first four to six hours of treatment, followed by 45 mL per pound taken over the next 18–24 hours. Freezer pops may be given to children older than one year as often as the child desires.

- Oral rehydration formulae. The WHO form of oral rehydration liquid is made by adding the full contents of one packet of powdered oral rehydration salts to a quart of drinking water. The solution should not be boiled. A fresh quart of solution should be mixed each day. Infants and young children should be given the solution in small amounts by spoon as often as possible. Adults and teenagers should take the WHO formula according to the doctor's directions.

- Multiple electrolyte injections. Basic TPN solutions are usually made up in liter batches and adjusted to each individual patient's needs. The standard adult dosage is 2 L per day, usually administered by drip through a needle or catheter placed in the patient's vein for a 10–12-hour period once a day or five days per week. The patient may be given several units of premixed TPN fluid to store at home in the refrigerator or freezer. Each dose should be taken from the refrigerator 4–6 hours prior to use to allow it to warm to room temperature. TPN solution stored in a freezer should be moved to a refrigerator 24 hours before use.

Precautions

Sports drinks should not be given to rehydrate children with vomiting or diarrhea, as they do not contain the proper balance of carbohydrates and electrolytes needed by children's bodies.

Over-the-counter powders and tablets should always be taken with adequate amounts of water and kept out of the reach of children.

Over-the-counter electrolyte replenishers for children should be stored out of the reach of children and away from heat and direct sunlight. In addition, they should not be given to patients with intestinal blockage.

WHO oral rehydration salts and packets of similar formulae should not be stored in damp places, as moisture can cause the contents to lose their effectiveness. These products should also be kept away from heat or direct sunlight. Unused oral rehydration solution should be discarded at the end of each day. As with electrolyte replenishers for children, oral rehydration formulae should not be given to patients with intestinal blockage.

Patients using multiple electrolyte injections as part of total parenteral nutrition should have their blood and urine checked at regular intervals while they are receiving these medicines. They should also be taught to recognize the signs of infection at the injection site (**pain**, swelling, redness, or a cold sensation). In addition, these patients should not use sports drinks, other electrolyte supplements, or over-the-counter medications (including herbal preparations) without consulting their doctor. The injections should not be used if the fluid looks cloudy, has solid particles floating in it, or has separated. The injections should be stored away from sunlight and moisture. In addition, patients receiving multiple electrolyte injections should not stop them suddenly without telling their doctor, as the dosage may need to be reduced slowly before the TPN is discontinued.

Side effects

Some people do not like the salty taste of many sports drinks. They may wish to consider products containing glycine, which is an amino acid that neutralizes the salty taste of the electrolytes themselves. A more serious side effect of sports drinks is **tooth decay**. An article published by researchers at the University of Maryland Dental School showed that sports drinks erode tooth enamel at a rate 3 to 11 times faster than cola-based soft drinks.

No side effects have been reported for over-the-counter powders and tablets.

Side effects from children's electrolyte replenishers may include allergic reactions, including **hives**, swelling of the face or hands, trouble breathing, and **tingling** in the mouth or throat. Other side effects may include signs of too much sodium in the body, such as **dizziness**, seizures, muscle twitching, or restlessness. The doctor should be notified immediately if any of these side effects occur. A less serious side effect that occurs in some children is mild vomiting.

Oral rehydration formulae may produce the same side effects as electrolyte replenishers for children.

Minor side effects from multiple electrolyte injections may include increased frequency of urination, dry mouth, increased thirst, or drowsiness. Serious side effects include rapid weight gain, yellowing of the skin or eyes, fruity odor on the breath, **numbness** or tingling in the hands or feet, uneven heartbeat, shortness of breath, confusion, or weakness with muscle twitching. Patients should notify their doctor immediately if they notice any of these side effects.

Interactions

Sports drinks may raise blood electrolyte levels in patients receiving total parenteral nutrition. They should not be consumed by patients receiving multiple electrolyte injections.

Children receiving premixed forms of electrolyte replenishers should not eat food with added salt or drink fruit juices until the diarrhea has stopped.

No interactions with other medications have been reported with oral rehydration formulae for adults or over-the-counter powders and tablets. However, the doctor should be informed of all other medications the patient is taking in case a dosage adjustment is necessary.

Resources

BOOKS

Beals, K., and M. Manore. "Nutritional Considerations for the Female Athlete." In *Advances in Sports and Exercise Science Series.* Philadelphia: Elsevier, 2007.

Otten, J., J. Hellwig, and L. Meyers, eds. *Dietary Reference Intakes: The Essential Guide to Nutrient Requirements.* Washington, DC: The National Academies Press, 2006.

PERIODICALS

Almond, Christopher S. D., et al. "Hyponatremia among Runners in the Boston Marathon." *New England Journal of Medicine* 352 (April 14, 2005): 1550–1556.

Bender, B.J., P.O. Ozuah, and E.F. Crain. "Oral Rehydration Therapy: Is Anyone Drinking?" *Pediatric Emergency Care* 23 no. 9 (September 2007): 624–6.

Diggins, K.C. "Treatment of Mild to Moderate Dehydration in Children with Oral Replacement Therapy." *Journal of the American Academy of Nurse Practitioners* 20 no. 8 (August 2008): 402–6.

Messahel, S., and T. Hussain. "Oral Rehydration Therapy: A Lesson from the Developing World." *Archives of Disease in Childhood* 93 no. 2 (February 2008): 183–4.

Sawka, M.N., et al. "American College of Sports Medicine Position Stand: Exercise and Fluid Replacement." *Medicine & Science in Sports & Exercise* 39 (2007): 377–90.

von Frauenhofer, J. A., and M. M. Rogers. "Effects of Sports Drinks and Other Beverages on Dental Enamel." *General Dentistry* 53 (January-February 2005): 28–31.

Woolley, W.L., and J.H. Burton. "Pediatric Acute Gastroenteritis: Clinical Assessment, Oral Rehydration, and Antiemetic Therapy." *Pediatric Health* 3 no. 2 (2009): 191–7.

OTHER

Rodriguez, Nancy, Nancy DiMarco, and Susie Langley. "Nutrition and Athletic Performance." Medscape Today March 1, 2010, http://www.medscape.com/viewarticle/717046 (accessed October 3, 2010).

ORGANIZATIONS

American College of Sports Medicine (ACSM), P.O. Box 1440, Indianapolis, IN, 46206-1440, (317) 637-9200, (317) 634-7817, http://www.acsm.org.

American Society of Health-System Pharmacists (ASHP), 7272 Wisconsin Avenue, Bethesda, MD, 20814, (301) 657-3000, (866)279-0681, http://www.ashp.org.

Rebecca J. Frey, PhD
Melinda G. Oberleitner, RN, DNS, APRN, CNS

Electronic fetal monitoring

Definition

The electronic fetal monitor (EFM) is a device that records a fetus's heart rate and the presence or absence of the mother's uterine contractions.

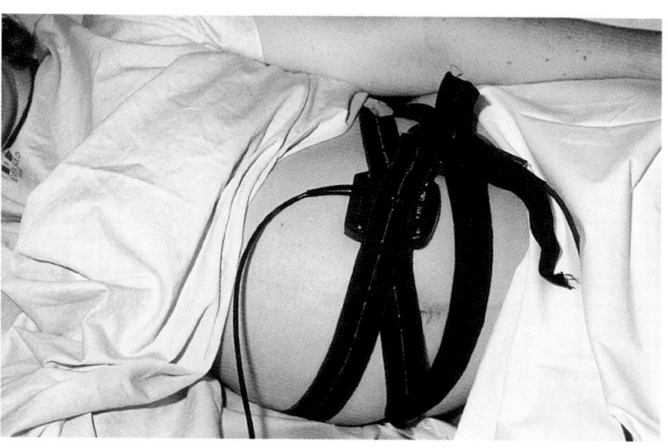

Fetal monitor belt around a pregnant woman's torso to record the heart rate of her baby. *(Custom Medical Stock Photo, Inc. Reproduced by permission.)*

Purpose

The EFM is used to assess fetal well being during routine prenatal visits. It is also used during labor and delivery when high-risk factors exist or when a clinical condition develops beforehand that places the fetus at risk. High-risk factors for EFM during labor include:

- low gestational age
- high maternal age
- placenta or cord problems
- meconium in the amniotic fluid
- maternal hypertension
- protein in the urine (proteinuria)

A fetus having trouble in labor often exhibits characteristic changes in heart rate after a contraction (late decelerations). Trouble also is indicated by significant slowing of the heart rate during a contraction (variable deceleration). If the fetus is not receiving enough oxygen to withstand the stress of labor, and delivery is many hours away, a **cesarean section** (C-section) may be necessary.

Description

The monitor produces a continuous paper record of the fetal heart rate (FHR) and records uterine contractions. FHR is captured on the top part of the paper printout; uterine activity, when monitored, appears on the lower part of the tracing.

Electronic fetal monitoring can be performed externally or internally. The external ultrasound approach is non-invasive and uses sensors (electrodes) placed on the mother's abdomen with an elastic belt. Another belt holds the contraction monitor.

External electronic fetal monitoring includes a non-stress test, which measures fetal heart rate (FHR) accelerations with normal movement of the fetus. Sometimes the fetal movement is encouraged by giving the mother a small meal or something to drink. Fetal acoustic stimulation and moving the fetus by rubbing the abdomen gently also may be used.

Two contraction stress tests, which measure the placenta's ability to provide enough oxygen to the fetus during pressure, are also used with electronic fetal monitoring. The nipple stimulation contractions stress test involves the mother self-stimulating her nipple while contractions and FHR are monitored. Another test, called oxytocin stimulation, involves the administration of the hormone oxytocin intravenously until three uterine contractions are observed within 10 minutes, during which time the FHR is monitored.

Sometimes it is difficult to hear the fetus's heartbeat with the monitoring device. Other times, the monitor may show subtle signs of a developing problem. In either case, the physician may recommend the use of an internal monitor, which provides a more accurate record of the fetus's heart rate. The internal monitor (or fetal scalp electrode) uses an electrode attached to the fetus's scalp through the cervix during an internal vaginal exam. The internal monitor can only be used when the cervix is dilated. In complicated pregnancies, continuous EFM is recommended during labor.

Benefits

Electronic fetal monitoring allows the physician to judge the well being of the fetus before and during delivery. Should the fetus appear to be in distress, the physician can recommend immediate delivery via cesarean section. EFM also allows an evaluation of the strength of the mother's contractions. Should labor not be progressing normally, medical intervention can be ordered.

Precautions

In general, no risks are associated with external fetal monitoring. However, the test can initiate labor and is generally not given to mothers at risk for preterm labor or with a condition that requires a cesarean section. Internal monitoring poses risks associated with improper placement of the electrodes. Some data suggest that EFM leads to unnecessary cesarean sections. Another drawback includes loss of maternal mobility when used during labor, which may slow labor.

Preparation

There are no special preparations required for external fetal monitoring. Preparation for placement of an internal scalp lead (ISL) is the same as for a routine vaginal exam.

Aftercare

No special preparations is required electronic fetal monitoring.

Risks

Fetal monitoring is not a perfect test. Fetal assessment in labor is subject to differences in interpretation and consequent intervention; therefore, institutional policies and procedures should be followed.

Results

The normal fetal heart rate ranges from 120–160 beats per minute (bpm). Just as an adult's heart rate increases with movement, FHR increases when the fetus moves. A reactive heart rate tracing (also known as a reactive non-stress test, or NST) is considered a positive sign of fetal well being. A non-reactive NST may or may not imply fetal well being. The monitor strip is considered to be reactive when the FHR rises at least 15–20 bpm above the baseline heart rate for at least 20 seconds. This must occur at least twice in a 20-minute period.

Results are considered abnormal if the FHR drops below 120 or rises above 160 for sustained periods. In either of these cases the fetus may be exhibiting fetal distress. A mean FHR of less than 110 bpm may indicate bradycardia (slow heart beat). A mean FHR of over 160 bpm may indicate a tachycardia (rapid beating of the heart). However, some babies who are having problems may not exhibit such clear signs.

KEY TERMS

Cesarean section—Also called a C-section; delivery of a baby through an incision in the mother's abdomen instead of through the vagina.

Late deceleration—Transient slowing of the fetal heart bradycardia, which reaches its height more than 30 seconds after the peak of the uterine contraction and may indicate the fetus is not receiving enough oxygen (hypoxia).

Non-stress test—A record of the fetal heart rate in the absence of contractions (stress).

Reactive stress test—A positive sign of fetal well being. The FHR rises at least 20 beats per minute above the baseline heart rate for at least 20 seconds, occurring at least twice in a 20-minute period.

Variable deceleration—Fetal bradycardia below 100 beats per minute denoting compression of the umbilical cord at the height of a uterine contraction.

During a contraction, the flow of oxygen from the mother through the placenta to the fetus is temporarily stopped. It is as if the fetus has to hold its breath during each contraction. Both the placenta and the fetus are designed to withstand this condition. Between contractions, the fetus should be receiving more than enough oxygen to do well during the contraction.

One sign that a fetus is not getting enough oxygen between contractions is a drop in the FHR after the contraction (late deceleration). The heart rate recovers to a normal level between contractions, only to drop again after the next contraction. This is a subtler sign of distress. Trouble is also indicated by significant slowing during a contraction (variable decelerations).

Training and certification

Electronic fetal monitoring is primarily conducted by specialists in obstetrics and gynecology. Qualified registered nurses and advanced practice nurses may assist in or conduct electronic fetal monitoring.

Applying the external monitor is simple, but requires practice in the proper placement of the monitoring devices. The interpretation of the tracings, however, requires continued vigilance in education and clinical practice. Training should include instruction

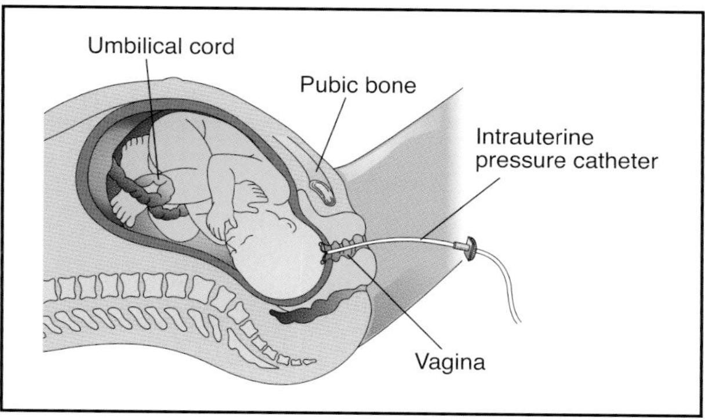

Electronic fetal monitoring (EFM) is performed late in pregnancy or continuously during labor to ensure normal delivery of a healthy baby. EFM can be utilized either externally or internally in the womb. This illustration shows the internal procedure, in which an electrode is attached directly to the baby's scalp to monitor the heart rate. Uterine contractions are recorded using an intrauterine pressure catheter that is inserted through the cervix into the uterus. *(Illustration by Electronic Illustrators Group. Reproduced by permission of Gale, a part of Cengage Learning.)*

electronic FHR monitoring and evaluation of uterine activity.

Resources

OTHER

Fetal Heart Monitoring. *MedlinePlus Encyclopedia.* May 8, 2008, http://www.nlm.nih.gov/medlineplus/ency/article/003405.htm.

Jocoy, Sandy. Electronic Fetal Monitoring. WebMD. June 28, 2008, http://www.webmd.com/baby/electronic-fetal-heart-monitoring.

ORGANIZATIONS

American College of Nurse-Midwives, 8403 Colesville Rd, Suite 1550, Silver Spring, MD, 20919, (240) 485-1800, (240) 485-1818, http://www.midwife.org.

American College of Obstetricians and Gynecologists, P.O. Box 96920, Washington, DC, 20090-6920, (202) 638-5577, http://www.acog.org.

Association of Women's Health, Obstetric, and Neonatal Nurses, 2000 L St. NW, Suite. 740, WashingtonDC , 20036, (202) 261-2400, (800) 673-8499. Toll free in Canada (800) 245-0231, (202) 728-0575, customer service@awhonn.org, http://www.awhonn.org.

Society for Maternal-Fetal Medicine, 409 12th Street, SW, Washington, DC, 20024, (202) 863-2476, (202) 554-1132, smfm@smfm.org, https://www.smfm.org.

Maggie Boleyn, R.N., B.S.N.
Tish Davidson, A.M.

Elimination diets

Definition

Elimination diets are diets in which people stop eating specific foods for a period and then challenge their body by adding the food back into their diet and evaluating how the body responds. Elimination diets are used to detect **food allergies** and food intolerances. They are not nutritionally balanced and are intended to be used only for diagnostic purposes.

Origins

For centuries it has been known that some people develop unpleasant symptoms (adverse reactions) to certain foods that other people can eat without any problems. However, it was not until the 1900s that food **allergies** began to be investigated in rigorous and scientific ways, and studies on food allergies started appearing in reputable medical journals. Elimination diets developed out of this scientific interest in the effects of food on the body.

Description

Adverse reactions to food fall into two main categories, food allergies, and food intolerances. Food allergies cause a response by the **immune system**. When a person has a food allergy, his or her body responds to something in food by treating it like a threatening foreign material. Immune system cells produce proteins called antibodies that act to disable this material. This process often causes inflammation and results undesirable symptoms that range from mild and annoying to life threatening. The reason why some people respond to certain foods and others do not is probably genetically based.

Food intolerances, on the other hand, also cause adverse reactions, but these reactions do not involve the immune system and are not life threatening. Lactose (milk sugar) intolerance is an example of a food intolerance. It is caused by the body producing too little of the enzyme needed to digest lactose. Interestingly, although surveys show that in the United States up to 30% of families believe they have at least one member with a food allergy, the actual documented rate of food allergies is about 6% in infants and children and 3.7% in adults. On the other hand, in Hispanic, Jewish, and Southern European populations, the rate of **lactose intolerance** is about 70%, and it reaches 90% or more in Asian and African populations. Food intolerances are much more common, but true food allergies tend to be much more severe. In this article, food sensitivities are used to include both food allergies and food intolerance.

The most common symptoms of food sensitivities are nausea, **diarrhea**, bloating, excessive gas, **hives**, **rashes**, **eczema**, headaches, migraine, **asthma**, wheezing, and hay fever-like symptoms. These symptoms may occur immediately after eating the trigger food or may not develop for hours. Most immediate reactions are severe allergic responses that can result in anaphylactic shock, a condition in which the airways swell shut and the person cannot breathe. One study found that in about one-third of individuals in anaphylactic shock who were brought for treatment to the emergency room at the at the Mayo Clinic in Minnesota, the shock trigger had been a food. Foods most likely to cause immediate reactions are peanuts, tree nuts, and shellfish.

Delayed symptoms are difficult to detect and are sometimes called "masked" food sensitivities. The most common causes of delayed sensitivities are dairy products, egg, wheat, and soy, however, sensitivities vary widely and can be caused by many foods. The amount of a trigger food that it takes to cause a response varies considerably from person to person.

A true elimination diet is very rigorous and needs to be implemented under the direction of a physician often in consultation with a dietitian or nutritionist. For the elimination diet to be useful, the patient must follow the diet strictly. Cheating invalidates the results.

For 2–3 weeks, a person on the elimination diet eats only the following foods (This list may be modified by the physician):

- grains: rice and rice products, sago, tapioca, buckwheat products, millet products
- proteins: veal, lamb, chicken, turkey, rabbit, tuna, bream, whiting, dried peas, lentils
- fruit: peeled pears, peeled apples, pawpaw
- vegetables: potatoes, sweet potatoes, lettuce, parsley, bamboo shoots, celery, cabbage
- sweeteners and seasonings: sugar, maple syrup, sunflower oil, safflower oil, salt, garlic
- beverages: water, fresh pear juice

The individual must avoid all medicines containing aspirin (salicylates) and food colorings. After several weeks on these restricted foods, one new food is introduced in larger than normal amounts. This is the challenge food, and it is eaten for three days in a row. If no symptoms appear, the dieter continues to eat that food in normal amounts and adds another challenge food. If symptoms appear, the challenge food is stopped immediately and no new challenge food is introduced until symptoms disappear. During this time the dieter keeps a food journal, writing down everything that is eaten and any symptoms, either physical or emotional, that appear. It can take 2 to 3 months to work through all challenge foods.

Function

Elimination diets are the first part of a diagnostic technique for determining what foods are causing undesirable symptoms. Their purpose is to prepare the patient for the second part of the diagnostic process, the food challenge by cleansing the body of all possible foods that could be causing the symptoms. During the challenge phase, the patient eats the suspect food and waits to see if symptoms reappear. Elimination and challenge give healthcare professionals a way to reproducibly pinpoint exactly which foods are causing an adverse reactions so that the patient can exclude these foods from their diet.

Benefits

People with symptoms that interfere with their daily life benefit greatly from pinpointing which foods are causing the symptoms so that these foods can be eliminated from the diet. People with less severe symptoms may find the process of elimination and challenge too costly and disruptive to make it worthwhile.

Precautions

Many people who suspect that certain foods are causing their symptoms try modified elimination diets found on the Internet or elimination diets they devise themselves. These diets have varying degrees of success. For example, many people try eliminating all dairy products to see if their symptoms of lactose intolerance—bloating, cramping, diarrhea, and gas—improve. This do-it-yourself approach may be adequate for people with mild sensitivities to only one food or food group, but it is risky for people with severe intolerances. People with moderate to severe sensitivities need professional guidance to eliminate non-obvious sources of the potential problem food.

Risks

One risk of all elimination diets is that they are not nutritionally balanced. They increase the risk that vitamin and mineral deficiencies will develop. Anyone going on a full elimination regimen needs to consult a dietitian or nutritionist about how to use dietary supplements to assure adequate, balanced **nutrition**

A second risk is that people who self-diagnose symptoms as food intolerances using a non-medically-supervised elimination diet may be ignoring symptoms of more serious and progressive diseases, such as **celiac disease**, Crohn's disease, **gastroesophageal reflux disease**, irritable syndrome, and other health problems that need medical treatment.

Finally, anyone suspected of having a moderate to severe food allergy should be under the care of a physician. Any food challenging must be done in a healthcare setting, as severe reactions can cause anaphylactic shock and **death**.

Research and general acceptance

The medical community accepts elimination diets as a standard way to diagnose food sensitivities. A true elimination diet is quite restrictive, takes a long time to implement, and should be supervised by a healthcare professional. Many short cut do-it-yourself elimination-style diets are available on the Internet. Although people who believe they have a food intolerance often try these diets, they are not accepted by healthcare professionals as diagnostically accurate, and they may cause short-term vitamin and mineral deficiencies.

Resources

BOOKS

Carter, Jill, and Alison Edwards. *The Allergy Exclusion Diet: The 28-Day Plan to Solve Your Food Intolerances.* Carlsbad, CA: Hay House, 2003.

——— *The Elimination Diet Cookbook.* Rockport, MA: Element,1997.

Scott-Moncrieff, Christina. *Overcoming Allergies: Home Remedies-Elimination and Rotation Diets-Complementary Therapies.* London: Collins & Brown, 2002.

OTHER

Atkins, Dan. "Food Allergies." eMedicine.com, June 13, 2006, http://www.emedicine.com/med/topic.htm.

Harvard School of Public Health. "Interpreting News on Diet." Harvard University, 2007, http://www.hsph.harvard.edu/nutritionsource/media.html.

Manners, Deborah. "The Elimination Diet The Detection Diet." Foodintol.com, February 11, 2006, http://www.foodintol.com/eliminationdiet.asp.

Meyers, Suzzanne. "The Elimination Diet." http://www.eliminationdiet.com/. (accessed April 24, 2007).

WebMD. "Allergies: Elimination Diet and Food Challenge Test." http://www.webmd.com/allergies/allergies-elimination-diet.

"Allergy Avoidance Diet. World's Healthiest Foods." Whfoods.org, http://www.whfoods.com (accessed April 21, 2007).

ORGANIZATIONS

American Dietetic Association, 120 S. Riverside Plaza, Suite 2000, Chicago, IL, 60606, (800) 877-1600, http://www.eatright.org.

Chronic Fatigue and Immune Dysfunction Syndrome Association of America (CFIDS), P. O. Box 220398, Chapel Hill, NC, 20222-0398, http://www.cfids.org.

Tish Davidson, A.M.

Emotional development

Definition

Emotional development refers to the process by which infants and children begin developing the capacity to experience, express, interpret, and understand emotions.

Description

The study of the emotional development of infants and children is relatively new, having been studied empirically only since the mid-twentieth century. Researchers have approached this area from a variety of theoretical perspectives, including those of social constructionism, differential emotion theory, and social learning theory. Each of these approaches explores the way infants and children develop emotionally, differing mainly on the question of whether emotions are learned or biologically predetermined, as well as debating the way infants and children manage their emotional experiences and behavior.

Early infancy (birth-six months)

Emotional expressivity

To formulate theories about the development of human emotions, researchers focus on observable display of emotion, such as facial expressions and public behavior. A child's private feelings and experiences cannot be studied by researchers, so interpretation of emotion must be limited to signs that can be observed. Although many descriptions of facial patterns appear intuitively to represent recognizable emotions, psychologists differ in the their views on the range of emotions experienced by infants. It is not clear whether infants actually experience these emotions, or if adults, using adult facial expressions as the standard, simply superimpose their own understanding of the meaning of infant facial expressions.

Between 6 and 10 weeks, a social smile emerges, usually accompanied by other pleasure-indicative actions and sounds, including cooing and mouthing. This social smile occurs in response to adult smiles and interactions. It derives its name from the unique process by which the infant engages a person in a social act, doing so by expressing pleasure (a smile), which consequently elicits a positive response. This cycle brings about a mutually reinforcing pattern in which both the infant and the other person gain pleasure from the social interaction.

As infants become more aware of their environment, smiling occurs in response to a wider variety of contexts. They may smile when they see a toy they have previously enjoyed, or they may smile when receiving praise for accomplishing a difficult task. Smiles such as these, like the social smile, are considered to serve a developmental function.

Laughter, which begins at around three or four months, requires a level of **cognitive development** because it demonstrates that the child can recognize incongruity. That is, laughter is usually elicited by actions that deviate from the norm, such as being kissed on the abdomen or a **caregiver** playing peek-a-boo. Because it fosters reciprocal interactions with others, laughter promotes social development.

Later infancy (7–12 months)

Emotional expressivity

During the last half of the first year, infants begin expressing **fear**, disgust, and anger because of the maturation of cognitive abilities. Anger, often expressed by crying, is a frequent emotion expressed by infants. As is the case with all emotional expressions, anger serves an adaptive function, signaling to caregivers of the infant's discomfort or displeasure, letting them know that something needs to be changed or altered. Although some infants respond to distressing events with sadness, anger is more common.

Fear also emerges during this stage as children become able to compare an unfamiliar event with what they know. Unfamiliar situations or objects often elicit fear responses in infants. One of the most common is the presence of an adult stranger, a fear that begins to appear at about seven months. The degree to which a child reacts with fear to new situations is dependent on a variety of factors. One of the most significant is the response of its mother or caregiver. Caregivers supply infants with a secure base from which to explore their world, and accordingly an exploring infant will generally not move beyond eyesight of the caregiver. Infants repeatedly check with their caregivers for emotional cues regarding **safety** and security of their explorations. If, for instance, they wander too close to something their caregiver perceives as dangerous, they will detect the alarm in the caregiver's facial expression, become alarmed themselves, and retreat from the potentially perilous situation. Infants look to caregivers for facial cues for the appropriate reaction to unfamiliar adults. If the stranger is a trusted friend of the caregiver, the infant is more likely to respond favorably, whereas if the stranger is unknown to the caregiver, the infant may respond with **anxiety** and distress. Another factor in expressing anxiety is the infant's innate **temperament**.

A second fear of this stage is called **separation anxiety**. Infants 7–12 months old may cry in fear if the mother or caregiver leaves them in an unfamiliar place.

Many studies have been conducted to assess the type and quality of emotional communication between caregivers and infants. Parents are one of the primary sources that socialize children to communicate emotional experience in culturally specific ways. That is, through such processes as modeling, direct instruction, and imitation, parents teach their children which emotional expressions are appropriate to express within their specific sub-culture and the broader social context.

Socialization of emotion begins in **infancy**. Research indicates that when mothers interact with their infants they demonstrate emotional displays in an exaggerated slow motion and that these types of display are highly interesting to infants. It is thought that this process is significant in the infant's acquisition of cultural and social codes for emotional display, teaching them how to express their emotions, and the degree of acceptability associated with different types of emotional behaviors.

Another process that emerges during this stage is **social referencing**. Infants begin to recognize the emotions of others, and use this information when reacting to novel situations and people. As infants explore their world, they generally rely on the emotional expressions of their mothers or caregivers to determine the safety or appropriateness of a particular endeavor. Although this process has been established by several studies, there is some debate about the intentions of the infant concerning whether the infants simply imitating their mother's emotional responses or actually experience a change in mood purely from the expressive visual cues of the mother. What is known, however, is that as infants explore their environment, their immediate emotional responses to what they encounter are based on cues portrayed by their mother or primary caregiver, to whom they repeatedly reference as they explore.

Toddlerhood (1–2 years)

Emotional expressivity

During the second year, infants express emotions of shame or embarrassment and pride. These emotions mature in all children, and adults contribute to their development. However, the reason for the shame or pride is learned. Different cultures value different actions. One culture may teach its children to express pride upon winning a competitive event, whereas another may teach children to dampen their pride or even to feel shame at another person's loss.

Emotional understanding

During this stage of development, toddlers acquire language and are learning to verbally express their feelings. In 1986, Inge Bretherton and colleagues found that 30% of 20-month-olds in the United States correctly labeled a series of emotional and physiological states, including sleep-fatigue, pain, distress, disgust, and affection. This ability, rudimentary as it is during early toddlerhood, is the first step children in the development of emotional self-regulation skills.

Although there is debate concerning an acceptable definition of emotion regulation, it is generally thought to involve the ability to recognize and label emotions, and to control emotional expression in ways that are consistent with cultural expectations. In infancy, children largely rely on adults to help them regulate their emotional states. If they are uncomfortable they may be able to communicate this state by crying, but have little hope of alleviating the discomfort on their own. In toddlerhood, however, children begin to develop skills to regulate their emotions with the emergence of language providing an important tool to assist in this process. Being able to articulate an emotional state in itself has a regulatory effect in that it enables children to communicate their feelings to a person capable of helping them manage their emotional state. Speech also enables children to self-regulate, using soothing language to talk themselves through difficult situations.

Empathy, a complex emotional response to a situation, also appears in toddlerhood, usually by age two. The development of empathy requires that children read others' emotional cues, understand that other people are entities distinct from themselves, and take the perspective of another person (put themselves in the position of another). These cognitive advances typically are not evident before the first birthday. The first sign of empathy in children occurs when they try to alleviate the distress of another using methods that they have observed or experienced themselves. Toddlers will use comforting language and initiate physical contact with their mothers if the mother is distressed, supposedly modeling their own early experiences when feeling upset.

Preschool (3–6 years)

Emotional expressivity

Children's capacity to regulate their emotional behavior continues to advance during this stage of development. Parents help preschoolers acquire skills to cope with negative emotional states by teaching and modeling use of verbal reasoning and explanation. For example, when preparing a child for a potentially emotionally evocative event, such as a trip to the doctor's office or weekend at their grandparents' house, parents will often offer comforting advice, such as "the doctor only wants to help" or "grandma and grandpa have all kinds of fun plans for the weekend." This kind of emotional preparation is crucial for children if they are to develop the skills necessary to regulate their own negative emotional states. Children who have trouble learning and/or enacting these types of coping skills often exhibit **acting out** types of behavior, or, conversely, can become withdrawn when confronted with fear or anxiety-provoking situations.

Beginning at about age four, children acquire the ability to alter their emotional expressions, a skill of high value in cultures that require frequent disingenuous social displays. Psychologists call these skills emotion display rules. They are culture-specific rules regarding the appropriateness of expressing in certain situations. These rules teach that one's external emotional expression need not match one's internal emotional state. For example, in Western culture, we teach children that they should smile and say thank you when receiving a gift, even if they really do not like the present. The ability to use display rules is complex. It requires that children understand the need to alter emotional displays, take the perspective of another, know that external states need not match internal states, have the muscular control to produce emotional expressions, be sensitive to social contextual cues that alert them to alter their expressivity, and have the motivation to enact such discrepant displays in a convincing manner.

It is thought that in the **preschool** years, parents or regular caregivers are the primary socializing force, teaching appropriate emotional expression in children. Moreover, children learn at about age three that expressions of anger and aggression are to be controlled in the presence of adults. Around peers, however, children are much less likely to suppress negative emotional behavior. These differences seem to arise because of the different consequences they have received for expressing negative emotions in front of adults as opposed to their peers. Furthermore this distinction made by children as a function of social context demonstrates that preschoolers have begun to internalize society's rules governing the appropriate expression of emotions.

Carolyn Saarni, an innovator in the exploration of emotional development, has identified two types of emotional display rules, prosocial and self-protective. Prosocial display rules involve altering emotional displays in order to protect another's feelings. For example, a child might not like the sweater she received from her aunt, but would appear happy because she did not want to make her aunt feel unhappy. On the other hand, self-protective display rules involve masking emotion in order to save face or to protect oneself from negative consequences. For instance, a child may feign toughness when he trips in front of his peers and scrapes his knee, in order to avoid teasing and further embarrassment. Research findings are mixed concerning the order in which prosocial and self-protective display rules are learned. Some studies demonstrate that knowledge of self-protective display rules emerges first, whereas other studies show the opposite effect.

There also has been research examining how children alter their emotional displays. Researchers Jackie Gnepp and Debra Hess found that there is greater pressure on children to modify their verbal rather than facial emotional expressions. It is easier for preschoolers to control their verbal utterances than their facial muscles.

Emotional understanding

Beginning at about age four or five, children develop a more sophisticated understanding of others' emotional states. Although it has been demonstrated that empathy emerges at quite a young age, with rudimentary displays emerging during toddlerhood, increasing cognitive development enables preschoolers to arrive at a more complex understanding of emotions. Through repeated experiences, children begin to develop their own theories of others' emotional states by referring to causes and consequences of emotions, and by observing and being sensitive to behavioral cues that indicate emotional distress. For instance, when asked why a playmate is upset, a child might respond "because the teacher took his toy" or by reference to some other external cause, usually one that relates to an occurrence familiar to them. Children of this age are also beginning to make predictions about others' experience and expression of emotions, such as predicting that a happy child will be more likely to share his or her **toys**.

Middle childhood (7–11 years)

Emotional expressivity

Children ages seven to eleven display a wider variety of self-regulation skills. Sophistication in understanding and enacting cultural display rules has increased dramatically by this stage, such that by now children begin to know when to control emotional expressivity as well as have a sufficient repertoire of behavioral regulation skills allowing them to effectively mask emotions in socially appropriate ways. Research has indicated that children at this age have become sensitive to the social contextual cues that serve to guide their decisions to express or control negative emotions. Several factors influence their emotion management decisions, including the type of emotion experienced, the nature of their relationship with the person involved in the emotional exchange, child age, and child gender. Moreover, it appears that children have developed a set of expectations concerning the likely outcome of expressing emotion to others. In general, children report regulating anger and sadness more with friends than mothers and fathers because they expect to receive a negative response, such as teasing or belittling, from friends. With increasing age, however, older children report expressing negative emotions more often to their mothers than their fathers, expecting fathers to respond negatively to an emotional display. These emotion regulation skills are considered to be adaptive and deemed essential to establishing, developing, and maintaining social relationships.

Children at this age also demonstrate that they possess rudimentary cognitive and behavioral coping skills that serve to lessen the impact of an emotional event and in so doing, may in fact alter their emotional experience. For example, when experiencing a negative emotional event, children may respond by employing rationalization or minimization cognitive coping strategies, in which they re-interpret or reconstruct the scenario to make it seem less threatening or upsetting. Upon having their bicycle stolen or being deprived of television for a weekend, they might tell themselves, "It's only a bike, at least I didn't get hurt." or "Maybe mom and dad will make up something fun to do instead of watching TV."

Emotional understanding

During middle childhood, children begin to understand that the emotional states of others are not as simple

KEY TERMS

Cognitive ability—The ability to think and reason.

Empathy—The ability to imagine and understand what another person is feeling.

as they imagined in earlier years, and that they often are the result of complex causes, some of which are not externally obvious. They also come to understand that it is possible to experience more than one emotion at a time, although this ability is somewhat restricted and evolves slowly. As Susan Harter and Nancy Whitsell demonstrated, seven-year-old children are able to understand that a person can feel two emotions simultaneously, even if the emotions are positive and negative. Children can feel happy and excited that their parents bought them a bicycle or angry and sad that a friend had hurt them, but they deny the possibility of experiencing "mixed feelings." It is not until age 10 that children are capable of understanding that one can experience two seemingly contradictory emotions, such as feeling happy that they were chosen for a team but also nervous about their responsibility to play well.

Displays of empathy also increase in frequency during this stage. Children from families that regularly discuss the complexity of feelings will develop empathy more readily than those whose families avoid such topics. Furthermore, parents who set consistent behavioral limits and who themselves show high levels of concern for others are more likely to produce empathic children than parents who are punitive or particularly harsh in restricting behavior.

Adolescence (12–18 years)

Emotional expressivity

Adolescents have become sophisticated at regulating their emotions. They have developed a wide vocabulary with which to discuss, and thus influence, emotional states of themselves and others. Adolescents are adept at interpreting social situations as part of the process of managing emotional displays.

By **adolescence**, children are widely believed to have developed a set of expectations, referred to as scripts, about how various people will react to their emotional displays, and regulate their displays in accordance with these scripts. Research in this area has found that in early adolescence, children begin breaking the emotionally intimate ties with their parents and begin forming them with peers. In one study, for instance, eighth-grade students, particularly boys, reported regulating (hiding) their emotions to (from) their mothers more than did either fifth- or eleventh-grade adolescents. This dip in emotional expressivity expression towards mothers appeared to be due to the boys' expectations of receiving less emotional support from their mothers. This particular finding demonstrates the validity of the script hypothesis of self-regulations; children's expectations of receiving little emotional support from their mothers, perhaps based on past experience, guide their decisions to regulate emotions more strictly in their mothers' presence.

Another factor that plays a significant role in the ways adolescents regulate emotional displays is their heightened sensitivity to others' evaluations of them, a sensitivity that can result in acute self-awareness and self-consciousness as they try to blend into the dominant social structure. David Elkind has described adolescents as operating as if they were in front of an imaginary audience in which every action and detail is noted and evaluated by others. As such, adolescents become very aware of the impact of emotional expressivity on their social interactions and fundamentally, on obtaining peer approval. Because guidelines concerning the appropriateness of emotional displays is highly culture-specific, adolescents have the difficult task of learning when and how to express or regulate certain emotions.

As expected, gender plays a significant role in the types of emotions displayed by adolescents. Boys are less likely than girls to disclose their fearful emotions during times of distress. This reluctance was similarly supported by boys' belief that they would receive less understanding and, in fact, probably be belittled, for expressing both aggressive and vulnerable emotions.

Resources

BOOKS

Landy, Sarah. *Pathways to Competence: Encouraging Healthy Social and Emotional Development in Young Children,* 2nd ed. Baltimore: Paul H. Brookes Pub., 2009.

Schiller, Pamela B. *Seven Skills For School Success: Activities to Develop Social & Emotional Intelligence in Young Children.* Beltsville, MD: Gryphon House, 2009.

OTHER

"Social and Emotional Development." Merck Manuals Online. May 2006, http://www.merck.com/mmhe/sec23/ch268/ch268d.html (accessed July 9, 2010).

"Social and Emotional Development." Nebraska Department of Education. Undated, http://www.nde.state.ne.us/ech/elgse.pdf (accessed July 9, 2010).

"Stages of Social-Emotional Development in Children and Teenagers." Child Development Institute, http://www.childdevelopmentinfo.com/development/erickson.shtml (accessed July 9, 2010).

ORGANIZATIONS

American Academy of Child and Adolescent Psychiatry, 3615 Wisconsin Avenue, NW, Washington, DC, 20016-3007, (202) 966-7300, (202) 966-2891, http://www.aacap.org.

American Academy of Pediatrics, 141 Northwest Point Boulevard, Elk Grove Village, IL, 60007-1098, (847) 434-4000, (847) 434-8000, http://www.aap.org.

American Psychological Association, 750 First Street, NE, Washington, DC, 20002-4242, (202) 336-5500; TDD/ TTY: (202) 336-6123, (800) 374-2721, apa@psych.org, http://www.apa.org.

National Association for the Education of Young Children, 1313 L Street, NW, Suite 500, Washington, DC, 20005, (202)232-8777, (800) 424-2460 or (866) NAEYC-4U, (202) 328-1846, http://www.naeyc.org.

Janice Zeman
Tish Davidson, AM

Encephalitis

Definition

Encephalitis is an inflammation of the brain, usually caused by a direct viral infection or a hypersensitivity reaction to a virus or foreign protein. Brain inflammation caused by a bacterial infection is sometimes called cerebritis. When both the brain and spinal cord are involved, the disorder is called encephalomyelitis. An inflammation of the brain's covering, or meninges, is called **meningitis**.

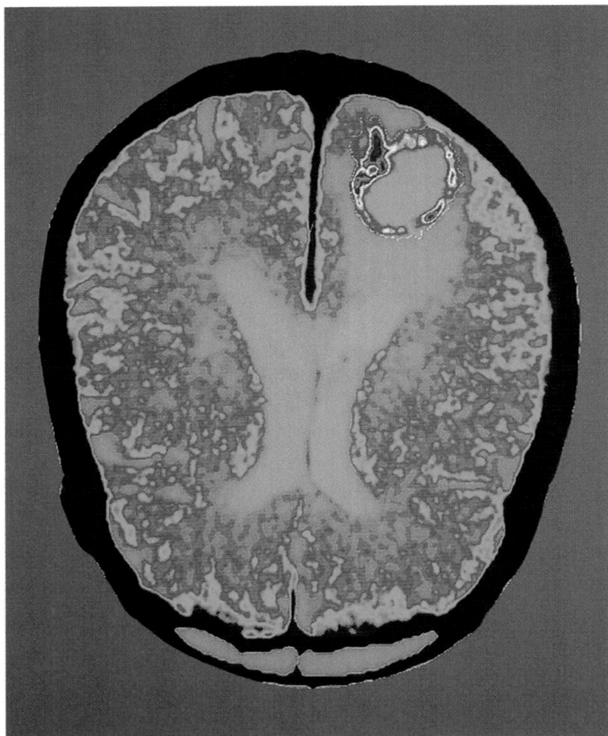

Computed tomography scan (CT scan) of a child with encephalitis. The right side of the brain shows abnormal dilation of the ventricles (orange). *(Airelle-Joubert/Photo Researchers, Inc.)*

Description

Encephalitis is an inflammation of the brain. The inflammation is a reaction of the body's **immune system** to infection or invasion. During the inflammation, the brain's tissues become swollen. The combination of the infection and the immune reaction to it can cause **headache** and a **fever**, as well as more severe symptoms in some cases.

Approximately 2,000 cases of encephalitis are reported to the Centers for Disease Control in Atlanta, Georgia, each year. The viruses causing primary encephalitis can be epidemic or sporadic. The **polio** virus is an epidemic cause. Arthropod-borne viral encephalitis is responsible for most epidemic viral encephalitis. The viruses live in animal hosts and mosquitos that transmit the disease. The most common form of non-epidemic or sporadic encephalitis is caused by the **herpes simplex** virus, type 1 (HSV-1), and has a high rate of **death**. **Mumps** is another example of a sporadic cause.

Causes and symptoms

Causes

There are more than a dozen viruses that can cause encephalitis, spread by either human-to human contact or by animal **bites**. Encephalitis may occur with several common viral infections of childhood. Viruses and viral diseases that may cause encephalitis include:

- chickenpox
- measles
- mumps
- Epstein-Barr virus (EBV)
- cytomegalovirus infection
- HIV
- herpes simplex
- herpes zoster (shingles)
- herpes B
- polio
- rabies
- mosquito-borne viruses (arboviruses)

Primary encephalitis is caused by direct infection by the virus, while secondary encephalitis is due to a post-infectious immune reaction to viral infection elsewhere in the body. Secondary encephalitis may occur with **measles**, **chickenpox**, mumps, **rubella**, and EBV. In secondary encephalitis, symptoms usually begin 5 to 10 days after the onset of the disease itself and are related to the breakdown of the myelin sheath that covers nerve fibers.

In rare cases, encephalitis may follow **vaccination** against some of the viral diseases listed above. Creutzfeldt-Jakob disease, a very rare brain disorder caused by an infectious particle called a prion, may also cause encephalitis.

Mosquitoes spread viruses responsible for equine encephalitis (eastern and western types), St. Louis encephalitis, California encephalitis, and **Japanese encephalitis**. **Lyme disease**, spread by ticks, can cause encephalitis, as can Colorado tick fever. **Rabies** is most often spread by animal bites from dogs, cats, mice, raccoons, squirrels, and bats and may cause encephalitis.

Equine encephalitis is carried by mosquitoes that do not normally bite humans but do bite horses and birds. It is occasionally picked up from these animals by mosquitoes that do bite humans. Japanese encephalitis and St. Louis encephalitis are also carried by mosquitoes. The risk of contracting a mosquito-borne virus is greatest in mid- to late summer, when mosquitoes are most active, in those rural areas where these viruses are known to exist. Eastern equine encephalitis occurs in eastern and southeastern United States; western equine and California encephalitis occur throughout the West; and St. Louis encephalitis occurs throughout the country. Japanese encephalitis does not occur in the United States, but is found throughout much of Asia. The viruses responsible for these diseases are classified as arbovirus and these diseases are collectively called arbovirus encephalitis.

Herpes simplex encephalitis, the most common form of sporadic encephalitis in western countries, is a disease with significantly high mortality. It occurs in children and adults and both sides of the brain are affected. It is theorized that brain infection is caused by the virus moving from a peripheral location to the brain via two nerves, the olfactory and the trigeminal (largest nerves in the skull).

Herpes simplex encephalitis is responsible for 10% of all encephalitis cases and is the main cause of sporadic, fatal encephalitis. In untreated patients, the rate of death is 70% while the mortality is 15–20% in patients who have been treated with acyclovir. The symptoms of herpes simplex encephalitis are fever, rapidly disintegrating mental state, headache, and behavioral changes.

Symptoms

The symptoms of encephalitis range from very mild to very severe and may include:

- headache
- fever
- lethargy (sleepiness, decreased alertness, and fatigue)
- malaise
- nausea and vomiting
- visual disturbances
- tremor
- decreased consciousness (drowsiness, confusion, delirium, and unconsciousness)
- stiff neck
- seizures

Symptoms may progress rapidly, changing from mild to severe within several days or even several hours.

Diagnosis

Diagnosis of encephalitis includes careful questioning to determine possible exposure to viral sources. Tests that can help confirm the diagnosis and rule out other disorders include:

- Blood tests. These are to detect antibodies to viral antigens, and foreign proteins.
- Cerebrospinal fluid analysis (spinal tap). This detects viral antigens and provides culture specimens for the virus or bacteria that may be present in the cerebrospinal fluid.
- Electroencephalogram (EEG).
- CT and MRI scans.

A brain biopsy (surgical gathering of a small tissue sample) may be recommended in some cases where treatment to date has been ineffective and the cause of the encephalitis is unclear. Definite diagnosis by biopsy may allow specific treatment that would otherwise be too risky.

Treatment

Choice of treatment for encephalitis will depend on the cause. Bacterial encephalitis is treated with **antibiotics**. Viral encephalitis is usually treated with **antiviral drugs**, including acyclovir, ganciclovir, foscarnet, ribovarin, and AZT. Viruses that respond to acyclovir include herpes simplex, the most common cause of sporadic (non-epidemic) encephalitis in the United States.

The symptoms of encephalitis may be treated with a number of different drugs. Corticosteroids, including prednisone and dexamethasone, are sometimes prescribed to reduce inflammation and brain swelling. Anticonvulsant drugs, including dilantin and phenytoin, are used to control seizures. Fever may be reduced with **acetaminophen** or other fever-reducing drugs.

A person with encephalitis must be monitored carefully, since symptoms may change rapidly. Blood tests may be required regularly to track levels of fluids and salts in the blood.

Prognosis

Encephalitis symptoms may last several weeks. Most cases of encephalitis are mild, and recovery is usually quick. Mild encephalitis usually leaves no residual neurological problems. Overall, approximately 10% of those with encephalitis die from their infections or complications such as secondary infection. Some forms of encephalitis have more severe courses, including herpes encephalitis, in which mortality is 15–20% with treatment, and 70–80% without. Antiviral treatment is ineffective for eastern equine encephalitis, and mortality is approximately 30%.

Permanent neurological consequences may follow recovery in some cases. Consequences may include personality changes, memory loss, language difficulties, seizures, and partial paralysis.

Prevention

Because encephalitis is due to infection, it may be prevented by avoiding the infection. Minimizing contact with others who have any of the viral illness listed above may reduce the chances of becoming infected. Most infections are spread by hand-to-hand or hand-to-mouth contact; frequent hand washing may reduce the likelihood of infection if contact cannot be avoided.

Mosquito-borne viruses may be avoided by preventing mosquito bites. Mosquitoes are most active at dawn and dusk, and are most common in moist areas with standing water. Minimizing exposed skin and use of mosquito repellents on other areas can reduce the chances of being bitten.

Vaccines are available against some viruses, including polio, herpes B, Japanese encephalitis, and equine encephalitis. **Rabies vaccine** is available for animals; it is also given to people after exposure. Japanese **encephalitis vaccine** is recommended for those traveling to Asia and staying in affected rural areas during transmission season.

ORGANIZATIONS

Centers for Disease Control and Prevention (CDC), 1600 Clifton Road, Atlanta, GA, 30333, (404) 498-1515, (800) 311-3435, http://www.cdc.gov.

Richard Robinson

KEY TERMS

Cerebrospinal fluid analysis—A analysis that is important in diagnosing diseases of the central nervous system. The fluid within the spine will indicate the presence of viruses, bacteria, and blood. Infections such as encephalitis will be indicated by an increase of cell count and total protein in the fluid.

Computerized tomography (CT) Scan—A test to examine organs within the body and detect evidence of tumors, blood clots, and accumulation of fluids.

Electroencephalagram (EEG)—A chart of the brain waves picked up by the electrodes placed on the scalp. Changes in brain wave activity can be an indication of nervous system disorders.

Inflammation—A response from the immune system to an injury. The signs are redness, heat, swelling, and pain.

Magnetic Resonance Imaging (MRI)—MRI is diagnostic radiography using electromagnetic energy to create an image of the central nervous system (CNS), blood system, and musculoskeletal system.

Vaccine—A prepartation containing killed or weakened microorganisms used to build immunity against infection from that microorganism.

Virus—A very small organism that can only live within a cell. They are unable to reproduce outside that cell.

Encephalitis vaccine

Definition

Japanese encephalitis (JE) vaccine is a vaccine designed to prevent Japanese **encephalitis**. Two vaccines are available in the United States for immunization against JE. Additional vaccines are successfully used in Asia but are not licensed for use in the United State.

Purpose

JE is an infection of the brain caused by a virus that is transmitted to humans by the bite of a mosquito. The disease is found primarily in rural areas of Japan, Korea, China, India, Thailand, Indonesia, Malaysia, Vietnam, Taiwan, and the Philippines. A risk assessment for JE in countries where it has been reported can be found in the

United States Centers for Disease Control and Prevention (CDC) Yellow Book.

Description

About 45,000 cases of Japanese encephalitis are reported each year, but the disease is thought to be seriously underreported. Not all infections cause severe symptoms. In many cases the only symptoms are a **fever** and **headache**; however, of those who develop severe symptoms, 20–30% die and another 30–50% develop permanent neurological or psychiatric complications. No specific treatment exists for JE. The disease can be prevented by **vaccination** with JE vaccine and good mosquito control procedures. Cases of JE in the United States are exceedingly rare (less than one case per year) and usually occur in military personnel or others who have returned home after living in affected areas.

Two types of JE vaccine are approved for use in the United States. Because the need for JE vaccine in the United States is extremely limited, physicians do not keep this vaccine on hand and generally access it through the CDC.

Inactivated vero cell culture-derived JE vaccine (JE-VC)

JE-VC is known by the brand name IXIARO. It is made of a strain of attenuated JE virus that is grown in a laboratory in vero cells. The finished vaccine contains no gelatin stabilizers, **antibiotics**, or thimerosal and must be stored at 35–46°F (2–8°C). JE-VC was approved for use in individuals age 17 years and older by the U. S. Food and Drug Administration (FDA) in March 2009. As of April 2010, it was not approved in the United States for use in children. JE-VC is manufactured by Intercell Biomedical in the United Kingdom and is about 96% effective in inducing immunity in healthy individuals.

Inactivated mouse brain-derived JE vaccine (JE-MB)

JE-MB is known by the brand name JE-VAX. It is made by injecting a strain of JE virus into the brains of mice where it reproduces and can be harvested to make the vaccine. The finished vaccine contains gelatin stabilizers and thimerosal and must be stored at 35-46°F (2-8°C). JE-MB has been approved for use in the United States since 1992 for both children over one year of age and adults. It is the only JE vaccine approved by the FDA for children. Until 2006, JE-MB was manufactured by Sanofi Pasteur. In that year, manufacture of JE-MB was discontinued. The remaining vaccine stockpile is restricted for use in children; adults should be vaccinated with JE-VC, which is equally effective.

KEY TERMS

Attenuated—Weakened, so as to reduce the ability to cause a disease. Attenuated viruses are used to create vaccines.

Pregnancy category—A system of classifying drugs according to their established risks for use during pregnancy. Category A: Controlled human studies have demonstrated no fetal risk. Category B: Animal studies indicate no fetal risk, but no human studies; or adverse effects in animals, but not in well-controlled human studies. Category C: No adequate human or animal studies; or adverse fetal effects in animal studies, but no available human data. Category D: Evidence of fetal risk, but benefits outweigh risks. Category X: Evidence of fetal risk. Risks outweigh any benefits.

Recommended dosage

Because JE vaccine is not kept on hand by most physicians and complete immunity takes about 40 days to develop, individuals who need to be vaccinated should allow plenty of time to complete the process. Immunization against JE is recommended only for a very limited number of people, including:

- Travelers going to a region where there is a current JE outbreak. (See the CDC Yellow Book for current information.)
- Travelers who expect to spend a month or more in rural areas where JE is common.
- Travelers to areas where JE is found who expect to spend a lot of time outdoors, especially around rice paddies and bodies of water that support large mosquito populations.
- Laboratory workers who may be exposed to the JE virus at work.

Short-term travelers to affected countries and those who expect to remain in urban areas generally do not need to be immunized. Individuals who plan long-term travel to countries where JE is found should, in consultation with a knowledgeable physician, weigh the risk of developing the disease against the possibility of adverse side effects of vaccination.

JE-VC is given as an injection to individuals age 17 and older in two doses that are spaced 28 days apart. The final dose should be given at least seven days before travel to an infected area. Because this vaccine is relatively new, as of 2010, there is no information on when a booster shot is needed.

JE-MB is given as an injection in a three-dose series to children ages one through 16 years. Doses are at days 0, 7, and 30. The final dose must be given at least 10 days before travel to an infected area. A booster shot is needed after two years.

Precautions

People who should not receive the vaccine include those who have had allergic reactions to any of the components of the vaccine or to a previous dose of JE vaccine.

JE-VC is a Pregnancy Category B drug, meaning that animal studies have shown that it does not harm the fetus, but that no controlled studies have been done on pregnant women. It is not known whether JE-VC is excreted in breast milk.

JE-MB is a Pregnancy Category C drug, meaning no adequate studies have been performed on pregnant or **breastfeeding** women.

Children infected with HIV have a reduced immune response to JE-MB.

Side effects

Mild side effects are similar for both vaccines. About 1 in five people develop redness, soreness, and swelling at the injection site after vaccination. About one in 10 people develop headache, fever, chills, rash, muscle **pain**, or gastrointestinal upset after vaccination.

More serious side effects, although uncommon, are allergic reactions. These usually manifest as an itchy rash, swelling of the extremities, and sometimes swelling of the throat and have been reported with JE-MB. Swelling of the throat may cause difficulty breathing. These reactions normally occur 24–48 hours after vaccination and are treated with **antihistamines** and corticosteroids. About 10% of people with a serious allergic reaction require hospitalization, and a few deaths have occurred.

As of 2010, no serious allergic reactions had been seen in people receiving JE-VC. The number of people receiving the vaccine as of 2010 was small, so rare serious allergic reactions are still possible.

Interactions

JE-VC can safely be given with **Hepatitis A** vaccine. Other drug and vaccine interactions have not yet been studied as of 2010. JE-MB can be safely given with other vaccines.

Resources

BOOKS

Miller, Neil Z. *Vaccine Safety Manual for Concerned Families and Health Practitioners,* 2nd ed. Santa Fe, NM: New Atlantean Press, 2010.

PERIODICALS

Fisher, Marc. "Japanese Encephalitis Vaccines: Recommendations of the Adivsory Committee on Immunization Practices (ACIP)." *Morbidity and Mortality Weekly* 59 no 1 (March 12, 2010): 1–27, http://www.cdc.gov/mmwr/preview/mmwrhtml/rr5901a1.htm (accessed June 3, 2010).

OTHER

Fisher, Marc, Anne Griggs, and J. Erin Staples. "Chapter 2—The Pre-Travel Consultation: Travel-related Vaccine Preventable Diseases." *Travelers' Health–Yellow Book.* Centers for Disease Control and Prevention. April 19, 2010, http://wwwnc.cdc.gov/travel/yellowbook/2010/chapter-2/japanese-encephalitis.aspx (accessed June 3, 2010).

Jani, Asim A., and Alexander J. Kallen. "Japanese Encephalitis." eMedicine. May 6, 2009, http://emedicine.medscape.com/article/233802-overview (accessed June 3, 2010).

ORGANIZATIONS

National Network for Immunization Information, 301 University Blvd, Galveston. TX, 77555-0351, (409) 772-0199, (409)772-5208, http://www.immunizationinfo.org.

National Vaccine Program Office, 200 Independence Avenue, SW Room 715-H, Washington. DC, 20201, (202) 619-0257, (877) 696-6775, (409) 772-5208, http://www.hhs.gov/nvpo.

United States Centers for Disease Control and Prevention (CDC), 1600 Clifton Road, Atlanta, GA, 30333, (404) 639-3534, (800) CDC-INFO (800-232-4636). TTY: (888) 232-6348, inquiry@cdc.gov, http://www.cdc.gov.

World Health Organization, Avenue Appia 20, 1211 Geneva, 27 Switzerland, +22 41 791 21 11, +22 41 791 31 11, info@who.int, http://www.who.int.

Tish Davidson, AM
Paul Checchia, MD

Encopresis

Definition

Encopresis is repeatedly having bowel movements in places other than the toilet after the age when bowel control can normally be expected.

Description

Most children have established bowel control by the time they are four years old. After that age, when they repeatedly have bowel movements in inappropriate places, they may have encopresis. In the United States, encopresis affects 1–2% of children under age 10. About 80% of these are boys.

Encopresis can be either involuntary or voluntary. Involuntary encopresis is related to **constipation**, passing hard painful feces, and difficult bowel movements. Often children with involuntary encopresis stain their underpants with liquid feces. They are usually unaware that this has happened. Voluntary encopresis is much less common and is associated with behavioral or psychological problems. Both types of encopresis occur most often when the child is awake, rather than at night.

Causes and symptoms

Although a few children experience encopresis because of malformations of the lower bowel and anus or irritable bowel disease, most have no physical problems to explain this disorder. Constipation is present in about 80% of children who experience involuntary encopresis. As feces moves through the large intestine, water is removed. The longer the feces stays in the large intestine, the more water is removed, and the harder the feces becomes. The result can be hard or painful bowel movements. In response, children may start to hold back when they feel the urge to eliminate in order to avoid pain. This starts a cycle of constipation that results in retentive encopresis.

Once elimination is avoided, the bowel becomes full of hard feces. This stretches the large intestine. Eventually the intestine becomes so stretched that liquid feces backed up behind the blockage is able to leak around the hard feces. Children with this type of encopresis do not feel the urge to have a bowel movement and are often surprised when their pants are stained with foul smelling liquid feces. This leakage of feces is called overflow incontinence. Parents sometimes mistake this soiling for **diarrhea**, because the feces expelled is liquid. Every so often, children with involuntary encopresis may pass large stools, sometimes with volumes big enough to clog the toilet, but the relief this brings is temporary.

Although about 95% of encopresis is involuntary, some children intentionally withhold bowel movements. The American Psychiatric Association (APA) recognizes voluntary encopresis without constipation as a psychological disorder. This disorder is said to occur when a child who has control over his bowel movements chooses to have them in an inappropriate place. The feces is a normal consistency, not hard. Sometimes it is smeared in an obvious place, but it may also be hidden from adults.

Voluntary encopresis may result from a power struggle between caregivers and the child during **toilet training**, or the child may have developed an unusual **fear** of the toilet. It is also associated with **oppositional defiant disorder** (ODD), **conduct disorder**, **sexual abuse**, and high levels of psychological stress. For example, children who were separated from their parents during World War II were reported to have a high rate of encopresis. However, parents and caregivers should be aware that very few children soil intentionally and most do not have a behavioral or psychological problem, so they should not be punished for their soiling accidents.

Diagnosis

Diagnosis is based primarily on the child's history of inappropriate bowel movements. Physical examinations are almost always normal, except for a mass of hard feces blocking the lower intestine. Other physical causes of soiling, such as illness, reaction to medication, **food allergies**, and physical disabilities, may also be ruled out through history and a physical examination. In addition, to be diagnosed with encopresis the child must be old enough to establish regular bowel control—usually chronologically and developmentally at least four years of age.

Treatment

The goal of treatment is to establish regular, soft, pain free bowel movements in the toilet. First the physician tries to determine the cause of encopresis, whether physical or psychological. Regardless of the cause, the bowel must be emptied of hard, impacted feces This can be done using an enema, **laxatives**, and/or stool softeners such as mineral oil. Enemas and laxatives should be used only at a doctor's recommendation.

Next, the child is given stool softeners to keep feces soft and to give the stretched intestine time to shrink back to its normal size. This shrinking process may take several months, during which time stool softeners may need to be used regularly. Children also need two or three regularly scheduled toilet sits daily in an effort to establish consistent bowel habits. These toilet sits are often more effective if done after meals. Maintaining soft, easy-to-pass stools is also important if the child is afraid of the toilet because of past painful bowel movements. A child psychologist or psychiatrist can suggest treatment for the rare child with serious behavioral problems such as smearing or hiding feces.

KEY TERMS

Feces—Waste products eliminated from the large intestine; excrement.

Incontinence—The inability to control the release of urine or feces.

Laxative—Material that encourages a bowel movement.

Stools—feces, bowel movements.

Alternative treatment

Many herbal stool softeners and laxatives are available as both tablets and liquids. Psyllium, the seed of several plants of the genus *Plantago* is one of the most effective. Other natural remedies for constipation include castor seed oil (*Ricinus communis*), senna (*Cassia senna* or *Senna alexandrina*), and dong quai *Angelica polymorpha* or *Angelica sinensis*).

Prognosis

For almost all children, once constipation is controlled, the problem of soiling disappears. This may take several months, and relapses may occur, but with effective prevention strategies, encopresis can be eliminated. Children who are in a power struggle over toileting usually outgrow their desire to have bowel movements in inappropriate places. The prognosis for children with serious behavioral and psychological problems that result in smearing or hiding feces depends largely on resolving the underlying problems.

Prevention

The best way to prevent encopresis is to prevent constipation. Methods of preventing constipation include:

- increasing the amount of liquids, especially water, the child drinks
- adding high fiber foods to the diet (e.g. dried beans, fresh fruits and vegetables, whole wheat bread and pasta, popcorn)
- establishing regular bowel habits
- limiting the child's intake of dairy products (e.g. milk, cheese, yogurt, ice cream) that promote constipation.
- treating constipation promptly with stool softeners, so that it does not become worse.

Parental concerns

Parents should work with their children to establish appropriate stooling behaviors and institute a system of rewards for successful toileting.

Resources

BOOKS

American Psychiatric Association. *Diagnostic and Statistical Manual of Mental Disorders*, 4th ed. text revision. Washington, D.C.: American Psychiatric Association, 2000.

PERIODICALS

Kuhn, Brett R., Bethany A. Marcus, and Sheryl L. Pitner. "Treatment Guidelines for Primary Nonretentive Encopresis and Stool Toileting Refusal." *American Family Physician*, 59 no. 8 (15 April 1999) 2171-2183. Available from http://www.aafp.org (accessed February 16, 2005).

OTHER

Borowitz, Stephen. *Encopresis,* 14 June 2004, http://www.emedicine.com/ped/topics670.html (accessed February 20, 2005).

ORGANIZATIONS

American Academy of Child and Adolescent Psychiatry (AACAP), 3615 Wisconsin Ave. NW, Washington, DC, 20016, (202) 966-7300, http://www.aacap.org.

Tish Davidson, A.M.

Enterobacterial infections

Definition

Enterobacterial infections are disorders of the digestive tract and other organ systems produced by a group of gram-negative, rod-shaped bacteria called Enterobacteriaceae. Gram-negative means that the organisms do not retain the violet color of the dye used to make Gram stains. The most troublesome organism in this group is *Escherichia coli*. Other enterobacteria are species of *Salmonella*, *Shigella*, *Klebsiella*, *Enterobacter*, *Serratia*, *Proteus*, and *Yersinia*.

Description

Enterobacterial infections can be produced by bacteria that normally live in the human digestive tract without causing serious disease or by bacteria that enter from the outside. In many cases these infections are nosocomial, which means that they can be acquired in the hospital. *Klebsiella* and *Proteus* sometimes cause **pneumonia**, ear and sinus infections, and urinary tract infections. *Enterobacter* and *Serratia* often cause bacterial infection of the blood (bacteremia), particularly in patients with weakened immune systems.

Diarrhea caused by enterobacteria is a common problem in the United States. It is estimated that each person in the general population has an average of 1.5 episodes of diarrhea each year, with higher rates in children, institutionalized people, and Native Americans. This type of enterobacterial infection can range from a minor nuisance to a life-threatening disorder, especially in infants, elderly persons, **AIDS** patients, and malnourished people. Enterobacterial infections are one of the two leading killers of children in developing countries.

Causes and symptoms

Causes

Enterobacterial infections in the digestive tract typically start when the organisms invade the mucous tissues that line the digestive tract. They may be bacteria that are already present in the stomach and intestines, or they may be transmitted by contaminated food and water. It is also possible for enterobacterial infections to spread by person-to-person contact. The usual incubation period is 12–72 hours.

***ESCHERICHIA COLI* INFECTIONS** *E. coli* infections cause most of the enterobacterial infections in the United States. The organisms are categorized according to whether they are invasive or noninvasive. Noninvasive types of *E. coli* include what are called enteropathogenic *E. coli*, or EPEC, and enterotoxigenic *E. coli*, or ETEC. EPEC and ETEC types produce a bacterial poison (toxin) in the stomach that interacts with the digestive juices and causes the patient to lose large amounts of water through the intestines.

The invasive types of *E. coli* are called enterohemorrhagic *E. coli*, or EHEC, and enteroinvasive *E. coli,* or EIEC. These subtypes invade the stomach tissues directly, causing tissue destruction and bloody stools. EHEC can produce complications leading to hemolytic-uremic syndrome (HUS), a potentially fatal disorder marked by the destruction of red blood cells and kidney failure. EHEC has become a growing problem in the United States because of outbreaks caused by contaminated food. A particular type of EHEC known as O157:H7 has been identified since 1982 in undercooked hamburgers, unpasteurized milk, and apple juice. Between 2–7% of infections caused by O157:H7 develop into HUS.

Symptoms

The symptoms of enterobacterial infections are sometimes classified according to the type of diarrhea they produce.

WATERY DIARRHEA Patients infected with ETEC, EPEC, some types of *Salmonella*, and some types of *Shigella* develop a watery diarrhea. These infections are located in the small intestine, result from bacterial toxins interacting with digestive juices, do not produce inflammation, and do not usually need treatment with **antibiotics**.

BLOODY DIARRHEA (DYSENTERY) Bloody diarrhea is sometimes called dysentery. It is produced by EHEC, EIEC, some types of *Salmonella*, some types of *Shigella*, and *Yersinia*. In dysentery, the infection is located in the colon, cells and tissues are destroyed, inflammation is present, and antibiotic therapy is usually required.

NECROTIZING ENTEROCOLITIS (NEC) **Necrotizing enterocolitis** (NEC) is a disorder that begins in newborn infants shortly after **birth**. Although NEC is not yet fully understood, it is thought that it results from a bacterial or viral invasion of damaged intestinal tissues. The disease organisms then cause the death (necrosis) of bowel tissue or gangrene of the bowel. NEC is primarily a disease of **prematurity**; 60–80% of cases occur in high-risk preterm infants. NEC is responsible for 2–5% of cases in newborn intensive care units (NICU). Enterobacteriaceae that have been identified in infants with NEC include *Salmonella*, *E. coli*, *Klebsiella*, and *Enterobacter*.

Diagnosis

Patient history

The diagnosis of enterobacterial infections is complicated by the fact that viruses, protozoa, and other types of bacteria can also cause diarrhea. In most cases of mild diarrhea, it is not critical to identify the organism because the disorder is self-limiting. Some groups of patients, however, should have stool tests. They include:

- patients with bloody diarrhea
- patients with watery diarrhea who have become dehydrated
- patients with watery diarrhea that has lasted longer than three days without decreasing in amount
- patients with disorders of the immune system

The patient history is useful for public health reasons as well as helping the doctor determine what type of enterobacterium may be causing the infection. The doctor will ask about the frequency and appearance of the diarrhea as well as other digestive symptoms. If the patient is nauseated and **vomiting**, the infection is more likely to be located in the small intestine. If the patient is running a **fever**, a diagnosis of dysentery is more likely. The doctor will also ask if anyone else in the patient's family or workplace is sick. Some types of enterobacteriaceae are more likely to cause group outbreaks than others. Other questions include the patient's food intake over the last few days and whether he or she has recently traveled to countries with **typhoid fever** or cholera outbreaks.

Physical examination

The most important parts of the physical examination are checking for signs of severe fluid loss and examining the abdomen to rule out typhoid fever. The doctor will look at the inside of the patient's mouth and evaluate the skin for signs of **dehydration**. The presence of a skin rash and an enlarged spleen suggests typhoid rather than a bacterial infection. If the patient's abdomen hurts when the doctor examines it, a diagnosis of dysentery is more likely.

Laboratory tests

The most common test that is used to identify the cause of diarrhea is the stool test. Examining a stool sample under a microscope can help to rule out parasitic and protozoal infections. Routine stool cultures, however, cannot be used to identify any of the four types of *E. coli* that cause intestinal infections. ETEC, EPEC, and EIEC are unusual in the United States and can usually be identified only by specialists in research laboratories. Because of concern about EHEC outbreaks, however, most laboratories in the United States can now screen for O157:H7 with a test that identifies its characteristic toxin. All patients with bloody diarrhea should have a stool sample tested for *E. coli* O157:H7.

Treatment

The initial treatment of enterobacterial diarrhea is usually empiric. Empiric means that the doctor treats the patient on the basis of the visible symptoms and professional experience in treating infections without waiting for laboratory test results. Since the results of stool cultures can take as long as two days, it is important to prevent dehydration. The patient will be given fluids to restore the electrolyte balance and paregoric to relieve abdominal cramping.

Newborn infants and patients with **immune system** disorders will be given antibiotics intravenously once the organism has been identified. Gentamicin, tobramycin, and amikacin are being used more frequently to treat enterobacterial infections because many of the organisms are becoming resistant to ampicillin and cephalosporin antibiotics.

Alternative treatment

Alternative treatments for diarrhea are intended to relieve the discomfort of abdominal cramping. Most alternative practitioners advise consulting a medical doctor if the patient has sunken eyes, dry eyes or mouth, or other signs of dehydration.

Herbal medicine

Herbalists may recommend cloves taken as an infusion or ginger given in drop doses to control intestinal cramps, eliminate gas, and prevent vomiting. Peppermint (*Mentha piperita*) or chamomile (*Matricaria recutita*) tea may also ease cramps and intestinal spasms.

Homeopathy

Homeopathic practitioners frequently recommend *Arsenicum album* for diarrhea caused by contaminated food, and *Belladonna* for diarrhea that comes on suddenly with mucus in the stools. *Veratrum album* would be given for watery diarrhea, and *Podophyllum* for diarrhea with few other symptoms.

Prognosis

The prognosis for most enterobacterial infections is good; most patients recover in about a week or 10 days without needing antibiotics. HUS, on the other hand, has a mortality rate of 3–5% even with intensive care. About

KEY TERMS

Dysentery—A type of diarrhea caused by infection and characterized by mucus and blood in the stools.

Empirical treatment—Medical treatment that is given on the basis of the doctor's observations and experience.

Escherichia coli—A type of enterobacterium that is responsible for most cases of severe bacterial diarrhea in the United States.

Hemolytic-uremic syndrome (HUS)—A potentially fatal complication of *E. coli* infections characterized by kidney failure and destruction of red blood cells.

Necrotizing enterocolitis (NEC)—A disorder in newborns caused by bacterial or viral invasion of vulnerable intestinal tissues.

Nosocomial infections—Infections acquired in hospitals.

Toxin—A poison produced by certain types of bacteria.

a third of the survivors have long-term problems with **kidney function**, and another 8% develop high blood pressure, seizure disorders, and blindness.

Prevention

The World Health Organization (WHO) offers the following suggestions for preventing enterobacterial infections, including *E. coli* O157:H7 dysentery:

- Cook ground beef or hamburgers until the meat is thoroughly done. Juices from the meat should be completely clear, not pink or red. All parts of the meat should reach a temperature of 70°C (158°F) or higher.
- Do not drink unpasteurized milk or use products made from raw milk.
- Wash hands thoroughly and frequently, especially after using the toilet.
- Wash fruits and vegetables carefully, or peel them. Keep all kitchen surfaces and serving utensils clean.
- If drinking water is not known to be safe, boil it or drink bottled water.
- Keep cooked foods separate from raw foods, and avoid touching cooked foods with knives or other utensils that have been used with raw meat.

ORGANIZATIONS

Centers for Disease Control and Prevention (CDC), 1600 Clifton Road, Atlanta, GA, 30333, (404) 498-1515, (800) 311-3435, http://www.cdc.gov.

Rebecca J. Frey, PhD

Enuresis

Also known as **bedwetting**, the inability to control urination during periods of **sleep**.

Enuresis is a common problem that is estimated to affect between 5 and 7 million children in the United States each year. At some point around the age of three, children typically begin to exhibit bladder control during the day and make the transition from diapers to toileting. For most children, nighttime bladder control follows. The term enuresis, which comes from the Greek phrase, "to make water," is often thought of as the technical term for bedwetting, but rather refers to the continued involuntary passage of urine after an age at which control is expected.

When daytime wetting persists beyond the age of four, or nighttime wetting persists beyond the age of six, the child is considered to have *primary enuresis*. When the ability to stay dry has developed normally and without intervention but is followed by a period of wetting that lasts for three months or more, the child is considered to have *secondary enuresis*. The distinction between these two types is based on the child's physiological ability to control his or her urinary output. In cases of primary enuresis, this ability is usually compromised. In cases of secondary enuresis, the child often has no physical problems impairing bladder control but may be reacting to some emotional or psychological issues. Most cases of enuresis–about 90 percent–are of the primary type.

Enuresis may interfere significantly with the social and emotional aspects of normal development. This interference is one reason why the American Psychiatric Association's *Diagnostic and Statistical Manual of Mental Disorders*, fourth edition (DSM-IV) defines enuresis as an "Elimination Disorder" in its chapter on "Disorders Usually First Diagnosed in **Infancy**, Childhood, or Adolescence." Consider the plight of the 10-year-old who still wets the bed regularly. He or she may avoid such activities as camping out or attending pajama parties because of the potential humiliation of wetting in the presence of friends and acquaintances. Bedwetting may also present a stressor to **family** functioning by adding daily loads of sheets, blankets, and pajamas to be washed. Limited laundry facilities or crowded living conditions can make this extra task even more difficult.

Children may also develop a sense of failure and helplessness with regard to the inability to control nighttime wetting. Some studies have shown that bedwetters show lower scores on indices of **self-esteem**, and tend to be underachievers compared to non-bedwetting peers. More importantly, these same studies showed that successful treatment of enuresis is associated with increased self-confidence and outgoing behavior at school.

Who becomes enuretic? Approximately 30 percent of four-year-old and 10 percent of six-year-old children wet their beds. By age 10, about 5 percent of children have primary enuresis, and 1 percent continue to show the disorder until age 18, with a few cases persisting into adulthood. Boys are three times more likely at all ages to be enuretic than girls.

Genetic factors play a role in who becomes enuretic. In 1995 a gene associated with enuresis was discovered on chromosome 22; other genes have since been identified on chromosomes 8, 12, and 16. Most children with primary enuresis have a relative-either a parent or an aunt or uncle-who wet the bed as a child. Many parents report that their bedwetting child is an extremely sound sleeper compared to their other children, an observation not supported by recent studies that suggest that parents' impressions may be due to the fact that they are not *trying* to wake their other children during the night. In fact, bedwetting may occur in any stage of sleep.

What causes enuresis? On occasion, enuresis turns out to be the result of a serious medical condition that causes increased urinary output, such as diabetes or sickle-cell **anemia**. A small number of enuretic children have a history of snoring and may have episodes of sleep apnea (interrupted breathing) that contribute to their bedwetting. Most cases of primary enuresis, however, are caused by smaller than normal functional bladder capacity and bladder irritability.

Functional bladder capacity refers to the number of fluid ounces that can be held in the bladder before one feels an urge to urinate as the result of wavelike contractions of the bladder. These contractions push fluid down past the inner sphincter, a ring-like muscle that keeps the bladder closed when it is tensed. Contractions are normally triggered when the bladder is full. In children with small functional bladder capacity, however, contractions are triggered by a smaller amount of fluid. Children who also have irritable bladders experience more and stronger contractions than normal at this lower volume. Both bladder contractions and the action of the inner sphincter are involuntary and are not under conscious control.

Only the action of the outer sphincter of the bladder is under voluntary control. We normally use this muscle to hold back urination in between the first urge of bladder contractions and the time that we are able to get to a bathroom. In deep sleep states, however, voluntary muscles relax. If a child reaches his or her functional capacity and experiences bladder contractions while the outer sphincter is relaxed in deep sleep, bedwetting may occur. This is not a problem for a child with normal bladder capacity. However, the enuretic child with a small functional bladder capacity and an irritable bladder is unable to hold the fluid that accumulates during a 10- or 12-hour period of nighttime sleep. When this child's functional bladder capacity is reached and many intense contractions push fluid beyond the relaxed outer sphincter, bedwetting occurs.

Although the most common causes of primary bedwetting are physical, psychological factors may also be involved. It can become a complex cycle as the child and family react to the bedwetting in ways that might exacerbate the problem.

The causes of secondary enuresis can be more difficult to pinpoint. It is a common reaction in children who have experienced trauma and may persist even after the incidents of physical, sexual, or emotional abuse have ceased. It may also be associated with urinary tract infections (UTIs). Even normal developmental changes in the family or the child's situation may result in a period of secondary enuresis, such as the bedwetting associated with the **birth** of a younger sibling or a child's entry to kindergarten. Bedwetting will resolve in most cases when the underlying emotional issues have been adequately addressed.

Can primary enuresis be treated? Yes. Many myths have surrounded the challenge of treating enuresis, dating from A.D. 77, when Pliny the Elder recommended feeding supplements of boiled mice to enuretic children. Fortunately, modern research has clarified factors that contribute to the causes of enuresis, thereby outlining the components of sound treatment.

Unfortunately, old myths occasionally appear in contemporary professional advice and health plan policy. One such myth is that "Enuresis is a self-limiting condition, and treatment is not necessary." While about 15 percent of children do grow out of enuresis, without intervention a substantial number remain enuretic into **adolescence** and a smaller number into adulthood. "Don't drink anything after dinner" is another myth. While the enuretic child should not drink a quart of soda before bedtime, excessive curtailing of liquids can be counterproductive by prompting an urge to urinate at even lower volumes of bladder pressure. Another common myth is "He could stay dry if only he tried harder." While *motivation* must be a part of any thorough treatment program, it is difficult for effort alone to accomplish anything when one is fast asleep.

No treatment plan should begin without a thorough evaluation designed to identify factors contributing to the problem. The basic assessment should include a complete physical examination, urinalysis and a urine specific gravity, evaluation of the urinary stream, neurologic examination, the assessment of bladder habits (e.g., the amount and frequency of urine produced each day, whether leakage occurs with laughter or effort), bedtime habits (e.g., evening consumption of such products as caffeinated colas or chocolate that may act as a diuretic, whether the child is overtired at bedtime), and urodynamic studies as needed.

The treatment program that follows may include the use of wetness alarms to heighten the child's awareness of the signals that his or her bladder is full, exercises to increase sphincter control and bladder capacity, pharmacological interventions for short-term use, and psychological support. The use of wetness alarms combined with exercises to improve sphincter control and increase bladder capacity provides the best long-term treatment results; reported success rates have ranged from 65 percent to 85 percent.

Wetness alarms condition the child to awaken at the sensation of impending urination, especially when they are paired with sphincter control exercises. By awakening the child with a loud noise immediately upon urinating, the alarm eventually conditions the child to awaken prior to the sound and urinate in the bathroom. The alarm can also be used during daily exercises as a signal to interrupt the stream of urination, helping the child to learn an association between "hearing the buzzer" and "holding it." Newer alarms are smaller and lighter, and include models that awaken the child with a buzzer rather than disturbing the entire family with a loud alarm.

Increasing functional bladder capacity by consuming a large amount of fluid and then waiting as long as possible before urinating is another component to being able to sleep through the night and remain dry. How much fluid should a child be able to retain? A child's normal bladder capacity in ounces may be estimated by adding two to the child's age in years. Martin Scharf recommends measuring the child's output during bladder stretching exercises twice weekly to chart improvement in the bladder capacity. Long-term success in treating enuresis is always accompanied by significant increase in bladder capacity that is evidenced in decreased frequency of daytime urination regardless of the type of treatment program used.

Pharmacological agents have been used to treat enuresis, which provide good results in the short term while the child is taking the medication, but poor effectiveness once the drug is removed. Desmopressin acetate (DDAVP) is an antidiuretic hormone that is administered by nasal spray. One drawback to DDAVP is that it is effective when nasal passages are clear and absorption is maximal, making it useless during cold and flu season. Imipramine (Tofranil) is an antidepressant that also has anticholinergic effects and suppresses the body's response to the neurochemical acetylcholine, thereby reducing bladder irritability. Both DDAVP and imipramine have spontaneous success rates of about 70 to 75 percent and are often prescribed for children going on camping trips or in need of a short-term treatment. As with any drug, there can be side effects, warranting careful monitoring of dosage and administration.

Urinary tract infections, if present, should be treated promptly with **antibiotics**. Enuresis caused by UTIs almost always goes away once the infection has been treated.

Finally, treatment programs must attend to the psychological needs of the child and family. Providing information, setting realistic goals, structuring reinforcement, and addressing any of the child's negative feelings engendered by his or her experience with enuresis will enhance the effectiveness of any treatment method. Richard Ferber stresses the need for responsibility training and reinforcement in helping the child take responsibility for staying dry through reinforcement rather than punishment. With reinforcement and support, the child is able to take pride in his or her accomplishments as wetness begins to decrease in amount and frequency.

Successful treatment of enuresis is seldom an overnight event. Progress is often slow and hampered by relapses. Parents who are well informed and able to maintain positive attitudes in support of their child are better able to help the entire family cope with the problem of enuresis.

Resources

BOOKS

American Psychiatric Association. *Diagnostic and Statistical Manual of Mental Disorders*, fourth edition, text revision. Washington, DC: American Psychiatric Association, 2000.

Azrin, N. H., and V. A. Besalel. *A Parent's Guide to Bedwetting Control*. New York: Pocket Books, 1981.

Ferber, Richard. *Solve Your Child's Sleep Problems*. New York: Simon & Schuster, 1985.

Kolvin, I., R. C. MacKeith, and S. R. Meadow, eds. *Bladder Control and Enuresis*. London: Heinemann Medical Books, 1973.

Rushton, G. "Enuresis." In *Clinical Pediatric Urology*. P. O. Kelalis, L. R. King, and A. B. Belman. eds. Philadelphia: W.B. Saunders, 1992.

Schaefer, C. K. *Childhood Encopresis and Enuresis*. New York: Von Nostrand Reinhold, 1979.

Scharf, M. B. *Waking Up Dry*. Cincinnati: Writer's Digest Books, 1986.

PERIODICALS

Koff, S. A. "Estimating Bladder Capacity in Children." *Urology* 21 (1988): 248.

Robson, William M. L., MD. "Enuresis." *eMedicine*. topic 689, September 22, 2005. Available online at http://www.emedicine.com/ped/topic689.htm.

Thiedke, C. Carolyn, MD. "Nocturnal Enuresis." *American Family Physician* 67 (April 1, 2003): 1499-1510.

ORGANIZATIONS

American Academy of Pediatrics (AAP), 141 Northwest Point Boulevard, Elk Grove Village, IL, 60007, (847) 434-4000, http://www.aap.org.

Doreen Arcus, Ph.D.
University of Massachusetts Lowell

Eosinophilic gastroenteropathies

Definition

Eosinophilic gastroenteropathies are a group of gastrointestinal (GI) diseases (enteropathies) in which one or more layers of the GI tract (most commonly the stomach and small intestine) are selectively infiltrated with a type of white blood cell called eosinophils, as part of an allergic response.

Demographics

Eosinophilic **gastroenteritis** is very rare in North America, and the incidence is difficult to estimate. However, since R. Kaijser's first description in 1937, more than 300 cases have been reported in the medical literature as of 2010. Although cases have also been reported worldwide, the exact incidence is unclear because of a lack of diagnostic precision. Cases of EG are reported mostly in Caucasians, with some cases occurring among Asians. A slight male preponderance has also been documented. People in their late 20s to late 40s are more likely to be diagnosed with EG than those in other age groups; however, cases of EG have been reported in infants and in adults in their 60s.

Eosinophilic esophagitis was long thought to be a variant of stomach reflux disease. It is now known to be a distinct disorder predominately occurring in children; it is thought to occur in approximately 1 in every 10,000 children. The exact incidence and prevalence of EC and ED are not known, but these diseases are occurring or being diagnosed with increasing frequency and are especially prominent in children.

Description

Eosinophilic gastroenteropathies are characterized by the accumulation of an abnormally large number of eosinophils (eosinophilic infiltration, defined as the presence of 20 or more eosinophils per high-power field) in one or more specific places anywhere in the digestive system and associated lymph nodes, resulting in nausea, difficulty swallowing, abdominal **pain**, **vomiting** and **diarrhea**, excessive loss of proteins in the GI tract, and **failure to thrive**. All gastroenteropathies are characterized by the presence of abnormal GI symptoms, eosinophilic infiltration in one or more areas of the GI tract, and the absence of an identified cause for the formation of an abnormally large number of eosinophils in the blood (eosinophilia). Some patients also suffer loss of protein from the body that often results in low blood levels of albumin and total protein (protein-losing enteropathy) due to increased GI tract permeability. As the GI tract wall becomes infiltrated with large numbers of eosinophils, its normal architecture is disrupted, and so is its function. Eosinophils themselves are **immune system** white blood cells that destroy parasitic organisms and play a major role in allergic reactions. For this reason, the gastroenteropathies are often considered food-related gastrointestinal allergy syndromes.

Eosinophilic gastroenteropathies have a specific name corresponding to the area of the digestive system where the highest numbers of eosinophils are found. They include the following disorders:

- osinophilic gastroenteritis (EG), in which eosinophilic infiltration occurs in one or more layers of the stomach and/or small intestine
- osinophilic esophagitis (EE), in which eosinophilic infiltration is confined to the muscular tube that carries food from the throat to the stomach (esophagus)
- osinophilic colitis (EC), in which the infiltration is confined to the large intestine (colon)
- osinophilic duodenitis (ED), in which the infiltration is confined to the small intestine

Eosinophilic gastroenteritis

Eosinophilic gastroenteritis (EG) is the best characterized gastroenteropathy. It is classified according to the layer of the GI tract involved, and mixed forms also occur. The walls of the GI tract have four layers of tissue, called mucosa, submucosa, muscularis externa, and serosa. The innermost layer is the mucosa, a membrane that forms a continuous lining of the GI tract from the mouth to the anus. In the large bowel, this tissue contains cells that produce mucus to lubricate and protect the smooth inner surface of the bowel wall. Connective tissue and muscle separate the mucosa from the second layer, the submucosa, which contains blood vessels, lymph vessels, nerves, and glands. Next to the submucosa is the muscularis externa, consisting of two layers of muscle fibers, one that runs lengthwise and one that encircles the bowel. The fourth layer, the serosa, is a thin membrane that produces fluid to lubricate the outer surface of the bowel so that it can slide against adjacent organs. The different types of EG are:

- Pattern I eosinophilic gastroenteritis. Children affected with Pattern I EG have extensive infiltration of eosinophils in the area below the submucosa and muscularis layers. It is more commonly seen in the stomach (gastric antrum) but may also affect the small intestine or colon. Patients typically have intestinal obstruction. Cramping and abdominal pain associated with nausea and vomiting occur frequently. Food allergy and past history of allergy are less common in these patients than in patients with Pattern II EG.

- Pattern II eosinophilic gastroenteritis. Pattern II is the most prevalent form of EG. It is characterized by extensive infiltration of eosinophils in the mucosal and submucosal layers. These patients have colicky abdominal pain, nausea, vomiting, diarrhea, and weight loss. Infants with Pattern II EG also commonly have a history of allergy. The condition may also be associated with protein-losing enteropathy, low levels of iron in the blood serum or in the bone marrow (iron-deficiency anemia), or impaired absorption of nutrients by the intestines (malabsorption). Growth retardation, delayed puberty, or abnormal menstruation has also been reported in children and adolescents with Pattern II EG.
- Pattern III eosinophilic gastroenteritis. This is the least common form of eosinophilic gastroenteropathy. It involves the serosal layer, and the entire GI wall is usually affected. Its inflammation leads to an accumulation of fluid in the abdomen (ascites). This fluid contains many eosinophils and can infiltrate the membrane of the lungs (pleural effusion). A history of allergy also appears to be common in this group. Symptoms may include chest pain, fever, shortness of breath, and limited motion of the chest wall.

Eosinophilic esophagitis

Eosinophilic esophagitis (EE) is characterized by the abnormal accumulation of eosinophils localized in the esophagus. In EE, high levels of eosinophils are detected in the esophagus but not in any other parts of the digestive tract. The presence of the eosinophils in the esophagus causes inflammation of its walls, which makes digestion extremely painful. Unlike that of normal children, the esophagus of an individual with EE does not have a smooth and uniform pink surface but displays lines (furrowing) and white patches. Children with EE have classic signs of gastroesophageal reflux (abdominal pain, difficulty swallowing, and vomiting) but fail to respond to antireflux medications. The danger of failing to diagnose this disorder is that children may be referred for unnecessary surgery because of their reflux symptoms.

Eosinophilic colitis

Eosinophilic colitis (EC) is characterized by eosinophilic infiltration localized only in the large bowel, resulting in **fever**, diarrhea, bloody stools, **constipation**, obstruction/strictures, acute abdominal pain, and tenderness often localized in the right lower abdomen. EC often follows the onset of EG.

Eosinophilic duodenitis

Eosinophilic duodenitis (ED) is characterized by eosinophilic inflammation of the small bowel that results in the production of leukotrienes—substances that participate in defense reactions and contribute to hypersensitivity and inflammation. Malabsorption of nutrients always results, along with severe cramping, bowel obstruction, and intestinal bleeding with passage of bloody stools.

Related enteropathies

Other diseases feature enteropathies with symptoms similar to those associated with eosinophilic gastroenteropathies:

- Whipple's disease. This rare digestive disease of unknown origin affects the lining of the small intestine and results in malabsorption of nutrients. It may also affect other organs of the body.
- Celiac disease(celiac sprue). This chronic hereditary malabsorption disorder is caused by an intolerance to gluten, the insoluble component of wheat and other grains. Clinical improvement of symptoms follows withdrawal of gluten-containing grains in the diet.
- Mastocytosis. This genetic disorder is characterized by abnormal accumulations of a type of cell (mast cells) normally found in connective tissue. The liver, spleen, lungs, bone, skin, and sometimes the membrane surrounding the brain and spine (meninges) may be affected.
- Tropical sprue. This disorder of unknown cause is characterized by malabsorption, multiple nutritional deficiencies, and abnormalities in the small bowel mucosa. It appears to be acquired and related to environmental and nutritional conditions. Tropical sprue is most prevalent in the Caribbean, South India, and Southeast Asia.
- Crohn's disease. Also known as ileitis, regional enteritis, or granulomatous colitis, this disease is a form of inflammatory bowel disease characterized by severe chronic inflammation of the wall of the GI tract.
- Dietary protein enteropathy. This disease is characterized by persistent diarrhea and vomiting with resulting malabsorption and failure to thrive with onset most commonly in infancy. Protein-losing enteropathy may lead to abnormally large amounts of fluid in the intercellular tissue spaces of the body (edema), abdominal distension, and lack of red blood cells (anemia).

- Dietary protein-induced proctocolitis. In generally healthy infants this disease of unknown origin causes visible specks or streaks of blood mixed with mucus in the stool. Blood loss is usually minimal, and anemia is rare. The disorder appears in the first months of life, with a mean age at diagnosis of two months.

Risk factors

Risk factors for these disorders include a history of **allergies**, **eczema**, or seasonal **asthma**, and a close relative diagnosed with an eosinophilic gastroenteropathy. About 50% of patients diagnosed with an eosinophilic gastroenteropathy have a history of hay fever, asthma, or **food allergies**.

Causes and symptoms

Causes

The eosinophil is a component of the immune system and is particularly involved with defense against parasites, but as of 2010 no parasite had been found responsible for any of the eosinophilic gastroenteropathies. The cause or mechanism of eosinophilic infiltration is also unknown, although some scientists suspect that the condition, first identified in Europe in the mid-1940s, is genetic, as it seems that in about 16 percent of known cases, an immediate family member is also diagnosed with an eosinophilic GI disorder. In the spring of 2010, a group of researchers in Ohio identified an association between eosinophilic esophagitis and a locus on the long arm of chromosome 5 at 5q22. The most likely candidate gene in this locus is *TSLP*, which is a gene that encodes a cytokine known as thymic stromal lymphopoetin.

Various factors have been shown to trigger eosinophilic infiltration of the GI tract, and it has been shown that this development in turn causes tissue damage by loss of cell granules (degranulation) and the untimely release of small proteins specialized for cell-to-cell communication (cytokines), which directly damages the GI tract wall. Examples of factors that are believed to have an incriminating role in triggering a flare-up include foods that trigger an allergic reaction (allergens) and **immunodeficiency** disorders caused by very low levels of immunoglobulins that result in an increased susceptibility to infection.

Honey intolerance and bee pollen administration have also been suggested as a causative agent for EG. Researchers have confirmed a familial pattern to EE, which suggests either a genetic predisposition or exposure relationship to an unknown environmental trigger.

Symptoms

Gastroenteropathy symptoms vary depending on where the eosinophils are found and in what layer of the digestive system their numbers are highest. Symptoms therefore tend to be highly specific to each individual case. They may only appear when certain foods are ingested, or only during certain seasons of the year, or every few weeks, or in severe cases, every time any food is eaten. Infants with eosinophilic gastroenteropathies usually have acute reactions after food intake (within minutes to in one to two hours) that generally include nausea, vomiting, and severe abdominal pain, later followed by diarrhea. These symptoms may occur alone or as part of a shock reaction. Symptoms vary depending on the type of gastroenteropathy (EG, EE, EC, or ED) and on the precise location of eosinophilic infiltration within the digestive system, as well as which layer or layers of the digestive system wall is infiltrated by eosinophils. Symptoms include but are not limited to the following:

- abdominal pain (EG, EE, ED)
- anorexia (EG, EE)
- asthma (EE)
- bloating (EG, ED, EC)
- cramps (EG, EC, ED)
- milk/formula regurgitation (EG, EE)
- nausea, vomiting (EG, EE, EC, ED)
- weight loss (EG, EE, EC, ED)
- diarrhea (EG, EC, ED)
- presence of fluid (edema) in ankles (EG, EE)
- choking (EE)
- difficulty swallowing (dysphagia) (EG, EE)
- strictures (EE, EC)
- passage of dark stools (melena) (EG, EC, ED)
- constipation (EC, ED)
- bowel obstruction (EC, ED)
- intestinal bleeding (EC, ED)

Diagnosis

Eosinophilic gastroenteropathies are diseases that can be easily misdiagnosed. EE has long been misdiagnosed as gastroesophageal reflux disorder (GERD), another digestive disease in which partially digested food from the stomach regurgitates and backs up (reflux). EE differs from esophageal reflux, however, in the large numbers of eosinophils that are present in the GI tract. Diagnosis for eosinophilic gastroenteropathies is therefore established only by microscopic analysis of a tissue specimen (biopsy) revealing eosinophilic infiltration.

KEY TERMS

Allergic reaction—An immune system reaction to a substance in the environment. Symptoms include rash, inflammation, sneezing, itchy watery eyes, and runny nose.

Anemia—A condition in which there is an abnormally low number of red blood cells in the bloodstream. It may be due to loss of blood, an increase in red blood cell destruction, or a decrease in red blood cell production. Major symptoms are paleness, shortness of breath, unusually fast or strong heart beats, and fatigue.

Antibody—A special protein made by the immune system as a defense against foreign material (bacteria, viruses, etc.) that enters the body. It is uniquely designed to attack and neutralize the specific antigen that triggered the immune response.

Antigen—A substance (usually a protein) identified as foreign by the immune system, triggering the release of antibodies as part of the body's immune response.

Ascites—Abnormal accumulation of fluid within the abdominal cavity.

Biopsy—The surgical removal and microscopic examination of living tissue for diagnostic purposes or to follow the course of a disease. Most commonly the term refers to the collection and analysis of tissue from a suspected tumor to establish malignancy.

Complete blood count (CBC)—A routine analysis performed on a sample of blood taken from a vein with a needle and vacuum tube. The measurements taken in a CBC include a white blood cell count, a red blood cell count, the red cell distribution width, the hematocrit (ratio of the volume of the red blood cells to the blood volume), and the amount of hemoglobin (the blood protein that carries oxygen).

Corticosteroids—A group of hormones produced naturally by the adrenal gland or manufactured synthetically. They are often used to treat inflammation. Examples include cortisone and prednisone.

Cytokines—Chemicals made by the cells that act on other cells to stimulate or inhibit their function. They are important controllers of immune functions.

Dysphagia—Difficulty in swallowing.

Elemental diet—A diet (or formula) in which no form of protein is allowed, either in whole or in incomplete (hydrolyzed or predigested) forms.

Enteropathy—Any disease of the intestinal tract.

Eosinophil—A type of white blood cell containing granules that can be stained by eosin, a chemical that leaves a red stain. Eosinophils increase in response to parasitic infections and allergic reactions.

Eosinophilia—An abnormal increase in the number of eosinophils in the blood.

Gastroesophageal reflux disease (GERD)—A disorder of the lower end of the esophagus in which the lower esophageal sphincter does not open and close normally. As a result the acid contents of the stomach can flow backward into the esophagus and irritate the tissues.

Glucocorticoids—A general class of adrenal cortical hormones that are mainly active in protecting against stress and in protein and carbohydrate metabolism. They are widely used in medicine as anti-inflammatory and immunosuppresive agents.

Immunodeficiency disease—A disease characterized chiefly by an increased susceptibility to infection. It is caused by very low levels of immunoglobulins that result in an impaired immune system. Affected people develop repeated infections.

Immunoglobulin G (IgG)—Immunoglobulin type gamma, the most common type found in the blood and tissue fluids.

Leukotrienes—Substances produced by white blood cells in response to antigens and contribute to inflammatory and asthmatic reactions.

Malabsorption—The inability of the digestive tract to absorb all the nutrients from food due to some malfunction or disability.

Melena—The passage of dark stools stained with blood pigments or with altered blood.

Protein-losing enteropathy—Excessive loss of plasma and proteins in the gastrointestinal tract.

Shock—A medical emergency in which the organs and tissues of the body are not receiving an adequate flow of blood. This inadequacy deprives the organs and tissues of oxygen and allows the build-up of waste products. Shock can be caused by certain diseases, serious injury, or blood loss.

Stricture—Abnormal narrowing or tightening of a body tube or passage.

Because of the high risk of misdiagnosis of eosinophilic gastroenteropathies, parents of infants who have persistent feeding problems and do not respond well to classical digestive disorder medications should request biopsies to test for possible eosinophilic involvement.

Tests

Additionally, diagnosis is based on the following laboratory and imaging tests, and possible surgical procedures:

- Complete blood count (CBC). CBC reveals the presence of blood eosinophilia, found in 20–80% percent of cases. CBC also appears to differentiate between different types of eosinophilic gastroenteropathies, since they have different total eosinophil counts.
- Mean corpuscular volume test. This test can determine the presence of iron-deficiency anemia and serum albumin levels that vary according to disorder type.
- Fecal protein loss test. This test is used to identify the inability to digest and absorb proteins in the GI tract.
- Stool test. At least three separate stool specimens should be obtained to rule out intestinal parasites.
- Imaging tests. Ultrasound and CT scan may show thickened intestinal walls and ascitic fluid in patients with Pattern III EG, as well as the degree of involvement of the different layers.
- Barium studies. In this test, the patient ingests a barium sulfate solution that makes a contrast on x rays. Barium studies can reveal mucosal edema and thickening of the small intestinal wall in EC and ED.
- Exploratory abdominal surgery (laparotomy). In some cases, laparotomy may be indicated, especially in patients with Pattern III EG.

Treatment

There was no cure for these disorders as of 2010. Treatment is supportive and aimed at relieving symptoms. Certain lifestyle changes are usually required, such as avoidance of certain foods or making sure that medication is taken every day. Parents of children with these disorders should also be aware that commonly prescribed corticosteroid medications have side effects that are potentially serious. People who use them tend to become overweight with swollen faces. Long-term use of these drugs has also been shown to damage kidneys.

Traditional

Drugs

Medications are used to relieve symptoms and prevent full-blown attacks (or flares). The only known medication to successfully stop eosinophilic inflammation is the corticosteroid drug prednisone. Oral glucocorticosteroids are usually prescribed for those with EC or ED obstructive symptoms. Children with Pattern II EG may benefit from anti-inflammatory medications (for example, oral glucocorticoids or oral cromolyn) and specialized diet therapy, particularly in the case of food intolerance or allergy. Fluticasone propionate (Flonase, Flovent) is reported to be helpful in most cases of EG, if the medicine is swallowed so that it comes directly in contact with the esophageal tissues that are infiltrated by eosinophils. Another anti-inflammatory medication that works well for patients with EG is budesonide (Pulmicort Respule, Entocort), which is available as an inhalant, a thick oral suspension, or an oral timed-release capsule. There is also reported success with the use of an oral drug (montelukast; trade name Singulair) that stops the production of the inflammatory leukotrienes associated with EC. Elemental formulas are also very effective. Cromolyn sodium (Gastrocrom) has been used with some success but does not work in all cases.

Surgery

Surgery may be necessary in severe EC cases in which there is an obstruction of the intestines.

Alternative

Some traditional Chinese medicines have been tried on patients with EG, but without success.

Diet

It is believed that whole food proteins are the most common triggers of an EG attack. Most infants with this condition are therefore put on a restricted diet and provided with elemental formulas containing no whole food proteins, such as Neocate or Elecare.

For older children, physicians usually start by recommending a trial elimination diet that excludes milk, eggs, wheat, gluten, soy, and beef, because a link has been established with food intolerance and food allergy. Most patients improve significantly on diets avoiding foods to which they are allergic. Radioallergosorbent assay test (RAST) or skin testing can identify food hypersensitivity. If an exceptionally high number of food reactions are found, an amino-acid-based diet or elemental diet is often considered. Some patients with EE/EG/EC are even fed elemental formulas via a gastrostomy tube or are limited to TPN (total parenteral nutrition or blood-vessel feeding) if the disease is severe with many complications.

Prognosis

Because there is no cure for eosinophilic gastroenteropathies, outcomes depend on the specific enteropathy. A small subset of patients are partly or totally disabled by the effects of their disorder, but most can have active and fulfilling lives. Eosinophilic gastroenteropathies are rarely reported to cause **death**, but some types cause such severe bleeding or nutritional deficiency that the condition may be life-threatening if not treated with appropriate medications and support measures. These disorders do not, however, increase the patient's risk of **cancer** in later life.

Children with EG have a good prognosis. Some younger children who have been diagnosed at an early age have been known to outgrow the most severe symptoms. Mild and sporadic symptoms can be managed with observation, and disabling GI flare-ups can be controlled with prednisone. Most patients (about 90%) also respond well to oral glucocorticosteroids.

Prevention

There was no known way to prevent eosinophilic gastroenteropathies as of 2010 because the causes of these disorders are not yet understood.

Resources

BOOKS

Banerjee, Bhaskar, ed. *Nutritional Management of Digestive Disorders*. Boca Raton, FL: Taylor and Francis Group, 2010.

Chesterton, Carrie M., ed. *Food Allergies: New Research*. New York: Nova Science Publishers, 2008.

PERIODICALS

Bischoff, S.C. "Food Allergy and Eosinophilic Gastroenteritis and Colitis." *Current Opinion in Allergy and Clinical Immunology* 10 (June 2010): 238–45.

Erwin, E.A., et al. "Serum IgE Measurement and Detection of Food Allergy in Pediatric Patients with Eosinophilic Esophagitis." *Annals of Allergy, Asthma and Immunology* 104 (June 2010): 496–502.

Feuling, M.B., and R.J. Noel. "Medical and Nutrition Management of Eosinophilic Esophagitis in Children." *Nutrition in Clinical Practice* 25 (April 2010): 166–74.

Genevay, M., et al. "Do Eosinophil Numbers Differentiate Eosinophilic Esophagitis from Gastroesophageal Reflux Disease?" *Archives of Pathology and Laboratory Medicine* 134 (June 2010): 815–25.

Holroyd, D.J., et al. "Transmural Eosinophilic Gastritis with Gastric Outlet Obstruction: Case Report and Review of the Literature." *Annals of the Royal College of Surgeons of England* 92 (May 2010): W18–W20.

Oh, H.E., and R. Chetty. "Eosinophilic Gastroenteritis: A Review." *Journal of Gastroenterology* 43 (October 2008): 741–50.

Rothenberg, M.E., et al. "Common Variants at 5q22 Associate with Pediatric Eosinophilic Esophagitis." *Nature Genetics* 42 (April 2010): 289–91.

White, S.B., et al. "The Small-caliber Esophagus: Radiographic Sign of Idiopathic Eosinophilic Esophagitis." *Radiology* 256 (July 2010): 127–34.

OTHER

American Partnership for Eosinophilic Disorders (APFED). "About EGID." http://www.apfed.org/index.htm.

Canadian Council on Eosinophilic Disorders (CCOED). "About EGIDs (Eosinophilic Gastrointestinal Disorders), http://www.ccoed.ca/index_files/Page410.html.

Nguyen, MyNgoc T., and Jean-Luc Szpakowski. "Eosinophilic Gastroenteritis." eMedicine, June 15, 2009, http://emedicine.medscape.com/article/174100-overview.

ORGANIZATIONS

American College of Gastroenterology (ACG), P.O. Box 342260, Bethesda, MD, 20827-2260, 301-263-9000, http://www.acg.gi.org/.

American Partnership for Eosinophilic Disorders (APFED), P.O. Box 29545, Atlanta, GA, 30359, 713-493-7749, mail@apfed.org, http://www.apfed.org/index.htm.

National Institute of Allergy and Infectious Diseases (NIAID), 6610 Rockledge Drive, MSC 6612, Bethesda, MD, 20892-6612, 301-496-5717, 866-284-4107, 301-402-3573, http://www3.niaid.nih.gov.

National Institute of Diabetes and Digestive and Kidney Diseases (NIDDK), Building 31. Rm 9A06, 31 Center Drive, MSC 2560, Bethesda, MD, 20892-2560, 301-496-3583, http://www2.niddk.nih.gov/Footer/ContactNIDDK.htm, http://www2.niddk.nih.gov/.

Canadian Council of Eosinophilic Disorders (CCOED), Box 1777, Crossfield, Alberta, Canada, T0M 0S0, 403-921-2170, info@ccoed.ca, http://www.ccoed.ca/.

Monique Laberge, PhD
Rebecca J. Frey, PhD

Epigastric hernia **see Abdominal wall defects**

Epiglottitis

Definition

Epiglottitis is an infection of the epiglottis, which can lead to severe airway obstruction.

Description

When air is inhaled (aspired), it passes through the nose and the nasopharynx or through the mouth and the oropharynx. These are both connected to the larynx, a tube made of cartilage. The air continues down the larynx to the trachea. The trachea then splits into two branches, the left and right bronchi (bronchial tubes). These bronchi branch into smaller air tubes that run within the lungs, leading to the small air sacs of the lungs (alveoli).

Either food, liquid, or air may be taken in through the mouth. While air goes into the larynx and the respiratory system, food and liquid are directed into the tube leading to the stomach, the esophagus. Because food or liquid in the bronchial tubes or lungs could cause a blockage or lead to an infection, the airway is protected. The epiglottis is a leaf-like piece of cartilage extending upwards from the larynx. The epiglottis can close down over the larynx when someone is eating or drinking, preventing these food and liquids from entering the airway.

Epiglottitis is an infection and inflammation of the epiglottis. Because the epiglottis may swell considerably, there is a danger that the airway will be blocked off by the very structure designed to protect it. Air is then unable to reach the lungs. Without intervention, epiglottitis has the potential to be fatal.

Epiglottitis is primarily a disease of two to seven-year-old children, although older children and adults can also contract it. Boys are twice as likely as girls to develop this infection. Because epiglottitis involves swelling and infection of tissues, which are all located at or above the level of the epiglottis, it is sometimes referred to as supraglottitis (*supra,* meaning "above"). About 25% of all children with this infection also have **pneumonia**.

Causes and symptoms

The most common cause of epiglottitis is infection with the bacteria called *Haemophilus influenzae type b.* Other types of bacteria are also occasionally responsible for this infection, including some types of *Streptococcus* bacteria and the bacteria responsible for causing **diphtheria**.

A patient with epiglottitis typically experiences a sudden **fever** and begins having severe throat and neck **pain**. Because the swollen epiglottis interferes significantly with air movement, every breath creates a loud, harsh, high-pitched sound referred to as **stridor**. Because the vocal cords are located in the larynx just below the area of the epiglottis, the swollen epiglottis makes the patient's voice sound muffled and strained. Swallowing becomes difficult, and the patient may drool. The patient often leans forward and juts out his or her jaw, while struggling for breath.

Epiglottitis strikes suddenly and progresses quickly. A child may begin complaining of a **sore throat**, and within a few hours be suffering from extremely severe airway obstruction.

Diagnosis

Diagnosis begins with a high level of suspicion that a quickly progressing illness with fever, sore throat, and airway obstruction is very likely to be epiglottitis. If epiglottitis is suspected, no efforts should be made to look at the throat, or to swab the throat in order to obtain a culture for identification of the causative organism. These maneuvers may cause the larynx to go into spasm (laryngospasm), completely closing the airway. These procedures should only be performed in a fully-equipped operating room, so that if laryngospasm occurs, a breathing tube can be immediately placed in order to keep the airway open.

An instrument called a laryngoscope is often used in the operating room to view the epiglottis, which will appear cherry-red and quite swollen. An x-ray picture taken from the side of the neck should also be obtained. The swollen epiglottis has a characteristic appearance, called the "thumb sign."

Treatment

Treatment almost always involves the immediate establishment of an artificial airway: inserting a breathing tube into the throat (intubation); or making a tiny opening toward the base of the neck and putting a breathing tube into the trachea (tracheostomy). Because the patient's apparent level of distress may not match the actual severity of the situation, and because the disease's progression can be quite surprisingly rapid, it is preferable to go ahead and place the artificial airway, rather than adopting a wait-and-see approach.

Because epiglottitis is caused by a bacteria, **antibiotics** such as cefotaxime, ceftriaxone, or ampicillin with sulbactam should be given through a needle placed in a vein (intravenously). This prevents the bacteria that are circulating throughout the bloodstream from causing infection elsewhere in the body.

Prognosis

With treatment (including the establishment of an artificial airway), only about 1% of children with epiglottitis die. Without the artificial airway, this figure jumps to 6%. Most patients recover form the infection and can have the breathing tube removed (extubation) within a few days.

KEY TERMS

Epiglottis—A leaf-like piece of cartilage extending upwards from the larynx, which can close like a lid over the trachea to prevent the airway from receiving any food or liquid being swallowed.

Extubation—Removal of a breathing tube.

Intubation—Putting a breathing tube into the airway.

Laryngospasm—Spasm of the larynx.

Larynx—The part of the airway lying between the pharynx and the trachea.

Nasopharynx—The part of the airway into which the nose leads.

Oropharynx—The part of the airway into which the mouth leads.

Supraglottitis—Another term for epiglottitis.

Trachea—The part of the airway that leads into the bronchial tubes.

Tracheostomy—A procedure in which a small opening is made in the neck and into the trachea. A breathing tube is then placed through this opening.

Prevention

Prevention involves the use of a vaccine against *H. influenzae type b* (called the **Hib vaccine**). It is given to babies at two, four, six, and 15 months. Use of this vaccine has made epiglottitis a very rare occurrence.

ORGANIZATIONS

American Academy of Otolaryngology—Head and Neck Surgery, One Prince Street, Alexandria, VA, 22314-3357, (703) 836-4444, http://www.entnet.org.

Rosalyn Carson-DeWitt, MD

Epilepsy

Definition

Epilepsy is a chronic (persistent) disorder of the nervous system. The primary symptoms of this disease are periodic or recurring seizures that are triggered by sudden episodes of abnormal electrical activity in the brain. The term "seizure" refers to any unusual body functions or activities that are under the control of the nervous system.

Demographics

Epilepsy affects about one percent of the population. Approximately 2.3 million people in the United States and 40 million people throughout the world have epilepsy. It is the second most common neurological disorder. According to the Epilepsy Foundation, about 30% of the 200,000 new cases reported every year begin in childhood, particularly in early childhood and around the time of **adolescence**. Another period of relatively high incidence is in people over the age of 65.

Description

The word epilepsy is derived from the Greek term for seizure. Seizures can involve a combination of sensations, muscle contractions, and other abnormal body functions. Seizures may appear spontaneously—without any apparent cause—or can be triggered by a specific type of stimulus such as a flashing light. Specific cases of epilepsy may result from known causes, such as brain injury, or may have no apparent cause (ideopathic epilepsy). Ideopathic epilepsy may be initiated by a combination of genetic and environmental factors.

An epileptic seizure involves a transient (temporary) episode of abnormal electrical activity in the brain. During a seizure, many nerve cells within a specific region of the brain may begin to fire at the same time. This activity may then spread out over other parts of the brain. In addition to abnormal physical symptoms, seizures can bring on emotions ranging from **fear**, anger, and rage, to joy or happiness. During a seizure, patients may experience disorientation, spontaneous sensations of sounds, smells, visions, and distorted visual perception—such as misshapen objects and places.

Epilepsy can be caused by some event or condition that results in damage to the brain such as strokes, tumors, abscesses, trauma (physical injury), or infections, such as **meningitis**. Epilepsy can also be triggered by inherited (genetic) factors or some form of injury or trauma at **birth**. Epilepsy cases that seem to have no readily identifiable cause are referred to as "idiopathic" cases in medical terminology. Symptoms of this disease can appear at any age. Seizures can damage and destroy brain cells and scar tissue can develop in the section of brain tissue where seizures originate.

There are many forms of epileptic seizures. The parts of the body that are affected by a seizure and the distinctive characteristics, duration, and severity of the symptoms can distinguish each type of epilepsy. Patients can experience more than one type of seizure. The nature of the symptoms depends on where in the brain the seizure originated and how much of the brain is involved. Seizures can be classified as either "generalized" or "partial." Partial seizures involve abnormal activity in a specific region of the brain.

Generalized (also called tonic–clonic) seizures last about two minutes and are the result of abnormal electrical activity that spreads out over both sides or hemispheres of the brain. They were formerly referred to as grand mal seizures. The patient will usually lose consciousness and fall during the episode. The term "tonic" refers to the first phase of a generalized seizure in which the body muscles become taunt or stiff. This is followed by strong, rhythmic muscular contractions (convulsions) of the "clonic" phase. Sometimes a patient's breathing may be hampered by a brief stoppage of the respiratory muscles, causing the skin to develop a bluish tinge due to lack of oxygen.

Epileptic seizures can also be classified as complex or simple. Complex seizures generally involve a loss of consciousness, whereas simple seizures do not. Simple partial seizures can begin as a localized (focal) seizure and then evolve into a secondary generalized episode in which the initial abnormal electrical activity spreads to involve other parts of the brain. Patients may actually remember the physical and psychological events that occur during a simple seizure, such as the types of movement, emotions, and sensations, but frequently are completely unaware of the event. Partial seizures are more common in adults.

An absence seizure (once called *petit mal*) typically results in brief periods of lack of awareness and some abnormal muscle movement. The patient generally remains conscious during the seizure episode, but may become absent–minded and unresponsive. They may also appear to be starring. Absence seizures last about 5–10 seconds.

How seizures affect a person's memory depends where in the brain seizures occur. Seizures can interfere with learning, storage, and retrieval of new information. For example, a form of epilepsy that produces seizures in the temporal lobe of the brain can cause a serious deterioration (loss) of memory function. Early treatment can help prevent or reduce memory loss.

In some forms of epilepsy, seizures can be triggered by a particular mental—or cognitive—activity. For example, the simple activity of reading aloud can trigger a seizure in patients with reading epilepsy. Symptoms include face **muscle spasms**. In medical terms, this type of epilepsy is referred to as idiopathic localization-related epilepsy. This means that seizures occur in one part of the brain (in this case, the temporal lobes) and that there is no apparent cause that brought on the disease.

Risk factors

Certain factors may increase the risk of epilepsy. The Mayo Clinic lists the following:

- Age: the onset of epilepsy is most common during early childhood and after age 65, but the condition can occur at any age.
- Sex: men are slightly more at risk of developing epilepsy than are women.
- Family history: a family history of epilepsy may increase the risk of developing a seizure disorder.
- Head injuries: head injuries injuries are responsible for many cases of epilepsy.
- Stroke and other vascular diseases: these conditions can lead to brain damage that may trigger epilepsy.
- Brain infections: infections like meningitis, which causes an inflammation in the brain or spinal cord, can increase the risk of epilepsy.
- Prolonged seizures in childhood: high fevers in childhood can sometimes be associated with prolonged seizures and subsequent epilepsy later in life.

Causes and symptoms

Epilepsy has many causes that have an effect on the clinical presentation of symptoms. In order for epilepsy to occur, there must be an underlying physical problem in the brain. The problem can be so mild that a person can be perfectly normal aside from having seizures. The brain has roughly 50–100 billion neurons. Each neuron can have up to 10,000 contacts with neighboring neurons. Hence, trillions of connections exist. However, only a very small area of dysfunctional brain tissue is necessary to create a persistent generator of seizures and, hence, epilepsy. The following are potential causes of epilepsy:

- genetics and/or inherited
- perinatal neurological insults
- trauma with brain injury
- stroke
- brain tumors
- infections such as meningitis and encephalitis
- multiple sclerosis
- ideopathic (unknown or genetic)

Any of the above conditions has the potential for causing the brain or a portion of it to be dysfunctional and produce recurrent seizures. Regardless of the exact cause, epilepsy is a paroxysmal (sudden) condition. It involves the synchronous discharging of a population of neurons. This is an abnormal event that, depending on the location in the brain, will correspond to the particular symptoms of a seizure. The International League Against Epilepsy (ILAE) issued a classification of types of seizures. Individual seizure types are based on the clinical behavior (semiology) and electrophysiological characteristics as seen on an electroencephalogram (EEG). Generalized seizures included in the list include:

- tonic-clonic seizures (includes variations beginning with a clonic or myoclonic phase)
- clonic seizures, including without tonic features and with tonic features
- typical absence seizures
- atypical absence seizures
- myoclonic absence seizures
- tonic seizures
- spasms
- myoclonic seizures
- eyelid myoclonia, including without absences and with absences
- myoclonic atonic seizures
- negative myoclonus
- atonic seizures
- reflex seizures in generalized epilepsy syndromes

Partial (or focal) seizures included in the ILAE list are:

- focal sensory seizures with elementary sensory symptoms (e.g., occipital and parietal lobe seizures) and experiential sensory symptoms (e.g., temporo-parieto-occipital junction seizures)
- focal motor seizures with elementary clonic motor signs, asymmetrical tonic motor seizures (e.g., supplementary motor seizures), typical (temporal lobe) automatisms (e.g., mesial temporal lobe seizures), hyperkinetic automatisms, focal negative myoclonus, and inhibitory motor seizures
- gelastic seizures
- hemiclonic seizures
- secondarily generalized seizures
- reflex seizures in focal epilepsy syndromes

The International League Against Epilepsy has also issued the following classification of epilepsies and epileptic syndromes:

- benign familial neonatal seizures
- early myoclonic encephalopathy
- Ohtahara syndrome
- migrating partial seizures of infancy (syndrome in development)
- West syndrome
- benign myoclonic epilepsy in infancy
- benign familial and non-familial infantile seizures
- Dravet's syndrome
- HH syndrome
- myoclonic status in nonprogressive encephalopathies (syndrome in development)
- benign childhood epilepsy with centrotemporal spikes
- early onset benign childhood occipital epilepsy (Panayiotopoulos type)
- late-onset childhood occipital epilepsy (Gastaut type)
- epilepsy with myoclonic absences
- epilepsy with myoclonic-astatic seizures
- Lennox-Gastaut syndrome
- Landau-Kleffner syndrome (LKS)
- epilepsy with continuous spike-and-waves during slow-wave sleep (other than LKS)
- childhood absence epilepsy
- progressive myoclonus epilepsies
- idiopathic generalized epilepsies with variable phenotypes include juvenile absence epilepsy, juvenile myoclonic epilepsy, and epilepsy with generalized tonic-clonic seizures only
- reflex epilepsies
- idiopathic photosensitive occipital lobe epilepsy
- other visual sensitive epilepsies
- primary reading epilepsy
- startle epilepsy
- autosomal dominant nocturnal frontal lobe epilepsy
- familial temporal lobe epilepsies
- generalized epilepsies with febrile seizures plus (syndrome in development)
- familial focal epilepsy with variable foci (syndrome in development)
- symptomatic focal epilepsies
- limbic epilepsies
- mesial temporal lobe epilepsy with hippocampal sclerosis
- mesial temporal lobe epilepsy defined by specific etiologies
- neocortical epilepsies
- Rasmussen syndrome

Classifying epilepsy is used in the evaluation and management of patients with seizure disorders. The combination of seizure type(s), etiology (cause), age of onset, family history, and other medical or neurological conditions can help identify an epilepsy syndrome. Syndrome classification schemes are revised periodically as individual components of particular categories are better understood.

The term idiopathic refers to a cause that is unknown. Cryptogenic is a term that suggests that an underlying cause is suspected, but not yet fully understood. Symptomatic is a term that is applied to epilepsies that are a result of understood underlying pathologies.

The management and prognosis vary considerably among these differing syndromes. Epilepsies that have a genetic basis can be inherited or occur spontaneously. A detailed family history can often identify other family members who have had seizures. However, because seizures are common, it is possible to have more than one family member with epilepsy, though the causes may not be related. To say that a particular type of epilepsy is genetic does not mean that it is necessarily transmitted by heredity. Often disorders can have a genetic cause, but may be spontaneously occurring in only one member of a family. In this case, there may simply be a random mutation in that particular person's genes.

Genetic factors contribute to about 40% of all epilepsy cases. Most of the generalized epilepsy syndromes and some of the partial epilepsy syndromes have an inherited component. Medical researchers suggest that at least 500 genes may somehow be involved in the development of various forms of epilepsy. It is believed that some of these genes can make people with epilepsy more susceptible or sensitive to environmental factors that initiate or start seizures. Only a few types of epilepsy are thought to be caused by just one type of gene.

Gene mutations can cause a variety of nervous system abnormalities that are associated with epilepsy. Different mutations may lead to abnormal brain development or progressive degeneration of brain tissue. Some gene mutations make nerve cells hyperexcitable. These abnormal nerve cells can trigger outbursts of abnormal patterns of electrical activity that can initiate an epileptic seizure.

Specific gene locations (called gene markers) have been linked to various forms of the disease, such as juvenile myoclonic epilepsy. However, researchers have discovered that some individuals who possess this gene do not develop symptoms of this disease. In some pairs of identical **twins** with this gene, one twin may appear normal while the other develops typical symptoms of epilepsy. Thus, genetics seems to be just one of many factors that influence the possibility of developing epilepsy symptoms.

Some genetic mutations may also reduce the effectiveness of antiepileptic medication. One of the major goals of epilepsy research is to determine how a patient's genetic makeup can influence their drug therapy.

With epilepsy, symptoms vary considerably depending on the type. The common link among the epilepsies is, of course, seizures. The different epilepsies can sometimes be associated with more than one seizure type. This is the case with Lennox-Gastaut syndrome.

The specific symptoms of epilepsy accordingly depend in part on the particular seizures that occur and other medical problems that may be associated. Seizures themselves can take on a variety of features. A simple sustained twitching of an extremity could be a partial seizure. If a seizure arises in the occipital lobes of the brain, then a visual experience can occur. Aura is a term often used to describe symptoms that a person may feel prior to the loss of consciousness of a seizure. However, auras are, themselves, small partial seizures that have not spread in the brain to involve consciousness. Smells, well formed hallucinations, **tingling** sensations, or nausea have all occurred in auras. The particular sensation can be a clue as to the location in the brain where a seizure starts. Partial seizures can then spread to involve other areas of the brain and lead to an alteration of consciousness, and possibly convulsions. In certain epilepsy syndromes such as Lennox Gastaut, there can be more than one type of seizure experienced, such as atonic, atypical absence, and tonic axial seizures.

Diagnosis

Examination

The diagnosis of epilepsy is relatively straightforward: when people suffer two or more seizures, they are considered to have epilepsy. However, diagnosing the specific epilepsy syndrome is much more complex. The first step in the evaluation process is to obtain a very detailed history of the illness, not only from the patient but also from the family. In a child, this includes birth history, complications, if any, maternal history, and developmental milestones. At any age, other medical problems are also considered. Medications that have been taken or currently being prescribed are documented. Since seizures can impair consciousness, the patient may not be able to recall specifics. In these cases, family or friends that have witnessed the episodes can fill in the gaps about the particulars of the seizure. The description of the behaviors during a seizure helps to categorize the type of seizure and with the overall diagnosis.

KEY TERMS

Aura—A sensation of a cold breeze or bright light that precedes the onset of a seizure.

Automatisms—Movements during a seizure that are semi-purposeful but involuntary.

Clonic—Referring to clonus, rapid contractions and relaxations of a muscle.

Convulsion—Involuntary contractions of body muscles that accompany a seizure episode.

Gelastic seizures—Seizures manifesting with brief involuntary laughter.

Gray matter—The portion of the brain that contains neurons, as opposed to white matter, which contains nerve tracts.

Infantile spasms—Clusters of rapid jerks followed by stiffening or jackknife movements. Usually starts in the first year of life and stops by age four.

Ideopathic—Of unknown origin.

Lesion—A defective or injured section or region of the brain (or other body organ).

Magnetic resonance imaging (MRI)—A technique that employs magnetic fields and radio waves to create detailed images of internal body structures and organs, including the brain.

Myoclonic—A rapid, involuntary muscle contraction, particularly near the eye.

Myoclonus—Jerking, involuntary movements of the arms and legs. These may occur normally during sleep.

Neuron—A unique type of cell found in the brain and body that is specialized to process and transmit information.

Partial seizure—A seizure that starts in one particular part of the brain. The abnormal electrical activity may remain confined to that area, or may spread to the entire brain. Also called a focal seizure.

Reflex seizure—Seizure brought on by specific sensory stimuli.

Seizure—Any unusual body functions or activity that is under the control of the nervous system.

Spike wave discharge—Characteristic abnormal wave pattern in the electroencephalogram that is a hallmark of an area that has the potential of generating a seizure.

A complete physical examination is performed, especially a **neurological exam**. Because seizures are an episodic disorder, abnormal neurological findings may not be present. Frequently, people with epilepsy have a normal exam. However, in some, there can be abnormal findings that can provide clues to the underlying cause of epilepsy. For example, if someone has had a **stroke** that subsequently caused seizures, then the neurological exam can be expected to reveal a focal neurological deficit such as weakness or language difficulties. In some children with seizures, there can be a variety of associated neurologic abnormalities such as **mental retardation** and **cerebral palsy** that are themselves non-specific but indicate that the brain has suffered, at some point in development, an injury or malformation. Also, subtle findings on examination can lead to a diagnosis of tuberous sclerosis. This is an autosomal dominantly inherited disorder associated with infantile spasms in 25% of cases. On examination, patients have so-called ash-leaf spots and adenoma sebaceum on the skin. There can also be a variety of systemic abnormalities that involve the kidneys, retina, heart, and gums, depending on severity.

Tests

In the course of evaluating epilepsy, a number of tests are typically ordered. Usually, **magnetic resonance imaging** (MRI) of the brain is performed. This is a scan that can help to find causes of epilepsy such as tumors, strokes, trauma, and congenital malformations. However, while MRI can reveal incredible brain details, it cannot image the presence of abnormalities in the microscopic neuronal environment. Another test that is routinely ordered is an electroencephalogram (EEG). Unlike the MRI scan, this can be considered a functional test of the brain. The EEG measures the electrical activity of the brain. Some seizure disorders or epilepsies have a characteristic EEG with particular abnormalities that can help in diagnosis. Blood tests are also frequently ordered to help screen for abnormalities that could be a factor in the cause of seizures. Occasionally, **genetic testing** is performed in those instances where a known genetic cause is suspected and can be tested. A major concern in the course of an evaluation of epilepsy is to identify the presence of life-threatening causes such as brain tumors, infections, and cerebrovascular disease.

Treatment

Traditional

Currently, no cure exists for epilepsy. However, a wide range of treatment programs are available that provide varying degrees of success in controlling the symptoms of epilepsy.

Drugs

Medication is the most effective and widely used treatment for the symptoms of epilepsy. Most medications work by interfering with or stopping the abnormal electrical activity in nerve cells that cause seizures. This form of treatment is generally referred to as anticonvulsant therapy. Medication is considered effective if the patient is free of seizures for at least one year.

As with any medication, individuals can have very different experiences with same drug. Consequently, it is difficult to predict the efficacy of treatment. A key concept of treatment is to first strive for monotherapy (or single drug therapy). This simplifies treatment and minimizes the chance of side effects. Sometimes, however, two or more drugs may be necessary to achieve satisfactory control of seizures. As with any treatment, potential side effects can be worse than the disease itself. Moreover, there is little point in controlling seizures if severe side effects limit quality of life. If a **seizure disorder** is characterized by mild, focal, or brief symptoms that do not interfere with routine activities, then aggressive treatments may not be advisable. Epilepsy medications do not cure epilepsy; the medications can only control the frequency and severity of seizures. A list of the most commonly used medications in the management of epilepsy includes:

- phenobarbital
- phenytoin (Dilantin, Phenytek)
- clonazepam (Klonipin)
- ethosuxamide (Zarontin)
- carbamazepine (Tegretol, Carbatrol)
- divalproex sodium (Depakote, Depakene)
- felbamate (Felbatol)
- gabapentin (Neurontin)
- lamotrigine (Lamictal)
- topiramate (Topamax)
- tiagabine (Gabatril)
- zonisamide (Zonegran)
- oxcarbazepine (Trileptal)
- leviteracetam (Keppra)

Anticonvulsants are powerful drugs that can produce a variety of side effects, including nausea, fatigue, **dizziness**, and weight change. They can also increase the risk of **birth defects**, especially involving the early stages of embryonic development of the nervous system if taken during pregnancy.

Doctors prefer to put their patients on just one type of anticonvulsant drug. Some patients, however, experience more effective relief from their epilepsy symptoms by taking a combination of two different but complementary forms of medication. The choice of medication depends on the type of seizure that affects a patient, the patient's medical history—including response to other drug therapies, their age, and gender. For example, the drug Carbamazepine is one of the most effective medications and has little impact on important cognitive functions such as thinking, memory, and learning.

Newer medications generally produce fewer side effects than their predecessors. Research into gene therapy may ultimately be the most effective form of epilepsy treatment, but is still in the very early stages.

Unfortunately, medication is ineffective for more than one-third of known cases of epilepsy. More than 30% of patients with epilepsy cannot maintain adequate control of their seizures. Some genetic mutations may reduce the effectiveness of antiepileptic medications.

Alternative

Surgery is recommended for some patients for whom medication cannot effectively control the frequency or severity of their seizures. Surgery is a treatment option only in extreme cases where doctors can identify the specific site in the brain where seizures originate. The most promising candidates for surgery are those with a single lesion on the temporal, frontal, or occipital lobes of the brain.

Prior to surgery, the patient must complete extensive testing to determine the precise patterns of seizures and to locate their point of origin in the brain. Patients spend extended stays in hospital during which their seizures are recorded on video and with the aid of EEGs. This machine records patterns of electrical activity in the brain using sensors (referred to as "electrodes") attached to various parts of the body.

The surgical procedure involves the removal of a small part of brain tissue in the "suspected" region. The anterior temporal lobe and hippocampus are the most common areas in which tissue is removed. In some studies, more than 83% of patients become free of seizures following surgery. Ninety–seven percent show significant improvement in their condition.

Vagus Nerve Stimulation (VNS) is another form of treatment for some cases of epilepsy that are unresponsive (referred to as refractory epilepsy) to other forms of medical therapy. VNS may also be recommended for patients who cannot tolerate the side effects of medication. This procedure involves implanting a device that stimulates the Vagus nerve, located in the left side of the neck. In one study, this treatment reduced seizures by 78%.

A special dietary program is another treatment option for patients who are not good candidates for surgery or who have had little success with anticonvulsant medication. This form of treatment called the Ketogenic Diet can be effective for many types of epilepsy. It is most appropriate for young children whose parents can follow the rigid requirements of the diet. Older children and adults tend to have greater difficulty in sticking to the dietary rules for an extended period of time. The Ketogenic Diet is a stringent diet that is very high in fat, but low in proteins, carbohydrates, and calories. The excessive fat produces high levels of a substance called ketones (which the body makes when it breaks down fat for energy). Somehow these ketones help reduce the incidence of epileptic seizures. The success of this form of treatment varies. For some patients, the high fat diet is the best form of treatment. For others, the diet is less effective.

As of 2009, 153 clinical trials for the study and treatment of epilepsy were being sponsored by the National Institutes of Health (NIH) and other agencies.

A few examples include:

- The effectiveness and safety of diazepam for patients with epilepsy who receive antiepileptic drugs. (NCT00319501)
- The role played by the brain chemical serotonin in seizures. (NCT00439387)
- The effectiveness and dose requirements of levetiracetam in subjects with newly diagnosed childhood absence epilepsy. (NCT00361010)
- The effectiveness of electrical brain stimulation to reduce epileptic seizures. (NCT00344877)
- The use of simultaneous EEG and functional magnetic resonance imaging (fMRI) to study the different brain regions involved in child absence seizures and how they are related to attention and cognition. (NCT00393666)
- The effectiveness and safety of seletracetam when it is used in addition to other anti-epileptic medications by patients with partial onset seizures. (NCT00422110)
- The evaluation of standard diagnostic tests and treatments for patients with epilepsy. (NCT00013845)
- The collection of brain tissue samples for research purposes from patients undergoing surgery to treat epilepsy. (NCT00025714)
- The use of functional magnetic resonance imaging (fMRI) and diffusion tensor imaging (DTI) to examine how the brain processes tasks involving language and emotion in normal volunteers and in patients with epilepsy. (NCT00081432)

Clinical trial information is constantly updated by NIH and the most recent information on epilepsy trials can be found at:http://clinicaltrials.gov.

Prognosis

The prognosis of epilepsy varies widely depending on the cause, severity, and patient's age. Even individuals with a similar diagnosis may have different experiences with treatment. For example, in benign epilepsy of childhood with centrotemporal spikes (also called benign rolandic epilepsy), the prognosis is excellent with nearly all children experiencing remission by their teens. With childhood absence epilepsy, the prognosis is variable. In this case, the absence seizures become less frequent with time, but almost half of patients may eventually develop generalized tonic-clonic seizures. Overall, the seizures are responsive to an appropriate anticonvulsant. On the other hand, the seizures in Lennox-Gastaut syndrome are very difficult to control. In this case, however, the ketogenic diet can help. In seizures that begin in adulthood, one can expect that medications will control seizures in up to 60–70% of cases. However, in some of the more than 30% of medically intractable cases, epilepsy surgery can improve or even cure the problem.

Overall, most patients have a good chance of controlling seizures with the available treatment options. The goal of treatment is complete cessation of seizures since a mere reduction in seizure frequency and/or severity may continue to limit patients' quality of life. For instance, they may not be able to drive, sustain employment, or be productive in school.

Prevention

Head injuries are associated with many epilepsy cases. The risk can be reduced by always wearing a seat belt while riding in a car and by wearing a helmet while bicycling, skiing, riding a motorcycle or engaging in other activities with a high risk of **head injury**. Vascular disease may also lead to epilepsy. Limiting alcohol intake, avoiding cigarettes, eating a healthy diet, and exercising regularly can reduce the risk for these diseases.

Resources

BOOKS

Browne, Thomas R., and Gregory L. Holmes. *Handbook of Epilepsy,* 4th edition, Philadelphia, PA: Lippincott Williams & Wilkins, 2008.

Devinsky, Orrin. *Epilepsy: Patient and Family Guide.* 3rd edition, New York, NY: Demos Health, 2007.

Gay, Kathlyn. *Epilepsy: The Ultimate Teen Guide.* Lanham, MD: Scarecrow Press, 2007.

Karia, Roopal. *The Why and What of Epilepsy: A Book for Children and Teens.* Frederick, MD: PublishAmerica, 2008.

Reuber, Markus, et al. *Epilepsy Explained: A Book for People. Who Want to Know More.* New York, NY: Oxford University Press, 2009.

Shorvon, Simon D., et al., eds. *The Treatment of Epilepsy,* 3rd edition,New York, NY: Wiley-Blackwell, 2009.

Wilner, Andrew N. *Epilepsy: 199 Answers: A Doctor Responds to His Patients' Questions,* 3rd edition, New York, NY: Demos Health, 2007.

Wyllie, Elaine, et al., eds. *The Treatment of Epilepsy: Principles and Practice,* 4th edition, Philadelphia, PA: Lippincott Williams & Wilkins, 2005.

Zelenka, Yvonne. *Let's Learn with Teddy about Epilepsy.* Leonia, NJ: Medicus Press, 2008.

PERIODICALS

Arts, W. F., and A. T. Geerts. "When to start drug treatment for childhood epilepsy: the clinical-epidemiological evidence." *European Journal of Paediatric Neurology* 13 no. 2 (March 2009): 93–101.

Beenhakker, M. P., and J. R. Huguenard. "Neurons that fire together also conspire together: is normal sleep circuitry hijacked to generate epilepsy?" *Neuron* 62 no. 5 (June 2009): 612–632.

Brodie, M. J., et al. "Epilepsy in later life." *Lancet Neurology* 8 no. 11 (November 2009): 1019–1030.

Fastenau, P. S., et al. "Neuropsychological status at seizure onset in children: risk factors for early cognitive deficits." *Neurology* 73 no. 7 (August 2009): 526–534.

Hamani, C., et al. "Deep brain stimulation for the treatment of epilepsy." *International Journal of Neural Systems* 19 no. 3 (June 2009): 213–226.

Hughes, J. R. "Absence seizures: a review of recent reports with new concepts." *Epilepsy & Behavior* 15 no. 4 (August 2009): 404–412.

McCagh, J., et al. "Epilepsy, psychosocial and cognitive functioning." *Epilepsy Research* 86 no. 1 (September 2009): 1–14.

McElroy-Cox, C. "Alternative approaches to epilepsy treatment." *Current Neurology and Neuroscience Reports* 9 no. 4 (July 2009): 313–318.

Rodin, E., et al. "Spikes and epilepsy." *Clinical EEG and Neuroscience* 40 no. 4 (October 2009): 288–299.

Sherman, E. M. "Maximizing quality of life in people living with epilepsy." *Canadian Journal of Neurological Sciences* 36 suppl. 2 (August 2009): S17–S24.

Vining, E. P. "Tonic and atonic seizures: medical therapy and ketogenic diet." *Epilepsia* 50 suppl. 8 (September 2009): 21–24.

Wheless, J. W. "Managing severe epilepsy syndromes of early childhood." *Journal of Child Neurology* 24 suppl. 8 (August 2009): 24S–32S.

OTHER

"Epilepsy." FamilyDoctor.org Information Page, http://familydoctor.org/online/famdocen/home/common/brain/disorders/214.printerview.html (accessed November 15, 2009).

"Epilepsy." Mayo Clinic. Information Page, http://www.mayoclinic.com/print/epilepsy/DS00342/DSECTION=all&METHOD=print (accessed November 15, 2009).

"Epilepsy." MedlinePlus. Health Topics, http://www.nlm.nih.gov/medlineplus/epilepsy.html (accessed November 15, 2009).

"Epilepsy." NINDS. Information Page, http://www.ninds.nih.gov/disorders/epilepsy/epilepsy.htm (accessed November 15, 2009).

"Facts about Epilepsy." Epilepsy Institute. Information Page, http://www.epilepsyinstitute.org/facts/index.htm (accessed November 15, 2009).

"Seizures and Epilepsy: Hope Through Research." *NINDS.* Information Page, http://www.ninds.nih.gov/disorders/epilepsy/detail_epilepsy.htm (accessed November 15, 2009).

"What is Epilepsy?" Epilepsy Foundation. Information Page, http://www.epilepsyfoundation.org/about (accessed November 15, 2009).

ORGANIZATIONS

Antiepileptic Drug Pregnancy Registry, MGH East, CNY-149, 10th Floor 149 13th Street, Charlestown, MA, 02129-2000, (800) 233-2334, (617) 724-8307, info@aedpregnancyregistry.org, http://www2.massgeneral.org/aed.

Charlie Foundation to Help Cure Pediatric Epilepsy, 1223 Wilshire Blvd., Suite 815, Santa Monica, CA, 90403, (310) 393-2347, (310) 453-4585, ketoman@aol.com, http://www.charliefoundation.org.

Citizens United for Research in Epilepsy (CURE), 730 North Franklin Street, Suite 404, Chicago, IL, 60654, (312) 255-1801, (312) 255-1809, info@CUREepilepsy.org, http://www.CUREepilepsy.org.

Epilepsy Foundation, 8301 Professional Place, Landover, MD, 20785-7223, (301) 459-3700, (800) 332-1000, (301) 577-2684, postmaster@efa.org, http://www.epilepsyfoundation.org.

Epilepsy Institute, 257 Park Avenue South, New York, NY, 10010, (212) 677-8550, , (212) 677-5825 website@epilepsyinstitute.org, http://www.epilepsyinstitute.org.

Epilepsy Therapy Project, P.O. Box 742, Middleburg, VA, 20118, (540) 687-8077, , (540) 687-8066, epilepsytherapy@epilepsytherapy.org, http://www.epilepsy.com.

National Institute of Neurological Disorders and Stroke (NINDS), PO Box 5801, Bethesda, MD, 20824, (301) 496-5751, (800) 352-9424, http://www.ninds.nih.gov.

People Against Childhood Epilepsy (PACE), 7 East 85th Street, Suite A3, New York, NY, 10028, (212) 665-PACE,

(212) 327-3075, pacenyemail@aol.com, http://www.paceusa.org.

Monique Laberge, PhD
Marshall G. Letcher, MA
Roy Sucholeiki, MD

Erb's palsy **see Brachial plexopathy, obstetric**

Erythema **see Fifth disease**

Erythroblastosis fetalis

Definition

Erythroblastosis fetalis refers to two potentially disabling or fatal blood disorders in infants: Rh incompatibility disease and ABO incompatibility disease. Either disease may be apparent before **birth** and can cause fetal **death** in some cases. The disorder is caused by incompatibility between a mother's blood and her unborn baby's blood. Because of the incompatibility, the mother's **immune system** may launch an immune response against the baby's red blood cells. As a result, the baby's blood cells are destroyed, and the baby may suffer severe **anemia** (deficiency in red blood cells), brain damage, or death.

Description

Red blood cells carry several types of proteins, called antigens, on their surfaces. The A, B, and O antigens are used to classify a person's blood as type A, B, AB, or O. Each parent passes one A, B, or O antigen gene to their child. How the genes are paired determines the person's blood type.

A person who inherits an A antigen gene from each parent has type A blood; receiving two B antigen genes corresponds with type B blood; and inheriting A and B antigen genes means a person has type AB blood. If the O antigen gene is inherited from both parents, the child has type O blood; however, the pairing of A and O antigen genes corresponds with type A blood; and if the B antigen gene is matched with the O antigen gene, the person has type B blood.

Another red blood cell antigen, called the Rh factor, also plays a role in describing a person's blood type. A person with at least one copy of the gene for the Rh factor has Rh-positive blood; if no copies are inherited, the person's blood type is Rh-negative. In blood typing, the presence of A, B, and O antigens, a the presence or absence of the Rh-factor, determine a person's specific blood type, such as A-positive, B-negative, and so on.

A person's blood type has no effect on health. However, an individual's immune system considers only that person's specific blood type, or a close match, acceptable. If a radically different blood type is introduced into the bloodstream, the immune system produces antibodies, proteins that specifically attack and destroy any cell carrying the foreign antigen.

Determining a woman blood type is very important if she becomes pregnant. Blood cells from the unborn baby (fetal red blood cells) can cross over into the mother's bloodstream, especially at delivery. If the mother and her baby have compatible blood types, the crossover does not present any danger. However, if the blood types are incompatible, the mother's immune system manufactures antibodies against the baby's blood.

Usually, this incompatibility is not a factor in a first pregnancy, because few fetal blood cells reach the mother's bloodstream until delivery. The antibodies that form after delivery cannot affect the first child. In later pregnancies, fetuses and babies may be in grave danger. The danger arises from the possibility that the mother's antibodies will attack the fetal red blood cells. If this happens, the fetus or baby can suffer severe health effects and may die.

There are two types of incompatibility diseases: Rh incompatibility disease and ABO incompatibility disease. Both diseases have similar symptoms, but Rh disease is much more severe because anti-Rh antibodies cross over the placenta more readily than anti-A or anti-B antibodies. (The immune system does not form antibodies against the O antigen.) Therefore, a greater percentage of the baby's blood cells are destroyed by Rh disease.

Both incompatibility diseases are uncommon in the United States due to medical advances over the last 60 years. For example, prior to 1946 (when newborn blood transfusions were introduced) 20,000 babies were affected by Rh disease yearly. Further advances, such as suppressing the mother's antibody response, have reduced the incidence of Rh disease to approximately 4,000 cases per year.

Rh disease only occurs if a mother is Rh-negative and her baby is Rh-positive. For this situation to occur, the baby must inherit the Rh factor gene from the father. Most people are Rh-positive. Only 15% of the Caucasian population is Rh-negative, compared to 5–7% of the

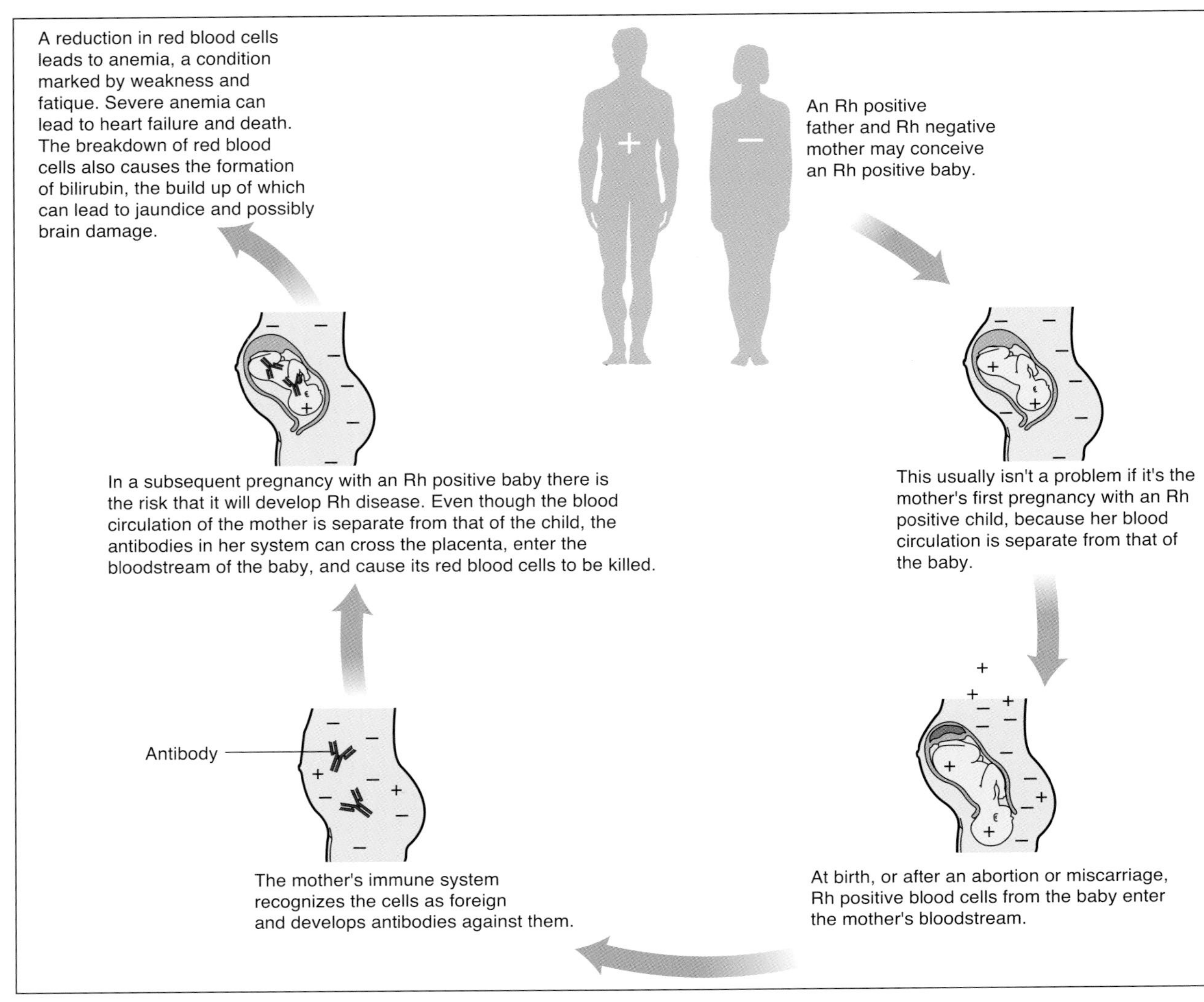

Flow chart demonstrating how RH disease is carried to a fetus through the mother. *(Illustration by Hans & Cassady, Inc. Reproduced by permission of Gale, a part of Cengage Learning.)*

African-American population and virtually none of Asian populations.

ABO incompatibility disease is almost always limited to babies with A or B antigens whose mothers have type O blood. Approximately one-third of these babies show evidence of the mother's antibodies in their bloodstream, but only a small percentage develop symptoms of ABO incompatibility disease.

Cause and symptoms

Rh disease and ABO incompatibility disease are caused when a mother's immune system produces antibodies against the red blood cells of her unborn child. The antibodies cause the baby's red blood cells to be destroyed and the baby develops anemia. The baby's body tries to compensate for the anemia by releasing immature red blood cells, called erythroblasts, from the bone marrow.

The overproduction of erythroblasts can cause the liver and spleen to become enlarged, potentially causing liver damage or a ruptured spleen. The emphasis on erythroblast production is at the cost of producing other types of blood cells, such as platelets and other factors important for blood clotting. Since the blood lacks clotting factors, excessive bleeding can be a complication.

The destroyed red blood cells release the blood's red pigment (hemoglobin) which degrades into a yellow substance called bilirubin. Bilirubin is normally produced as red blood cells die, but the body is only equipped to handle a certain low level of bilirubin in the bloodstream at one time. Erythroblastosis fetalis overwhelms the removal system, and high levels of bilirubin accumulate, causing hyperbilirubinemia, a condition in which the baby becomes jaundiced. The **jaundice** is apparent from the yellowish tone of the baby's eyes and skin. If hyperbilirubinemia cannot be controlled, the baby develops kernicterus. The term kernicterus means that bilirubin is being deposited in the brain, possibly causing permanent damage.

Other symptoms that may be present include high levels of insulin and low blood sugar, as well as a condition called hydrops fetalis. Hydrops fetalis is characterized by an accumulation of fluids within the baby's body, giving it a swollen appearance. This fluid accumulation inhibits normal breathing because the lungs cannot expand fully and may contain fluid. If this condition continues for an extended period, it can interfere with lung growth. Hydrops fetalis and anemia can also contribute to heart problems.

Diagnosis

Erythroblastosis fetalis can be predicted before birth by determining the mother's blood type. If she is Rh-negative, the father's blood is tested to determine whether he is Rh-positive. If the father is Rh-positive, the mother's blood will be checked for antibodies against the Rh factor. A test that demonstrates no antibodies is repeated at week 26 or 27 of the pregnancy. If antibodies are present, treatment is begun.

In cases in which incompatibility is not identified before birth, the baby suffers recognizable characteristic symptoms such as anemia, hyperbilirubinemia, and hydrops fetalis. The blood incompatibility is uncovered through blood tests such as the Coombs test, which measures the level of maternal antibodies attached to the baby's red blood cells. Other blood tests reveal anemia, abnormal blood counts, and high levels of bilirubin.

Treatment

When a mother has antibodies against her unborn infant's blood, the pregnancy is watched very carefully. The antibodies are monitored and if levels increase, **amniocentesis**, fetal umbilical cord blood sampling, and ultrasound are used to assess any effects on the baby. Trouble is indicated by high levels of bilirubin in the amniotic fluid or baby's blood or if the ultrasound reveals hydrops fetalis. If the baby is in danger, and the pregnancy is at least 32–34 weeks along, labor is induced. Under 32 weeks, the baby is given blood transfusions while still in the mother's uterus.

There are two techniques that are used to deliver a blood transfusion to a baby before birth. In the first, a needle is inserted through the mother's abdomen and uterus, and into the baby's abdomen. Red blood cells injected into the baby's abdominal cavity are absorbed into its bloodstream. In early pregnancy or if the baby's bilirubin levels are gravely high, cordocentesis is performed. This procedure involves sliding a very fine needle through the mother's abdomen and, guided by ultrasound, into a vein in the umbilical cord to inject red blood cells directly into the baby's bloodstream.

After birth, the severity of the baby's symptoms are assessed. One or more transfusions may be necessary to treat anemia, hyperbilirubinemia, and bleeding. Hyperbilirubinemia is also treated with phototherapy, a treatment in which the baby is placed under a special light. This light causes changes in how the bilirubin molecule is shaped, which makes it easier to excrete. The baby may also receive oxygen and intravenous fluids containing electrolytes or drugs to treat other symptoms.

Prognosis

In many cases of blood type incompatibility, the symptoms of erythroblastosis fetalis are prevented with careful monitoring and blood type screening. Treatment of minor symptoms is typically successful and the baby will not suffer long-term problems.

Nevertheless, erythroblastosis is a very serious condition for approximately 4,000 babies annually. In about 15% of cases, the baby is severely affected and dies before birth. Babies who survive pregnancy may develop kernicterus, which can lead to deafness, speech problems, **cerebral palsy**, or **mental retardation**. Extended hydrops fetalis can inhibit lung growth and contribute to heart failure. These serious complications are life threatening, but with good medical treatment, the fatality rate is very low. According to the U.S. Centers for Disease Control and Prevention, there were 21 infant deaths in the United States during 1996 that were attributable to hemolytic disease (erythroblastosis fetalis) and jaundice.

Prevention

With any pregnancy, whether it results in a live birth, miscarriage, stillbirth, or **abortion**, blood typing is a universal precaution against blood compatibility disease. Blood types cannot be changed, but adequate forewarning allows precautions and treatments that limit the danger to unborn babies.

If an Rh-negative woman gives birth to an Rh-positive baby, she is given an injection of immunoglobulin G, a type of antibody protein, within 72 hours of the birth. The immunoglobulin destroys any fetal blood cells in her bloodstream before her immune system can react to them. In cases where this precaution is not taken, antibodies are created and future pregnancies may be complicated.

Resources

PERIODICALS

Bowman, John. "The Management of Hemolytic Disease in the Fetus and Newborn." *Seminars in Perinatology* 21 no. 1 (February 1997): 39.

Julia Barrett

Erythromycins and macrolide antibiotics

Definition

Macrolides are **antibiotics** that kill bacteria or prevent their growth.

Purpose

Macrolides are used to treat bacterial infections in various sites:

- middle and inner ear
- eyes
- sinuses
- tonsils
- throat and larynx (voice box)
- lungs (pneumonia and bronchitis)
- skin (infected eczema, acne, psoriasis)
- genitalia, sexually transmitted diseases (Chlamydia, gonorrhea)

These antibiotics are used to prevent infections prior to dental and other procedures for patients at risk for developing infections of the heart valves (endocarditis).

Macrolide antibiotics can be used as alternatives to penicillin for people with penicillin **allergies**.

These antibiotics will *not* cure colds, flu, and other viral infections.

Description

Members of the macrolide antibiotic family include erythromycin (Erythrocin, Ery-C, E-Mycin, azithromycin (Zithromax), and clarithromycin (Biaxin). They are

KEY TERMS

Amniocentesis—A procedure in which a needle is inserted through a pregnant woman's abdomen and into her uterus to withdraw a small sample of amniotic fluid. The amniotic fluid can be examined for sign of disease or other problems afflicting the fetus.

Amniotic fluid—The fluid that surrounds a fetus in the uterus.

Anemia—A condition in which there is an abnormally low number of red blood cells in the bloodstream. Major symptoms are paleness, shortness of breath, unusually fast or strong heart beats, and tiredness.

Antibody—A protein molecule produced by the immune system in response to a protein that is not recognized as belonging in the body.

Antigen—A protein that can elicit an immune response in the form of antibody formation. With regard to red blood cells, the major antigens are A, B, O, and the Rh factor.

Bilirubin—A yellow-colored end-product of hemoglobin degradation. It is normally present at very low levels in the bloodstream; at high levels, it produces jaundice.

Cordocentesis—A procedure for delivering a blood transfusion to a fetus. It involves a fine needle being threaded through a pregnant woman's abdomen and into the umbilical cord with the aid of ultrasound imaging.

Hemoglobin—A molecule in red blood cells that transports oxygen and gives the cells their characteristic color.

Hydrops fetalis—A condition in which a fetus or newborn baby accumulates fluids, causing swollen arms and legs and impaired breathing.

Hyperbilirubinemia—A condition in which bilirubin accumulates to abnormally high levels in the bloodstream

Placenta—A protective membrane that surrounds and protects the fetus during pregnancy.

Platelet—A blood factor that is important in forming blood clots.

Rh factor—An antigen that is found on the red blood cells of most people. If it is present, the blood type is referred to as Rh-positive; if absent, the blood type is Rh-negative.

available by prescription as capsules, tablets (including chewable), liquids, and for injection.

Recommended dosage

Dosage depends on the drug used and the reason for its use.

Antibiotics should always be taken exactly as directed, for as long as they are prescribed. Do not stop antibiotics if symptoms begin improving.

Precautions

These drugs should be used with caution by patients with liver or kidney disease

People who have inherited blood disorders, like porphyria, should not take these antibiotics.

Macrolides increase the risk of heart arrhythmia in patients who have prolonged Q-T interval on EKG.

These antibiotics may aggravate muscle weakness in patients with Myasthenia Gravis.

ALLERGIES Anyone who has had unusual reactions to a macrolide antibiotic previously should avoid taking it again.

PREGNANCY There are no well controlled studies on these antibiotics and pregnancy.

BREASTFEEDING Macrolide antibiotics pass into breast milk, though no specific dangers have been identified.

Side effects

Macrolide antibiotics may widen the Q-T interval on EKG. People who are at risk for developing severe heart arrhythmias or who take drugs that widen the Q-T interval should avoid taking these antibiotics.

The more common side effects from macrolides include mild **diarrhea**, nausea, **vomiting**, and stomach or abdominal cramps that go away as the body adjusts to the drug.

Less commonly, sore mouth or tongue and vaginal **itching** may occur. These rarely require medical attention.

If these, more serious, side effects occur, seek medical help:

- severe abdominal pain, and continued nausea, vomiting, or diarrhea
- fever
- skin rash, redness, or itching

KEY TERMS

Bronchitis—Infection of the air passages in the lungs.

Gonorrhea—A sexually transmitted infection with fever and a pussy penile discharge in males and abdominal pain and vaginal discharge in females.

Bacteria—Organisms that can only be seen under a microscope.

Pneumonia—Infection of the lungs caused by bacteria, viruses, or chemical irritants.

Sinus—Air-filled cavities in the bones of the skull.

- unusual tiredness or weakness
- swelling of the lips, face, or neck

Interactions

Prescribers need to know the medications their patients take; this class of antibiotics may interact with many drugs.

Food may change the effects of erythromycin and clarithromycin (Biaxin), increasing the risks of side or adverse effects.

Grapefruit juice may increase the absorption of macrolide antibiotics, possibly increasing the possibility of adverse or side effects.

St. John's wort may decrease blood levels of erythromycin.

The effectiveness of combined **oral contraceptives** may be reduced when macrolide antibiotics are taken. It would be wise to use an additional method of preventing pregnancy for up to seven days after discontinuing these antibiotics.

Taking quinolone antibiotics (Tequin, Levaquin, Avelox) with erythromycin increases the potential for fatal heart arrhythmias.

Macrolide antibiotics increase the risk of fatal heart arrhythmias when taken with medications to treat heart arrhythmias (Cordarone, Norpace, Tikosyn, Sotalol, Bretylium, and Quinidine).

Macrolide antibiotics increase the blood-thinning effects of warfarin (Coumadin).

Macrolide antibiotics increase the adverse, muscle wasting effects of cholesterol-reducing medications (Lipitor, Zocor, Mevacor).

People who take digoxin (Lanoxin) and macrolide antibiotics together risk developing digoxin toxicity.

People who take carbamazepine (Tegretol) for seizures, **schizophrenia**, ethanol withdrawal, restless-leg syndrome, or post-traumatic stress disorder (PTSD) risk developing carbamazepine toxicity when they take macrolide antibiotics.

Macrolide antibiotics increase the effects of Colchicine used to treat Gout, increasing the risk of toxicity.

Macrolide antibiotics increase the effects, and toxicity, of ergot drugs used to treat migraine headaches.

Macrolide antibiotics increase the effects and toxicity of pimozide (Orap) and clozapine (Clozaril) used to treat psychosis.

Macrolide antibiotics increase the effects and toxicity of verapamil (Calan) used to treat angina (heart **pain**) and rapid heartbeats.

Macrolide antibiotics increase the sedative effects of anti-anxiety medications Buspar and benzodiazepines Xanax, Valium, and Halcion.

Taken together, macrolide antibiotics and theophyllines (Choledyl, Theo-Dur and Uniphyl), used to treat chronic **asthma** and asthma-like conditions, adversely effect each other. Theophyllin levels increase in the blood, increasing the chance of toxicity, and macrolide effectiveness is reduced.

Resources

OTHER

"Antibiotics, macrolide." NHS Choices. Nation Health Service (NHS). http://www.nhs.uk/ (accessed July 29, 2009).

James Waun, MD, RPh

Esophageal atresia

Definition

Esophageal atresia is a serious **birth** defect in which the esophagus, the long tube that connects the mouth to the stomach, is segmented and closed off at any point. This condition usually occurs with **tracheoesophageal fistula**, a condition in which the esophagus is improperly attached to the trachea, the nearby tube that connects the nasal area to the lungs. Esophageal atresia occurs in approximately 1 in 4,000 live births.

Description

Failure of an unborn child (fetus) to develop properly results in **birth defects**. Many of these defects involve organs that do not function, or function only incidentally, before birth, and, as a result, go undetected until the baby is born. In this case, the digestive tract is unnecessary for fetal growth, since all **nutrition** comes from the mother through the placenta and umbilical cord.

During fetal development, the esophagus and the trachea arise from the same original tissue. Normally, the two tubes would form separately (differentiate); however, in cases of esphageal atresia and tracheoesophageal fistulas, they do not, resulting in various malformed configurations. The most common configuration is the "C" type, in which the upper part of the esophagus abruptly ends in a blind pouch, while the lower part attaches itself to the trachea. This configuration occurs in 85–90% of cases. Esophageal atresia without involvement of the trachea occurs in only 8% of cases.

Causes and symptoms

The cause of esophageal atresia, like that of most birth defects, is unknown.

An infant born with this defect will at first appear all right, swallowing normally. However, the blind pouch will begin to fill with mucus and saliva that would normally pass through the esophagus to the stomach. These secretions back up into the mouth and nasal area, causing the baby to drool excessively. When fed, the baby will also immediately regurgitate what he or she has eaten. **Choking** and coughing may also occur as the baby breaths in the fluid backing up from the esophagus. Aspiration **pneumonia**, an infection of the respiratory system caused by inhalation of the contents of the digestive tract, may also develop.

Diagnosis

Physicians who suspect esophageal atresia after being presented with the above symptoms diagnose the condition using x-ray imaging or by passing a catheter through the nose and into the esophagus. Esophageal atresia is indicated if the catheter hits an obstruction 4–5 in (10–13 cm) from the nostrils.

Treatment

Infants with esophageal atresia are unlikely to survive without surgery to reconnect the esophagus. The procedure is done as soon as possible; however,

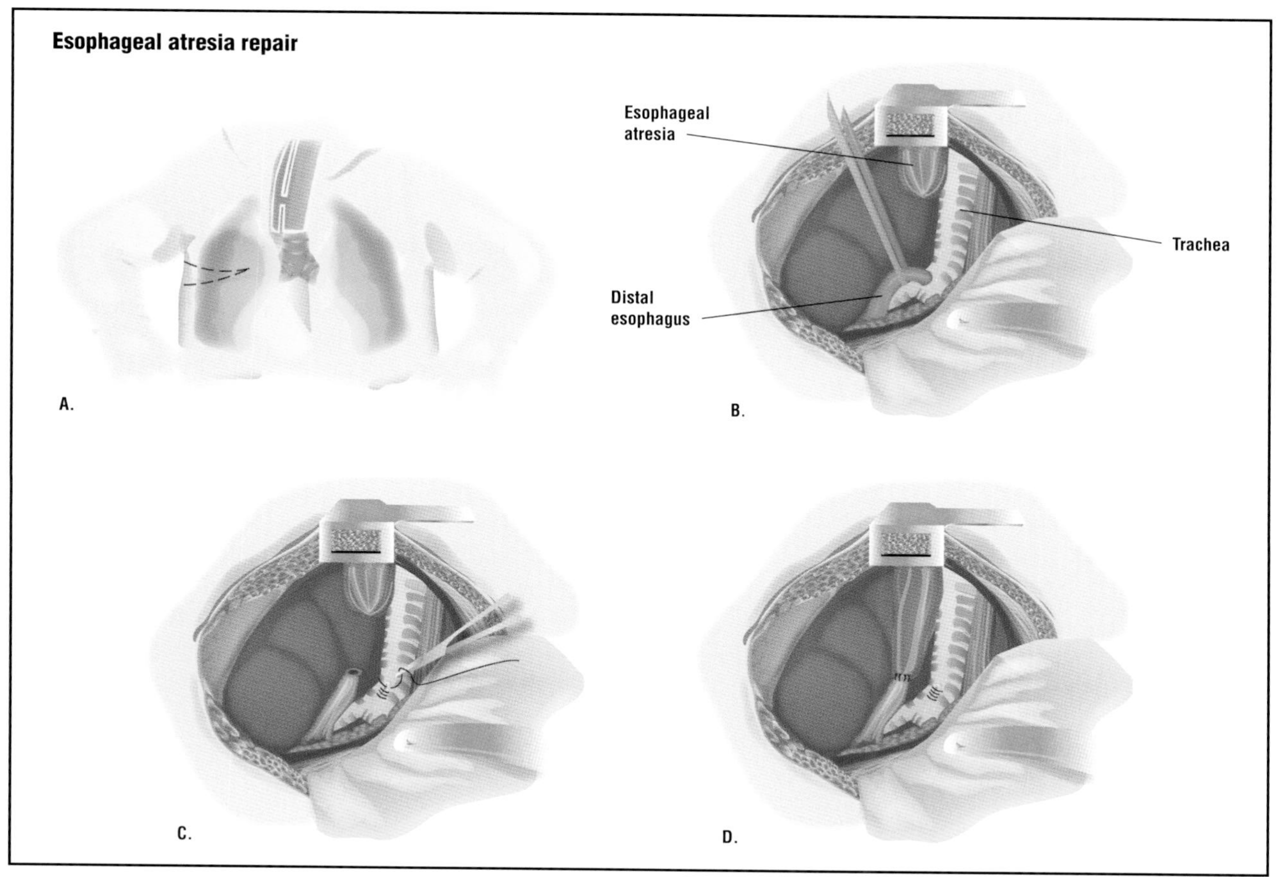

To repair esophageal atresia, an opening is cut into the chest (A). The two parts of the existing esophagus are identified (B). The lower esophagus is detached from the trachea (C) and connected to the upper part of the esophagus (D). *(Illustration by PreMediaGlobal. Reproduced by permission of Gale, a part of Cengage Learning.)*

prematurity, the presence of other birth defects, or complications of apiration pneumonia may delay surgery. Once diagnosed, the baby will be fed intraveneously until he or she has recovered sufficiently from the operation. Mucus and saliva will also be continuously removed via a catheter until recovery has occured. When surgery is performed, the esophagus is reconnected and, if neccessary, separated from the trachea. If the two ends of the esophagus are too far apart to be reattached, tissue from the large intestine is used to join them.

Prognosis

Surgery to correct esophageal atresia is usually successful. Post-operative complications may include difficulty swallowing, since the esophagus may not contract efficiently, and gastrointestinal reflux, in which the acidic contents of stomach back up into the lower part of the esophagus, possibly causing ulcers.

Resources

BOOKS

Long, John D., and Roy Orlando. "Anatomy and Development and Acquired Anomalies of the Esophagus." In *Sleisenger & Fordtran's Gastrointestinal and Liver Disease*, edited by Mark Feldman, et al. Philadelphia: W. B. Saunders Co., 1998.

J. Ricker Polsdorfer, MD

Exercise

Definition

Exercise can be defined as physical activity that involves planned, structured, and repetitive bodily movements for the purpose of maintaining or improving physical fitness and overall health. Exercise includes cardiovascular training, muscle-strength training, and stretching activities for flexibility and to prevent injury. Typical exercise activities include walking, running, cycling, **swimming**, weight training, aerobics, and individual and team **sports**.

Purpose

Regular exercise is important for the physical, mental, and emotional health of people of all ages—from young children to the elderly. Exercise promotes:

- weight maintenance or weight loss
- cardiovascular efficiency
- musculoskeletal strength and flexibility
- improved functioning of the metabolic, endocrine, and immune systems
- bone density
- lower cholesterol levels
- recovery from illness, injury, or surgery
- mental and emotional wellbeing

The beneficial effects of exercise diminish within two weeks of substantially reducing physical activity. Physical fitness is lost completely if exercise is not resumed within two to eight months.

Demographics

The National Institutes of Health (NIH) has identified inactivity as a major public health problem in the United States, and most North American adults would benefit from increasing their level of physical activity. More than 60% of adults in the United States do not get enough physical activity to provide health benefits and more than 25% are inactive during their leisure time. Lack of exercise is a major contributor to the current epidemic of obesity, since people burn fewer calories than they take in, resulting in weight gain. Sedentary lifestyles and unhealthy eating patterns are responsible for at least 300,000 deaths from chronic disease each year in the United States. Likewise, a recent survey in the United Kingdom found that only one-third of adults meet recommended goals for physical activity.

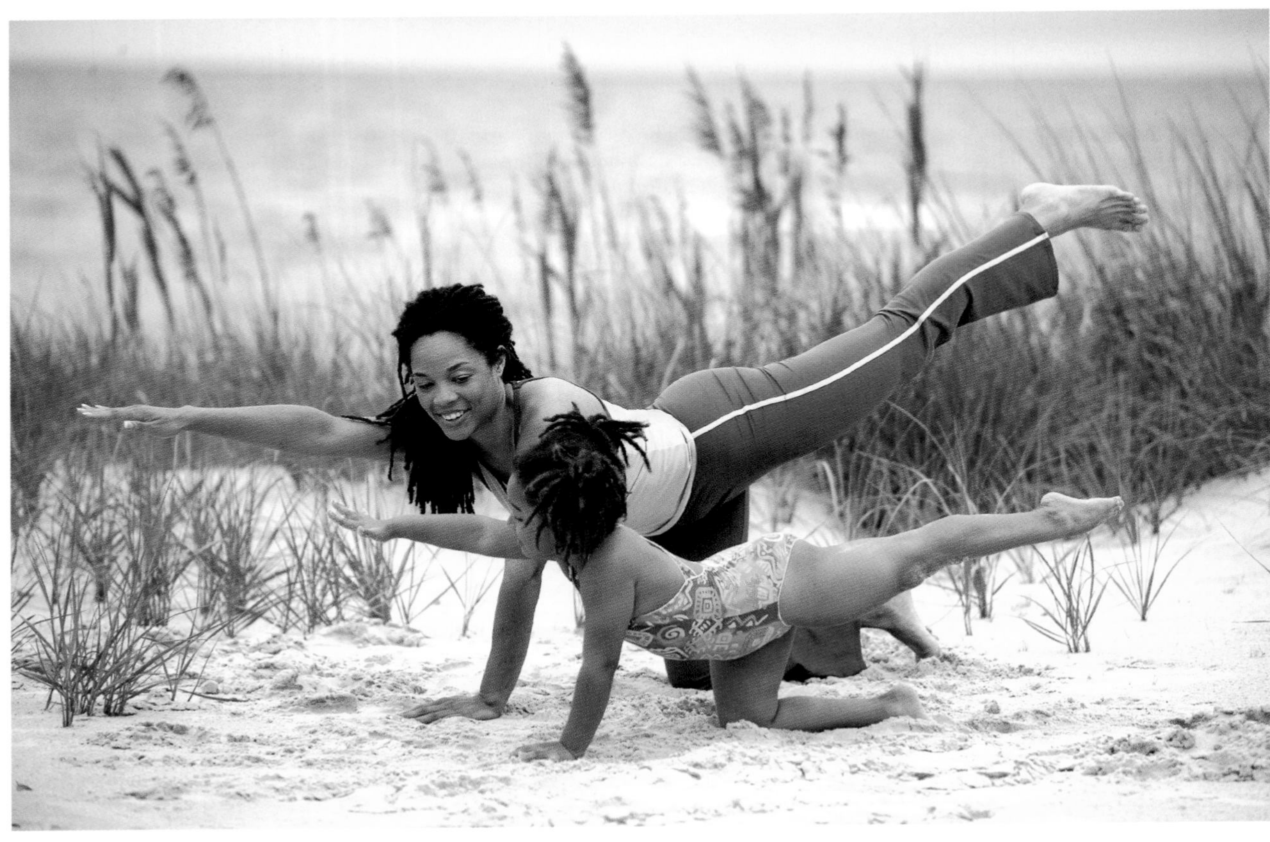

Mother and daughter practicing yoga. *(© Ariel Skelley/Corbis.)*

Percentage of high school students who were physically active during the past week,* by sex, race/ethnicity, and grade, 2009

	Physically active at least 60 minutes/day on all 7 days			Physically active at least 60 minutes/day on 5 or more days		
	Female %	Male %	Total %	Female %	Male %	Total %
Race/ethnicity						
White[†]	12.4	26.2	**19.7**	31.3	47.3	**39.9**
Black[†]	10.0	24.4	**17.2**	21.9	43.3	**32.6**
Hispanic	10.5	20.7	**15.6**	24.9	41.3	**33.1**
Grade						
9	13.6	28.0	**21.3**	30.8	47.5	**39.7**
10	12.7	25.3	**19.3**	30.5	47.4	**39.3**
11	10.3	23.3	**17.0**	26.0	46.2	**36.4**
12	8.6	21.9	**15.3**	22.4	40.4	**31.6**
Total %	**11.4**	**24.8**	**18.4**	**27.7**	**45.6**	**37.0**

*Were physically active during the 7 days before the survey, doing any kind of physical activity that increased their heart rate and made them breathe hard some of the time
[†]Non-Hispanic

SOURCE: Centers for Disease Control and Prevention. Youth Risk Behavior Surveillance—United States, 2009. Surveillance Summaries, June 4, 2010. *MMWR* 2010;59(No. SS-5).

(Table by PreMediaGlobal. Reproduced by permission of Gale, a part of Cengage Learning.)

Pediatric

Exercise is essential for improving overall health, maintaining fitness, and helping to prevent the development of obesity, hypertension, and cardiovascular disease. Surveys conducted by the Centers for Disease Control and Prevention (CDC) indicate that 61.5 percent of children aged nine to 13 years do not participate in any organized physical activity (for example, sports, dance classes) and 22.6 percent are not physically active during their free time. According to the American Obesity Association, approximately 30 percent of children and adolescents aged six to 19 years are overweight and 15 percent are obese.

A sedentary lifestyle and excess caloric consumption are the primary causes of this increase in overweight and obesity; regular exercise is considered an important factor in controlling weight. Overweight and obese children and adolescents are at higher risk of developing severe medical conditions.

Description

Exercise programs should include three types of exercise: strengthening, including weight or resistance training, stretching and flexibility exercises, and cardiovascular exercise. Recent studies have indicated that muscle strength and aerobic fitness make independent contributions to health and that more muscle strength correlates with lower **death** rates, regardless of aerobic fitness. The American College of Sports Medicine recommends two strength-training workouts per week, each consisting of about 10 repetitions of 10 exercises for strengthening all of the major muscle groups. **Yoga** is often recommended for stretching, bending, and improving overall flexibility.

Chosen exercises should be interesting and appealing. Studies have found that people are more likely to stick with an exercise program when they enjoy the activity, whether as an individual, with a partner, or with a group or team. Convenience is also an important consideration. Exercise can take place at home, outdoors, at a health club or fitness center, school, church, or community center. Taking a class, working out with a friend, competing, or setting personal goals can help maintain motivation. Walking for exercise can be combined with various enjoyable activities, such as bird watching, museum visits, window shopping, or exercising the dog. Group exercises and team sports are good ways to socialize. Varying exercise routines every few weeks can benefit different muscle groups and help prevent **boredom**. In addition, since the human body adjusts rapidly to most exercises, continuing the same routine for too long can result in decreased benefits.

The most efficient cardiovascular exercises for improving physical fitness include:

- brisk walking (3–4 mph), whether outside, in a mall, or on a treadmill

- jogging
- running
- bicycling, either outside or on a stationary bike
- stair climbing
- elliptical cross-training on exercise machines
- aerobics
- swimming
- water exercise or aerobics
- rowing
- cross-country (Nordic) skiing
- jumping rope—a particularly good exercise for children

Other exercises that provide cardiovascular conditioning—but are less endurance-promoting because they usually require frequent starting and stopping—include:

- dancing
- basketball
- soccer
- softball
- badminton
- racquetball
- squash
- tennis
- table tennis
- volleyball
- skating
- golfing, if walking and carrying clubs

Teenagers can get cardiovascular exercise through school sports including:

- baseball
- cross country
- track and field
- cheerleading
- drill team
- field hockey
- football
- lacrosse
- wrestling

People who are generally sedentary can still get exercise through their occupation, housework, home repair, gardening, using stairs instead of an elevator, and various recreational pursuits. People with health problems can find exercises that accommodate their injuries or disorders. The American Council on Exercise suggests specific exercises for the elderly and for adults with problems such as **asthma**, chronic pain, bad knees, shoulder injuries, arthritis, and flat feet.

Regularity and intensity are key elements of exercise. It has generally been recommended that all adults get at least 30 minutes of moderate-intensity exercise on most days of the week. However, the most recent consensus is to aim for 150 minutes per week, regardless of how it is divided up. The latest evidence suggests that three 10-minute bouts of exercise are as beneficial as one 30-minute workout. Improving cardiovascular endurance requires at least 20–60 minutes of cardiovascular exercise three to five days per week. The U.S. Department of Health and Human Services recommends at least 60 minutes of physical activity for children and teens on most or all days of the week.

Defining "moderate intensity" can be tricky. Until recently exercise intensity was generally gauged by increased heart rate. However, intensity is more accurately measured by metabolic rate, as represented by units of metabolic equivalents (METS). MET is an individual's metabolic rate during exercise divided by the metabolic rate when sitting still. The latter is defined as 1 kilocalorie per kilogram (kg) of body weight per hour or an oxygen uptake of 3.5 milliliters per kg per minute. Moderate activity is defined as 3–6 METS. Although a precise measurement requires determining oxygen intake in a laboratory, charts of average METS for various activities are available. Examples of METS include:

- walking, 2–8
- running, 8–18
- bicycling, 4–16
- stationary bicycling, 3–12.5
- general health-club exercise, 5.5
- calisthenics, 3–8
- weight lifting, 3–6
- swimming, 6–11
- cross-country skiing, 7–16.5
- downhill skiing, 5–8
- volleyball, 3–8
- dancing, 3–10
- basketball, 4.5–8
- tennis, 5–8
- tai chi, 4
- stretching, hatha yoga, 2.5
- household tasks, 2–9
- mowing with a hand mower, 6

Exercise geared to a target heart rate is typically about 70% of the maximum heart rate for one's age. Heart rate is calculated by counting the pulse, usually about halfway through a 20–30-minute workout. Fingers are placed firmly but lightly over the inside of the wrist or on the neck just below the angle of the jaw;

however, too much pressure on the neck can slow down the heart rate. The palm also can be placed over the heart to count the number of beats. A zero is added to a six-second count or a 10-second count is multiplied by six to obtain the beats per minute (bpm). Maximum bpm is calculated by subtracting one's age from 220. For example:

- The target heart rate during cardiovascular exercise for a healthy 50-year-old might be 170 multiplied by 70% or 119 bpm.
- A particularly fit 50-year-old might have a target heart rate of 80% of maximum or 136 bpm.
- A 50-year-old with a medical condition may have a target exercising heart rate of only 50% or 85 bpm. A bpm above the target rate indicates a need to slow down, whereas a bpm below the target indicates a need to speed up the pace of exercise.

There are other methods for measuring the intensity of cardiovascular exercise:

- Classes and DVDs usually include a timed heart-rate check and a chart of target rates by age.
- Electronic exercise pulse monitors are available.
- A simple "talk test"is based on speaking a complete sentence. The pace of exercise is too high if the sentence cannot be completed and too low if it is overly easy to speak the sentence.
- Cardiovascular exercise usually involves sweating; therefore, people who no longer sweat during their exercise routine may need to increase the intensity, duration, or frequency of their workouts.

Improved fitness in response to exercise appears to be genetically determined and to run in families. Some previously sedentary people show less improvement in fitness than would be expected following weeks of a vigorous exercise program and about 10% show no improvement at all. However, even those who show no improvement in fitness measures still respond to exercise with lowered blood pressure and **cholesterol**, improved insulin levels, and less abdominal fat.

Benefits

Exercise promotes:

- cardiovascular fitness, including improved heart function and increased heart, lung, and muscle endurance
- muscle strength and mass
- flexibility
- weight loss
- lowered blood pressure
- bone density and strength, which reduces the risk of fractures and osteoporosis
- mental health and psychological and emotional wellbeing from the release of brain hormones called endorphins

Additional benefits of cardiovascular exercise include:

- improved immune system function
- improved utilization and control of blood sugar
- decreased cholesterol and triglycerides
- decreased abdominal fat
- increased energy levels
- less fatigue
- improved appetite
- improved sleep
- reduced stress
- pain reduction

Regular exercise lowers the risk of a heart attack by 50–80%. Exercise also has been shown to reduce the risk of:

- stroke
- cancer
- diabetes
- liver and kidney disease
- osteoporosis
- depression
- dementia

Even those who are overweight or obese can become aerobically fit with exercise. Studies have found that the risk of dying is more closely related to fitness than to weight. In fact people who are fit but obese have a lower risk of dying than people who are unfit but of normal weight.

More than 30 million people in the United States undergo surgery each year. Each patient's surgical risk, complications, and outcome depend, at least in part, on their physical fitness: how well their cardiovascular and pulmonary systems withstand the stress of anesthesia; how quickly their bones and muscles recover after surgical procedures; and how well their metabolic and immune systems respond to surgery and the risk of infection.

Precautions

- Everyone should have a physical examination before embarking on an exercise program for the first time or after a long period of inactivity.
- Exercise intensity and duration should be increased gradually.

- People who are very weak may need to build strength before they can participate in cardiovascular exercise.
- Warming up before and stretching after exercise are very important.
- People should pace themselves and check their heart rate or otherwise judge their level of exertion.
- If exercising becomes "very hard" or worse, it is important to slow the pace.
- Although some discomfort, such as aches or stiffness, are to be expected during the first few days of a new exercise program, if pain is intrusive it is important to stop the activity or get instruction on technique.
- Strenuous cardiovascular exercise should never be halted abruptly without a cool-down, since blood that has concentrated in the working muscles can pool and cause dizziness or lightheadedness.
- Cardiovascular exercise requires a healthy diet with plenty of vegetables.
- It is best to wait up to two hours after a full meal before exercising and about an hour after exercising before having a meal, although a small healthy snack before exercising can boost energy levels.
- It is important to drink enough fluid to replace water that is lost as sweat; however, coffee, tea, colas, chocolate, or alcohol can cause the body to lose fluid.
- Simple home exercises, such as a balance board, can reduce the risk of recurrent sprained ankles.
- Taking a few days off from cardiovascular exercise every month can help rejuvenate the body.

Geriatric

Both maximum heart rate and cardiac output are lower in older adults, in part due to a decrease in the beta-adrenergic response. Older adults should have a stress test before embarking on a cardiovascular exercise program. A good result on a stress test is a bpm that is 80% of the age-adjusted maximum, with 90% considered excellent.

Other conditions

Various medical conditions can affect exercise. For example people with back problems should avoid exercises that require twisting or vigorous forward movements, such as aerobic dancing or rowing. People with spinal disk disease should avoid high-impact activities.

Preparation

Exercise should begin with a light or very light warm-up of 5–10 minutes that may include gentle stretching to loosen muscles and joints and help prevent injury. The warm-up may involve slowly beginning the conditioning activity—warming up for a brisk walk or jog by walking slowly or strolling, or warming up to ride a stationary bike by pedaling slowly with no resistance. Warming up increases blood flow to the muscles, increases muscle temperature, and prepares them to work harder.

Aftercare

Cardiovascular exercise should be followed by a light or very light 5 or 10 -minute cool-down to allow the heart and circulation to gradually return to a resting state. The cool-down can include the same activity as the conditioning phase at a slower pace—slower walking or pedaling with reduced resistance on a stationary bike.

Risks

Exercise poses a risk of injury, particularly if exercises are inappropriate or improperly performed. Too much exercise can be as harmful as too little; overuse of certain muscles and joints can lead to problems such as tennis elbow or shin splints. High-intensity exercises, such as high-impact aerobics and jogging, are not recommended as frequently as in the past. Running, in particular, is hard on the knees and ankle joints, and there is a risk of sprained ankles and injuries from falls. About one-half of all regular runners and players of team sports suffer some type of musculoskeletal injury each year.

Inadequate rest increases the risk of **stroke** and circulatory problems. Injury or illness from overtraining is sometimes indicated by a high resting heart rate, sleeping difficulties, or exhaustion.

For children and adolescents who perform high-impact activities, such as running, stress **fractures** may occur. **Dehydration** is a risk during longer activities that involve sweating; children and adolescents should be supplied with water during and after activity.

Parental concerns

Given the increasing prevalence of overweight and obesity in children and adolescents, it is important for parents to encourage regular exercise and also serve as role models by exercising themselves. Television, computers, and **video games** have replaced physical activity for playtime for the majority of children. Parents should make a commitment to replacing sedentary activities with active indoor and outdoor games. For busy families, exercise can be performed in multiple 10- to 15-minute sessions throughout the day.

For children aged two to five years, physical activities should emphasize basic movement skills,

KEY TERMS

Aerobic exercise—Any exercise that increases the body's oxygen consumption and improves the functioning of the cardiovascular and respiratory systems.

Cholesterol—A fat-soluble steroid alcohol (sterol) found in animal fats and oils and produced in the body from saturated fats. High cholesterol levels contribute to the development of cardiovascular disease.

Endorphins—A class of peptides in the brain that are produced during exercise and bind to opiate receptors, resulting in pleasant feelings and pain relief.

Metabolic equivalent of task; MET—The energy cost of a physical activity, measured as a multiple of the resting metabolic rate, which is defined as 3.5 milliliters of oxygen consumed per kilogram (kg) of body weight per minute, equivalent to 1 kilocalorie per kg per hour.

Obesity—Excessive weight due to accumulation of fat, usually defined as a body mass index (BMI) of 30 or above or body weight greater than 30% above normal on standard height-weight tables.

Physical activity—Any activity that involves moving the body and burning calories.

Physical fitness—A combination of muscle strength, cardiovascular health, and flexibility that is usually attributed to regular exercise and good nutrition.

Sedentary—Inactivity and lack of exercise; a lifestyle that is a major risk factor for becoming overweight or obese and developing chronic diseases.

Stress test—An electrocardiogram recorded before, during, and after a period of increasingly strenuous cardiovascular exercise, usually on a treadmill or stationary bicycle.

Target heart rate—The heart rate, in beats per minute (bpm), that should be maintained during cardiovascular exercise by an individual of a given age.

Triglycerides—Neutral fats; lipids formed from glycerol and fatty acids that circulate in the blood as lipoprotein. Elevated triglyceride levels contribute to the development of cardiovascular disease.

imagination, and **play**. Examples of appropriate activities for this age group include rolling and bouncing a ball, jumping, hopping, skipping, mimicking animal movements, and pedaling a tricycle.

For children aged five to eight years, physical activities should emphasize basic motor skills and more complex movements (eye-hand coordination). Noncompetitive group sports or classes are appropriate for this age, and parents should focus on helping their children find an enjoyable physical activity.

Resources

BOOKS

Harper, Bob. *Are You Ready! Take Charge, Lose Weight, Get in Shape, and Change Your Life Forever.* New York: Broadway Books, 2008.

Manocchia, Pat. *Anatomy of Exercise: A Trainer's Inside Guide to Your Workout.* Richmond Hill, Ontario, Canada: Firefly Books, 2008.

Ratey, John J., and Eric Hagerman. *Spark: The Revolutionary New Science of Exercise and the Brain.* New York: Little, Brown, 2008.

Silver, J. K., and Christopher Morin. *Understanding Fitness: How Exercise Fuels Health and Fights Disease.* Westport, CT: Praeger, 2008.

PERIODICALS

Centers for Disease Control and Prevention. "Prevalence of Regular Physical Activity Among Adults—United States, 2001 and 2005." *MMWR: Morbidity and Mortality Weekly Report* 56 (November 23, 2007): 1209–1212.

Ignelzi, R. J. "Survival of the Fitness: Staying in Shape Without the Gym Easily Doable if You're Disciplined." *San Diego Union-Tribune* (March 24, 2009): D1.

Vanderburg, Helen. "Put Your Heart Health to the Test; Undergo a Stress Test Before Starting Cardiovascular Exercises." *Vancouver Sun* (September 14, 2009): C1.

"What's Your Function?" *Current Health 2* 36 no. 2 (October 2009): 6–7.

OTHER

Hatfield, Heather. "Kick It Up With Cardio Exercise." WebMD Web site, http://www.webmd.com/fitness-exercise/guide/kick-up-with-cardio-exercise.

"Health and Wellness: Battling Boredom in Your Workout." American Osteopathic Association, http://www.osteopathic.org/index.cfm?PageID=you_workout boredom.

"Let's Get Physical: Nine Facts About Fitness." *NewScientist,* http://www.newscientist.com/special/get-physical-nine-facts-about-fitness.

"Physical Activity." Centers for Disease Control and Prevention, http://www.cdc.gov/physicalactivity/.

"Target Heart Rate Calculator." *WebMD Web site*, http://www.webmd.com/fitness-exercise/healthtool-target-heart-rate-calculator.

Wilkerson, Rick, ed. "Sports & Exercise." Your Orthopaedic Connection, http://orthoinfo.aaos.org/menus/sports.cfm.

ORGANIZATIONS

American College of Sports Medicine, PO Box 1440, Indianapolis, IN, 46202-1440, (317) 637-9200, (317) 634-7817, http://www.acsm.org.

American Council on Exercise, 4851 Paramount Drive, San Diego, CA, 92123, (858) 279-8227, (888) 825-3636, (858) 576-6564, support@acefitness.org, http://www.acefitness.org.

American Heart Association, 7272 Greenville Avenue, Dallas, TX, 75231, (800) 242-8721, http://www.americanheart.org.

National Institute of Arthritis and Musculoskeletal and Skin Diseases, Information Clearinghouse, 1 AMS Circle, Bethesda, MD, 20892-3675, (301) 495-4484, (877) 22-NIAMS (226-4267), (301) 718-6366, NIAMSinfo@mail.nih.gov, http://www.niams.nih.gov.

U.S. Centers for Disease Control and Prevention, 1600 Clifton Road, Atlanta, GA, 30333, (800) CDC-INFO (232-4636), cdcinfo@cdc.gov, http://www.cdc.gov.

Margaret Alic, PhD

Expectorants

Definition

Expectorants are drugs that loosen and clear mucus and phlegm from the respiratory tract.

Purpose

The drug described here, guaifenesin, is a common ingredient in **cough** medicines. It is classified as an expectorant, a medicine that helps clear mucus and other secretions from the respiratory tract. However, it has not been fully tested on children in a controlled study to determine its effectiveness. In addition, some cough medicines contain other ingredients that may cancel out guaifenesin's effects. **Cough suppressants**, such as codeine, for example, work against guaifenesin because they discourage coughing up the secretions that the expectorant loosens.

There are other ways to loosen and clear the respiratory secretions associated with colds. These include using a humidifier and drinking six to eight glasses of water a day.

Description

Guaifenesin is an ingredient in many cough medicines, such as the brand names Anti-Tuss, Dristan Cold & Cough, Guaifed, GuaiCough, and some Robitussin products. Some products that contain guaifenesin are available only with a physician's prescription; others can be bought without a prescription. They come in several forms, including capsules, tablets, and liquids.

Recommended dosage

Adults and children 12 and over

Children 6–11

The FDA is deciding whether or not to remove cold medications for children up to 12 years of age. This would include expectorants and is due to lack of pediatric-specific studies and the number of accidental pediatric overdoses.

100–200 mg every four hours. No more than 1,200 mg in 24 hours.

Children under four

Not recommended. The FDA has removed many cold treatments from the shelves for children under 2. Manufacturers have taken the additional step to discourage use for children under 4.

Precautions

Do not take more than the recommended daily dosage of guaifenesin.

Guaifenesin is not meant to be used for coughs associated with **asthma**, or chronic **bronchitis**. It also should not be used for coughs that are producing a large amount of mucus.

A lingering cough could be a sign of a serious medical condition. Coughs that last more than seven days or are associated with **fever**, rash, **sore throat**, or lasting **headache** should have medical attention. Call a physician as soon as possible.

Some studies suggest that guaifenesin causes **birth defects**. Women who are pregnant or plan to become pregnant should check with their physicians before using any products that contain guaifenesin. Whether guaifenesin passes into breast milk is not known, but no ill effects have been reported in nursing babies whose mothers used guaifenesin.

KEY TERMS

Asthma—A disease in which the air passages of the lungs become inflamed and narrowed.

Bronchitis—Inflammation of the air passages of the lungs.

Chronic—A word used to describe a long-lasting condition. Chronic conditions often develop gradually and involve slow changes.

Cough suppressant—Medicine that stops or prevents coughing.

Emphysema—An irreversible lung disease in which breathing becomes increasingly difficult.

Mucus—Thick fluid produced by the moist membranes that line many body cavities and structures.

Phlegm—Thick mucus produced in the air passages.

Respiratory tract—The air passages from the nose into the lungs.

Secretion—A substance, such as saliva or mucus, that is produced and given off by a cell or a gland.

Side effects

Side effects are rare, but may include **vomiting**, **diarrhea**, stomach upset, headache, skin rash, and **hives**.

Interactions

Guaifenesin is not known to interact with any foods or other drugs. However, cough medicines that contain guaifenesin may contain other ingredients that do interact with foods or drugs. Check with a physician or pharmacist for details about specific products.

Nancy Ross-Flanigan

Extracorporeal membrane oxygenation

Definition

Extracorporeal membrane oxygenation (ECMO) is a special procedure that uses an artificial heart-lung machine to take over the work of the lungs and sometimes also the heart.

Purpose

In newborns, ECMO is used to support or replace an infant's undeveloped or failing lungs by providing oxygen and removing carbon dioxide waste products so the lungs can rest. Infants who need ECMO may include those with:

- meconium aspiration syndrome, (breathing in of a newborn's first stool by a fetus or newborn, which can block air passages and interfere with lung expansion)
- persistent pulmonary hypertension, (a disorder in which the blood pressure in the arteries supplying the lungs is abnormally high)
- respiratory distress syndrome (a lung disorder usually of premature infants that causes increasing difficulty in breathing, leading to a life-threatening deficiency of oxygen in the blood)
- congenital diaphragmatic hernia, (the profusion of part of the stomach through an opening in the diaphragm)
- pneumonia
- blood poisoning

ECMO also is used to support a child or adult patient's damaged, infected, or failing lungs for a few hours to allow treatment or healing. It is effective for those patients with severe, but reversible, heart or lung problems who have not responded to treatment with a ventilator, drugs, or extra oxygen. Adults and children who need ECMO usually have one of these problems:

- heart failure
- pneumonia
- respiratory failure caused by trauma or severe infection

The ECMO procedure can help a patient's lungs and heart rest and recover, but it will not cure the underlying disease. Any patient who requires ECMO is seriously ill and will likely die without the treatment. Because there is some risk involved, this method is used only when other means of support have failed.

Demographics

ECMO is used most often in newborns and young children, but it also can be used as a last resort for adults whose heart or lungs are failing.

Description

There are two types of ECMO. Venoarterial (V-A) ECMO supports the heart and lungs, and is used for patients with blood pressure or heart functioning problems in addition to respiratory problems. Venovenous (V-V) ECMO supports the lungs only.

V-A ECMO requires the insertion of two tubes, one in the jugular and one in the carotid artery. In the V-V ECMO procedure, the surgeon places a plastic tube into the jugular vein through a small incision in the neck.

Once in place, the tubes are connected to the ECMO circuit, and then the machine is turned on. The patient's blood flows out through the tube and may look very dark because it contains very little oxygen. A pump pushes the blood through an artificial membrane lung, where oxygen is added and carbon dioxide is removed. The size of the artificial lung depends on the size of the patient; sometimes adults need two lungs. The blood is then warmed and returned to the patient. A steady amount of blood (called the flow rate) is pushed through the ECMO machine every minute. As the patient improves, the flow rate is lowered. Many patients require heavy sedation while they are on ECMO to lessen the amount of oxygen needed by the muscles.

If the patient improves, the amount of ECMO support is decreased gradually until the machine is turned off for a brief trial period. If the patient does well without ECMO, the treatment is stopped.

Typically, newborns remain on ECMO for three to seven days, although some babies need more time (especially if they have a diaphragmatic **hernia**). Once the baby is off ECMO, he or she will still need a ventilator (breathing machine) for a few days or weeks. Adults may remain on ECMO for days to weeks, depending on the condition of the patient, but treatment may be continued for a longer time depending on the type of heart or lung disease, the amount of damage to the lungs before ECMO was begun, and the presence of any other illnesses or health problems.

KEY TERMS

Carotid artery—Two main arteries (passageway carrying blood from the heart to other parts of the body) that carry blood to the brain.

Congenital diaphragmatic hernia—The profusion of part of the stomach through an opening in the diaphragm.

Meconium aspiration syndrome—Breathing in of meconium (a newborn's first stool) by a fetus or newborn, which can block air passages and interfere with lung expansion.

Membrane oxygenator—The artificial lung that adds oxygen and removes carbon dioxide.

Pulmonary hypertension—A disorder in which the blood pressure in the arteries supplying the lungs is abnormally high.

Respiratory distress syndrome—A lung disorder usually of premature infants that causes increasing difficulty in breathing, leading to a life-threatening deficiency of oxygen in the blood.

Venoarterial (V-A) bypass—The type of ECMO that provides both heart and lung support, using two tubes (one in the jugular vein and one in the carotid artery).

Venovenous (V-V) bypass—The type of ECMO that provides lung support only, using a tube inserted into the jugular vein.

Benefits

ECMO can be a life-saving procedure when time is needed for the lungs to recover.

Precautions

Typically, ECMO patients have daily chest **x rays** and blood work, as well as and constant vital sign monitoring. They are usually placed on a special rotating bed that is designed to decrease pressure on the skin and help move secretions from the lungs.

After the patient is stable on ECMO, the breathing machine settings will be lowered to "rest" settings, which allow the lungs to rest without the risk of too much oxygen or pressure from the ventilator.

Preparation

Before ECMO is begun, the patient receives medication to ease **pain** and restrict movement.

Aftercare

Because infants on ECMO may have been struggling with low oxygen levels before treatment, they may be at higher risk for developmental problems. They will need to be monitored as they grow.

Risks

Bleeding is the biggest risk for ECMO patients, since blood thinners are given to guard against blood clots. Bleeding can occur anywhere in the body, but is most serious when it occurs in the brain. This is why doctors periodically perform ultrasound brain scans of anyone on ECMO. **Stroke**, which may be caused by bleeding or blood clots in the brain, has occurred in some patients undergoing ECMO.

If bleeding becomes a problem, the patient may require frequent blood transfusions or operations to control the bleeding. If the bleeding cannot be stopped, ECMO will be withdrawn.

Other risks include infection or vocal cord injury. Some patients develop severe blood infections that cause irreversible damage to vital organs.

There is a small chance that some part of the complex equipment may fail, which could introduce air into the system or affect the patient's blood levels, causing damage or **death** of vital organs (including the brain). For this reason, the ECMO circuit is constantly monitored by a trained technologist.

Resources

OTHER

Introduction to ECMO for Parents. Stanford Medical Center, http://lane.stanford.edu/portals/cvicu/HCP_CV_Tab_1/ecmo_for_parents.pdf (accessed June 25, 2010).

Rodriguez-Cruz, Edwin and Henry Waters, III. "Extracorporeal membrane Oxygenation." eMedicine.com, February 19, 2010, http://emedicine.medscape.com/article/1818617-overview.

ORGANIZATIONS

American Society of Extra-Corporeal Technology, 2209 Dickens Road, Richmond, VA, 23230-2005, (804) 565-636, (804) 282-0090, amsect@amsect.org, http://www.amsect.org.

Extracorporeal Life Support Organization (ELSO), 2600 Plymouth Road, Building 300, Room 303, Ann Arbor, MI, 48109-2800, (734) 998-6601, (734) 998-6602, http://www.elso.med.umich.edu.

Carol A. Turkington
Tish Davidson, AM

Extracurricular activities

Activities sponsored by and usually held at school, but that are not part of the academic curriculum.

Extracurricular activities, which are programs offered by a school system that do not form part of the academic curriculum, range from **sports** to newspaper editing to music and theater. Many, like football and drama, enjoy extreme longevity, serving as a part of their school's program over a number of years. Others, like a recycling club or writer's workshop, may be offered for a shorter time span to reflect a community interest or involvement by a particular sponsoring faculty member. For many students, extracurricular activities present an opportunity to practice social skills and to experiment in activities that may represent a career interest.

Extracurricular activities also help to form a student's profile for consideration in college admissions. A student's academic record and scores on standardized tests form the core of his or her college application profile. However, admissions officers consider other factors, such as a demonstrated talent and participation in athletics or the arts, or leadership in school or extracurricular activities. Many schools like to see well-rounded students, so participating in extracurricular activities helps improve a student's chances with some colleges.

Sometimes students take on too much, however. Even at the elementary level, a child may begin participating in so many activities that grades, **sleep**, or **family** life suffer. Many experts recommend that a child narrow down his or her choices to help prevent burnout. Selecting just two activities to begin with instead of four or more may help. Following a routine and helping students learn to prioritize their time will help use extracurricular activities to teach valuable skills. It also helps to allow for some downtime, when kids can be kids, just relaxing and using their **creativity** and imagination. Parents can help by being alert to signs of burnout and by allowing a child to quit an activity when he or she asks to do so.

Resources

BOOKS

Miracle, Andres, and C. Roger Rees. *Lessons of the Locker Room.* New York: Prometheus Books, 1994.

PERIODICALS

Couts, Cherylann. "How Busy Should Your Kid Be?" *Family Life* (October 1, 2001):35.

James, Chantal. "Time Tips." *Choices* (October 2005):33.

"Knock for Jocks." *Psychology Today* 27, (November-December 1994) pp. 12+.

Townsend-Butterworth, Diana. "It's 3:15–Is Your Child Having Fun Yet?" *Family Circle* 108, September 1, 1995, pp. 60+.

Eye abrasion **see** **Corneal abrasion**

Eye and vision development

Definition

Eye and vision development refers to the process of the eye's formation before **birth** and its growth and maturation after birth. The visual system is the part of the central nervous system that enables humans to see. The visual system consists of the eye, the optic nerve, and other pathways to the visual cortex, which is the part of the brain that processes visual images.

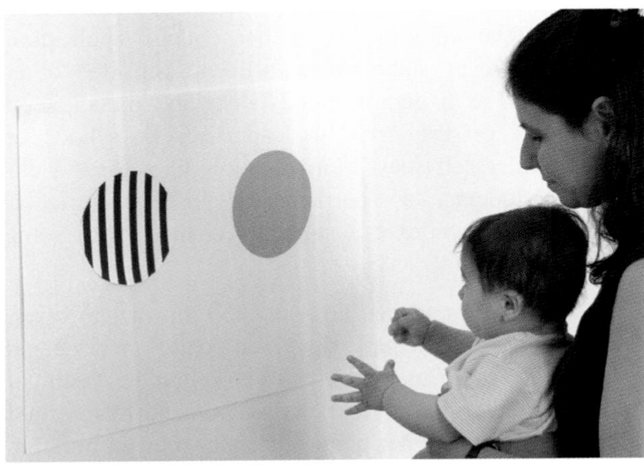

Child being tested for visual acuity. *(© Laura Dwight/Corbis.)*

The human eye itself is often compared to a camera. Light enters the eye through the cornea, the transparent front part of the eye. It then passes through the pupil, an opening in the center of the iris, which is the thin circular structure that governs the size of the pupil and gives the eye its color. The light is further refracted by the lens of the eye, which lies behind the iris. The cornea and lens together act like a compound lens, focusing the image of the object on the retina, the light-sensitive layer of cells at the back of the eyeball. The lens can change its shape to maintain its focus on an object as the viewer's distance from the object changes. This ability to change focus to allow for changes in distance from an object is called accommodation. The information about the image is conveyed from the retina to the visual cortex in the brain via the optic nerve.

Vision disorders can result from diseases or injuries affecting any part of the visual system, or from what are called refractive errors. Refractive errors are not eye diseases in the strict sense but are vision problems resulting from the eye's inability to focus light reflected from an object precisely on the retina at the back of the eyeball. Refractive errors can result from irregularities in the shape of the cornea or lens or an overly long or overly short eyeball.

Demographics

In general, eye problems in developed countries are more common in adults than in children because of the effects of aging and diseases like diabetes on the human eye. According to the World Health Organization (WHO), about 2.6% of the population of the world is considered legally blind (20/200 vision or less). In the United States, about 600,000 people are considered legally blind. Most are over age 60. The leading causes of blindness in the United States—age-related macular degeneration and diabetic retinopathy—are both associated with aging.

Most people have developed one or more refractive errors by the time they are adults. There are three major types of refractive errors: **myopia** (nearsightedness), hyperopia (farsightedness), and astigmatism. In the United States, the rate of myopia in the general population severe enough to require corrective lenses is thought to be between 20 and 25 percent. While a few children are born with myopia, the condition is most likely to appear between age 5 and age 20; about 25 percent of Americans in this age group are nearsighted.

Hyperopia affects about 25% of the general North American population and is often found together with astigmatism. Most babies are mildly hyperopic at birth. Hyperopia in children is usually less severe than hyperopia in adults, partly because the eyeball in many children lengthens as they grow older and allows the eye to focus normally. It is thought that between 6 and 9% percent of children in the United States may have mild hyperopia. As many as a third of the general U.S. population has some degree of astigmatism. Mild astigmatism is considered normal and may not require corrective lenses

Refractive errors tend to run in families. In addition, some times of refractive errors affect some racial and ethnic groups more than others. While astigmatism is equally common in men and women and in all races and ethnic groups, Asian Americans are far more likely to develop nearsightedness than are members of other racial groups. About 78% of Asian Americans have myopia, followed by Hispanics (13%), African Americans (7%), and Caucasians (5%). As far as is known, myopia is equally common in men and women. With regard to farsightedness, Native Americans, African Americans, and Pacific Islanders have higher than average rates of hyperopia.

Description

The human eye begins to develop within two weeks after conception. By six weeks, all the major structures of the eye are formed in the unborn child. The optic nerve completes its development during the last seven months of pregnancy. The infant eye is only partially developed at birth, however; it is only 75% of the size of an adult eye. Newborns are generally very far-sighted—they can see light and shapes and notice movement, but the eyes focus only 8–15 in (20–38 cm) away. This focus corresponds to about 20/400 vision. Eye movements are not coordinated in the newborn, and the eyes may not begin to move together until four weeks or after. Infants are also relatively insensitive to the contrast between bright and dim light. Binocular vision develops between two and six months of age, and by five months, the infant's vision has generally improved to about 20/100. By the age of two, a normal child's vision is still only about 20/60, and 20/20 vision is not approached until the child is between four and five years old, or later.

The newborn eye appears different from the adult eye. The iris lacks pigment, so many Caucasian babies are born with grayish-blue eyes—the mature eye color does not develop for at least six months. The cornea of the infant eye is also relatively large compared to the adult eye. The sclera (the white outer part of the eye) is thin and undeveloped in the newborn and may appear bluish until the scleral fibers develop and thicken. In rare instances, infant cataracts may be present in one or both eyes. The lachrymal glands, which produce tears, generally do not begin to function until the child is about four weeks old, so a newborn may cry without tears. The size and shape of the eyeball changes rapidly during the first years of life, and the optic nerve and the visual parts of the brain are also developing.

Before an infant develops the muscular coordination to move the eyes together, the eyes may move randomly, and the baby may appear intermittently cross-eyed. This is normal for a child under the age of two months. Between two and three months, the infant's eyes begin to move together, and can track a moving object. At around four months, the infant can usually detect and reach for a nearby object. The infant can usually distinguish between objects by six months. Vision improves during the next six months as control of binocular vision develops. In binocular vision, the information transmitted from each eye to the brain along the optic nerve is transformed into a single image. Binocular vision depends on the ability of the eyes to align properly. Precise movement of the eyes is controlled by small muscles around the eye.

Common eye problems in children may result from problems in these muscles (**strabismus**, **amblyopia**), defects of a part of the eye itself (retinal disorders, corneal disorders), or structural defects of the eye (myopia, hyperopia, astigmatism) related to the curvature of the lens or the distance between the lens and the retina at the back of the eyeball. Myopia (nearsightedness), hyperopia (farsightedness), and astigmatism are all considered refractive errors. According to the American Association for Pediatric Ophthalmology and Strabismus (AAPOS), between 2 and 4% of young children have eye problems requiring treatment.

Risk factors

Risk factors for vision problems include a number of genetic and environmental factors:

- Heredity. Refractive errors tend to run in families.
- Race or ethnicity. Different ethnic groups have different rates of refractive errors, as noted above.
- Age. The ability of the lens to accommodate changes in distance declines with age, one reason that many older adults need bifocal corrective lenses. Other age-related problems include gradual drying of the tear ducts that lubricate the eye and increased sensitivity to glare caused by cataracts.
- Diabetes. Diabetes is a risk factor for several serious eye disorders and eventual blindness.
- Being born to a mother with untreated gonorrhea or chlamydia. These sexually transmitted infections can lead to blindness in the infant.
- Premature birth. Premature newborns are at risk of an eye disorder called retinopathy of prematurity (ROP), characterized by disorganized growth of blood vessels in the retina. It may lead to the formation of scar tissue and detachment of the retina.
- Long periods of computer work. Since the 1970s, computers have been increasingly recognized as a factor in what is now called computer vision syndrome (CVS). As many as one out of six persons receiving an eye examination have a computer-related vision problem.

Causes and symptoms

Causes of eye and vision problems range from heredity (a factor in many refractive errors) and infectious diseases to aging, traumatic injury, and systemic diseases such as **cancer** or diabetes.

Parents of young children should be alert to signals of possible eye problems, including crossed eyes, red or swollen eyes or eyelids, drooping eyelids, squinting, shutting or covering one eye, holding the head at an angle, sensitivity to light, holding objects close to the eye, or random or jerky eye movements (in a child older than two months). An older child may complain of inability to see clearly, seeing double, or headaches or nausea after doing close work, and these all may be signs of an eye or vision problem.

Eye problems in adults may include cloudy vision or sensitivity to glare (common symptoms of cataracts); dry eye, neck spasms, and sensitivity to bright lights (computer vision syndrome); discharge, **itching**, or **pain** (infections); blurry vision (side effect of diabetes); severe pain, nausea, **vomiting**, and seeing halos or rainbows around lights (glaucoma).

Diagnosis

Examination

A **pediatrician** will normally examine a child's eyes as part of a regular health checkup. Children aged three or older can be screened for vision by family practitioners, nurses, and technicians at regular well care office visits. In addition, many **day care** programs, churches, schools, and health departments offer vision screening programs for children. Some states require vision screening before the child can enter school. Vision screening at this age includes checking the cornea for irregular shape or structure, checking the pupil of the eye for irregular shape, checking for misalignment of the eyes, and checking the child's distance vision with a simple eye chart designed for children. Children with known risk factors for eye disease, a family history of pediatric eye disease, or signs or symptoms suspicious for a vision problem should have a comprehensive eye examination.

If the child requires a comprehensive visual examination, he or she should be taken to an optometrist, an eye professional who holds the doctor of optometry (OD) degree. Optometrists are trained and licensed to perform examinations of the visual system, diagnose refractive errors, and prescribe corrective lenses.

If a parent or pediatrician suspects that a child has an eye injury or disease requiring surgery, the child should be examined by an ophthalmologist (doctor who specializes in diagnosing and treating eye disorders) or pediatric ophthalmologist (eye doctor specially trained to work with children).

Tests

Initial comprehensive testing of a child or adult's visual system is usually done by an optometrist.

- Patient history. This is the first step in a complete eye examination. The optometrist will ask about the person's general health, history of eye problems (if any), family history of eye disorders, any medications the patient is taking, and any allergies, environmental, or occupational factors that may affect the eyes.

KEY TERMS

Accommodation—The eye's ability to change its focus automatically for viewing objects at different distances.

Amblyopia—Dimness of sight in one eye without any change in the structure of the eye.

Astigmatism—A refractive error caused by irregularities in the shape of the cornea or the lens of the eye.

Cornea—The transparent front part of the eye where light enters the eye.

Hyperopia—Farsightedness.

Myopia—Nearsightedness.

Ophthalmologist—A doctor who specializes in diagnosing and treating eye disorders and can perform eye surgery.

Optic nerve—The nerve that transmits visual information from the retina at the back of the eyeball to the brain. It is also known as cranial nerve II.

Optician—An eye care professional who fills prescriptions for eyeglasses and corrective lenses.

Optometrist—An eye care professional who diagnoses refractive errors and other eye problems and prescribes corrective lenses.

Phoropter—A device positioned in front of a patient's eyes during an eye examination that allows the examiner to place various lenses in front of the eyes to determine the strength of corrective lenses required.

Refractive error—A general term for vision problems caused by the eye's inability to focus light correctly.

Retina—The light-sensitive layer of tissue at the back of the eyeball.

Snellen chart—A series of letters arranged in lines on a chart to be viewed from a distance of 20 feet. It is used to measure visual acuity (clearness of vision). It is named for Hermann Snellen, a Dutch ophthalmologist who invented it in 1862.

Strabismus—A condition in which the eyes are not properly aligned with each other.

Visual cortex—The part of the brain that interprets visual images. It is located at the back of the brain above the cerebellum.

- Visual acuity. Visual acuity refers to the clearness of vision in each eye. It is tested by measuring distance vision, using either a Snellen chart, which uses all the letters of the alphabet arranged in rows of gradually decreasing size, or an Allen chart, which uses the letter E arranged in different positions for children who have not yet learned all the letters of the alphabet. The Allen chart is also known as the Tumbling E chart.

- Specific visual functions. The optometrist will evaluate the patient's color vision, depth perception, ability to move the eye muscles, peripheral (side) vision, and the way the pupils respond to changes in light intensity.
- Keratometry. Keratometry is a measurement of the curvature of the patient's cornea, an important measurement if the person is being fitted for contact lenses. Keratometry is done by focusing a circle of light on the cornea and measuring its reflection.
- Refraction. This part of the examination evaluates the patient for refractive errors. The optometrist uses a phoropter, a device positioned in front of a patient's eyes that allows the examiner to place various lenses in front of the eyes to determine the strength of corrective lenses required. In some cases the optometrist may use eye drops to keep the patient's eyes from changing focus during the testing.
- General eye health. The optometrist may again use eye drops in order to obtain a better view of the internal structures of the eye. Another test commonly performed on adult patients is a measurement of the fluid pressure inside the eye. Normal eye pressures range from 10–21 millimeters of mercury (mm Hg), averaging about 14–16 mm Hg. Anyone with eye pressure greater than 22 mm Hg is at an increased risk of developing glaucoma, a disorder that can lead to blindness.

Treatment

Traditional

For people with normal vision, including mild astigmatism, no treatment is necessary. People with refractive errors may be given a prescription for corrective lenses by the optometrist. The lenses are usually designed and fitted to the patient by an optician, another type of eye care professional who specializes in corrective lenses, both **contact lenses** and eyeglasses.

Patients with evidence of glaucoma, cataract, trauma to the eye, or other disorders requiring eye surgery are usually referred to an ophthalmologist for surgery or other specialized treatment.

Drugs

Some eye disorders, like dry eye, infections of the eye, or high fluid pressure inside the eye, can be treated with various types of eye drops.

Prognosis

The prognosis of vision problems depends on the cause. Almost all refractive errors can be corrected by the use of eyeglasses or contact lenses. Most eye infections can be treated with the use of antibiotic eye drops. Computer vision syndrome can usually be treated with a combination of moisturizing eye drops and changes in the lighting and positioning of the person's computer desk. Cataracts can be safely removed through surgery; about three million such procedures were performed each year in the United States as of 2010. Glaucoma and diabetic retinopathy, however, can lead to eventual blindness if not diagnosed and treated.

Prevention

Refractive errors cannot always be prevented because many are hereditary, and eye disorders associated with aging cannot always be prevented either. People can, however, lower their risk of serious eye disorders or blindness by having regular visual checkups, keeping diabetes and other systemic diseases under control, and seeing their doctor promptly if they develop headaches, dry eyes, pain in the eyes, or other symptoms of a vision problem.

Resources

BOOKS

Bakri, Sophie J., ed. *Mayo Clinic Guide to Better Vision*. Rochester, MN: Mayo Clinic, 2007.

Lueder, Gregg T., ed. *Pediatric Practice: Ophthalmology*. New York: McGraw-Hill, 2011.

Pavan-Langston, Deborah. *Manual of Ocular Diagnosis and Therapy*, 6th ed. Philadelphia: Wolters Kluwer Health/ Lippincott Williams and Wilkins, 2008.

Viegas, Jennifer. *The Eye: Learning How We See*. New York: Rosen Publishing Group, 2002.

PERIODICALS

Augusteyn, R.C. "On the Growth and Internal Structure of the Human Lens." *Experimental Eye Research* 90 (June 2010): 643–54.

Brown, A.M., and D.T. Lindsey. "Contrast Insensitivity: the Critical Immaturity in Infant Visual Performance." *Optometry and Visual Science* 86 (June 2009): 572–76.

Cringle, S.J., and D.Y. Yu. "Oxygen Supply and Consumption in the Retina: Implications for Studies of Retinopathy of Prematurity." *Documenta Ophthalmologica* 120 (February 2010): 99–109.

Frick, K.D., et al. "The Cost of Visual Impairment: Purposes, Perspectives, and Guidance." *Investigative Ophthalmology and Visual Science* 51 (April 2010): 1801–05.

Jancevski, M., and C.S. Foster. "Cataracts and Uveitis." *Current Opinion in Ophthalmology* 21 (January 2010): 10–14.

McKeefry, D.J., et al. "The Noninvasive Dissection of the Human Visual Cortex: Using FMRI and TMS to Study the Organization of the Visual Brain." *Neuroscientist* 15 (October 2009): 489–506.

OTHER

American Academy of Ophthalmology (AAO). "Refractive Errors." http://geteyesmart.org/eyesmart/diseases/refractive–errors.cfm (accessed September 25, 2010).

American Association for Pediatric Ophthalmology and Strabismus (AAPOS). "Vision Screening." http://www.aapos.org/terms_faqs/faq_list/vision_screening (accessed September 25, 2010).

American Optometric Association (AOA). "Comprehensive Eye and Vision Examination." http://www.aoa.org/x4725.xml (accessed September 25, 2010).

American Optometric Association (AOA). "Good Vision Throughout Life." http://www.aoa.org/x9419.xml (accessed September 25, 2010).

Izquierdo, Natalio J., and William Townsend. "Computer Vision Syndrome." eMedicine (May 3, 2010). http://emedicine.medscape.com/article/1229858–overview (accessed September 25, 2010).

National Eye Institute (NEI). "Diagram of the Eye." http://www.nei.nih.gov/health/eyediagram/index.asp (accessed September 25, 2010).

National Eye Institute (NEI). "Facts about Refractive Errors." http://www.nei.nih.gov/CanWeSee/qa_refractive.asp (accessed September 25, 2010).

ORGANIZATIONS

American Academy of Ophthalmology (AAO), PO Box 7424, San Francisco, CA, 94120 (415) 561-8500 (415) 561-8533 eyesmart@aao.org, http://www.aao.org/.

American Association for Pediatric Ophthalmology and Strabismus (AAPOS) aapos@aao.org, http://www.aapos.org/.

American Optometric Association (AOA), 243 N. Lindbergh Blvd., St. Louis, MO, 63141 (800) 365-2219, http://www.aoa.org/.

National Eye Institute (NEI), Information Office, 31 Center Dr., MSC 2510, Bethesda, MD, 20892 (301) 496-5248 2020@nei.nih.gov, http://www.nei.nih.gov/index.asp.

A. Woodward
Rebecca J. Frey, PhD

Eye cancer **see Retinoblastoma**

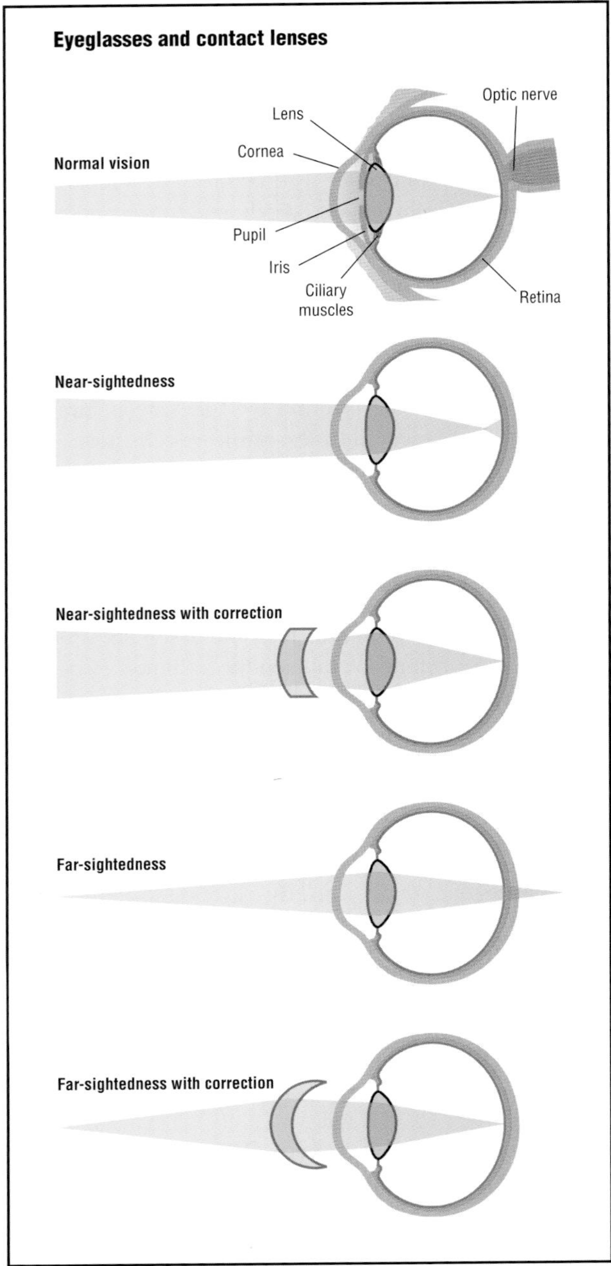

When the eyes function properly, the lens can focus images perfectly on the retina. However, nearsightedness causes the image to focus before it reaches the retina, and farsightedness causes the image to focus past the retina. In each case, a corrective lens is used to adjust the focus of the image to bring a clear picture to the retina, optic nerve, and eventually to the brain. *(Illustration by PreMediaGlobal. Reproduced by permission of Gale, a part of Cengage Learning.)*

Eyeglasses and contact lenses

Definition

Eyeglasses and contact lenses are devices that correct refractive errors in vision. Eyeglass lenses are mounted in frames worn on the face, sitting mostly on the ears and nose, so that the lenses are positioned in front of the eyes. Contact lenses appear to be worn in direct contact with the cornea, but they actually float on a layer of tears that separates them from the cornea.

Purpose

The purpose of eyeglasses and contact lenses is to correct or improve the vision of people with nearsightedness (**myopia**), farsightedness (hyperopia), presbyopia, and astigmatism.

Precautions

People allergic to certain plastics should not wear contact lenses or eyeglass frames or lenses manufactured from that type of plastic. People allergic to nickel should not wear Flexon frames. People at risk of being in accidents that might shatter glass lenses should wear plastic lenses, preferably polycarbonate. (Lenses made from polycarbonate, the same type of plastic used for the space shuttle windshield, are about 50 times stronger than other lens materials.) Also, people at risk of receiving electric shock should avoid metal frames.

People employed in certain occupations may be prohibited from wearing contact lenses or may be required to wear safety eyewear over the contact lenses. Some occupations, such as construction or auto repair, may require safety lenses and safety frames. Physicians and employers should be consulted for recommendations.

Description

Eyes are examined by optometrists (O.D.) or by ophthalmologists (M.D. or D.O.—doctor of osteopathy). Prescriptions, if necessary, are then given to patients for glasses. The glasses are generally made by an optician. A separate contact lens-fitting exam is necessary if the patient wants contact lenses, because an eyeglass prescription is not the same as a contact lens prescription.

Eyeglasses

More than 140 million people in the United States wear eyeglasses. People whose eyes have refractive errors do not see clearly without glasses, because the light emitted from the objects they are observing does not come into focus on their retinas. For people who are farsighted, images come into focus behind the retina; for people who are nearsighted, images come into focus in front of the retina.

LENSES Lenses work by changing the direction of light so that images come into focus on the retina. The greater the index of refraction of the lens material and the greater the difference in the curvature between the two surfaces of the lens, the greater the change in direction of light that passes through it, and the greater the correction.

Lenses can be unifocal, with one correction for all distances, or they can be correct for more than one distance (multifocal). One type of multifocal, the bifocal, has an area of the lens (usually at the bottom) that corrects for nearby objects (about 14 in from the eyes); the remainder of the lens corrects for distant objects (about 20 ft from the eyes). Another type of multifocal, a trifocal, has an area in-between that corrects for intermediate distances (usually about 28 in). Conventional bifocals and trifocals have visible lines between the areas of different correction; however, lenses where the correction gradually changes from one area to the other, without visible lines, have been available since the 1970s. Such lenses are sometimes called progressives or no-line bifocals.

To be suitable for eyeglass lenses, a material must be transparent, without bubbles, and have a high index of refraction. The greater the index of refraction, the thinner the lens can be. Lenses are made from either glass or plastic (hard resin). The advantage of plastic is that it is lightweight and more impact resistant than glass. The advantage of glass is that it is scratch resistant and provides the clearest possible vision.

Glass was the first material to be used for eyeglass lenses and was used for several hundred years before plastic was introduced.

Optical-quality acrylic was introduced for eyeglass use in the early 1940s, but because it was easily scratched, brittle, and discolored rapidly, it did not supplant glass as the material of choice. Furthermore, it wasn't suitable for people with large refractive errors. A plastic called CR-39, introduced in the 1960s, was more suitable. Today, eyeglass wearers can choose between polycarbonate, which is the most impact-resistant material available for eyewear, and polyurethane, which has exceptional optical qualities and higher refraction than the conventional plastics even glass. Patients with high prescriptions should ask about high index material options for their lenses. Aspheric lenses are also useful for high prescriptions. They are flatter and lighter than conventional lenses.

There are many lenses and lens-coating options for individual needs, including coatings that block the ultraviolet (UV) light or UV and blue light, which have been found to be harmful to the eyes. Such coatings are not needed on polycarbonate lenses, which already have UV protection. UV coatings are particularly important on sunglasses and ski goggles. Sunglasses, when nonprescription, should be labeled with an indication that they block out 99–100% of both UV-A and UV-B rays.

There are anti-scratch coatings that increase the surface hardness of lenses (an important feature when using plastic lenses) and anti-reflective (AR) coatings that eliminate almost all glare and allow other people to see the eyes of the wearer. AR coatings may be particularly helpful to people who use computers or who drive at night. Mirror coatings that prevent other people from seeing the wearer's eyes are also available. There is a whole spectrum of tints, from light tints to darker tints, used in sunglasses. Tint, however, does not block out UV rays, so a UV coating is needed. Polaroid lenses that block out much of the reflected light also allow better vision in sunny weather and are helpful for people who enjoy boating. Photosensitive (photochromatic) lenses that darken in the presence of bright light are handy for people who don't want to carry an extra set of glasses. Photochromatic lenses are available in glass and plastic.

FRAMES Frames can be made from metal or plastic, and they can be rimless. There is an almost unlimited variety of shapes, colors, and sizes. The type and degree of refractive correction in the lens determine to some extent the type of frame most suitable. Some lenses are too thick to fit in metal rims, and some large-correction prescriptions are best suited to frames with small-area lenses.

Rimless frames are the least noticeable type, and they are lightweight because the nosepiece and temples are attached directly to the lenses, eliminating the weight of the rims. They tend to not be as sturdy as frames with rims, so they are not a good choice for people who frequently remove their glasses and put them on again. They are also not very suitable for lenses that correct a high degree of farsightedness, because such lenses are thin at the edges.

Metal frames are less noticeable than plastic, and they are lightweight. They are available in solid gold, gold-filled, anodized aluminum, nickel, silver, stainless steel, and now titanium and titanium alloy. Until the late 1980s, when titanium-nickel alloy and titanium frames were introduced, metal frames were, in general, more fragile than plastic frames. The titanium frames, however, are very strong and lightweight. An alloy of titanium and nickel, called Flexon, is not only strong and lightweight, but returns to its original shape after being twisted or dented. It is not perfect for everyone, however, because some people are sensitive to its nickel. Flexon frames are also relatively expensive.

Plastic frames are durable, can accommodate just about any lens prescription, and are available in a wide range of prices. They are also offered in a variety of plastics (including acrylic, epoxy, cellulose acetate, cellulose propionate, polyamide, and nylon) and in different colors, shapes, and levels of resistance to breakage. Epoxy frames are resilient and return to their original shape after being deformed, so they do not need to be adjusted as frequently as other types. Nylon frames are almost unbreakable. They revert to their original shape after extreme trauma and distortion; because of this property, however, they cannot be readjusted after they are manufactured.

FIT The patient should have the distance between the eyes (PD) measured, so that the optical centers of the lenses will be in front of the patient's pupils. Bifocal heights also have to be measured with the chosen frame in place and adjusted on the patient. Again, this is so the lenses will be positioned correctly. If not positioned correctly, the patient may experience eyestrain or other problems. This can occur with over-the-counter reading glasses. The distance between the lenses is for a "standard" person. Generally, this will not be a problem, but if a patient is sensitive or has more closely set eyes, for example, it may pose a problem. Persons buying ready-made sunglasses or reading glasses should hold them up to see if they appear clear. They should also hold the lenses to see an object with straight lines reflected off of the lenses. If the lines don't appear straight, the lenses may be warped or inferior.

Patients may sometimes need a few days to adjust to a new prescription; however, problems should be reported, because the glasses may need to be rechecked.

Contact lenses

More than 32 million people in the United States wear these small lenses that fit on top of the cornea. They provide a field of view unobstructed by eyeglass frames; they do not fog up or get splattered, so it is possible to see well while walking in the rain; and they are less noticeable than any eyeglass style. On the other hand, they take time to get accustomed to; require more measurements for fitting; require many follow-up visits to the eye doctor; can lead to complications, such as infections and corneal damage; and may not correct astigmatism as well as eyeglasses, especially if the astigmatism is severe.

Originally, hard contact lenses were made of a material called PMMA. Although still available, the more common types of contact lenses are listed below:

- Rigid gas-permeable (RGP) daily-wear lenses are made of plastic that does not absorb water but allows oxygen to get from the atmosphere to the cornea. (This is important because the cornea has no blood supply and needs to get its oxygen from the atmosphere through the film of tears that moves beneath the lens.) They must be removed and cleaned each night.

KEY TERMS

Astigmatism—Assymetric vision defects due to irregularities in the cornea.

Cornea—The clear outer covering of the front of the eye.

Index of refraction—A constant number for any material for any given color of light that is an indicator of the degree of the bending of the light caused by that material.

Lens—A device that bends light waves.

Permeable—Capable of allowing substances to pass through.

Polycarbonate—A very strong type of plastic often used in safety glasses, sport glasses, and children's eyeglasses. Polycarbonate lenses have approximately 50 times the impact resistance of glass lenses.

Polymer—A substance formed by joining smaller molecules. For example, plastic, acrylic, cellulose acetate, cellulose propionate, nylon, etc.

Presbyopia—A condition affecting people over the age of 40 where the system of accommodation that allows focusing of near objects fails to work because of age-related hardening of the lens of the eye.

Retina—The inner, light-sensitive layer of the eye containing rods and cones; transforms the image it receives into electrical messages sent to the brain via the optic nerve.

Ultraviolet (UV) light—Part of the electromagnetic spectrum with a wavelength just below that of visible light. It is damaging to living material, especially eyes and DNA.

- Rigid gas-permeable (RGP) extended-wear lenses are made from plastic that also does not absorb water but is more permeable to oxygen than the plastic used for daily-wear lenses. They can be worn up to a week.
- Daily wear soft lenses are made of plastic that is permeable to oxygen and absorbs water; therefore, they are soft and flexible. These lenses must be removed and cleaned each night, and they do not correct all vision problems. Soft lenses are easier to get used to than rigid lenses, but are more prone to tears and do not last as long.
- Extended-wear soft lenses are highly permeable to oxygen, are flexible by virtue of their ability to absorb water, and can usually be worn for up to one week. They do not correct all vision problems. There is more of a risk of infection with extended-wear lenses than with daily-wear lenses.
- Extended-wear disposable lenses are soft lenses worn continually for up to six days and then discarded, with no need for cleaning.
- Planned-replacement soft lenses are daily wear lenses that are replaced on a regular schedule, which is usually every two weeks, monthly, or quarterly. They must also be cleaned.

Soft contact lenses come in a variety of materials. There are also different kinds of RGP and soft multifocal contact lenses available. Monovision, where one contact lens corrects for distance vision while the other corrects for near vision, may be an option for presbyopic patients. Monovision, however, may affect depth perception and may not be appropriate for everyone. Contact lenses also come in a variety of tints. Soft contacts are available that can make eyes appear a different color. Even though such lenses have no prescription, they must still be fitted and checked to make sure that an eye infection does not occur. People should never wear someone else's contact lenses. This can lead to infection or damage to the eye.

Tiny, surgically implanted contact lenses may one day replace eyeglasses, contact lenses and laser surgery for some patients with extreme nearsightedness. Called intraocular lenses, they were approved by the FDA in 2008.

Aftercare

Contact lens wearers must be examined periodically by their eye doctors to make sure that the lenses fit properly and that there is no infection. Infection and lenses that do not fit properly can damage the cornea. Patients can be allergic to certain solutions that are used to clean or lubricate the lenses. For that reason, patients should not randomly switch products without speaking with their doctor. Contact lens wearers should seek immediate attention if they experience eye **pain**, a burning sensation, red eyes, intolerable sensitivity to light, cloudy vision, or an inability to keep the eyes open.

To avoid infection, it is important for contact lens wearers to exactly follow their instructions for lens insertion and removal, as well as cleaning. Soft contact lens wearers should never use tap water to rinse their lenses or to make up solutions. All contact lens wearers should also always have a pair of glasses and a carrying case for their contacts with them, in case the contacts have to be removed due to eye irritation.

Risks

Wearing contact lenses increases the risk of corneal damage and eye infections.

Normal results

The normal expectation is that people will achieve 20/20 vision while wearing corrective lenses. A new technology for customized eyeglasses patented in 2004 claimed to achieve exceptional vision assessment and 20/10 acuity by using wavefront measurements and precise parameters to produce measurements, such as pupil size and distance, along with other customized lens and frame features.

Resources

PERIODICALS

Asp, Karen. "Implanted Contact Lenses." *Prevention* (June 2004): 68.

"Patent Issued for Z-lens Wavefront Guided, Customized Eyeglasses." *Medical Devices & Surgical Technology Week* (April 18, 2004): 150.

OTHER

Contact Lens Council, http://www.contactlenscouncil.org

ORGANIZATIONS

American Academy of Ophthalmology (AAO), P. O. Box 7424, San Francisco, CA, 94120-7424, (415) 561-8500, (415) 561-8533, http://www.aao.org.

American Optometric Association, 243 North Lindbergh Blvd, St. Louis, MO, 63141, (314) 991-4100, http://www.aoanet.org.

Optician Association of America, 7023 Little River Turnpike, Suite 207, Annandale, VA, 22003, (703) 916-8856, http://www.opticians.org.

Lorraine Lica, PhD
Teresa G. Odle

Eyelid disorders

Definition

An eyelid disorder is any abnormal condition that affects the eyelids.

Description

Eyelids consist of thin folds of skin, muscle, and connective tissue. The eyelids protect the eyes and spread tears over the front of the eyes. The inside of the eyelids are lined with the conjunctiva of the eyelid (the palpebral conjunctiva), and the outside of the lids are covered with the body's thinnest skin. Some common lid problems include stye, blepharitis, chalazion, entropion, ectropion, eyelid edema, and eyelid tumors.

Stye

A stye is an infection of one of the three types of eyelid glands near the lid margins at the base of the lashes.

Chalazion

A chalazion is an enlargement of a meibomian gland (an oil-producing gland in the eyelid), usually not associated with an infectious agent. More likely, the gland opening is clogged. Initially, a chalazion may resemble a stye, but it usually grows larger. A chalazion may also be located in the middle of the lid and be internal.

Blepharitis

Blepharitis is the inflammation of the eyelid margins, often with scales and crust. It can lead to eyelash loss, chalazia, styes, ectropion, corneal damage, excessive tearing, and chronic **conjunctivitis**.

Entropion

Entropion is a condition where the eyelid margin (usually the lower one) is turned inward; the eyelashes touch the eye and irritate the cornea.

Ectropion

Ectropion is a condition where one or both eyelid margins turn outward, exposing both the conjunctiva that covers the eye and the conjunctiva that lines the eyelid.

Eyelid edema

Eyelid edema is a condition where the eyelids contain excessive fluid.

Eyelid tumors

Eyelids are susceptible to the same skin tumors as the skin over the rest of the body, including noncancerous tumors and cancerous tumors (basal cell carcinoma, squamous cell carcinoma, malignant melanoma, and sebaceous gland carcinoma). Eyelid muscles are susceptible to sarcoma.

Causes and symptoms

Stye

Styes are usually caused by bacterial **staphylococcal infections**. The symptoms are **pain** and inflammation in one or more localized regions near the eyelid margin.

Chalazion

A chalazion is caused by a blockage in the outflow duct of a meibomian gland. Symptoms are inflammation and swelling in the form of a round lump in the lid that may be painful.

Blepharitis

Some cases of blepharitis are caused by bacterial infection and some by head lice, but in some cases, the cause is unclear. It may also be caused by an overproduction of oil by the meibomian glands. Blepharitis can be a chronic condition that begins in early childhood and can last throughout life. Symptoms can include **itching**, burning, a feeling that something is in the eye, inflammation, and scales or matted, hard crusts surrounding the eyelashes.

Entropion

Entropion usually results from aging, but sometimes can be due to a congenital defect, a spastic eyelid muscle, or a scar on the inside of the lid from surgery, injury, or disease. It is accompanied by excessive tearing, redness, and discomfort.

Ectropion

Similar to entropion, the usual cause of ectropion is aging. It also can be due to a spastic eyelid muscle or a scar, as in entropion. It also can be the result of **allergies**. Symptoms are excessive tearing and hardening of the eyelid conjunctiva.

Eyelid edema

Eyelid edema is most often caused by allergic reactions, for example, allergies to eye makeup, eyedrops or other drugs, or plant allergens such as pollen. Trichinosis, a disease caused by eating undercooked meat, also causes eyelid edema. However, swelling can also be caused by more serious causes, such as infection, and can lead to orbital cellulitis which can threaten vision. Symptoms can include swelling, itching, redness, or pain.

Eyelid tumors

Tumors found on the eyelids are caused by the same conditions that cause these tumors elsewhere on the body. They are usually painless and may or may not be pigmented. Some possible causes include **AIDS** (Kaposi's sarcoma) or increased exposure to ultraviolet (UV) rays which may lead to skin **cancer**.

Diagnosis

An instrument called a slit lamp is generally used to magnify the structures of the eyes. The doctor may press on the lid margin to see if oil can be expressed from the meibomian glands. The doctor may invert the lid to see the inside of the lid. Biopsy is used to diagnose cancerous tumors.

Treatment

Stye

Styes are treated with warm compresses for 10–15 minutes, three to four times a day. Chloramphenicol ointment may be used as well. Sometimes **topical antibiotics** may be prescribed if the infection is spreading.

Chalazion

About 25% of chalazia will disappear spontaneously, but warm compresses may speed the process. Chloramphenicol ointment may be used as well. Because chalazia are inside the lid, topical medications are generally of no benefit. Medication may need to be injected by the doctor into the chalazion or if that doesn't help the chalazion may need to be excised. If what appears to be a chalazion recurs on the same site as any previous one, the possibility of sebaceous gland carcinoma should be investigated by biopsy.

Blepharitis

Blepharitis is treated with hot compresses, with antibiotic ointment, and by cleaning the eyelids with a moist washcloth and then with baby shampoo. Good hygiene is essential. Patients can try to keep rooms dry, such as by placing a bowl of water on top of a radiator. Tear film supplements such as hypromellose can help moisten the eyes when dry. If itching, soreness, or redness occurs from the tear film drops, they should be stopped. Topical or systemic **antibiotics** also may be prescribed. If the blepharitis doesn't clear up with treatment or if it seems to be a chronic problem, the patient may have **acne** rosacea. These patients may need to see a dermatologist as well.

Entropion and ectropion

Both entropion and ectropion can be surgically corrected. Prior to surgery, the lower lid of entropion can be taped down to keep the lashes off the eye, and both can be treated with lubricating drops to keep the cornea moist.

Eyelid edema

Patients with swollen eyelids should contact their eye doctor. A severely swollen lid can press on the eye and possibly increase the intraocular pressure. An infection needs to be ruled out, or something as simple as an allergy to nail polish and then touching the eyes can cause swelling. The best treatment for allergic eyelid edema is to find and remove the substance causing the allergy. When that is not possible, as in the case of plant allergens, cold compresses and immunosuppresesive drugs such as corticosteroid creams are helpful. However, **steroids** can cause cataracts and increase intraocular pressure and patients must be very careful not to get the cream in their eyes. This should not be done unless under a doctor's care. For edema caused by trichinosis, the trichinosis must be treated.

Eyelid tumors

Cancerous tumors should be removed upon discovery, and noncancerous tumors should be removed before they become big enough to interfere with vision or eyelid function. Eyelid tumors require special consideration because of their sensitive location. It is important that treatment not compromise vision, eye movement, or eyelid movement. Accordingly, eyelid reconstruction will sometimes accompany tumor excision.

Prognosis

The prognosis for styes and chalazia is good to excellent. With treatment, blepharitis, ectropion, and entropion usually have good outcomes. The prognosis for nonmalignant tumors, basal cell carcinoma, and squamous cell carcinoma is good once they are properly removed. Survival rate for malignant melanoma depends upon how early it was discovered and if it was completely removed. Sebaceous carcinomas are difficult to detect, so poor outcomes are more frequent.

All of these eyelid disorders, if not treated, can lead to other, possibly serious vision problems—dry eye, astigmatism, or even vision loss, for example. An ophthalmologist or optometrist should be consulted.

Prevention

Good lid hygiene is very important. Regular eyelid washing with baby shampoo helps prevent styes, chalazia, blepharitis, and eyelid edema. To avoid these problems, it's also important to refrain from touching and rubbing the eyes and eyelids, especially with hands that have not just been washed.

Blepharitis is associated with dandruff, which is caused by a kind of bacteria that is one of the causes of blepharitis. Controlling dandruff by washing the hair, scalp, and eyebrows with shampoo containing selenium sulfide to kill the bacteria helps control the blepharitis. When using anything near the eyes, it is important to read the label or consult with a doctor first.

Avoiding allergens helps prevent allergic eyelid edema. Staying inside as much as possible when pollen counts are high and eliminating the use of eye makeup or removing it thoroughly or even using hypo-allergenic makeup may help if the person is sensitive to those substances.

Sunscreen, UV-blocking sunglasses, and wide brimmed hats can help prevent eyelid tumors.

Entropian and ectropian seem to be unpreventable.

KEY TERMS

Allergen—A substance capable of inducing an allergic response.

Allergic reaction—An immune system reaction to a substance in the environment; symptoms include rash, inflammation, sneezing, itchy watery eyes, and runny nose.

Conjunctiva—The mucous membrane that covers the white part of the eyes and lines the eyelids.

Edema—A condition where tissues contain excessive fluid.

Meibomian gland—Oil-producing glands in the eyelids that open near the eyelid margins.

Resources

PERIODICALS

"At a Glance: Chalazion Versus Stye." *GP* May 3, 2004: 52.

"Practical Ophthalmology for GPs: The Treatment of Blepharitis." *Pulse* (May 10, 2004): 60.

OTHER

"Eyelid Abnormalities." *Eye Clinic of Fairbanks,* http://www.eyeclinicfbks.com/ECFLID.htm.

RxMed, http://www.rxmed.com

ORGANIZATIONS

American Academy of Ophthalmology (AAO), P. O. Box 7424, San Francisco, CA, 94120-7424, (415) 561-8500, (415) 561-8533, http://www.aao.org.

American Optometric Association, 243 North Lindbergh Blvd, St. Louis, MO, 63141, (314) 991-4100, http://www.aoanet.org.

American Society of Ophthalmic Plastic and Reconstructive Surgery, 1133 West Morse Blvd, #201, Winter Park, FL, 32789, (407) 647-8839, http://www.asoprs.org.

Lorraine Lica, PhD
Teresa G. Odle

Eyelid problems

Eyelid problems include conditions or diseases that affect the eyelid.

There are a few common conditions that can affect a child's eyelids. A stye is a common problem that is easily treated. It appears as a red bump on the edge of the eyelid and is caused by a bacterial infection in a hair follicle or sweat gland on the lid margin. Warm, moist compresses applied several times a day are a successful treatment. If the stye is stubborn, a **pediatrician** may prescribe an antibiotic ointment.

A chalazion is an inflammation of an oil gland in the underside of the eyelid. It appears as a small bump beneath the eyelid, accompanied by redness and mild discomfort. Like styes, chalazions can be treated with application of warm, moist compresses. Prescription antibiotic ointment or drops may also be necessary. Chalazions often recur, and if they are problematic, a pediatrician may recommend surgery to remove the affected gland.

Ptosis is a condition in which the eyelid or eyelids droop. In some cases it is present from **birth** as the result of incomplete development of the muscles which hold up the lid. Rarely, it is the result of trauma to the cranial nerves at birth. Ptosis may also develop after birth because of some trauma to the eyelid, or because of an underlying disease, such a myasthenia gravis. Ptosis may appear as a droopy, partially lowered lid, as a heavy or enlarged upper lid, or the lid may completely cover the eye. In the rare case of congenital ptosis in which the drooping lid covers the entire eye or pupil, the child may need immediate surgery to correct the condition, so vision will develop normally. In a milder case, surgery is also the advised treatment, but it is usually not done until the child is three or four years old.

Resources

BOOKS

Collins, James F. *Your Eyes: An Owner's Guide.* Englewood Cliffs, NJ: Prentice-Hall, 1995.

Savage, Stephen. *Eyes.* New York: Thomson Learning, 1995.

Showers, Paul. *Look at Your Eyes.* New York: HarperCollins Publishers, 1992.

Zinn, Walter J., and Herbert Solomon. *Complete Guide to Eyecare, Eyeglasses and Contact Lenses.* Hollywood, FL: Lifetime Books, 1995.

ORGANIZATIONS

American Academy of Ophthalmology (AAO), P. O. Box 7424, San Francisco, CA, 94120-7424, (415) 561-8500, (415) 561-8533, http://www.aao.org.

National Eye Institute, Building 31, Room 6A32., Bethesda, MD, 20892, (301) 496-5248

A. Woodward

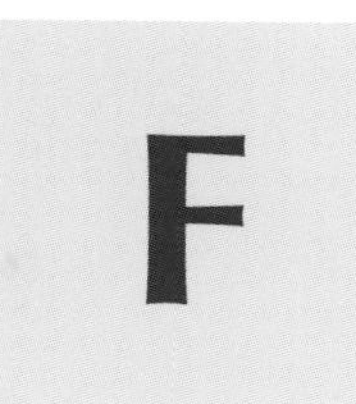

Fabry's disease *see* **Lipidoses**

Facial nerve palsy *see* **Bell's palsy**

Factor VIII deficiency *see* **Hemophilia**

Factor IX deficiency *see* **Hemophilia**

Failing a grade *see* **Retention in school**

Failure to thrive

Definition

Failure to thrive (FTT) is used to describe a serious delay in a child's growth or development. This diagnosis usually is applied to infants and children up to two years of age who do not gain or maintain weight as they should. Failure to thrive is not a specific disease, but rather a cluster of symptoms that may come from a variety of sources.

Demographics

Premature infants are at greatest risk for failure to thrive. As many as 10% of hospitalized young children show some signs of failure to thrive. The rate of failure to thrive for non-specific physiological reasons (nonorganic failure to thrive) is higher in the United Sates than in other developed countries. Internationally **malnutrition** is the most common cause of failure to thrive.

Description

Shortly after **birth** most infants lose some weight. After that expected loss, infants normally gain weight at a steady and predictable rate. When an infant does not gain weigh as expected, or continues to lose weight, it is not thriving. Failure to thrive may be due to one or more conditions.

Organic failure to thrive (OFTT) implies that the organs involved with digestion and absorption of food are malformed or incomplete so the baby cannot digest its food. Nonorganic failure to thrive (NOFTT) is the most common cause of FTT and implies the baby is not receiving enough food due to economic factors parental neglect, or psychosocial problems.

Causes and symptoms

Occasionally, underlying physical conditions inhibit an infant's ability to take in, digest, or process food. These defects can occur anywhere in the digestive tract—in the esophagus, stomach, small or large intestine, rectum or anus. Usually the defect is an incomplete development of the organ, and it must be surgically corrected. Other physical causes of FTT include hormonal abnormalities, chromosomal abnormalities, **cystic fibrosis**, and metabolic disorders. Most physical defects can be detected shortly after birth.

Failure to thrive may also result from lack of available food or the quality of the food offered. This can be due to economic factors in the **family**, parental beliefs and concepts of **nutrition**, or neglect of the child. In addition, if the infant is breast fed, the quality or quantity of the mother's milk may be the source of the problem.

Psychosocial problems, often stemming from lack of a nurturing parent-child relationship can lead to a failure to thrive. The child may exhibit poor appetite due to depression from insufficient attention from parents.

Infants and toddlers whose growth is substantially less than expected, are considered to be suffering from FTT.

Diagnosis

Infants are weighed at birth, and that weight is used as a baseline in future well-baby check-ups. If the infant is not gaining weight at a predictable rate, the doctor will do a more extensive examination. If there are no apparent physical deformities in the digestive tract, the doctor will

KEY TERMS

Esophagus—The muscular tube that leads from the back of the throat to the stomach. Coated with mucus and surrounded by muscles, it pushes food to the stomach by contraction.

Psychosocial—A term referring to the mind's ability to, consciously or unconsciously, adjust and relate the body to its social environment.

examine the child's environment. As part of that examination, the doctor will look at the family history of height and weight. In addition, the parents will be asked about feedings, illnesses, and family routines. If the mother is **breastfeeding** the doctor will also evaluate her diet, general health, and well being as it affects the quantity and quality of her milk.

Treatment

If there is an underlying physical reason for failure to thrive, such as a disorder of swallowing mechanism or intestinal problems, correcting that problem should reverse the condition. If the condition is caused by environmental factors, the physician will suggest several ways parents may provide adequate food for the child. Maternal education and parental counseling may also be recommended. In extreme cases, hospitalization or a more nurturing home may be necessary.

Prognosis

The first year of life is important as a foundation for growth and physical and intellectual development in the future. Children with extreme failure to thrive in the first year may never catch up to their peers, even if their physical growth improves. In about one-third of these extreme cases, mental development remains below normal and roughly half will continue to have psychosocial and eating problems throughout life.

When failure to thrive is identified and corrected early, most children catch up to their peers and remain healthy and well developed.

Prevention

Initial failure to thrive caused by physical defects cannot be prevented but can often be corrected before they become a danger to the child. Maternal education and emotional and economic support systems all help to prevent failure to thrive in those cases where there is no physical deformity.

Parental concerns

Parents who note any of the symptoms of failure to thrive should report them to their child's physician so that treatment can begin.

Resources

OTHER

"Failure to Thrive." MedlinePlus Encyclopedia. August 2, 2009, http://www.nlm.nih.gov/medlineplus/ency/article/000991.htm.

"Failure to Thrive." The Merck Manuals Online. January 2007, http://www.merck.com/mmhe/sec23/ch267/ch267j.html.

Rabinowitz, Simon S., Madhavi Katturupalli, and Genie Rogers. Failure to Thrive. emedicine.com. May 4, 2010, http://emedicine.medscape.com/article/985007-overview.

ORGANIZATIONS

American Academy of Family Physicians, P. O. Box 11210, Shawnee Mission KS, 66207, (913)906-6000, (800) 274-2237, (913) 906-6075, http://familydoctor.org.

American Academy of Pediatrics, 141 Northwest Point Boulevard, Elk Grove Village IL, 60007-1098, (847) 434-4000, (847) 434-8000, http://www.aap.org.

American College of Gastroenterology (ACG), P.O. Box 34226, Bethesda MD, 20827-2260, (301) 263-9000, http://www.acg.gi.org.

American Gastroenterological Association (AGA), 4930 Del Ray Avenue, Bethesda MD, 20814, (310) 654-2055, (301) 654-5920, http://www.gastro.org.

March of Dimes Foundation, 1275 Mamaroneck Avenue, White Plains NY, 10605, (914)997-4488, askus@march-ofdimes.com, http://www.marchofdimes.com.

Dorothy Elinor Stonely
Tish Davidson, A.M.

Familial Mediterranean fever

Definition

Familial Mediterranean **fever** (FMF) is an inherited disorder of the inflammatory response characterized by recurring attacks of fever, accompanied by intense **pain** in the abdomen, chest, or joints. Attacks usually last 12–72 hours, and can occasionally involve a skin rash. Kidney disease is a serious concern if the disorder is not treated. FMF is most prevalent in people of Armenian, Sephardic-Jewish, Arabic, and Turkish ancestry.

Description

FMF could be described as a disorder of "inappropriate" inflammation. That is, an event that in a normal situation causes a mild or unnoticeable inflammation might cause a severe inflammatory response in someone with FMF. Certain areas of the body are at risk for FMF-related symptoms. A serosa is a serous (fluid-producing) membrane that can be found inside the abdominal cavity (peritoneum), around the lungs (pleura), around the heart (pericardium), and inside the joints (synovium). The symptoms of FMF are due to inflammation of one or more of the serosal membranes (serositis). Thus, FMF is also sometimes called recurrent polyserositis.

During an attack, large numbers of neutrophils, a type of white blood cell, move into the affected areas causing painful inflammation and fever. These episodes may be accompanied by a skin rash or joint pain. In a few cases, chronic arthritis is a problem. Amyloidosis is a potentially serious condition in which proteins called amyloids are mistakenly produced and deposited in organs and tissues throughout the body. Left untreated, amyloidosis often leads to kidney failure, which is the major long-term health risk in FMF.

In most cases, the attacks of fever and pain are first noticed in childhood or **adolescence**. The interval between these episodes may be days or months, and is not predictable. However, during these intervals people with FMF typically lead normal lives. It is not entirely clear what brings on an attack, but people with FMF often report mild physical trauma, physical exertion, or emotional stress just prior to the onset of symptoms. Treatment for FMF involves an oral medication called colchicine, which is highly effective for the episodes of fever and pain, as well as for amyloidosis and the kidney disease that can result from it.

FMF is most common in certain ethnic groups from the eastern Mediterranean region, but cases in other ethnic groups in other parts of the world are increasingly being reported. FMF is also known by many other names. They include: recurrent hereditary polyserositis, benign paroxysmal peritonitis, familial paroxysmal polyserositis, paroxysmal polyserositis, familial recurrent polyserositis, periodic fever, periodic amyloid syndrome, periodic peritonitis syndrome, Reimann periodic disease, Reimann syndrome, Siegel-Cattan-Mamou syndrome, and Armenian syndrome.

Estimates of the incidence of FMF in specific eastern Mediterranean populations range from 1 in 2000 to 1 in 100, depending on the population studied. Specific mutations in the MEFV gene are more common in certain ethnic groups, and may cause a somewhat different course of the disease. A few mutations in the MEFV gene likely became common in a small population in the eastern Mediterranean several thousand years ago. It is postulated that carrying a single copy of a mutated gene produced a modified (but not abnormal) inflammatory response that may have been protective against some infectious agent at that time. Those who carried a single "beneficial" mutation in the MEFV gene were more likely to survive and reproduce, which may explain the high carrier frequency (up to one in five) in some populations. People of Armenian, Sephardic-Jewish, Arabic, and Turkish ancestry are at greatest risk for FMF. However, a better understanding and recognition of the symptoms of FMF in recent years has resulted in more reports of the condition in other ethnic groups, such as Italians and Armenian-Americans.

Causes and symptoms

FMF is a genetic condition inherited in an autosomal recessive fashion. Mutations in the MEFV gene (short for Mediterranean Fever) on chromosome number 16 are the underlying cause of FMF. Autosomal recessive inheritance implies that a person with FMF has mutations in both copies of the MEFV gene. All genes come in pairs, and one copy of each pair is inherited from each parent. If neither parent of a child with FMF has the condition, it means they carry one mutated copy of the MEFV gene, but also one normal copy, which is enough to protect them from disease. If both parents carry the same autosomal recessive gene, there is a one in four chance in each pregnancy that the child will inherit both recessive genes, and thus have the condition.

The MEFV gene carries the instructions for production of a protein called pyrin, named for pyrexia, a medical term for fever. The research group in France that co-discovered the protein named it marenostrin, after ancient Latin words that referred to the Mediterranean Sea. The movement of neutrophils into an area of the body where trauma or infection has occurred is the major cause of inflammation, which is a normal process. Research has shown that pyrin has some function in controlling neutrophils. In a situation where minor trauma or stress occurs, some initial inflammation may follow, but a functional pyrin protein is responsible for shutting-down the response of neutrophils once they are no longer needed. An abnormal pyrin protein associated with FMF may be partly functional, but unstable. In some instances, the abnormal pyrin itself seems to be "stressed", and loses its ability to regulate neutrophils and inflammation. Left unregulated, a normal, mild inflammation spirals out of control. Exactly what causes pyrin in FMF to lose its ability to control neutrophils in some situations is not known.

The recurrent acute attacks of FMF typically begin in childhood or adolescence. Episodes of fever and painful inflammation usually last 12–72 hours. About 90% of people with FMF have their first attack by age 20. The group of symptoms that characterizes FMF includes the following:

Fever

An FMF attack is nearly always accompanied by a fever, but it may not be noticed in every case. Fevers are typically 100–104 °F (38–40 °C). Some people experience chills prior to the onset of fever.

Abdominal pain

Nearly all people with FMF experience abdominal pain at one point or another, and for most it is the most common complaint. The pain can range from mild to severe, and can be diffuse or localized. It can mimic **appendicitis**, and many people with undiagnosed FMF have had appendectomies or exploratory surgery of the abdomen done, only to have the fever and abdominal pain return.

Chest pain

Pleuritis, also called pleurisy, occurs in up to half of the affected individuals in certain ethnic groups. The pain is usually on one side of the chest. Pericarditis would also be felt as chest pain.

Joint pain

About 50% of people with FMF experience joint pain during attacks. The pain is usually confined to one joint at a time, and often involves the hip, knee, or ankle. For some people, however, the recurrent joint pain becomes chronic arthritis.

Myalgia

Up to 20% of individuals report muscle pain. These episodes typically last less than two days, and tend to occur in the evening or after physical exertion. Rare cases of muscle pain and fever lasting up to one month have been reported.

Skin rash

A rash, described as erysipelas-like erythema, accompanies attacks in a minority of people, and most often occurs on the front of the lower leg or top of the foot. The rash appears as a red, warm, swollen area about 4–6 in (10–15 cm) in diameter.

Amyloidosis

FMF is associated with high levels in the blood of a protein called serum amyloid A (SAA). Over time, excess SAA tends to be deposited in tissues and organs throughout the body. The presence and deposition of excess SAA is known as amyloidosis. Amyloidosis may affect the gastrointestinal tract, liver, spleen, heart, and testes, but effects on the kidneys are of greatest concern. The frequency of amyloidosis varies among the different ethnic groups, and its overall incidence is difficult to determine because of the use of colchicine to avert the problem. Left untreated, however, those individuals who do develop amyloidosis of the kidneys may require a renal transplant, or may even die of renal failure. The frequency and severity of a person's attacks of fever and serositis seem to have no relation to whether they will develop amyloidosis. In fact, a few people with FMF have been described who have had amyloidosis but apparently no other FMF-related symptoms.

Other symptoms

A small percentage of boys with FMF develop painful inflammation around the testes, headaches are a common occurrence during attacks, and certain types of vasculitis (inflammation of the blood vessels) seem to be more common in FMF.

Diagnosis

Individually, the symptoms that define FMF are common. Fevers occur for many reasons, and nonspecific pains in the abdomen, chest, and joints are also frequent ailments. Several infections can result in symptoms similar to FMF (Mallaret **meningitis**, for instance), and many people with FMF undergo exploratory abdominal surgery and ineffective treatments before they are finally diagnosed. Membership in a less commonly affected ethnic group may delay or hinder the correct diagnosis.

In general, symptoms involving one or more of the following broad groups should lead to suspicion of FMF: Unexplained recurrent fevers, polyserositis, skin rash, and/or joint pain; abnormal blood studies (see below); and renal or other disease associated with amyloidosis. A family history of FMF or its symptoms would obviously be an important clue, but the recessive nature of FMF means there usually is no family history. The diagnosis may be confirmed when a person with unexplained fever and pain responds to treatment with colchicine since colchicine is not known to have a beneficial effect on any other condition similar to FMF. Abnormal results on a blood test typically include leukocytosis (elevated number of neutrophils in the blood), an increased erythrocyte sedimentation rate (rate at which red blood cells form a sediment in a blood sample), and increased levels of proteins associated with inflammation (called acute phase reactants) such as SAA.

Direct analysis of the MEFV gene for FMF mutations is the only method to be certain of the diagnosis. However, it is not yet possible to detect all MEFV gene mutations that might cause FMF. Thus, if DNA analysis is negative, clinical methods must be relied upon. If both members of a couple were proven to be FMF carriers through **genetic testing**, highly accurate prenatal diagnosis would be available in any subsequent pregnancy.

Similar syndromes of periodic fever and inflammation include familial Hibernian fever and hyperimmunoglobulinemia D syndrome, but both are more rare than FMF.

Treatment

Colchicine is a chemical compound that can be used as a medication, and is frequently prescribed for gout. Some years ago, colchicine was discovered to also be effective in reducing the frequency and severity of attacks in FMF. Treatment for FMF at this point consists of taking colchicine daily. Studies have shown that about 75% of FMF patients achieve complete remission of their symptoms, and about 95% show marked improvement when taking colchicine. Lower effectiveness has been reported, but there is some question about the number of FMF patients who choose not to take their colchicine between attacks when they are feeling well, and thus lose some of the ability to prevent attacks. Compliance with taking colchicine every day may be hampered by its side effects, which include **diarrhea**, nausea, abdominal bloating, and gas. There is a theoretical risk that colchicine use could damage chromosomes in sperms and eggs, or in an embryo during pregnancy, or that it might reduce fertility. However, studies looking at reproduction in men and women who have used colchicine have so far not shown any increased risks. Colchicine is also effective in preventing, delaying, or reversing renal disease associated with amyloidosis.

Other medications may be used as needed to deal with the pain and fever associated with FMF attacks. Dialysis and/or renal transplant might become necessary in someone with advanced kidney disease. Given its genetic nature, there is no cure for FMF, nor is there likely to be in the near future. Any couple that has a child diagnosed with FMF, or anyone with a family history of the condition (especially those in high-risk ethnic groups), should be offered genetic counseling to obtain the most up-to-date information on FMF and testing options.

KEY TERMS

Acute phase reactants—Blood proteins whose concentrations increase or decrease in reaction to the inflammation process.

Amyloid—A waxy translucent substance composed mostly of protein, that forms plaques (abnormal deposits) in the brain.

Amyloidosis—Accumulation of amyloid deposits in various organs and tissues in the body such that normal functioning of an organ is compromised.

Colchicine—A compound that blocks the assembly of microtubules–protein fibers necessary for cell division and some kinds of cell movements, including neutrophil migration. Side effects may include diarrhea, abdominal bloating, and gas.

Leukocyte—A white blood cell. The neutrophils are a type of leukocyte.

Leukocytosis—An increase in the number of leukocytes in the blood.

Neutrophil—The primary type of white blood cell involved in inflammation. Neutrophils are a type of granulocyte, also known as a polymorphonuclear leukocyte.

Pericarditis—Inflammation of the pericardium, the membrane surrounding the heart.

Peritonitis—Inflammation of the peritoneum, the membrane surrounding the abdominal contents.

Pleuritis—Inflammation of the pleura, the membrane surrounding the lungs.

Pyrexia—A medical term denoting fevers.

Serositis—Inflammation of a serosal membrane. Polyserositis refers to the inflammation of two or more serosal membranes.

Synovitis—Inflammation of the synovium, a membrane found inside joints.

Prognosis

For those individuals who are diagnosed early enough and take colchicine consistently, the prognosis is excellent. Most will have very few, if any, attacks of fever and polyserositis, and will likely not develop serious complications of amyloidosis. The problem of misdiagnosing FMF continues, but education attempts directed at both the public and medical care providers should improve the situation. Future research should provide a better understanding of the inflammation process, focusing on how neutrophils are genetically regulated. That information could then be used to develop treatments for FMF with fewer side effects, and might also assist in developing therapies for other diseases in which abnormal inflammation and immune response are a problem.

ORGANIZATIONS

National Institute of Arthritis and Musculoskeletal and Skin Diseases, 1 AMS Circle, Bethesda MD, 20892, (877) 226-4267, http://www.niams.nih.gov.

National Organization for Rare Disorders (NORD), 55 Kenosia Avenue, P. O. Box 1968 Danbury CT, 06813-1968 (203) 744-0100, (800) 999-6673, http://www.rarediseases.org.

National Society of Genetic Counselors, 233 Canterbury Dr., Wallingford PA, 19086-6617, (610) 872-1192, http://www.nsgc.org/GeneticCounselingYou.asp.

Scott J. Polzin, M.S.

Family

Definition

Family is broadly defined as any two people who are related to each other through a genetic connection, **adoption**, marriage, or by mutual agreement.

Description

Family members share emotional and economic bonds. The term *nuclear family* is used to refer to family members who live together and share emotional, economic, and social responsibilities. The nuclear family is often comprised of a married couple who are parents to their biological or adopted children; all members live together in one household. This type of nuclear family is increasingly referred to by social scientists as an *intact family,* signifying that the family had not been through a **divorce**, separation, or **death** of a member. The U.S. Bureau of Census statistics on families are presented in the accompanying tables. The data are based on past census information and future projections.

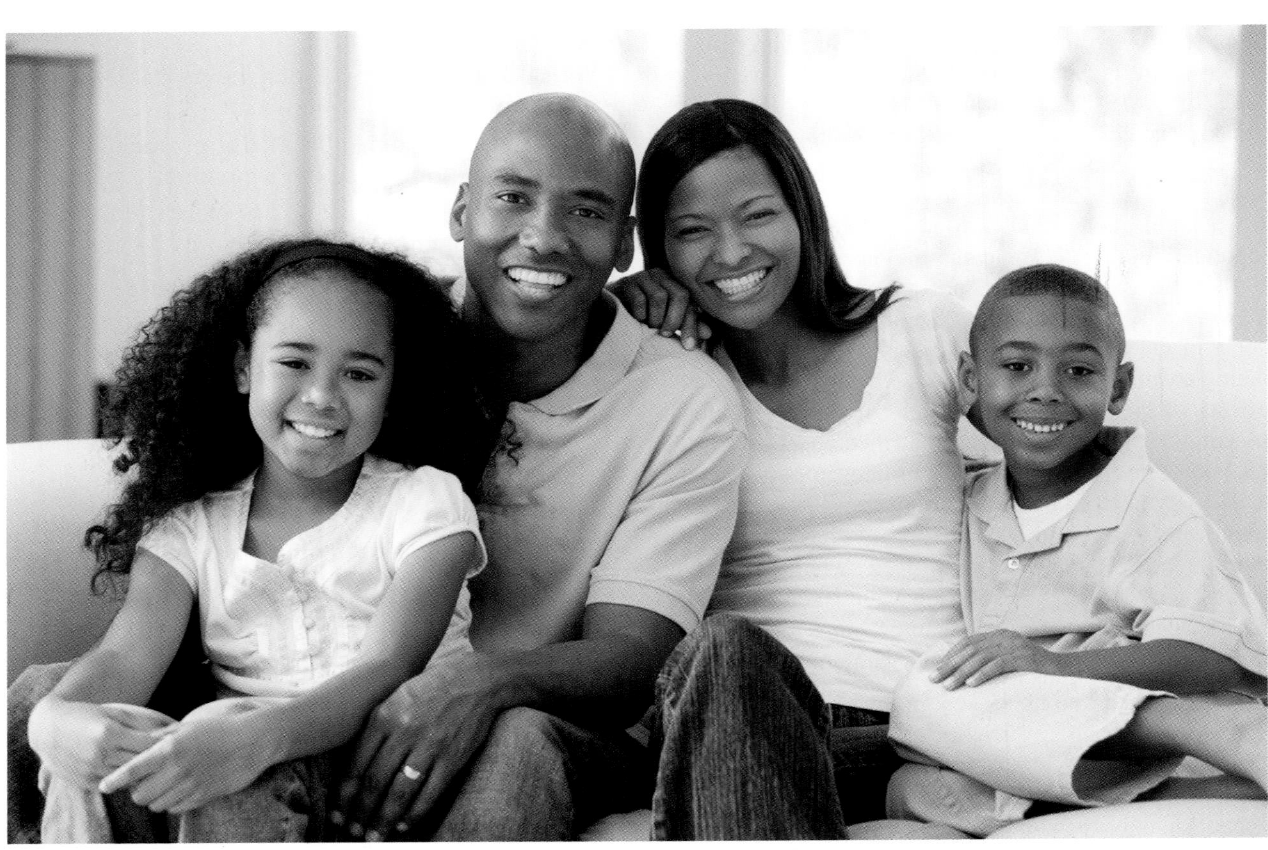

A family consisting of a mother, a father, a daughter, and a son. *(© iStockPhoto.com/Catherine Yeulet.)*

In addition to the nuclear family, other complex and diverse combinations of individuals lead to what social scientists call blended or nontraditional families. When a family has experienced divorce or death leaving one parent to be primarily responsible for raising the children, they become a *single-parent family*. (The terms *broken family* and *broken home* are no longer widely used because of their negative connotations.)

Following the end of one marriage, one or both of the ex-spouses may enter a new marriage. Through this process of remarriage, stepfamilies are formed. The second spouse becomes a step-parent to the children from the first marriage. In the family formed by the second marriage, the children from each spouse's first marriage become step-siblings. Children born or adopted by the couple of the second marriage are half-siblings to the children from the first marriage, since they share one parent in common.

In some cases, a step-parent will legally adopt his or her spouse's children from a previous marriage. The biological father or mother must either be absent with no legal claim to **custody**, or must grant permission for the step-parent to adopt.

In situations where a single parent lives with someone outside of marriage, that person may be referred to as a co-parent. Co-parent is also the name that may be given to the partner in a homosexual relationship who shares the household and parenting responsibilities with a child's legal adoptive or **biological parent**. The focus on families with homosexual heads of household increased in 2004 to 2006 as gay marriage became a heated political issue. Nationwide, the number of self-identified same sex couples sharing a household surged 30% in 2005 to reach 1.5 million people. About one-third of the homes include children.

The home that was owned by the family prior to a divorce or separation is referred to as the *family home* in many state laws. In court settlements of divorce and child custody issues, the sale of the family home may be prohibited as long as the minor children are still living there with the custodial parent. The sale of the home may be permitted (or required to pay the noncustodial parent his or her share of its value) if the custodial parent moves or remarries, or when the children leave home to establish their own residences.

The term *extended family* traditionally meant the biological relatives of a nuclear family; i.e., the parents, sisters, and brothers of both members of a married couple. It was sometimes used to refer to the people living in the household beyond the parents and children. As family relationships and configurations have become more complex due to divorce and remarriage, extended family has come to refer to all the biological, adoptive, step-, and half-relatives.

Family structure of children ages 0–17 by presence of parents in household, 2009

Parent(s) living in household	Percentage of families
Two married parents	69.8
Two unmarried parents	3.0
Mother only	22.8
Father only	3.4
No parent	4.0

SOURCE: U.S. Census Bureau, Current Population Survey, "America's Families and Living Arrangements: 2009." Available online at: http://www.census.gov/population/www/socdemo/hh-fam/cps2009.html (accessed September 2, 2010).

(Table by PreMediaGlobal. Reproduced by permission of Gale, a part of Cengage Learning.)

Government agencies and other statistics-gathering organizations use the term *head of household* to refer to the person who contributes more than half of the necessary support of the family members (other than the spouse); in common usage, the head of household is the person who provides primary financial support for the family.

Resources

BOOKS

Bernardes, Jon. *Family Studies: An Introduction.* New York: Routledge, 1997.

PERIODICALS

Michels, Scott. "For Gays, New Math." *U.S. News and World Report* (August 14, 2006): 34-36.

Seckler, Valerie. "Census Reveals More Diversity in Gay Market." *WWD* (October 12, 2006): 11.

ORGANIZATIONS

Family Service Association of America (FSA), 11600 West Lake Park Drive, Milwaukee WI, 53244, (414) 359-1040, (800) 221-3726

Step Family Foundation (SFF), 333 West End Avenue, New York NY, 10023, (212) 877-3244

Family therapy

Definition

Family therapy is a form of psychotherapy that involves all the members of a nuclear or extended family. It may be conducted by a pair or team of therapists. In many cases the team consists of a man and a woman in order to treat gender-related issues or serve as role models for family members. Although some forms of family therapy are based on behavioral or psychodynamic principles, the most widespread form is based on family systems theory. This approach regards the family, as a whole, as the unit of treatment, and emphasizes such factors as relationships and communication patterns rather than traits or symptoms in individual members.

Family therapy is a relatively recent development in psychotherapy. It began shortly after World War II, when doctors, who were treating schizophrenic patients, noticed that the patients' families communicated in disturbed ways. The doctors also found that the patients' symptoms rose or fell according to the level of tension between their parents. These observations led to considering a family as an organism or system with its own internal rules, patterns of functioning, and tendency to resist change. The therapists started to treat the families of schizophrenic patients as whole units rather than focusing on the hospitalized member. They found that in many cases the family member with **schizophrenia** improved when the "patient" was the family system. (This should not be misunderstood to mean that schizophrenia is caused by family problems, although family problems may worsen the condition.) This approach of involving the entire family in the treatment plan and therapy was then applied to families with problems other than the presence of schizophrenia.

Family therapy is becoming an increasingly common form of treatment as changes in American society are reflected in family structures. It has led to two further developments: couples therapy, which treats relationship problems between marriage partners or gay couples; and the extension of family therapy to religious communities or other groups that resemble families.

Purpose

Family therapy is often recommended in the following situations:

- Treatment of a family member with schizophrenia or multiple personality disorder (MPD). Family therapy helps other family members understand their relative's disorder and adjust to the psychological changes that may be occurring in the relative.
- Families with problems across generational boundaries. These would include problems caused by parents sharing housing with grandparents, or children being reared by grandparents.
- Families that deviate from social norms (common-law relationships, gay couples rearing children, etc.). These families may not have internal problems but may be troubled by outsiders' judgmental attitudes.
- Families with members from a mixture of racial, cultural, or religious backgrounds.
- Families who are scapegoating a member or undermining the treatment of a member in individual therapy.
- Families where the identified patient's problems seem inextricably tied to problems with other family members.
- Blended families with adjustment difficulties.

Most family therapists presuppose an average level of **intelligence** and education on the part of adult members of the family.

Precautions

Some families are not considered suitable candidates for family therapy. They include:

- families in which one, or both, of the parents is psychotic or has been diagnosed with antisocial or paranoid personality disorder,
- families whose cultural or religious values are opposed to, or suspicious of, psychotherapy,
- families with members who cannot participate in treatment sessions because of physical illness or similar limitations,
- families with members with very rigid personality structures. (Here, members might be at risk for an emotional or psychological crisis),
- families whose members cannot or will not be able to meet regularly for treatment,
- families that are unstable or on the verge of breakup.

Description

Family therapy tends to be short-term treatment, usually several months in length, with a focus on resolving specific problems such as **eating disorders**, difficulties with school, or adjustments to bereavement or geographical relocation. It is not normally used for long-term or intensive restructuring of severely dysfunctional families.

In family therapy sessions, all members of the family and both therapists (if there is more than one) are present at most sessions. The therapists seek to analyze the process of family interaction and communication as a whole; they do not take sides with specific members. They may make occasional comments or remarks intended to help family members become more conscious of patterns or structures that had been previously taken for granted. Family therapists, who work as a team, also model new behaviors for the family through their interactions with each other during sessions.

Family therapy is based on family systems theory, which understands the family to be a living organism that is more than the sum of its individual members. Family therapy uses "systems" theory to evaluate family members in terms of their position or role within the system as a whole. Problems are treated by changing the way the system works rather than trying to "fix" a specific member. Family systems theory is based on several major concepts:

Family therapy can be and is usually provided by clinical social workers or licensed therapists known as marriage and family therapists. Many of these therapists have postgraduate degrees and often become credentialed by the American Association for Marriage and Family Therapy (AAMFT).

The identified patient

The identified patient (IP) is the family member with the symptom that has brought the family into treatment. The concept of the IP is used by family therapists to keep the family from scapegoating the IP or using him or her as a way of avoiding problems in the rest of the system.

Homeostasis (balance)

The concept of homeostasis means that the family system seeks to maintain its customary organization and functioning over time. It tends to resist change. The family therapist can use the concept of homeostasis to explain why a certain family symptom has surfaced at a given time, why a specific member has become the IP, and what is likely to happen when the family begins to change.

The extended family field

The extended family field refers to the nuclear family, plus the network of **grandparents** and other members of the extended family. This concept is used to explain the intergenerational transmission of attitudes, problems, behaviors, and other issues.

Differentiation

Differentiation refers to the ability of each family member to maintain his or her own sense of self, while remaining emotionally connected to the family. One mark of a healthy family is its capacity to allow members to differentiate, while family members still feel that they are "members in good standing" of the family.

Triangular relationships

Family systems theory maintains that emotional relationships in families are usually triangular. Whenever any two persons in the family system have problems with each other, they will "triangle in" a third member as a way of stabilizing their own relationship. The triangles in a family system usually interlock in a way that maintains family homeostasis. Common family triangles include a child and its parents; two children and one parent; a parent, a child, and a grandparent; three siblings; or, husband, wife, and an in-law.

Preparation

In some instances the family may have been referred to a specialist in family therapy by their **pediatrician** or other primary care provider. It is estimated that as many as 50% of office visits to pediatricians have to do with developmental problems in children that are affecting their families. Some family doctors use symptom checklists or psychological screeners to assess a family's need for therapy.

Family therapists may be either psychiatrists, clinical psychologists, or other professionals certified by a specialty board in marriage and family therapy. They will usually evaluate a family for treatment by scheduling a series of interviews with the members of the immediate family, including young children, and significant or symptomatic members of the extended family. This process allows the therapist(s) to find out how each member of the family sees the problem, as well as to form first impressions of the family's functioning. Family therapists typically look for the level and types of emotions expressed, patterns of dominance and submission, the roles played by family members, communication styles, and the locations of emotional triangles. They will also note whether these patterns are rigid or relatively flexible.

Preparation also usually includes drawing a genogram, which is a diagram that depicts significant persons and events in the family's history. Genograms also include annotations about the medical history and major personality traits of each member. Genograms help in uncovering intergenerational patterns of behavior, marriage choices, family alliances and conflicts, the existence of family secrets, and other information that sheds light on the family's present situation.

KEY TERMS

Blended family—A family formed by the remarriage of a divorced or widowed parent. It includes the new husband and wife, plus some or all of their children from previous marriages.

Differentiation—The ability to retain one's identity within a family system while maintaining emotional connections with the other members.

Extended family field—A person's family of origin plus grandparents, in-laws, and other relatives.

Family systems theory—An approach to treatment that emphasizes the interdependency of family members rather than focusing on individuals in isolation from the family. This theory underlies the most influential forms of contemporary family therapy.

Genogram—A family tree diagram that represents the names, birth order, sex, and relationships of the members of a family. Therapists use genograms to detect recurrent patterns in the family history and to help the members understand their problem(s).

Homeostasis—The tendency of a family system to maintain internal stability and resist change.

Identified patient (IP)—The family member in whom the family's symptom has emerged or is most obvious.

Nuclear family—The basic family unit, consisting of father, mother, and their biological children.

Triangling—A process in which two family members lower the tension level between them by drawing in a third member.

Risks

The chief risk in family therapy is the possible unsettling of rigid personality defenses in individuals, or couple relationships that had been fragile before the beginning of therapy. Intensive family therapy may also be difficult for psychotic family members.

Normal results

Normal results vary, but in good circumstances, they include greater insight, increased differentiation of individual family members, improved communication within the family, loosening of previously automatic behavior patterns, and resolution of the problem that led the family to seek treatment.

Resources

BOOKS

Gurman AS, et al. Family Therapy and Couple Therapy. In: Sadock BJ, et al. *Kaplan & Sadock's Comprehensive Textbook of Psychiatry. 8th ed.* Philadelphia, Pa.: Lippincott Williams & Wilkins; 2005.

OTHER

Marriage and Family Therapists: The Family-Friendly Mental Health Professionals. American Association for Marriage and Family Therapy (AAMFT), http://www.aamft.org/Press_Room/MFT%20Brochure%207-03.htm. Accessed July 20, 2010.

Rebecca J. Frey, PhD
Karl Finley

FAS **see Fetal alcohol syndrome**

Father-child relationships **see Parent-child relationships**

Fear

Definition

Fear is an emotional and physical reaction related to a person, place, activity, event, or object that causes emotional distress and often avoidance behavior.

Description

Biological dimension of fear

Children and adolescents experience the same physical reactions to fear as adults. In humans, the biochemical response to fear is known as the "fight–or–flight" reaction. It begins with the activation of a section of the brain called the hypothalamic–pituitary–adrenal system, or HPA. This system first activates the release of steroid hormones, also known as glucocorticoids. These hormones include cortisol, the primary stress hormone in humans.

The HPA system then releases a set of neurotransmitters called catecholamines. The catecholamines include dopamine, norepinephrine, and epinephrine (also known as adrenaline). Catecholamines have three important effects:

- They activate the amygdala, an almond–shaped structure in the limbic system that triggers an emotional response of fear.

- They signal the hippocampus, another part of the limbic system, to store the emotional experience in long–term memory. This storage helps to explain why memories can trigger fear reactions as well as a present situation or object.
- Catecholamines also suppress activity in parts of the brain associated with short–term memory, concentration, and rational thinking. This suppression allows a human to react quickly to a stressful situation, but it also lowers ability to deal with complex social or intellectual tasks that may be part of the situation.

Fear causes heart rate and blood pressure to rise. The person breathes more rapidly, which allows the lungs to take in more oxygen. Blood flow to the muscles, lungs, and brain may increase by 300–400 percent. The spleen releases more blood cells into the circulation, which increases the blood's ability to transport oxygen. The **immune system** redirects white blood cells to the skin, bone marrow, and lymph nodes because these are areas where injury or infection is most likely to occur.

At the same time, nonessential body systems shut down. The skin becomes cool and sweaty as blood is drawn away from it toward the heart and muscles. The mouth becomes dry, and the digestive system slows down. These physical responses help to explain the headaches, nausea, **vomiting**, chest pains, **dizziness**, and cold sweats that many people feel when they experience fear.

Not all humans experience fear with the same degree of physical intensity. The differences among people in this regard are genetic. A person who seems to have unusually strong reactions to fear may well have inherited this characteristic from his or her parents.

The range of children's fears

Symptoms of fear may include stiffening and crying in the newborn; crying and avoidance of the feared person or object in toddlers; such bodily symptoms as a **stomachache** or **headache** in children or adolescents (especially regarding school or separation anxieties); anger, avoidance, and denial of the fear in adolescents and adults; and panic reactions—sweating, trembling, and a racing heartbeat. While normal fears tend to be experienced in phases and tend to be outgrown by adulthood, unwarranted abnormal fears are those that are persistent and recurrent, or fears that interfere with daily activities for at least a month. Abnormal fears, including extreme **separation anxiety**, **school refusal** (being afraid to go to school), or extreme social fears, may indicate the presence of an **anxiety** disorder.

Children's fears exist along a continuum from what are called age–appropriate anxious variations to anxiety problems to full–blown anxiety disorders. Anxiety problems are distinguished from anxiety disorders by two characteristics: the degree of the person's distress and whether the fear subsides when the stimulus is removed. A person with an anxiety problem has a higher degree of fear of a specific object or situation than is considered age–appropriate, but is able to function and usually feels relief from the fear as soon as he or she has left the feared situation or avoided the feared object. A person with an anxiety disorder, on the other hand, is so fearful that he or she cannot carry out normal activities of daily life (ADLs), and removal of the feared object does not always relieve the anxiety.

More than 50 percent of children experience simple **phobias** (fear of a specific object) or anxieties (more general worries) before they are 18 years old. For adults it may be helpful to distinguish between rational fears, such as fear of snakes or guns, which are survival mechanisms and serve to protect a person from danger, and irrational fears (phobias) which cannot be traced to any reasonable cause. Many childhood fears fall somewhere between the rational and irrational, occurring in phases as the child or adolescent is exposed to new experiences and as both cognitive reasoning and the capacity for imagination develop. Whether a child's fear is considered normal generally depends on his or her age, background, and most importantly by the extent to which the fear interferes with his or her normal daily activities. Fear of water may be considered normal in a child who has never learned to swim, but it might be considered abnormal in the adolescent son of a swimming coach.

There are many avenues that parents, guardians, and teachers can follow in responding to childhood or adolescent fears. The first step is to assess whether the fear is age–normal. Following are some normal fears of **infancy**, toddlerhood, and **preschool** years and their approximate ages of occurrence.

- Infants: fear of being dropped or of falling; most are also afraid of loud noises
- Toddlerhood/Preschool: fear of strangers, animals, insects, storms, darkness, people with masks, monsters, "bad" people; fear of being separated from parents or attachment figures (i.e., age–appropriate separation anxiety); fear of being left alone, especially at night.
- School–age years: separation anxiety; fear of death and violence (war, murder, kidnapping); anxiety about school achievement.
- Adolescence: anxiety about school achievement; fear of social rejection and related worries; sexual anxieties; fear of other new experiences (public speaking, musical performance, learning to drive)

KEY TERMS

Anxiety—Worry or tension in response to real or imagined stress, danger, or dreaded situations. Physical reactions, such as fast pulse, sweating, trembling, fatigue, and weakness may accompany anxiety.

Catecholamines—Family of neurotransmitters containing dopamine, norepinephrine and epinephrine, produced and secreted by cells of the adrenal medulla and the brain. Catecholamines have excitatory effects on smooth muscle cells of the vessels that supply blood to the skin and mucous membranes and have inhibitory effects on smooth muscle cells located in the wall of the gut, the bronchial tree of the lungs, and the vessels that supply blood to skeletal muscle. There are two different main types of receptors for these neurotransmitters, called alpha and beta adrenergic receptors. The catecholamines are therefore are also known as adrenergic neurotransmitters.

Desensitization—A treatment for phobias which involves exposing the phobic person to the feared situation. It is often used in conjunction with relaxation techniques. Also used to describe a technique of pain reduction in which the painful area is stimulated with whatever is causing the pain.

Neurotransmitter—One of a group of chemicals secreted by a nerve cell (neuron) to carry a chemical message to another nerve cell, often as a way of transmitting a nerve impulse. Examples of neurotransmitters include acetylcholine, dopamine, serotonin, and norepinephrine.

Phobia—An intense, abnormal, or illogical fear of something specific, such as heights or open spaces.

Other fears not associated with any specific age are fear of visiting the doctor or dentist; fear of traveling by car, boat, or plane; and fear of going to school, sometimes called school refusal. School refusal often results in a refusal to attend school and is caused either by a deeper separation anxiety or fear of some aspect of the school environment. It is not considered a separate type of anxiety disorder but rather a complex syndrome with many causes and characterized by a high level of fear and anxiety. Many children experience a mild temporary form of school refusal. If refusal to attend school lasts longer than three days in a row, however, parents might want to seek the help of a school counselor in addressing the underlying problem(s). In earlier grades the many new experiences of school may contribute to school refusal—being with strange authority figures, older children, submitting to a new rule system, publicly performing or speaking. In later grades the social and academic or extracurricular pressures may create additional fears. The child may also be afraid of bullying at school. It is thought that between one and five percent of school–age children and adolescents have school refusal.

The most significant factors in overcoming fear are identifying the fear, developing a sense of control over the feared environment (autonomy), and envisioning alternatives to the feared negative outcomes. Forcing children to perform activities they are afraid to do destroys rather than builds autonomy and self–confidence. If a child refuses to do something or explicitly voices fear, the feelings should be taken seriously and explored through questioning and discussion. Ask the child or adolescent what change can be made to accommodate the fear and make him or her feel more in control of the situation.

Some theories hold that reading scary picture books functions as a courage–building tool for children and helps them face their fears in a controlled environment; they are free to turn the page or to remind themselves that the monster is not real. Horror stories or movies may serve the same purpose for teens (although children do not have the same level of choice in leaving the theater and should not be exposed to disturbing movies). Controlled exposure, which involves gradually introducing the child to the source of fear, often provides the necessary structure for addressing most fears. For instance, treating a child's fear of water might begin by incrementally filling the bathtub higher and working up to wading in a small stream or baby pool. This approach is sometimes called desensitization. Treating or preventing school phobias may require repeated short visits to the school accompanied by the parent, and brief meetings or gatherings with teachers and/or groups of other children before leaving the child alone.

Before, during, and after exposure to the source of fear, the child can begin to imagine controlling the environment and his own reactions in other ways. Creative visualization can be used, for example, to imagine a switch the child can use to control his fear when visiting the doctor or dentist. A comforting ritual, a familiar object, or thoughts of a beloved person can be used as a good luck charm before embarking on a scary trip or performing a task such as speaking in class or sleeping alone. Relaxation techniques can also be taught.

In some cases the child's fears may be related to and reinforced by **family** members. Children are understandably afraid of adults who subject them to physical, verbal, emotional, or **sexual abuse**. One form of verbal abuse that is common in troubled families is terrorization, which means that the parent makes frightening threats in order to scare the child into obedience or compliance. Such threats may range from threatening to abandon the child in a strange place to giving the child away or even killing the child. In some families older siblings may think it is amusing to frighten or scare younger children. Sometimes parents who may not be abusive may nonetheless arouse fear in their children by talking a great deal about their own fears and worries, whether personal or related to world events. For example, one study of people's reactions to the events of September 11, 2001 found that the amount of fear experienced by children living at a distance from the East Coast was in direct proportion to the intensity of fear expressed by their parents.

Anxiety disorders

A child or adolescent who is unable to function socially or academically because of fear or has severe physical symptoms caused by fear should be evaluated by a doctor. The doctor will first want to make sure that the nausea, dizziness, chest pains, headaches, or other symptoms are not caused by a disease or physical injury. Some heart conditions, blood disorders, or thyroid imbalances can cause the same symptoms as high levels of emotional fear. The doctor will then spend time talking with the child and the parents to find out whether there are any areas of stress in the child's life, whether he or she is taking medications that may affect mood, and the child's school history. The doctor may then give the child a diagnostic interview to determine what specific type of anxiety disorder the child may have.

Specific anxiety disorders that may be diagnosed in a child or teenager include:

- Generalized anxiety disorder (two to five percent of children in the United States)
- Social anxiety disorder (three to 18 percent)
- Selective mutism (inability to speak in stressful situations; 1 percent)
- Specific phobias (three to 20 percent)
- Separation anxiety (three to five percent)
- Panic disorder (one percent)
- Post–traumatic stress disorder (six percent)

Treatment

As of 2010, most doctors recommend behavioral forms of treatment for dealing with school refusal, anxiety problems, and anxiety disorders in children and adolescents. Tranquilizers and antidepressant medications may be prescribed for short–term treatment, to relieve headaches and vomiting or other physical symptoms related to the fear, but they should not be used as the sole form of treatment. The best intervention is one that helps the child to master the skills he or she will need to cope with difficult experiences in the future. If the family's interaction patterns are part of the child's problem, **family therapy** may be recommended as well.

Prognosis

Most children outgrow their fears or learn to control them to the degree that they do not interfere with daily life. Anxiety disorders are much more difficult to treat. The outcome depends on how early treatment is begun, the degree of anxiety, and the response to treatment.

Prevention

Although everyone experiences fears, and certain fears in childhood are developmentally normal, parents and family members can help prevent children from developing abnormal fears by controlling their own responses to situations they find fearful. For example, a parent who is irrationally afraid of thunder should attempt to avoid showing this fear to his or her child.

Resources

BOOKS

American Psychiatric Association.*Diagnostic and Statistical Manual of Mental Disorders,* 4th edition, text revision. Washington, DC: American Psychiatric Association, 2000.

Gower, Paul L., editor. *New Research on the Psychology of Fear.* Hauppauge, NY: Nova Science Pubs., 2005.

Rapee, Ronald M. *Helping Your Anxious Child: A Step–by–step Guide for Parents,* 2nd ed. Oakland, CA: New Harbinger, 2008.

OTHER

"Phobias." MedlinePlus. (April 21, 2010), http://www.nlm.nih.gov/medlineplus/phobias.html (accessed September 25, 2010).

Smith, Melinda. "Phobias and Fears." HelpGuide.org. (May 2010), http://helpguide.org/mental/phobia_symptoms_types_treatment.htm (accessed September 25, 2010).

"Understanding Children: Fears." Iowa State University. Undated, http://www.extension.iastate.edu/Publications/PM1529D.pdf (accessed September 25, 2010).

ORGANIZATIONS

American Academy of Child and Adolescent Psychiatry (AACAP), 3615 Wisconsin Ave., NW, Washington DC, 20016–3007 (202) 966–7300 (202) 966–2891, http://www.aacap.org.

American Academy of Pediatrics (AAP), 141 Northwest Point Blvd., Elk Grove Village IL, 60007–1098 (847) 434–4000 (847) 434–8000, http://www.aap.org.

American Psychological Association (APA), 750 First St., NE, Washington DC, 20002–4242 (202) 336–5500; TDD/TTY: (202) 336–6123 (800) 374–2721 apa@psych.org, http://www.apa.org.

Tish Davidson, AM

Febrile seizures

Definition

Febrile seizures are convulsions of sudden onset due to abnormal electrical activity in the brain caused by **fever**. Fever is a condition in which body temperature is elevated above normal, generally above 100.4°F (38°C). Febrile seizures are also known as febrile convulsions or fever fits.

Demographics

Febrile seizures are the most common **seizure disorder** in children, occurring in 2 to 5 percent of children from six months to five years of age throughout Europe and North America. The incidence elsewhere in the world varies between 5% and 10% for India; 8.8% for Japan; 14% for Guam; 0.35% for Hong Kong; and 0.5–1.5% for China.

First onset usually occurs by two years of age, with the risk decreasing after age three; most children stop having febrile seizures by the age of five or six. Boys have been shown to have a higher incidence of febrile seizures than girls. The majority of children who experience a febrile seizure will have only one in their lifetime; but approximately 33 percent will go on to have more than one.

According to the National Institute of Neurological Disorders and Stroke (NINDS), children below the age of 12 months at the time of their first simple febrile seizure have a 50% probability of having a second seizure. In those older than 12 months, the probability decreases to 30%.

Description

Febrile seizures were first distinguished from epileptic seizures in the twentieth century. The National Institutes of Health (NIH) defined febrile seizures in 1980 as "an event in **infancy** or childhood usually occurring between three months and five years of age, associated with fever, but without evidence of intracranial infection or defined cause."

There are three major subtypes of febrile seizures. The simple febrile seizure accounts for 70 to 75 percent of febrile seizures. It is one in which the affected child is between six months and five years of age and has no history or evidence of neurological abnormalities. The seizure is generalized (affects multiple parts of the brain); lasts less than 15 minutes; and the fever is not caused by such brain illnesses as **meningitis** or **encephalitis**.

The complex febrile seizure is similar to the simple febrile seizure, with the exception that the seizure lasts longer than 15 minutes or is local (affects a localized part of the brain); or multiple seizures take place. About 20 to 25 percent of all febrile seizures are complex febrile seizures.

Lastly, about 5 percent of febrile seizures are diagnosed as symptomatic. These account for cases in which the child has a history or evidence of a neurological abnormality, or has an acute illness.

In a febrile seizure, the seizure activity itself is generally characterized as clonic (consisting of rhythmic jerking movements of the arms and/or legs), or tonic-clonic (commencing with a stiffening of the body followed by a clonic phase).

Risk factors

There are two major risk factors for febrile seizures in general. The first is age: these seizures are unusual in infants less than 6 months old or in children older than 3 years. Most febrile seizures occur in children between 6 months and 5 years of age. The older a child is when the first febrile seizure occurs, the less likely that child is to have additional seizures.

The other major factor is heredity. Children from families with a history of febrile seizures are at increased risk. In addition, several specific genes have been linked as of 2010 to an increased susceptibility to febrile seizures. These genes include *SCN1A*, *SCN9A*, *GPR98*, and *GABRG2*. All four genes are related in some way to the transmission of electrical signals and the levels of various neurotransmitters in the central nervous system.

Other risk factors that have been reported to affect the onset and frequency of febrile seizures include placement in a **day care** center and a history of the mother's **smoking** and drinking during pregnancy.

Causes and symptoms

Causes

Under normal circumstances, information is transmitted in the brain by means of electrical discharges from brain cells. A seizure occurs when the normal electrical patterns of the brain become disrupted. A febrile seizure is caused by fever, most commonly a high fever that has risen quickly. The average temperature at which febrile seizures take place is 104°F (40°C). Conversely, a healthy person's body temperature fluctuates between 97°F (36.1°C) and 100°F (37.8°C). As of 2010, however, researchers do not fully understand the precise way in which fevers trigger seizures in some children.

Fevers in young children are caused in most cases by viral or bacterial infections, such as **otitis media** (ear infection), upper respiratory infection, pharyngitis (throat infection), **pneumonia**, **chickenpox**, and urinary tract infection. Other conditions can induce a fever, including allergic reactions, ingestion of toxins, **teething**, autoimmune disease, trauma, **cancer**, excessive sun exposure, or certain drugs. In some cases no cause of the fever can be determined.

Symptoms

Febrile seizures generally last between one and ten minutes. A child experiencing a febrile seizure may exhibit some or all of the following behaviors:

- stiffening of the body
- twitching or jerking of the extremities or face
- rolled-back eyes
- unconsciousness
- difficulty breathing
- inability to talk
- involuntary urination or defecation
- vomiting
- confusion, sleepiness, or irritability after the seizure

About one-third of children who have had a febrile seizure will experience recurrent seizures. Several risk factors are associated with recurrent febrile seizures; children who exhibit all four have a 70 percent chance of developing recurrent seizures, while those who have none of the risk factors have only a 20 percent chance. The risk factors for recurrent seizures include:

- family history of febrile seizures
- child is younger than 18 months at the time of the first seizure
- seizure occurs soon after or with onset of fever
- the fever associated with the seizure is relatively low

Diagnosis

A healthcare provider should be contacted after a febrile seizure. A visit to the emergency room is warranted if the accompanying fever is greater than 103°F (39.4°C) in a child older than three months; or 100.5°F (38°C) in an infant of three months or younger; or if the seizure is the child's first. Emergency medical personnel (telephone 911) should be called if a febrile seizure lasts more than five minutes; if the child stops breathing; if the child's skin starts to turn blue; or if the fever is greater than 105.8°F (41°C), a condition called hyperpyrexia.

Examination

A key focus of the diagnostic evaluation will be to determine the underlying cause of the fever. A comprehensive medical history, including the fever's duration and course; other symptoms the child is experiencing; prior or current medical conditions; recent vaccinations or exposure to communicable diseases; and the child's current behaviors may point to the fever's origin. Vaccines against **measles**, or combination vaccines containing measles vaccine, appear to increase the risk of febrile seizures in the 10-day period following administration of the vaccine. A temperature below 100.4°F (38°C) suggests another cause for the seizure. The **caregiver** who was present with the child while he or she was having the seizure will be asked questions related to the child's behaviors in an attempt to determine the type of seizure.

KEY TERMS

Anticonvulsants—A class of drugs given to treat seizures.

Antipyretics—A class of drugs given to reduce fever.

Autoimmune disorders—A group of disorders, like rheumatoid arthritis and systemic lupus erythematosus, in which the immune system is overactive and has lost the ability to distinguish between self and non-self. The body's immune cells turn against the body, attacking various tissues and organs.

Encephalitis—Inflammation of the brain, usually caused by a virus. The inflammation may interfere with normal brain function and may cause seizures, sleepiness, confusion, personality changes, weakness in one or more parts of the body, and even coma.

Febrile—The medical term for feverish or pertaining to a fever.

Hyperpyrexia—Fever greater than 105.8°F (41°C).

Meningitis—An infection or inflammation of the membranes that cover the brain and spinal cord. It is usually caused by bacteria or a virus.

Tests

Physicians may administer blood or urine tests to rule out conditions other than fever that could have caused the seizure, such as **epilepsy**, meningitis, or encephalitis. Children who suffer from recurrent febrile seizures are not diagnosed with epilepsy, a seizure disorder that is not caused by fever. In the case of children under 18 months of age, a lumbar puncture (spinal tap) may be recommended to rule out meningitis because symptoms are often lacking or subtle in children of that age. Because of the benign nature of the simple febrile seizure, such tests as computed tomography (CT) scans, **magnetic resonance imaging** (MRI), or electroencephalograms (EEG) are not usually recommended.

Treatment

Traditional

During a febrile seizure, parents or caregivers need to remain calm and take steps to make sure the child remains safe. During the period after the seizure (called the postictal state) the child may be disoriented and/or sleepy; however, quick recovery from this state is normal, and medical treatment is not normally needed.

When a parent or caregiver observes a child having a seizure, there are a number of measures that they should take to ensure the child's **safety**. These include:

- remain calm
- position the child on his or her side or front to prevent vomited matter from being aspirated into the lungs
- loosen any tight clothing or items that could constrict breathing
- mark the start and end times of the seizure
- try to note which part or parts of the child's body begin to shake first
- clear the surrounding area of unsafe items
- attend the child for the duration of the seizure
- clear the child's airway if it becomes obstructed with vomited material or other objects

Parents or caregivers should not attempt to stop the seizure or slap or shake the child in attempt to wake him/her. The child may move around during the seizure, and parents should not try to hold the child down. If the child vomits, a suction bulb can be used to help clear the airway.

After the seizure, a healthcare professional should be called immediately in the event that further treatment or tests are required. Hospitalization is not normally required unless the child is suffering from a serious infection or illness or the seizure itself was abnormally long. Parents or caregivers may be instructed to take certain measures at home to reduce the child's fever, such as administering such fever-reducing drugs (called antipyretics) as **acetaminophen** (Tylenol) or ibuprofen (Advil). There is, however, no evidence that shows fever-reducing therapies reduce the risk of another febrile seizure occurring. If the child is suffering from a bacterial infection that is the cause of the fever, he or she may be placed on **antibiotics**.

Drugs

Medications are the mainstay of treatment for fevers in children. The treatment of pediatric fever varies according to the age of the child and the fever's cause, if known. Physicians recommend that newborns less than four weeks of age with fever be admitted to the hospital and administered antibiotics until a complete workup can be done to rule out bacterial infection or other serious illness. The same is recommended for infants between 4 and 12 weeks of age if they appear ill. Infants of this age who otherwise appear well can often be managed on an outpatient basis with antipyretics and antibiotics in the case of bacterial infection.

For children ages three months and older, the course of treatment depends on the extent and cause of the fever. Most fevers and associated conditions can be managed on an outpatient basis. Low-grade fevers often do not need to be treated in otherwise healthy children. Antipyretics may be suggested to lower a fever and make the child more comfortable but will not affect the course of an underlying infectious disease. Aspirin should not be given to a child or adolescent with a fever since this drug has been linked to an increased risk of the serious condition called Reye's syndrome. Antibiotics may be prescribed if the child has a known or suspected bacterial infection.

Home remedies

There are some outpatient treatments that parents or caregivers may administer to reduce their febrile child's discomfort, although there is no evidence that indicates such treatments reduce the risk of febrile seizures. These include dressing the child lightly, applying cold wash-cloths to the face and neck, providing plenty of fluids to avoid **dehydration**, and giving the child a lukewarm bath or sponging the child in lukewarm water.

Prognosis

Complications from a febrile seizure are uncommon but may include falling down, biting the tongue, or aspirating vomitus into the lungs. In a few cases children develop complications from the underlying cause of the fever.

Children who have simple febrile seizures are at an increased risk for epilepsy. The rate of epilepsy in these children by age 25 years is approximately 2.4%, which is about twice the risk in the general population. There is no indication, however, that simple febrile seizures lower a child's **intelligence** or lead to a shortened lifespan.

Prevention

In some cases, a febrile seizure may be the first indication that a child is ill. Prevention is therefore not always possible. While the use of such anticonvulsants as phenobarbital or valproate has been shown to prevent recurrent febrile seizures, these drugs are associated with such significant side effects as adverse behaviors, allergic reaction, and organ injury, and have not been shown to benefit simple febrile seizures. Only rarely is anticonvulsant therapy recommended for a child with febrile seizures because of the generally benign nature of the seizures and the risk of side effects from the drugs. In some cases oral diazepam (Valium) can be administered at the first sign of fever to reduce the risk of febrile seizures; about two-thirds of children who receive this drug experience such side effects as sleepiness and loss of coordination. The majority of children who have had a febrile seizure do not need drug therapy. Parents may be directed to administer over-the-counter antipyretics at the first sign of fever.

Parental concerns

A febrile seizure can be a frightening experience for both the child and his or her parents. It is important that parents be educated about the low risk of simple febrile seizures and the measures that can be taken to ensure their child's safety during and after a seizure.

Resources

BOOKS

Baram, Tallie Z., and Shlomo Shinnar, eds. *Febrile Seizures.* San Diego, CA: Academic Press, 2002.

Kliegman, Robert M. et al., eds. *Nelson Textbook of Pediatrics*, 18th ed. Philadelphia: Saunders Elsevier, 2007.

Rowland, Lewis P., and Timothy A. Pedley, eds. *Merritt's Neurology*, 12th ed. Philadelphia: Lippincott Williams and Wilkins, 2010.

PERIODICALS

Friese, G., and K.T. Collopy. "Febrile Seizures. Learn to Distinguish Simple Febrile Seizures from Complex Seizures." *EMS Magazine* 39 (May 2010): 52–57.

Klein, N.P., et al. "Measles-Mumps-Rubella-Varicella Combination Vaccine and the Risk of Febrile Seizures." *Pediatrics* 126 (July 2010): e1–e8.

Li, N., et al. "Novel Mutation of SCN1A in Familial Generalized Epilepsy with Febrile Seizures Plus." *Neuroscience Letters* 480 (August 23, 2010): 211–214.

Lloyd, M.B., et al. "Rotavirus Gastroenteritis and Seizures in Young Children." *Pediatric Neurology* 42 (June 2010): 404–08.

Reid, A.Y., et al. "Febrile Seizures: Current Views and Investigations." *Canadian Journal of Neurological Sciences* 36 (November 2009): 679–86.

Shi, X., et al. "Mutational analysis of GABRG2 in a Japanese Cohort with Childhood Epilepsies." *Journal of Human Genetics* 55 (June 2010): 375–78.

OTHER

Bauman, Robert. "Febrile Seizures." *eMedicine*, January 8, 2010, http://emedicine.medscape.com/article/1176205-overview.

Epilepsy Foundation. *Epilepsy Syndromes*, http://www.epilepsyfoundation.org/about/types/syndromes/index.cfm.

International League Against Epilepsy (ILAE). *Epilepsy Syndromes and Related Conditions* Febrile seizures are listed under "Conditions with Epileptic Seizures That Do Not Require a Diagnosis of Epilepsy." http://www.ilaeepilepsy.org/Visitors/Centre/ctf/syndromes.html.

Mayo Clinic. *Febrile Seizure*, http://www.mayoclinic.com/health/febrile-seizure/DS00346.

National Institute of Neurological Disorders and Stroke (NINDS). *Febrile Seizures Fact Sheet*, http://www.ninds.nih.gov/disorders/febrile_seizures/detail_febrile_seizures.htm.

Tejani, Nooruddin R. "Pediatrics, Febrile Seizures." *eMedicine*, February 5, 2010, http://emedicine.medscape.com/article/801500-overview.

ORGANIZATIONS

American Academy of Pediatrics (AAP), 141 Northwest Point Boulevard, Elk Grove Village IL, 60007, 847-434-4000, 847-434-8000, http://www.aap.org/.

American College of Emergency Physicians (ACEP), 1125 Executive Circle, Irving TX, 75038-2522, 972-550-0911, 800-798-1822, 972-580-2816, http://www.acep.org/.

Epilepsy Foundation, 8301 Professional Place, Landover MD, 20785, 800-332-1000, 301-577-2684, info@efa.org, http://www.epilepsyfoundation.org/.

National Institute of Neurological Disorders and Stroke (NINDS), P.O. Box 5801, Bethesda MD, 20824, 800-352-9424 301-496-5751, http://www.ninds.nih.gov/index.htm.

International League Against Epilepsy (ILAE), 342 North Main Street, West Hartford CT United States, 06117, 860-586-7547, 860-586-7550, http://www.ilae-epilepsy.org/.

Stephanie Dionne Sherk
Rebecca J. Frey, PhD

Fetal alcohol syndrome

Definition

Fetal alcohol syndrome (FAS) is a pattern of **birth defects**, learning, and behavioral problems affecting individuals whose mothers drank alcohol during pregnancy.

Demographics

The occurrence FAS/FASD is independent of race, ethnicity, or gender of the individual. Individuals from different genetic backgrounds exposed to similar amounts of alcohol during pregnancy may show different symptoms of FAS. The reported rates of FAS vary widely among different populations studied depending on the degree of alcohol use within the population and the monitoring methods used. Studies by the Centers for Disease Control (CDC) show that, as of 2008, FAS occurs in 0.2 to 1.5 per 1,000 live births in different areas of the United States. FASDs are believed to occur approximately three times as often as FAS.

Description

FAS is the most severe of a range of disorders represented by the term fetal alcohol spectrum disorder (FASD). FAS/FASD is caused by exposure of a developing fetus to alcohol. FASD is used to describe individuals with some, but not all, of the features of FAS. Other terms used to describe specific types of FASD are alcohol-related neurodevelopmental disorder (ARND) and alcohol-related **birth** defects (ARBD).

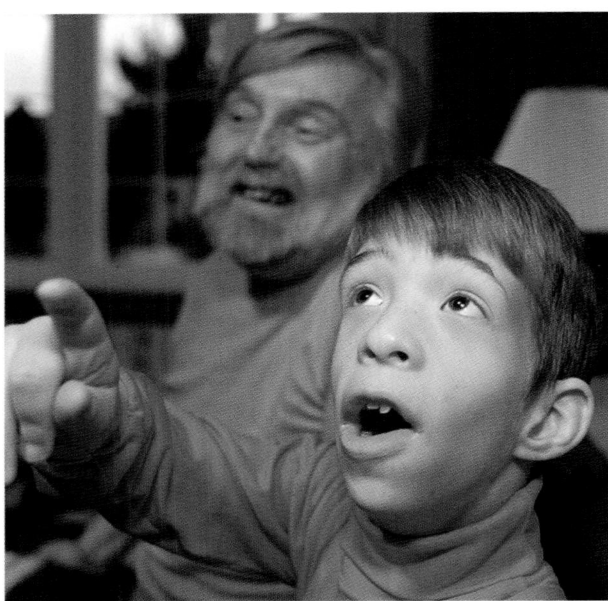

A boy with fetal alcohol syndrome, a birth defect caused by his mother consuming alcohol during her pregnancy. *(© David H. Wells/Corbis.)*

FAS is the most common preventable cause of **mental retardation**. This condition was first recognized and reported in the medical literature in 1968 in France and in 1973 in the United States. Alcohol is a teratogen, the term used for any drug, chemical, maternal disease, or other environmental exposure that can cause birth defects or functional impairment in a developing fetus. Some features of FAS that may be present at birth include low birth weight, **prematurity**, and microcephaly. Characteristic facial features may be present at birth or may become more obvious over time. Signs of brain damage include delays in development, behavioral abnormalities, and mental retardation, but affected individuals exhibit a wide range of abilities and disabilities.

FAS is a life-long condition. It is not curable and has serious long-term consequences. Learning, behavioral, and emotional problems are common in adolescents and adults with FAS/FASD. The costs of FAS to the American economy were estimated in 2006 as $321 million annually.

Risk factors

The only risk factor for a child to develop FAS is the consumption of alcohol by a women who is pregnant. There is no known amount of alcohol use that is safe during pregnancy, nor is there a particular stage of pregnancy during which alcohol use is safe.

Causes and symptoms

The only cause of FAS is maternal use of alcohol during pregnancy. FAS is not a genetic or inherited disorder. Alcohol drunk by the mother freely crosses the placenta and damages the developing fetus. Alcohol use by the father cannot cause FAS. Not all offspring who are exposed to alcohol during pregnancy have signs or symptoms of FAS; individuals of different genetic backgrounds may be more or less susceptible to the damage that alcohol can cause. The amount of alcohol, stage of development of the fetus, and the pattern of alcohol use create the range of symptoms that encompass FASD.

Classic features of FAS include short stature, low birth weight, poor weight gain, microcephaly, and a characteristic pattern of abnormal facial features. These facial features in infants and children may include small eye openings (measured from inner corner to outer corner), epicanthal folds (folds of tissue at the inner corner of the eye), small or short nose, low or flat nasal bridge, smooth or poorly developed philtrum (the area of the upper lip above the colored part of the lip and below the nose), thin upper lip, and small chin. Some of these features are nonspecific, meaning they can occur in other conditions, or be appropriate for age, racial, or family background.

Other major and minor birth defects that have been reported to occur in conjunction with FAS/FASD include **cleft palate**, congenital heart defects, **strabismus**, hearing loss, defects of the spine and joints, alteration of the hand creases, small fingernails, and toenails. Since FAS was first described in infants and children, the diagnosis is sometimes more difficult to recognize in older adolescents and adults. Short stature and microcephaly remain common features, but weight may normalize, and the individual may actually become overweight for his/her height. The chin and nose grow proportionately more than the middle part of the face, and dental crowding may become a problem. The small eye openings and the appearance of the upper lip and philtrum may continue to be characteristic. Pubertal changes typically occur at the normal time.

Newborns with FAS may have difficulty nursing due to a poor sucking response, have irregular sleep-wake cycles, decreased or increased muscle tone, seizures or tremors. Delays in achieving developmental milestones such as rolling over, **crawling**, walking, and talking may become apparent in **infancy**. Behavior and learning difficulties typical in the **preschool** or early school years include poor attention span, hyperactivity, poor motor skills, and slow **language development**. Attention deficit-hyperactivity disorder (**ADHD**) is often associated with FASD. Learning disabilities or mental retardation may be diagnosed during this time.

During middle school and high school years the behavioral difficulties and learning difficulties can be significant. Memory problems, poor judgment, difficulties with daily living skills, difficulties with abstract reasoning skills, and poor social skills are often apparent by this time. It is important to note that animal and human studies have shown that neurologic and behavioral abnormalities can be present without characteristic facial features. These individuals may not be identified as having FAS, but may fulfill criteria for alcohol-related neurodevelopmental disorder (ARND).

FASD continues to affect individuals into adulthood. One study looked at FAS adults and found that about 95% had mental health problems, 82% lacked the ability to live independently, 70% had problems staying employed, 60% had been in trouble with the law, and 50% of men and 70% of women were alcohol or drug abusers.

Another long-term study found that the average **IQ** of the group of adolescents and adults with FAS in the study was 68 (70 is lower limit of the normal range). However, the range of IQ was quite large, ranging from a low of 20 (severely retarded) to a high of 105 (normal). Academic abilities and social skills were also below normal levels. The average achievement levels for reading, spelling, and arithmetic were fourth grade, third grade, and second grade, respectively. The Vineland Adaptive Behavior Scale was used to measure adaptive functioning in these individuals. The composite score for this group showed functioning at the level of a seven-year-old. Daily living skills were at a level of nine years, and social skills were at the level of a six-year-old.

KEY TERMS

Cleft plate—A congenital malformation in which there is an abnormal opening in the roof of the mouth that allows the nasal passages and the mouth to be improperly connected.

IQ—Abbreviation for Intelligence Quotient. Compares an individual's mental age to his/her true or chronological age and multiplies that ratio by 100.

Microcephaly—An abnormally small head.

Miscarriage—Spontaneous pregnancy loss.

Placenta—The organ responsible for oxygen and nutrition exchange between a pregnant mother and her developing baby.

Strabismus—An improper muscle balance of the ocular muscles resulting in crossed or divergent eyes.

Teratogen—Any drug, chemical, maternal disease, or exposure that can cause physical or functional defects in an exposed embryo or fetus.

Diagnosis

In 1996, the Institute of Medicine suggested a five-level system to describe the birth defects, learning problems, and behavioral difficulties in offspring of women who drank alcohol during pregnancy. This system contains criteria including confirmation of maternal alcohol exposure, characteristic facial features, growth problems, learning and behavioral problems, and birth defects known to be associated with prenatal alcohol exposure.

FAS is a clinical diagnosis, which means that there is no blood, x ray or psychological test that can be performed to confirm the suspected diagnosis. The diagnosis is made based on the history of maternal alcohol use, and detailed physical examination for the characteristic major and minor birth defects and characteristic facial features. It is often helpful to examine siblings and parents of an individual suspected of having FAS, either in person or by photographs, to determine whether findings on the examination might be familial, of if other siblings may also be affected. Sometimes, genetic tests are performed to rule out other conditions that may present with **developmental delay** or birth defects. Individuals with developmental delay, birth defects, or other unusual features are often referred to a clinical geneticist, developmental **pediatrician**, or neurologist for evaluation and diagnosis of FAS. Psychoeducational testing to determine IQ and/or the presence of learning disabilities may also be part of the evaluation process.

Treatment

There is no cure for FAS. The disorder is irreversible. Nothing can change the physical features or brain damage associated with maternal alcohol use during the pregnancy. Children should have psychoeducational evaluation to help plan appropriate educational interventions. Common associated diagnoses such ADHD, depression, or **anxiety** can be recognized and treated. The disabilities that present during childhood persist into adult life. However, some of the behavioral problems mentioned above may be avoided or lessened by early and correct diagnosis, better understanding of the life-long complications of FAS, and intervention. The goal of treatment is to help the individual affected by FAS become as independent and successful in school, employment, and social relationships as possible.

Prognosis

The prognosis for FAS/FASD depends on the severity of birth defects and the brain damage present at birth. Miscarriage, stillbirth, or **death** in the first few weeks of life may be outcomes in very severe cases. Generally individuals with FAS have a long list of mental health problems and associated social difficulties: alcohol and drug problems, inappropriate sexual behavior, problems with employment, trouble with the law, inability to live independently, and often confinement in prison, drug or alcohol treatment centers, or psychiatric institutions.

Some of the factors that have been found to reduce the risk of learning and behavioral disabilities in FAS individuals include diagnosis before the age of six years, stable and nurturing home environments, never having experienced personal violence, and referral and eligibility for disability services. Some physical birth defects associated with FAS are treatable with surgery. The long-term data help in understanding the difficulties that individuals with FAS encounter throughout their lifetime and can help families, caregivers, and professionals provide the care, supervision, education and treatment geared toward their special needs.

Prevention

FAS and FASD are completely preventable by avoiding all use of alcohol while pregnant. Prevention efforts include public education efforts aimed at the entire population, not just women of child bearing age, appropriate treatment for women with high-risk drinking habits, and increased recognition and knowledge about FAS/FASD by professionals, parents, and caregivers.

Resources

BOOKS

Golden, Janet. *Message in a Bottle: The Making of Fetal Alcohol Syndrome.* Cambridge, MA: Harvard University Press, 2006.

Kulp, Jodie. *The Best I Can Be: Living with Fetal Alcohol Syndrome—Effects.* Brooklyn Park, MN: Better Endings New Beginnings, 2006.

Lawryk, Liz. *Finding Perspective: Raising Successful Children Affected by Fetal Alcohol Spectrum Disorders.* Bragg Creek, AB (Canada): OBD Triage Institute, 2005.

Soby, Jeanette M. *Prenatal Exposure to Drugs/Alcohol: Characteristics and Educational Implications of Fetal Alcohol Syndrome and Cocaine/Polydrug Effects,* 2nd ed. Springfield, IL: Charles C Thomas, 2006.

PERIODICALS

Franklin, L., et al. "Children With Fetal Alcohol Spectrum Disorders: Problem Behaviors and Sensory Processing." *American Journal of Occupational Therapy* 62, no. 3 (May–June 2008): 265–273.

Green, J. H. "Fetal Alcohol Spectrum Disorders: Understanding the Effects of Prenatal Alcohol Exposure and Supporting Students." *Journal of School Health* 77, no. 3 (March 2007): 103–108.

OTHER

Chambers, Christine and Keith Vaux. "Fetal Alcohol Syndrome." eMedicine.com, October 20, 2006. [accessed August 29, 2009], http://emedicine.medscape.com/article/974016-overview.

"Fetal Alcohol Spectrum Disorders (FASDs)." United States Centers for Disease Control and Prevention. August 24, 2009 [accessed August 29, 2009], http://www.cdc.gov/ncbddd/fasd/index.html.

"Fetal Alcohol Syndrome." Medline Plus August 17, 2009 [accessed August 29, 2009], http://www.nlm.nih.gov/medlineplus/fetalalcoholsyndrome.html.

ORGANIZATIONS

Fetal Alcohol Spectrum Disorders Center for Excellence, 2101 Gaither Road., Suite 600, Rockville MD, 20850, (866) STOP-FAS (786-7327), http://fasdcenter.samhsa.gov.

Fetal Alcohol Syndrome (FAS) World Canada, 250 Scarborough Golf Club Road, Toronto ON Canada, M1J 3G8, (416) 264-8000, (416) 264-8222, info@fasworld.com, http://www.fasworld.com.

March of Dimes Foundation, 1275 Mamaroneck Avenue, White Plains NY, 10605, (914) 997-4488, askus@marchofdimes.com, http://www.marchofdimes.com.

National Institute on Alcohol Abuse and Alcoholism (NIAAA), 5635 Fishers Lane, MSC 9304, Bethesda MD, 20892-9304, (301) 443-3860, http://www.niaaa.nih.gov.

National Organization on Fetal Alcohol Syndrome (NOFAS), 900 17th St., NW, Suite 910, Washington DC, 20006, (202) 785-4585, (800) 66-NOFAS, (202) 466-6456, http://www.nofas.org.

Laurie Heron Seaver, M.D.
Tish Davidson, A.M.

Fetal hemoglobin test

Definition

Fetal hemoglobin (Hemoglobin F), Alkali-resistant hemoglobin, HBF (or Hb F), is the major hemoglobin component in the bloodstream of the fetus. After **birth**, it decreases rapidly until only traces are found in normal children and adults.

Purpose

The determination of fetal hemoglobin is an aid in evaluating low concentrations of hemoglobin in the blood (**anemia**), as well as the hereditary persistence of fetal hemoglobin, and a group of inherited disorders affecting hemoglobin, among which are the thalassemias and sickle cell anemia.

Description

At birth, the newborn's blood is comprised of 60%–90% of fetal hemoglobin. The fetal hemoglobin then rapidly decreases to 2% or less after the second to fourth years. By the time of adulthood, only traces (0.5% or less) are found in the bloodstream.

In some diseases associated with abnormal hemoglobin production (see Hemoglobinopathy, below), fetal hemoglobin may persist in larger amounts. When this occurs, the elevation raises the question of possible underlying disease.

For example, HBF can be found in higher levels in hereditary hemolytic anemias, in all types of leukemias, in pregnancy, diabetes, thyroid disease, and during anticonvulsant drug therapy. It may also reappear in adults when the bone marrow is overactive, as in the disorders of pernicious anemia, multiple myeloma, and metastatic **cancer** in the marrow. When HBF is increased after age four, it should be investigated for cause.

Hemoglobinopathy

Hemoglobin is the oxygen-carrying pigment found in red blood cells. It is a large molecule made in the bone marrow from two components, heme and globin.

Defects in hemoglobin production may be either genetic or acquired. The genetic defects are further subdivided into errors of heme production (porphyria), and those of globin production (known collectively as the hemoglobinopathies).

There are two categories of hemoglobinopathy. In the first category, abnormal globin chains give rise to abnormal hemoglobin molecules. In the second category, normal hemoglobin chains are produced but in abnormal amounts. An example of the first category is the disorder of sickle cell anemia, the inherited condition characterized by curved (sickle-shaped) red blood cells and chronic hemolytic anemia. Disorders in the second category are called the thalassemias, which are further divided into types according to which amino acid chain is affected (alpha or beta), and whether there is one defective gene (**thalassemia** minor) or two defective genes (thalassemia major).

Preparation

This test requires a blood sample. The patient is not required to be in a fasting state (nothing to eat or drink for a period of hours before the test).

Risks

Risks for this test are minimal, but may include slight bleeding from the blood-drawing site, fainting or feeling lightheaded after venipuncture, or hematoma (blood accumulating under the puncture site).

Normal results

Reference values vary from laboratory to laboratory but are generally found within the following ranges:

- six months to adult: up to 2% of the total hemoglobin
- ewborn to six months: up to 75% of the total hemoglobin

KEY TERMS

Anemia—A disorder characterized by a reduced blood level of hemoglobin, the oxygen-carrying pigment of blood.

Hemolytic anemia—A form of anemia caused by premature destruction of red cells in the blood stream (a process called hemolysis). Hemolytic anemias are classified according to whether the cause of the problem is inside the red blood cell (in which case it is usually an inherited condition), or outside the cell (usually acquired later in life).

Abnormal results

Greater than 2% of total hemoglobin is abnormal.

Resources

BOOKS

Pagana, Kathleen Deska. *Mosby's Manual of Diagnosticand Laboratory Tests.* St. Louis: Mosby, Inc., 1998.

Janis O. Flores

Fetal monitoring, electronic **see Electronic fetal monitoring**

Fever

Definition

A fever is any body temperature elevation over 100 °F (37.8 °C).

Description

A healthy person's body temperature fluctuates between 97 °F (36.1 °C) and 100 °F (37.8 °C), with the average being 98.6 °F (37 °C). The body maintains stability within this range by balancing the heat produced by the metabolism with the heat lost to the environment. The "thermostat" that controls this process is located in the hypothalamus, a small structure located deep within the brain. The nervous system constantly relays information about the body's temperature to the thermostat, which in turn activates different physical responses designed to cool or warm the body, depending on the circumstances. These responses include: decreasing or

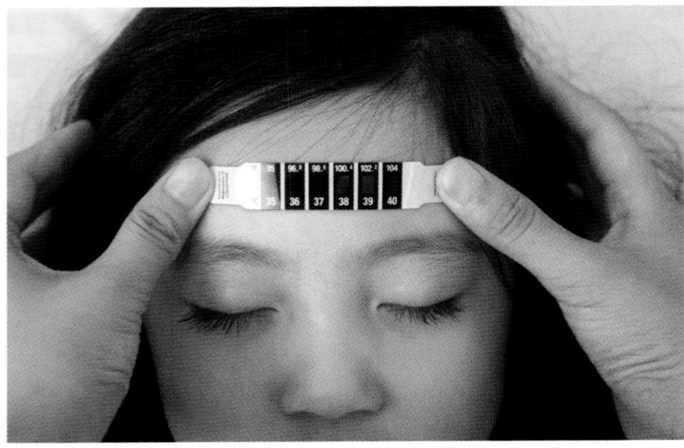

Young girl having her temperature taken with a forehead thermometer. *(© Blue Jean Images/Alamy.)*

increasing the flow of blood from the body's core, where it is warmed, to the surface, where it is cooled; slowing down or speeding up the rate at which the body turns food into energy (metabolic rate); inducing shivering, which generates heat through muscle contraction; and inducing sweating, which cools the body through evaporation.

A fever occurs when the thermostat resets at a higher temperature, primarily in response to an infection. To reach the higher temperature, the body moves blood to the warmer interior, increases the metabolic rate, and induces shivering. The "chills" that often accompany a fever are caused by the movement of blood to the body's core, leaving the surface and extremities cold. Once the higher temperature is achieved, the shivering and chills stop. When the infection has been overcome or drugs such as aspirin or **acetaminophen** (Tylenol) have been taken, the thermostat resets to normal and the body's cooling mechanisms switch on: the blood moves to the surface and sweating occurs.

Fever is an important component of the immune response, though its role is not completely understood. Physicians believe that an elevated body temperature has several effects. The **immune system** chemicals that react with the fever-inducing agent and trigger the resetting of the thermostat also increase the production of cells that fight off the invading bacteria or viruses. Higher temperatures also inhibit the growth of some bacteria, while at the same time speeding up the chemical reactions that help the body's cells repair themselves. In addition, the increased heart rate that may accompany the changes in blood circulation also speeds the arrival of white blood cells to the sites of infection.

Causes and symptoms

Fevers are primarily caused by viral or bacterial infections, such as **pneumonia** or **influenza**. However, other conditions can induce a fever, including allergic reactions; autoimmune diseases; trauma, such as breaking a bone; **cancer**; excessive exposure to the sun; intense **exercise**; hormonal imbalances; certain drugs; and damage to the hypothalamus. When an infection occurs, fever-inducing agents called pyrogens are released, either by the body's immune system or by the invading cells themselves, that trigger the resetting of the thermostat. In other circumstances, the immune system may overreact (allergic reactions) or become damaged (autoimmune diseases), causing the uncontrolled release of pyrogens. A **stroke** or tumor can damage the hypothalamus, causing the body's thermostat to malfunction. Excessive exposure to the sun or intensely exercising in hot weather can result in heat stroke, a condition in which the body's cooling mechanisms fail. Malignant hyperthermia is a rare, inherited condition in which a person develops a very high fever when given certain anesthetics or muscle relaxants in preparation for surgery.

How long a fever lasts and how high it may go depends on several factors, including its cause, the age of the patient, and his or her overall health. Most fevers caused by infections are acute, appearing suddenly and then dissipating as the immune system defeats the infectious agent. An infectious fever may also rise and fall throughout the day, reaching its peek in the late afternoon or early evening. A low-grade fever that lasts for several weeks is associated with autoimmune diseases such as lupus or with some cancers, particularly leukemia and lymphoma.

Diagnosis

A fever is usually diagnosed using a thermometer. A variety of different thermometers are available, including traditional glass and mercury ones used for oral or rectal temperature readings and more sophisticated electronic ones that can be inserted in the ear to quickly register the body's temperature. For adults and older children, temperature readings are usually taken orally. Younger children who cannot or will not hold a thermometer in their mouths can have their temperature taken by placing an oral thermometer under their armpit. Infants generally have their temperature taken rectally using a rectal thermometer.

As important as registering a patient's temperature is determining the underlying cause of the fever. The presence or absence of accompanying symptoms, a patient's medical history, and information about what he or she may have ingested, any recent trips taken, or possible exposures to illness help the physician make a diagnosis. Blood tests can aid in identifying an infectious agent by detecting the presence of antibodies against it or providing samples for growth of the organism in a culture. Blood tests can also provide the doctor with white blood cell counts. Ultrasound tests, **magnetic resonance imaging** (MRI) tests, or computed tomography (CT) scans may be ordered if the doctor cannot readily determine the cause of a fever.

Treatment

Physicians agree that the most effective treatment for a fever is to address its underlying cause, such as through the administration of **antibiotics**. Also, because a fever helps the immune system fight infection, it usually should be allowed to run its course. Drugs to lower fever (antipyretics) can be given if a patient (particularly a child) is uncomfortable. These include aspirin, acetaminophen (Tylenol), and ibuprofin (Advil). Aspirin, however, should not be given to a child or adolescent with a fever since this drug has been linked to an increased risk of **Reye's syndrome**. Bathing a patient in cool water can also help alleviate a high fever.

A fever requires emergency treatment under the following circumstances:

- newborn (three months or younger) with a fever over 100.5 °F (38 °C)
- infant or child with a fever over 103 °F (39.4 °C)
- fever accompanied by severe headache, neck stiffness, mental confusion, or severe swelling of the throat

A very high fever in a small child can trigger seizures (**febrile seizures**) and therefore should be treated immediately. A fever accompanied by the above symptoms can indicate the presence of a serious infection, such as **meningitis**, and should be brought to the immediate attention of a physician.

Prognosis

Most fevers caused by infection end as soon as the immune system rids the body of the pathogen and do not produce any lasting effects. The prognosis for fevers associated with more chronic conditions, such as autoimmune disease, depends upon the overall outcome of the disorder.

Resources

BOOKS

Gelfand, Jeffrey. "Fever, Including Fever of Unknown Origin." In *Harrison's Principles of Internal Medicine*, edited by Anthony S. Fauci, et al. New York: McGraw-Hill, 1997.

Bridget Travers

KEY TERMS

Antipyretic—A drug that lowers fever, like aspirin or acetaminophen.

Autoimmune disease—Condition in which a person's immune system attacks the body's own cells, causing tissue destruction.

Febrile seizure—Convulsions brought on by fever.

Malignant hyperthermia—A rare, inherited condition in which a person develops a very high fever when given certain anesthetics or muscle relaxants in preparation for surgery.

Meningitis—A potentially fatal inflammation of the thin membrane covering the brain and spinal cord.

Metabolism—The chemical process by which the body turns food into energy, which can be given off as heat.

Pyrogen—A chemical circulating in the blood that causes a rise in body temperature.

Reye's syndrome—A disorder principally affecting the liver and brain, marked by the rapid development of life-threatening neurological symptoms.

Fever blister ***see* Cold sore**

Fever of unknown origin

Definition

Fever of unknown origin (FUO) refers to the presence of a documented fever for a specified time, for which a cause has not been found after a basic medical evaluation. The classic criteria developed in 1961 included: temperature greater than 101 °F (38.3 °C), for at least three weeks, and inability to find a cause after one week of study. Within the past decade, a revision has been proposed that categorizes FUO into classic, hospital acquired FUO, FUO associated with low white blood counts, and HIV associated FUO (**AIDS** related).

Description

Fever is a natural response of the body that helps in fighting off foreign substances, such as microorganisms, toxins, etc. Body temperature is set by the thermoregulatory center, located in an area in the brain called hypothalamus. Body temperature is not constant all day, but actually is lowest at 6 A.M. and highest around 4–6 P. M. In addition, temperature varies in different regions of the body; for example, rectal and urine temperatures are about one degree Fahrenheit higher than oral temperature and rectal temperature is higher than urine. It is also important to realize that certain normal conditions can effect body temperature, such as pregnancy, food ingestion, age, and certain hormonal changes.

Substances that cause fever are known as "pyrogens." There are two types of pyrogens; exogenous and endogenous. Those that originate outside the body, such as bacterial toxins, are called "exogenous" pyrogens. Pyrogens formed by the body's own cells in response to an outside stimulus (such as a bacterial toxin) are called "endogenous" pyrogens.

Researchers have discovered that there are several "endogenous" pyrogens. These are made up of small groups of amino acids, the building blocks of proteins. These natural pyrogens have other functions in addition to inducing fever; they have been named "cytokines." When cytokines are injected into humans, fever and chills develop within an hour. Interferon, tumor necrosis factor, and various interleukins are the major fever producing cytokines.

The production of fever is a very complex process; somehow, these cytokines cause the thermoregulatory center in the hypothalamus to reset the normal temperature level. The body's initial response is to conserve heat by vasoconstriction, a process in which blood vessels narrow and prevent heat loss from the skin and elsewhere. This alone will raise temperature by two to three degrees. Certain behavioral activities also occur, such as adding more clothes, seeking a warmer environment, etc. If the hypothalamus requires more heat, then shivering occurs.

Fever is a body defense mechanism. It has been shown that one of the effects of temperature increase is to slow bacterial growth. However, fever also has some downsides; the body's metabolic rate is increased and with it, oxygen consumption. This can have a devastating effect on those with poor circulation. In addition, fever can lead to seizures in the very young.

When temperature elevation occurs for an extended period of time and no cause is found, the term FUO is then used. The far majority of these patients are eventually found to have one of several diseases.

Causes and symptoms

The most frequent cause of FUO is still infection, though the percentage has decreased in recent years. **Tuberculosis** remains an important cause, especially when it occurs outside the lungs. The decrease in infections as a cause of FUO is due in part to improved culture techniques. In addition, technological advances have made it easier to diagnose non-infectious causes. For example, tumors and autoimmune diseases in particular are now easier to diagnose. (An autoimmune disease is one that arises when the body tolerance for its own cell antigenic cell markers disappears.)

Allergies to medications can also cause prolonged fever; sometimes patients will have other symptoms suggesting an allergic reaction, such as a rash.

There are many possible causes of FUO; generally though, a diagnosis can be found. About 10% of patients will wind up without a definite cause, and about the same percentage have "factitious fevers" (either self induced or no fever at all).

Some general symptoms tend to occur along with fever; these are called constitutional symptoms and consist of myalgias (muscle aches), chills, and **headache**.

Diagnosis

Few symptoms in medicine present such a diagnostic challenge as fever. Nonetheless, if a careful, logical, and thorough evaluation is performed, a diagnosis will be found in most cases. The patient's past medical history as well as travel, social, and family history should be carefully searched for important clues.

Usually the first step is to search for an infectious cause. Skin and other screening tests for diseases such as tuberculosis, and examination of blood, urine, and stool, are generally indicated. Antibody levels to a number of infectious agents can be measured; if these are rising, they may point to an active infection.

Various x-ray studies are also of value. In addition to standard examinations, recently developed radiological techniques using ultrasound, computed tomography scan (CT scan) and **magnetic resonance imaging** (MRI) scans are now available. These enable physicians to examine areas that were once accessible only through surgery. Furthermore, new studies using radioactive materials (nuclear medicine), can detect areas of infection and inflammation previously almost impossible to find, even with surgery.

Biopsies of any suspicious areas found on an x-ray exam can be performed by either traditional or newer surgical techniques. Material obtained by biopsy is then examined by a pathologist to look for clues as to the cause of the fever. Evidence of infection, tumor or other diseases can be found in this way. Portions of the biopsy are also sent to the laboratory for culture in an attempt to grow and identify an infectious organism.

KEY TERMS

AIDS—Acquired immune deficiency syndrome is often represented by these initials. The disease is associated with infection by the human immunodeficiency virus (HIV), and has the main feature of repeated infections, due to failure of certain parts of the immune system. Infection by HIV damages part of the body's natural immunity, and leads to recurrent illnesses.

Antibiotic—A medication that is designed to kill or weaken bacteria.

Computed tomography scan (CT Scan)—A specialized x-ray procedure in which cross-sections of the area in question can be examined in detail. This allows physicians to examine organs such as the pancreas, bile ducts, and others which are often the site of hidden infections.

Magnetic Resonance Imaging (MRI)—This is a new technique similar to CT Scan, but based on the magnetic properties of various areas of the body to compose images.

NSAID—Nonsteroidal anti-inflammatory drugs are medications such as aspirin and ibuprofen that decrease pain and inflammation. Many can now be obtained without a doctor's prescription.

Ultrasound—A non-invasive procedure based on changes in sound waves of a frequency that cannot be heard, but respond to changes in tissue composition. It is very useful for diagnosing diseases of the gallbladder, liver, and hidden infections, such as abscesses.

Patients with HIV are an especially difficult problem, as they often suffer from many unusual infections. HIV itself is a potential cause of fever.

Treatment

Most patients who undergo evaluation for FUO do not receive treatment until a clear-cut cause is found. **Antibiotics** or medications designed to suppress a fever (such as NSAIDs) will only hide the true cause. Once physicians are satisfied that there is no infectious cause, they may use medications such as NSAIDs, or corticosteroids to decrease inflammation and diminish constitutional symptoms.

The development of FUO in certain settings, such as that acquired by patients in the hospital or in those with a low white blood count, often needs rapid treatment to avoid serious complications. Therefore, in these instances patients may be placed on antibiotics after a minimal number of diagnostic studies. Once test results are known, treatment can be adjusted as needed.

Prognosis

The outlook for patients with FUO depends on the cause of the fever. If the basic illness is easily treatable and can be found rather quickly, the potential for a cure is quite good. Some patients continue with temperature elevations for 6 months or more; if no serious disease is found, medications such as NSAIDs are used to decrease the effects of the fever. Careful follow-up and reevaluation is recommended in these cases.

Resources

BOOKS

Gelfand, Jeffrey A., and Charles A. Dinarello. "Fever of Unknown Origin." In *Harrison's Principles of Internal Medicine*, edited by Anthony S. Fauci, et al. New York: McGraw-Hill, 1997.

David Kaminstein, MD

Fever seizures ***see*** **Febrile seizures**

Fifth disease

Definition

Fifth disease is a mild childhood illness caused by the human parvovirus B19 that causes flu–like symptoms and a rash.

Demographics

Anyone can get the disease, but it occurs more frequently in school–aged children. Outbreaks most often occur in the winter and spring, peaking every four to seven 7 years. About 60% of adults have had the disease by age 20.

Description

Fifth disease got its name because it was fifth on a list of common childhood illnesses that are accompanied by a rash, including measles, **rubella** or German measles, **scarlet fever** (or scarlatina), and scarlatinella, a variant of scarlet **fever**. The Latin name for the disease is *erythema infectiosum*, meaning infectious redness. It is also called the "slapped cheek disease" because, when the bright red rash first appears on the cheeks, it looks as if the face has been slapped. The disease is usually mild, and both children and adults normally recover quickly without complications. In fact, some individuals exhibit no symptoms and never feel ill.

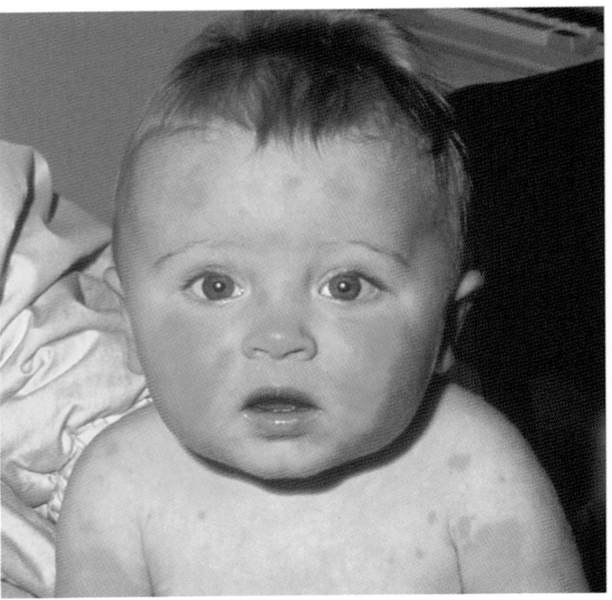

Infant with a rash caused by fifth disease, or *erythema infectiosum*. *(Custom Medical Stock Photo, Inc. Reproduced by permission.)*

Causes and symptoms

Fifth disease is caused by the human parvovirus B19, a member of the Parvoviridae family of viruses that lives in the nose and throat of the infected person. The virus is spread through the air by coughing and sneezing. Because the virus needs a rapidly dividing cell in order to multiply, it attacks the red blood cells of the body. Once infected, a person is believed to be immune to re–infection.

Symptoms appear four to 21 days after exposure to the virus. Initial symptoms are flu–like and include **headache**, body ache, **sore throat**, a mild fever of 101 °F (38.3 °C), and chills. It is at this time, before development of the rash, that individuals are contagious. These symptoms last for two to three days. In children, a bright red rash that looks like a slap mark develops suddenly on the cheeks. The rash may be flat or raised and may or may not be itchy. Sometimes, the rash spreads to the arms, legs, and trunk, where it has a lace–like or net–like appearance. The rash can also involve the palms of the hands and soles of the feet. By the time the rash appears, individuals are no longer infectious. On average, the rash lasts for 10–11 days, but may last for as long as five to six weeks. The rash may fade away and then reappear upon exposure to sunlight, hot baths, emotional distress, or vigorous **exercise**.

Adults generally do not develop a rash, but instead may have swollen and painful joints, especially in the hands and feet. In adults, symptoms such as sore throat, headache, muscle and joint pain, abdominal pain, **diarrhea**, and **vomiting** occur more frequently than in children and usually are more severe. Joint pain can be arthritis–like and last for several months, especially in women, but the disease does not appear to progress to rheumatoid arthritis.

The virus causes the destruction of red blood cells; therefore, a deficiency in the oxygen–carrying capacity of the blood (**anemia**) can result. In healthy people, the anemia is mild and lasts only a short while. In people with weakened immune systems, either because they have a chronic disease such as HIV infection/AIDS or **cancer** (immunocompromised), or they are receiving medication to suppress the **immune system** (immunosuppressed), (e. g., organ transplant recipients), this anemia can be severe and last long after the infection has subsided. Symptoms of anemia include fatigue, lack of healthy color, lack of energy, and shortness of breath. Some individuals with **sickle cell disease**, iron deficiency, a number of different hereditary blood disorders, and those who have received bone marrow transplantations may be susceptible to developing a potentially life–threatening complication called a transient aplastic crisis, in which the body is temporarily unable to form new red blood cells.

In very rare instances, the virus can cause inflammation of different areas of the body, including the brain (**encephalitis**), the covering of the brain and spinal cord (**meningitis**), the lungs (pneumonitis), the liver (hepatitis), and the heart muscle (myocarditis). The virus also can aggravate symptoms for people with an autoimmune disease called systemic lupus erythematosus (SLE).

There is some concern about fifth disease in pregnant women. Although no association with an increased number of **birth defects** or **mental retardation** has been demonstrated, there is concern that infection during the first three months of pregnancy may slightly increase the risk of miscarriage. There is also some concern that infection later in pregnancy may involve a very small risk of premature delivery or stillbirth. As a result, women who get fifth disease while they are pregnant should be monitored closely by a physician.

Diagnosis

Examination

Fifth disease usually is suspected based on a patient's symptoms, including the typical appearance of the bright red rash on the cheeks, patient history, age, and time of year. The physician will exclude other potential causes for the symptoms and rash, including rubella, **infectious mononucleosis**, bacterial infections such as **Lyme disease**, allergic reactions, and SLE.

KEY TERMS

Anemia—A congenital or acquired deficiency in the iron–carrying capacity of the blood.

Antibody—A specific protein produced by the immune system in response to a specific foreign protein or particle called an antigen.

Immunocompromised—A state in which the immune system is weakened or is not functioning properly due to chronic disease.

Immunosuppressed—A state in which the immune system is suppressed by medications during the treatment of other disorders, such as cancer, or following an organ transplantation.

Reye's syndrome—A very serious, rare disease, most common in children, that involves an upper respiratory tract infection followed by brain and liver damage.

Sickle cell disease—A hereditary blood disorder in which red blood cells are misshapen into crescent or sickle shapes resulting in a reduced oxygen–carrying capacity of the lungs.

Systemic lupus erythematosus (SLE)—A chronic, inflammatory, autoimmune disorder in which the individual's immune system attacks, injures, and destroys the body's own organs and tissues. It may affect many organ systems including the skin, joints, lungs, heart, and kidneys.

Tests

In addition, there is a blood test for fifth disease, but it is generally used only for pregnant women and for people who have weakened immune systems or who have blood disorders, such as sickle cell disease. The test involves measuring for a particular antibody or protein that the body produces in response to infection with the human parvovirus B19. The test is 92–97% specific for this disease.

Because fifth disease can pose problems for an unborn fetus exposed to the disease through the mother, testing may also be conducted while a fetus is still in the uterus. This test uses fluid collected from the sac around the fetus (amniotic fluid) instead of blood to detect the viral DNA.

Treatment

In general, no specific treatment for fifth disease is required. The symptoms can be treated using over–the counter medications, such as **acetaminophen** (Tylenol) or ibuprofen (Motrin, Advil). If the rash itches, calamine lotion can be applied. Aspirin is not given to children under the age of 18 to prevent the development of a serious illness called **Reye's syndrome**.

Patients who are receiving medications to suppress the immune system in the treatment of some other condition may be allowed to temporarily decrease the medications in order to allow the immune system to combat the infection and recover from the anemia. Those with weakened (not suppressed) immune systems, such as HIV/AIDS patients, may be given immunoglobulin intravenously to help the immune system fight the infection. People with severe anemia or who experience an aplastic crisis may require hospitalization and blood transfusions.

Prognosis

Generally, fifth disease is mild, and patients tend to improve without any complications. In cases where the patient is either immunocompromised or immunosuppressed, a life–threatening aplastic crisis can occur. With prompt treatment, however, the prognosis is good. Mothers who develop the infection while pregnant can pass the infection on to their fetus, and as such, stand a very small increased risk of miscarriage and stillbirth. There are tests and treatments, however, that can be performed on the fetus while still in the uterus that can reduce the risk of anemia or other complications.

Prevention

Currently, there is no vaccine against fifth disease. Because people with fifth disease are contagious before definitive symptoms appear, it is very difficult to prevent infection. Avoiding contact with persons who exhibit symptoms of a cold and maintaining good personal hygiene by regularly washing hands may minimize the chances of an infection. Pregnant women should avoid exposure to persons infected with the disease and notify their obstetrician immediately if they are exposed so that they can be tested and monitored closely.

Resources

OTHER

"Fifth Disease." MedlinePlus. (May 4, 2010). http://www.nlm.nih.gov/medlineplus/fifthdisease.html (accessed September 17, 2010).

"Parvovirus B19 Infection and Pregnancy." (January 21, 2005). United States Centers for Disease Control and Prevention, http://www.cdc.gov/ncidod/dvrd/revb/respiratory/B19&preg.htm (accessed September 17, 2010).

Zellerman, Glenn. "Erythema Infectiosum (Fifth Disease)" eMedicine.com. (December 8, 2009), http://emedicine.medscape.com/article/1132078-overview (accessed September 17, 2010).

ORGANIZATIONS

National Institute of Allergy and Infectious Diseases, Office of Communications and Government Relations, 6610 Rockledge Dr., MSC 6612, Bethesda MD, 20892–6612, (301) 496–5717, (866) 284–4107 or TDD: (800)877–8339 (for hearing impaired), (301) 402–3573, http://www3.niaid.nih.gov.

Centers for Disease Control and Prevention (CDC), 1600 Clifton Rd., Atlanta GA, 30333, (404) 639–3534, (800) CDC–INFO (800–232–4636). TTY: (888) 232–6348, inquiry@cdc.gov, http://www.cdc.gov.

Lata Cherath, PhD
Tish Davidson, AM

Fighting **see** Acting out

Finding a pediatrician

Definition

Pediatricians provide primary healthcare for newborns, infants, children, adolescents, and young adults through age 21. Many parents find a **pediatrician** before the **birth** of their first child. However a family physician, physician's assistant (PA), or pediatric nurse practitioner (PNP) may fulfill many of the same roles as a pediatrician.

Purpose

Finding a pediatrician is very important for new parents, because children will visit their pediatrician often during the early years of life. There should be at least eight well–baby visits during the first two years. In addition, young children can be particularly susceptible to minor illnesses, such as **strep throat**, fevers, and earaches. A good pediatrician provides preventive care, diagnosis and treatment of minor and major illnesses and chronic disorders, referrals to pediatric specialists or surgeons as necessary, and overall coordination of a child's healthcare. Pediatricians also monitor a child's development and offer advice on everything from **breastfeeding** newborns to **toilet training** toddlers to teenage sexuality. Therefore it is essential that parents trust and feel comfortable with their pediatrician. Ideally, the pediatrician will come to know the child well over many years, and it is equally important that children are at ease with their pediatrician.

Description

Finding an available pediatrician with whom parents feel comfortable—and who is appropriate for the family's needs—may take some time. Many parents begin the process as early as three months before the baby's due date. It is useful to have the pediatrician examine the newborn at birth—and many babies are born before their due date. The hospital will notify the pediatrician of the birth. If the baby's pediatrician is not available, a staff pediatrician or neonatologist may conduct the initial examination. In any case, newborns should visit their own pediatrician within two or three days of leaving the hospital. This initial visit is very important, especially for breastfed babies. The pediatrician will ensure that the baby is receiving adequate **nutrition** and will check for **jaundice**, which affects many newborns.

There are various methods for compiling a list of potential pediatricians:

- Trusted friends can explain what they like—or do not like—about their pediatricians.
- The mother's obstetrician can make recommendations.
- The American Academy of Pediatrics (AAP) provides a list of board–certified pediatricians. Board credentials also can be checked on the AAP web site.
- A local hospital, medical school, or county medical society can provide a list of local pediatricians.
- Managed healthcare plans often limit the choice of pediatricians. Checking the plan's on–line listing of participating doctors should provide an up–to–date list. If a chosen pediatrician is not on the list, or if a child has medical needs that require a particular pediatrician, parents should call their plan directly.

Interviewing two or three prospective pediatricians can be very helpful. Many pediatricians and family doctors are accustomed to interview requests. Some may even allow as much as one hour for the interview, without charging for their time. Some pediatricians conduct group classes for expectant parents, in which they discuss their pediatric practices, as well as newborn care. Many healthcare plans pay for prenatal appointments or classes. If possible, both parents should attend the interview or class, since they may have different concerns.

Before choosing pediatricians to interview, parents should determine that:

- The pediatricians are accepting new patients covered by their health plan.
- Their offices are conveniently located.
- They are associated with hospitals that are preferred by the parents and that accept their health insurance.

Some families have a preference for a male or a female pediatrician. Some prefer to take their boys to a male pediatrician and their girls to a female, especially once they become teenagers; however most pediatricians treat teens of either gender. Some families may have a preference for younger or older pediatricians. Solo practitioners may be able to provide more personalized attention; however those in group practices are more likely to have back–up pediatricians to cover for them when they are unavailable.

The pediatrician's office staff can answer some basic—but important—questions, including:

- office hours
- fee schedules for office, after–hours, home, and hospital visits
- how billing, payment plans, and insurance claims are handled
- when and how routine phone calls are handled
- whether the pediatrician communicates by e–mail
- how urgent calls are handled
- the average wait time for a routine or more urgent appointment
- whether there are other pediatricians in the practice
- whether the child will sometimes be seen by a nurse, PA, or PNP, instead of the pediatrician
- whether the pediatrician makes house calls

While waiting for their interview, parents can ask other parents about their experiences with the pediatrician. The interview is also an opportunity to observe the pediatrician's office:

- Is the waiting room clean, accommodating, and child–friendly?
- Does the waiting room seem peaceful or chaotic?
- Is there a separate waiting area for sick children?
- If the waiting room is crowded, is this because the pediatrician is overbooked or because special circumstances required more time with a particular patient?
- Is the staff polite and considerate to the waiting patients and to those on the phone?

Pediatricians differ in their policies and philosophies. Interviews are an opportunity for parents to learn about some of these differences and determine their own preferences. Relationships between a family and their pediatrician may last two decades or more, so it is important that both parents are comfortable with the choice of pediatrician. In addition to having compatible philosophies, parents should like and trust their pediatrician and feel confident that the pediatrician will care deeply for their child and listen carefully to all of their concerns. Parents should come prepared with a list of questions and should not hesitate or feel embarrassed about asking anything that seems important to them. The pediatrician should be friendly, easy to talk to, and respectful. Questions may include:

- the pediatrician's philosophies on parenting, breast-feeding, immunizations, vegetarianism, circumcision, antibiotics and other medications, complementary, alternative, and integrative medicine, and any other healthcare issues of importance to the family
- the pediatrician's degree of concern with preventive care, child safety, and nutrition
- whether the pediatrician offers advice and other assistance with non–medical problems, including toilet training, developmental issues, school and behavioral issues, or family problems
- how the pediatrician handles teenage sexuality issues
- guidelines for issues that can be handled with a phone call or by e–mail versus those that require an office visit
- procedures for a child who is injured or suddenly becomes seriously ill
- whether the pediatrician accepts emergency after–hours calls or sees a seriously ill or injured child in the office after–hours or whether the child must be taken to an emergency department or urgent care center
- the pediatrician's ability to recommend and work with various pediatric specialists, if required

In addition to specific information, parents can get a sense of the pediatrician's personality. The pediatrician should not be intimidating. Parents should feel comfortable with the pediatrician, the office staff, and any other doctors in the practice. Most parents want a pediatrician who will:

- listen carefully and respond to their information, questions, and concerns
- partner with them in their child's care
- take the time to explain issues carefully
- be supportive of their seeking a second opinion

Common problems

There may be many reasons for finding a new pediatrician, including relocation, changes in health insurance, or a pediatrician's retirement. Families may also find that they are dissatisfied with their pediatrician for any of a number of reasons. Although parents should discuss problems directly with the pediatrician, if the pediatrician is not responsive to their concerns or if the problem cannot be resolved, the family should find another doctor. Parents may want to return to their original list of potential pediatricians and resume the interviewing process. This time around, they may have a better idea of their concerns and what they should look for in a pediatrician.

Before traveling, parents should consider what to do if their child requires a pediatrician while away from home. Before leaving, they may want to identify pediatricians in the areas where they will be traveling.

Parental concerns

The process of finding appropriate care for their child is the same, regardless of whether a pediatrician, a family doctor, or a PNP is chosen. However the training and certifications for these professions are different.

Pediatrics is a medical specialty that focuses on the physical, developmental, emotional, and social health of children from birth through **adolescence**, with a primary focus on preventive healthcare. Following four years of medical school and at least three years of pediatric residency, a pediatrician can choose to take a written examination for board certification every seven years. Board–certified pediatricians use the initials FAAP, for Fellow of the **American Academy of Pediatrics**. Certification ensures that the pediatrician has kept current on pediatric medical advances. In addition, state licensure requires that pediatricians complete annual continuing medical education (CME) courses. Some pediatricians have an additional one to three years of training in a subspecialty, such as neonatology, pediatric cardiology, hematology, or critical care or emergency medicine. Board certification in a pediatric subspecialty usually requires an additional three years of training after residency.

Many children receive their health care from family physicians. Family physicians complete three years of residency after medical school, usually spending several months training in each of several medical specialties, including pediatrics. They can take exams to be certified by the American Board of Family Medicine and are required to complete CME courses. Family physicians can care for all family members and can continue to treat children after they reach adulthood. Family physicians may have the advantage of being well–acquainted with the medical histories of all family members, as well as familiarity with any emotional and social issues within the family. However some family physicians accept only a few children as patients or care only for older children.

PNPs usually have a master's degree in nursing and special training in pediatrics. They take medical histories, perform physical examinations, diagnose and treat

KEY TERMS

Board–certified—A physician who has completed medical school, a residency, trained in a specialty, and passed a qualifying exam administered by a medical specialty board.

Circumcision—A procedure in which the prepuce—the skin covering the tip of the penis—is cut away, usually soon after birth.

Neonatologist—A specialist in the medical care of newborns.

Newborn jaundice—Physiological jaundice; a usually harmless condition in newborns, characterized by yellowing of the skin and eyes due to excess bilirubin in the blood.

Pediatric nurse practitioner; PNP—A nurse with at least a master's degree and advanced training in pediatrics, who takes medical histories and performs examinations, diagnoses, treatments, and counseling of children, in collaboration with physicians.

Physician's assistant; physician assistant; PA—A specially trained practitioner who provides basic medical services, such as diagnosis and treatment of minor illnesses, usually under the supervision of a physician.

Strep throat—A sore throat caused by hemolytic Group A streptococci bacteria.

illnesses, and counsel patients. Some PNPs have pediatric specialties, such as neurology or endocrinology. PNPs work closely with pediatricians and family physicians in private practices, clinics, and hospitals. PNPs may have more time to spend with children and parents than pediatricians.

Resources

BOOKS

Shelov, Steven P., editor. *Caring For Your Baby and Young Child: Birth to Age 5,* 5th ed. New York: Bantam, 2009.

PERIODICALS

Palfrey, Judith. "The Doc Dossier: Get to Know Your Pediatrician Before Your Baby's First Appointment." *Baby Talk* 75(5) (June–July 2010): 52–53.

OTHER

American Academy of Pediatrics. "Finding a Pediatrician." HealthyChildren.org. (June 22, 2010), http://www.healthychildren.org/English/ages-stages/prenatal/decisions-to-make/pages/Finding-a-Pediatrician.aspx (accessed September 17, 2010).

"Finding a Doctor for Your New Baby." KidsHealth. (September 2008), http://kidshealth.org/parent/system/doctor/find_ped.html#a_Your%20Options (accessed September 17, 2010).

ORGANIZATIONS

American Academy of Pediatrics (AAP), 141 Northwest Point Blvd., Elk Grove Village IL, 60007–1098, (874) 434–4000, (874) 434–8000, kidsdocs@aap.org, http://www.aap.org.

American Board of Pediatrics (ABP), 111 Silver Cedar Ct., Chapel Hill NC, 27514, (919) 929–0461, (919) 929–9255, abpeds@abpeds.org, https://www.abp.org.

Margaret Alic, PhD

Fine motor skills

Definition

Fine motor skills are the ability to make smooth, controlled movements using the small muscles in the fingers, hand, and wrist.

Description

Fine motor skills involve deliberate and controlled movements requiring both muscle development and maturation of the central nervous system. Although newborn infants can move their hands and arms, these motions are reflexes that an infant cannot consciously start or stop. The development of fine motor skills is crucial to an infant's ability to experience and learn about the world. It thus plays a central role in the development of **intelligence**. Like **gross motor skills**, fine motor skills develop in an orderly progression, but at an uneven pace characterized by both rapid spurts and, at times, frustrating but harmless delays. In most cases, difficulty with certain fine motor skills is temporary and does not indicate a serious problem. Medical help should be sought, however, if a child is significantly behind his peers in multiple aspects of fine motor development or if he regresses, losing previously acquired skills.

Infancy

The hands of newborns are closed most of the time and, like the rest of their body, they have little control over them. If the palm is touched, the newborn will make a very tight fist, but this is an unconscious action called the Darwinian reflex, and it disappears within two to three

Fine motor skills

Age	Skill
One to three months	Reflexively grasps finger or toy placed in hand.
Three months	Grasping reflex gone. Briefly holds small toy voluntarily when it is placed in the hand.
Four months	Holds and shakes rattle. Brings hands together to play with them. Reaches for objects but frequently misses them.
Five months	Grasps objects deliberately. Splashes water. Crumples paper.
Six months	Holds bottle. Grasps at own feet. May bring toes to mouth.
Seven months	Transfers toy from hand to hand. Bangs objects on table. Puts everything into the mouth. Loves playing with paper.
Nine months	Able to grasp small objects between thumb and forefinger.
Ten months	Points at objects with index finger. Lets go of objects deliberately.
Eleven months	Places object into another's hand when requested, but does not release.
Twelve months	Places and releases object into another's hand when requested. Rolls ball on floor. Starts to hold crayon and mark paper with it.
Fifteen months	Builds tower of two blocks. Repeatedly throws objects on floor. Starts to be able to take off clothing, starting with shoes.
Eighteen months	Builds tower of three blocks. Starts to feed self well with spoon. Turns book pages two or three at a time. Scribbles on paper.
Two years	Builds tower of six or seven blocks. Turns book pages one at a time. Turns door knobs and unscrews jar lids. Washes and dries hands. Uses spoon and fork well.
Two and a half years	Builds tower of eight blocks. Holds pencil between fingers instead of grasping with fist.
Three years	Builds tower of nine or ten blocks. Puts on shoes and socks. Can button and unbutton. Carries containers with little spilling or dropping.
Four years	Dresses self except for tying. Cuts with scissors, but not well. Washes and dries face.
Five years	Dresses without help. Ties shoes. Prints simple letters.

SOURCE: *Miller-Keane Encyclopedia and Dictionary of Medicine, Nursing, and Allied Health, 7th ed.*, and Child Development Institute, http://www.childdevelopmentinfo.com.

(Table by PreMediaGlobal. Reproduced by permission of Gale, a part of Cengage Learning.)

months. Similarly, the infant will grasp at an object placed in his or her hand, but without any awareness that she is doing so. At some point, the hand muscles will relax, and the infant will drop the object, equally unaware that it has been dropped. Babies may begin flailing at objects that interest them by two weeks of age but cannot grasp them. By eight weeks, they begin to discover and play with their hands, at first solely by touch, and then, at about three months, by sight as well. At this age, however, the deliberate grasp remains largely undeveloped.

Hand-eye coordination begins to develop between the ages of two and four months, inaugurating a period of trial-and-error practice at sighting objects and grabbing at them. At four or five months, most infants can grasp an object that is within reach, looking only at the object and not at their hands. Referred to as "top-level reaching," this achievement is considered an important milestone in fine motor development. At the age of six months, infants typically can hold on to a small block briefly, and many have started banging objects. Although their grasp is still clumsy, they have acquired a fascination with grabbing small objects and trying to put them in their mouths. At first, babies will indiscriminately try to grasp things that cannot be grasped, such as pictures in a book, as well as those that can, such as a rattle or ball. During the latter half of the first year, they begin exploring and testing objects before grabbing, touching them with an entire hand and eventually poking them with an index finger.

One of the most significant fine motor accomplishments is the pincer grip, which typically appears between the ages of 12 and 15 months. Initially, an infant can hold an object, such as a rattle, only in his palm, wrapping his fingers (including the thumb) around it from one side. This is an awkward position called the palmar grasp, which makes it difficult to hold on to and manipulate the object. By the age of eight to ten months, the infant begins to use a finger grasp, but can grasp objects only with all four fingers pushing against the thumb, which still makes it awkward to pick up and hold small objects. The development of the pincer grip, defined as the ability to hold objects between the thumb and index finger, gives the infant a more sophisticated ability to grasp and manipulate objects, and also to deliberately drop them. By about the age of one year, an infant can drop an object into a receptacle, compare objects held in both hands, stack objects, and nest them within each other.

Toddlerhood

Toddlers develop the ability to manipulate objects with increasing sophistication, including using their fingers to twist dials, pull strings, push levers, turn book pages, and use crayons to produce crude scribbles. **Handedness**, the dominance of either the right or left hand, usually emerges during this period as well. Toddlers also add a new dimension to touching and manipulating objects by simultaneously being able to name them. Instead of random scribbles, their **drawings** include such patterns as circles. Their play with blocks is more elaborate and purposeful than that of infants, and they can stack as many as six blocks. They are also able to fold a sheet of paper in half (with supervision), string

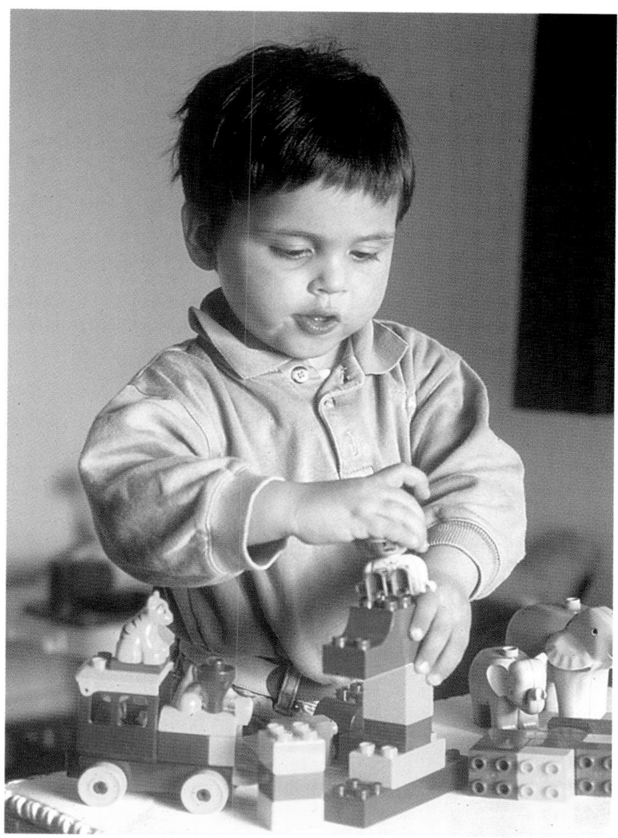

A toddler demonstrates his fine motor skills by grasping and manipulating building blocks. *(S. Villeger/Explorer/Photo Researchers, Inc.)*

large beads, manipulate snap **toys**, play with clay, unwrap small objects, and pound pegs.

Preschool

The delicate tasks facing **preschool** children, such as handling silverware or tying shoelaces, represent more of a challenge than most of the gross motor activities learned during this period of development. The central nervous system is still in the process of maturing sufficiently for complex messages from the brain to get to the child's fingers. In addition, small muscles tire more easily than large ones, and the short stubby fingers of preschoolers make delicate or complicated tasks more difficult. Finally, gross motor skills call for energy, which often seems endless in preschoolers, while fine motor skills require patience, which is in shorter supply. Thus, there is considerable variation in fine motor development among children in this age group.

By the age of three, many children have good control of a pencil. Three-year-olds can often draw a circle, although their attempts at drawing people are still very primitive. It is common for four year olds to be able to use scissors, copy geometric shapes and letters, button large buttons, and form clay shapes with two or three sections. Some can print their own names in capital letters. A human figure drawn by a four year old is typically a head atop two legs with one arm radiating from each leg.

School-age children

By the age of five, most children have clearly advanced beyond the fine motor skill development of the preschool age. They can draw recognizably human figures with facial features and legs connected to a distinct trunk. Besides drawing, five year olds can also cut, paste, and trace shapes. Their right- or left-handedness is well established, and they use the preferred hand for writing and drawing.

By age four or five years, children have begun to acquire the fine motor skills needed for daily self-care (e.g., dressing, washing, toileting, eating with spoons and forks). They can fasten visible buttons (as opposed to those at the back of clothing), and many can tie bows, including shoelace bows. By age six, most children can spread jelly or butter on bread with a knife, and cut the bread.

Encouraging fine motor development

Encouraging gross motor skills requires a safe, open play space, peers to interact with, and some adult supervision. Nurturing the development of fine motor skills is considerably more complicated. Helping a child succeed in fine motor tasks requires planning, time, and a variety of play materials. Fine motor development can be encouraged by activities that youngsters enjoy and that involve manipulating objects or materials with the hands, including crafts, puzzles, making **music** on percussion instruments, and playing with building blocks. There is also considerable evidence that studying a keyboard instrument (i.e., piano, organ, harpsichord, electric keyboard) leads to great improvement in a child's fine motor skills.

Helping parents with such everyday domestic activities as baking can be fun for the child in addition to developing fine motor skills. For example, stirring batter provides a good workout for the hand and arm muscles, and cutting and spooning out cookie dough requires hand-eye coordination. Even a computer keyboard and mouse can provide practice in finger, hand, and hand-eye coordination. Because the development of fine motor skills plays a crucial role in school readiness and **cognitive development**, it is considered an important part of the preschool curriculum. The Montessori schools, in particular, were early leaders in emphasizing the significance of fine motor tasks and the use of such learning aids as pegboards and puzzles in early childhood education. The development of fine motor skills in children of low-income parents, who often lack the time or knowledge required to foster these abilities, is a key ingredient in the success of such programs as Head Start.

School-age children who have difficulty with writing or drawing may be suffering from weakness in the shoulder girdle. In mature writing, only the person's wrist moves, while the other arm joints remain steady. Children with a weak shoulder girdle, however, must move the entire arm instead of just the wrist in order to write. As a result, they tire quickly when asked to write or draw. A child whose problems in writing or drawing are severe enough to interfere with schoolwork should be evaluated for neurological or musculoskeletal problems that may be contributing to his or her difficulties with fine motor skills. In general, boys are more likely than girls to have problems with fine motor coordination. **Occupational therapy** is available for children with fine motor difficulties, and there are many good school-based occupational therapists who specialize in working with these children.

Children also can be helped to develop fine motor skills by modification of tools and writing equipment and choosing desks and chairs of the proper size and height. Large thick crayons, brushes, and pencils are easier for young artists to use than smaller or thinner ones. A child's desk chair should allow him or her to sit with feet firmly on the floor and hips, knees, and ankles at 90 degree angles. The surface of the desk should be about 2 inches above the elbows when the child's arms are resting at his side. It is easier for children to move their arms, hands, and fingers effectively and smoothly when the trunk of the body is stable.

KEY TERMS

Central nervous system (CNS)—Part of the nervous system consisting of the brain, cranial nerves and spinal cord. The brain is the center of higher processes, such as thought and emotion and is responsible for the coordination and control of bodily activities and the interpretation of information from the senses. The cranial nerves and spinal cord link the brain to the peripheral nervous system, that is the nerves present in the rest of body.

Gross motor skills—Controlled movement of large muscle groups allowing activities such as walking or throwing a ball.

Resources

BOOKS

Piek, Jan P. *Infant Motor Development*. Champaign, IL: Human Kinetics, 2006.

Thomas, Jerry R., Jack K. Nelson, and Stephen J. Silverman. *Research Methods in Physical Activity*, 5th ed. Champaign, IL: Human Kinetics, 2005.

PERIODICALS

Costa-Giomi, E. "Does Music Instruction Improve Fine Motor Abilities?" *Annals of the New York Academy of Sciences* 1060 (December 2005): 262–264.

OTHER

Logsdon, Anne. Fine Motor Skills. About.com. 2010. [accessed July 15, 2010], http://learningdisabilities.about.com/od/df/p/finemotorskills.htm.

Ready for Kindergarten: Fine Motor Activities. Education.com. Undated. [accessed July 15, 2010], http://www.education.com/reference/article/Ref_Ready_Fine_Motor.

ORGANIZATIONS

American Academy of Family Physicians, P. O. Box 11210, Shawnee Mission KS, 66207, (913)906-6000, (800) 274-2237, (913) 906-6075, http://familydoctor.org.

American Academy of Pediatrics, 141 Northwest Point Boulevard, Elk Grove Village IL, 60007-1098, (847) 434-4000, (847) 434-8000, http://www.aap.org.

American Occupational Therapy Association, PO Box 31220, Bethesda MD, 20824-1220, (301) 652-2682, TDD: (800) 377-8555, (301) 652-7711, http://www.1.aota.org.

Tish Davidson, AM

Fingertip injuries

Definition

Fingertip trauma covers cuts, accumulation of blood (hematoma), bone breakage, or amputation in the fingertip.

Description

The fingertips are specialized areas of the hand with highly developed sensory and manipulative functions. Large sensory and motor areas located in the brain regulate the precise and delicate functions of fingertips. The fingertip is the site where extensor and flexor tendons insert. Fingertip injuries are extremely common since the hands hold a wide array of objects. In 2001, the approximately 10% of all accidents in the United States referred for Emergency Room consults involve the hand. Hand injuries are frequently the result of job injuries and account for 11–14% of on-the-job injuries and 6% of compensation paid injuries. Injury to the nail bed occurs in approximately 15–24% of fingertip injuries.

Fingertip injuries can result in amputation or tissue loss. The injury is assessed whether the bone and underlying tissue are intact and the size of the wound area. The pulp is the area of skin opposite the fingernail and is usually very vulnerable to injury. Pulp injuries commonly occur in persons who use or are in close contact with fast moving mechanical devices. These injuries can crush, cut, and puncture. The fingertips can also be injured by common crushing accidents. This could cause the development of a subungal hematoma (an accumulation of blood under the nail). At the base of the distal phalanx (the first circular skin fold from the tip) injuries can occur that can fracture the underlying bone in the area. Quite commonly a hammer, closing a door, or sport accidents usually cause these injuries. These **fractures** can be simple, requiring little treatment or more complicated involving the joint. The accident may involve the point of insertion of a tendon. Usually this occurs when the terminal joint is being forced to flex while held straight. This motion typically occurs when tucking in sheets during bed making, a common cause of tendon injury. This injury causes a loss of extension (straightening the finger) ability.

Causes and symptoms

Accidental amputations will usually result in profuse bleeding and tissue loss. Injuries to the pulp can occur as from fast moving mechanical instruments, such as drills. These injuries may puncture the pulp. Injuries such as a subungal hematoma are caused by a crushing type injury. Fractures typically occur as the result of crushing injuries or tendon avulsion. These crushing injuries are frequently caused during sport injury and can be treated by simple interventions such as **immobilization** or more complex procedures if tendons are affected (the trauma is then treated as a tendon injury). Fractures can cause **pain** and, depending on the extent of swelling, there may be some restriction of movement. Tendon injuries can be caused when the terminal joint is exposed to force flexing motion (moving the finger toward the palm) while held straight.

Diagnosis

The attending clinician should evaluate the injury in a careful and systematic manner. The appearance of the hand can provide valuable information concerning presence of fractures, vascular status, and tendon involvement. Bones and joints should be evaluated for motion and tenderness. Nerves should be examined for sensory (feeling sensations) and motor (movement) functioning. Amputations usually profusely bleed and there is tissue loss. The wound is treated based on loss of tissue, bone, and wound area. Injuries to the pulp can be obvious during inspection. Subungal hematoma usually present a purplish-black discoloration under the nail. This is due to a hematoma underneath the nail. Radiographs may be required to assess the alignment of fractures or detect foreign bodies. Patients usually suffer from pain since injuries to the fingertip bone are usually painful and movement may be partially restricted due to swelling of the affected area. Tendon injuries usually result in the loss of ability to straighten or bend the finger.

Treatment

Amputation with bone and underlying tissue intact and a wound area 1 cm or less should be cleaned and treated with a dressing. With these types of **wounds** healthy tissue will usually grow and replace the injured area. Larger wounds may require surgical intervention. Puncture wounds should be cleaned and left open to heal. Patients typically receive **antibiotics** to prevent infection. A procedure called trephining treats subungal hematomas. This procedure is usually done with a straight cutting needle positioned over the nail. The clinician spins the needle with forefinger and thumb until a hole is made through the nail.

Patients who have extensive crush injuries or subungal hematomas involving laceration to skin folds or nail damage should have the nail removed to examine the underlying tissue (called the matrix). Patients who have a closed subungal hematoma with an intact nail and no other damage (no nail disruption or laceration) are treated conservatively. If the fracture is located two-thirds below the fingertip immobilization using a splint may be needed. Conservative treatment is recommended for crush injuries that fracture the terminal phalanx if a subungal hematoma is not present. Severe fractures near the fist circular skin crease may require surgical correction to prevent irregularity of the joint surface, which can cause difficulty with movement. Injury to a flexor tendon usually requires surgical repair. If this is not possible, the finger and wrist should be placed in a splint with specific positioning to prevent further damage.

Prognosis

Prognosis depends on the extent of traumatic damage to the affected area. Nail lacerations that are

KEY TERMS

Distal—Movement away from the origin.

Flex—To bend.

Laceration—A cut in the skin

Phalanx—A bone of the fingers or toes.

Tendon—A structure that connects a skeletal muscle to bone.

not treated may cause nail deformities. When amputation is accompanied with loss of two-thirds of the nail, half of the fingers develop beaking, or a curved nail. Aftercare and follow up are important components of treatment. The patient is advised to keep the hand elevated, check with a clinician two days after treatment, and to splint fractures for two weeks in the extended position. Usually a nail takes about 100 days to fully grow. Healing for an amputation takes about 21 to 27 days. This markedly decreases in elderly patients, primarily due to a compromised circulation normally part of advancing age.

Resources

BOOKS

Townshend, Courtney M., et al. *Sabiston Textbook of Surgery*. 16th ed. W. B. Saunders Company, 2001.

Laith Farid Gulli, M.D.

Firearm safety

Definition

Firearms are weapons that use the controlled explosion of a propellant to shoot projectiles at high velocity. The term "firearms" is generally taken to mean guns and rifles. Firearm **safety** involves both proper handling and proper storage of firearms. With firearms present in more than one third of all American households, safe storage and handling is a critical issue for families, especially those with children.

Purpose

The purpose of firearm safety is prevent accidental injury and **death**, suicides committed in moments of temporary despair, and crimes committed out of emotional or mental derangement. Thousands of Americans are seriously injured or killed every year because:

- children accidentally fire guns that they have found or are showing off to friends
- a depressed teen or adult becomes suicidal
- an argument goes out of control
- a family member or friend is mistaken for an intruder

Even children in households without guns should learn about firearm safety and what to do if they come across a gun. Children younger than about eight are unable to tell the difference between a real gun and a toy gun and a three–year–old may be strong enough pull a trigger.

Demographics

On average, an American child under age ten is killed or disabled by a gun every other day. Firearm–related injuries are second only to motor–vehicle accidents as the most common cause of fatal injury in children and adults. The majority of firearm fatalities in childen (more than 60%) are homicides, with the remainder classified as suicides (about 30%) and accidents (eight percent). More than half of all unintentional shootings are committed by children and teenagers, and for every child killed with a firearm, five more are injured.

Among American teens aged 13 through 19, **suicide** is one of the three leading causes of death, with an average of four teens committing suicide every day. More adolescent suicides are committed with firearms than by any other method, in part because suicide attempts with guns are much more likely to be fatal. The risk of suicide is four to 10 times higher in homes with firearms, and even higher if the firearm is a handgun or is loaded and unlocked. Likewise, many injuries and deaths could be prevented if firearms were not within easy reach at moments of anger or perceived danger.

Many firearm injuries and deaths occur because children and teens obtain improperly stored household firearms. One third of all American families with children and almost 40% of homes with children have firearms, and more than 40% of families with both children and firearms do not keep the firearms locked up. The majority of these families have not talked to their children about firearm safety, and although many patients and physicians believe that firearm safety counseling should be a part of family practice, the vast majority of family physicians have never discussed firearm safety with their patients, nor do they feel competent to do so.

Overall, 42% of men and 25% of women in the United States report having a gun, pistol, or rifle in their home. Women are less likely than men to be aware of a firearm kept in the household and, if they are aware of the firearm, to know how it is stored. Studies have shown that twice as many firearm deaths among children occur in states where a higher percentage of firearms are stored loaded, with the greatest risk occurring when loaded firearms are more likely to be unlocked.

Description

Homes without firearms are safer than those with firearms. Before bringing a firearm into the home for protection, parents should consider less dangerous methods, such as window locks, dogs, or burglar alarms. No one should have a firearm unless he or she knows how to handle and store it safely and have completed a firearm safety course.

Rules for safe handling of firearms include:

- always keeping firearms unloaded until ready for use
- always assuming that all firearms are loaded at all times
- keeping the muzzle pointed in a safe direction at all times
- keeping the finger off the trigger and out of the trigger guard until ready to shoot
- always being sure of the target and what is beyond the target

Children are naturally curious and given to exploring. This makes the safe storage of firearms even more urgent in households with children or where children visit. Firearms should always be stored unloaded and in the uncocked position; locked up in a rack, case, or safe; and out of the sight and reach of children. Ammunition should be locked up separately from firearms, and supplies for cleaning firearms should also be locked up, since they are often poisonous.

Although trigger locks or other childproof devices, which are applied to unloaded firearms, can be useful as an additional precaution, some trigger locks can be removed in as little as six seconds. Revolvers can be made childproof with a padlock that prevents the cylinder from being locked in place, but all keys or combinations to firearm and ammunition locks should be hidden out of children's reach. Adults who **sleep** with an unlocked gun under their pillows should always lock it first thing upon rising.

Firearms should never be kept in a home with an individual who is depressed, has a mental illness, has Alzheimer's disease, abuses alcohol or drugs, or is abusive to others or has the potential for violent behavior.

Even families without firearms need to ensure that their children are safe in homes that they visit. Some families do not let their children visit homes with firearms or homes in which firearms are not stored safely.

Firearm safety includes hearing protection. Noise–induced hearing loss (NIHL) is permanent hearing damage that can be caused by a one–time exposure to a loud sound, such as a shotgun firing at close range, or repeated exposures to harmful sounds over an extended period, such as from hunting. Earmuffs or earplugs should always be worn when shooting a firearm.

Laws governing the disposal of firearms differ among states and locales. Local police should be contacted if a firearm is found or if an individual owns an unwanted firearm. Some communities have firearm buy–back or amnesty programs. Generally, turned–in firearms are checked to ensure that they are not part of a criminal investigation and then made unusable or destroyed.

Common problems

Some children and teens may respond aggressively or violently when faced with situations that they do not know how to handle. Many communities have laws against teenagers possessing firearms or other weapons. Firearms and ammunition should never be kept in households with young people who are at risk for violent behaviors. Signs that a child or adolescent is at high risk for violent behavior may include:

- physical fights
- a history of inflicting violent injury
- having been a victim of violence
- dropping out of school
- having delinquent friends
- being a gang member
- using drugs or alcohol or selling drugs
- having a criminal record

Shootings have become increasingly common on the streets of American cities and even in schools. It is very important that teenagers are able to recognize signs of potential violence. Any signs or threats should be taken seriously. Warning signs that an individual may be more likely to become violent can include:

- cruelty to pets or other animals
- frequent talk of weapons and violence
- preoccupation with violent movies, television, or video games
- isolation from family and friends
- threatening or bullying behavior

Teens—and even younger children—should know what to do if they encounter someone with a firearm or suspect that someone may have a gun. They should first move quickly and quietly away from the situation, and then immediately tell a responsible adult—such as a school principal, teacher, counselor, coach, or parent—what they saw. All details should be relayed, including the type of weapon, when and where the incident occurred, and who was involved. If a trustworthy adult is not available, or if teens are afraid that their identity will not be protected, they can call the school office anonymously or call 911 and ask that their identity be kept confidential. As soon as possible, the witness should write down all of the details of the incident, so that they have a written record if they are asked about it later.

Pellet guns and BB guns can cause serious injury. They are not regulated by the government, but the U.S. Consumer Product Safety Commission (CPSC) advises that children under the age of 16 not be allowed to use high–velocity BB guns or pellet guns. Children and teens who have BB or pellet guns, or who are likely to come in contact with them, should know never to point the gun at themselves or anyone else.

KEY TERMS

Alzheimer's disease—A progressive, neurodegenerative disease characterized by loss of function and death of nerve cells in several areas of the brain, leading to loss of mental functions, such as memory and learning. Alzheimer's disease is the most common cause of dementia.

Muzzle—The mouth or discharge end of the barrel of a firearm.

Noise–induced hearing loss (NIHL)—Permanent hearing damage caused by one–time or repeated exposure to loud sounds such as firearms.

Trigger—A small, projecting tongue on a firearm that, when pressed with a finger, activates the mechanism that discharges the weapon.

Trigger lock—A device that prevents a firearm from being discharged.

Parental concerns

Many children grow up with firearms in the home, especially in families that hunt. All children should be taught firearm safety, even if there are no guns in the home. First and foremost, children should be taught that firearms are dangerous and should never be touched without permission. If children find a firearm—even if they are not sure whether it is real or a toy—they should not touch it; rather they should immediately leave the area and tell an adult. The National Rifle Association (NRA) rules for children are: "Stop! Don't touch; remove yourself from the area; tell an adult." Leaving the area is especially important because someone else may pick up the gun. If a child knows that a fellow student possesses a gun at school, he or she should know to immediately report the information to an adult.

Parents may choose to prevent their children from watching violent television or movies, playing violent **video games**, or playing with toy or pretend weapons. However, since playmates may have toy guns or violent media, it is important that parents clearly explain the difference between **toys** and weapons. Parents should also talk with their children about the differences between screen violence and real–life violence in which people are injured or killed. Parents can model peaceful and respectful behaviors for their children, and teenagers may participate in programs for safe rifle handling.

Parents should discuss firearm safety with the parents of their children's friends. Before a child goes to the home of a friend or a **babysitter**, parents should ask whether the home has firearms and, if so, whether they are unloaded and locked away.

Teenagers who are troubled or depressed often act impulsively. Many teens who attempt suicide are upset about a temporary problem, such as a failed romance. It is dangerous to have firearms in homes with a teenager who is depressed or has severe mood swings. Keys to locked–up firearms and ammunition should be kept away from teenagers. In addition to depression, risk factors for adolescent suicide include:

- psychiatric illness or a family history of mental disorders or depression
- drug or alcohol abuse
- a traumatic loss or event
- suicide of a friend or family member
- chronic or debilitating physical disorders
- previous suicide attempts

Resources

BOOKS

Canino, Kate. *Turkey Hunting.* New York: Rosen Central, 2011.

Wheeler, Timothy W., and E. John Wipfler. *Keeping Your Family Safe: The Responsibilities of Firearm Ownership.* Bellevue, WA: Merril Press, 2009.

PERIODICALS

Carroll, Matt. "License to Shoot; A Course in Firearms Safety is Basic in Massachusetts if You Want to Handle a Gun." *Boston Globe* (March 21, 2010): 1.

Zarbock, Sarah. "Ready! Fire! Aim! Firearm Safety is Every Physician Assistant's Job." *Journal of the American*

Academy of Physicians Assistants 22(12) (December 2009): 11.

OTHER

Editorial Staff. "Gun Safety." FamilyDoctor.org. July 2010, http://familydoctor.org/online/famdocen/home/healthy/safety/crisis/228.pr interview.html (accessed September 26, 2010).

"Gun Safety." FBI Kids K–5th Grade, http://www.fbi.gov/kids/k5th/safety5.htm (accessed September 26, 2010).

"Gun Safety." KidsHealth. July 2008, http://kidshealth.org/parent/firstaid_safe/home/gun_safety.html# (accessed September 26, 2010).

"Gun Safety." MedlinePlus. August 24, 2010, http://www.nlm.nih.gov/medlineplus/gunsafety.html (accessed September 26, 2010).

"Parent's Firearm Safety Checklist." Injury Free Coalition for Kids, http://www.injuryfree.org/resources/FirearmInjuryPreventionChecklist.pdf (accessed September 26, 2010).

ORGANIZATIONS

American Academy of Family Physicians (AAFP), 11400 Tomahawk Creek Pkwy., Leawood KS, 66211–2680 (913) 906–6000 (800) 274–6000 (913) 906–6075, http://www.aafp.org.

American Academy of Pediatrics (AAP), 141 Northwest Point Blvd., Elk Grove Village IL, 60007–1098 (874) 434–4000 (874) 434–8000 kidsdocs@aap.org, http: //www.aap.org.

Injury Free Coalition for Kids (IFCK), Columbia University, Department of Epidemiology, School of Public Health, 722 W. 168th St., Room 821 H–I, New York NY, 10032 (212) 342–0514 info@injuryfree.org, http://www.injuryfree.org

Margaret Alic, PhD

First aid

Definition

First aid is the treatment of minor injuries or conditions or immediate care or treatment for a medical emergency that is administered while awaiting professional help.

Purpose

First aid ranges from cleaning and bandaging a minor scrape to saving a life with **cardiopulmonary resuscitation** (CPR). It is often required to stop bleeding or to stabilize and protect an ill or injured person until they can get to a hospital or emergency help arrives on the scene. First aid may be used to treat:

- cuts, scrapes, and scratches
- nosebleeds
- severe bleeding
- heat exhaustion and heatstroke
- frostnip and frostbite
- burns
- poisoning
- choking
- a foreign object in the eye or nose
- injured or broken bones
- head or spinal injuries
- seizures
- shock
- unconsciousness
- respiratory or heart failure

Demographics

Every year millions of children require first aid for minor injuries, serious accidents, or life-threatening emergencies. For this reason, every home, automobile, daycare, and school should be equipped with a well-stocked first-aid kit and every parent, **caregiver**, and teacher should be trained in first aid and CPR.

Description

First aid for a minor scrape, cut, or puncture wound may include:

- using sterile gauze, tissue, or a clean, soft cloth to apply gentle, firm pressure to stop bleeding
- cleaning with cool running water or soaking the wound
- using a soft cloth and gentle soap to clean around the injury
- using a soft, damp cloth or tweezers cleaned with rubbing alcohol to remove dirt or debris
- applying antibiotic ointment
- covering with butterfly tape, adhesive strips, or sterile gauze and adhesive tape, if the injury is in an area that could get dirty or rubbed by clothing
- changing bandages daily

For severe bleeding:

- lie down and cover the injured person to prevent loss of body heat

- if possible, elevate the legs to increase blood flow to the brain and prevent fainting or elevate the injured area above the level of the heart to slow bleeding
- apply firm, gentle pressure to the wound for at least 20 minutes
- add more gauze or cloth if needed, without removing the lower layers
- pressure may be applied to a main artery leading to the injured area
- tightly wrap the wound with a bandage or clean cloth and tape
- immobilize the injured part and leave bandages in place once the bleeding has stopped

For a nosebleed:

- sit, leaning slightly forward to drain the blood out of the nose, but with the head above the level of the heart
- squeeze the soft part of the nose, using the thumb and index finger, until the bleeding stops or for at least five minutes
- do not do anything to make the bleeding restart, such as bending over or blowing through the nose

For heat exhaustion or heatstroke:

- rest in a cool, shady spot, with unnecessary clothing removed
- drink plenty of water or other fluids
- be bathed or sprayed with cool water
- be cooled by evaporating water from the skin

For **frostnip** or **frostbite**:

- dress in dry clothing in a warm environment and drink warm fluids
- if emergency help is not immediately available for frostbite, the frozen parts should be immersed in warm water (100°F, 38°C) or treated with warm compresses for 30 minutes
- if warm water is unavailable, gently wrap the affected person in blankets
- thawed areas should be kept still and wrapped to prevent refreezing

For **burns**:

- clothing should be gently removed from around the burn, unless it is stuck to the skin
- first-degree burns should be soaked in cool water for at least five minutes and loosely wrapped with a dry gauze bandage or a clean soft towel or sheet
- second-degree burns should be soaked in cool water for 15 minutes and covered with a dry nonstick dressing that is changed daily
- third-degree burns should be covered with a cool, wet, sterile bandage or clean cloth, without first soaking the burn; if possible, the burned area should be raised above the level of the heart until medical assistance is available
- electrical burns should be covered with gauze without rinsing
- for chemical burns, any contaminated clothing or jewelry should be removed and any dry chemical brushed off the skin; the burn should be gently rinsed with cool, running water for at least 20 minutes; loosely wrapped with a dry, sterile, dressing or gauze or a clean cloth; and rewashed if the pain worsens

If someone begins **choking**, they should be given abdominal thrusts—the **Heimlich maneuver**. For an infant under one year:

- place the infant face down over the rescuer's forearm with the head lower than the chest and the neck and head supported with the rescuer's fingers
- apply five quick blows to the infant's back, between the shoulders, with the heel of the free hand
- if no object is ejected, place the infant face-up on a table or floor and give five quick chest thrusts, with two fingers in the middle of the breastbone just below the level of the nipples
- repeat the five back blows and five chest thrusts until the object is dislodged and the infant starts breathing
- if the infant becomes unresponsive or unconscious, CPR must be performed; check the mouth for the object before each rescue breath

To perform the Heimlich maneuver on someone over one year of age (including adults):

- wrap the rescuer's arms around the choking person's waist from behind
- make a fist with one hand and grasp it with the other hand with the thumb just above the person's navel; quickly thrust upward and inward until the object is dislodged or the person begins breathing
- if the person loses consciousness, lower them to the floor for CPR

For a foreign object in the eye:

- sit in a well-lit area.
- pull down the lower lid while the individual looks up and then pull the upper lid while they look down to look for the object
- if the object is floating in the tear film, it can be flushed out with lukewarm water or a saline solution, using an eyecup or small glass

For a foreign object lodged in the nose:

- blow out gently through the nose, but not hard or repeatedly
- if only one nostril is affected, gentle pressure can be used to close the other nostril while blowing out
- if the object is visible, it may be removed with tweezers

For a bone injury:

- remove clothing from the injured limb without moving it
- apply an ice pack wrapped in cloth
- make a simple splint—use anything firm and padded with something soft—to prevent the limb from moving or bending; the splint must extend beyond the joints above and below the injury

A fall from a distance greater than a person's height or a bicycle or automobile accident can result in a head or spinal injury. The injured person should not be moved and the head, neck, and spine should be stabilized until help arrives.

A person having a seizure should:

- be laid on the ground or floor, preferably on the right side, with no nearby objects
- have clothing around the head and neck loosened
- be comforted and remain lying down until fully recovered

A person in shock should:

- be laid face-up, unless a head or spinal injury is suspected
- have the legs elevated about 12 in (30 cm), if possible
- have tight clothing loosened
- be covered with a blanket
- be kept warm, still, and comfortable
- may have the lips moistened with water, but should be given nothing by mouth
- be raised to a half-sitting position if vomiting or having trouble breathing, unless there is a head or spinal injury
- should be turned to the side if the child vomits or bleeds from the mouth

An unconscious person should be placed in the recovery position if there is no possibility of a spinal injury. While lying face-up:

- the arm closest to the rescuer is placed by the person's side and tucked under the buttock
- the other arm is placed across the person's chest
- the ankles are crossed with the far leg over the near leg
- the person is rolled over toward the rescuer by pulling on clothing at the hip, while supporting the head with the other hand
- one arm is bent up and the other down to support the upper and lower body
- the head is tilted back to allow air to move freely in and out of the mouth

If there is **vomiting** or bleeding from the mouth, the person should be rolled to the side in one move, while supporting the neck and back. They should be kept warm and gently restrained if awakened.

CPR should be performed on a someone who is not breathing and is unconscious or unresponsive. The technique used is slightly different for infants, children, and adults.

To perform CPR on an infant:

- place the infant face-up on a hard, flat surface
- tilted back and lift the chin so the mouth opens
- completely cover the mouth and nose of an infant under one year of age and give two rescue breaths
- check to see if the infant's chest rises with each breath; if it does, then begin chest compressions, otherwise repeat breathing
- give the infant 30 chest compressions using two fingers in the middle of the breastbone just below nipple level
- continue the cycle of two breaths and 30 chest compressions until emergency help arrives or the child begins breathing

To perform CPR on a child or an adult:

- place the person face-up on a hard, flat surface
- tilted back and lift the chin so the mouth opens
- completely cover the mouth and give two long rescue breaths
- check to see if the person's chest rises with each breath; if it does, then begin chest compressions, otherwise repeat breathing
- give 30 chest compressions using the heel of the hand on the lower half of the chest for children; for adults, place the heel of one hand on the center of the chest just below the nipples and the other hand on top of the first with the rescuer's body weight over the arms
- continue the cycle of two breaths and 30 chest compressions until emergency help arrives or the child begins breathing

Benefits

First aid can save lives. It can also prevent injuries from worsening or becoming infected and can speed healing.

Precautions

Serious injuries or emergency medical situations require summoning emergency responders, usually by calling 911, or rushing the child to a hospital emergency room or other critical care facility. Precautions for administering first aid depend on the type of injury. The most important precautions include never:

- moving a person if there is any possibility of spinal injury
- applying a tourniquet to stop bleeding
- attempting to remove a deeply imbedded object
- attempting to replace organs
- using direct heat on frostbite or rubbing frostbitten skin
- thawing frostbitten skin if there is a risk of refreezing
- breaking burn blisters or applying ice or any ointment or lotion to burns except under a doctor's direction
- giving anything to someone who may have ingested a toxin and never inducing vomiting, unless directed by the poison control center
- attempting to remove an object embedded in the eyeball or rubbing the eyes
- probing the nose for an object that is not visible and easily grasped
- washing or moving bone injuries
- restraining movement or putting anything in the mouth of a person having a seizure
- attempting to awake an unconscious person by shaking, slapping, or using cold water
- putting a pillow under an unconscious person's head, as this can block an airway

If possible, wear gloves and wash hands before and after administering first aid. It is also a good idea to ensure that a child's **tetanus** shots are current.

Preparation

An individual can prepare for first-aid by taking first-aid classes, learning CPR and renewing CPR certification at least every two years, and by learning to use an automatic external defibrillator (AED).

Basic first aid can be taught to children. It is a good idea for babysitters to also receive training in first aid and CPR.

KEY TERMS

Aloe vera—An extract from the plant *Aloe barbadensis* that is used in skin creams and for treating burns.

Automatic external defibrillator (AED)—An electronic device for restoring regular heart rhythm.

Cardiopulmonary resuscitation (CPR)—A procedure for restoring normal breathing following cardiac arrest. It includes clearing the air passages, mouth-to-mouth artificial respiration, and heart massage by exerting pressure on the chest.

Heimlich maneuver—The application of sudden upward pressure on the upper abdomen to force a foreign object from the trachea of a choking victim; developed by the American surgeon Henry Jay Heimlich.

Shock—Severe depression of vital physiological processes, characterized by paleness, a rapid but weak pulse, rapid and shallow breathing, and low blood pressure; typically caused by injury, severe bleeding, or burns.

Tetanus—An acute infectious disease caused by a toxin produced by the bacterium *Clostridium tetani* and usually introduced into the body through a wound.

Every home and automobile should have a well-stocked first-aid kit. Use a container that is clean, strong, and easy to carry and open to store items. First-aid kits are often designed for specific activities, such as hiking, camping, or boating, and should include items geared toward those activities. For example, include ointment for mosquito **bites** in a camping kit. A first-aid manual should also be stored in the kit.

Keep the container out of the reach of young children, but easily accessible to adults and anyone trained in its use. The contents should be checked every three months for missing items and expired medicines. Medicines should be in their original containers and marked with dosage and instructions.

A general purpose first-aid kit should contain:

- emergency and physician phone numbers
- a list of allergies and medications for all family members
- medical consent and medical history forms
- a first-aid manual
- a waterproof flashlight and batteries

- a cell phone and charger
- duct tape
- scissors, tweezers, needles, and safety pins
- a non-mercury, non-glass, oral thermometer
- sterile, disposable gloves
- eye goggles or eye shield
- a breathing barrier or mouthpiece for CPR
- a mylar emergency blanket
- aluminum finger splints
- a tooth-saver kit
- a bulb suction device for flushing out wounds
- instant cold packs
- assorted adhesive bandages, gauze pads, roller gauze, and compress dressings
- adhesive cloth tape
- an elastic (Ace) bandage
- sterile cotton balls and cotton-tipped swabs
- plastic bags for waste
- soap, hand sanitizer, and alcohol wipes
- antiseptic solution or wipes
- sterile eyewash or saline solution
- petroleum jelly or other lubricant
- aloe vera gel
- calamine lotion
- antibiotic ointment or cream
- hydrocortisone ointment or cream
- a medicine cup or spoon and oral medicine syringe
- aspirin, acetaminophen, and ibuprofen
- anti-diarrhea medication
- antihistamines
- decongestant
- cough suppressant
- antacid
- laxatives
- sunscreen
- prescription medications that do not need refrigeration
- any prescribed medical supplies

Aftercare

Most small cuts, scrapes, and abrasions heal without any special care, although it may be necessary to apply an antibiotic ointment. Bandages should be changed daily or whenever they become wet or dirty. After a bone injury is treated, the area should be elevated and ice packs or cold compresses should be applied every few hours for 20-minute periods.

Risks

An individual should be cautious about providing first-aid and must assess the situation before getting involved. If the situation is dangerous, such as the scene of an accident, the individual should not intervene and instead contact emergency personnel by dialing 9-1-1.

When coming in contact with blood or other bodily fluids, there may be a risk of infection with HIV or hepatitis virus. Wearing latex gloves can help prevent disease transmission. A mouth-to-mouth barrier device may not protect against contracting an infection when giving rescue breaths.

Resources

BOOKS

American Academy of Pediatrics. *Pediatric First Aid for Parents.* Sudbury, MA: Jones and Bartlett, 2008.

American Red Cross. *First Aid and Safety for Babies and Children.* Yardley, PA: StayWell, 2009.

Borgenicht, David, Justin Heimberg, and Chuck Gonzales. *The Worst-Case Scenario Survival Handbook: Extreme Junior Edition.* San Francisco: Chronicle, 2008.

National Safety Council. *Pediatric First Aid, CPR, and AED.* 2nd ed. Boston: McGraw-Hill Higher Education, 2008.

Porter, Robert S., et al. *The Merck Manual Home Health Handbook.* 3rd ed. Whitehouse Station, NJ: Merck Research Laboratories, 2009.

Subbarao, Italo, Jim Lyznicki, and James J. James. *American Medical Association Handbook of First Aid and Emergency Care.* Rev. and updated ed. New York: Random House Reference, 2009.

PERIODICALS

Onderko, Patty. “How to Save Your Child’s Life.” *Parenting. Early Years* 24, no. 3 (April 2010): 97–100.

“Qwik Sheet: Teaching Your Kids First Aid.” *Pediatrics for Parents* 26, no. 3/4 (March/April 2010): 33–34.

OTHER

American College of Emergency Physicians. “Fast Aid First.” Patient Center, http://www.acep.org/patients.aspx (accessed August 18, 2010).

American College of Emergency Physicians. “Home First Aid Kits.” Patient Center, http://www3.acep.org/patients.aspx?id=26036 (accessed August 18, 2010).

“Anatomy of a First Aid Kit.” American Red Cross, http://www.redcross.org/services/hss/lifeline/fakit.html (accessed August 18, 2010).

“Choking First Aid—Adult or Child Over 1 Year—Series.” MedlinePlus. July 8, 2009, http://www.nlm.nih.gov/medlineplus/ency/presentations/100222_1.htm (accessed August 18, 2010).

“First-Aid Kit.” KidsHealth. September 2007, http://kidshealth.org/parent/firstaid_safe/home/firstaid_kit.html (accessed August 18, 2010).

"First-Aid Kits: Stock Supplies That Can Save Lives." MayoClinic.com. January 16, 2010, http://www.mayoclinic.com/health/first-aid-kits/FA00067 (accessed August 18, 2010).

"First Aid: Burns." FamilyDoctor.org. November 2009, http://familydoctor.org/online/famdocen/home/healthy/firstaid/after-injury/638.printerview.html (accessed August 18, 2010).

"First Aid: Cuts, Scrapes and Stitches." FamilyDoctor.org. November 2009, http://familydoctor.org/online/famdocen/home/healthy/firstaid/after-injury/041.printerview.html (accessed August 18, 2010).

"First Aid." MedlinePlus. July 9, 2010, http://www.nlm.nih.gov/medlineplus/firstaid.html (accessed August 18, 2010).

ORGANIZATIONS

American Academy of Family Physicians, 11400 Tomahawk Creek Parkway, Leawood KS, 66211-2680, (913) 906-6000, (800) 274-6000, (913) 906-6075, http://www.aafp.org.

American College of Emergency Physicians, PO Box 619911, Dallas TX, 75261-9911, (972) 550-0911, (800) 798-1822, (972) 580-2816, membership@acep.org, http://www3.acep.org.

American Red Cross, 2025 E Street, NW, Washington DC, 20006, (202) 3035000, http://www.redcross.org.

Ready Campaign, Federal Emergency Management Agency, 500 C Street, SW, Washington DC, 20024, (202) 646-3272, ready@dhs.gov, http://www.ready.gov.

Margaret Alic, PhD

5p minus syndrome ***see* Cri du chat syndrome**

Flu ***see* Influenza**

Flu shot ***see* Influenza vaccine**

Fluoridation

Fluoridation is the process of adding the element fluoride to drinking water or another substance in order to reduce the occurrence of **tooth decay**. Fluoridation was first introduced into the United States in the 1940s in an attempt to combat the serious problem of tooth decay. Today, more than half of the population of the United States drinks fluoridated water from public water supplies.

Tooth decay (dental caries) occurs when food acids dissolve the protective enamel surrounding each tooth and create a hole, or cavity, in the tooth. Acids are present in food and can also be formed by acid-producing bacteria that convert sugars into acids in the mouth.

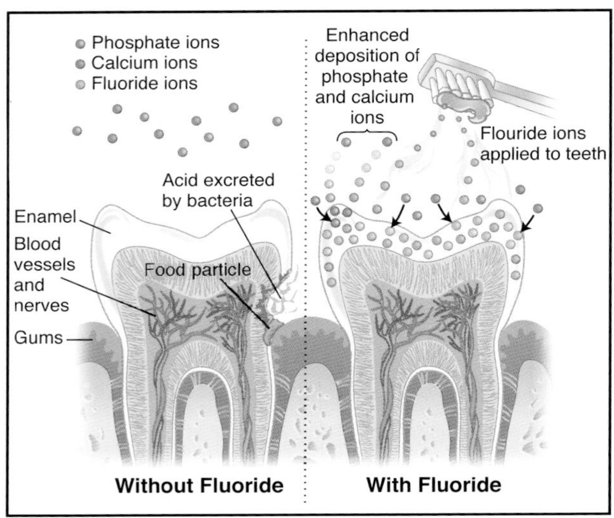

Fluoride helps protect teeth from decay. (*Illustration by Electronic Illustrators Group. Reproduced by permission of Gale, a part of Cengage Learning.*)

There is overwhelming evidence that fluoride can substantially reduce tooth decay. When ingested, fluoride concentrates in bones and in dental enamel making the tooth enamel more resistant to decay. It is also believed that fluoride may inhibit the bacteria that convert sugars into acidic substances that attack the enamel. Fluoride is present in most water supplies at low levels and nearly all food contains traces of fluoride. Toothpaste and mouthwash also contain added fluoride. Fluoride supplements are also available for children who drink non-fluoridated water from sources such as wells.

Opponents of fluoridation are not been convinced of its effectiveness, and are concerned by possible side effects. Opponents of fluoridation are also disturbed by the moral issues of personal rights that are raised by the addition of a chemical substance to an entire city's water supply. The decision to fluoridate drinking water has generally rested with local governments and communities and has always been a controversial issue.

The issue of fluoridation became controversial in the 1950s and 1960s, when heated debate surrounded the issue across the country. The debate continues today. Critics pointed to the known harmful effects of large doses of fluoride that led to bone damage and to the special risks for people with kidney disease or those who were particularly sensitive to toxic substances. Large doses of fluoride can also lead to fluoridosis. Fluoridosis is an irregular browning of the teeth caused by the presence of too much fluoride during tooth development. While fluoridosis can be unsightly, there is no evidence it weakens the positive effects of fluoride. Recent research also suggests that direct application of a fluoride gel to teeth with braces can ease bleeding of the gums and plaque buildup.

Between the 1950s and 1980s, some scientists suggested that fluoride may have a mutagenic effect (that is, it may be capable of causing human **birth defects**). Controversial claims that fluoride can cause cancerwere also raised. These claims have been disproved by numerous studies. However, some scientists still argue that fluoridation is not without health risks that may outweigh the benefits of fluoridation of public water supplies, especially when other sources of fluoride (e.g. toothpaste, mouthwash) are available. Others argue that fluoridation of public water supplies improves both dental health and reduces the cost of dental care, especially for children in low socioeconomic groups.

It also remains unclear what, if any, side-effects are of one ppm levels of fluoride in water ingested over many years. In 1993, the National Research Council published a report on the health effects of ingested fluoride and attempted to determine if the maximum recommended level of four ppm for fluoride in drinking water should be modified. The report concluded that this level was appropriate but that further research may indicate a need for revision. With fluoride increasingly being added to toothpaste and mouthwash, there is concern that some children may be exposed to fluoride in excess of the recommended level.

Infants who do not receive adequate amounts of fluoride in the water or formula they drink routinely have been given fluoride supplements beginning at about one month of age. In 1995, the **American Academy of Pediatrics** (AAP) recommended delaying such supplements until six months of age. Along with the American Dental Association, the AAP also revised downward the minimum level of fluoride at which supplementation is necessary.

Resources

BOOKS

Bryson, Christopher. *The Fluoride Deception*, new ed. New York: Seven Stories Press, 2006.

Fawell, J., K Bailey, and J Chilton, eds. *Fluoride in Drinking-water*. Seattle, WA: IWA Pub., 2006.

Fluoride in Drinking Water: A Scientific Review of EPA's Standards. Washington, DC: National Academies Press, 2006.

PERIODICALS

Bebermeyer, Richard D. "Fluoridation of Drinking Water Reduces Caries Prevalence." *Evidence-Based Dentistry* 3(2002): 39.

Centers for Disease Control. "Recommendations for Using Fluoride to Prevent and Control Dental Caries in the United States." *Mortality and Morbidity Weekly Review Recomm Rep 2001*. 50(RR-14) (Aug 17, 2001): 1-42. Also available at National Guideline Clearinghouse, http://www.guideline.gov/.

Keels, Martha A. "Guidelines Advise Pediatricians on Judicious Use of Fluoride in Children." *AAP News*. 19 (2001): 226.

OTHER

National Cancer Institute. "Fluoridated Water: Questions and Answers." undated; accessed November 11, 2006, http://www.cancer.gov/cancertopics/factsheet/Risk/fluoridated water.

ORGANIZATIONS

American Academy of Pediatric Dentistry, 211 East Chicago Ave., Ste. 700, Chicago IL, 60611-2616, (312) 337-2169, http://www.aapd.org.

Safe Drinking Water Coalition, P. O. Box 443, Lehi UT, 84043, (801) 766-8825, (801) 776-8826, http://www.stopfluoridation.homestead.com.

Tish Davidson, A.M.

Folate **see Folic acid**

Folic acid

Definition

Folic acid is a water-soluable vitamin belonging to the B-complex group of **vitamins**. These vitamins help the body break down complex carbohydrates into simple sugars to be used for energy. Excess B vitamins are excreted from the body rather than stored for later use. This is why sufficient daily intake of folic acid is necessary.

Description

Folic acid is also known as folate, or folacin. It is one of the nutrients most often found to be deficient in the Western diet, and there is evidence that deficiency is a problem on a worldwide scale. Folic acid is found in leafy green vegetables, beans, peas and lentils, liver, beets, brussel sprouts, poultry, nutritional yeast, tuna, wheat germ, mushrooms, oranges, asparagus, broccoli, spinach, bananas, strawberries, and cantaloupes. In 1998, the U.S. Food and Drug Administration (FDA) required food manufacturers to add folic acid to enriched bread and grain products to boost intake and to help prevent neural tube defects (NTD).

Purpose

Folic acid works together with vitamin B_{12} and vitamin C to metabolize protein in the body. It is important for the formation of red and white blood cells. It is necessary for the proper differentiation and growth of cells and for the development of the fetus. It is also used to form the nucleic acid of DNA and RNA. It increases the appetite and stimulates the production of stomach acid for digestion and it aids in maintaining a healthy liver. A deficiency of folic acid may lead to **anemia**, in which there is decreased production of red blood cells. This reduces the amounts of oxygen and nutrients that are able to get to the tissues. Symptoms may include fatigue, reduced secretion of digestive acids, confusion, and forgetfulness. During pregnancy, a folic acid deficiency may lead to preeclampsia, premature **birth**, and increased bleeding after birth.

People who are at high risk of strokes and heart disease may greatly benefit by taking folic acid supplements. An elevated blood level of the amino acid homocysteine has been identified as a risk factor for some of these diseases. High levels of homocysteine have also been found to contribute to problems with osteoporosis. Folic acid, together with vitamins B_6 and B_{12}, helps break down homocysteine, and may help reverse the problems associated with elevated levels.

Pregnant women have an increased need for folic acid, both for themselves and their child. Folic acid is necessary for the proper growth and development of the fetus. Adequate intake of folic acid is vital for the prevention of several types of **birth defects**, particularly NTDs. The neural tube of the embryo develops into the brain, spinal cord, spinal column, and the skull. If this tube forms incompletely during the first few months of pregnancy a serious, and often fatal, defect results in **spina bifida** or anencephaly. Folic acid, taken from one year to one month before conception through the first four months of pregnancy, can reduce the risk of NTDs by 50–70%. It also helps prevent a **cleft lip and palate**.

Research shows that folic acid can be used to successfully treat cervical dysplasia, a condition diagnosed by a Pap smear, of having abnormal cells in the cervix. This condition is considered to be a possible precursor to cervical **cancer**, and is diagnosed as an abnormal Pap smear. Daily consumption of 1,000 mcg of folic acid for three or more months has resulted in improved cervical cells upon repeat Pap smears.

Studies suggest that long-term use of folic acid supplements may also help prevent lung and colon cancer. Researchers have also found that alcoholics who have low folic acid levels face a greatly increased possibility of developing colon cancer.

KEY TERMS

Homocysteine—An amino aid involved in the breakdown and absorption of protein in the body.

Preeclampsia—A serious disorder of late pregnancy in which the blood pressure rises, there is a large amount of retained fluids, and the kidneys become less effective and excrete proteins directly into the urine.

Raynaud's disease—A symptom of various underlying conditions affecting blood circulation in the fingers and toes and causing them to be sensitive to cold.

Recommended Dietary Allowance (RDA)—Guidelines for the amounts of vitamins and minerals necessary for proper health and nutrition established by the National Academy of Sciences in 1989.

Water-soluble vitamins—Vitamins that are not stored in the body and are easily excreted. They must, therefore, be consumed regularly as foods or supplements to maintain health.

Preparations

To correct a folic acid deficiency, supplements are taken in addition to food. Since the functioning of the B vitamins is interrelated, it is generally recommended that the appropriate dose of B-complex vitamins be taken in place of single B vitamin supplements. The Recommended Dietary Allowances (**RDA**) for folate is 400 mcg per day for adults, 600 mcg per day for pregnant women, and 500 mcg for nursing women. Medicinal dosages of up to 1,000-2,000 mcg per day may be prescribed.

Precautions

Folic acid is not stable. It is easily destroyed by exposure to light, air, water, and cooking. Therefore, the supplement should be stored in a dark container in a cold, dry place, such as a refrigerator. Many medications interfere with the body's absorption and use of folic acid. This includes sulfa drugs, sleeping pills, estrogen, anticonvulsants, birth control pills, antacids, quinine, and some **antibiotics**. Using large amounts of folic acid (e.g., over 5,000 mcg per day) can mask a vitamin B_{12} deficiency and thereby risk of irreversible nerve damage.

Side effects

At levels of 5,000 mcg or less, folic acid is generally safe for use. Side effects are uncommon. However, large doses may cause nausea, decreased appetite, bloating, gas, decreased ability to concentrate, and insomnia. Large doses may also decrease the effects of phenytoin (Dilantin), a seizure medication.

Interactions

As with all B-complex vitamins, it is best to take folic acid with the other B vitamins. Vitamin C is important to the absorption and functioning of folic acid in the body.

Resources

OTHER

Adams, Suzanne L. *The Art of Cytology: Folic Acid/ B-12 Deficiency.* suzann@concetric.net, http://www.concentric.net/~Suza2/page22.htm.

"Folic Acid: Coming to A Grocery Store Near You." http://www.mayohealth.org/mayo/9710/htm/folic.htm.

"Folic Acid." http://www.cybervitamins.com/folicacid.htm.

"Folic acid (oral/injectible)." Dr. Koop.com.Inc. 700 N. Mopac, Suite 400, Austin, TX 48731, http://www.drkoop.com/hcr/drugstore/pharmacy/leaflets/english/d00241a1.asp.

Pregnancy and Nutrition Update, http://www.mayohealth.org/mayo/9601/htm/pregvit.htm.

ORGANIZATIONS

Centers for Disease Control and Prevention (CDC), 1600 Clifton Road, Atlanta GA, 30333, (404) 498-1515, (800) 311-3435, http://www.cdc.gov.

Patience Paradox

Food allergies

Definition

Food **allergies** are the body's abnormal responses to harmless foods; the reactions are caused by the immune system's reaction to some food proteins.

Description

Food allergies are often confused with food intolerance. However, the two conditions have different causes and produce different symptoms. A food allergy is also known as food hypersensitivity. The allergy is caused when a person eats something that the **immune system** incorrectly identifies as harmful.

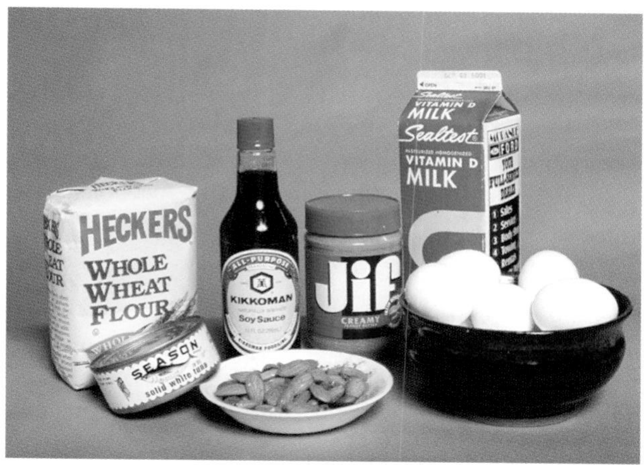

Foods such as whole-wheat flour, tuna, soy sauce, eggs, peanut butter, almonds, and milk are common causes of food allergies. *(© Erik Freeland/Corbis.)*

Food allergies

About 4% of adults have food allergies according to the National Institute of Allergy and Infectious Diseases (NIAID). The condition affects approximately 6 to 8% of children age 4 and younger.

The immune system works to protect the body and creates food-specific antibodies. The antibodies are proteins that battle antigens, substances that are foreign or initially outside the body. The introduction of an antigen produces the immune response. Antibodies are created to destroy the antigen or counteract its effectiveness.

The food that triggered that reaction is called an allergen. The antibodies are like an alarm system coded to detect the food regarded as harmful. The next time the person eats that food, the immune system discharges a large amount of histamine and chemicals. This process meant to protect the body against the allergen causes an allergic reaction that can affect the respiratory tract, digestive tract, skin, and cardiovascular system.

Allergic reactions can occur in minutes or in up to two hours after the person ate the food. Symptoms include swelling of the tongue, **diarrhea**, and **hives**. In severe cases, the allergic reaction can be fatal. The most severe reaction is **anaphylaxis**, which could be life-threatening.

Food intolerance

While food allergies involve the immune system, food intolerance is not related to the immune system. For example, a person who is lactose intolerant has a shortage of lactose, the digestive enzyme that breaks down the sugar in milk and dairy products. That person could experience stomach **pain** or bloating several hours after drinking milk.

People who are food-intolerant can sometimes consume that food and not experience intolerance symptoms. Those diagnosed with food allergies must avoid the foods that produce the allergic reactions.

Allergy-producing foods

Although approximately 160 foods produce allergic reactions, approximately 90% of reactions are caused by some or all items within eight food families. These are milk, eggs, peanuts, tree nuts, fish, shellfish, wheat, and soy. These foods can cause severe reactions. The most adverse reactions are caused by peanuts and tree nuts. According to NIAID, about 0.6% of Americans are impacted by peanut allergies. Approximately 0.4% of Americans have allergic reactions to tree nuts.

Food allergy demographics

Most children have allergies to eggs, milk, peanuts or tree nuts, and soy, according to the American Dietetic Association (ADA). The young generally outgrow their allergies. They are more likely to outgrow milk and soy allergies, according to NIAID. However, children and adults usually allergic to peanuts and tree nuts for life. The most frequent causes of food allergies in adulthood are peanuts, tree nuts, fish, and shellfish.

Allergies are hereditary. There is a tendency for the immune system to create IgE antibodies in people with family histories of allergies and allergic conditions like hay **fever** and **asthma**, according to NIAID. The likelihood of a child having food allergies increases when both parents are allergic.

Furthermore, people are allergic to the foods that are eaten frequently in their countries. A rice allergy is more common in Japan, and codfish allergies occur more in Scandinavian countries, according to NIAID.

Causes and symptoms

Food allergies are caused by the immune system's reaction to a food item that it believes is harmful. When the food is digested, the immune system responds by creating immunoglobulin E (IgE) antibodies as a defense. The antibodies are proteins found in the bloodstream. Formed to protect the body against harmful substances, the antibodies are created after the person's first exposure to the allergen.

The majority of food allergies are caused by foods in eight families. In some families, every food causes an allergic reaction. In other families like shellfish, a person may be allergic to one species, but able to eat others. The allergy-inducing foods include:

- Milk. The dairy family includes milk, ice cream, yogurt, butter, and some margarines. Nondairy foods that contain casein must be avoided. Prepared foods that contain milk range from breads and doughnuts to sausage and soup, according to the ADA.
- Eggs. Although a person may be allergic to either the egg white or yolk, the entire egg must be avoided because there is a risk of cross-contamination. Eggs are an ingredient in mayonnaise. Moreover, products such as baked goods, breads, pasta, yogurt, and batter on fried foods may contain eggs. In addition, some egg-substitute products contain egg whites.
- Peanuts grow in the ground and are legumes like lentils and chickpeas. A person with a peanut allergy may not be allergic to other legumes or tree nuts. Products to be avoided include peanuts, peanut butter, peanut oil, and some desserts and candy. In addition, some Asian dishes are prepared with a peanut sauce. Tree nuts include almonds, cashews, pecans, walnuts, Brazil nuts, chestnuts, hazelnuts, macadamia nuts, pine nuts, pistachios, and hickory nuts. Products containing tree nuts include nut oil, nut oil, desserts, candy, crackers, and barbecue sauce. A person may be allergic to one type of nut but able to eat other nuts. That should be determined after consulting with a doctor.
- Fish allergy is generally diagnosed as an allergy to all fish species because the allergen is similar among the different species.
- Shellfish species include lobster, crab, shrimp, clams, oysters, scallops, mollusks, and crawfish. An allergy to one type of shellfish may indicate an allergy to others.
- Wheat is a grain found in numerous foods including breads, cereals, pastas, lunch meats, desserts, and bulgar. It is also found in products such as enriched flour and farina.
- Soy. The soybean is a legume, and people who have this allergy are rarely allergic to peanuts or other legumes. Soy is an ingredient in many processed foods including crackers and baked goods, sauces, and soups. There is also soy in canned tuna, according to the ADA.

The chemical reaction

During the initial exposure, many IgE antibodies are created. These attach to mast cells. These cells are located in tissue throughout the body, especially in areas such as the nose, throat, lungs, skin, and gastrointestinal tract. These are also the areas where allergic reactions occur.

The antibodies are in place, and a reaction is triggered the next time the person eats the food regarded as harmful. As the allergen reacts with the IgE, the body releases histamine and other chemicals. Histamine is a chemical located in the body's cells. When released during an allergic reaction, histamine and other chemicals cause symptoms like inflammation.

The type of allergic reaction depends on where the antibodies are released, according to NIAID. Chemicals released in the ears, nose, and throat could cause the mouth to itch. The person may also have difficulty breathing or swallowing. If the allergen triggers a reaction in the gastrointestinal tract, the person could experience stomach pain or diarrhea. An allergic reaction that affects skin cells could produce hives. This condition also known as urticaria is an allergic reaction characterized by **itching**, swelling, and the presence of patchy red areas called wheals.

Severe allergic reaction

Anaphylaxis is a severe allergic reaction that is potentially life-threatening. Also known as an anaphylactic reaction, this condition requires immediate medical attention. The reaction occurs within seconds or up to several hours after the person ate the allergy-inducing food.

Symptoms can include difficulty breathing, a **tingling** feeling in the mouth, and a swelling in the tongue and throat. The person may experience hives, **vomiting**, abdominal cramps, and diarrhea. There is also a sudden drop in blood pressure. Anaphylaxis could be fatal if not treated promptly.

Each year, some 150 Americans die from food-induced anaphylaxism, according to NIAID. The casualties are generally adolescents and young adults. The risk increases for people who have allergies and asthma. Also at increased risk are people who experienced previous episodes of a naphylaxis.

The peanut is one of the primary foods that trigger an anaphylactic reaction. Tree nuts also cause the reaction. The nuts generally linked to anaphylaxis are almonds, Brazil nuts, cashews, chestnuts, hazelnuts, macadamia nuts, pecans, pine nuts, pistachios and walnuts. Fish, shellfish, and eggs can also set off the reaction, according to the ADA.

Cross-reactivity

Cross-reactivity is the tendency of a person with one allergy to reaction to another allergen. A person allergic to crab might also be allergic to shrimp. In addition, someone with ragweed sensitivity could experience sensations when trying to eat melons during ragweed pollinating season, according to NIAID. The person's mouth would start itching, and the person wouldn't be able to eat the melon. The cross-reaction happens frequently with cantaloupes. The condition is known as oral allergy syndrome.

Diagnosis

Food allergies are diagnosed by first determining whether a person has an allergy or if symptoms are related to a condition like food intolerance. The medical professional may be a board-certified allergist, a doctor with education and experience in treating allergies. However, some health plans may require that the patient first see a family practice doctor.

If food allergies are suspected, the doctor will take a detailed case history. The doctor asks the patient if there is a family history of allergies. Other questions are related to the patient's adverse reactions.

The doctor's questions include how the food was prepared, the amount eaten and what time the reaction happened. The patient describes the symptoms and actions taken to relieve them. The doctor also asks if the patient had other similar experiences when eating that food.

The patient receives a physical exam. In addition, the doctor may ask the patient to keep a food diary, a log of what the person eats for one to two weeks. The medical history and the food diary are used in conjunction with testing to diagnose the patient.

Allergy tests

Doctors generally start the testing process with a skin test or a blood test. The prick skin test, which is also known as the scratch test, examines the patient's reaction to a solution containing a protein that triggers allergies.

The doctor places a drop of the substance on the patient's arm or back. The doctor then uses a needle to prick or scratch the skin. This allows the potential allergen to enter the patient's skin. If more than one food allergy is suspected, the test is repeated with other proteins applied to the skin. After about 15 minutes, the doctor can read the reactions on the patient's skin.

If there is no reaction, the patient is probably not allergic to that food. The possibility of an allergy is indicated by the presence of a wheal, a bump that resembles a mosquito bite. The wheal signifies a positive reaction to the test. However, the test may show a false positive, which is a reaction to a food that does not cause allergies.

The skin test is not appropriate for people who are severely allergic or have skin conditions like **eczema**. Those people are given the RAST (radioallergosorbent test). This test measures the presence of food-specific IgE in the blood. After a sample of the patient's blood is taken, it is sent to a laboratory. The sample is tested with different foods. Levels of antibodies are measured, and the reactions to different proteins are ranked. While measurement systems may vary, a high ranking indicates a high number of antibodies. Lab results are generally completed within a week.

Results to this test may not be conclusive. A negative test may not have identified antibodies in the patient's blood. Positive results make it probable but not definite that the patient has allergies.

Costs for blood and skin tests will vary, with fees ranging from $10 to more than $300. Insurance may cover some of the cost. While both tests are reliable, they aren't 100% accurate. If questions remain, the diagnosis takes into account the patient's medical history and the food diary. If necessary, the patient is put on a special diet.

Elimination diet

If the skin or blood test shows strong positive results, the doctor may put the patient on an elimination diet. This is done when needed to narrow the list of suspected allergens. The person stops eating the foods suspected of causing the allergic reaction. That food is eliminated from the diet for from two to four weeks. If allergy symptoms improve, the food is probably an allergen.

If more confirmation is needed, the doctor may ask the patient to start eating the food again. The elimination diet procedure is generally not utilized if the patient initially had a severe reaction.

Food challenges

Other tests called food challenges may be performed. The challenges are done in a medical setting, with a doctor present. The patient is given capsules that each contain a different food. Some capsules contain allergy-producing foods. Other capsules may be placebos that won't produce a reaction.

The patient swallows the capsule, and the doctor watches for an allergic reaction. In an open food challenge, doctor and patient are aware of the capsule contents. In a single-blind food challenge, only the doctor knows. In a double-blind challenge, neither doctor nor patient knows the contents.

Challenges are rarely authorized by health care providers. Testing is time-consuming and many allergens are difficult to evaluate with the challenges, according to NIAID.

Treatment

The treatment for food allergies is to avoid eating the food that causes the allergy. This preventive treatment includes reading food labels. Manufacturers are required by the U.S. Food and Drug Administration to list a product's ingredients on the label. However, if there is a question about an ingredient, the person should contact the manufacturer before eating the food. When dining out, people should ask if food contains the allergen or ingredients contain the allergy-inducing foods.

When reading food labels, people with food allergies should know that:

- Words indicating the presence of milk include lactose, ghee, and whey.
- Words signifying eggs in a product include albumin, globulin, and ovomucin.
- While it is apparent that peanuts are an ingredient in a product like peanut butter, there could be peanuts in hydrolyzed plant protein and hydrolyzed vegetable protein.
- People with tree nut allergies should carefully read the labels of products such as cereals and barbecue sauce.
- The American Dietetic Association cautions that surimi, an ingredient in imitation seafood, is made from fish muscle. Furthermore, fish in the form of anchovies is sometimes an ingredient in Worcestshire sauce.
- Words on labels that signal the presence of wheat include gluten, sietan, and vital gluten.

Allergies and children

Parents of children with food allergies need to monitor their children's food choices. They also must know how to care for the child if there is an allergic reaction. Parents need to notify the child's school about the condition. Caregivers should be informed, too. Both the school and caregivers should know how to handle an allergic reaction. Care must be taken because a highly allergic person could react to a piece of food as small as 1/44,000 of a peanut kernel, according to NIAID.

Living with severe allergies

Despite precautions, people may accidentally eat something that causes an allergic reaction. People with severe allergies must be prepared to treat the condition and prevent an anaphylactic reaction. A medical alert bracelet should be worn. This informs people that the person has a food allergy and could have severe reactions.

To reduce the risks from an anaphylactic reaction, the person carries a syringe filled with epinephrine, which is adrenaline. This is a prescription medication sold commercially as the EpiPen auto injector. While prices vary, one syringe costs about $50.

The person with allergies must know how to inject the epinephrine. It is helpful for other family members to know how to do this, and parents of an allergic child must be trained in the procedure.

The person is injected at the first sign of a severe reaction. Medical attention is required, and the person should be taken to an emergency room. The person will be treated and monitored because there could be a second severe reaction about four hours after the initial one.

Allergy treatment research

There was no cure for food allergies as of the spring of 2005. That could change, with some relief available for people diagnosed with peanut allergies. According to a study reported on in 2003 in the *New England Journal of Medicine*, 84 people who took the drug TNX-901 had a decrease in their IgE antibody levels.

Organizations including the Food Allergy & Anaphylaxis Network (FAAN) lauded the results of the study that was conducted from July of 1999 through March of 2002. Work on that study was stopped in 2004 when biotechnology companies Genentech, Novartis, and Tanox concentrated efforts instead on use of an asthma medication for treating peanut allergies. Research started in June of 2004 on omalizumab, a medication sold commercially as Xolair. The study of Xolair's effectiveness was expected to take from two to three years.

Alternative treatment

The only treatment for food allergies is for a person to stop eating the food that causes the allergies. Some alternative treatments may be helpful in easing the symptoms caused by allergies. However, people should check with their health care providers before embarking on an alternative treatment.

Prognosis

Food allergies cannot be cured, but they can be managed. The allergen-inducing foods should be avoided. These foods should be replaced with others that provide the **vitamins** and nutrients needed for a healthy diet. Organizations including the American Dietetic Association recommend the following dietetic changes:

- Milk is a source of calcium and vitamins A and D. For people with milk allergies, alternate choices of calcium include calcium-fortified orange juice and cereal.
- Since eggs are an ingredient in products like bread, egg-free sources of grains are an alternate source of vitamin B.
- Peanuts are a source of vitamin E, niacin, and magnesium. Other sources of these nutrients include other legumes, meat, and grains.
- Fish is a source of protein and nutrients like B vitamins and niacin. Alternate sources of these nutrients should be sought.
- Wheat is a source of many nutrients including niacin and riboflavin. The person allergic to wheat should substitute products made from grains such as oat, corn, rice and barley.
- Although soybeans are rich in nutrients, very little soy is used in commercial products. As a result, a person with this food allergy would not need to find a safe substitute in order to get needed nutrients.

Prevention

People prevent the return of food allergies by following treatment guidelines. These include avoiding the foods that cause allergic reactions, reading food labels, and taking measures to prevent an anaphylactic reaction.

Anaphylaxis is a major concern after a diagnosis of severe food allergies. To reduce the risks associated this reaction, people with food allergies should wear medical alert bracelets and never go anywhere without epinephrine. If possible, family members or friends of adults with allergies should learn how to administer this medication.

The American Dietetic Association advises people to develop an emergency plan. ADA recommendations include preparing a list of the foods the person is allergic to, three emergency contacts, the doctor's name, and a description of how to treat the reaction. This list is kept with the epinephrine syringe.

Parental concerns

Because children can come into contact with food allergens at school and during extracurricular activities, parents should meet with school officials to discuss procedures for keeping their children safe. Parents and school personnel should develop an action plan for dealing with allergens in the school and handling an emergency. Not only should the cafeteria staff be notified about the food allergy, but parents should also ask about snack time, birthdays and holiday celebrations, field trips, and arts and crafts projects. Arrangements should be made to keep medications to treat accidental exposure at the school, and personnel should be trained in their use.

Due to the seriousness of nut allergies and other allergies that can cause anaphylaxis, some school districts have created policies that forbid nuts on school premises and do not allow students to trade food at lunch. Some parents have lobbied school boards for such restrictions.

Avoiding the trigger food may be very problematic, even at home. Parents need to become proficient label readers, especially if the allergen is a nut or other food that may cause anaphylaxis. Understanding what the ingredient names mean is critical to total food avoidance. For example, dairy products can be listed as milk, casein, whey, and sodium caseinate. If a child is allergic to corn, it can be found not only as corn and corn syrup, but also cornstarch, which is a binding agent in a number of medications, including acetaminophen (Tylenol). Consultation with a dietitian can help parents understand food labels.

Peanut allergies in the United States doubled between 1997 and 2002. A controversial British study, reported in 2003, found a peanut/soy link, which is clinically rare. The study reported a link between early use of soy formula and peanut oil baby lotion in the later diagnosis of peanut food allergy. Soy formula may sensitize an infant to legumes, and therefore to peanuts. Peanut oil, known by doctors and nurses as arachis oil, is found in baby lotion and creams, especially those used to treat diaper rash, eczema, and dry skin.

Children who have severe reactions to a trigger food should wear a medical alert bracelet. Parents should also have on hand an emergency epinephrine-filled syringe like those found in bee-sting kits, or an epinephrine pen.

Parents should also notify day-care providers, Girl Scout and Boy Scout leaders, religious education teachers, sports coaches, and parents of their child's friends. They should explain what foods their child is allergic to, how the child reacts to the food, and how adults can help, either by making sure these foods are not served as snacks or by giving emergency care or support during an allergic reaction. In addition, parents can teach their child how to ask for help.

Resources

BOOKS

Freund, Lee and Rejaunier, Jeanne. *The Complete Idiot's Guide to Food Allergies.*Penguin Group, USA, 2003.

OTHER

Food Allergy An Overview. National Institute of Allergy and Infectious Diseases. July 2004. [accessed March 30, 2005], http://www.niaid.nih.gov/publications/pdf/foodallergy.pdf.

Peanut Anti-IgE Study Update. The Food Allergy & Anaphylaxis Network. September 2, 2004 [accessed April 5], http://www.foodallergy.org/Research/antiigetherapy.html.

ORGANIZATIONS

American Dietetic Association, 120 S. Riverside Plaza, Suite 2000, Chicago IL, 60606, (800) 877-1600, http://www.eatright.org.

National Institute of Allergy and Infectious Disease, 31 Center Drive MSC 2520, Building 31, Room 7A-50, Bethesda MD, 20892-2520, (301) 496-5717, (800) 877-8339 (TTY), http://www.niaid.nih.gov/default.htm.

The Food Allergy & Anaphylaxis Network, 11781 Lee Jackson Highway, Suite 160, Fairfax VA, 22033, (800) 929-4040. http://www.foodallergy.org.

Liz Swain

Food poisoning

Definition

Food poisoning is a general term for health problems arising from eating contaminated food. Food may be contaminated by bacteria, viruses, environmental toxins, or toxins present within the food itself, such as the poisons in some mushrooms or certain seafood. Symptoms of food poisoning usually involve nausea, **vomiting** and/or **diarrhea**. Some food-borne toxins can affect the nervous system.

Description

Each year in the United States, one to two bouts of diarrheal illness occur in every adult. The Centers for Disease Control and Prevention (CDC) estimates that there are from six to 33 million cases of food poisoning in the United States annually. Many cases are mild and pass so rapidly that they are never diagnosed. Occasionally a severe outbreak creates a newsworthy public health hazard.

Classical food poisoning, sometimes incorrectly called ptomaine poisoning, is caused by a variety of different bacteria. The most common are *Salmonella*, *Staphylococcus aureus*, *Escherichia coli* O157:H7 or other E. coli strains, *Shigella*, and *Clostridium botulinum*. Each has a slightly different incubation period and duration, but all except *C. botulinum* cause inflammation of the intestines and diarrhea. Sometimes food poisoning is called bacterial **gastroenteritis** or infectious diarrhea. Food and water can also be contaminated by viruses (such as the Norwalk agent that causes diarrhea and the viruses of **hepatitis A** and E), environmental toxins (heavy metals), and poisons produced within the food itself (mushroom poisoning or fish and shellfish poisoning).

Careless food handling during the trip from farm to table creates conditions for the growth of bacteria that make people sick. Vegetables that are eaten raw, such as lettuce, may be contaminated by bacteria in soil, water, and dust during washing and packing. Home canned and commercially canned food may be improperly processed at too low a temperature or for too short a time to kill the bacteria.

Raw meats carry many food-borne bacterial diseases. The United States Food and Drug Administration (FDA) estimates that 60% or more of raw poultry sold at retail carry some disease-causing bacteria. Other raw meat products and eggs are contaminated to a lesser degree. Thorough cooking kills the bacteria and makes the food harmless. However, properly cooked food can become re-contaminated if it comes in contact with plates, cutting boards, countertops, or utensils that were used with raw meat and not cleaned and sanitized.

Cooked foods can also be contaminated after cooking by bacteria carried by food handlers or from bacteria in the environment. It is estimated that 50% of healthy people have the bacteria *Staphylococcus aureus* in their nasal passages and throat, and on their skin and hair. Rubbing a runny nose, then touching food can introduce the bacteria into cooked food. Bacteria flourish at room temperature, and will rapidly grow into quantities capable of making people sick. To prevent this growth, food must be kept hot or cold, but never just warm.

Although the food supply in the United States is probably the safest in the world, anyone can get food poisoning. Serious outbreaks are rare. When they occur, the very young, the very old, and those with **immune system** weaknesses have the most severe and life-threatening cases. For example, this group is 20 times more likely to become infected with the *Salmonella* bacteria than the general population.

Travel outside the United States to countries where less attention is paid to sanitation, water purification, and good food handling practices increases the chances that a person will get food poisoning. People living in institutions such as nursing homes are also more likely to get food poisoning.

Causes and symptoms

The symptoms of food poisoning occur when food-borne bacteria release toxins or poisons as a byproduct of their growth in the body. These toxins (except those from *C. botulinum*) cause inflammation and swelling of the stomach, small intestine and/or large intestine. The result is abdominal muscle cramping, vomiting, diarrhea, **fever**, and the chance of **dehydration**. The severity of symptoms depends on the type of bacteria, the amount consumed, and the individual's general health and sensitivity to the bacterial toxin.

Salmonella

According to a 2001 report from the CDC, *Salmonella* caused almost 50,000 culture-confirmed cases of food poisoning in the United States annually. However, between two and four million probably occur each year. *Salmonella* is found in egg yolks from infected chickens, in raw and undercooked poultry and in other meats, dairy products, fish, shrimp, and many more foods. The CDC estimates that one out of every 50 consumers is exposed to a contaminated egg yolk each year. However, thorough cooking kills the bacteria and makes the food harmless. *Salmonella* is also found in the feces of pet reptiles such as turtles, lizards, and snakes.

About one out of every 1,000 people get food poisoning from *Salmonella*. Of these, two-thirds are under age 20, with the majority under age nine. Most cases occur in the warm months between July and October.

Symptoms of food poisoning begin eight to 72 hours after eating food contaminated with *Salmonella*. These include traditional food poisoning symptoms of abdominal **pain**, diarrhea, vomiting, and fever. The symptoms generally last one to five days. Dehydration can be a complication in severe cases. People generally recover without antibiotic treatment, although they may feel tired for a week after the active symptoms subside.

Staphylococcus aureus

Staphylococcus aureus is found on humans and in the environment in dust, air, and sewage. The bacteria is spread primarily by food handlers using poor sanitary practices. Almost any food can be contaminated, but salad dressings, milk products, cream pastries, are likely candidates.

It is difficult to estimate the number of cases of food poisoning from *Staphylococcus aureus* that occur each year, because its symptoms are so similar to those caused by other foodborne bacteria. Many cases are mild and the victim never sees a doctor.

Symptoms appear rapidly, usually one to six hours after the contaminated food is eaten. The acute symptoms of vomiting and severe abdominal cramps without fever usually last only three to six hours and rarely more than 24 hours. Most people recover without medical assistance. Deaths are rare.

Escherichia coli (E. coli)

There are many strains of *E. coli*, and not all of them are harmful. The strain that causes most severe food poisoning is *E. coli O157:H7*. Food poisoning by *E. coli* occurs in three out of every 10,000 people. Foodborne *E. coli* is found and transmitted mainly in food derived from cows such as raw milk, raw or rare ground beef and fruit or vegetables that are contaminated.

Symptoms of food poisoning from *E. coli* are slower to appear than those caused by some of the other foodborne bacteria. *E. coli* produces toxins in the large intestine rather than higher up in the digestive system. This accounts for the delay in symptoms and the fact that vomiting rarely occurs in *E. coli* food poisoning.

One to three days after eating contaminated food, the victim with *E. coli O157:H7* begins to have severe abdominal cramps and watery diarrhea that usually becomes bloody within 24 hours. There is little or no fever, and rarely does the victim vomit. The bloody, watery diarrhea lasts from one to eight days in uncomplicated cases.

Campylobacter jejuni (C. jejuni)

According to the FDA, *C. jejuni* is the leading cause of bacterial diarrhea in the United States. It is responsible for more cases of bacterial diarrhea than *Shigella* and *Salmonella* combined. Anyone can get food poisoning from *C. jejuni*, but children under five and young adults between the ages of 15 and 29 are more frequently infected.

C. jejuni is carried by healthy cattle, chickens, birds, and flies. It is not carried by healthy people in the United States or Europe. The bacteria is also found ponds and stream water. The ingestion of only a few hundred *C. jejuni* bacteria can make a person sick.

Symptoms of food poisoning begin two to five days after eating food contaminated with *C. jejuni*. These symptoms include fever, abdominal pain, nausea, **headache**, muscle pain, and diarrhea. The diarrhea can be watery or sticky and may contain blood. Symptoms last from seven to 10 days, and relapses occur in about one quarter of people who are infected. Dehydration is a common complication. Other complications such as arthritis-like joint pain and hemolytic-uremic syndrome (HUS) are rare.

Shigella

Shigella is a common cause of diarrhea in travelers to developing countries. It is associated with contaminated food and water, crowded living conditions, and poor sanitation. The bacterial toxins affect the small intestine.

Symptoms of food poisoning by *Shigella* appear 36–72 hours after eating contaminated food. These symptoms are slightly different from those associated with most foodborne bacteria. In addition to the familiar watery diarrhea, nausea, vomiting, abdominal cramps, chills and fever occur. The diarrhea may be quite severe with cramps progressing to classical dysentery. Up to 40% of children with severe infections show neurological symptoms. These include seizures caused by fever, confusion, headache, lethargy, and a stiff neck that resembles **meningitis**.

The disease runs its course usually in two to three days but may last longer. Dehydration is a common complication. Most people recover on their own, although they may feel exhausted, but children who are malnourished or have weakened immune systems may die.

Clostridium botulinum (C. botulinum)

C. botulinum, which causes both adult **botulism** and infant botulism, is unlike any of the other foodborne bacteria. First, *C. botulinum* is an anaerobic bacterium in that it can only live in the absence of oxygen. Second, the toxins from *C. botulinum* are neurotoxins. They poison the nervous system, causing paralysis without the vomiting and diarrhea associated with other foodborne illnesses. Third, toxins that cause adult botulism are released when the bacteria grows in an airless environment outside the body. They can be broken down and made harmless by heat. Finally, botulism is much more likely to be fatal even in tiny quantities.

Adult botulism outbreaks are usually associated with home canned food, although occasionally commercially canned or vacuum packed foods are responsible for the disease. *C. botulinum* grows well in non-acidic, oxygen-free environments. If food is canned at too low heat or for too brief a time, the bacteria is not killed. It reproduces inside the can or jar, releasing its deadly neurotoxin. The toxin can be made harmless by heating the contaminated food to boiling for ten minutes. However, even a very small amount of the *C. botulinum* toxin can cause serious illness or **death**.

Symptoms of adult botulism appear about 18–36 hours after the contaminated food is eaten, although there are documented times of onset ranging from four hours to eight days. Initially a person suffering from botulism feels weakness and **dizziness** followed by double vision. Symptoms progress to difficulty speaking and swallowing. Paralysis moves down the body, and when the respiratory muscles are paralyzed, death results from asphyxiation. People who show any signs of botulism poisoning must receive immediate emergency medical care to increase their chance of survival.

Infant botulism is a form of botulism first recognized in 1976. It differs from food-borne botulism in its causes and symptoms. Infant botulism occurs when a child under the age of one year ingests the spores of *C. botulinum*. These spores are found in soil, but a more common source of spores is honey.

The *C. botulinum* spores lodge in the baby's intestinal tract and begin to grow, producing their neurotoxin. Onset of symptoms is gradual. Initially the baby is constipated. This is followed by poor feeding, lethargy, weakness, drooling, and a distinctive wailing cry. Eventually, the baby loses the ability to control its head muscles. From there the paralysis progresses to the rest of the body.

Diagnosis

One important aspect of diagnosing food poisoning is for doctors to determine if a number of people have eaten the same food and show the same symptoms of illness. When this happens, food poisoning is strongly suspected. The diagnosis is confirmed when the suspected bacteria is found in a stool culture or a fecal smear from the person. Other laboratory tests are used to isolate bacteria from a sample of the contaminated food. Botulism is usually diagnosed from its distinctive neurological symptoms, since rapid treatment is essential. Many cases of food poisoning go undiagnosed, since a definite diagnosis is not necessary to effectively treat the symptoms. Because it takes time for symptoms to develop, it is not necessarily the most recent food one has eaten that is the cause of the symptoms.

Treatment

Treatment of food poisoning, except that caused by *C. botulinum,* focuses on preventing dehydration by replacing fluids and electrolytes lost through vomiting and diarrhea. Electrolytes are salts and **minerals** that form electrically charges particles (ions) in body fluids. Electrolytes are important because they control body fluid balance and are important for all major body reactions. Pharmacists can recommend effective, pleasant-tasting, electrolytically balanced replacement fluids that are available without a prescription. When more fluids are being lost than can be consumed, dehydration may occur. Dehydration more likely to happen in the very young, the elderly, and people who are taking diuretics. To prevent dehydration, a doctor may give fluids intravenously.

In very serious cases of food poisoning, medications may be given to stop abdominal cramping and vomiting. Anti-diarrheal medications are not usually given. Stopping the diarrhea keeps the toxins in the body longer and may prolong the infection.

People with food poisoning should modify their diet. During period of active vomiting and diarrhea they should not try to eat and should drink only clear liquids frequently but in small quantities. Once active symptoms stop, they should eat bland, soft, easy to digest foods for two to three days. One example is the BRAT diet of bananas, rice, applesauce, and toast, all of which are easy to digest. Milk products, spicy food, alcohol and fresh fruit should be avoided for a few days, although babies should continue to breastfeed. These modifications are often all the treatment that is necessary.

Severe bacterial food poisonings are sometimes treated with **antibiotics**. Trimethoprim and sulfamethoxazole (Septra, Bactrim), ampicillin (Amcill, Polycill) or ciprofloxacin (Ciloxan, Cipro) are most frequently used.

Botulism is treated in a different way from other bacterial food poisonings. Botulism antitoxin is given to adults, but not infants, if it can be administered within 72 hours after symptoms are first observed. If given later, it provides no benefit.

Both infants and adults require hospitalization, often in the intensive care unit. If the ability to breathe is impaired, patients are put on a mechanical ventilator to assist their breathing and are fed intravenously until the paralysis passes.

Alternative treatment

Alternative practitioners offer the same advice as traditional practitioners concerning diet modification. In addition they recommend taking charcoal tablets, *Lactobacillus acidophilus*, *Lactobacillus bulgaricus*, and citrus seed extract. An electrolyte replacement fluid can be made at home by adding one teaspoon of salt and four teaspoons of sugar to one quart of water. For food poisoning other than botulism, two homeopathic remedies, either *Arsenicum album* or *Nux vomica*, are strongly recommended.

Prognosis

Most cases of food poisoning (except botulism) clear up on their own within one week without medical assistance. The ill person may continue feel tired for a few days after active symptoms stop. So long as the ill person does not become dehydrated, there are few complications. Deaths are rare and usually occur in the very young, the very old and people whose immune systems are already weakened.

Complications of *Salmonella* food poisoning include arthritis-like symptoms that occur three to four weeks after infection. Although deaths from *Salmonella* are rare, they do occur. Most deaths caused by *Salmonella* food poisoning have occurred in elderly people in nursing homes.

Adults usually recover without medical intervention, but many children need to be hospitalized as the result of *E. coli* food poisoning. *E. coli* toxins may be absorbed into the blood stream where they destroy red blood cells and platelets. Platelets are important in blood clotting. About 5% of victims develop hemolytic-uremic syndrome which results in sudden kidney failure and makes dialysis necessary. (Dialysis is a medical procedure used to filter the body's waste product when the kidneys have failed).

Botulism is the deadliest of the bacterial food-borne illnesses. With prompt medical care, the death rate is less than 10%.

Prevention

Food poisoning is almost entirely preventable by practicing good sanitation and good food handling techniques. These include:

- keep hot foods hot and cold foods cold
- cook meat to the recommended internal temperature, use a meat thermometer to check and cook eggs until they are no longer runny
- refrigerate leftovers promptly, do not let food stand at room temperature
- avoid contaminating surfaces and other foods with the juices of uncooked meats
- wash fruits and vegetables before using
- purchase pasteurized dairy products and fruit juices
- throw away bulging or leaking cans or any food that smells spoiled
- wash hands well before and during food preparation and after using the bathroom
- sanitize food preparation surfaces regularly

KEY TERMS

Diuretic—Medication that increases the urine output of the body.

Electrolytes—Salts and minerals that produce electrically charged particles (ions) in body fluids. Common human electrolytes are sodium chloride, potassium, calcium, and sodium bicarbonate. Electrolytes control the fluid balance of the body and are important in muscle contraction, energy generation, and almost all major biochemical reactions in the body.

Lactobacillus acidophilus—This bacteria is found in yogurt and changes the balance of the bacteria in the intestine in a beneficial way.

Platelets—Blood cells that help the blood to clot.

Resources

OTHER

U. S. Food and Drug Administration. Center for Food Safety and Applied Nutrition. *Bad Bug Book*, http://vm.cfsan.fda.gov.

Suzanne M. Lutwick, MPH

Foreign objects

Definition

Foreign means "originating elsewhere" or simply "outside the body." Foreign objects, also known as foreign bodies, typically become lodged in the eyes, ears, nose, airways, and rectum of human beings.

Demographics

Swallowing foreign bodies is a fairly common pediatric emergency; about 80,000 cases involving persons 19 years old or younger are reported each year to the 67 poison control centers in the United States. In a recent survey of the parents of 1,500 children, 4% reported that their children had swallowed a foreign object of some kind. The highest incidence of swallowed foreign bodies is in children between the ages of six months and four years.

The type of object most frequently swallowed varies somewhat across different historical periods and cultures. A recent study comparing the Jackson collection of foreign bodies removed from children between 1920 and 1932 with data collected from North American children's hospitals between 1988 and 2000 found that coins have replaced **safety** pins as the objects most commonly swallowed by American children. In Asia, fish bones are a frequent offender because fish is a dietary staple in most countries of the Far East.

In younger children, boys are at slightly greater risk than girls (53–47%) of swallowing foreign objects. Among teenagers, males are at a much higher risk than females of swallowing foreign bodies or inserting them into the rectum.

Younger children usually swallow or insert foreign objects into their bodies accidentally, usually as a result of play or exploring their environment. Adolescents are more likely to swallow or insert foreign bodies intentionally as a risk-taking behavior, a bid for attention, or while under the influence of drugs or alcohol. A small minority of teenagers who harm themselves by swallowing or inserting foreign bodies have **schizophrenia** or another psychotic disorder.

Description

Both children and adults experience problems caused by foreign objects getting stuck in their bodies. Young children are naturally curious and may intentionally put shiny objects, such as coins or button batteries, into their mouths. They also like to stick things in their ears and up their noses. Adults may accidentally swallow a non-food object or inhale a foreign body that gets stuck in the throat. Even if an object like a toothpick successfully passes through the esophagus and into the stomach, it can get stuck inside the rectum. Airborne particles can lodge in the eyes of people at any age.

Foreign bodies can be in hollow organs (like swallowed batteries) or in tissues (like bullets). They can be inert or irritating. If they irritate, they will cause inflammation and scarring. They can bring infection with them or acquire it and protect it from the body's immune defenses. They can obstruct passageways either by their size or by the scarring they cause. Some can be toxic.

Causes and symptoms

Eyes

Dust, dirt, sand, or other airborne material can lodge in the eyes, causing minor irritation and redness. More serious damage can be caused by hard or sharp objects that penetrate the surface and become embedded in the cornea or conjunctiva (the mucous membranes around the inner surface of the eyelids). Swelling, redness, bleeding from the surface blood vessels, sensitivity to light, and sudden vision problems are all symptoms of foreign matter in the eyes.

Ears and nose

Children will sometimes put things into their noses, ears, and other openings. Beans, popcorn kernels, raisins, and beads are just a few of the many items that have been found in these bodily cavities. On occasion, insects may fly into the ears and nose. **Pain**, hearing loss, and a sense of something stuck in the ear are symptoms of foreign bodies in the ears. A smelly, bloody discharge from one nostril is a symptom of foreign bodies in the nose.

Airways and stomach

At a certain age children will eat anything. A very partial list of items recovered from young stomachs includes: coins, chicken bones, fish bones, beads, rocks, plastic toys, pins, keys, round stones, marbles, nails, rings, batteries, ball bearings, screws, staples, washers, a heart pendant, a clothespin spring, and a toy soldier. Some of these items pass right on through and come out the other end. The progress of metal objects has been successfully followed with a metal detector. Others, like sharp bones, can get stuck and cause trouble. Batteries are corrosive and must be removed immediately.

Some objects can be inhaled unintentionally. The most commonly inhaled item is probably a peanut. A crayon and a cockroach have been found in a child's windpipes. These items always cause symptoms (difficulty swallowing and spitting up saliva, for instance) and may elude detection for some time while the child is being treated for **asthma** or recurring **pneumonia**.

Adults are not exempt from unusual inedibles. Dental devices are commonly swallowed. Adults with mental illness or subversive motives may swallow inappropriate objects, such as toothbrushes.

Rectum

Sometimes a foreign object will successfully pass through the throat and stomach only to get stuck at the juncture between the rectum and the anal canal. Items may also be self-introduced to enhance sexual stimulation and then get stuck. Sudden sharp pain during elimination may signify that an object is lodged in the rectum. Other symptoms vary depending upon the size of the object, its location, how long it has been in place, and whether or not infection has set in.

Diagnosis

The symptoms are as diverse as the objects and their locations. The most common manifestation of a foreign object anywhere in the body is infection. Even if the object started out sterile, germs may still be introduced. Blockage of passageways—breathing, digestive or excretory—is another result. Pain is common.

Treatment

Eyes

Small particles like sand may be removable without medical help, but if the object is not visible or cannot be retrieved, prompt emergency treatment is necessary. Trauma to the eyes can lead to loss of vision. Before attempting any treatment, the person should move to a well-lit area where the object can be better viewed. Hands should be washed and only clean, preferably sterile, materials should make contact with the eyes. If the particle is small, it may be dislodged by blinking or pulling the upper lid over the lower lid and flushing out the speck. A clean cloth can also be used to remove the particle. Once the object is removed, the eye should be rinsed with clean, lukewarm water or an opthalmic wash.

If the foreign object cannot be removed at home, the eye should be lightly covered with sterile gauze to discourage rubbing. A physician will use a strong light and possibly special eye drops to locate the object. Surgical tweezers can effectively remove many objects. An antibiotic sterile ointment and a patch may be prescribed. If the foreign body has penetrated the deeper layers of the eye, an ophthalmic surgeon will be consulted for emergency treatment.

Ears and nose

A number of ingenious extraction methods have been devised for removing foreign objects from the nose and ears. A bead in a nostril, for example, can be popped out by blowing into the mouth while holding the other nostril closed. Insects can be floated out of the ear by pouring warm (not hot) mineral oil, olive oil, or baby oil into the ear canal. Items that are lodged deep in the ear canal are more difficult to remove because of the possibility of damaging the ear drum. These require emergency treatment from a qualified physician.

Airways and stomach

Mechanical obstruction of the airways, which commonly occurs when food gets lodged in the throat, can be treated by applying the **Heimlich maneuver**. If the object is lodged lower in the airway, a bronchoscope (a special instrument to view the airway and remove obstructions) can be inserted. If the object is blocking the entrance to the stomach, a fiberoptic endoscope (an illuminated instrument that views the interior of a body cavity) may be used. The physician typically administers a sedative and anesthetizes the throat. The foreign object will then either be pulled out or pushed into the stomach, depending on whether or not the physician thinks it will pass through the digestive tract on its own. Objects in the digestive tract that are not irritating, sharp, or large may be followed as they continue on through. Sterile objects that are not causing symptoms may be left in place. Surgical removal of the offending object is necessary if it is causing symptoms.

Rectum

A rectal retractor can remove objects that a physician can feel during physical examination. Surgery may be required for objects deeply lodged within the recturm.

Prevention

Using common sense and following safety precautions are the best ways to prevent foreign objects from entering the body. Parents and other child care providers should toddler-proof their homes. Batteries should be stored in a locked cabinet and properly disposed of after use. To minimize the chance of youngsters inhaling food, parents should not allow children to eat while walking or playing. Adults should chew food thoroughly and not talk while chewing. Many eye injuries can be prevented by wearing safety glasses while using tools

KEY TERMS

Bronchoscope—An illuminated instrument that is inserted into the airway to inspect and retrieve objects from the bronchial tubes.

Conjunctiva—Mucous membranes around the inner surface of the eyelid.

Cornea—The rounded, transparent portion of the eye that covers the pupil and iris and lets light into the interior

Endoscopy—The surgical use of long, thin instruments that have both viewing and operating capabilities.

Heimlich maneuver—An emergency procedure for removing a foreign object lodged in the airway that is preventing the person from breathing.

Resources

PERIODICALS

Al-Sebeih, Khalid, Khairy-Alhag Abu-Shara, and Amro Sobeih. "Extraluminal Perforation Complicating Foreign

Bodies in the Upper Aerodigestive Tract." *The Annals of Otology, Rhinology & Laryngology* 119, no. 5 (May 1, 2010): 284-8.
Shivakumar, A., et al. "Foreign Bodies in Upper Digestive Tract." *Indian Journal of Otolaryngology and Head and Neck Surgery* 58, no. 1 (January-March 2006): 63-68.

J. Ricker Polsdorfer, MD
Karl Finley

Foster care

Definition

Foster care is full-time substitute care of children outside their own homes by people other than the biological parents.

Description

Children are placed in foster care for a number of reasons. Some are being protected from abuse at home; others have been neglected by their parents, or have parents who are unable to take care of them. A small percentage of children are in foster care because their parents feel unable to control them, and their behavior may have led to delinquency. In all cases, the child's natural parents temporarily give up legal **custody** of the child. A child may be placed in foster care with the natural parents' consent. In a clear case of abuse or neglect, a court can order a child into foster care without the parents' consent. Foster care does not necessarily mean care by strangers. If a government agency decides a child must be removed from her home, the child may be placed with relatives or with a family friend. Children may also be placed in a group home, where several foster children live together. State social service agencies are usually in control of foster care decisions, though they may also work with private foundations.

Federal money supports most foster care programs, and a federal law governs foster care policy. This law, the **Adoption** Assistance and Child Welfare Reform Act of 1980, emphasizes two aims of foster care. One is to preserve the child's biological family if at all possible. Children are placed in foster care only after other options have failed, and social service agencies work with the biological family to resolve its problems, so that children can return to their homes. The second aim of the Child Welfare Reform Act is to support "permanency planning." This means that if a child must be removed from her home, the social service agency handling the case tries to decide as quickly as is reasonable whether the child will ever be returned. If it seems likely that parents will not be able to care for their children again, their parental rights may be terminated so that the child is free to be adopted. This policy is articulated in this law in order to prevent children from living too long in an unstable situation. Today about two-thirds of all children in foster care are returned to their original homes within two years. Nevertheless, some children remain in foster care for many years.

There are more than 400,000 children in foster care in the United States. Children from economically disadvantaged families are more likely to be in foster care children from middle-class families. Often this is due fewer available resources to help care for the children in case of illness or loss of a job. African American children make up about two-thirds of all children in foster care. They are also more likely to stay in foster care longer, or to have been in foster care since **infancy**. Also, children of alcoholics or drug addicts are more likely to be in foster care.

In most cases, children who have been placed in foster care have been subjected to some form of abuse or neglect, and being removed from familiar surroundings is, in itself, usually highly traumatic. Children in foster care may have **nightmares**, problems sleeping or eating, and may be depressed, angry, and confused. Many young children in foster care are unable to understand why they have been taken from their parents. Even if a child is in some sense relieved to be out of a home that was dangerous to her, she may still miss her parents, and imagine that there is something she must do to get back to them. Though there is evidence that children from abusive and neglectful homes start to feel better in foster care, separation is almost always difficult for children.

Foster care can be difficult for foster parents as well. A child who has been neglected or abused suffers psychological damage that may make the child withdrawn, immature, aggressive, or otherwise difficult to reach. Foster placements sometimes fail because the parents simply cannot handle the demands of a troubled foster child. Despite the stress of foster parenting, more than 100,000 homes in the United States take in foster children. A foster parent may be a couple or a single person, and may or may not have their own biological children at home along with the foster child or children.

Foster parents must be licensed by the agency that handles foster care in their area. The foster parent or parents' home must pass an inspection for health and **safety**, and in most states, the parents must attend training sessions covering issues of foster care and how to deal with problems. When a child is placed, the foster family has responsibility for feeding and clothing the child, getting the child to school and to appointments, and doing any of the usual things a child's parents might be called on to do. The foster parents might also need to meet with the foster child's therapist, and will meet regularly with the child's caseworker as well. The foster parent aims to help the foster child develop normally in a family situation.

Foster parents usually receive money for taking in foster children. With this money they are expected to buy the child's food and clothing, and take care of incidental expenses. In many cases this money does not cover all of the child's expenses however, and foster parents spend some of their own money as well. Most of the foster parent's responsibilities toward the foster child are clearly defined in a legal contract. Foster parents do not become the guardians of foster children; legal guardianship remains with the state agency. Foster placements may last for a few days or weeks, or even years. If the biological parents give up their rights or their rights to their child are severed, the foster family may wish to adopt the foster child. Foster parenting is meant to be an in-between stage, while a permanent placement for the child is settled. As such, it is stressful and uncertain, but for many families very rewarding.

Resources

BOOKS

Barber, James G. and Paul H. Delfabbro. *Children in Foster Care.* New York: Routledge, 2004.

Libal, Joyce. *A House Between Homes: Youth in the Foster Care System.* Broomall, PA: Mason Crest Publishers, 2004.

PERIODICALS

"Fewer U.S. kids in foster care." Burlington, Vermont: Burlington Free Press. 1 September 2010. pp. 1A, http://www.google.com/hostednews/ap/article/ALeqM5gq1yhAPK8txoVpGAPujSMUK9wz5gD9HULPCG4.

A. Woodward

Fractures

Definition

A fracture is a complete or incomplete break in a bone resulting from the application of excessive force.

Description

A fracture usually results from traumatic injury to bones causing the continuity of bone tissues or bony cartilage to be disrupted or broken. Fracture classifications include simple, compound, incomplete and complete. Simple fractures (more recently called "closed") are not obvious as the skin has not been ruptured and remains intact. Compound fractures (now commonly called "open") break the skin, exposing bone and causing additional soft tissue injury and possible infection. A single fracture means that one fracture only has occurred and multiple fractures refer to more than one fracture occurring in the same bone. Fractures are termed complete if the break is completely through the bone and described as incomplete or "greenstick" if the fracture occurs partly across a bone shaft. This latter type of fracture is often the result of bending or crushing forces applied to a bone.

Fractures are also named according to the specific part of the bone involved and the nature of the break. Identification of a fracture line can further classify fractures. Types include linear, oblique, transverse, longitudinal, and spiral fractures. Fractures can be further subdivided by the positions of bony fragments and are described as comminuted, non-displaced, impacted, overriding, angulated, displaced, avulsed, and segmental. Additionally, an injury may be classified as a fracture-

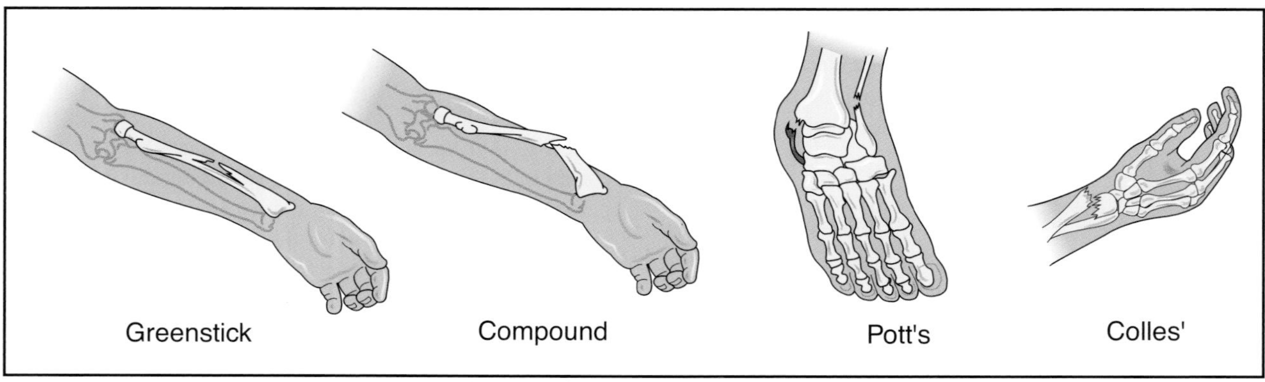

Fractures usually result from a traumatic injury to a bone where the continuity of bone tissues or bony cartilage is disrupted or broken. The illustrations above feature common sites where fractures occur. *(Illustration by Electronic Illustrators Group. Reproduced by permission of Gale, a part of Cengage Learning.)*

dislocation when a fracture involves the bony structures of any joint with associated dislocation of the same joint.

Fractures line identification

Linear fractures have a break that runs parallel to the bone's main axis or in the direction of the bone's shaft. For example, a linear fracture of the arm bone could extend the entire length of the bone. Oblique and transverse fractures differ in that an oblique fracture crosses a bone at approximately a 45° angle to the bone's axis. In contrast, a transverse fracture crosses a bone's axis at a 90° angle. A longitudinal fracture is similar to a linear fracture. Its fracture line extends along the shaft but is more irregular in shape and does not run parallel to the bone's axis. Spiral fractures are described as crossing a bone at an oblique angle, creating a spiral pattern. This break usually occurs in the long bones of the body such as the upper arm bone (humerus) or the thigh bone (femur).

Bony fragment position identification

Comminuted fractures have two or more fragments broken into small pieces, in addition to the upper and lower halves of a fractured bone. Fragments of bone that maintain their normal alignment following a fracture are described as being non-displaced. An impacted fracture is characterized as a bone fragment forced into or onto another fragment resulting from a compressive force. Overriding is a term used to describe bony fragments that overlap and shorten the total length of a bone. Angulated fragments result in pieces of bone being at angles to each other. A displaced bony fragment occurs from disruption of normal bone alignment with deformity of these segments separate from one another. An avulsed fragment occurs when bone fragments are pulled from their normal position by forceful muscle contractions or resistance from ligaments. Segmental fragmented positioning occurs if fractures in two adjacent areas occur, leaving an isolated central segment. An example of segmental alignment is when the arm bone fractures in two separate places, with displacement of the middle section of bone.

Causes and symptoms

Individuals with high activity levels appear to be at greater risk for fractures. This group includes children and athletes participating in contact **sports**. Because of an increase in bone brittleness with aging, elderly persons are also included in this high-risk population. Up to the age of 50, more men suffer from fractures than women due to occupational hazards. However, after the age of 50, women are more prone to fractures than men. Specific diseases causing an increased risk for fractures include Paget's disease, rickets, **osteogenesis imperfecta**, osteoporosis, bone **cancer** and tumors, and prolonged disuse of a nonfunctional body part such as after a **stroke**.

Symptoms of fractures usually begin with **pain** that increases with attempted movement or use of the area and swelling at the involved site. The skin in the area may be pale and an obvious deformity may be present. In more severe cases, there may be a loss of pulse below the fracture site, such as in the extremities, accompanied by **numbness**, **tingling**, or paralysis below the fracture. An open or compound fracture is often accompanied by bleeding or bruising. If the lower limbs or pelvis are fractured, pain and resistance to movement usually accompany the injury causing difficulty with weight bearing.

Diagnosis

Diagnosis begins immediately with an individual's own observation of symptoms. A thorough medical history and physical exam by a physician often reveals the presence of a fracture. An x-ray of the injured area is the most common test used to determine the presence of a bone fracture. Any x ray series performed involves at least two views of the area to confirm the presence of the fracture because not all fractures are apparent on a single x ray. Some fractures are often difficult to see and may require several views at different angles to see clear fracture lines. In some cases, CT, MRI or other imaging tests are required to demonstrate fracture. Sometimes, especially with children, the initial x ray may not show any fractures but repeat seven to 14 days later may show changes in the bone(s) of the affected area. If a fracture is open and occurs in conjunction with soft tissue injury, further laboratory studies are often conducted to determine if blood loss has occurred.

In the event of exercise-related stress fractures (micro-fractures due to excessive stress), a tuning fork can provide a simple, inexpensive test. The tuning fork is a metal instrument with a stem and two prongs that vibrate when struck. If an individual has increased pain when the tuning fork is placed on a bone, such as the tibia or shinbone, the likelihood of a stress fracture is high. Bone scans also are helpful in detecting stress fractures. In this diagnostic procedure, a radioactive tracer is injected into the bloodstream and images are taken of specific areas or the entire skeleton by CT or MRI.

Treatment

Treatment depends on the type of fracture, its severity, the individual's age and general health. The first priority in treating any fracture is to address the entire medical status of the patient. Medical personnel are trained not allow a painful, deformed limb to distract them from potentially life-threatening injury elsewhere or shock. If an open fracture is accompanied by serious soft tissue injury, it may be necessary to control bleeding and the shock that can accompany loss of blood.

First aid is the appropriate initial treatment in emergency situations. It includes proper splinting, control of blood loss, and monitoring vital signs such as breathing and circulation.

Immobilization

Immobilization of a fracture site can be done internally or externally. The primary goal of immobilization is to maintain the realignment of a bone long enough for healing to start and progress. Immobilization by external fixation uses splints, casts, or braces. This may be the primary and only procedure for fracture treatment. Splinting to immobilize a fracture can be done with or without traction. In emergency situations if the injured individual must be moved by someone other than a trained medical person, splinting is a useful form of fracture management. It should be done without causing additional pain and without moving the bone segments. In a clinical environment, plaster of Paris casts are used for immobilization. Braces are useful as they often allow movement above and below a fracture site. Treatments for stress fractures include rest and decreasing or stopping any activity that causes or increases pain.

Fracture reduction

Fracture reduction is the procedure by which a fractured bone is realigned in normal position. It can be either closed or open. Closed reduction refers to realigning bones without breaking the skin. It is performed with manual manipulation and/or traction and is commonly done with some kind of anesthetic. Open reduction primarily refers to surgery that is performed to realign bones or fragments. Fractures with little or no displacement may not require any form of reduction.

Traction is used to help reposition a broken bone. It works by applying pressure to restore proper alignment. The traction device immobilizes the area and maintains realignment as the bone heals. A fractured bone is immobilized by applying opposing force at both ends of the injured area, using an equal amount of traction and countertraction. Weights provide the traction pull needed or the pull is achieved by positioning the individual's body weight appropriately. Traction is a form of closed reduction and is sometimes used as an alternative to surgery. Since it restricts movement of the affected limb or body part, it may confine a person to bed rest for an extended period of time.

A person may need open reduction if there is an open, severe, or comminuted fracture. This procedure allows a physician to examine and surgically correct associated soft tissue damage while reducing the fracture and, if necessary, applying internal or external devices. Internal fixation involves the use of metallic devices inserted into or through bone to hold the fracture in a set position and alignment while it heals. Devices include plates, nails, screws, and rods. When healing is complete, the surgeon may or may not remove these devices. Virtually any hip fracture requires open reduction and internal fixation so that the bone will be able to support the patient's weight.

Alternative treatment

In addition to the importance of calcium for strong bones, many alternative treatment approaches recommend use of mineral supplements to help build and maintain a healthy, resilient skeleton. Some physical therapists use electro-stimulation over a fractured site to promote and expedite healing. Chinese traditional medicine may be helpful by working to reconnect chi through the meridian lines along the line of a fracture. Homeopathy can enhance the body's healing process. Two particularly useful homeopathic remedies are *Arnica* (*Arnica montana*) and *Symphytum* (*Symphytum officinalis*). If possible, applying contrast hydrotherapy to an extremity (e.g., a hand or foot) of a fractured area can assist healing by enhancing circulation.

Prognosis

Fractures involving joint surfaces almost always lead to some degree of arthritis of the joint. Fractures can normally be cured with proper first aid and appropriate aftercare. If determined necessary by a physician, the fractured site should be manipulated, realigned, and immobilized as soon as possible. Realignment has been shown to be much more difficult after six hours. Healing time varies from person to person with the elderly generally needing more time to heal completely. A non-union fracture may result when a fracture does not heal, such as in the case of an elderly person or an individual with medical complications. Recovery is complete when there is no bone motion at the fracture site, and **x rays** indicate complete healing. Open fractures may lead to bone infections, which delay the healing process. Another possible complication is compartment syndrome, a painful condition resulting from the expansion of enclosed tissue and that may occur when a body part is immobilized in a cast.

KEY TERMS

Avulsion fracture—A fracture caused by the tearing away of a fragment of bone where a strong ligament or tendon attachment forcibly pulls the fragment away from the bone tissue.

Axis—A line that passes through the center of the body or body part.

Comminuted fracture—A fracture where there are several breaks in a bone creating numerous fragments.

Compartment syndrome—Compartment syndrome is a condition in which a muscle swells but is constricted by the connective tissue around it, which cuts off blood supply to the muscle.

Contrast hydrotherapy—A series of hot and cold water applications. A hot compress (as hot as an individual can tolerate) is applied for three minutes followed by an ice cold compress for 30 seconds. These applications are repeated three times each and ending with the cold compress.

Osteogenesis imperfecta—A genetic disorder involving defective development of connective tissues, characterized by brittle and fragile bones that are easily fractured by the slightest trauma.

Osteoporosis—Literally meaning "porous bones," this condition occurs when bones lose an excessive amount of their protein and mineral content, particularly calcium. Over time, bone mass and strength are reduced leading to increased risk of fractures.

Paget's disease—Chromic disorder of unknown cause, usually affecting middle aged and elderly people, characterized by enlarged and deformed bones. Excessive breakdown and formation of bone tissue occurs with Paget's disease and can cause bone to weaken, resulting in bone pain, arthritis, deformities, and fractures.

Reduction—The restoration of a body part to its original position after displacement, such as the reduction of a fractured bone by bringing ends or fragments back into original alignment. The useof local or general anesthesia usually accompanies a fracture reduction. If performed by outside manipulation only, the reduction is described as closed; if surgery is necessary, it is described as open.

Rickets—A condition caused by the dietary deficiency of vitamin D, calcium, and usually phosphorus, seen primarily in infancy and childhood, and characterized by abnormal bone formation.

Traction—The process of placing a bone, limb, or group of muscles under tension by applying weights and pulleys. The goal is to realign or immobilize the part or to relieve pressure on that particular area to promote healing and restore function.

Prevention

Adequate calcium intake is necessary for strong bones and can help decrease the risk of fractures. People who do not get enough calcium in their diets can take a calcium supplement. **Exercise** can help strengthen bones by increasing bone density, thereby decreasing the risk of fractures from falls. A University of Southern California study reported that older people who exercised one or more hours per day had approximately half the incidence of hip fractures as those who exercised fewer than 30 minutes per day or not at all.

Fractures can be prevented if **safety** measures are taken seriously. These measures include using seat belts in cars and encouraging children to wear protective sports gear. Estrogen replacement for women past the age of 50 has been shown to help prevent osteoporosis and the fractures that may result from this condition. In one study, elderly women on estrogen replacement therapy demonstrated the lowest occurrence of hip fractures when compared to similar women not on estrogen replacement therapy.

Parental concerns

Parents should ensure that their children get an adequate intake of calcium. Children should also participate in regular physical exercise.

Resources

BOOKS

Burr, David B. *Musculoskeletal Fatigue and Stress Fracture.* Boca Raton, FL: CRC Press, 2001.

Jupiter, J. *Fractures and Dislocations of the Hand.* St. Louis: Mosby, 2001.

Moehring, H. David, and Adam Greenspan. *Fractures: Diagnosis and Treatment.* New York: McGraw Hill, 2000.

Ogden, John A. *Skeletal Injury in the Child.* New York: Springer Verlag, 2000.

OTHER

"About the Human." http://orthopedics.about.com/health/orthopedics/blhipfracture.htm.

Family Practice Notebook.com, http://www.fpnotebook.com/FRA.htm

National Library of Medicine, http://medlineplus.adam.com/ency/article/000001.htm.

University of Iowa, http://www.vh.org/Providers/ClinRef/FPHandbook/Chapter06/18-6.html.

ORGANIZATIONS

American Academy of Orthopaedic Surgeons, 6300 North River Road, Rosemont IL, 60018-4262, (847) 823-7186, (800) 346-2267, (847) 823-8125, http://orthoinfo.aaos.org.

American College of Sports Medicine (ACSM), 401 West Michigan Street, Indianapolis IN, 46202, (317) 637-9200, (317) 634-7817, http://www.acsm.org.

Children's Orthopedics of Atlanta, 5445 Meridian Mark Road, Suite 250, Atlanta GA, 30342, (404) 255-1933, (404) 256-7924, http://www.childrensortho.com.

L. Fleming Fallon, Jr., MD, DrPH

Fragile X syndrome

Definition

Fragile X syndrome is the most common form of inherited **mental retardation**. Individuals with this condition have **developmental delay**, variable levels of mental retardation, and behavioral and emotional difficulties. They may also have characteristic physical traits. Generally, males are affected with moderate mental retardation and females with mild mental retardation.

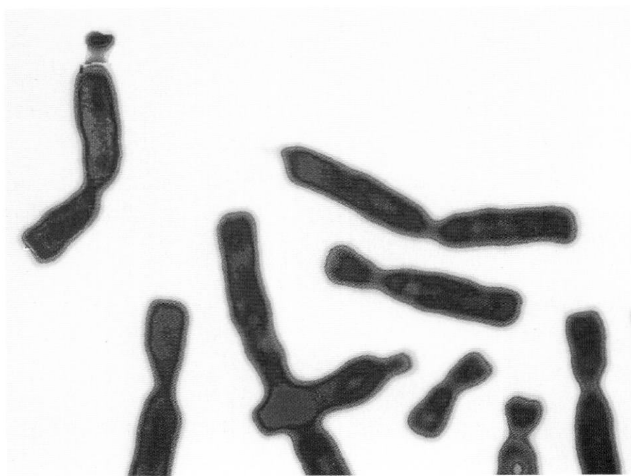

Fragile X chromosome, shaded in purple at upper left corner, is shown among other chromosomes. *(Custom Medical Stock Photo, Inc. Reproduced by permission.)*

Description

Fragile X syndrome is also known as Martin-Bell syndrome, Marker X syndrome, and FRAXA syndrome. It is the most common form of inherited mental retardation. Fragile X syndrome is caused by a mutation in the FMR-1 gene, located on the X chromosome. The role of the gene is unclear, but it is probably important in early development.

In order to understand fragile X syndrome it is important to understand how human genes and chromosomes influence this condition. Normally, each cell in the body contains 46 (23 pairs of) chromosomes. These chromosomes consist of genetic material (DNA) needed for the production of proteins, which lead to growth, development, and physical/intellectual characteristics. The first 22 pairs of chromosomes are the same in males and females. The remaining two chromosomes are called the sex chromosomes (X and Y). The sex chromosomes determine whether a person is male or female. Males have only one X chromosome, which is inherited from the mother at conception, and they receive a Y chromosome from the father. Females inherit two X chromosomes, one from each parent. Fragile X syndrome is caused by a mutation in a gene called FMR-1. This gene is located on the X chromosome. The FMR-1 gene is thought to play an important role in the development of the brain, but the exact way that the gene acts in the body is not fully understood.

Fragile X syndrome affects males and females of all ethnic groups. It is estimated that there are about one in 4,000 to one in 6,250 males affected with fragile X syndrome. There are approximately one-half as many females with fragile X syndrome as there are males. The carrier frequency in unaffected females is one in 100 to one in 600, with one study finding a carrier frequency of one in 250.

Causes and symptoms

For reasons not fully understood, the CGG sequence in the FMR-1 gene can expand to contain between 54 and 230 repeats. This stage of expansion is called a premutation. People who carry a premutation do not usually have symptoms of fragile X syndrome, although there have been reports of individuals with a premutation and subtle intellectual or behavioral symptoms. Individuals who carry a fragile X premutation are at risk to have children or grandchildren with the condition. Female premutation carriers may also be at increased risk for earlier onset of menopause; however, premutation carriers may exist through several generations of a family and no symptoms of fragile X syndrome will appear.

The size of the premutation can expand over succeeding generations. Once the size of the premutation exceeds 230 repeats, it becomes a full mutation and the FMR-1 gene is disabled. Individuals who carry the full mutation may have fragile X syndrome. Since the FMR-1 gene is located on the X chromosome, males are more likely to develop symptoms than females. This is because males have only one copy of the X chromosome. Males who inherit the full mutation are expected to have mental impairment. A female's normal X chromosome may compensate for her chromosome with the fragile X gene mutation. Females who inherit the full mutation have an approximately 50% risk of mental impairment. The phenomenon of an expanding trinucleotide repeat in successive generations is called anticipation. Another unique aspect of fragile X syndrome is that mosaicism is present in 15–20% those affected by the condition. Mosaicism is when there is the presence of cells of two different genetic materials in the same individual.

The mutation involves a short sequence of DNA in the FMR-1 gene. This sequence is designated CGG. Normally, the CGG sequence is repeated between six to 54 times. People who have repeats in this range do not have fragile X syndrome and are not at increased risk to have children with fragile X syndrome. Those affected by fragile X syndrome have expanded CGG repeats (over 200) in the first exon of the FMR1 gene (the full mutation)

Fragile X syndrome is inherited in an X-linked dominant manner (characters are transmitted by genes on the X chromosome). When a man carries a premutation on his X chromosome, it tends to be stable and usually will not expand if he passes it on to his daughters (he passes his Y chromosome to his sons). Thus, all of his daughters will be premutation carriers like he is. When a woman carries a premutation, it is unstable and can expand as she passes it on to her children, therefore a man's grandchildren are at greater risk of developing the syndrome. There is a 50% risk for a premutation carrier female to transmit an abnormal mutation with each pregnancy. The likelihood for the premutation to expand is related to the number of repeats present; the higher the number of repeats, the greater the chance that the premutation will expand to a full mutation in the next generation. All mothers of a child with a full mutation are carriers of an FMR-1 gene expansion. Ninety-nine percent of patients with fragile X syndrome have a CGG expansion, and less than one percent have a point mutation or deletion on the FMR1 gene.

Individuals with fragile X syndrome appear normal at **birth** but their development is delayed. Most boys with fragile X syndrome have mental impairment. The severity of mental impairment ranges from learning disabilities to severe mental retardation. Behavioral problems include attention deficit and hyperactivity at a young age. Some may show aggressive behavior in adulthood. Short attention span, poor eye contact, delayed and disordered speech and language, emotional instability, and unusual hand mannerisms (hand flapping or hand biting) are also seen frequently. Characteristic physical traits appear later in childhood. These traits include a long and narrow face, prominent jaw, large ears, and enlarged testes. In females who carry a full mutation, the physical and behavioral features and mental retardation tend to be less severe. About 50% of females who have a full mutation are mentally retarded. Other behavioral characteristics include whirling, spinning, and occasionally **autism**.

Children with fragile X syndrome often have frequent ear and sinus infections. Nearsightedness and lazy eye are also common. Many babies with fragile X syndrome may have trouble with sucking and some experience digestive disorders that cause frequent gagging and **vomiting**. A small percentage of children with fragile X syndrome may experience seizures. Children with fragile X syndrome also tend to have loose joints which may result in joint dislocations. Some children develop a curvature in the spine, flat feet, and a heart condition known as mitral valve prolapse.

Diagnosis

Any child with signs of developmental delay of speech, language, or motor development with no known cause should be considered for fragile X testing, especially if there is a family history of the condition. Behavioral and developmental problems may indicate fragile X syndrome, particularly if there is a family history of mental retardation. Definitive identification of the fragile X syndrome is made by means of a genetic test to assess the number of CGG sequence repeats in the FMR-1 gene. Individuals with the premutation or full mutation may be identified through **genetic testing**. Genetic testing for the fragile X mutation can be done on the developing baby before birth through **amniocentesis** or chorionic villus sampling (CVS), and is 99% effective in detecting the condition due to trinucleotide repeat expansion. Prenatal testing should only be undertaken after the fragile X carrier status of the parents has been confirmed and the couple has been counseled regarding the risks of recurrence. While prenatal testing is possible to do with CVS, the results can be difficult to interpret and additional testing may be required.

Treatment

Presently there is no cure for fragile X syndrome. Management includes such approaches as **speech therapy**, **occupational therapy**, and physical therapy. The expertise of psychologists, **special education** teachers, and genetic counselors may also be beneficial. Drugs may be used to treat hyperactivity, seizures, and other problems. Establishing a regular routine, avoiding over-stimulation, and using calming techniques may also help in the management of behavioral problems. Children with a troubled heart valve may need to see a heart specialist and take medications before surgery or dental procedures. Children with frequent ear and sinus infections may need to take medications or have special tubes placed in their ears to drain excess fluid. Mainstreaming of children with fragile X syndrome into regular classrooms is encouraged because they do well imitating behavior. Peer tutoring and positive reinforcement are also encouraged.

Prognosis

Early diagnosis and intensive intervention offer the best prognosis for individuals with fragile X syndrome. Adults with fragile X syndrome may benefit from vocational training and may need to live in a supervised setting. Life span is typically normal.

A 2004 study found that men who are carriers of the fragile X gene but have not have the mutation severe enough to have fragile X syndrome may begin to show signs of tremor disorder, gait instability and memory impairment as they age. The higher prevalence of these symptoms among grandfathers of children with fragile x syndrome was noted so a study was done to investigate their symptoms compared to men of the same age without the mutation. About 17% of the grandfathers in their 50s had the condition, 37% of those in their 60s, 47% of men in their 70s and 75% of men in their 80s. Often, these men have been diagnosed with other diseases such as Parkinson's or Alzheimer's rather than with fragile X-associated tremor/ataxia syndrome, the name which has been given to these late symptoms from the fragile x mutation.

KEY TERMS

Amniocentesis—A procedure performed at 16–18 weeks of pregnancy in which a needle is inserted through a woman's abdomen into her uterus to draw out a small sample of the amniotic fluid from around the baby. Either the fluid itself or cells from the fluid can be used for a variety of tests to obtain information about genetic disorders and other medical conditions in the fetus.

CGG or CGG sequence—Shorthand for the DNA sequence: cytosine-guanine-guanine. Cytosine and guanine are two of the four molecules, otherwise called nucleic acids, that make up DNA.

Chorionic villus sampling (CVS)—A procedure used for prenatal diagnosis at 10-12 weeks gestation. Under ultrasound guidance a needle is inserted either through the mother's vagina or abdominal wall and a sample of cells is collected from around the early embryo. These cells are then tested for chromosome abnormalities or other genetic diseases.

Chromosome—A microscopic thread-like structure found within each cell of the body that consists of a complex of proteins and DNA. Humans have 46 chromosomes arranged into 23 pairs. Changes in either the total number of chromosomes or their shape and size (structure) may lead to physical or mental abnormalities.

FMR-1 gene—A gene found on the X chromosome. Its exact purpose is unknown, but it is suspected that the gene plays a role in brain development.

Mitral valve prolapse—A heart defect in which one of the valves of the heart (which normally controls blood flow) becomes floppy. Mitral valve prolapse may be detected as a heart murmur but there are usually no symptoms.

Premutation—A change in a gene that precedes a mutation; this change does not alter the function of the gene.

X chromosome—One of the two sex chromosomes (the other is Y) containing genetic material that, among other things, determine a person's gender.

Resources

PERIODICALS

Kirn, Timothy F. "New Fragile X Often Misdiagnosed as Parkinson's." *Clinical Psychiatry News* March 2004: 84.

OTHER

"Fragile X Site Mental Retardation 1; FMR1." *Online Mendelian Inheritance in Man.* March 6, 2001, http://www3.ncbi.nlm.nih.gov/Omim/.

Tarleton, Jack, and Robert A. Saul. "Fragile X Syndrome." *GeneClinics* March 6, 2001, http://www.geneclinics.org.

ORGANIZATIONS

Arc of the United States (formerly Association for Retarded Citizens of the US), 500 East Border St., Suite 300, Arlington TX, 76010, (817) 261-6003, http://thearc.org.

National Fragile X Foundation PO Box 190488, San Francisco CA, 94119-0988 (800) 688-8765 (510) 763-6030, natlfx@sprintmail.com http://nfxf.org.

National Fragile X Syndrome Support Group 206 Sherman Rd., Glenview IL, 60025 (708) 724-8626

Nada Quercia, MS, CCGC
Teresa G. Odle

Friedreich's ataxia

Definition

Friedreich's ataxia (FA) is an inherited, progressive nervous system disorder causing loss of balance and coordination.

Description

Ataxia is a condition marked by impaired coordination. Friedreich's ataxia is the most common inherited ataxia, affecting between 3,000–5,000 people in the United States. FA is an autosomal recessive disease, which means that two defective gene copies must be inherited to develop symptoms, one from each parent. A person with only one defective gene copy will not show signs of FA, but may pass along the gene to offspring. Couples with one child affected by FA have a 25% chance in each pregnancy of conceiving another affected child.

Causes and symptoms

Causes

The gene for FA codes for a protein called frataxin. Normal frataxin is found in the cellular energy structures known as mitochondria, where it is thought to be involved in regulating the transport of iron. In FA, the frataxin gene on chromosome 9 is expanded with nonsense information known as a "triple repeat." This extra DNA interferes with normal production of frataxin, thereby impairing iron transport. Normally, there are 10-21 repeats of the frataxin gene. In FA, this sequence may be repeated between 200-900 times. The types of symptoms and severity of FA seems to be associated with the number of repetitions. Patients with more copies have more severe symptomatology. Researchers are still wrestling with how frataxin and the repeats on chromosome 9 are involved in causing FA. One theory suggests that FA develops in part because defects in iron transport prevent efficient use of cellular energy supplies.

The nerve cells most affected by FA are those in the spinal cord involved in relaying information between muscles and the brain. Tight control of movement requires complex feedback between the muscles promoting a movement, those restraining it, and the brain. Without this control, movements become uncoordinated, jerky, and inappropriate to the desired action.

Symptoms

Symptoms of FA usually first appear between the ages of 8 and 15, although onset as early as 18 months or as late as age 25 is possible. The first symptom is usually gait incoordination. A child with FA may graze doorways when passing through, for instance, or trip over low obstacles. Unsteadiness when standing still and deterioration of position sense is common. Foot deformities and walking up off the heels often results from uneven muscle weakness in the legs. **Muscle spasms and cramps** may occur, especially at night.

Ataxia in the arms follows, usually within several years, leading to decreased **hand-eye coordination**. Arm weakness does not usually occur until much later. Speech and swallowing difficulties are common. **Diabetes mellitus** may also occur. **Nystagmus**, or eye tremor, is common, along with some loss of visual acuity. Hearing loss may also occur. A side-to-side curvature of the spine (**scoliosis**) occurs in many cases, and may become severe.

Heartbeat abnormalities occur in about two thirds of FA patients, leading to shortness of breath after exertion, swelling in the lower limbs, and frequent complaints of cold feet.

Diagnosis

Diagnosis of FA involves a careful medical history and thorough **neurological exam**. Lab tests include electromyography, an electrical test of muscle, and a nerve conduction velocity test. An electrocardiogram may be performed to diagnose heart arrhythmia.

Direct DNA testing is available, allowing FA to be more easily distinguished from other types of ataxia. The

KEY TERMS

Ataxia—A condition marked by impaired coordination.

Scoliosis—An abnormal, side-to-side curvature of the spine.

same test may be used to determine the presence of the genetic defect in unaffected individuals, such as siblings.

Treatment

There is no cure for FA, nor any treatment that can slow its progress. Amantadine may provide some limited improvement in ataxic symptoms, but is not recommended in patients with cardiac abnormalities. Physical and **occupational therapy** are used to maintain range of motion in weakened muscles, and to design adaptive techniques and devices to compensate for loss of coordination and strength. Some patients find that using weights on the arms can help dampen the worst of the uncoordinated arm movements.

Heart arrhythmias and diabetes are treated with drugs specific to those conditions.

Prognosis

The rate of progression of FA is highly variable. Most patients lose the ability to walk within 15 years of symptom onset, and 95% require a wheelchair for mobility by age 45. Reduction in lifespan from FA complications is also quite variable. Average age at **death** is in the mid-thirties, but may be as late as the mid-sixties. As of mid-1998, the particular length of the triple repeat has not been correlated strongly enough with disease progression to allow prediction of the course of the disease on this basis.

Prevention

There is no way to prevent development of FA in a person carrying two defective gene copies.

Resources

BOOKS

Feldman, Eva L. "Hereditary Cerebellar Ataxias and Related Disorders." In *Cecil Textbook of Medicine*, edited by Russel L. Cecil, et al. Philadelphia: W.B. Saunders Company, 2000.

Isselbacher, Kurt J., et al. "Spinocerebellar Degeneration (Friedreich's Ataxia)." In *Harrison's Principles of Internal Medicine*. New York: McGraw-Hill, 2001.

ORGANIZATIONS

Muscular Dystrophy Association, 3300 East Sunrise Dr., Tucson AZ, 85718, (520) 529-2000, (800) 572-1717, http://www.mdausa.org.

Rosalyn Carson-DeWitt, MD

Frostbite and frostnip

Definition

Frostbite is the term for damage to the skin and other tissues caused by freezing. Frostnip is a milder form of cold injury; it is sometimes described as the first stage of frostbite.

Demographics

Frostbite is most likely to occur among military personnel, people who work outdoors in cold weather, mountain climbers, skiers and other winter **sports** participants, homeless people, travelers stranded outside in cold weather, and people who live close to the polar regions. In a few cases frostbite is caused by industrial accidents, when workers who must handle liquid nitrogen or other liquefied gases fail to protect their hands or use proper **safety** equipment. It is estimated that frostbite in North America and northern Europe causes 2.5 hospital admissions per 100,000 people per year. The true rate is unknown because there is no standardized reporting system for this disorder.

Most frostbite victims are male, but this ratio is thought to reflect occupational choices and interest in high-risk outdoor sports rather than a genetic factor.

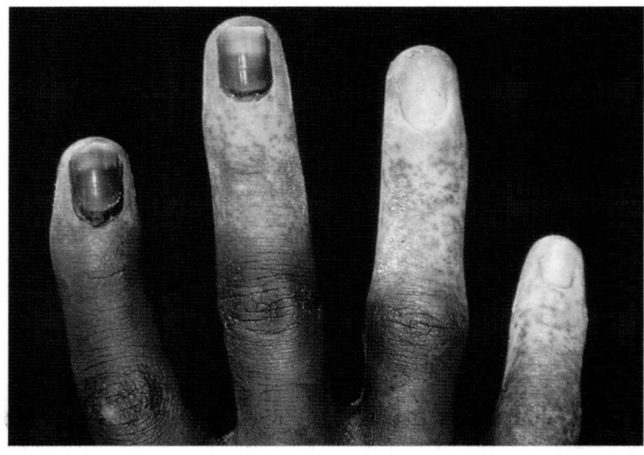

Hand with effects of frostbite. *(SIU/Photo Researchers, Inc.)*

According to U.S. military statistics, African American male soldiers are 4 times as likely and African American female soldiers 2.2 times as likely to suffer frostbite as their Caucasian or Native American counterparts. Pacific Islanders and other ethnic and racial groups from warmer climates are also thought to be more likely to suffer frostbite. British Army findings are similar. In addition to race, certain diseases, including diabetes, thyroid disorders, arthritis, and some infections increase a person's risk of developing frostbite during exposure to cold.

Most frostbite victims are middle-aged adults between the ages of 35 and 50; one study found the average age of patients treated for frostbite is 41.

Description

Frostbite is most likely to affect the face, hands, and feet; however, the shins, knees, and the outer portions of the eyes may also be affected. Freezing of exposed tissues results in the formation of ice crystals inside the cell wall. There is a variation of frostbite known as mountain frostbite, which affects mountain climbers and others exposed to extremely cold temperatures at high altitude. It combines tissue freezing with oxygen deprivation and general body **dehydration**.

Risk factors

Risk factors for frostbite and frostnip include:

- Military service or employment that requires being outdoors for long periods of time in cold weather or cold climates.
- Participation in mountain climbing, alpine skiing, or other winter sports.
- Homelessness.
- Alcohol or substance abuse.
- Mental illness.
- Previous exposure to frostbite or cold injury.
- Smoking. Nicotine causes blood vessels to constrict, thus lowering the body's ability to circulate blood to the hands, feet, and face.
- Malnutrition.
- Underlying infection.
- Medical conditions that affect a person's ability to feel or respond to cold, including dehydration, exhaustion, diabetes, or circulatory disorders.

Causes and symptoms

Causes

Frostbite is caused by exposure of skin and underlying tissues to extreme cold, usually environmental. When the skin is exposed to temperatures at or below 32°F (0°C), the blood vessels in the skin start to constrict. This closing down of the blood flow in the extremities is the body's protective strategy for preserving normal body temperature in the body core (the heart and other internal organs).

Skin exposed to temperatures a little below the freezing mark can take hours to freeze, but very cold skin can freeze in minutes or seconds. Air temperature, wind speed, and moisture all affect how cold the skin becomes. A strong wind can lower skin temperature considerably by dispersing the thin protective layer of warm air that surrounds our bodies. Wet clothing readily draws heat away from the skin because water is a potent conductor of heat. The evaporation of moisture on the skin also produces cooling. For these reasons, wet skin or clothing on a windy day can lead to frostbite even if the air temperature is above the freezing mark.

Three nearly simultaneous physiological processes underlie frostbite injury: tissue freezing, tissue **hypoxia**, and the release of inflammatory mediators. Tissue freezing causes ice crystal formation and other changes that damage and eventually kill cells. Much of this harm occurs because the ice produces pressure changes that cause water (crucial for cell survival) to flow out of the cells. Tissue hypoxia (oxygen deficiency) occurs when the blood vessels in the hands, feet, and other extremities narrow in response to cold. Among its many tasks, blood transfers body heat to the skin, which then dissipates the heat into the environment. Blood vessel narrowing is the body's way of protecting vital internal organs at the expense of the extremities by reducing heat flow away from the core. However, blood also carries life-sustaining oxygen to the skin and other tissues, and narrowed vessels result in oxygen starvation. Narrowing also causes acidosis (an increase in tissue acidity) and increases blood viscosity (thickness). Ultimately, blood stops flowing through the capillaries (the tiny blood vessels that connect the arteries and veins) and blood clots form in the arterioles and venules (the smallest arteries and veins). Damage also occurs to the endothelial cells that line the blood vessels. Hypoxia, blood clots, and endothelial damage lead, in turn, to the release of inflammatory mediators (substances that act as links in the inflammatory process), which promote further endothelial damage, hypoxia, and cell destruction.

Symptoms

The early stage of frostbite is sometimes called frostnip. Short-term symptoms include loss of feeling or aching **pain** in the affected part, followed by redness of the skin and tissue swelling. Unfortunately, a victim is

KEY TERMS

Amputation—Surgical removal of a limb.

Debridement—The medical term for the surgical removal of dead or damaged soft tissue.

Dermis—The layer of skin just below the epidermis.

Epidermis—The outermost layer of the skin.

Gangrene—Decay and death of soft tissue due to loss of blood supply.

Hypoxia—The medical term for deprivation of an adequate oxygen supply, either to specific tissues or to the entire organism.

often unaware of frostbite until someone else points it out because the frozen tissues are numb. Long-term symptoms include intense pain in the affected part, **tingling** sensations, cracks in the skin, dry skin, loss of fingernails, joint stiffness, loss of bone or muscle tissue, and increased sensitivity to cold. If left untreated, frostbitten skin gradually darkens and blisters after a few hours. Skin destroyed by frostbite is completely black, looks burnt, and may hang loosely from the underlying tissues.

Diagnosis

Diagnosis of frostbite is usually made in the field on the basis of the appearance of the frostbitten parts of the body. Some doctors use a four-degree classification of injuries:

- First-degree: The epidermis (outermost layer of the skin) is reddened, swollen, and may look waxy. There is also a loss of sensation in the affected skin.
- Second-degree: The skin is reddened, swollen, and has formed blisters filled with a clear or milky fluid.
- Third-degree: The blisters are filled with blood and the skin begins to turn black.
- Fourth-degree: The epidermis, dermis, and underlying muscles, tendons, and bones are damaged.

Examination

Examination of the patient usually has to be done at the scene rather than in a doctor's office, although it can also be conducted in an ambulance, helicopter, or other emergency medical transport. The doctor will examine the condition of the affected parts, including skin color, the presence of blisters, and other features. If the patient has also been injured in an accident, the doctor will also evaluate the patient for **sprains**, broken bones, and internal injuries.

Tests

A technique that can be used to diagnose the extent of soft-tissue injury after frostbite is technetium scintigraphy. This is a technique in which radioactive technetium is administered intravenously. The radioactive element is taken up differently by healthy and damaged tissue, and the pattern of "hot spots" and "cold spots" as traced by a scanner allows the doctor to tell whether and where deep tissues have been damaged by frostbite. Scintigraphy can also be used to monitor the recovery of the injured tissues following emergency treatment.

X rays and other imaging studies will not help in diagnosing frostbite but may be used to evaluate the injured person for broken or fractured bones.

Treatment

Traditional

FROSTBITE Emergency medical help should always be summoned whenever frostbite is suspected. While waiting for help to arrive, one should, if possible, remove wet or tight clothing and put on dry, loose clothing or wraps. A splint and padding are used to protect the injured area. The patient should not be allowed to walk on frostbitten toes or feet, as the weight of the body will cause further damage to tissue—unless walking is the only way the patient can get to shelter.

Rubbing the area with snow or anything else is dangerous. The key to prehospital treatment is to avoid partial thawing and refreezing, which releases more inflammatory mediators and makes the injury substantially worse. For this reason, the affected part must be kept away from such heat sources as campfires and car heaters. In addition, the injured person should not be given alcohol or tranquilizers, as these will increase loss of body heat. Experts advise rewarming in the field only when emergency help will take more than two hours to arrive and refreezing can be prevented.

Because the outcome of a frostbite injury cannot be predicted at first, all hospital treatment follows the same route. Treatment begins by rewarming the affected part for 15–30 minutes in water at a temperature of 104–108 °F (40–42.2 °C). This rapid rewarming halts ice crystal formation and dilates narrowed blood vessels. Aloe vera (which acts against inflammatory mediators) is applied to the affected part, which is then splinted, elevated, and wrapped in a dressing. Depending on the extent of injury, blisters may be debrided (cleaned by removing foreign material) or simply covered with aloe vera. Except when injury is minimal, treatment generally requires a hospital stay of several days, during which hydrotherapy and physical therapy are used to restore the affected part to health. Experts recommend a cautious approach to tissue removal, and advise that 22–45 days must pass before a decision on amputation can safely be made.

If frostbitten skin is not treated and its blood vessels are affected, gangrene may set in. Gangrene is the death of soft tissue due to loss of blood supply. It may be treated by surgical removal of the affected tissue if caught early; otherwise, the surgeon may have to amputate the affected digit or limb to prevent bacterial infections from spreading from the dead tissue to the rest of the body.

FROSTNIP Frostnipped fingers are helped by blowing warm air on them or holding them under one's armpits. Other frostnipped areas can be covered with warm hands. The injured areas should never be rubbed.

Drugs

The goals of medical therapy for frostbite are pain control and prevention of such complications as further tissue damage or infection. Patients being treated in the hospital for severe frostbite may be given morphine for **pain management** as **narcotics** are needed in most cases to reduce the excruciating pain that occurs as sensation returns during rewarming. A **tetanus** shot and penicillin G are used to prevent infection, and the patient is given ibuprofen or another NSAID to combat inflammation.

Alternative

Alternative practitioners suggest several kinds of treatment to speed recovery from frostbite after leaving the hospital. Bathing the affected part in warm water or using contrast hydrotherapy can help enhance circulation. Contrast hydrotherapy involves a series of hot and cold water applications. A hot compress (as hot as the patient can stand) is applied to the affected area for three minutes followed by an ice cold compress for 30 seconds. These applications are repeated three times each, ending with the cold compress. Nutritional therapy to promote tissue growth in damaged areas may also be helpful.

Homeopathic and botanical therapies may also assist recovery from frostbite. Homeopathic *Hypericum* (*Hypericum perforatum*) is recommended when nerve ending are affected (especially in the fingers and toes) and *Arnica* (*Arnica montana*) is prescribed for shock. Cayenne pepper (*Capsicum frutescens*) can enhance circulation and relieve pain. Drinking hot ginger (*Zingiber officinale*) tea also aids circulation. Other possible approaches include acupuncture to avoid permanent nerve damage and oxygen therapy.

Prognosis

Patients with early recovery of sensation in the affected part, blisters filled with clear fluid, and healthy-appearing skin color have a better prognosis for full recovery than those whose skin has turned bluish, has blood-filled blisters, and looks frozen.

People who have recovered from frostbite have an increased risk of another episode during future exposures to cold. They should take extra precautions to dress properly for extreme cold or avoid it altogether. They may also notice that the frostbitten parts of their body are more sensitive to ordinary cold weather, and ache or tingle whenever they are outdoors.

The extreme throbbing pain that many frostbite sufferers endure for days or weeks after rewarming is not the only prolonged symptom of frostbite. Other possible consequences of frostbite include skin—color changes, nail deformation or loss, joint stiffness and pain, **hyperhidrosis** (excessive sweating), and heightened sensitivity to cold. For everyone, a degree of sensory loss lasting at least four years—and sometimes a lifetime—is inevitable. About 65 percent of people with severe frostbite will eventually develop arthritis in the affected hand, foot, or leg.

Prevention

With the appropriate knowledge and precautions, frostbite can be prevented even in the coldest and most challenging environments. Appropriate clothing and footwear are essential. To prevent heat loss and keep the blood circulating properly, clothing should be worn loosely and in layers. Covering the hands, feet, and head is also crucial for preventing heat loss; mittens are better than gloves for keeping hands warm. Outerwear should be wind- and water-resistant; and wet clothing and footwear must be replaced as quickly as possible. People should also be aware of the early warning signs of frostbite, which include redness of the skin, prickling sensations, and **numbness**.

Alcohol and drugs should be avoided because of their harmful effects on judgment and reasoning. Experts also warn against alcohol use and **smoking** in the cold because of the circulatory changes they produce. Paying close attention to the weather report before venturing outdoors and avoiding such unnecessary risks as driving in isolated areas during a blizzard are also important precautionary measures. In addition, when traveling in cold weather, people should carry emergency supplies and warm clothing in case they become stranded. Last, people who are hiking or skiing in cold temperatures should use a buddy system in case one person is injured and must be evacuated quickly.

Resources

BOOKS

Auerbach, Paul S., Howard J. Donner, and Eric A. Weiss. *Field Guide to Wilderness Medicine*, 3rd ed. Philadelphia: Mosby/Elsevier, 2008.

Forgey, William W., ed. *Wilderness Medical Society Practice Guidelines for Wilderness Emergency Care*, 5th ed. Guilford, CT: Falcon Guide, 2006.

Giesbrecht, Gordon G. *Hypothermia, Frostbite, and Other Cold Injuries: Prevention, Survival, Rescue and Treatment*, 2nd ed. Seattle, WA: Mountaineers Books, 2006.

PERIODICALS

Bruen, K.G., and W.F. Gowski. "Treatment of Digital Frostbite: Current Concepts." *Journal of Hand Surgery* 34 (March 2009): 553–54.

Burgess, J.E., and F, Macfarlane. "Retrospective Analysis of the Ethnic Origins of Male British Army Soldiers with Peripheral Cold Weather Injury." *Journal of the Royal Army Medical Corps* 155 (March 2009): 11–15.

Imray, C., et al. "Cold Damage to the Extremities: Frostbite and Non-freezing Cold Injuries." *Postgraduate Medical Journal* 85 (September 2009): 481–88.

Mohr, W.J., et al. "Cold Injury." *Hand Clinics* 25 (November 2009): 481–96.

Rehman, H., and A. Seguin. "Images in Clinical Medicine: Frostbite." *New England Journal of Medicine* 361 (December 17, 2009): 2461.

Schlagenhauf, P., et al. "Sex and Gender Differences in Travel-associated Disease." *Clinical Infectious Diseases* 50 (March 15, 2010): 826–32.

Sheridan, R.L., et al. "Case Records of the Massachusetts General Hospital: Case 41-2009. A 16-year-old Boy with Hypothermia and Frostbite." *New England Journal of Medicine* 362 (December 31, 2009): 2654–2662.

OTHER

Centers for Disease Control and Prevention (CDC). *Winter Weather: Frostbite*, http://emergency.cdc.gov/disasters/winter/staysafe/frostbite.asp.

Mayo Clinic. *Frostbite*, http://www.mayoclinic.com/health/frostbite/DS01164.

Mechem, C. Crawford. "Frostbite." *eMedicine*, February 5, 2010, http://emedicine.medscape.com/article/770296-overview.

MedlinePlus Medical Encyclopedia. *Frostbite*, http://www.nlm.nih.gov/medlineplus/ency/article/000057.htm.

ORGANIZATIONS

American College of Emergency Physicians (ACEP), 1125 Executive Circle, Irving TX, 75038-2522, 972-550-0911, 800-798-1822, 972-580-2816, http://www.acep.org/.

Centers for Disease Control and Prevention (CDC), 1600 Clifton Road, Atlanta GA, 30333, 800-232-4636, cdcinfo@cdc.gov, http://www.cdc.gov.

Wilderness Medical Society (WMS), 2150 S 1300 E, Suite 500, Salt Lake City UT, 84106, 801-990-2988, 801-990-2987, wms@wms.org, http://www.wms.org/.

International Society of Travel Medicine (ISTM), 2386 Clower Street, Suite A-102, Snellvile GA, United States, 30078, +1 770 736 060, +1-770 736 0313, istm@istm.org, https://www.istm.org/.

Howard Baker
Rebecca J. Frey, PhD

Frostig developmental test of visual perception

Definition

The Frostig Developmental Test of Visual Perception is a widely used **assessment** of visual perception skills and eye-hand coordination in children aged four through ten. It is sometimes called the Marianne Frostig Developmental Test of Visual Perception and is abbreviated DTVP or FDTVP.

Purpose

The DTVP is commonly used to diagnose possible learning disabilities or neurological disorders in prekindergarten through third-grade children. Children are usually referred for testing by a **special education** teacher, occupational therapist, or psychologist. The DTVP estimates overall visual perception ability and identifies specific visual perception problems that require training. The DTVP is usually one component of a battery of assessments for evaluating the development of visual-perceptual skills. The DTVP has also been widely used in research studies. Over the years, the DTVP has been administered to more than six million children.

The second edition of the Developmental Test of Visual Perception (DTVP-2) is a more comprehensive battery than the original DTVP. It includes additional tests for specific visual perception problems and is used to document both the existence of difficulties with visual perception and/or visual-motor development and the degree of the problem in individual children. Thus, the DTVP-2 may be significantly more useful than the original DTVP for diagnosing specific deficits. The DTVP-2 is used:

- to identify children who are candidates for referrals for special services
- to assess the effectiveness of school intervention programs
- as a research tool

Description

Marianne Frostig first developed the DTVP in the late 1950s for use with children aged four through eight. She guided it through several editions and revisions. The DTVP consists of five subtests for measuring visual acuity or clarity of vision. These subtests have been thought to measure five distinct visual-perceptual skills:

- eye-motor or eye-hand coordination, as assessed by the ability to draw continuous straight lines and curved and angular shapes
- constancy of shape—the ability to distinguish common geometric shapes
- position in space—the ability to identify reversed positions
- spatial relationships, as in the ability to connect dots to form shapes and patterns
- figure-ground—exemplified by the ability to distinguish between foreground and background shapes in an image and to detect embedded figures

The five subtests of the DTVP consist of 41 tasks, arranged on demonstration cards in the order of increasing difficulty. The DTVP can be administered to individual children or to groups of children in 30–45 minutes. Versions of the DTVP have been adapted for testing hearing-impaired and non-English-speaking children.

The DTVP-2 was developed by Donald D. Hammill, Nils A. Pearson, and Judith K. Voress in 1993, to incorporate advances in theories of visual-perceptual development and to add more visual-motor integration skills to the DTVP. Visual perception and visual-motor integration are considered to be distinct but interrelated abilities. The DTVP-2 consists of eight subtests:

- eye-hand coordination
- form constancy
- position in space
- spatial relations
- figure-ground
- copying
- visual closure
- visual-motor speed

The DTVP-2 is appropriate for children aged four through ten years. It requires 30–60 minutes to administer. Young children may need more than one session to complete the DTVP-2. The complete DTVP-2 kit includes:

- examiner's manual
- picture book
- 25 profile/examiner record forms
- 25 response booklets
- storage box

Origins

Marianne Frostig (1906–1985) was born in Vienna, Austria, where she trained as a social worker and gymnastics and eurhythmics teacher. After emigrating to the United States in 1939, Frostig earned a Master's degree from Claremont College and a doctorate in education psychology from the University of Southern California.

Frostig founded the internationally recognized Frostig School, at the Marianne Frostig Center of Educational Therapy in Los Angeles, in 1951. It was one of the very few programs specifically designed to serve children with learning disabilities who do not also have serious emotional disturbances. The Frostig School, now located in Pasadena, California, continues to offer a full range of academic and support services for first- through twelfth-grade students.

Along with her colleagues at the Frostig Center, Marianne Frostig developed an individualized, holistic approach to teaching children with specific learning disabilities. This program became known as the Frostig Approach. In addition to the DTVP, she developed the Frostig Movement Skills Test Battery. She also developed a movement education program called the MGL—Move-Grow-Learn—and the Developmental Program in Visual Perception for improving visual-perceptual skills. Although Frostig retired as director of the Center in 1972, she continued to teach, publish, and lecture on the education of learning-disabled children until her **death**. In 1986, her colleagues in Germany founded the International Frostig Society, dedicated to teacher training.

Results

Raw scores are obtained for each subtest of the DTVP. These are converted to age equivalents, called perceptual age (PA), and to scale scores (SS). The scaled scores of the subtests are combined for a total test score, which is expressed as a perceptual quotient (PQ)—the total scaled score divided by the child's age—and as a

KEY TERMS

Age equivalent—A decimal number that indicates the age of a typical child who earns a given score on a standardized test.

Figure-ground—The cognitive ability to separate elements in an image based upon contrast, such as foreground and background, or dark and light.

Learning disability—Any of various disorders that interfere with a child's ability to learn, resulting in problems with verbal language, reasoning, and academic skills; believed to be caused by deficits in processing and integrating information.

Norm—A standard of achievement, usually derived from the average or median achievement of a large representative group of a particular age.

Percentile—A rank in a population that has been divided into 100 equal groups; thus, test results in the 50th percentile indicate that half of those who took the test scored higher and half scored lower.

Perceptual quotient (PQ)—A measure of perceptual level relative to age; the perceptual developmental age divided by chronological age.

Reliability—The extent to which a test or measure yields the same results with repeated trials.

Standardized—A test with established procedures and norms that serve as the standard for future test results.

Validity—The extent to which a test measures the trait that it is designed to assess.

Visual acuity (VA)—Clarity or acuteness of vision, which depends on the sharpness of the retinal focus within the eye and on the brain's interpretive abilities.

Visual-motor integration (VMI)—Eye-hand coordination, such as the ability to accurately perceive and reproduce designs.

Visual-perceptual skills—The ability of the mind and the eye to perceive something as it objectively exists.

percentile rank. Guidelines are supplied for the score levels that are considered to indicate readiness for the first grade. The DTVP provides scores both for pure visual perception on items that do not involve any motor response and for visual-motor integration ability.

Test-retest reliability of the original DTVP at two–three-week intervals was not particularly high. The figure-ground subtest had the highest reliability and the position-in-space subtest had the lowest. However the reliability of the DTVP-2 is significantly higher than the original DTVP for all age groups. Correlations between scores on the original DTVP and teacher ratings of a child's classroom adjustment, motor coordination, and intellectual functioning were also not particularly high. However the DTVP-2 is considered to have higher validity.

The original DTVP was standardized with norms from a population of 2,116 schoolchildren with normal abilities between the ages of three and nine. This sample population was from a relatively small geographic area and was 93% middle class. There were very few children from low socioeconomic groups, very few Hispanics and Asians, and no black children in the population. In contrast, the DTVP-2 was standardized with 1,972 children from 12 states. It has been shown to be unbiased with regard to gender, race, and **handedness**.

Parental concerns

Although the DTVP can be an effective tool for identifying possible learning disabilities, it is not a definitive diagnostic indicator and the validity of the DTVP for diagnostic purposes has been questioned. For example, visual perception difficulties do not necessarily lead to problems with **learning to read**. The ability of the DTVP to assess specific areas of visual perception has also been called into question. Some researchers have further argued that there is only a single perceptual factor, rather than independent factors represented by the subtests of the DTVP. Finally, high scores on the DTVP do not rule out the existence of learning disabilities. For these reasons, the DTVP should be used only as one component of a battery of assessment tests.

Resources

BOOKS

Frostig, Marianne. *Marianne Frostig Developmental Test of Visual Perception.* Palo Alto, CA: Consulting Psychologists Press, 1961–1966.

Hammill, Donald D., Nils A. Pearson, and Judith K. Voress. *Developmental Test of Visual Perception: DTVP-2.* 2nd ed. Austin, TX: Pro-Ed, 1993.

OTHER

"Frostig—Developmental Test of Visual Perception." Paediatric Assessment Tools, Saetra HEALTH, http://www.saetrahealth.co.za/paediatric_assessment/dtvp.html (accessed September 29, 2010).

"Frostig Developmental Test of Visual Perception." Center for Psychological Studies, Nova Southeastern University, http://www.cps.nova.edu/~cpphelp/FDTVP.html (accessed September 29, 2010).

"Marianne Frostig PhD." Frostig Site, http://www.frostig.com/html/marianne.html (accessed October 1, 2010).

ORGANIZATIONS

American Psychological Association, 750 First St., NE, Washington DC, 20002-4242, (202) 336-5500, (800) 374-2721, http://www.apa.org.

Center for Psychological Studies, Nova Southeastern University, 3301 College Ave., Fort Lauderdale-Davie FL, 33314-7796, (954) 262-5790, (800) 541-6682 x25790, http://www.cps.nova.edu.

Margaret Alic, PhD

Fructose intolerance ***see*** **Hereditary fructose intolerance**

Fugue disorder ***see*** **Dissociative disorders**

Fused fingers and toes ***see*** **Polydactyly and syndactyly**

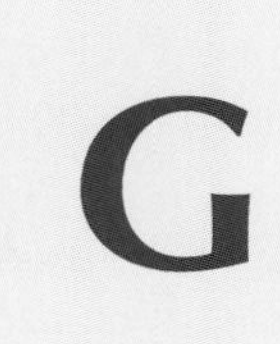

Galactosemia

Definition

Galactosemia is an inherited disease in which the transformation of galactose to glucose is blocked, allowing galactose to increase to toxic levels in the body. If galactosemia is untreated, high levels of galactose cause **vomiting**, **diarrhea**, lethargy, low blood sugar, brain damage, **jaundice**, liver enlargement, cataracts, susceptibility to infection, and **death**.

Galactosemia: Foods and ingredients to avoid

Butter	Milk
Buttermilk	Milk chocolate
Buttermilk solids	Milk derivatives
Calcium caseinate	Milk solids
Casein	MSG (monosodium glutamate)****
Cheese	Nonfat milk
Cream	Nonfat dry milk
Dough conditioners*	Nonfat dry milk solids
Dried cheese	Organ meats (liver, heart, kidney, brains, sweetbreads, pancreas)
Dry milk	Sodium caseinate
Dry milk protein	Soy sauce*****
Hydrolyzed protein**	Sour cream
Lactalbumin	Tragacanth gum
Lactose	Whey and whey solids
Lactostearin	Yogurt
Margarine***	

Note: Lactate, lactic acid and lactylate do not contain lactose and are acceptable ingredients.
*Dough conditioners may include caseinates; most labels specify the name of the conditioner that is added to the product.
**Hydrolyzed protein is unacceptable to eat and is commonly found in canned meats, like tuna. Hydrolyzed vegetable protein, however, is acceptable.
***A few diet margarines do not contain milk; check labels before using any brand. If "margarine" is listed as an ingredient in any processed food, consider the product unacceptable.
****MSG or monosodium glutamate itself is acceptable; however, some MSGs contain lactose extenders, so it is best to avoid MSG whenever possible.
*****Soy sauce is unacceptable if it is fermented.

SOURCE: Parents of Galactosemic Children, Inc. (PGC), "Unacceptable Ingredients List." Available online at: http://www.galactosemia.org (accessed September 28, 2010).

(Table by PreMediaGlobal. Reproduced by permission of Gale, a part of Cengage Learning.)

Description

Galactosemia is a rare but potentially life-threatening disease that results from the inability to metabolize galactose. Serious consequences from galactosemia can be prevented by screening newborns at **birth** with a simple blood test.

Galactosemia is an inborn error of metabolism. "Metabolism" refers to all chemical reactions that take place in living organisms. A metabolic pathway is a series of reactions where the product of each step in the series is the starting material for the next step. Enzymes are the chemicals that help the reactions occur. Their ability to function depends on their structure, and their structure is determined by the deoxyribonucleic acid (DNA) sequence of the genes that encode them. Inborn errors of metabolism are caused by mutations in these genes which do not allow the enzymes to function properly.

Sugars are sometimes called "the energy molecules," and galactose and glucose are both sugars. For galactose to be utilized for energy, it must be transformed into something that can enter the metabolic pathway that converts glucose into energy (plus water and carbon dioxide). This is important for infants because they typically get most of their nutrient energy from milk, which contains a high level of galactose. Each molecule of lactose, the major sugar constituent of milk, is made up of a molecule of galactose and a molecule of glucose, and galactose makes up 20% of the energy source of a typical infant's diet.

Three enzymes are required to convert galactose into glucose-1-phosphate (a phosphorylated glucose that can enter the metabolic pathway that turns glucose into energy). Each of these three enzymes is encoded by a separate gene. If any of these enzymes fail to function, galactose build-up and galactosemia result. Thus, there are three types of galactosemia with a different gene responsible for each.

Every cell in a person's body has two copies of each gene. Each of the forms of galactosemia is inherited as a recessive trait, which means that galactosemia is only present in individuals with two mutated copies of one of the three genes. This also means that carriers, with only one copy of a gene mutation, will not be aware that they are carrying a mutation (unless they have had a genetic test), as it is masked by the normal gene they also carry and they have no symptoms of the disease. For each step in the conversion of galactose to glucose, if only one of the two copies of the gene controlling that step is normal (i.e., for carriers), enough functional enzyme is made so that the pathway is not blocked at that step. If a person has galactosemia, both copies of the gene coding for one of the enzymes required to convert glucose to galactose are defective and the pathway becomes blocked. If two carriers of the same defective gene have children, the chance of any of their children getting galactosemia (the chance of a child getting two copies of the defective gene) is 25% (one in four) for each pregnancy.

Classic galactosemia occurs in the United States about one in every 50,000–70,000 live births.

Causes and symptoms

Galactosemia I

Galactosemia I (also called classic galactosemia), the first form to be discovered, is caused by defects in both copies of the gene that codes for an enzyme called galactose-1-phosphate uridyl transferase (GALT). There are 30 known different mutations in this gene that cause GALT to malfunction.

Newborns with galactosemia I appear normal at birth, but begin to develop symptoms after they are given milk for the first time. Symptoms include vomiting, diarrhea, lethargy (sluggishness or fatigue), low blood glucose, jaundice (a yellowing of the skin and eyes), enlarged liver, protein and amino acids in the urine, and susceptibility to infection, especially from gram negative bacteria. Cataracts (a grayish-white film on the eye lens) can appear within a few days after birth. People with galactosemia frequently have symptoms as they grow older even though they have been given a galactose-free diet. These symptoms include **speech disorders**, cataracts, ovarian atrophy and infertility in females, learning disabilities, and behavioral problems.

Galactosemia II

Galactosemia II is caused by defects in both copies of the gene that codes for an enzyme called galactokinase (GALK). The frequency of occurrence of galactosemia II is about one in 100,000–155,000 births.

Galactosemia II is less harmful than galactosemia I. Babies born with galactosemia II will develop cataracts at an early age unless they are given a galactose-free diet. They do not generally suffer from liver damage or neurologic disturbances.

Galactosemia III

Galactosemia III is caused by defects in the gene that codes for an enzyme called uridyl diphosphogalactose-4-epimerase (GALE). This form of galactosemia is very rare.

There are two forms of galactosemia III, a severe form, which is exceedingly rare, and a benign form. The benign form has no symptoms and requires no special diet. However, newborns with galactosemia III, including the benign form, have high levels of galactose-1-phosphate that show up on the initial screenings for elevated galactose and galactose-1-phosphate. This situation illustrates one aspect of the importance of follow-up enzyme function tests. Tests showing normal levels of GALT and GALK allow people affected by the benign form of galactosemia III to enjoy a normal diet.

The severe form has symptoms similar to those of galactosemia I, but with more severe neurological problems, including seizures. Only two cases of this rare form have been reported as of 1997.

Diagnosis

The **newborn screening** test for classic galactosemia is quick and straightforward; all but three states require testing on all newborns. Blood from a baby who is two to three days old is usually first screened for high levels of galactose and galactose-1-phosphate. If either of these compounds is elevated, further tests are performed to find out which enzymes (GALT, GALK, or GALE) are present or missing. DNA testing may also be performed to confirm the diagnosis.

If there is a strong suspicion that a baby has galactosemia, galactose is removed from the diet right away. In this case, an initial screen for galactose or galactose-1-phosphate will be meaningless. In the absence of galactose in the diet, this test will be negative whether or not the baby has galactosemia. In this case, tests to measure enzyme levels must be given to find out if the suspected baby is indeed galactosemic.

In addition, galactosemic babies who are refusing milk or vomiting will not have elevated levels of galactose or galactose phosphate, and their condition will not be detected by the initial screen. Any baby with symptoms of galactosemia (for example, vomiting) should be given enzyme tests.

Treatment

Galactosemia I and II are treated by removing galactose from the diet. Since galactose is a break-down product of lactose, the primary sugar constituent of milk, this means all milk and foods containing milk products must be totally eliminated. Other foods like legumes, organ meats, and processed meats also contain considerable galactose and must be avoided. Pills that use lactose as a filler must also be avoided. Soy-based and casein hydrolysate-based formulas are recommended for infants with galactosemia.

Treatment of the severe form of galactosemia III with a galactose-restricted diet has been tried, but this disorder is so rare that the long-term effects of this treatment are unknown.

Prognosis

Early detection in the newborn period is the key to controlling symptoms. Long-term effects in untreated babies include severe **mental retardation**, cirrhosis of the liver, and death. About 75% of the untreated babies die within the first two weeks of life. On the other hand, with treatment, a significant proportion of people with galactosemia I can lead nearly normal lives, although speech defects, learning disabilities, and behavioral problems are common. A 2004 study revealed that children and adolescents with classic galactosemia often have lower quality of life than peers without the disease, exhibiting problems with cognition (thinking and intellectual skills) and social function. In addition, cataracts due to galactosemia II can be completely prevented by a galactose-free diet.

Prevention

Since galactosemia is a recessive genetic disease, the disease is usually detected on a newborn screening test, since most people are unaware that they are carriers of a gene mutation causing the disease. For couples with a previous child with galactosemia, prenatal diagnosis is available to determine whether a pregnancy is similarly affected. Families in which a child has been diagnosed with galactosemia can have DNA testing that can enable other more distant relatives to determine their carrier status. Prospective parents can then use that information to conduct family planning or to prepare for a child with special circumstances. Children born with galactosemia should be put on a special diet right away to reduce the symptoms and complications of the disease.

KEY TERMS

Casein hydrolysate—A preparation made from the milk protein casein, which is hydrolyzed to break it down into its constituent amino acids. Amino acids are the building blocks of proteins.

Catalyst—A substance that changes the rate of a chemical reaction, but is not physically changed by the process.

Enzyme—A protein that catalyzes a biochemical reaction or change without changing its own structure or function.

Galactose—One of the two simple sugars, together with glucose, that makes up the protein, lactose, found in milk. Galactose can be toxic in high levels.

Glucose—One of the two simple sugars, together with galactose, that makes up the protein, lactose, found in milk. Glucose is the form of sugar that is usable by the body to generate energy.

Lactose—A sugar made up of of glucose and galactose. It is the primary sugar in milk.

Metabolic pathway—A sequence of chemical reactions that lead from some precursor to a product, where the product of each step in the series is the starting material for the next step.

Metabolism—The total combination of all of the chemical processes that occur within cells and tissues of a living body.

Recessive trait—An inherited trait or characteristic that is outwardly obvious only when two copies of the gene for that trait are present.

Resources

PERIODICALS

Bosch, Annet M., et al. "Living With Classical Galactosmeia: Health-related Quality of Life Consequences." *Pediatrics* May 2004: 1385–1387.

OTHER

"GeneCards: Human Genes, Proteins and Diseases." http://bioinfo.weizmann.ac.il/cards/.

"Vermont Newborn Screening Program: Galactosemia." http://www.vtmednet.org/~m145037/vhgi_mem/nbsman/galacto.htm.

ORGANIZATIONS

Association for Neuro-Metabolic Disorders, 5223 Brookfield Lane, Sylvania, OH, 43560, (419) 885-1497.

Metabolic Information Network, PO Box 670847, Dallas, TX, 75367-0847, (214) 696-2188, (800) 945-2188.

Parents of Galactosemic Children, Inc., 2148 Bryton Dr., Powell, OH, 43065, http://www.galactosemia.org/index.htm.

Amy Vance, MS, CGC
Teresa G. Odle

Gangs

Definition

A gang is group of people recognized as a distinct entity and involved in antisocial, rebellious, or illegal activities.

Demographics

In 2008, the United States Department of Justice estimated that there were 27,900 gangs and about 774,000 gang members in the United States. From the mid-1990s to 2001, there was a decrease in gang activity. This has been followed by a slow increase through the 2000s. The National Gang Youth Survey, completed by the United States Department of Justice, found that in 2008, about 32% of the jurisdictions they surveyed had a gang problem. This compares to 40% of jurisdictions in 1996, but is a increase of 15% since 2001.

The gang problem is most prevalent in large cities, with 86% of large cities reporting gang activity in 2007. Fifty percent of suburban counties reported gang activity, followed by 35% of small cities and 15% of rural counties. However, the greatest increase in gang activity between 2002 and 2007 occurred in suburban counties, which reported a 33% increase during this time period.

The rate of gang membership varies by ethnicity and location, with most large city gangs composed of Hispanic/Latino or African-American youths, while many rural gangs are largely made up of white youths. Asian gangs have established themselves in certain East and West Coast cities.

Description

A youth gang is a group of young people whose members recognize themselves as a distinct entity and are recognized as such by their community. Their involvement in antisocial, rebellious, and illegal activities draws a negative response from the community and from law enforcement officials. Other characteristics of gangs include:

- a recognized leader
- formal membership with initiation requirements and rules for its members
- its own territory, or turf
- standard clothing or tattoos
- private slang and hand signals
- a group name

The United States Department of Justice has divided gangs into several types. Territorial ("turf" or "hood") gangs are concerned with controlling a specific geographical area. Organized, or corporate, gangs are mainly involved in illegal activities, such as drug dealing. Scavenger gangs are more loosely organized than the other two types and are identified primarily by common group behavior.

Today's gangs are more involved in serious criminal activities than their predecessors. Gang-related violence, especially violence involving firearms, has risen and tends to involve younger perpetrators who are increasingly ready to use deadly force to perpetuate rivalries or carry out drug activities. In addition, the scope of gang activities has increased, often involving links to drug suppliers or customers in distant locations.

Youth gangs are found among virtually all ethnic groups. Mexican-American gangs, whose members are sometimes referred to as *cholos*, have long been active in the Southwest and are now spreading to other parts of the country. Today Hispanic/Latino gangs include not only the traditional Mexican-American groups but also gangs of immigrants from Central American countries, such as El Salvador. The most visible Hispanic gangs on the East Coast have traditionally been the Puerto Rican gangs in New York City, originally formed by the children of immigrants who came to this country in the 1940s and 1950s. African-American gang affiliations often center on the Crips and Bloods, Los Angeles gangs that are bitter rivals, or the Vice Lords and Folk Nation, which are Chicago gangs. Chinese gangs, which began in New York in the 1960s and 1970s, prey on the Asian community, extorting money in return for protection. With the wave of immigration from Southeast Asia following the Vietnam War, Vietnamese and Cambodian gangs have formed, also terrorizing their own communities.

The most visible white gangs are the skinheads (named for their close-shaven heads), who typically embrace a racist, anti-Semitic, and anti-gay philosophy, often involving neo-Nazi symbolism and beliefs. There are thought to be between 3,000 and 4,000 skinheads in the United States, including such groups as the Aryan Youth Movement, Blitz Krieg, and White Power.

Skinhead activities have included painting racial slurs on buildings, damaging synagogues and the homes of Jews and blacks, and sometimes fatal assaults on members of minority groups.

Possible signs indicating that a teenager has joined a gang include lower grades and disciplinary problems in school; nervous, hostile, or uncommunicative behavior at home; new friends who are not introduced to the **family**; reduced amounts of time spent at home; unexplained possession of money; and possession of a weapon.

Causes

A variety of factors have been cited as causes for teen involvement in gangs. Social problems associated with gang activity include poverty, racism, high unemployment rates, and the disintegration of the nuclear family. Some critics claim that gangs are glamorized in the media and by the entertainment industry. On a personal level, adolescents whose families are not meeting their emotional needs turn to gangs as substitute families where they can find acceptance, intimacy, and approval. Gangs can also provide the sense of identity that young people crave as they confront the dislocations of **adolescence**.

Some youths join gangs because of social pressure from friends. Others feel physically unsafe in their neighborhoods if they do not join a gang. For some youths, the connection to a gang is through family members who belong—sometimes even several generations of a single family. Yet another incentive for joining is money from the gangs' lucrative drug trade. Drug profits can be so exorbitant as to dwarf the income from any legitimate job.

Gang structure

The basic unit in gangs, whatever their origin or larger structure, is a clique of members who are about the same age; these groups are also called posses or sets. A gang may consist entirely of such a clique, or it may be allied with similar groups as part of a larger gang. The Crips and Bloods, for example, consist of many sets, with names such as the Playboy Gangster Crips, the Bounty Hunters, and the Piru Bloods. It is to their clique or set that members feel the greatest loyalty. These neighborhood groups have leaders, who may command as many as 200 followers. In groups affiliated with larger gangs, these local leaders are accountable to chiefs higher up in the gang hierarchy. At the top is the kingpin, generally an adult, who has the ultimate say on how the gang conducts its financial operations and oversees its members.

The lowest level at which a young person may be associated with a gang is as a lookout—the person who watches for the police during drug deals or other criminal activities. Lookouts, who are commonly between 7 and 12 years old, can be paid as much as $300 a week. At the next level are "wannabes," older children or preteens who identify themselves with a gang although they are still too young for membership. They may wear clothing resembling that of the gang they aspire to join and try to ingratiate themselves with its members. Sometimes they cause trouble in or out of school as a way of drawing the gang's attention. Once wannabes are being considered for entrance into a gang, they undergo some form of initiation. Often it includes the commission of a specified crime as a way of proving themselves suitable for membership. In addition, gangs generally practice certain initiation rituals, such as "walking the line," in which initiates have to pass between two lines of members who beat them. In other cases, initiation brutalities follow a less orderly course, with a succession of gang members randomly perpetrating surprise beatings that initiates have to withstand without attempting to defend themselves. Other rituals, such as cutting initiates and mixing their blood with that of older members, are also practiced.

Gang identification

Gangs adopt certain dress codes by which members show their unity and make their gang affiliation visible both to members of other gangs and to the community at large. Gang members are usually identifiable by both the style and color of their clothing. The Crips are strongly associated with the color blue, typically wearing blue jackets, running shoes with blue stripes and laces, and blue bandannas, either tied around their heads or hanging prominently from a back pocket. The color of the rival Bloods is red. Two rival African-American gangs in Chicago wear hats tilted in different directions to signal their affiliation. With the increased use of deadly force by today's gang members, gang clothing codes can be very dangerous; nonmembers have been killed for accidentally wandering onto gang turf wearing the colors of a rival group. Many schools have responded by banning certain colors or styles of clothing. In addition to their clothing, gang members express solidarity by adopting street names and using secret symbols and codes, often in graffiti spray painted in public places.

Girls and gangs

Although most gang members are male, young women do join gangs—either mixed-gender or all-female gangs (which are sometimes satellites of male gangs and sometimes independent of them). Traditionally they have played a subservient role in mixed gangs, assisting the males in their activities and forming sexual attachments within the gang. Traditionally, girls engage in less serious criminal activities more serious than shoplifting or fighting girls from other gangs. To be initiated into a mixed-sex gang, female members often are required to have sex with multiple gang members. Today girl gang members are more apt than in the past to participate in serious violence, such as drive-by shootings, armed robbery, and "wildings," savage group attacks on innocent victims in public places, often involving **sexual assault**.

Perhaps the most troubling feature of gang activity in the 2000s is the increased level of firearm violence, which often victimizes not only gang members themselves but also innocent bystanders who unwittingly find themselves in its path. Thousands of young people with no gang connections have been killed because they were in the wrong place at the wrong time. Most gang-related killings are linked to fights over turf (including drug turf), "respect" (perceived threats to a gang member's status), or revenge. As many as 90% of drive-by shootings are thought to be committed by gang members. A major factor that has raised the level of gang violence is easy access to such weapons as automatic rifles, rapid-fire pistols, and submachine guns.

Leaving the gang

A common feature of membership in youth gangs is the difficulty encountered by young people who want to quit. They are virtually always punished in some way, ranging from ritualized beatings (mirroring the initiation ceremony) to murder. Sometimes the member's entire family is terrorized. Many young people—and sometimes even their families—have had to relocate to a different city in order to safely end gang affiliations. In some cities, there are organizations (some staffed by ex-gang members) that help young people who want to leave gangs.

Prevention

Prevention involves many parts of the community, including parents, schools, law enforcement agencies, and social clubs, such as the Boys and Girls Club or the Police Athletic League. Intervention must begin early, as children as young as age seven may be used by gangs as lookouts. Ultimately, prevention involves alleviating the social conditions, such as fractured families, unemployment, poverty, **boredom**, and a sense of hopelessness and aloneness, that make gangs attractive.

KEY TERMS

Wilding—Savage random public beatings or sexual assaults of innocent individuals by a group of young people (usually male) often associated with a gang.

Resources

BOOKS

Hagedorn, John M. *A World of Gangs: Armed Young Men and Gangsta Culture.* Minneapolis: University of Minnesota Press, 2008.

Jackson, Robert K., and Wesley D. McBride. *Understanding Street Gangs.* Incline Village, NV: Copperhouse, 2000.

Klein, Malcolm W. *Street Gang Patterns and Policies.* New York: Oxford University Press, 2006.

OTHER

Egley, Arlen, James C. Howell, and John P. Moore. Highlights of the 2008 National Youth Gang Survey. United States Department of Justice, http://www.ncjrs.gov/pdffiles1/ojjdp/229249.pdf (accessed July 13, 2010).

Gang Reduction Through Intervention, Prevention & Education (GRIPE). East Coast Gang Investigators Association, http://www.gripe4rkids.org/index.html (accessed July 14, 2010).

National Gang Threat Assessment 2009. National Gang Intelligence Center. 2009, http://www.justice.gov/ndic/pubs32/32146/32146p.pdf (accessed July 14, 2010).

"Teen Violence." MedlinePlus. May 17, 2010, http://www.nlm.nih.gov/medlineplus/teenviolence.html (accessed July 11, 2010).

"Violent Gangs." Federal Bureau of Investigation. May 17, 2010, http://www.fbi.gov/hq/cid/ngic/violent_gangs.htm (accessed July 14, 2010).

ORGANIZATIONS

National Gang Center, P. O. Box 12729, Tallahassee, FL, 32317-2729, (850) 385-0600, (850) 422-3529, information@nationalgangcenter.gov, http://www.nationalgangcenter.gov.

Tish Davidson, AM

Gastroenteritis

Definition

Gastroenteritis is a catchall term for infection or irritation of the digestive tract, particularly the stomach and intestine. It is frequently referred to as the stomach or intestinal flu, although the **influenza** virus is not associated with this illness. Major symptoms include nausea and **vomiting**, **diarrhea**, and abdominal cramps. These symptoms are sometimes also accompanied by **fever** and overall weakness. Gastroenteritis typically lasts about three days. Adults usually recover without problem, but children, the elderly, and anyone with an underlying disease are more vulnerable to complications, such as **dehydration**.

Demographics

Gastroenteritis is an uncomfortable and inconvenient ailment, but it is rarely life-threatening in the United States and other developed nations. However, an estimated 220,000 children younger than age five are hospitalized with gastroenteritis symptoms in the United States annually. Of these children, 300 die as a result of severe diarrhea and dehydration. In developing nations, diarrheal illnesses are a major source of mortality. Worldwide, inadequate treatment of gastroenteritis kills 5 to 8 million people per year and is a leading cause of **death** among infants and children under the age of five. Annually, worldwide, rotaviruses are estimated to cause 800,000 deaths in children below age five.

Description

Typically, children are more vulnerable to rotaviruses, the most significant cause of acute watery diarrhea. For this reason, much research has gone into developing a vaccine to protect children from this virus. Adults can be infected with rotaviruses, but these infections typically have minimal or no symptoms. Children are also susceptible to adenoviruses and astroviruses, which are minor causes of childhood gastroenteritis. Adults experience illness from astroviruses as well, but the major causes of adult viral gastroenteritis are the caliciviruses and SRSVs. These viruses also cause illness in children. The SRSVs are a type of calicivirus and include the Norwalk, Southhampton, and Lonsdale viruses. These viruses are the most likely to produce vomiting as a major symptom.

Bacterial gastroenteritis is frequently a result of poor sanitation, the lack of safe drinking water, or contaminated food—conditions common in developing nations. Natural or man-made disasters can make underlying problems in sanitation and food **safety** worse. In developed nations, the modern food production system potentially exposes millions of people to disease-causing bacteria through its intensive production and distribution methods. Common types of bacterial gastroenteritis can be linked to *Salmonella* and *Campylobacter* bacteria; however, *Escherichia coli* 0157 and *Listeria monocytogenes* are creating increased concern in developed nations. Cholera and Shigella remain two diseases of great concern in developing countries, and research to develop long-term vaccines against them is underway.

Causes and symptoms

Gastroenteritis arises from ingestion of viruses, certain bacteria, or parasites. Food that has spoiled may also cause illness. Certain medications and excessive alcohol can irritate the digestive tract to the point of inducing gastroenteritis. Regardless of the cause, the symptoms of gastroenteritis include diarrhea, nausea and vomiting, and abdominal **pain** and cramps. Sufferers may also experience bloating, low fever, and overall tiredness. Typically, the symptoms last only two to three days, but some viruses may last up to a week.

A usual bout of gastroenteritis shouldn't require a visit to the doctor. However, medical treatment is essential if symptoms worsen or if there are complications. Infants, young children, the elderly, and persons with underlying disease require special attention in this regard.

The greatest danger presented by gastroenteritis is dehydration. The loss of fluids through diarrhea and vomiting can upset the body's electrolyte balance, leading to potentially life-threatening problems such as heart beat abnormalities (arrhythmia). The risk of dehydration increases as symptoms are prolonged. Dehydration should be suspected if a dry mouth, increased or excessive thirst, or scanty urination is experienced.

If symptoms do not resolve within a week, an infection or disorder more serious than gastroenteritis may be involved. Symptoms of great concern include a high fever (102° F [38.9°C] or above), blood or mucus in the diarrhea, blood in the vomit, and severe abdominal pain or swelling. These symptoms require prompt medical attention.

Diagnosis

The symptoms of gastroenteritis are usually enough to identify the illness. Unless there is an outbreak affecting several people or complications are encountered in a particular case, identifying the specific cause of the illness is not a priority. However, if identification of the infectious agent is required, a stool sample will be collected and analyzed for the presence of viruses, disease-causing (pathogenic) bacteria, or parasites.

Treatment

Gastroenteritis is a self-limiting illness which will resolve by itself. However, for comfort and convenience, a person may use over-the-counter medications, such as

Pepto-Bismol, to relieve the symptoms. These medications work by altering the ability of the intestine to move or secrete spontaneously, absorbing toxins and water, or altering intestinal microflora. Some over-the-counter medicines use more than one element to treat symptoms.

If over-the-counter medications are ineffective and medical treatment is sought, a doctor may prescribe a more powerful anti-diarrheal drug, such as motofen or lomotil. Should pathogenic bacteria or parasites be identified in the patient's stool sample, medications such as **antibiotics** will be prescribed.

It is important to stay hydrated and nourished during a bout of gastroenteritis. If dehydration is absent, the drinking of generous amounts of nonalcoholic fluids, such as water or juice, is adequate. **Caffeine**, since it increases urine output, should be avoided. The traditional BRAT diet—bananas, rice, applesauce, and toast—is tolerated by the tender gastrointestinal system, but it is not particularly nutritious. Many, but not all, medical researchers recommend a diet that includes complex carbohydrates (e.g., rice, wheat, potatoes, bread, and cereal), lean meats, yogurt, fruit, and vegetables. Milk and other dairy products shouldn't create problems if they are part of the normal diet. Fatty foods or foods with a lot of sugar should be avoided. These recommendations are based on clinical experience and controlled trials, but are not universally accepted.

Minimal to moderate dehydration is treated with oral rehydrating solutions that contain glucose and electrolytes. These solutions are commercially available under names such as Naturalyte, Pedialyte, Infalyte, and Rehydralyte. Oral rehydrating solutions are formulated based on physiological properties. Fluids that are not based on these properties, such as cola, apple juice, broth, and sports beverages, are not recommended to treat dehydration. If vomiting interferes with oral rehydration, small frequent fluid intake may be better tolerated. Should oral rehydration fail or severe dehydration occur, medical treatment in the form of intravenous (IV) therapy is required. IV therapy can be followed with oral rehydration as the patient's condition improves. Once normal hydration is achieved, the patient can return to a regular diet.

Alternative treatment

Symptoms of uncomplicated gastroenteritis can be relieved with adjustments in diet, herbal remedies, and homeopathy. An infusion of meadowsweet (*Filipendula ulmaria*) may be effective in reducing nausea and stomach acidity. Once the worst symptoms are relieved, slippery elm (*Ulmus fulva*) can help calm the digestive tract. Of the homeopathic remedies available, *Arsenicum album*, ipecac, or *Nux vomica* are three said to relieve the symptoms of gastroenteritis.

Probiotics, bacteria that are beneficial to a person's health, are recommended during the recovery phase of gastroenteritis. Specifically, live cultures of *Lactobacillus acidophilus* are said to be effective in soothing the digestive tract and returning the intestinal flora to normal. *L. acidophilus* is found in live-culture yogurt, as well as in capsule or powder form at health food stores. The use of probiotics is found in folk remedies and has some support in the medical literature. Castor oil packs to the abdomen can reduce inflammation and also reduce spasms or discomfort.

KEY TERMS

Dehydration—A condition in which the body lacks the normal level of fluids, potentially impairing normal body functions.

Electrolyte—An ion, or weakly charged element, that conducts reactions and signals in the body. Examples of electrolytes are sodium and potassium ions.

Glucose—A sugar that serves as the body's primary source of fuel.

Influenza—A virus that affects the respiratory system, causing fever, congestion, muscle aches, and headaches.

Intravenous (IV) therapy—Administration of intravenous fluids.

Microflora—The bacterial population in the intestine.

Pathogenic bacteria—Bacteria that produce illness.

Probiotics—Bacteria that are beneficial to a person's health, either through protecting the body against pathogenic bacteria or assisting in recovery from an illness.

Prognosis

Gastroenteritis is usually resolved within two to three days and there are no long-term effects. If dehydration occurs, recovery is extended by a few days.

Prevention

There are few steps that can be taken to avoid gastroenteritis. Ensuring that food is well-cooked and unspoiled can prevent bacterial gastroenteritis, but may not be effective against viral gastroenteritis.

Resources

BOOKS

Craig, S. A., and D. K. Zich. "Gastroenteritis." In: *Rosen's Emergency Medicine: Concepts and Clinical Practice*. 7th ed., edited by J. A. Marx. Chapter 92. Philadelphia, PA: Mosby Elsevier, 2009.

Sodha, S. V., P. M. Griffin, and J. M. Hughes. "Foodborne Disease." In: *Principles and Practice of Infection Diseases*. 7th ed. Chapter 99. Philadelphia, PA: Elsevier Churchill Livingstone, 2009.

PERIODICALS

Hart, C. Anthony, and Nigel A. Cunliffe. "Viral Gastroenteritis." *Current Opinion in Infectious Diseases* 10 (1997): 408.

Moss, Peter J., and Michael W. McKendrick. "Bacterial Gastroenteritis." *Current Opinion in Infectious Diseases* 10 (1997): 402.

OTHER

Centers for Disease Control and Prevention. "Investigation Update: Outbreak of Salmonella Typhimurium Infections, 2008–2009." Available at http://www.cdc.gov/salmonella/typhimurium/update.html (accessed June 20, 2010). *Current Opinion in Infectious Diseases* 10 (1997): 408.

Julia Barrett
Karl Finley

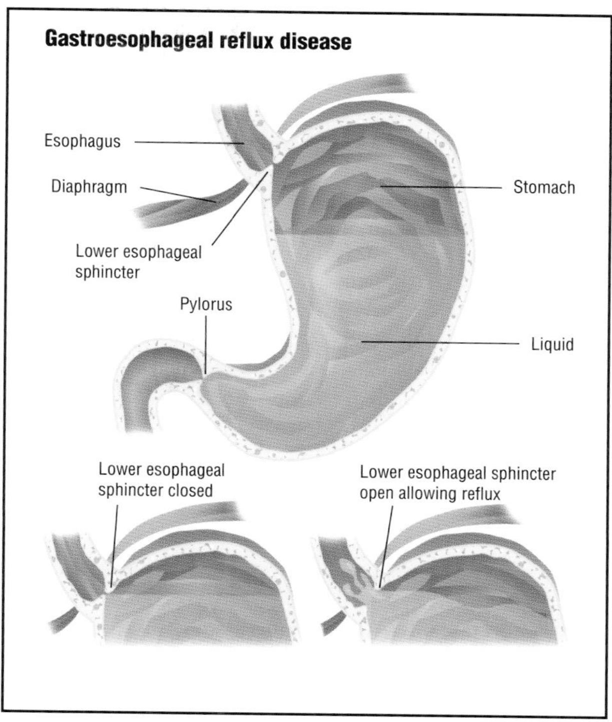

Normally, the lower esophageal sphincter keeps the stomach contents contained with the stomach (top). However, with gastroesophageal reflux disease, the sphincter opens, allowing the acidic contents to flow up the esophagus. *(Illustration by PreMediaGlobal. Reproduced by permission of Gale, a part of Cengage Learning.)*

Gastroesophageal reflux disease

Definition

Gastroesophageal reflux disease (GERD) is a condition in which stomach acids and other stomach contents backflow into the esophagus, the tube leading from the mouth to the stomach, causing a burning sensation in the middle of the chest known as heartburn.

Demographics

Estimates of the number of people in the United States with GERD may be significantly under-reported because some people who experience heartburn self-treat through over-the-counter medications and are never officially diagnosed with GERD unless a more serious condition occurs. The American College of Gastroenterology estimates that about 60 million people in the United States experience heartburn at least once a month; of these, 15 million experience the condition daily. Other estimates suggest that 7% of the population has heartburn daily, and of these individuals, 20–40% have GERD, while heartburn in the remaining individuals arises from other causes. GERD occurs in all races and at all ages but is most common in people over age 40. Men and women are equally affected, although white men are 10 times more likely to develop Barrett's esophagus (a precursor of esophageal **cancer**) than women.

Description

The mechanism behind GERD is a weakness in the lower esophageal sphincter (LES), causing stomach acids to back into the esophagus. The LES is a muscle located at the bottom of the esophagus that acts as a doorkeeper to the stomach. Normally, when food is eaten, it passes through the esophagus into the stomach, and the LES closes to keep the highly acidic stomach contents from washing back into the esophagus. Although a malfunctioning LES can be present from **birth** and can cause infants and children to complain of stomachaches and have frequent bouts of **vomiting**, GERD is most often seen in adults.

The esophagus risks being damaged every time stomach acids wash into it. Constant irritation by stomach acids can cause esophagitis, a condition in which the esophagus becomes red and irritated. Because the lining of the esophagus is thinner and less acid-resistant than the stomach or the intestines, untreated GERD over many years can cause ulcers to develop in the esophagus. These can bleed and can, in turn, result in **anemia**. Scar tissue can also build up.

The body may try to protect the esophagus by developing a thick lining made up of cells like those in the stomach and intestine. This is known as Barrett's esophagus and is a pre-cancerous condition that can lead to cancer of the esophagus.

Some people have trouble eating because there is a feeling that something is in their throats or that their food keeps getting stuck when they eat. This may be a serious condition called dysphagia, which develops from long-term GERD. It is a narrowing of the esophagus caused by a thickening of the lining in response to acids from the stomach. When swallowing hurts, the condition is called odynophagia. This type of GERD often is referred to as silent reflux because no other symptoms are reported.

Everyone experiences heartburn occasionally, especially after overeating or eating fatty foods. Continued heartburn, however can disrupt **sleep**. Moreover, if stomach acids keep bathing the esophagus, chronic inflammation of the lower esophagus can occur. In addition, if stomach material from the esophagus finds its way into the windpipe (trachea), it can enter the lungs, leading to **asthma** and **pneumonia**. For elderly individuals who are bedridden, aspiration of stomach contents can cause **choking**, infection, and even suffocation and **death**.

Causes and symptoms

Causes

Often, a structural abnormality called a hiatal **hernia** is the cause of constant reflux and GERD. In a hiatal hernia, a part of the stomach protrudes through a hole in the diaphragm (a sheet of muscle that separates the abdominal cavity from the chest cavity). This condition is more common in older individuals. Impaired motility in the stomach also can be a factor in GERD. In this case, the stomach nerves or muscles do not allow the stomach and the esophagus to contract normally, thereby allowing acid to build up in the esophagus. Scleroderma, a disease that causes muscular tissue to thicken, can affect digestive muscles and keep the LES open.

Lifestyle factors affect the development of GERD. Being overweight or pregnant increases abdominal pressure, and can cause the LES to remain open, thus allowing the stomach contents to squeeze into the esophagus. Wearing tight clothing around the abdomen, eating large meals, and lying down after eating can keep the LES open. Some foods may act as triggers for GERD, including chocolate, peppermint, high fat foods, citrus foods, tomato products, and onions. **Smoking** can stimulate acid production in the stomach and also can relax the LES. Consuming alcoholic, caffeinated, and carbonated drinks also can contribute to GERD.

Some medications have been linked to the development of GERD. They include high blood pressure medications such as calcium channel blockers, nitrate heart medications, asthma drugs such as theophylline, antidepressants, sedatives such as diazepam (Valium), and corticosteroid drugs. Nitrates in foods also may trigger GERD. Non-steroidal anti-inflammatory drugs (NSAIDs), such as aspirin, ibuprofen, and naproxen, can irritate the stomach and lead to GERD.

Symptoms

Although heartburn is the characteristic symptom of GERD, people with this condition also may experience other symptoms. Regurgitation of stomach acid into the mouth (sometimes called water brash) is often present. Some individuals report abdominal **pain**, difficulty in swallowing, nausea, morning hoarseness, **sore throat**, coughing, wheezing, or a need to repeatedly clear the throat. Others experience vomiting or frequent burping or **hiccups**. A few note weight loss or snoring.

Some people do not experience noticeable symptoms. This is particularly common in older adults. In a 2006 study, researchers found that people over age 65 years had fewer or milder forms of common GERD symptoms, but they experienced more instances of difficulty swallowing, vomiting, anemia, and weight loss. The study also found that abdominal pain and heartburn seemed to decrease with age, and that GERD in the elderly most often was related to nonsteroidal anti-inflammatory drug (NSAID) use.

Having heartburn several times a week or waking up with heartburn at night is a good indicators that an appointment should be made for evaluation by a physician. If symptoms disturb sleep or interfere with work or leisure activities, a doctor should be consulted. Losing weight, breathing difficulties, vomiting blood, or producing black, tarry stool, indicate that a doctor should be seen immediately. In addition, if an individual has been treated by a family physician for GERD for more than two years, a consultation with a gastroenterologist (a doctor specializing in diseases of the digestive system) usually is recommended.

Diagnosis

Examination

Because GERD is common, it often will be diagnosed after the doctor takes a thorough medical history, listens carefully for GERD symptoms, and does a physical examination. If the patient responds positively to treatment, no further tests are ordered. However, if the patient has serious symptoms, such as intense pain, vomiting blood, or rapid weight loss, the doctor will investigate through a series of tests. In addition, if the patient has been complaining of heartburn for a long time or has been treated for GERD for more than two years, other tests will likely be ordered to gauge the extent of damage done to the esophagus.

Procedures

The most common procedures are the upper gastrointestinal (GI) series and the upper GI endoscopy. The upper GI series examines the esophagus, stomach, and the duodenum (the first section of the small intestine). The patient drinks a cup of barium (barium swallow), a metallic, chalky liquid that coats the digestive track and makes it show up on **x rays**. X rays or images are then taken as the barium flows down the esophagus, into the stomach, and into the duodenum. The patient may be asked to turn to the side so that the technician can gently massage the stomach to move the barium into the duodenum. Images are sent to a video monitor where the doctors and technicians observe the behavior of the upper digestive tract and snap still images from the monitor.

The upper GI series can reveal anatomical changes in the esophagus, such as a hiatal hernia or esophageal narrowing. It also can assess damage to the esophagus, detect stomach ulcers or ulcers in the duodenum, and determine whether an intestinal blockage is present.

The upper GI endoscopy, also called the esophagogastroduodenoscopy (EGD), offers a more complete picture of what is happening in the upper digestive tract. It is the test of choice for many gastroenterologists. Before the endoscopy, the patient receives a mild sedative, and then the doctor inserts a small, flexible tube down the patient's throat. At the end of the tube is a light, a tiny camera, and a small instrument used to take tissue samples (biopsies). The camera broadcasts live images from the esophagus and stomach to a video monitor. Using these tools, the doctor can capture still images for further diagnosis and can examine suspicious areas more closely with the camera or by taking tissue samples. The EGD allows the doctor to determine the extent of damage to the esophagus and to rule out serious complications, such as Barrett's esophagus. Mild GERD may show no damage to the esophagus at all.

Another test, esophageal manometry, measures pressure within the esophagus and how well the LES functions. A thin tube is inserted through the nose and down the throat. Coupled with the 24-hour pH probe study, esophageal manometry becomes the best determinant of GERD because it monitors how often the patient has reflux into the esophagus during a full day. One episode of acid reflux is considered having a pH of less than 4.0 for at least 15–30 seconds. This test can determine if there is a correlation between episodes of acid reflux and other symptoms, such as chronic **cough**, wheezing, or sleep apnea.

To do a pH probe study, a small computer is attached to the outside end of the thin tube in the patient's nose, and the computer is worn around the waist or over the shoulder. The patient goes home, carries on a normal routine, then comes back to have the probe removed and the results analyzed.

A more comfortable form of the 24-hour pH probe study is the Bravo pH probe that is placed in the esophagus during endoscopy. This tiny probe transmits data to a miniature recorder the size of a paper clip that is worn around the waist. Eventually, the probe makes its way through the digestive system and is passed in the patient's stool in a week to 10 days.

Sometimes, chest x rays are ordered to check for pneumonia or lung damage due to aspiration of stomach contents.

Treatment

The preferred treatments for GERD are lifestyle changes and drugs.

Lifestyle changes

Either prescribed alone or in combination with drug therapy, lifestyle changes can ease many GERD symptoms. Food choices, the timing of meals, and the size of meals are key lifestyle factors. Individuals should avoid foods that trigger GERD and eat smaller, more frequent meals. Doing so helps to control the amount of acid in the stomach. Individuals also should stop eating three hours before lying down. Lying down after eating can cause stomach contents to backflow into the esophagus. In addition, elevating the head of the bed about six inches may help keep acid within the stomach. Losing weight and avoiding slumping will reduce pressure on the stomach.

Drugs

Drugs often are prescribed along with lifestyle changes, even in the early stages of the disease. Commonly, the first medications prescribed are over-the-counter antacids and/or histamine-2 receptor blockers (H2 blockers). Antacids, such as Gaviscon, Tums,

Maalox, and Mylanta, help neutralize acid already in the stomach or esophagus but do nothing to heal inflammation. Some have a foaming agent that helps prevent acid from backflowing into the esophagus. Unless otherwise instructed by a doctor, antacids can be used every day for three weeks. If taken longer, they can produce **diarrhea**, interfere with calcium absorption in the body, and increase levels of magnesium, which can damage the kidneys. Antacids are not recommended for individuals taking drugs to correct **hypothyroidism**.

Common H2 blockers are nizatidine (Axid), ranitidine (Zantac), famotidine (Pecid), and cimetidine (Tagamet). At half the strength of their prescription counterparts, these over-the-counter medications block acid production, but they have no effect on acid already present in the stomach. These drugs should be taken 30 minutes to one hour before meals. H2 blockers do not work as quickly as antacids, but they produce longer relief and are effective in reducing acid reflux at night. These drugs can heal mild esophageal damage but are not strong enough to heal serious injury. Standard dosage for 6–12 weeks has been found to relieve symptoms in half of GERD patients using H2 blockers.

If symptoms do not improve, proton-pump inhibitors (PPIs) may be given. PPIs can be bought without a prescription and, like H2 blockers, are also available in stronger strengths with a prescription. PPIs include esomeprazole (Nexium), omeprazole (Prilosec), lansoprazole (Prevacid), and rabeprazole (Aciphex). These drugs block the production of an enzyme that aids in acid formation. PPIs can reduce stomach acid by more than 95%. They are used to treat GERD and can heal some gastric and duodenal ulcers and prevent upper GI tract bleeding. PPIs are contraindicated for people with liver disease and may make the intestinal tract more susceptible to bacterial infections.

In addition to PPIs, the doctor may prescribe coating agents, such as sucralfate (Carfate), to cover the sores and mucous membranes of the esophagus and stomach. This acts as a protective barrier.

Some doctors also prescribe a prokinetic agent to tighten the LES and promote faster emptying of the stomach. Metaclopramide (Reglan) is the only prokinetic drug approved for use in the United States. Many doctors are reluctant to use prokinetic drugs because they have serious side effects.

Surgery

If all other treatments fail, surgery is a final option. A surgical procedure called fundoplication creates a one-way valve into the stomach. During surgery, the doctor wraps a part of the stomach around the esophagus and sews it down. This procedure can be done laparoscopically, a less invasive surgical method in which the doctor makes small cuts into the abdomen to insert a camera and the surgical instruments. Laparoscopic surgery produces very little scarring and has a faster recovery rate than traditional open surgery. However, the benefits of fundoplication have been challenged in some studies.

Certain endoscopy treatments can be used to repair the upper digestive tract instead of using surgery. Plication allows the doctor to stitch tears in the esophagus or narrow the LES. The Stretta procedure uses radiofrequency energy to cause the LES sphincter to tighten. The Enteryx procedure lets the doctor inject a bulking material into the LES to narrow it. As of 2010, these procedures were not widely available but were being used at some larger medical centers.

Alternative treatments

Alternative remedies include eating bananas or drinking chamomile or ginger tea. Chamomile should be avoided by people who have ragweed **allergies**. Some people eat licorice to balance the acid output in the stomach and to increase the mucous coating of the esophagus, but this is contraindicated for people with high blood pressure. Teas made from marsh mallow root, papaya, fennel, and catnip are also suggested treatments for heartburn, as well as eating papayas.

Homeopathic remedies most recommended are Nux vomica, Carbo vegetabilis, and Srsenicum album. Acupuncture and acupressure have also been used to treat heartburn.

Home Remedies

In addition to lifestyle changes a common home remedy offering temporary relief is drinking water with sodium bicarbonate (baking soda) in it. However, this remedy can also add uncomfortable gas to the stomach; more sodium to the diet, which can increase blood pressure; and the excessive bicarbonate can produce rebound hyperacidity with worsening symptoms.

Prognosis

In most cases, GERD is easily managed. Between 80% and 90% of individuals improve with drug therapy. However, the length of treatment varies. Some patients may not see improvement for several weeks or months. Some patients can experience relief after two to three months of treatment and are able to modify their lifestyle to minimize symptoms so that medications are reduced or discontinued. Many patients with serious, persistent

KEY TERMS

Calcium channel blocker—A drug that lowers blood pressure by regulating calcium-related electrical activity in the heart.

Dysphagia—Difficulty in swallowing, as if something is stuck in the throat.

Esophagogastroduodenoscopy (EGD)—A test that involves visually examining the lining of the esophagus, stomach, and upper duodenum with a flexible fiber-optic endoscope.

Esophagus—The muscular tube that leads from the back of the throat to the stomach. Coated with mucus and surrounded by muscles, it pushes food to the stomach by contraction.

Fundoplication—A surgical procedure that tightens the lower esophageal sphincter by stretching and wrapping the upper part of the stomach around the sphincter.

Gastroenterologist—A physician who specializes in diseases of the digestive system.

H2 Blockers—Medications used to treat some GERD symptoms, for example, Tagamet, Pepcid, Axid.

Heartburn—A burning sensation in the chest that can sometimes also be felt in the neck, throat, and face. It is the primary symptom of GERD.

Hiatal hernia—A condition in which part of the stomach protrudes above the diaphragm next to the esophagus.

Laparoscopic surgery—A minimally invasive surgery in which a camera and surgical instruments are inserted through a small incision.

Lower esophageal sphincter (LES)—A muscular ring at the base of the esophagus that keeps stomach contents from entering back into the esophagus.

Odynophagia—Pain felt when swallowing.

pH—A measure of the acidity of a fluid. On a scale of 1–14, a pH of 7 is neutral. Higher pH readings are alkaline and lower pH readings are acidic.

Silent reflux—An acid reflux problem that does not have marked symptoms but can cause chronic, recurrent respiratory symptoms much like asthma.

Sleep apnea—A sleep disorder in which breathing stop briefly then resumes on its own. These pauses can occur many times each night, resulting in poor quality sleep.

Water brash—The flow of saliva and stomach acid back up the esophagus and into the throat or lungs.

GERD may need to take medications for the rest of their lives.

Even with successful treatment, some patients experience acid breakthrough. This response occurs when symptoms appear even though the patient has faithfully taken medications. Some patients on PPIs may be symptom free during the day but wake up at night with heartburn. Sometimes an H2 blocker is given to the patient at night in addition to PPI medications. Some patients on H2 blockers may benefit from a combination pill that contains an antacid and an H2 blocker.

Untreated GERD can lead to the development of Barrett's esophagus. Barrett's is a pre-cancerous condition. Many times it can be reversed with proper treatment of GERD.

Prevention

Symptoms of GERD can be prevented by taking drugs as prescribed, avoiding alcohol, not smoking, eating smaller meals, limiting fatty foods, and eliminating trigger foods. Individuals should avoid belts and tight clothing around the waist and try to lose excess weight. Individuals may chew gum or suck on hard candies to increase saliva production, which can sooth the esophagus and wash the acid back to the stomach. People with heartburn should wait two hours after eating before exercising and plan not to eat anything at least three hours before lying down. Finally, elevating the head of the bed at least six inches and sleeping on the left side may reduce nighttime heartburn.

Resources

BOOKS

Burns, David L., and Neeral L. Shah. *100 Questions & Answers About Gastroesophageal Reflux Disease (GERD).* Sudbury, MA: Jones and Bartlett Publishers, 2007.

Wendland, Barbara E., and Lisa Marie Ruffolo. *Chronic Heartburn: Managing Acid Reflux and GERD Through Understanding, Diet, and Lifestyle.* Toronto, Ontario, Canada: Robert Rose, 2006.

PERIODICALS

Wellbery, Caroline. "GERD Symptoms Differ with Patient Age." *American Family Physician* (March 15, 2007): 906.

OTHER

"Gastroesophageal Reflux in Children and Adolescents." National Digestive Diseases Information Clearinghouse. August 2006, http://digestive.niddk.nih.gov/ddiseases/pubs/gerinchildren.

"GERD." MedlinePlus February 4, 2010, http://www.nlm.nih.gov/medlineplus/gerd.html.

"The Word on GERD." American College of Gastroenterology, http://www.acg.gi.org/patients/gerd/word.asp (accessed February 7, 2010).

ORGANIZATIONS

American College of Gastrolenterology (ACG), P.O. Box 34226, Bethesda, MD, 20827-2260, (301) 263-9000, http://www.acg.gi.org.

American Gastroenterological Association (AGA), 4930 Del Ray Avenue, Bethesda, MD, 20814, (310) 654-2055, (301) 654-5920, www.gastro.org.

International Foundation for Functional Gastrointestinal Disorders, P.O. Box 170864, Milwaukee, WI, 53217-8076, (414) 964-1799, (U.S. only) (888) 964-2001, (414) 964-7176, iffgdiffgd.org, http://www.iffgd.org.

National Digestive Diseases Information Clearinghouse (NDDIC), 2 Information Way, Bethesda, MD, 20892-3570, (800) 891-5389; TTY (866) 569-1162, (703) 738-4929, info@niddk.nih.gov, http://digestive.niddk.nih.gov.

Janie F. Franz
Tish Davidson, AM

Gastroschisis **see Abdominal wall defects**

Gates-MacGinitie reading tests (GMRT)

Definition

The Gates-MacGinitie reading tests (GMRT) are among the most widely used and most highly respected surveys of reading achievement for grades K-12 and for adult education.

Purpose

The GMRT are used by teachers and school districts throughout the United States to measure student reading achievement and to follow each student's progress through the grade levels. The pre-reading (PR) and beginning reading (BR) levels of the GMRT are designed to aid teachers in identifying specific concepts with which beginning readers may need additional help. Vocabulary and comprehension scores for levels 1–10/12 can identify students who require remedial help, those who are reading at grade level, and those who are ready for more challenging material. The fourth edition of the GMRT became available as on online test in August of 2010, enabling teachers and administrators to obtain results and start implementing strategies based on those results within 24 hours of testing.

The GMRT are used for a variety of purposes, including:

- monitoring student progress, both throughout the school year and from year to year
- obtaining a complete history of reading development for students who take the test each year, from preschool through high school
- screening for reading difficulties
- diagnosing specific reading problems or areas where students require additional help
- identifying students in need of further evaluation and special instruction
- choosing reading materials and instructional programs for individuals and groups
- adjusting teaching strategies for individual students and classrooms to improve student performance
- organizing students into instructional groups that are appropriate for their reading level, including remedial and accelerated programs
- placing new students in appropriate instructional groups
- designing individualized instruction
- advising students
- evaluating outcomes and the effectiveness of instructional programs, including school-wide and district-wide programs, using a common standard
- comparing different instructional methods for learning the alphabet and for vocabulary and reading comprehension
- reporting student progress to parents, teachers, and the community
- identifying underperforming classrooms, grade levels, schools, and districts
- conducting educational research

Various programs, including Reading Recovery and the Iowa Test of Basic Skills (ITBS), rely on the GMRT for program and test evaluation. The GMRT are also compatible with the Reading First and Striving Readers programs.

Description

The GMRT were first developed in the early 1960s by Arthur I. Gates, Walter H. MacGinitie, and Ruth K. MacGinitie. The fourth edition was published in 2000. The GMRT are short, timed, multiple-choice tests. They are administered to groups of students, usually twice each year in the fall and spring. More frequent testing can be accomplished by alternating the two test forms, S and T, or by using a lower- or higher-level test, within certain limits.

The PR and BR levels are pencil-paper tests only. The other levels can be either pencil-paper or online tests. For the pencil-paper levels 3 and below, the answers are marked directly in the test booklet. Students taking higher-level tests who have trouble maneuvering the test booklet and answer sheet may also mark their answers in the booklet.

Levels PR and BR are taken at a pace determined by the administrator, usually about 75–100 minutes. This pace allows students to attempt each question, but is fast enough that they do not become distracted or lose interest. The higher-level tests are timed at 55 minutes, except for level 2, which is 75 minutes. The time limits are designed to enable most students to attempt all of the questions.

The content of the fourth edition pencil-paper and online GMRT are nearly identical. The online form does not require computer proficiency. Students view one vocabulary item at a time and do not need to scroll down during the comprehension passages. Progress bars indicate the time remaining and the number of answered questions. Icons indicate questions answered and questions remaining. Online testing allows extended testing times for students whose individualized education programs (IEPs) require such accommodation.

Levels

Each GMRT level is designed to be appropriate for most students and most classes at the specified grade level or levels. Testing at one level higher is usually recommended for students whose raw scores are within four points of perfect. Testing at one level lower is usually recommended for students whose raw scores are less than six points above the chance-level score.

The PR level test, which utilizes pictures, is designed for preschoolers and kindergarteners. It measures background concepts that are important for building beginning reading skills at the end of kindergarten and start of the first grade. There are four subtests:

- literacy concepts, which evaluate understanding of the nature and uses of written language and words and phrases that are commonly used in beginning reading
- oral language concepts, or phonological awareness, which evaluate recognition of phonemes—the sounds of speech—and the basic structure of spoken English words
- knowledge of letters and letter/sound recognition and correspondences
- listening (story) comprehension, which evaluates understanding of elements in a connected text

The BR level test includes both pictures and basic story words and is especially appropriate for testing at the start and again at the end of first grade. It has both very easy questions for children just beginning to learn to read and more challenging questions that are appropriate for the end of first grade. The first three subtests evaluate decoding skills with combinations of consonants and vowels that make up English words. The fourth subtest evaluates the ability to identify common text words that are usually learned without decoding. The four subtests are:

- initial consonants and consonant clusters
- final consonants and consonant clusters
- vowels
- basic story words

Levels 1 and 2 are general assessments of early independent reading. Since they use the same sample questions and general procedures, they can be administered together in the same room. Both levels include a subtest to evaluate word decoding or recognition, in which the incorrect answer choices are common decoding errors. Both levels also have a comprehension test, which consists of extended written texts, including fiction and nonfiction and narrative and expository, in a variety of writing styles. All but the last passage have four text segments, for which the student chooses the picture that illustrates the text segment or answers a question about it. Level 2 has an additional 20-minute word knowledge test in which the incorrect answers are common errors in meaning. This subtest assesses beginning reading vocabulary and segues into the higher-level vocabulary tests.

Levels 3–10/12 are general reading assessments for grades 3 through 12, consisting of a vocabulary test and a comprehension test. Levels 4–10/12 can be administered at the same time in the same room. The vocabulary tests present each test word in a short context that suggests the part of speech, but not the meaning, and students select the word or phrase that is closest in meaning. The comprehension tests assess ability to read and understand different types of prose. The passages are from published fiction and nonfiction and vary in content and style, with the number of passages depending on the test level. The content of the passages reflect school and recreational reading. The questions assess comprehension of the literal or inferred meaning of the passages or require students to draw conclusions from a passage. Level 10/12 is the most difficult of the GMRT tests. It assesses a narrower range of abilities and is appropriate for tenth–twelfth graders.

The adult reading (AR) GMRT is designed to assess reading by students in colleges, adult education programs, general educational development (GED) programs, vocational and training schools, the military, and other post-secondary education. It is also used by businesses and other organizations. The format is the same as levels 3–10/12, with vocabulary and comprehension tests, but with content that is more appropriate for adults. The AR level test has a wide range of difficulty, with a ninth-grade median difficulty level.

Results

Levels PR-3 are available as machine-scored or hand-scored booklets. Levels 4-AR are available as machine-scored or self-scored answer sheets or hand-scored reusable test booklets. Machine-scored answer sheets can be sent to Riverside Scoring Service, scanned locally, or hand-scored with an acetate scoring template. A range of hand-scoring aids are available. A variety of score reports can be ordered from Riverside. Score converting and reporting software is available for hand-scored tests.

GMRT norms are from 1999 and 2006, depending on the test. Norms for the AR level are based on students entering community college. The types of available scores include:

- raw scores (RS)—the number of correctly answered questions
- national percentile rank (NPR)—the percentages of students nationwide in the same grade whose raw scores were lower or higher, on a scale of 1 to 99
- local percentile rank (LPR)
- national stanine (NS)–performance compared to students nationwide in the same grade, on a scale of 1–9
- local stanine (LS)
- normal curve equivalent (NCE)—level of achievement in relation to scores of other students in the same grade, on a scale of 1 to 99
- grade equivalent (GE)—the grade level of an average student who earned the same score
- extended scale score (ESS)—an individual's single continuous score scale or development scale over a period of years
- Lexile range—a measure that helps locate suitable reading material for a student's abilities

Student GMRT comprehension scores can be linked to Lexile measures for levels 1 through 10/12 via the Lexile website and the GMRT online Results Manager. Students can use Lexile measures to locate reading materials of appropriate difficulty.

KEY TERMS

Decoding skills—The systematic transformation of written words into spoken words by matching letters or letter clusters into oral sounds.

General Educational Development (GED)—General Education Diploma, General Equivalency Diploma, Graduate Equivalency Degree; a group of five subject tests leading to a credential that indicates that an individual has academic skills equivalent to a U.S. or Canadian high-school graduate.

Lexile—A registered trademark of the educational measurement company MetaMetrics. The Lexile Framework consists of the Lexile measure, which represents reading ability and text difficulty as a number, such as 1000L, and the Lexile scale, a developmental scale ranging from 200L for beginning readers and tests to 1700L for advanced readers and texts.

Literacy—The ability to efficiently comprehend and interpret written language and to communicate through written language.

Norm—A standard of achievement, usually derived from the average or median achievement of a large group of a particular age.

Percentile—A rank in a population that has been divided into 100 equal groups; thus, test results in the 50th percentile indicate that half of those who took the test scored higher and half scored lower.

Phoneme—A basic unit of sound in a language.

Phonological awareness—An awareness or appreciation of language sounds.

Reading First—A federal program that helps states and school districts implement scientifically based reading programs in kindergarten through the third grade.

Stanine—Normalized standard scores ranked into nine classes, with the bottom 4% ranked 1, the top 4% ranked 9, and the middle 20% ranked 5.

The GMRT includes support materials and services for helping teachers interpret test results and link the assessments to instruction. These services can also help teachers and administrator plan instruction, intervention, and enrichment, including identifying specific reading skills that are weak and techniques for developing those skills.

Parental concerns

Although the GMRT purports to be a diagnostic reading test, each test only assesses at a single grade level. The Diagnostic Online Reading **Assessment** (DORA) is an online test that is comparable to the GMRT. However the DORA is an adaptive test that adjusts in difficulty based on each student's responses. It assesses more reading sub-skills than the GMRT and is available in Spanish as well as English.

Resources

BOOKS

MacGinitie, Walter H., Ruth K. MacGinitie, Katherine Maria, and Lois G. Dreyer. *Gates-MacGinitie Reading Tests.* 4th ed. Itasca, IL: Riverside, 2000.

PERIODICALS

Guthrie, John T., et al. "Impacts of Comprehensive Reading Instruction on Diverse Outcomes of Low- and High-Achieving Readers." *Journal of Learning Disabilities* 42- no. 3 (May/June 2009): 195–214.

Yasuhiro, Ozuru, et al. "Where's the Difficulty in Standardized Reading Tests: The Passage or the Question?" *Behavior Research Methods* 40 (2008): 1001–1015.

OTHER

"DORA—Diagnostic Online Reading Assessment." Curriculum Associates, http://www.curriculumassociates.com/products/detail.asp?title=DORA (accessed October 3, 2010).

Fortson, Laura L. "How to Use the Gates-MacGinitie Reading Test Effectively." Middle Grades Reading Network, http://mgrn.evansville.edu/10w2006.htm (accessed October 2, 2010).

MacGinitie, Walter H., Ruth K. MacGinitie, Katherine Maria, and Lois G. Dreyer. "Gates-MacGinitie Reading Tests Online." Riverside Publishing. 2010, http://www.riversidepublishing.com/products/gmrtOnline (accessed October 2, 2010).

MacGinitie, Walter H., Ruth K. MacGinitie, Katherine Maria, Lois G. Dreyer, and Kay E. Hughes. "Gates-MacGinitie Reading Tests (GMRT) Fourth Edition Forms S and T—Paper-Pencil." Riverside Publishing. 2010, http://www.riversidepublishing.com/products/gmrt/index.html (accessed October 2, 2010).

ORGANIZATIONS

National Institute of Child Health and Human Development (NICHD) Information Resource Center, PO Box 3006, Rockville, MD, 20847, (800) 370-2943, (866) 760-5947, NICHDInformationResourceCenter@mail.nih.gov, http://www.nichd.nih.gov.

Margaret Alic, PhD

Gaucher's disease ***see* Lipidoses**

Gay issues ***see* Bisexuality; Homosexuality**

Gender constancy

Definition

Gender constancy is a term in psychology used to refer to a child's recognition that a person's biological sex is fixed and does not change over time. It is considered by some psychologists to represent a critical stage in the formation of **gender identity** in that it allows the child to organize his or her understanding of human sexuality on a stable basis.

Demographics

There is some debate among psychologists regarding the age at which children develop gender constancy, whether this age is the same across cultures, and whether it is affected by the child's mental age. Although some researchers maintain that children do not achieve gender constancy until the early elementary school years (age six or seven), others maintain that children can attain such constancy as early as age four. One possible explanation of the discrepancy is that several studies suggest that children with high IQs attain gender constancy at an earlier age than children of average or below-average **intelligence**.

Description

The concept of gender constancy, influenced by the **cognitive development** theory of Jean Piaget (1896–1980), was introduced in 1966 by Lawrence Kohlberg (1927–1987), a psychologist best known for his theory of stages of **moral development**. Addressing the formation of gender identity in terms of cognition, Kohlberg advanced the idea that the development of sex roles depends in large part on a child's understanding that gender remains constant throughout a person's lifetime. Children realize that they are male or female and are aware of the gender of others by the age of three. However, at these ages they still do not understand that people cannot change their sex the way they can change their clothes, names, or behavior. Kohlberg theorized that children do not learn to behave in gender-appropriate ways until they understand that gender is permanent, which occurs at about the age of seven. At this point they start modeling the behavior of members of their own sex. Although it has been supported by some research studies,

Kohlberg's theory has also been criticized on the grounds that children do show certain types of gender-associated behavior, such as toy and playmate selection, by the ages of two or three. These behaviors point to the fact that there are other factors, such as parental reinforcement, that influence the adoption of sex-typed behavior.

Kohlberg's cognitive theory of gender constancy was worked out in opposition to earlier theories of gender that made either biology (children's perception of anatomical differences between the sexes) or socialization (**family** members and other adults' transmission of gender roles) primary. In Kohlberg's own words, he "assume[d] that basic sexual attitudes are not patterned directly by either biological instincts or arbitrary cultural norms, but by the child's cognitive organization of his social world along sex-role dimensions." Following Piaget's notion of stages in childhood cognitive development, Kohlberg identified three stages in the child's cognitive understanding of gender:

- Gender identification or gender labeling. In this early stage, the child can identify him- or herself and other people as male or female. The child does not yet, however, understand gender as stable over time or as unaffected by such external matters as clothing or hair styles. Kohlberg thought that most children reach this stage by about three years.
- Gender stability. In this stage, the child recognizes that gender remains stable over time (for example, boys grow up to become fathers and girls grow up to become mothers). The child still does not understand gender as a permanent aspect of one's being, and may still think of gender as changeable depending on a person's occupation or other activity.
- Gender constancy. In the final stage of the child's cognitive understanding of gender, he or she recognizes that their sex is permanent, regardless of the passage of time, changes in social context, or alterations of physical features. Kohlberg thought that most children reach this stage at around six or seven years.

Common problems

Most common problems regarding gender constancy involve academic debates among psychologists that are still unresolved rather than agreed-upon findings that affect the general public. In the years following Kohlberg's definition of gender constancy and his three-stage outline of gender identity development, some researchers devised verbal questionnaires or other tests to evaluate the adequacy of Kohlberg's theory. There are two major instruments used for research purposes to measure gender constancy:

- Slaby and Frey (1975): Gender Constancy Interview Schedule. The GCIS is a verbal interview consisting of 13 questions and counterquestions. The first eight questions ask the child to identify the gender of four dolls (boy, girl, adult male, adult female) and four photographs of adults (two males and two females). Question 9 asks the child to identify his or her own gender. Questions 10 and 11 assess the child's attainment of gender stability by asking such questions as "When you were a little baby, were you a boy or a girl?", and questions 12 and 13 measure gender constancy by asking the child whether he or she would remain a boy or girl if they wore the clothes of the other sex or participated in an activity associated with the other sex.
- Emmerich et al. (1977): Boy-Girl Identity Task (BGIT). In this test, the child is shown a drawing of a child of his or her own sex and asked to suggest an appropriate name. The next two questions are verbal. Using the name suggested by the child, the examiner asks whether [name of boy] could be a girl if he wants to. For questions 3 through 5, the drawing is altered by the examiner to change the appearance of the child in the drawing. In the case of the boy, the examiner lifts part of the drawing to reveal the boy wearing a dress (question 3); another part of the drawing to reveal the boy's face with long hair (question 4); and both parts to reveal the boy wearing both long hair and a dress (question 5). For each of these changes, the examiner asks if [name of boy] puts on girl clothes (or hair or both clothes and hair), is he still a boy. If the child answers correctly (indicating gender stability or constancy), the examiner then asks the child to give a reason for the correct answer, which is then scored according to whether the child has attained gender constancy (the child comments that the child in the drawing was born a boy), is referring to a portion of the picture (the boy is still wearing pants even though he now has long hair), or cannot give a reason.

As of 2010, however, there is no widespread agreement about the adequacy of Kohlberg's concept of three stages in gender constancy formation; the role that gender constancy plays in later psychosexual maturation; the role of intelligence as well as age in gender constancy; the ability to distinguish between appearance and reality in the attainment of gender constancy; or the role of cognition in general in gender identity formation in comparison to biological and social factors. In recent years, however, both the GCIS and the BGIT have been used to evaluate children who show early signs of gender identity disorder as well as in academic research in the field of child development.

KEY TERMS

Cognitive—Referring to such human mental functions as reasoning, analysis, learning, memory, and judgment.

Mental age—A measure of a child's intelligence, expressed as the age at which the child is performing intellectually. A 10-year-old who reads at the level of an average ninth-grader would be said to have a mental age of 14. IQ is calculated by dividing the mental age by the chronological age and multiplying by 100. In the present example, the eight-year-old would have an IQ of 140.

Parental concerns

The primary concern for parents regarding gender constancy would be early signs of gender identity disorder (GID). Parents may wish to talk to the child's **pediatrician** for a possible evaluation by a clinical psychologist who may administer one or more of the gender constancy questionnaires or tests. Another possibility is a visit to the only clinic in North America as of 2010 that offers gender identity evaluations of young children (as opposed to clinics offering gender identity counseling to adults), which is located in Toronto, Ontario, Canada. The Gender Identity Service of the Centre for **Addiction** and Mental Health (CAMH) describes itself as offering "a comprehensive **assessment**, followed by treatment recommendations for children and adolescents age 2 to 18 when there is concern about a child's gender identity development; an adolescent's transvestic fetishism (cross-dressing associated with sexual arousal); or an adolescent who is struggling with sexual orientation."

Resources

BOOKS

Beere, Carole A. *Gender Roles: A Handbook of Tests and Measures*. New York: Greenwood Press, 1990.

Kohlberg, Lawrence, and Edward Zigler. *The Impact of Cognitive Maturity on the Development of Sex-role Attitudes in the Years 4 to 8*. Provincetown, MA: Genetic Psychology Monographs, 1967.

PERIODICALS

Arthur, A.E., et al. "An Experimental Test of the Effects of Gender Constancy on Sex Typing." *Journal of Experimental Child Psychology* 104 (December 2009): 427–46.

Ruble, D.N., et al. "The Role of Gender Constancy in Early Gender Development." *Child Development* 78 (July—August 2007): 1121–36.

Trautner, H.M., et al. "Appearance-Reality Distinction and Development of Gender Constancy Understanding in Children." *International Journal of Behavioral Development* 27 (March 2003): 275–283.

Zucker, K.J., et al. "Gender Constancy Judgments in Children with Gender Identity Disorder: Evidence for a Developmental Lag." *Archives of Sexual Behavior* 28 (December 1999): 475–502.

OTHER

"Course Extract: Cognition and Gender Development." BBC: The Open University. June 1, 2005, http://www.open2.net/healtheducation/family_childdevelopment/2005/extractone.html (accessed September 18, 2010).

"Gender Identity Service." Centre for Addiction and Mental Health (CAMH). June 22, 2010, http://www.camh.net/Care_Treatment/Program_Descriptions/Child_Youth_Family/Gender_Identity_Service/index.html (accessed September 18, 2010.

ORGANIZATIONS

American Psychological Association (APA), 750 First Street NE, Washington, DC, 20002, (202) 336-5500, (800) 374-2721, http://www.apa.org.

Centre for Addiction and Mental Health (CAMH), Gender Identity Service, 1001 Queen Street West, and 30-60 White Squirrel Way (Queen and Ossington), 1st floor, Toronto, Ontario, M6J 1H4, Canada, (416) 535-8501, ext. 4040, http://www.camh.net.

Rebecca J. Frey, PhD

Gender identity

Gender identity is the sense of identification with either the male or female sex as manifested in appearance, behavior, and other aspects of a person's life.

Influenced by a combination of biological and sociological factors, gender identity emerges by the age of two or three and is reinforced at **puberty**. Once established, it is generally fixed for life. Gender identity should not be confused with sexual identity, which is defined by a person's gonads whereas gender identity refers to a personal conception of oneself as male or female. The difference is sometimes explained that gender identity is located in the brain whereas sexual identity is located in the abdomen and parts further south.

Aside from sex differences, other biological contrasts between males and females are already evident in childhood. Girls mature faster than boys, are physically healthier, and are more advanced in developing oral and written linguistic skills. Boys are generally more advanced at envisioning and manipulating objects in space. They are more aggressive and more physically active, preferring noisy, boisterous forms of play that require larger groups and more space than the play of girls the same age. In spite of conscious attempts to reduce sex role stereotyping in recent decades, boys and girls are still treated differently by adults from the time they are born. The way adults play with infants has been found to differ according to gender: girls are treated more gently and approached more verbally than boys. As children grow older, many parents, teachers, and other authority figures still tend to encourage greater independence, competition, and exploration in boys and greater expressivity, nurturance, and obedience in girls.

A major step in the formation of gender identity occurs at about the age of three when children first become aware of anatomical differences between the sexes, usually through observation of siblings or peers. The awareness of physical differences is followed by awareness of the cultural differences between males and females and identification with the parent of the same sex, whose behavior the child begins to imitate. The most famous twentieth-century theory about the acquisition of gender identity at this stage of life is the Oedipus complex formulated by Sigmund Freud (1856–1939). Like its female counterpart, which Freud termed the Electra complex, the Oedipus complex revolves around a child's wish to possess the parent of the opposite sex while simultaneously wishing to eliminate the parent of the same sex, who is perceived as a rival.

In the Oedipus complex, the young boy develops incestuous desires toward his mother, while regarding his father as a rival for her affections. Fearing that the father will cut off his penis in retaliation—a phenomenon Freud called castration anxiety—the boy represses his forbidden desires and finally comes to identify with the father, internalizing his values and characteristics, which form the basis for the child's superego. In the female version of this theory, the young girl's discovery of sexual difference results in penis envy, which parallels castration **anxiety** in boys. The girl blames her mother for depriving her of a penis, and desires her father because he possesses one. As in the Oedipus complex, the girl eventually represses her incestuous desires and identifies with the same-sex parent (in this case, the mother).

The Oedipus complex has been widely criticized, especially by feminist critics who reject its assumption that "anatomy is destiny." One respected feminist theory is that of Nancy Chodorow, for whom the central factor in gender identity acquisition is the mother's role as primary **caregiver**. According to Chodorow, this maternal role leads to a greater sense of interrelatedness in girls, who identify with the mother and go on to reproduce the same patterns of mothering in their own adult lives, while boys, needing to identify with the parent of the opposite sex, acquire a defining sense of separateness and independence early in life. This "reproduction of mothering," being both biologically and sociologically determined, is at least theoretically open to the possibility of change if patterns of parenting can be altered.

The formation of gender identity has been approached in different terms by Lawrence Kohlberg (1927–1987), who formulated the concept of **gender constancy**, the awareness that gender remains fixed throughout a person's lifetime. Kohlberg noted that while children are aware of their own gender and the gender of others by the age of three, they do not really begin assuming appropriate gender-based behavior until the age of about seven, when they first understand that gender is permanent—that they cannot change gender the way they can change their clothes or their behavior. Kohlberg believed that children do not start systematically imitating the behavior of members of their own sex until that point.

While most children follow a predictable pattern in the acquisition of gender identity, some develop a gender identity inconsistent with their biological sex, a condition variously known as gender confusion, gender identity disorder (GID), gender dysphoria, or **transsexualism**. This condition affects about 1 in 20,000 males and 1 in 50,000 females. Researchers have found that both early socialization and hormonal factors may play a role in the development of gender identity disorder. In some children chromosomal abnormalities play a part, such as those that give rise to **Klinefelter syndrome** (XXY, XXXY, or XXXXY sex chromosome pattern) and **Turner syndrome** (X0 sex chromosome pattern). A condition that affects some girls is called **congenital adrenal hyperplasia** (CAH), which affects about 1 in 14,200 girl babies. In CAH, the fetus is exposed to abnormally high levels of cortisol produced by its own adrenal gland during pregnancy. The girl may be born with external genitalia resembling those of a male and develop the gender identity of a male. About one male infant in 20,000 has androgen insensitivity syndrome, which means that his genitals do not develop normally in utero even though he has a normal XY sex chromosome pattern. In some cases, children are born with malformed, unusually small, or partially absent genitals; these deformities very often affect their sense of gender identity as they mature.

Children with gender identity disorder usually feel from their earliest years that they are trapped in the wrong body and begin to show signs of gender confusion between the ages of two and four. They prefer playmates of the opposite sex at an age when most children prefer to spend time in the company of same-sex peers. They also show a preference for the clothing and typical activities of the opposite sex: transsexual boys like to play house and play with dolls. Girls with gender identity disorder are bored by ordinary female pastimes and prefer the rougher types of play typically associated with boys, such as contact **sports**.

Both male and female transsexuals believe and repeatedly insist that they actually are or will grow up to be members of the opposite sex. Girls cut their hair short, favor boys' clothing, and have negative feelings about maturing physically as they near **adolescence**. In childhood, girls with gender identity disorder experience less overall social rejection than boys, as it is more socially acceptable for a girl to be a tomboy than for a boy to be perceived as a "sissy." About five times more boys than girls are referred to therapists for this condition. Teenagers with gender identity disorder suffer social isolation and are vulnerable to depression and **suicide**. They have difficulty developing peer relationships with members of their own sex as well as romantic relationships with the opposite sex. They may also become alienated from their parents.

Most children eventually outgrow gender identity disorder. About 75 percent of boys with gender identity disorder develop a homosexual or bisexual orientation by late adolescence or adulthood, but without continued feelings of transsexuality. Most of the remaining 25 percent become heterosexuals (also without transsexuality). Those individuals in whom gender identity disorder persists into adulthood retain the desire to live as members of the opposite sex, sometimes manifesting this desire by cross-dressing, either privately or in public. In some cases, adult transsexuals (both male and female) have their primary and secondary sexual characteristics altered through a sex change operation, consisting of hormone treatments followed by surgery. One of the better-known personal accounts of undergoing a sex change operation is that by Jan (formerly James) Morris, a British journalist and military veteran who was married and the father of five children when he underwent surgery in 1972 at the age of 46.

There is no general agreement among medical professionals as of 2006 about the proper course of treatment for GID, in part because the various genetic, gestational, anatomical, and social contributions to the condition are so varied. One statistic that recurs in studies of youths of either sex with GID is the high rate of concurrent psychiatric disorders in this population. One group of researchers reported in 2005 that 71 percent of the patients interviewed had a lifetime diagnosis of either depression or an anxiety disorder, while 42 percent were diagnosed with one or more **personality disorders**. Boys with GID appear to be more likely to have comorbid mental disorders than girls. In any event, sex change operations have not been found to be an effective treatment for these other disorders. The chief of psychiatry at Johns Hopkins, Paul McHugh, summarized a group of studies of persons who had received a sex change operation. Although most subjects in these surveys said that they felt better about having changed their sex, none of them had resolved any of their other disorders or personality problems. Dr. McHugh's advice regarding children born with ambiguous genitalia is to surgically correct any problems they may have with urination, but not to otherwise change their sexual organs until they are older. They should be raised according to their genetic sex until they are old enough to have a sense of their own identity.

Resources

BOOKS

American Psychiatric Association. *Diagnostic and Statistical Manual of Mental Disorders*, 4th ed., text revision, Washington, DC: American Psychiatric Association, 2000.

Bamberg-Smith, Barbara A. *The Psychology of Sex and Gender*. Boston: Pearson/Allyn and Bacon, 2007.

Chodorow, Nancy. *The Reproduction of Mothering: Psychoanalysis and the Sociology of Gender.* Berkeley, CA: University of California Press, 1978.

Diamant, Louis, and Richard D. McAnulty, eds. *The Psychology of Sexual Orientation, Behavior, and Identity: A Handbook.* Westport, CT: Greenwood Press, 1995.

Golombok, Susan, and Robyn Fivush. *Gender Development.* Cambridge: Cambridge University Press, 1994.

Kohlberg, Lawrence. *Child Psychiatry and Childhood Education: A Cognitive-Developmental View.* New York: Longman, 1987.

Lee, Janice W., ed. *Focus on Gender Identity*. New York: Nova Science Publishers, 2005.

Morris, Jan. *Conundrum*. New York: Harcourt Brace Jovanovich, 1974.

PERIODICALS

Cohen-Kettenis, P. T., et al. "Demographic Characteristics, Social Competence, and Behavior Problems in Children with Gender Identity Disorder: A Cross-National, Cross-Clinic Comparative Analysis." *Journal of Abnormal Child Psychology* 31 (February 2003): 41–53.

Ghosh, Shuvo, MD, and Leslie Walker, MD. "Sexuality: Gender Identity." *eMedicine*, July 20, 2006. Available from http://www.emedicine.com/ped/topic2789.html.

Hepp, U., et al. "Psychiatric Comorbidity in Gender Identity Disorder." *Journal of Psychosomatic Research* 58 (March 2005): 259–261.

McHugh, Paul, MD. "Surgical Sex." *First Things* 147 (November 2004): 34–38.

ORGANIZATIONS

American Academy of Child and Adolescent Psychiatry (AACAP), 3615 Wisconsin Ave. NW, Washington, DC, 20016, (202) 966-7300, http://www.aacap.org.

Society for Adolescent Medicine (SAM), 1916 Copper Oaks Circle, Blue Springs, MO, 64015, (816) 224-8010, http://www.adolescenthealth.org.

Genetic disorders

Variations within the DNA sequence of a particular gene affect its function and may cause or predispose an individual a particular disease. Alterations in the genome may increase the frequency of disorder and disease with entire populations.

Although there are many types of genetic disorders, a specific disorder does not have to be inheritable to have a genetic basis. For example, non-heritable disorders can also arise from mutations in somatic cells resulting from exposure to mutagenic factors in the environment. Mutations, whether inherited mutations that appear in every cell of the body, or random mutations affecting a particular cell, can cause groups of cells to grow out of control, or inhibit the processes (contact inhibition processes) that normally prevent this from happening.

Some diseases and disorders are traced to the presence of a single form of a gene, as with a mutation in a specific normal gene. Other common conditions, including not only some cancers but also some forms of heart disease and diabetes, are polygenic. Variations in a number of genes, in combination with environmental conditions that determine the extent to which these genes are expressed, affect the risk that an individual will develop such conditions. The risk calculations associated with many of the disorders commonly regarded as genetic diseases are often predictable as functions of relatively simple Mendelian inheritance.

There are many types of genetic diseases, and disorders result from a few well-established mechanisms. Autosomal dominant disorders, in which one deleterious gene, or allele, expresses itself over a normal complementary allele, is the mechanism underlying Crouzon disease. In contrast, **phenylketonuria** is an autosomal recessive disorder in which both deleterious alleles must be present. There are also sex-linked diseases and disorders wherein the deleterious gene or genes lie on sex chromosomes (X and Y chromosomes). There are X-linked dominant disorders (e.g., hypoplastic amelogenesis imperfecta), X-linked recessive disorders (Menkes' syndrome), and Y-linked disorders, in which the only mechanism of transmission is from father to son.

Not all genetic disorders depend on alterations to nuclear DNA. There are disorders such as mitochondrial myopathy that can result from alterations to mitochondrial DNA.

Genetic counseling deals with the problems associated with the diagnosis of a genetic disorder, the probable disease course, and possible treatments and management. **Genetic testing** used to assess the risks of genetic disorders and the risks of recurrence. Options for dealing with the risk of a genetic disorder and its recurrence sometimes involve methods of **contraception**, **adoption**, insemination by donor sperm, and prenatal diagnosis.

Bayes' theorem is used in genetic epidemiology in order to obtain the probability of disease in a group of people with some characteristic. In addition, Bayes' theorem is able to calculate unknown conditional probabilities (PVP) from known conditional probabilities (detection rate or sensitivity). For example, biochemical and ultrasound marker-based screenings use a derivation of Bayes' theorem to select patients for whom further testing for a particular disease or disorder may be appropriate.

A variation of Bayes' theorem, termed the Bart's test, is very popular in prenatal screening. Bart's test allows an adjustment of the probability of the disease (expressed as 1/total) for an appropriate factor named likelihood ratio, or the ratio between the detection rate and the false positive rate.

Except for genes appearing on the X or Y chromosomes in males, there are usually two copies of each gene in humans. This redundancy provides a buffer to genetic diseases and disorders. In many cases, only one correctly functioning copy of a gene is necessary. Only when an individual has obtained two copies of an abnormal recessive gene will the corresponding disease manifest itself. Inheritance of this type is called homozygous recessive.

A heterozygous individual with one allele for such a condition may be completely unaffected. In other cases, the individual may even be at an advantage, which provides a clue as to why the mutation remains in the population. **Sickle cell disease**, relatively common among people of African descent, is an often-fatal condition in which red blood cells become sickle-shaped when the oxygen content of the blood decreases, as it does during physical exertion. The deformed blood cells block small blood vessels, causing tissue **death** (necrosis) in affected areas. Although only an individual with two alleles for sickle cell will have the disease, individuals with one sickle cell allele (type pf gene) have sickle cell trait. Trait carriers only experience disease-like symptoms at extreme low-oxygen conditions such as those found at very high altitudes. On the other hand, such an individual actually gains a significant advantage relative to malarial resistance.

Malaria is endemic in Africa, and the evolutionary benefit of having a large population of people who are heterozygous for the trait overcomes the disadvantage of a fatal condition affecting homozygotes with two copies of the allele. Therefore this type of genetic disease may persist at a relatively high frequency in a population over a long period of time even if the actual disorder is serious or potentially fatal.

With dominant alleles, one copy of a defective gene is enough to produce a disease or disorder. Genetic disorders with dominant inheritance that are lethal at an early age do not remain in the population because they kill the affected individual before he or she can reproduce. However, nonlethal dominant genetic disorders, such as the hand and foot malformation called camptobrachydactyly, do persist over time. Likewise, a lethal genetic disorder such as Huntington's disease that strikes after the individual has reached reproductive maturity can also be passed along to future generations.

If the gene associated with a disorder is found on the X chromosome, typically males are afflicted more often and/or more severely than females. That is because in females who are heterozygous for such an X-linked trait, there is a normal version of the gene to compensate. Males have only one X chromosome, so if a X-linked gene is mutated, it usually has a severe effect. X-linked genetic disorders include **hemophilia** and red-green **color blindness**.

Chromosome abnormalities, such as the addition or deletion of a chromosome, may result from errors that occur when gametes (sperm and egg) are formed, during fertilization, or during the early development of the zygote. Most chromosome aberrations are lethal, resulting in spontaneous **abortion** (miscarriage), or death in **infancy**. Only a few, including the extra copy of chromosome 21 that results in **Down syndrome**, produces individuals who, although affected by mental and physical abnormalities, can survive into adulthood.

Genetic testing

Definition

A genetic test seeks to identify changes in a person's chromosomes, genes, or proteins that are associated with inherited disorders. Genetic testing is performed to determine if a person has or will develop a certain disease or could pass a disease to his or her offspring. Genetic tests also determine whether or not couples are at a higher risk than the general population for having a child affected with a genetic disorder.

Purpose

Some families or ethnic groups have a higher incidence of a certain disease than does the population as a whole. For example, individuals from Eastern European Ashkenazi Jewish descent are at higher risk for carrying genes for rare conditions that occur much less frequently in populations from other parts of the world. Before having a child, a couple from such a family or ethnic group may want to know if their child would be at risk of having that disease. Genetic testing for this type of purpose is called genetic screening.

During pregnancy, the baby's cells can be studied for certain **genetic disorders** or chromosomal problems, such as **Down syndrome**. Chromosome testing is most commonly offered when the mother is 35 years or older at the time of delivery. When there is a family medical history of a genetic disease or there are individuals in a family affected with developmental and physical delays, genetic testing may also be offered during pregnancy. Genetic testing during pregnancy is called prenatal diagnosis.

Prior to becoming pregnant, couples who are having difficulty conceiving a child or who have suffered multiple miscarriages may be tested to see if a genetic cause can be identified.

A genetic disease may be diagnosed at **birth** by doing a physical evaluation of the baby and observing characteristics of the disorder. Genetic testing can help to confirm the diagnosis made by the physical evaluation. In addition, genetic testing is used routinely on all newborns to screen for certain genetic diseases which can affect a newborn baby's health shortly after birth.

There are several genetic diseases and conditions in which the symptoms do not occur until adulthood. One such example is Huntington's disease. This is a serious disorder affecting the way in which individuals walk, talk and function on a daily basis. Genetic testing may be able to determine if someone at risk for the disease will in fact develop the disease.

Some genetic defects may make a person more susceptible to certain types of **cancer**. Testing for these defects can help predict a person's risk. Other types of genetic tests help diagnose and predict and monitor the course of certain kinds of cancer, particularly leukemia and lymphoma.

Description

Gene tests

Gene tests look for signs of a disease by examining DNA taken from a person's blood, body fluids or tissues. The tests can look for large changes, such as a gene that has a section missing or added, or small changes, such as a missing, added, or altered chemical base within the DNA strand. Other important changes can be genes with too many copies, genes that are too active, genes that are turned off, or those that are lost entirely.

Various techniques are used for gene tests. Direct DNA sequencing examines the direct base pair sequence of a gene for specific gene mutations. Some genes contain more than 100,000 bases; a mutation of any one base can make the gene nonfunctional and cause disease. The more mutations possible, the less likely it is for a test to detect all of them. This test is usually done on white blood cells from a person's blood, but can also be performed on other tissues. There are different ways in which to perform direct DNA mutation analysis. When the specific genetic mutation is known, it is possible to perform a complete analysis of the genetic code, also called direct sequencing. There are several different lab techniques used to test for a direct mutation. One common approach begins by using chemicals to separate DNA from the rest of the cell. Next, the two strands of DNA are separated by heating. Special enzymes (called restriction enzymes) are added to the single strands of DNA; they then act like scissors and cut the strands in specific places. The DNA fragments are then sorted by size through a process called electrophoresis. A special piece of DNA, called a probe, is added to the fragments. The probe is designed to bind to specific mutated portions of the gene. When bound to the probe, the mutated portions appear on x-ray film with a distinct banding pattern.

Another gene test technique is indirect DNA testing. Family linkage studies are done to study a disease when the exact type and location of the genetic alteration is not known, but the general location on the chromosome has been identified. These studies are possible when a chromosome marker has been found associated with a disease. Chromosomes contain certain regions that vary in appearance between individuals. These regions are called polymorphisms and do not cause a genetic disease to occur. If a polymorphism is always present in family members with the same genetic disease and absent in family members without the disease, it is likely that the gene responsible for the disease is near that polymorphism. The gene mutation can be indirectly detected in family members by looking for the polymorphism.

To look for the polymorphism, DNA is isolated from cells in the same way it is for direct DNA mutation analysis. A probe is added that will detect the large polymorphism on the chromosome. When bound to the probe, this region will appear on x–ray film with a distinct banding pattern. The pattern of banding of a person being tested for the disease is compared to the pattern from a family member affected by the disease.

Linkage studies have disadvantages not found in direct DNA mutation analysis. These studies require multiple family members to participate in the testing. If key family members choose not to participate, the incomplete family history may make testing other members useless. The indirect method of detecting a mutated gene also causes more opportunity for error.

Chromosome tests

Various genetic syndromes are caused by structural chromosome abnormalities. To analyze a person's chromosomes, his or her cells are allowed to grow and multiply in the laboratory until they reach a certain stage of growth. The length of growing time varies with the type of cells. Cells from blood and bone marrow take one to two days; fetal cells from amniotic fluid take 7–10 days.

When the cells are ready, they are placed on a microscope slide using a technique to make them burst open, spreading their chromosomes. The slides are stained, and the stain creates a banding pattern unique to each chromosome. Under a microscope, the chromosomes are counted, identified, and analyzed based on their size, shape, and stained appearance.

Types of chromosome tests include the karyotype test and the FISH (fluorescent in situ hybridization) test. In a karyotype test, the chromosomes are counted, and a photograph is taken of the chromosomes from one or more cells as seen through the microscope. Then the chromosomes are cut out and arranged side-by-side with their partner in ascending numerical order, from largest to smallest. The karyotype is done either manually or using a computer attached to the microscope. The FISH test identifies specific regions on chromosomes using fluorescent DNA probes. FISH analysis can find small pieces of chromosomes that are missing or have extra copies and that can be missed by the karyotype test.

Biochemical tests

Genes contain instructions for making proteins and abnormal protein levels can be indicative of a genetic disorder. Biochemical tests look at the level of key proteins. This level can identify genes that are not working normally. These types of tests are typically used for **newborn screening**. For example, this screening can detect infants who have metabolic conditions such as **phenylketonuria** (PKU).

Applications of genetic testing

Newborn screening

In the United States, genetic testing is used most often for newborn screening, a major public health program which can find disorders in newborns that have long-term health effects. Newborn screening tests infant blood samples for abnormal or missing gene products. Every year, millions of newborn babies have their blood samples tested for potentially serious genetic diseases. As of 2009, newborn screening programs were testing for disorders that can cause infectious disease, premature **death**, hearing disorders, and heart problems. A new technology called tandem mass spectrometry allows screening of up to 30 other metabolic disorders.

Carrier testing

An individual who has a gene associated with a disease but never exhibits any symptoms of the disease is called a carrier. A carrier is a person who is not affected by the mutated gene he or she possesses, but can pass the gene to an offspring. Genetic tests have been developed that tell prospective parents whether or not they are carriers of certain diseases. If one or both parents are a carrier, the risk of passing the disease to a child can be predicted.

To predict the risk, it is necessary to know if the gene in question is autosomal or sex-linked. If the gene is carried on any one of chromosomes 1–22, the resulting disease is called an autosomal disease. If the gene is carried on the X or Y chromosome, it is called a sex-linked disease.

Sex-linked diseases, such as the bleeding condition **hemophilia**, are usually carried on the X chromosome. A woman who carries a disease-associated gene on one of her X chromosomes has a 50% chance of passing that gene to her son. A son who inherits that gene will develop the disease because he does not have another normal copy of the gene on a second X chromosome to compensate for the abnormal copy. A daughter who inherits the disease-associated gene from her mother will be at risk for having a son affected with the disease.

The risk of passing an autosomal disease to a child depends on whether the gene is dominant or recessive. A prospective parent carrying a dominant gene has a 50% chance of passing the gene to a child. A child needs to receive only one copy of the mutated gene to be affected by the disease.

If the gene is recessive, a child needs to receive two copies of the mutated gene, one from each parent, to be affected by the disease. When both parents are carriers, their child has a 25% chance of inheriting two copies of the mutated gene and being affected by the disease; a 50% chance of inheriting one copy of the mutated gene, and being a carrier of the disease but not affected; and a 25% chance of inheriting two normal genes. When only one parent is a carrier, a child has a 50% chance of inheriting one mutated gene and being an unaffected carrier of the disease and a 50% chance of inheriting two normal genes.

Cystic fibrosis is a disease that affects the lungs and pancreas and is discovered in early childhood. It is the most common autosomal recessive genetic disease found in the Caucasian population: one in 25 people of Northern European ancestry are carriers of a mutated cystic fibrosis gene. The gene, located on chromosome 7, was identified in 1989.

The gene mutation for cystic fibrosis is detected by a direct DNA test. Over 600 mutations of the cystic fibrosis gene have been found; each of these mutations cause the same disease. Tests are available for the most common mutations. Tests that check for the 86 of the most common mutations in the Caucasian population will detect 90% of carriers for cystic fibrosis. (The percentage of mutations detected varies according to the individual's ethnic background). If a person tests negative, it is likely, but not guaranteed, that he or she does not have the gene. Both parents must be carriers of the gene to have a child with cystic fibrosis.

Tay-Sachs disease, also autosomal recessive, affects children primarily of Ashkenazi Jewish descent. Children with this disease usually die between the ages of two and five. This disease was previously detected by looking for a missing enzyme. The mutated gene has now been identified and can be detected using direct DNA mutation analysis.

Presymptomatic testing

Not all genetic diseases show their effect immediately at birth or early in childhood. Although the gene mutation is present at birth, some diseases do not appear until adulthood. If a specific mutated gene responsible for a late-onset disease has been identified, a person from an affected family can be tested before symptoms appear.

Huntington disease is one example of a late-onset autosomal dominant disease. Its symptoms of mental confusion and abnormal body movements do not appear until middle to late adulthood. The chromosome location of the gene responsible for Huntington chorea was located in 1983 after studying the DNA from a large Venezuelan family affected by the disease. Ten years later the gene was identified. A test is now available to detect the presence of the expanded base pair sequence responsible for causing the disease. The presence of this expanded sequence means the person will develop the disease.

Another late onset disease, Alzheimer's, does not have as well an understood genetic cause as Huntington disease. The specific genetic cause of Alzheimer's disease is not as clear. Although many cases appear to be inherited in an autosomal dominant pattern, many cases exist as single incidents in a family. Like Huntington, symptoms of mental deterioration first appear in adulthood. Genetic research has found an association between this disease and genes on four different chromosomes. The validity of looking for these genes in a person without symptoms or without family history of the disease is still being studied.

CANCER SUSCEPTIBILITY TESTING Cancer can result from an inherited (germline) mutated gene or a gene that mutated sometime during a person's lifetime (acquired mutation). Some genes, called tumor suppressor genes, produce proteins that protect the body from cancer. If one of these genes develops a mutation, it is unable to produce the protective protein. If the second copy of the gene is normal, its action may be sufficient to continue production, but if that gene later also develops a mutation, the person is vulnerable to cancer. Other genes, called oncogenes, are involved in the normal growth of cells. A mutation in an oncogene can cause too much growth, which is the beginning of cancer.

Direct DNA tests are currently available to look for gene mutations identified and linked to several kinds of cancer. People with a family history of these cancers are those most likely to be tested. If one of these mutated genes is found, the person is more susceptible to developing the cancer. The likelihood that the person will develop the cancer, even with the mutated gene, is not always known because other genetic and environmental factors are also involved in the development of cancer.

Cancer susceptibility tests are most useful when a positive test result can be followed with clear treatment options. In families with familial polyposis of the colon, testing a child for a mutated APC gene can reveal whether or not the child needs frequent monitoring for the disease. In families with potentially fatal familial medullary thyroid cancer or multiple endocrine neoplasia type 2, finding a mutated RET gene in a child provides the opportunity for that child to have preventive removal of the thyroid gland. In the same way, MSH1 and MSH2 mutations can reveal which members in an affected family are vulnerable to familiar colorectal cancer and would benefit from aggressive monitoring.

In 1994, a mutation linked to early-onset familial breast and ovarian cancer was identified. BRCA1 is located on chromosome 17. Women with a mutated form of this gene have an increased risk of developing breast and ovarian cancer. A second related gene, BRCA2, was later discovered. Located on chromosome 13, it also carries increased risk of breast and ovarian cancer. Although both genes are rare in the general population, they are slightly more common in women of Ashkenazi Jewish descent.

When a woman is found to have a mutation in one of these genes, the likelihood that she will get breast or ovarian cancer increases, but not to 100%. Other genetic and environmental factors influence the outcome.

Testing for these genes is most valuable in families where a mutation has already been found. BRCA1 and BRCA2 are large genes; BRCA1 includes 100,000 bases. More than 120 mutations to this gene have been discovered, but a mutation could occur in any one of the bases. Studies show tests for these genes may miss 30% of existing mutations. The rate of missed mutations, the unknown disease likelihood in spite of a positive result, and the lack of a clear preventive response to a positive result make the value of this test for the general population uncertain.

Prenatal and postnatal chromosome analysis

Chromosome analysis is performed on fetal cells primarily when the mother is age 35 or older at the time of delivery, has experienced multiple miscarriages, or reports a family history of a genetic abnormality. Prenatal testing is done on the fetal cells from a chorionic villus sampling (from the baby's developing placenta) at 10–12 weeks or from the amniotic fluid (the fluid surrounding the baby) at 16–18 weeks of pregnancy. Cells from amniotic fluid grow for 7–10 days before they are ready to be analyzed. Chorionic villi cells have the potential to grow faster and can be analyzed sooner.

Chromosome analysis using blood cells is done on a child who is born with or later develops signs of **mental retardation** or physical malformation. In the older child, chromosome analysis may be done to investigate developmental delays.

Extra or missing chromosomes cause mental and physical abnormalities. A child born with an extra chromosome 21 (trisomy 21) has Down syndrome. An extra chromosome 13 or 18 also produce well known syndromes. A missing X chromosome causes **Turner syndrome** and an extra X in a male causes **Klinefelter syndrome**. Other abnormalities are caused by extra or missing pieces of chromosomes. **Fragile X syndrome** is a sex-linked disease that causes mental retardation in males.

Chromosome material may also be rearranged, such as the end of chromosome 1 moving to the end of chromosome 3. This is called a chromosomal translocation. If no material is added or deleted in the exchange, the person may not be affected. Such an exchange, however, can cause infertility or abnormalities if passed to children.

Evaluation of a man and woman's infertility or repeated miscarriages will include blood studies of both to check for a chromosome translocation. Many chromosome abnormalities are incompatible with life; babies with these abnormalities often miscarrry during the first trimester. Cells from a baby that died before birth can be studied to look for chromosome abnormalities that may have caused the death.

Diagnostic testing

This type of genetic testing is used to confirm a diagnosis when a person has signs or symptoms of a genetic disease. The genetic test used depends on the disease for which a person is tested. For example, if a patient has physical features indicative of Down syndrome, a chromosomal test is used. To test for Duchenne **muscular dystrophy**, a gene test is done to look for missing sections in the dystrophin gene.

Chromosome tests are also used to diagnose certain cancers, particularly leukemia and lymphoma, which are associated with changes in chromosomes: extra or missing complete chromosomes, extra or missing portions of chromosomes, or exchanges of material (translocations) between chromosomes. Studies show that the locations of the chromosome breaks are at locations of tumor suppressor genes or oncogenes.

Chromosome analysis on cells from blood, bone marrow, or solid tumor helps diagnose certain kinds of leukemia and lymphoma and often helps predict how well the person will respond to treatment. After treatment has begun, periodic monitoring of these chromosome changes in the blood and bone marrow gives the physician information as to the effectiveness of the treatment.

A well-known chromosome rearrangement is found in chronic myelogenous leukemia. This leukemia is associated with an exchange of material between chromosomes 9 and 22. The resulting smaller chromosome 22 is called the Philadelphia chromosome.

Pharmacogenetic testing

Among the latest types of genetic testing is pharmacogenetic testing. This test examines a person's genes to gain information on how drugs would be broken down by the body. Pharmacogenetic testing aims to design drug treatments that are specific to each person. For example, a test used in patients who have chronic myelogenous leukemia can show which patients would benefit from a medicine called Gleevac. Another test looks at a liver enzyme called cytochrome P450, which breaks down certain types of drugs. Gene mutations can affect the ability of the body to break down certain drugs and people with a less active form of P450 might be taking excessive levels of a drug. Pharmacogenetic testing seeks to help patients obtain the right amount of a medication.

Precautions

Because genetic testing is not always accurate and because there are privacy concerns for the individual receiving a genetic test, genetic counseling should always be performed prior to genetic testing. A genetic counselor is an individual with a master's degree in genetic counseling. A medical geneticist is a physician specializing and board certified in genetics.

A genetic counselor reviews the person's family history and medical records and the reason for the test. The counselor explains the likelihood that the test will detect all possible causes of the disease in question (known as the sensitivity of the test) and the likelihood that the disease will develop if the test is positive (known as the positive predictive value of the test).

Learning about the disease in question, the benefits and risks of both a positive and a negative result, and what treatment choices are available if the result is positive will help prepare the person undergoing testing. During the genetic counseling session, the individual interested in genetic testing will be asked to consider how the test results will affect his or her life, family, and future decisions.

After this discussion, the person should have the opportunity to indicate in writing that he or she gave informed consent to have the test performed, verifying that the counselor provided complete and understandable information.

A variety of genetic tests are now increasingly being offered directly to consumers, usually over the Internet. Such genetic testing usually involves scraping a few cells from inside the cheek and mailing the sample to a test laboratory, where the test is performed. People considering such genetic tests, should discuss the issue with their health-care provider or a genetic counselor.

Preparation

Most tests for genetic diseases of children and adults are done on blood. To collect the 5–10 mL of blood needed, a healthcare worker draws blood from a vein in the inner elbow region. Collection of the sample takes only a few minutes.

KEY TERMS

Autosomal disease—A disease caused by a gene mutation located on a chromosome other than a sex chromosome.

Karyotype—A photomicrograph (picture taken through a microscope) of a person's 46 chromosomes, lined up in 23 pairs, that is used to identify some types of genetic disorders.

Oncogene—A gene that causes normal cell growth, but if mutated or expressed at high levels, encourages normal cells to change into cancerous cells.

Sex-linked genetic disorder—A disease or disorder caused by a gene mutation located on the X (female) or Y (male) chromosome.

Translocation—The rearrangement or exchange of segments of chromosomes that does not alter the total number of chromosomes, but sometimes results in a genetic disorder or disease.

Prenatal testing is done either on amniotic fluid or a chorionic villus sampling. To collect amniotic fluid, a physician performs a procedure called **amniocentesis**. An ultrasound is done to find the baby's position and an area filled with amniotic fluid. The physician inserts a needle through the woman's skin and the wall of her uterus and withdraws 5–10 mL of amniotic fluid. Placental tissue for a chorionic villus sampling is taken through the cervix. Each procedure takes approximately 30 minutes.

Bone marrow is used for chromosome analysis in a person with leukemia or lymphoma. The person is given local anesthesia. Then the physician inserts a needle through the skin and into the bone (usually the sternum or hip bone). One-half to 2 mL of bone marrow is withdrawn. This procedure takes approximately 30 minutes.

Aftercare

After blood collection the person can feel discomfort or bruising at the puncture site or may become dizzy or faint. Pressure to the puncture site until the bleeding stops reduces bruising. Warm packs to the puncture site relieve discomfort.

The chorionic villus sampling, amniocentesis, and bone marrow procedures are all done under a physician's supervision. The person is asked to rest after the procedure and is watched for weakness and signs of bleeding.

Risks

Collection of amniotic fluid and chorionic villus sampling have the risk of miscarriage, infection, and bleeding; the risks are higher for the chorionic villus sampling. Because of the potential risks for miscarriage, 0.5% following the amniocentesis and 1% following the chorionic villus sampling procedure, both of these prenatal tests are offered to couples, but not required. A woman should tell her physician immediately if she has cramping, bleeding, fluid loss, an increased temperature, or a change in the baby's movement following either of these procedures.

After bone marrow collection, the puncture site may become tender and the person's temperature may rise. These are signs of a possible infection.

Genetic testing involves other nonphysical risks. Many people **fear** the possible loss of privacy about personal health information. Other family members may be affected by the results of a person's genetic test. Privacy of the person tested and the family members affected is a consideration when deciding to have a test and to share the results.

A positive result carries a psychological burden, especially if the test indicates the person will develop a disease later in life, such as Huntington's chorea. The news that a person may be susceptible to a specific kind of cancer, while it may encourage positive preventive measures, may also negatively shadow many decisions and activities.

A genetic test result may also be inconclusive, meaning no definitive result can be given to the individual or family. This may cause the individual to feel more anxious and frustrated and experience psychological difficulties.

Prior to undergoing genetic testing, individuals need to learn from the genetic counselor the likelihood that the test could miss a mutation or abnormality.

Results

A normal result for chromosome analysis is 46, XX or 46, XY. This means there are 46 chromosomes (including two X chromosomes for a female or one X and one Y for a male) with no structural abnormalities. A normal result for a direct DNA mutation analysis or linkage study includes no gene mutations found.

There can be some benefits from genetic testing when the individual tested is not found to carry a genetic mutation. Those who learn with great certainty they are no longer at risk for a genetic disease may choose not to undergo prophylactic therapies and may feel less anxious and relieved.

An abnormal chromosome analysis report will include the total number of chromosomes and will identify the abnormality found. Tests for gene mutations will report the mutations found.

There are many ethical issues to consider with an abnormal prenatal test result. Many of the diseases tested for during a pregnancy cannot be treated or cured. In addition, some diseases tested for during pregnancy may have a late-onset of symptoms or have minimal effects on the affected individual.

Before making decisions based on an abnormal test result, the person should meet again with a genetic counselor to fully understand the meaning of the results, learn what options are available based on the test results and what are the risks and benefits of each of those options.

Resources

BOOKS

Betta, Michella, ed. *The Moral, Social, and Commercial Imperatives of Genetic Testing and Screening: The Australian Case*. New York, NY: Springer, 2006.

Hart, Anne. *How to Safely Tailor Your Food, Medicines, & Cosmetics to Your Genes: A Consumer's Guide to Genetic Testing Kits from Ancestry to Nourishment*. Lincoln, NE: iUniverse, 2003.

Institute of Medicine of the National Academies. *Cancer–Related Genetic Testing and Counseling: Workshop Proceedings*.Washington, DC: National Academies Press, 2007.

Lemmens, Trudo, et al. *Reading the Future?: Legal and Ethical Challenges of Predictive Genetic Testing*. Montreal, Quebec, Canada: Editions Themis, 2007.

Sharpe, Neil F., and Ronald F. Carter. *Genetic Testing: Care, Consent and Liability*. New York, NY: Wiley-Liss, 2006.

Teichler, Doris Zallen. *To Test or Not To Test: A Guide to Genetic Screening and Risk*. Piscataway, NJ: Rutgers University Press, 2008.

PERIODICALS

Bandelt, H. J. "The Brave New Era of Human Genetic Testing." *Bioessays* 30-no. 11–12 (November 2008): 1246–1251.

Borry, P., et al. "Predictive Genetic Testing in Minors for Adult-Onset Genetic Diseases." *Mount Sinai Journal of Medicine* 75-no. 3 (May–June 2008): 287–296.

Clarke, A. J., and C. Gaff. "Challenges in the Genetic Testing of Children for Familial Cancers." *Archives of Disease in Childhood* 93-no. 11 (November 2008): 911–9141.

Goodeve, A. "Molecular Genetic Testing of Hemophilia A." *Seminars in Thrombosis and Hemostasis* 34-no. 6 (September 2008): 4911–501.

Innes, A. Micheil. "Molecular Genetic Testing and Genetic Counseling." *Handbook of Clinical Neurology* 87 (2007): 517–531.

Kuehn, B. M. "Risks and Benefits of Direct-to-Consumer Genetic Testing Remain Unclear." *Journal of the American Medical Association* 300-no. 13 (October 2008): 1503–1505.

Rich, T. A., and M. Salazar. "Genetic Risk Assessment, Counseling and Testing." *Surgical Oncology Clinics of North America* 18-no. 1 (January 2009): 19–38.

Tutt, A., and A. Ashworth. "Can Genetic Testing Guide Treatment in Breast Cancer?" *European Journal of Cancer* 44-no. 18 (December 2008): 2774–2780.

Valente, E. M., et al. "Genetic Testing for Pediatric Neurological Disorders." *Lancet Neurology* 7-no. 12 (December 2008): 1113–1126.

OTHER

Human Genome Project Information. "Pharmacogenitics." http://www.ornl.gov/sci/techresources/Human_Genome/medicine/pharma.shtml (accessed February 3, 2010).

March of Dimes. "Your First Tests." http://www.marchofdimes.com/pnhec/159_519.asp (accessed February 3, 2010).

National Human Genome Research Institute. "Frequently Asked Questions About Genetic Testing." http://www.genome.gov/19516567 (accessed February 3, 2010).

———. "Genetic Testing." http://www.genome.gov/10002335 (accessed February 3, 2010).

National Institutes of Health. "Genetic Testing." http://www.nlm.nih.gov/medlineplus/genetictesting.html (accessed February 3, 2010).

ORGANIZATIONS

EuroGentest, Gasthuisberg O&N, Herestraat 49, Box 602, Leuven, Belgium, 3000, (+32)16 345860, (+32) 16 34599, http://www.eurogentest.org.

March of Dimes Foundation, 1275 Mamaroneck Avenue, White Plains, NY, 10605, (914) 428-7100, (888) MODIMES (663-4637), (914) 428-8203, askus@marchofdimes.com, http://www.marchofdimes.com.

National Office of Public Health Genomics, 4770 Buford Highway Mailstop K-89, Atlanta, GA, (770) 488-8510, (770) 488-8355, genetics@cdc.gov, http://www.cdc.gov/genomics.

National Society of Genetic Counselors, 401 N. Michigan Ave., Chicago, IL, 60611, (312) 321-6834, (312) 673-6972, nsgc@nsgc.org, http://www.nsgc.org.

Katherine S. Hunt, MS
Brenda W. Lerner

Genital herpes

Definition

Genital herpes is a sexually transmitted disease caused by a herpes virus. The disease is characterized by the formation of fluid-filled, painful blisters in the genital area.

Description

Genital herpes (herpes genitalis, herpes progenitalis) is characterized by the formation of fluid-filled blisters on the genital organs of men and women. The word "herpes" comes from the Greek adjective *herpestes,* meaning *creeping,* which refers to the serpent-like pattern that the blisters may form. Genital herpes is a sexually transmitted disease, which means that it is spread from person to person only by sexual contact. Herpes may be spread by vaginal, anal, or oral sexual activity. It is not spread by objects (such as a toilet seat or doorknob), swimming pools, hot tubs, or through the air.

Genital herpes is a disease resulting from an infection by a **herpes simplex** virus. There are eight different kinds of human herpes viruses. Only two of these, herpes simplex types 1 and 2, can cause genital herpes. It has been commonly believed that herpes simplex virus type 1 infects above the waist (causing **cold sores**) and herpes simplex virus type 2 infects below the waist (causing genital sores). This is not completely true. Both herpes virus type 1 and type 2 can cause herpes lesions on the lips or genitals, but recurrent cold sores are almost always type 1. The two viruses seem to have evolved to infect better at one site or the other, especially with regard to recurrent disease.

To determine the occurrence of herpes type 2 infection in the United States, the Centers for Disease Control and Prevention (CDC) used information from a survey called the National Health and Nutrition Examination Survey III (1988–1994). This survey of 40,000 noninstitutionalized people found that 21.9% of persons age 12 or older had antibodies to herpes type 2. This means that 45 million people in the United States have been exposed at some point in their lives to herpes simplex virus type 2. More women (25.6%) than men (17.8%) had antibodies. The racial differences for herpes type 2 antibodies were whites, 17.6%; blacks, 45.9%; and Mexican Americans, 22.3%. Interestingly, only 2.6% of adults reported that they have had genital herpes. Over half (50% to 60%) of the white adults in the United States have antibodies to herpes simplex virus type 1. The occurrence of antibodies to herpes type 1 is higher in blacks.

Viruses are different from bacteria. While bacteria are independent and can reproduce on their own, viruses cannot reproduce without the help of a cell. Viruses enter human cells and force them to make more virus. A human cell infected with herpes virus releases thousands of new viruses before it is killed. The cell **death** and resulting tissue damage causes the actual sores. The highest risk for spreading the virus is the time period beginning with the appearance of blisters and ending with scab formation.

Herpes virus can also infect a cell and instead of making the cell produce new viruses, it hides inside the cell and waits. Herpes virus hides in cells of the nervous system called "neurons." This is called "latency." A latent virus can wait inside neurons for days, months, or even years. At some future time, the virus "awakens" and causes the cell to produce thousands of new viruses which causes an active infection. Sometimes an active infection occurs without visible sores. Therefore, an infected person can spread herpes virus to other people even in the absence of sores.

This process of latency and active infection is best understood by considering the genital sore cycle. An active infection is obvious because sores are present. The first infection is called the "primary" infection. This active infection is then controlled by the body's **immune system,** and the sores heal. In between active infections, the virus is latent. At some point in the future latent viruses become activated and once again cause sores. These are called "recurrent infections" or "outbreaks." Genital sores caused by herpes type 1 recur much less frequently than sores caused by herpes type 2.

Although it is unknown what triggers latent viruses to activate, several conditions seem to bring on infections. These include illness, tiredness, exposure to sunlight, **menstruation**, skin damage, food allergy, and hot or cold temperatures. Although many people believe that stress can bring on their genital herpes outbreaks, there is no scientific evidence that there is a link between stress and recurrences. However, at least one clinical study has shown a connection between how well people cope with stress and their belief that stress and recurrent infections are linked.

Newborn babies who are infected with herpes virus experience a very severe, and possibly fatal disease. This is called "neonatal herpes infection." In the United States, 1 in 3,000–5,000 babies born will be infected with herpes virus. Babies can become infected during passage through the **birth** canal, but can become infected during the pregnancy if the membranes rupture early. Doctors will perform a **Cesarean section** on women who go into labor with active genital herpes.

Causes and symptoms

While anyone can be infected by herpes virus, not everyone will show symptoms. Risk factors for genital herpes include early age at first sexual activity, multiple sexual partners, and a medical history of other sexually-transmitted diseases.

Most patients with genital herpes experience a prodrome (symptoms of oncoming disease) of **pain**, burning, **itching**, or **tingling** at the site where blisters will form. This prodrome stage may last anywhere from a few hours to one to two days. The herpes infection prodrome can occur for both the primary infection and recurrent infections. The prodrome for recurrent infections may be severe and cause a severe burning or stabbing pain in the genital area, legs, or buttocks.

Primary genital herpes

The first symptoms of herpes usually occur within two to seven days after contact with an infected person, but may take up to two weeks to appear. Symptoms of the primary infection are usually more severe than those of recurrent infections. For up to 70% of the patients, the primary infection causes symptoms which affect the whole body (called "constitutional symptoms"), including tiredness, **headache**, **fever**, chills, muscle aches, and loss of appetite, as well as painful, swollen lymph nodes in the groin. These symptoms are greatest during the first three to four days of the infection and disappear within one week. The primary infection is more severe in women than in men.

Following the prodrome are the herpes blisters, which are similar on men and women. First, small red bumps appear. These bumps quickly become fluid-filled blisters. In dry areas, the blisters become filled with pus and take on a white to gray appearance, become covered with a scab, and heal within two to three weeks. In moist areas, the fluid-filled blisters burst and form painful ulcers which drain before healing. New blisters may appear over a period of one week or longer and may join together to form very large ulcers. The pain is relieved within two weeks and the blisters and ulcers heal without scarring by three to four weeks.

Women can experience a very severe and painful primary infection. Herpes blisters first appear on the labia majora (outer lips), labia minora (inner lips), and entrance to the vagina. Blisters often appear on the clitoris, at the urinary opening, around the anal opening, and on the buttocks and thighs. In addition, women may get herpes blisters on the lips, breasts, fingers, and eyes. The vagina and cervix are almost always involved which causes a watery discharge. Other symptoms that occur in women are: painful or difficult urination (83%), swelling of the urinary tube (85%), **meningitis** (36%), and throat infection (13%). Most women develop painful, swollen lymph nodes (lymphadenopathy) in the groin and pelvis. About 1 in 10 women get a vaginal yeast infection as a complication of the primary herpes infection.

In men, the herpes blisters usually form on the penis but can also appear on the scrotum, thighs, and buttocks. Fewer than half of the men with primary herpes experience the constitutional symptoms. Thirty percent to 40% of men have a discharge from the urinary tube. Some men develop painful swollen lymph nodes (lymphadenopathy) in the groin and pelvis. Although less frequently than women, men also may experience painful or difficult urination (44%), swelling of the urinary tube (27%), meningitis (13%), and throat infection (7%).

Recurrent genital herpes

One or more outbreaks of genital herpes per year occur in 60–90% of those infected with herpes virus. About 40% of the persons infected with herpes simplex virus type 2 will experience six or more outbreaks each year. Genital herpes recurrences are less severe than the primary infection; however, women still experience more severe symptoms and pain than men. Constitutional symptoms are not usually present. Blisters will appear at the same sites during each outbreak. Usually there are fewer blisters, less pain, and the time period from the beginning of symptoms to healing is shorter than the primary infection. One out of every four women experience painful or difficult urination during recurrent infection. Both men and women may develop lymphadenopathy.

Diagnosis

Because genital herpes is so common, it is diagnosed primarily by symptoms. It can be diagnosed and treated by the family doctor, dermatologists (doctors who specialize in skin diseases), urologists (doctors who specialize in the urinary tract diseases of men and women and the genital organs of men), gynecologists (doctors who specialize in the diseases of women's genital organs) and infectious disease specialists. The diagnosis and treatment of this infectious disease should be covered by most insurance providers.

Laboratory tests may be performed to look for the virus. Because healing sores do not shed much virus, a sample from an open sore would be taken for viral culture. A sterile cotton swab would be wiped over open sores and the sample used to infect human cells in culture. Cells that are killed by herpes virus have a certain appearance under microscopic examination. The results of this test are available within 2–10 days. Other areas that may be sampled, depending upon the disease symptoms in a particular patient, include the urinary tract, vagina, cervix, throat, eye tissues, and cerebrospinal fluid.

Direct staining and microscopic examination of the lesion sample may also be used. A blood test may be performed to see if the patient has antibodies to herpes virus. The results of blood testing are available within one day. The disadvantage of this blood test is that it usually does not distinguish between herpes type 1 and 2, and only determines that the patient has had a herpes infection at some point in his or her life. Therefore, the viral culture test must be performed to be absolutely certain that the sores are caused by herpes virus.

Because genital sores can be symptoms of many other diseases, the doctor must determine the exact cause of the sores. Tests are performed to determine that herpes virus is causing the genital sores. Other diseases which may cause genital sores are syphilis, chancroid, lymphogranuloma venereum, granuloma inguinale, herpes zoster, erythema multiform, Behçet's syndrome, inflammatory bowel disease, **contact dermatitis**, **candidiasis**, and **impetigo**.

Because most newborns who are infected with herpes virus were born to mothers who had no symptoms of infection, it is important to check all newborn babies for symptoms. Any skin sore should be sampled to determine if it is caused by herpes simplex. Babies should be checked for sores in their mouth and for signs of herpes infection in their eyes.

Treatment

There is no cure for herpes virus infections. There are **antiviral drugs** available which have some effect in lessening the symptoms and decreasing the length of herpes outbreaks. There is evidence that some may also prevent future outbreaks. These antiviral drugs work by interfering with the replication of the viruses and are most effective when taken as early in the infection process as possible. For the best results, drug treatment should begin during the prodrome stage before blisters are visible. Depending on the length of the outbreak, drug treatment could continue for up to 10 days.

Acyclovir (Zovirax) is the drug of choice for herpes infection and can be given intravenously, taken by mouth (orally), or applied directly to sores as an ointment. Acyclovir has been in use for many years and only 5 out of 100 patients experience side effects. Side effects of acyclovir treatment include nausea, **vomiting**, itchy rash, and **hives**. Although acyclovir is the recommended drug for treating herpes infections, other drugs may be used including famciclovir (Famvir), valacyclovir (Valtrex), vidarabine (Vira-A), idoxuridine (Herplex Liquifilm, Stoxil), trifluorothymidine (Viroptic), and penciclovir (Denavir).

Acyclovir is effective in treating both the primary infection and recurrent outbreaks. When taken intravenously or orally, acyclovir reduces the healing time, virus shedding period, and duration of vesicles. The standard oral dose of acyclovir for primary herpes is 200 mg five times daily or 400 mg three times daily for a period of 10 days. Recurrent herpes is treated with the same doses for a period of five days. Intravenous acyclovir is given to patients who require hospitalization because of severe primary infections or herpes complications such as aseptic meningitis or sacral ganglionitis (inflammation of nerve bundles).

Patients with frequent outbreaks (greater than six to eight per year) may benefit from long term use of acyclovir which is called "suppressive therapy." Patients on suppressive therapy have longer periods between herpes outbreaks. The specific dosage used for suppression needs to be determined for each patient and should be reevaluated every few years. Alternatively, patients may use short term suppressive therapy to lessen the chance of developing an active infection during special occasions such as weddings or holidays.

There are several things that a patient may do to lessen the pain of genital sores. Wearing loose fitting clothing and cotton underwear is helpful. Removing clothing or wearing loose pajamas while at home may reduce pain. Soaking in a tub of warm water and using a blow dryer on the "cool" setting to dry the infected area is helpful. Putting an ice pack on the affected area for 10 minutes, followed by five minutes off and then repeating this procedure may relieve pain. A zinc sulfate ointment may help to heal the sores. Application of a baking soda compress to sores may be soothing.

Neonatal herpes

Newborn babies with herpes virus infections are treated with intravenous acyclovir or vidarabine for 10 days. These drugs have greatly reduced deaths and increased the number of babies who appear normal at one year of age. However, because neonatal herpes infection is so serious, even with treatment babies may not survive, or may suffer nervous system damage. Infected babies may be treated with long-term suppressive therapy.

Alternative treatment

An imbalance in the amino acids lysine and arginine is thought to be one contributing factor in herpes virus outbreaks. A ratio of lysine to arginine that is in balance (that is more lysine than arginine is present) seems to help the immune system work optimally. Thus, a diet that is rich in lysine may help prevent recurrences of genital herpes. Foods that contain high levels of lysine include most vegetables, legumes, fish, turkey, beef, lamb, cheese, and chicken. Patients may take 500 mg of lysine daily and increase to 1,000 mg three times a day during

KEY TERMS

Groin—The region of the body that lies between the abdomen and the thighs.

Latent virus—A nonactive virus that is in a dormant state within a cell. Herpes virus is latent in cells of the nervous system.

Prodrome—Symptoms which warn of the beginning of disease. The herpes prodrome consists of pain, burning, tingling, or itching at a site before blisters are visible.

Recurrence—The return of an active herpes infection following a period of latency.

Ulcer—A painful, pus-draining depression in the skin caused by an infection.

an outbreak. Intake of the amino acid arginine should be reduced. Foods rich in arginine that should be avoided are chocolate, peanuts, almonds, and other nuts and seeds.

Clinical experience indicates a connection between high stress and herpes outbreaks. Some patients respond well to stress reduction and relaxation techniques. Acupressure and massage may relieve tiredness and stress. Meditation, **yoga**, tai chi, and hypnotherapy can also help relieve stress and promote relaxation.

Some herbs, including echinacea (*Echinacea* spp.) and garlic (*Allium sativum*), are believed to strengthen the body's defenses against viral infections. Red marine algae (family Dumontiaceae), both taken internally and applied topically, is thought to be effective in treating herpes type I and type II infections. Other topical treatments may be helpful in inhibiting the growth of the herpes virus, in minimizing the damage it causes, or in helping the sores heal. Zinc sulphate ointment seems to help sores heal and to fight recurrence. Lithium succinate ointment may interfere with viral replication. An ointment made with glycyrrhizinic acid, a component of licorice (*Glycyrrhiza glabra*), seems to inactivate the virus. Topical applications of vitamin E or tea tree oil (*Melaleuca* spp.) help dry up herpes sores. Specific combinations of homeopathic remedies may also be helpful treatments for genital herpes.

Prognosis

Although physically and emotionally painful, genital herpes is usually not a serious disease. The primary infection can be severe and may require hospitalization for treatment. Complications of the primary infection may involve the cervix, urinary system, anal opening, and the nervous system. Persons who have a decreased ability to produce an immune response to infection (called "immunocompromised") due to disease or medication are at risk for a very severe, and possibly fatal, herpes infection. Even with antiviral treatment, neonatal herpes infections can be fatal or cause permanent nervous system damage.

Prevention

The only way to prevent genital herpes is to avoid contact with infected persons. This is not an easy solution because many people aren't aware that they are infected and can easily spread the virus to others. Avoid all sexual contact with an infected person during a herpes outbreak. Because the herpes virus can be spread at any time, condom use is recommended to prevent the spread of virus to uninfected partners.

Resources

BOOKS

Ebel, Charles. *Managing Herpes: How to Live and Love With a Chronic STD.* American Social Health Association, 1998.

Belinda Rowland, PhD

Genital warts

Definition

Genital **warts**, which are also called condylomata acuminata or venereal warts, are growths in the genital area caused by a sexually transmitted papillomavirus. A papillomavirus is a virus that produces papillomas, or benign growths on the skin and mucous membranes.

Description

Genital warts are the most common sexually transmitted disease (STD) in the general population. It is estimated that 1% of sexually active people between the ages of 18 and 45 have genital warts; however, polymerase chain reaction (PCR) testing indicates that as many as 40% of sexually active adults carry the human papillomavirus (HPV) that causes genital warts.

Genital warts vary somewhat in appearance. They may be either flat or resemble raspberries or cauliflower in appearance. The warts begin as small red or pink growths and grow as large as four inches across, interfering with intercourse and **childbirth**. The warts grow in the moist tissues of the genital areas. In women, they occur on the external genitals and on the walls of the vagina and cervix; in men, they develop in the urethra and on the shaft of the penis. The warts then spread to the area behind the genitals surrounding the anus.

Risk factors for genital warts include:

- multiple sexual partners
- infection with another STD
- pregnancy
- anal intercourse
- poor personal hygiene
- heavy perspiration

Causes and symptoms

There are about 80 types of human papillomavirus. Genital warts are caused by HPV types 1, 2, 6, 11, 16, and 18. HPV is transmitted by sexual contact. The incubation period varies from one to six months.

The symptoms include bleeding, **pain**, and odor as well as the visible warts.

Diagnosis

The diagnosis is usually made by examining scrapings from the warts under a darkfield microscope. If the warts are caused by HPV, they will turn white when a 5% solution of white vinegar is added. If the warts reappear, the doctor may order a biopsy to rule out **cancer**.

Treatment

No treatment for genital warts is completely effective because therapy depends on destroying skin infected by the virus. There are no drugs that will kill the virus directly.

Medications

Genital warts were treated until recently with applications of podophyllum resin, a corrosive substance that cannot be given to pregnant patients. A milder form of podophyllum, podofilox (Condylox), has been introduced. Women are also treated with 5-fluorouracil cream, bichloroacetic acid, or trichloroacetic acid. All of these substances irritate the skin and require weeks of treatment.

Genital warts can also be treated with injections of interferon. Interferon works best in combination with podofilox applications.

KEY TERMS

Condylomata acuminata—Another name for genital warts.

Papilloma—A benign growth on the skin or mucous membrane. Viruses that cause these growths are called human papillomaviruses (HPVs).

Podophyllum resin—A medication derived from the May apple or mandrake and used to treat genital warts.

Surgery

Surgery may be necessary to remove warts blocking the patient's vagina, urethra, or anus. Surgical techniques include the use of liquid nitrogen, electrosurgery, and laser surgery.

Prognosis

Genital warts are benign growths and are not cancerous by themselves. Repeated HPV infection in women, however, appears to increase the risk of later cervical cancer. Women infected with HPV types 16 and 18 should have yearly cervical smears. Recurrence is common with all present methods of treatment—including surgery—because HPV can remain latent in apparently normal surrounding skin.

Prevention

The only reliable method of prevention is sexual abstinence. The use of **condoms** minimizes but does not eliminate the risk of HPV transmission. The patient's sexual contacts should be notified and examined.

Resources

BOOKS

Foster, David C. "Vulvar and Vaginal Disease." In *Current Diagnosis*, edited by Rex B. Conn, et al., Vol. 9. Philadelphia: W. B. Saunders Co., 1997.

MacKay, H. Trent. "Gynecology." In *Current Medical Diagnosis and Treatment, 1998,* edited by Stephen McPhee, et al., 37th ed. Stamford: Appleton & Lange, 1997.

Rebecca J. Frey, PhD

GERD *see* Gastroesophageal reflux disease

Germ cell tumors

Definition

Germ cell tumors (GCTs) are solid tumors that are diagnosed in children, adolescents, and, less frequently, in adults. The term germ cell tumor alludes to the term "germinate" rather than to the term "germ" as it relates to bacterial or other related organisms that are capable of causing disease. These tumors arise from germ cells that develop into reproductive tissue such as testicular and ovarian cells. GCTs can be benign tumors or malignant (cancerous) tumors.

Demographics

The incidence of GCTs appears to be increasing. Malignant germ cell tumors account for about 3% of all cases of **cancer** occurring in children and adolescents prior to age 20 years. Malignant GCTs are more commonly diagnosed in adolescents between the ages of 15 and 19 years and account for about 14% of all cancers which occur in this age group.

Description

GCTs appear to arise from primitive germs cells. During embryo development, these germ cells migrate from the yolk sac down the midline of the body to the pelvis and eventually to the gonads, or reproductive organs. During fetal development, some of the cells may migrate to abnormal sites other than the gonads, however. Therefore, GCTs are classified as gonadal GCTs or extragonadal GCTs, meaning they occur in tissues that are not reproductive tissue. About 90% of GCTs are gonadal in origin.

Malignant GCTs can be further histologically classified according to the origin of the tumor. In young children, GCTs are classified as yolk sac tumors, which can arise from extragonadal, ovarian, or testicular tissue, or dysgerminoma, which arises from ovarian tissue and is rarely diagnosed in young children. In adolescents and in young adults, malignant GCTs can be classified as follows:

- seminoma-germinomas which arise from testicular tissue
- dysgerminoma-germinomas which arise from ovarian tissue
- germinoma-extagonadal origin
- yolk sac tumor-extragonadal, ovarian and testicular origin; also termed endodermal sinus tumors
- choriocarcinoma-extragonadal, ovarian, and testicular origin; a rare tumor type
- embryonal carcinoma-arises from testicular tissue
- mixed germ cell tumors-arises from extragonadal and ovarian tissue

Testicular and mediastinal seminomas are most likely to be diagnosed in adolescent and young adult males, while ovarian dysgerminomas are more likely to be diagnosed in adolescent and young adult females. Most children who are diagnosed with a malignant GCT are most likely to have a yolk sac component to their tumors.

Some of the malignant GSTs secrete abnormal proteins such as alpha-fetaprotein (AFP) and beta–human chorionic gonadotropin (b-HCG) which are considered to be tumor markers. For example, yolk sac tumors secrete AFP while germinomas (such as seminoma and dysgerminoma) and choriocarcinomas produce b-HCG. Serum levels of these tumor markers can be monitored during treatment to determine the response of the tumor to the treatment.

Risk factors

Specific risk factors related to the development of GCTs have not been identified. However, patients diagnosed with certain genetic or hereditary syndromes or disorders appear to be at higher risk for the development of some types of GCTs. For example, individuals with **Klinefelter syndrome** appear to be at increased risk for the development of extragonadal GCT and patients with Swyer syndrome may be at increased risk for the development of germinomas.

Causes and symptoms

The specific cause of most cases of GCTs is unknown at this time. Some individuals with certain genetic or hereditary syndromes and disorders appear to be at higher risk for the development of some types of GCTs. In addition, several chromosomal abnormalities are being studied to determine their exact role in causing GCTs.

Symptoms of GCTs are linked to the size and location of the tumor. Symptoms may include:

- a swelling or mass of tissue that can be palpated
- abnormal shape or size of the testicle
- excessive hair growth
- early puberty
- hormonal abnormalities such as diabetes
- headache
- weakness in the lower extremities
- constipation

KEY TERMS

Embryo—the human organism in the earliest stages of development.

Extragonadal—occurring outside of the gonads or outside of the reproductive organs.

Gonads—the reproductive organs; testes in males and ovaries in females.

Histology—the study of the structure, composition, and function of tissues of organs.

Tumor marker—a biochemical substance produced and released or secreted by a tumor.

Yolk sac—a sac made of membranous tissue which is attached to the embryo and which provides nutrition to the embryo.

Diagnosis

Examination

A complete history and physical examination will be conducted. The suspected tumor mass will be examined and palpated. A focused assessment and examination will be conducted based on the location of the suspected tumor.

Tests

Levels of tumor markers, such as AFP and b-HCG should be assessed prior to surgical intervention. Lactate dehydrogenase levels will also be determined. Tests which should be conducted prior to **chemotherapy** administration include a complete blood count (CBC) with differential and **platelet count**; tests to determine baseline **kidney function**, such as the glomerular filtration rate and creatinine clearance rate; uric acid levels; **liver function** tests; and electrolyte levels as well as the levels of calcium and magnesium in the body.

Radiologic procedures which may be utilized include chest xray and magnetic imaging scanning (MRI) to evaluate for metastasis to the lungs, computed tomography (CT) and/or MRI scanning of the abdomen and/or pelvis if a tumor is suspected in those locations, and bone scans to further determine the extent of metastasis. Other tests that may be done, depending on the location of the tumor, include CT or MRI scans of the brain, ultrasounds of the abdomen and pelvis, testicular ultrasounds, and positron emission tomography (PET) scans to detect relapse of tumor. In addition, **pulmonary function tests** may be done to establish baseline pulmonary function prior to the start of chemotherapy administration.

Treatment

Treatment for these relatively rare types of cancer should be conducted at pediatric cancer centers experienced in treating GCTs. Factors which play a role in determining optimum treatment for GCTs include the histology of the tumor, tumor stage, the location of the primary tumor, and the patient's age. Clinicians treating these children and adolescents will attempt to maximize the potential for survival while attempting to minimize the risk for adverse long-term side effects, such as the development of second cancers, and other serious physical and cognitive impairments.

Currently, multimodality therapy is utilized including surgery and administration of chemotherapy. Based on the factors described above, treatment options may include:

- surgical removal of the tumor followed by strict surveillance for tumor relapse
- biopsy of the tumor to obtain a definitive diagnosis, followed by preoperative chemotherapy administration which includes a platinum-based chemotherapy drug, followed by surgical removal of all remaining tumor
- surgical removal of the tumor followed by platinum–based chemotherapy administration.

Currently, the standard chemotherapy regimen for children and adults diagnosed with malignant nonseminomatous GCTs includes the drugs cisplatin, etoposide and bleomycin. However, children are given fewer doses of bleomycin than adults.

There are different treatment options for malignant testicular GCTs in boys than for adolescents and young adult males which vary by stage of disease at the time of diagnosis and age of the patient. Treatment options for childhood ovarian GCT includes a multimodality approach which may utilize surgery, observation, and chemotherapy. Current standard treatment options for childhood malignant extragonadal GCTs varies by patient age, tumor location, tumor histology, and stage at time of diagnosis and may include surgery and chemotherapy administration.

Prognosis

The five-year survival rate for gonadal GCTs increased from 89% to 98% in children younger than age 15 years between 1975 and 2002 according to the National Cancer Institute. The five-year survival rate for adolescents diagnosed with gonadal GCTs between the ages of 15 and 19 years increased from 70% to 95% during that same time.

The five-year survival rate for extragonadal GCTs increased from 42% to 83% in children younger than age 15 years between 1979 and 2002. The five-year survival rate for adolescents between the ages of 15 and 19 years increased from 80% to 95% during that same time period.

Prevention

As the cause of most cases of childhood GCTs is not currently known, there are no ways to prevent development of GCTs. Children diagnosed with specific congenital or hereditary syndromes or disorders which increase their risk of developing GCTs should be screened for GCTs.

Resources

PERIODICALS

Horton, Z., M. Schlatter, and S. Schultz. "Pediatric Germ Cell Tumors." *Surgical Oncology* (2007); 16(3): 205–13.

McIntyre, A., et al. "Genes, Chromosomes, and the Development of Testicular Germ Cell Tumors of Adolescents and Adults." *Genes Chromosomes and Cancer* (2008); 47(7): 547–57.

OTHER

Adkins, E. S. "Teratomas and Other Germ Cell Tumors." eMedicine. May 29, 2008, http://www.emedicine.medscape.com (accessed September 5, 2010).

"Childhood Extracranial Germ Cell Tumors Treatment (PDQ)." National Cancer Institute. June 24, 2010, http://www.cancer.gov (accessed September 5, 2010).

ORGANIZATIONS

Candlelighters Childhood Cancer Family Alliance, 8323 Southwest Freeway, Suite 435, Houston, Texas, 77074, (713) 270-4700, (713) 270-9802, http//www.candle.org.

CureSearch for Children's Cancer, National Childhood Cancer Foundation, 4600 East West Highway, Suite 600, Bethesda, MD, 20814-3457, (800)458–6223 (U.S. and Canada), info@curesearch.org, http://www.curesearch.org.

Genetic and Rare Disease Information Center (GARD), P.O. Box 8126, Gaithersburg, MD, 20898-8126, (888) 205-2311, (301) 251-4911, http://www.rarediseases.info.nih.gov/GARD.

St. Jude's Children's Research Hospital, 262 Danny Thomas Place, Memphis, TN, 38105, (901) 595-3300, http://www.stjude.org.

Melinda Granger Oberleitner, RN, DNS, APRN, CNS

German measles ***see* Rubella**

Gesell developmental schedules

Definition

The Gesell Developmental Schedules are timetables of developing skills for infants, toddlers, and preschoolers. They evaluate physical or motor and **language development** and adaptive and personal-social behaviors by observing a child's performance on a variety of tasks at specific ages. The Gesell Developmental Schedules strongly influenced subsequent tests and assessments of child development.

Purpose

The Gesell Developmental Schedules delineated the normal sequences of physical, cognitive, emotional, and social development in infants and young children, in order to identify developmental deficits and delays. For decades they were one of the most widely used assessments for detecting neurological problems, such as **cerebral palsy** in infants, and cognitive and social difficulties in young children, so that early intervention could be initiated. The Schedules continue to be used by pediatricians, child psychologists, and other child development professionals.

The Gesell Developmental Schedules serve as a basis for predicting and evaluating children's performances on various other tests and assessments that were developed by psychologist Arnold Gesell and his colleagues at the Gesell Institute of Human Development. In particular, the Schedules have been used to predict future performance on the Gesell Preschool Test and the Gesell School Readiness Test (GSRT).

Although the Gesell Developmental Schedules are no longer as widely used as in previous decades, they are still frequently used in research studies and have served as an important prototype for newer assessments of physical, cognitive, emotional, and social development in infants and children. These assessments have become increasingly important in recent years, as the focus has shifted from the study of normal development to the identification and evaluation of infants who are at risk for developmental delays. This is because advances in medical technologies have led to the survival of ever-increasing numbers of premature and medically challenged infants with cerebral palsy and developmental disabilities. Infant assessments are now most often used for identifying developmental delays, determining eligibility for early intervention services, and assessing whether interventions are effective in improving rates of development. Newer assessments that were significantly influenced by the Gesell Developmental Schedules include the Denver Developmental Screening Test (DDST) for children from **birth** to age six and the Early Language Milestone (ELM) Scale for children from birth to age three.

Description

The Gesell Developmental Schedules were first introduced in 1925 and have undergone periodic revisions. They provide a standardized procedure for observing and measuring the motor, cognitive, language, and social developmental progress of infants and children from four weeks of age to six years.

The Gesell Developmental Schedules evaluate typical behaviors that develop at specified ages. The tasks in the assessments are based on natural home and clinic situations and utilize objects and activities that are appealing to infants and young children. Examples include assessing:

- gross-motor skills by a baby reaching for an object or a toddler beginning to walk
- fine-motor skills by an infant grasping a string or a preschooler using scissors
- language development by a baby saying "da-da" upon seeing her daddy or a toddler using short sentences
- adaptive behavior by a baby pulling a string to reach a ring
- personal-social behavior by a toddler pushing his arm through a shirt sleeve or a five-year-old tying a bow

Two–six-year-olds

Between the ages of two and six years, the Gesell Developmental Schedules assess skills at six-month intervals. Task accomplishments at specified ages on the Motor Schedule include:

- age two—running, walking up and down stairs, kicking a large ball, turning the pages of a book
- age two-and-a-half—attempting to stand on one foot, holding crayons with fingers
- age three—walking on tiptoe, riding a tricycle, alternating feet on the stairs
- ages three to three-and-a-half—jumping down and landing on the feet
- age three-and-a-half—standing and hopping on one foot
- age four—skipping on one foot, catching a bean bag
- age four-and-a-half—overhand throwing with a bean bag
- age five—skipping with alternating feet
- age six—standing alternately on each foot, advanced catching and throwing with a bean bag
- ages three to six—successively longer broad jumps, placing pellets in a bottle of increasingly smaller openings

Tasks on the Adaptive Schedule include:

- age two—building a tower with six cubes, placing blocks separately on a formboard
- age two-and-a-half—building a tower of ten cubes, aligning two or more cubes, placing one color form, drawing V and H strokes by imitation
- age three—imitating a bridge with cubes, copying a circle, counting three objects, placing three color forms
- age three-and-a-half—building a bridge with cubes, copying a cross
- age four—imitating a gate with cubes, counting four objects
- age four-and-a-half—building a gate with cubes from a model, copying a square, recognizing one or two letters and numbers
- age five—printing first name, counting 10 objects, calculating within five
- ages five to five-and-a-half—copying a triangle
- age five-and-a-half—counting 12 objects
- ages six to six-and-a-half—printing first and last name, counting 13 or more objects, adding and subtracting within 10
- ages two-and-a-half to six—adding increasing numbers of body parts to a human figure
- ages three to six—placing pellets in a bottle of increasingly smaller openings

Tasks on the Language Schedule include:

- age two—using three-word sentences and "I," "me," and "you"
- age two-and-a-half—giving first name and gender in an interview, using one or two prepositions correctly, seven correct answers on a picture vocabulary
- age three—using plurals, knowing one's age, answering a comprehension question
- age three-and-a-half—knowing number of siblings, using four correct prepositions
- age four-and-a-half—non-infantile articulation, naming siblings, answering three comprehension questions
- age five—giving first and last name and 15 correct answers on a picture vocabulary
- age five-and-a-half—knowing month of birthday
- ages six to six-and-a-half—knowing birth date and 16 correct answers on a picture vocabulary

- ages three to six—repeating increasingly long series of numbers

Tasks on the Personal-Social Schedule include:

- age two—verbalizing the need to use the toilet, pulling on a simple garment, referring to self by name, temperamentally gentle and easy
- age two-and-a-half—helping to put toys away, using "me," using repetition, putting on coat, temperamentally opposite extremes
- age three—feeding self, pouring from a pitcher, putting on shoes, unbuttoning clothes, asking questions, understanding taking turns, knowing a few rhymes, temperamentally cooperative
- age three-and-a-half—washing and drying hands and face, using "I," using the toilet consistently, temperamentally vulnerable
- age four—buttoning clothes, brushing teeth, dressing and undressing with supervision, lacing shoes, performing errands outside the home, going out-of-bounds, asking "why" questions, temperamentally expansive
- age four-and-a-half—telling imaginative stories, temperamentally unpredictable
- age five—tying a bow, dressing and undressing, asking meaning of words, temperamentally gentle and friendly
- age five-and-a-half—identifying pennies and nickels
- age six—tying shoelaces, knowing morning and night and left and right, reciting numbers up to the 30s, temperamentally oppositional and emotional
- ages two to five-and-a-half—increasingly complex and cooperative play

Preschool and School Readiness Tests

The Gesell Preschool Test, which is administered individually to children aged two to six, involves tasks and activities similar to those in the Developmental Schedules:

- Oral tests—for assessing language skills, attention span, and personal knowledge—involve children talking about themselves and their families, naming animals, and relating their favorite activities.
- Pencil-and-paper activities, to evaluate fine-motor skills, handedness, neuromuscular development, and task-appropriate behaviors, include writing their names, copying geometric shapes, writing numbers, and completing a drawing.
- Children build increasingly complex structures with cubes to assess fine-motor skills, hand-eye coordination, and attention span.
- Other tasks include repeating numbers, recognizing shapes, and discriminating among prepositions.

Gesell believed that school readiness depends on the level of a child's inherent maturation processes. The Gesell School Readiness Test (GSRT) and the Gesell Developmental **Assessment** (GDA), another version of the Readiness Test, have been widely used to place children aged four to nine in kindergarten through the third grade. The Readiness Test consists of the Preschool Test and additional visual exercises, matching and drawing tests, and a labeling and naming exercise. During the 1980s and 1990s, the GSRT was used extensively in decisions about whether a child should enter kindergarten, remain at home for another year, or enter a developmental or early-five kindergarten. Many children were held back from school as a result of their performance on the GSRT and some states raised the minimum age for kindergarten entry on the basis of statewide GSRT scores.

Origins

Arnold Lucius Gesell (1880–1961), a U.S. psychologist and **pediatrician**, pioneered scientific research into child development. After earning a Ph.D. from Clark University in 1906, Gesell received his M.D. degree from Yale University in 1915. There he founded the Yale Clinic of Child Development, which eventually evolved into the Gesell Institute of Child Development, the premier center in the United States for the study of childhood development and behavior. Gesell directed the Institute from 1911 until his **death**.

Although Gesell's early research focused on developmentally disabled children, he came to believe that it was essential to first understand normal infant and child development. He was one of the first to develop methods of observation and measurement for quantifying infant and child development by age. He observed the responses of infants and children to stimulating objects, such as cubes, pellets, and bells. Beginning in the 1920s, Gesell filmed some 12,000 children, analyzing their responses and behaviors frame-by-frame.

Gesell's research led to his maturational philosophy—the concept that infants and children proceed through predetermined stages of mental development, comparable to sequential physical development, and that their progress through these stages can be quantitatively assessed. Although Gesell did not dismiss environmental effects on child development, he stressed biological imperatives that determined the maturational processes. Gesell believed that normal children all proceed through the same sequence of stages, albeit at somewhat varying rates. This provided a basis for comparing children and determining their school readiness. Thus, Gesell believed that children learned to read when they had reached a specific stage of mental development or mental age, whereas **literacy** research in the decades since Gesell has led to the conclusion that children learn to read, not only when they are developmentally ready to read, but also because of specific pre-reading experiences.

Over the years, in addition to the Developmental Schedules, Preschool Test, and GSRT, Gesell produced the Gesell Child Development Age Scale (GCDAS), the Gesell Developmental Observation, which determines developmental age for grade placement and formulation of instructional programs, and the Gesell System of Developmental Diagnosis. These measures were used in child development centers throughout the United States for most of the twentieth century. Gesell also authored and co-authored books on **infancy**, childhood, and **adolescence** that were widely read by parents and had a major impact on child-rearing practices during the 1940s and 1950s. Gesell devoted much of his energy to arousing public support for preschool education, better **foster care** for orphans, and **special education** for physically and mentally disabled children.

Results

The data from the Gesell Developmental Schedules were used to calculate the Gesell Development Quotient (DQ). Although Gesell did not believe that the DQ was a measure of **intelligence**, for a time it was widely taken as such, and many studies have indicated that the Developmental Schedules are effective for screening infants for risks of cognitive delays. The DQ is no longer used, and later researchers have argued that Gesell's conclusions about child development were based on studies of relatively few children, all of whom were white and middle class, from a single New England city. Researchers have further argued that Gesell underestimated both individual variations in development and cultural influences on child behavior. Nevertheless, comparisons among well-trained observers showed high agreement in the scoring of the Developmental Schedules. The Developmental Schedules have been used to evaluate children's performances on other Gesell tests and to assign children an overall developmental age (DA).

Parental concerns

Although the Gesell Developmental Schedules have proved to be exceptionally useful over the decades, more recent research has revealed their limits and they are no longer widely used for school placement. Although numerous studies have found

KEY TERMS

Adaptive behavior—The ability to accomplish tasks on one's own and adapt to and function in one's environment.

Cerebral palsy—Brain damage before, during, or just after birth that results in lack of muscle coordination and problems with speech.

Cognitive—Conscious intellectual activity, including thinking, imagining, reasoning, remembering, and learning.

Denver Developmental Screening Test (DDST)—A widely used developmental assessment for children from birth to age six.

Developmental quotient (DQ)—A measure of child development, derived from a child's age, as determined by test scores, divided by chronological age and multiplied by 100.

Early Language Milestone (ELM) Scale—A tool for assessing language development in children under age three.

Fine-motor skills—Control of the smaller muscles of the body, especially in the hands, feet, and head, for activities such as writing and drawing.

Gesell Preschool Test—An adaptation of the Gesell Developmental Schedules that measures relative maturity of preschool-age children in four basic areas of behavior.

Gesell School Readiness Test (GSRT)—A test developed by Arnold Gesell for assessing whether a child has reached a mental age that is adequate for success in school.

Gross-motor skills—Control of the large muscles of the body, including the arms, legs, back, abdomen, and torso, for activities such as sitting, crawling, walking, and running.

Intelligence quotient (IQ)—An expression of apparent relative intelligence; the ratio of mental age, as determined by a standardized test, relative to chronological age and multiplied by 100; a score on a standardized intelligence test relative to the average performance of others of the same age.

Mental age—A psychological test measure of an individual's mental attainment in terms of the number of years it would take an average child to reach that level.

Standardized—A test with established procedures and norms that serve as the standard for future test results.

strong correlations between scores on the GSRT and both **IQ** scores and academic achievement, other studies have found that the Gesell assessments routinely underestimate children's abilities. Some of the measures on the Schedules, such as **temperament**, are subjective and much more susceptible to individual variations than indicated by the Schedules. Undiagnosed visual or other perceptual problems, as well as individual differences in developmental rates, can result in children being assigned inappropriately low DAs.

Resources

BOOKS

Gesell School Age Assessment Kit. New Haven, CT: Gesell Institute of Human Development, 1978–1980.

The Gesell Developmental Observation. New Haven, CT: Gesell Institute of Human Development, 2007.

Walker, Richard N. *The Revised Gesell Preschool Examination Manual.* New Haven, CT: Gesell Institute of Human Development, 1991.

OTHER

"Gesell Developmental Schedules." Gesell Institute of Human Development. 1979, http://www.gesellinstitute.org/pdf/GesellSchedules.pdf (accessed October 5, 2010).

ORGANIZATIONS

Fair Test: The National Center for Fair and Open Testing, 15 Court Square, Suite 820, Boston, MA, 02108, (857) 350-8207, (857) 350-8209, http://www.fairtest.org.

Gesell Institute of Human Development, 310 Prospect St., New Haven, CT, 06511, (203) 777-3481, (800) 369-7709, (203) 776-5001, info@gesellinstitute.org, http://www.gesellinstitute.org.

Margaret Alic, PhD

Gingivitis *see* **Periodontal disease**

Gluten sensitive enteropathy *see* **Celiac disease**

GMRT *see* **Gates-MacGinitie reading tests (GMRT)**

Gonadal dysgenesis *see* **Turner syndrome**

Gonorrhea

Definition

Gonorrhea is a highly contagious sexually transmitted infection (STI) or disease (STD) caused by the bacterium *Neisseria gonorrhoeae*. These bacteria grow in the urethra and in warm, moist parts of the reproductive tract, including the cervix, uterus, and fallopian tubes of women. The bacteria also can infect the anus, mouth, throat, and eyes. Untreated gonorrhea can cause serious medical complications.

Demographics

For most of the twentieth century gonorrhea was the most common STD worldwide. The incidence of gonorrhea has declined steadily in the developed world since the mid-1970s, reaching an all-time low in 2004. This decline is largely due to increased public awareness of the risks and prevention of STDs such as herpes and HIV/AIDS. However, there are still about 200 million new cases of gonorrhea annually throughout the world, and gonorrhea rates in certain urban areas of the United States are once again on the rise.

Gonorrhea is the second most common reportable disease in the United States. More than 350,000 newly diagnosed cases were reported in 2007. Experts believe that the actual number is much higher since gonorrhea tends to be both under-diagnosed and underreported. Estimates of the actual number of annual cases in the United States range from 400,000 to one million. An estimated 40,000 pregnant women are infected with gonorrhea each year in the United States. **Pelvic inflammatory disease** (PID), the most common complication of gonorrhea, affects one million American women annually.

Although gonorrhea affects people of all ages, races, and socioeconomic levels, adolescents and young adults are at the highest risk. More than 80% of cases occur in those aged 15–29. Gonorrhea is most common among females aged 15–19 and males aged 20–24. Infection rates are higher in men than in women and highest in men who have sex with other men. African Americans and those living in urban areas and having multiple sex partners are at the greatest risk for infection.

Description

Commonly called "the clap," gonorrhea is transmitted through sexual contact, including oral, anal, and vaginal intercourse. The risk of contracting gonorrhea from a single sexual encounter with an infected partner is 60–90%. Gonorrhea also can be spread through contact with the bodily fluids of an infected person. There is some evidence for transmission of gonorrhea among children and from adults to children via unclean hands. However, gonorrhea infection in children is considered a warning flag for **sexual abuse**.

Gonorrhea usually affects the genitourinary tract, but can also spread to the rectum, throat, and eyes. Left untreated, gonorrhea can spread through the bloodstream and infect the reproductive system, joints, heart valves, skin, liver, and brain. As many as 10% of women infected with gonorrhea experience a pregnancy in a fallopian tube (ectopic pregnancy) or become infertile as a result of a PID. Gonorrhea also increases the risk of contracting and transmitting HIV/AIDS. Being cured of gonorrhea does not protect a person against re-infection.

Pregnant women with untreated gonorrhea are at increased risk for miscarriage, preterm **birth**, or membranes that rupture prematurely. An infected mother can transmit the disease to her infant as it passes through the birth canal during delivery, causing newborn conjunctivitis—an eye infection that can lead to blindness. The infant also is at risk for joint infection or a life-threatening blood infection.

Risk factors

Risk factors for gonorrhea are similar to those for other STDs. The primary risk factors are unprotected sex (without a condom) with multiple partners.

Causes and symptoms

Gonnorrhea is caused by the bacterium *N. gonorrhoeae*, which is transmitted through sexual contact. It can be transmitted to the eyes by touching an infected organ and then touching the eyes. *N. gonorrhoeae* cannot survive for any length of time outside of the human body. It cannot be transmitted via a toilet seat or by shaking hands.

Although most gonorrhea-infected males have symptoms, as many as 80% of infected females do not. Symptoms usually appear between 1 and 14 days following infection, but the incubation period can be as long as 30 days. Often the only symptom of gonorrhea is inflammation of mucous membranes in the genital region. Some people experience nausea, **vomiting**, **fever**, chills, and **pain** during intercourse.

In males the infection usually appears first in the urethra—the tube that carries urine and sperm to the outside of the body. About 95% of infected men have thick, cloudy, white, yellowish, green, or bloody discharge from the penis. Other common symptoms in males include frequent urination and burning or pain during urination. Complications of gonorrhea in males can affect the prostate, testicles, and surrounding glands. Epididymitis is a painful condition of the testicles that can lead to sterility if untreated.

In females gonorrhea usually infects the cervix—the lower narrow portion of the uterus that opens to the vagina—as well as the uterus and fallopian tubes. Symptoms can include:

- vaginal discharge that may be cloudy and yellow
- frequent, painful, or burning urination
- bleeding between menstrual periods (breakthrough bleeding or spotting)
- pain or bleeding during vaginal intercourse
- heavy bleeding during menstrual periods
- chronic abdominal pain

Women are more likely than men to suffer from complications of gonorrhea because the disease often progresses without symptoms. The most common complication of untreated gonorrhea is PID, which can occur in as many as 40% of infected women. PID can damage the ovaries and fallopian tubes, resulting in a pregnancy developing outside of the uterus or sterility. A less common complication is disseminated gonococcal infection (DGI), in which the bacteria travels through the blood to distant sites such as the skin or joints.

Newborn **conjunctivitis** caused by gonorrhea usually appears two to seven days after birth. Symptoms of eye infection include redness, **itching**, or discharge from the eye. Other symptoms of gonorrhea in infants and children include irritation, redness, swelling, or a pus-like discharge from the urethra and possibly painful urination.

Anal gonorrheal infection may cause rectal itching, discharge, a constant urge to move the bowels, painful bowel movements, or blood in the stool. However about 90% of anal infections are without symptoms. Oral gonorrheal infection may cause a **sore throat** or painful swallowing.

Diagnosis

Examination

An initial diagnosis of gonorrhea is based on symptoms, sexual history, and at-risk behavior. The diagnosis may be made by a family physician or STD specialist or at a public health clinic. Women may be diagnosed by an obstetrician/gynecologist, particularly if there are gynecological complications. Men may be diagnosed by a urologist. Physicians are required to report cases of gonorrhea to public health officials. Patients are asked to provide the names of all sexual partners who may have been exposed to the infection, so that they can be notified and tested for gonorrhea.

Tests

Many physicians use more than one test to confirm a diagnosis of gonorrhea:

KEY TERMS

Cervix—The lower, narrow part—or neck—of the uterus.

Chlamydia—The most common sexually transmitted bacterial infection in the United States. It often occurs along with gonorrhea. The majority of infected women have no symptoms.

Conjunctivitis—An inflammation of the eye that can be caused by gonorrhea or chlamydia.

Ectopic pregnancy—A pregnancy that develops outside of the uterus, such as in the fallopian tubes. The fetus dies and the mother's life may be threatened.

ELISA—Enzyme-linked immunosorbent assay; a screening test that uses antibodies to detect infections such as gonorrhea and HIV.

HIV/AIDS—Human immunodeficiency virus/acquired immunodeficiency syndrome; a sexually transmitted viral disease that is more likely to be transmitted or acquired in the presence of gonorrhea or another STD.

Neisseria gonorrhoeae—The bacterium that causes gonorrhea.

Nucleic acid amplification test (NAAT)—A screening test for gonorrhea that detects bacterial DNA in a urine sample or cervical swab.

Pelvic inflammatory disease (PID)—An infection of the female upper genital tract that can be a complication of gonorrhea. At least 25% of women with PID suffer long-term consequences such as infertility or an ectopic pregnancy.

Sexually transmitted disease (STD)—A disease that is transmitted by sexual contact, including gonorrhea, chlamydia, HIV/AIDS, genital herpes, syphilis, and genital warts.

Sexually transmitted infection (STI)—An infectious disease, such as gonorrhea, that is transmitted through sexual activity.

Sterility—Inability to conceive a child.

Urethra—The urine channel leading from the bladder to the outside of the body and, in men, the channel for semen.

Urethritis—Inflammation of the urethra.

- A nucleic acid amplifications test (NAAT) that detects bacterial DNA in a urine or cervical sample is the fastest and most accurate diagnostic test.
- An enzyme-linked immunosorbent assay (ELISA) that uses antibodies specific for *N. gonorrhoeae* is also fast and sensitive.
- Culturing bacteria from a discharge or sample obtained with a cotton swab can diagnose gonorrhea and determine whether the bacteria are drug resistant. Culturing takes for up to two days.
- Discharge from an infected area can Gram stained and examined under a microscope for the presence of *N. gonorrhoeae*; however, this test is only about 70% accurate in men and about 50% accurate in women.
- Since other STDs, such as chlamydia and syphilis, often occur along with gonorrhea, patients also may be tested for these infections.

Treatment

Traditional

Gonorrhea is treated with **antibiotics**. Patients should refrain from sexual intercourse until they and their partners have completed treatment and have had follow-up testing to ensure that the infection has been completely eradicated.

Drugs

In the past gonorrhea was usually treated with penicillin, a penicillin derivative, or tetracycline. However, since the 1940s *N. gonorrhoeae* has become increasingly resistant to these antibiotics. Resistance to fluoroquinolone antibiotics also has increased rapidly over the past decade. Therefore, as of 2009, the recommended treatments for gonorrhea are:

- a single 125-mg injection of ceftriaxone
- a single 400-mg dose of oral cefixime
- another single-dose cephalosporin antibiotic

Infants born to gonorrhea-infected mothers may be treated with intravenous ceftriaxone or another antibiotic. Infant conjunctivitis caused by gonorrhea is treated with an eye ointment containing polymyxin and bacitracin, erythromycin, or tetracycline.

If chlamydial infection is also present, a combination of antibiotics—such as ceftriaxone and doxycycline or azithromycin—is used to treat both infections simultaneously. Erythromycin is used to treat chlamydia in pregnant women.

Alternative

Antibiotic treatment for gonorrhea may be complemented with various alternative therapies:

- *Lactobacillus acidophilus* (live-culture yogurt) can help replace gastrointestinal flora that are killed by the antibiotics.
- Zinc, multivitamin/mineral complexes, vitamin C, and garlic (*Allium sativum*) may help improve immune system function.
- Kelp (*Macrocystis pyrifera* and related species) can supply vitamins and minerals.
- Teas or douches made with calendula (*Calendula officinalis*), myrrh (*Commiphora molmol*), and thuja (*Thuja occidentalis*) may reduce discharge and inflammation.
- The Chinese herb *Coptis chinensis*, used for "damp-heat"; infections, can be helpful for treating the genitourinary tract, especially if PID develops.
- Various other herbs can help treat reproductive and urinary system symptoms.
- With physician approval, a three-day juice fast may help cleanse the urinary and gastrointestinal systems and support healing.
- Acupuncture or acupressure can help cleanse body systems.

Home remedies

Antibiotic treatment is absolutely essential for gonorrhea. Hot baths can help reduce pain and inflammation.

Prognosis

Gonorrhea is curable with cephalosporin antibiotics and the prognosis is excellent with prompt treatment. However, many people, especially women, have no symptoms of the disease and are unaware that they are infected. Adolescent girls are at particular risk for untreated gonorrhea. Up to 40% of women who do not receive early treatment may develop PID, which can damage the fallopian tubes and result in sterility. Women who have had PID are six to ten times more likely to have an ectopic pregnancy. Although the risk of infertility is higher for women than for men, men also can become sterile if untreated gonorrhea causes inflammation of the urethra (urethritis).

Untreated gonorrhea can cause inflammation, abscesses, and scarring. In about 2% of patients with untreated gonorrhea, the infection spreads throughout the body, causing fever, arthritis-like joint pain, and skin lesions. The bacterium also can infect the heart valves and brain. In men, untreated gonorrhea can affect the prostate, testicles, and surrounding glands.

Prevention

The best prevention for gonorrhea is sexual abstinence or sexual activity that is confined to a mutually monogamous relationship in which both partners have been tested for gonorrhea and other STDs. If used properly and consistently for vaginal and anal sex, latex male **condoms** and polyurethane female condoms can reduce the risk of *N. gonorrhoeae* transmission. A dental dam may reduce the risk of transmission during oral sex. However, anyone who has multiple sexual partners should be tested regularly for gonorrhea and other STDs. It is recommended that all sexually active teenagers and young adults be screened regularly for gonorrhea. All pregnant women should be screened at their first prenatal visit.

All newborns are treated under the eyelids with an antibiotic ointment, such as silver nitrate or erythromycin, to prevent gonorrhea. Infants born to mothers with untreated gonorrhea are given a prophylactic dose of ceftriaxone.

Resources

BOOKS

Grimes, Jill. *Seductive Delusions: How Everyday People Catch STDs.* Baltimore: Johns Hopkins University Press, 2008.

Marr, Lisa. *Sexually Transmitted Diseases: A Physician Tells You What You Need to Know,* 2nd ed. Baltimore: Johns Hopkins University Press, 2007.

Michaud, Christopher. *Gonorrhea.* New York: Rosen, 2006.

Sutton, Amy. *Sexually Transmitted Diseases Sourcebook,* 3rd ed. Detroit: Omnigraphics, 2006.

PERIODICALS

Du, Ping, et al. "Changes in Community Economic Status and Racial Distribution Associated with Gonorrhea Rates: An Analysis at the Community Level." *Sexually Transmitted Diseases* 36 no. 7 (July 2009): 430–438.

Hosenfeld, Christina B., et al. "Repeat Infection with Chlamydia and Gonorrhea Among Females: A Systematic Review of the Literature." *Sexually Transmitted Diseases* 36 no. 8 (August 2009): 478–489.

Workowski, K. A., S. M. Berman, and J. M. Douglas, Jr. "Emerging Antimicrobial Resistance in *Neisseria gonorrhoeae*: Urgent Need to Strengthen Prevention Strategies." *Annals of Internal Medicine* 148 no. 9 (April 15, 2008): 606–613.

OTHER

Behrman, Amy J., and William H. Shoff. "Gonorrhea." eMedicine Web site, http://emedicine.medscape.com/article/782913-overview

"Gonorrhea." National Institute of Allergy and Infectious Diseases, http://www3.niaid.nih.gov/topics/gonorrhea.

"Gonorrhea: Frequently Asked Questions." WomensHealth.gov Web site, http://www.womenshealth.gov/faq/gonorrhea.cfm.

"Gonorrhea: Questions and Answers." American Social Health Association, http://www.ashastd.org/learn/learn_gonorrhea.cfm.

"Gonorrhea." *Sexually Transmitted Diseases Surveillance, 2007*, http://www.cdc.gov/std/stats07/gonorrhea.htm

"Updated Recommended Treatment Regimens for Gonococcal Infections and Associated Conditions—United States, April 2007." Centers for Disease Control and Prevention, http://www.cdc.gov/std/treatment/2006/updated-regimens.htm.

ORGANIZATIONS

American Social Health Association, P.O. Box 13827, Research Triangle Park, NC, 27709, (919) 361-8400, (800) 227-8922, (919) 361-8425, info@ashastd.org, http://www.ashastd.org.

National Institute of Allergy and Infectious Diseases (NIAID), Office of Communications and Public Liaison, 6610 Rockledge Drive, Bethesda, MD, 20892-66123, (866) 284-4107, http://www3.niaid.nih.gov.

U.S. Centers for Disease Control and Prevention (CDC), 1600 Clifton Road, Atlanta, GA, 30333, 800-CDC-INFO (232-4636), cdcinfo@cdc.gov, http://www.cdc.gov.

Teresa G. Odle
Margaret Alic, PhD

Goodenough-Harris drawing test

Definition

The Goodenough-Harris Drawing Test (GHDT or G-HDT) is a widely used, projective figure-drawing test that attempts to assess **intelligence** or mental maturity in children and adolescents without relying on verbal ability. Projective tests are **psychological tests** that are based on open-ended responses to ambiguous stimuli. Figure drawing is a commonly used projective diagnostic technique.

Purpose

The GHDT is used extensively in educational and clinical settings as a fast—albeit crude—estimate of intelligence or cognitive developmental level that is not significantly influenced by other factors, such as language or cultural barriers, special needs, or **hearing impairments**. It is designed for children aged 3 years to 15 years 11 months, but is most accurately administered to children between the ages of 3 and 10 years. The GHDT is not intended as a stand-alone test. Rather, it is usually one component of a battery of assessments.

The GHDT is widely used in research studies. It also is sometimes used for purposes other than as a cognitive measure. For example, it is sometimes used as a projective personality test or as a screen for emotional disorders. It has also been used as an indicator of **schizophrenia**. However the GHDT is validated only as an intelligence test.

Description

Figure-drawing tests, such as the GHDT, require the subject to create pictures; whereas with other projective tests, such as the Rorschach and the **Thematic Apperception Test** (TAT), the subject interprets pictures. Figure-drawing tests are usually administered to children, because they are simple, familiar, and non-threatening tasks that children usually enjoy.

The GHDT can be administered individually or to groups of children. It is usually given by an educator or psychologist. The child is provided with a pencil and unlined white paper and asked to draw the best pictures possible of a man and/or woman. The GHDT includes an optional Self-Drawing Test. Each drawing is done on a separate sheet of paper. The child is specifically told to draw the entire body, rather than just the head and shoulders. Other than that, no instructions are given, and children can draw the figures however they choose. Children can erase and start over. If the test is administered individually, the child may talk to the examiner about any of the **drawings**. The GHDT is not timed, but it usually takes about 10–15 minutes to complete all three drawings.

Origins

The original Goodenough Draw-a-Man Test, for children aged 2–13, was developed by Florence Laura Goodenough (1886–1959). She introduced it in her 1926 book *Measurement of Intelligence by Drawings*. It was the first formal psychological figure-drawing test.

Florence Goodenough earned her Ph.D. in psychology with Lewis Terman at Stanford University in 1924. Terman was the developer of the Stanford-Binet test for measuring **intelligence quotient (IQ)**. Goodenough, who spent her professional career at the Institute of Child Welfare at the University of Minnesota, was particularly interested in gifted children and in methods for assessing intelligence in young children. Her Draw-a-Man Test was shown to be highly reliable and to correlate well with the standard **IQ** tests of the day. Twenty years after its introduction, the Draw-a-Man Test remained the third most popular test in use by clinical psychologists. During the course of her career, Goodenough developed other alternative assessments of intelligence, as well as the Minnesota Preschool Scale. She was the author of nine psychology textbooks.

In the late 1940s, Goodenough and her colleague, Dale B. Harris, revised and expanded the Draw-a-Man Test as the Goodenough-Harris Drawing Test and developed a detailed scoring system. Harris described their test in detail in his 1963 *Children's Drawings as Measures of Intellectual Maturity.*

Results

The GHDT provides a nonverbal measure of intellectual ability and is believe to reflect a child's cognitive maturity. GHDT scoring is based on extensive research. The drawings are scored according to 73 specified criteria, usually with one point for each detail. For example, one point is given for a head alone with no facial features. Additional points are assigned for each facial feature and article of clothing. Points are also given for the proportionality of parts. The manual includes drawing samples and the scores awarded them. The drawings also can be compared with ranked drawings—called quality scale cards—12 each for the man and the woman. Studies have indicated fairly good agreement between point scores and quality scale comparisons. Scores are totaled for each of the three drawings.

Raw scores for the Draw-a-Man and Draw-a-Woman Tests, but not for the Self-Drawing Test, are converted to standardized scores with a mean of 100 and a standard deviation of 15. The standardized scores are converted to a percentile based on the child's age and used to determine mental age. Harris re-standardized the 1926 Goodenough Draw-a-Man Test and standardized the Draw-a-Woman Test in 1963. He also included an experimental Self-Drawing Scale. The standardizations were based on the characteristics of human figure drawings made by children of different ages. The norms were based on tests of 2,622 children nationwide, from a variety of racial and ethnic groups, and rated by 11 examiners who had high inter-rater reliability. There were no significant differences between African-American and white children on the test, although there was a slight difference between Hispanics and non-Hispanics in the 15–17-year age group. Male and female norms are provided because of a slight, but statistically significant, difference between the scores for boys and girls. The average test-retest reliability of the GHDT is good and, despite the decades-old norms, the GHDT correlates well with Wechsler IQ scores. Older children score higher on

KEY TERMS

Cognitive—Conscious intellectual activity, including thinking, imagining, reasoning, remembering, and learning.

Intelligence quotient (IQ)—An expression of apparent relative intelligence; the ratio of mental age, as determined by a standardized test, relative to chronological age and multiplied by 100; a score on a standardized intelligence test relative to the average performance of others of the same age.

Mental age—A psychological test measure of an individual's mental attainment, in terms of the number of years it would take an average child to reach that level.

Norm—A standard of achievement, usually derived from the average or median achievement of a large group of a particular age.

Percentile—A rank in a population that has been divided into 100 equal groups; thus, test results in the 50th percentile indicate that half of those who took the test scored higher and half scored lower.

Personality test—Various standardized tasks that are used to determine aspects of personality or emotional status.

Projective test—A psychological test for assessing thinking patterns, observational abilities, attitudes, and feelings, based on open-ended responses to ambiguous stimuli; often used to evaluate personality disorders.

Reliability—The extent to which a test or measure yields the same results with repeated trials and different examiners.

Rorschach test—A popular projective psychological test, in which a subject's interpretation of a series of ten standard inkblots are used to assess personality and emotional traits and diagnose disorders.

Schizophrenia—A psychotic disorder characterized by loss of contact with one's environment, deterioration of everyday functioning, and personality disintegration.

Standardized—A test with established procedures and norms that serve as the standard for future test results.

Thematic Apperception Test (TAT)—A clinical psychology projective test for diagnostic, psychodynamic, and personality assessments, based on responses to black and white pictures.

Validity—The extent to which a test measures the trait that it is designed to assess.

the GHDT because of more detail and higher accuracy and scores level off at age 14 or 15, so the test has higher validity for younger children.

Many clinicians do not use the scoring system for the GHDT; rather, they rely on their own subjective estimations and interpretations. A 2006 study found that measures of children's intellectual maturity using human figure drawings agreed fairly well with teachers' assessments of the children's mental ages.

Figure-drawing tests are sometimes used to evaluate a child's self-image and personality traits, since children often project themselves into the drawings. For example, body image concerns among young girls may be reflected in their drawings. Likewise, child victims of **sexual abuse** may emphasize sexual characteristics in their drawings. However figure-drawing tests are more often used to evaluate psychological or emotional problems in adults than in children.

Parental concerns

Because it is a simple, enjoyable, non-threatening, and nonverbal evaluation, the GHDT can eliminate various sources of bias that are often present in intelligence testing. These variables can include language, hearing, verbal skills, communication deficits, and **test anxiety**. Nevertheless, several factors should be considered when interpreting GHDT results:

- Figure-drawing tests can be useful for enhancing the observations of teachers and other professionals. However results on the GHDT alone, without corroborating assessments, can be very misleading.
- As with all projective tests, scoring of figure-drawing tests, such as the GHDT, is subjective, even when an established scoring system is used.
- Differences in the instructions given to the child, in questions and answers between the child and the examiner, and in the examiner's interpretations of the drawings can make it difficult to compare results among different children, even when the scoring is identical.
- Test results can be influenced by a child's previous drawing experience. It has been suggested that this may account for a tendency of middle-class children to score higher on the GHDT than children from lower socioeconomic backgrounds.
- The correlations between GHDT scores and standard IQ scores and academic achievement tend to be low, but statistically significant, reinforcing Goodenough's original disclaimer that figure-drawing tests should not be used as substitutions for established intelligence and achievement tests.
- There is relatively little evidence to support the use of figure-drawing tests for assessing self-image or specific personality characteristics or dysfunctions.
- It is easy to over-interpret figure-drawing characteristics. Although at times the GHDT has been administered routinely for diagnosing schizophrenia, it has not been validated for that use. Nevertheless, although not all patients with schizophrenia have problems with figure drawing, it is not uncommon for schizophrenics to draw distorted figures or omit anatomical parts such as hands and eyes.

Resources

BOOKS

Goodenough, Florence. *Measurement of Intelligence by Drawings.* New York: World Book Co., 1926.

Goodenough, Florence, and Dale B. Harris. *Goodenough-Harris Drawing Test.* New York: Harcourt, Brace & World, 1963.

Harris, Dale B. *Children's Drawings as Measures of Intellectual Maturity.* New York: Harcourt, Brace & World, 1963.

Harris, Dale B., and Glenn D. Pinder. *The Goodenough-Harris Drawing Test as a Measure of Intellectual Maturity of Youths 12–17 Years, United States.* Rockville, MD: National Center for Health Statistics, 1974.

Kaplan, Robert M., and Dennis P. Saccuzzo. *Psychological Testing: Principles, Applications, and Issues.* Belmont, CA: Wadsworth, 2008.

OTHER

Fahmy, Ali. "Figure Drawings." Encyclopedia of Mental Disorders, http://www.minddisorders.com/Del-Fi/Figure-drawings.html (accessed October 7, 2010).

"Goodenough-Harris Drawing Test." Center for Equity and Excellence in Education, http://r3cc.ceee.gwu.edu/standards_assessments/EAC/eac0103.htm (accessed October 7, 2010).

Health Services and Mental Health Administration. "Intellectual Maturity of Children as Measured by the Goodenough-Harris Drawing Test: United States." Education Resources Information Center. December 1970, http://www.eric.ed.gov/PDFS/ED068532.pdf (accessed October 7, 2010).

Plucker, Jonathan. "Florence Goodenough." Human Intelligence. July 25, 2007, http://www.indiana.edu/~intell/goodenough.shtml (accessed October 7, 2010).

ORGANIZATIONS

Education Resources Information Center, ERIC Program c/o CSC, 655 15th St. NW, Suite 500, Washington, DC, 20005, (800) LET-ERIC (538-3742), http://www.eric.ed.gov.

George Washington University, Center for Equity and Excellence in Education, 1555 Wilson Blvd., Suite

515, Arlington, VA, 22209-2004, (703) 528-3588, (800) 925-3223, (703) 528-5973, ceeeinfo@ceee.gwu.edu, http://ceee.gwu.edu.

Margaret Alic, PhD

Grandparents

Definition

The parents of one's mother and father.

Description

Grandparents can play an important role in children's lives, providing love and comfort as well as stability and a sense of **family** identity. There are about 60 million grandparents in the United States as of the early 2000s, and they are playing an increasingly important role in U.S. families. Modern medical advances have given grandparents better health and longer life expectancy, allowing them to participate more fully in the lives of their grandchildren, leading to greater closeness and a larger impact on their lives. In the past, many adults didn't live long enough to spend much, if any, time with their grandchildren. Today, for the first time in history, adults in this country usually have the chance to know most of their grandchildren, and children usually know most of their grandparents. In 1900 there was only a 25 percent chance that all four grandparents of a newborn child would be alive, and the odds decreased to 2 percent by the child's fifteenth birthday. By comparison, children born in 1976 had a one in six chance of having all four grandparents alive by the time they turned 15 and a 50 percent chance of having three out of four still living.

Grandparents have a unique role to play in the life of a family. They can provide their grandchildren with comfort and companionship in a relaxed atmosphere removed from most of the disciplinary tensions that are often unavoidable between parents and children. Grandparents can be a source of refuge and strength in times of crisis. They can also help relieve some of the everyday stress faced by working couples by offering babysitting, advice, and other forms of assistance. Their own work commitments, however, keep some grandparents in their forties and fifties as busy as their children. In other cases, though, a grandparent may have precious extra time, often lacking in busy dual-career families, to spend with grandchildren, talking with and reading to them, listening to their thoughts, and perhaps accompanying them on outings, such as a trip to the movies or the zoo. Grandparents can also help defuse tensions between parents and children. If they are able to avoid taking sides, they can serve as sympathetic and insightful listeners.

In addition to increased longevity, another major factor that has led to an increased role for many grandparents is the rising **divorce** rate. Many older people will see at least one of their grown children divorce. A divorce can bring grandparents closer to both their children and grandchildren. They may be called on for help ranging from moral support, advice, and babysitting, to financial assistance and a place to live. In most cases, maternal grandparents become closer to the children following a divorce, while the children's contact with paternal grandparents often decreases. Sometimes grandparents on the noncustodial side are placed in the uncomfortable position of trying to maintain good relations with the custodial parent at the risk of alienating their own child to ensure continuing contact with the grandchildren. In the past, grandparents had few legal rights when it came to their grandchildren and they could be denied contact at the whim of a daughter- or son-in-law who had **custody**. Today grandparents in all 50 states can petition for visitation rights in the event of a divorce. Such rights may be formally included in the final divorce settlement by the parents' lawyers or granted in court by the judge. In some states grandparents also have the right to petition for custody if a court finds both parents unfit to care for a child. However, the granting of such rights is rare and generally limited to extreme cases. Also, like other aspects of custody law, laws pertaining to grandparents vary from one state to another.

In addition to those few who are legally granted custody in divorce cases, an increasing number of grandparents are informally taking over the primary responsibility for raising their grandchildren due to parental military deployment; parental imprisonment, neglect, abuse, or **abandonment**; or following the **death** of a parent. The number of grandparents assuming full-time responsibility for their grandchildren rose 41 percent between 1980 and 1994; a large part of this increase had to do with the drug epidemic of the 1980s and early 1990s. The 2000 U.S. Census reported that 4.5 million children in the United States were living with their grandparents, a 30 percent increase over 1990. These 4.5 million children represented 6.3 percent of all children in the United States under the age of 18. As many as 60 percent of children in some Native American tribes are living with grandparents, compared to 13 percent of African American, 8 percent of Hispanic, and 4 percent of Caucasian and Asian American children.

The 2000 Census was the first census to count the number of grandparents who are responsible for meeting the basic needs of grandchildren living with them. About

2.4 million grandparents fall into this category; 35 percent of them do not have either of the child's parents present in the household, and 19 percent are living at poverty level. Seventy-one percent of these grandparents are younger than 60; most either still work or have gone back to work in order to meet their grandchildren's needs.

Suddenly finding themselves with young children at home at a time when they had expected to have leisure in their lives, as well as the burden of heavier financial responsibilities, is difficult for both middle-aged and elderly grandparents. Younger grandparents may find themselves "sandwiched" between taking care of their grandchildren and caring for their own aging parents, while elderly grandparents often have given up driving because of failing eyesight or have other chronic medical problems. The situation is further complicated by the fact that the grandchildren may arrive in the grandparents' home with such preexisting problems as a history of abuse or neglect, health problems, or mental disorders related to the mother's use of drugs or alcohol during pregnancy. Even when the grandchildren have not been exposed to these problems, the speeded-up pace of historical and technological change means that the gap between generations is wider than it was in the 1950s; thus both grandparents and grandchildren may have to deal with a kind of "culture shock" when they share a household. A network of support groups for grandparents who are their grandchildren's primary caretaker, Grandparents As Parents, was begun in California in the 1980s and has spread throughout the country.

Another current demographic trend that poses a challenge for grandparents is geographic mobility, which makes for many long-distance grandparenting relationships. There are a variety of ways that grandparents who live too far away for regular visits can still remain an active and visible part of their grandchildren's lives. Occasional visits both to and from one's grandchildren are, of course, the best means for establishing and maintaining a close relationship. Whether or not this is possible, there are other ways that contact can be maintained, including letters and audio or videotapes. Imaginative ideas for keeping in touch include joint projects, such as having a grandparent and grandchild plant matching gardens and compare their progress, or take turns composing a joint story and mailing the latest installment back and forth. Parents can mail or fax the children's **drawings** and keep grandparents up to date on the youngsters' latest interests so they can treat them to age-appropriate small gifts from time to time.

One of the most important roles a grandparent can fulfill is that of historian, passing on to grandchildren a sense of family history and identity. Even seemingly ordinary details of grandparents' lives, such as descriptions of everyday life when they were young or of famous historical events they remember, can be fascinating to children. Grandparents can also share family stories. Often they remember stories the children's own parents are familiar with but have never thought of telling their children. Grandparents can leave their grandchildren (and future generations) a unique legacy by creating a record of their recollections, either written or on tape. An enhanced sense of history can be imparted by including photographs, old letters, and other souvenirs, and also by recording lullabies or other songs that are part of the family's traditions. Yet another way that a grandparent can help keep the family in touch with its roots is by creating a family tree, complete with pictures if possible.

Resources

BOOKS

Carson, Lillian. *The Essential Grandparent: A Guide for Making a Difference.* Deerfield Beach, FL: Health Communications, 1996.

Dodson, Fitzhugh. *How to Grandparent.* New York: Harper & Row, 1981.

Kornhaber, Arthur, M. D. *The Grandparent Guide: The Definitive Guide to Coping with the Challenges of Modern Grandparenting.* Chicago: Contemporary Books, 2002.

———. *The Grandparent Solution: How Parents Can Build a Family Team for Practical, Emotional, and Financial Success.* San Francisco, CA: Jossey-Bass, 2004.

PERIODICALS

Brown-Standridge, M. D., and C. W. Floyd. "Healing Bittersweet Legacies: Revisiting Contextual Family Therapy for Grandparents Raising Grandchildren in Crisis." *Journal of Marital and Family Therapy* 26 (April 2000): 185-197.

Hayslip, B., Jr., and P. L. Kaminski. "Grandparents Raising Their Grandchildren: A Review of the Literature and Suggestions for Practice." *Gerontologist* 45 (April 2005): 262-269.

Thomas, J. L., L. Sperry, and M. S. Yarbrough. "Grandparents as Parents: Research Findings and Policy Recommendations." *Child Psychiatry and Human Development* 31 (Fall 2000): 3-22.

OTHER

American Academy of Child and Adolescent Psychiatry (AACA). "Facts for Families #77." *Grandparents Raising Grandchildren.* Washington, DC: AACAP, 2000, Available at http://www.aacap.org/.

Davies, Curt, and Dameka Williams. *Lean on Me: Support and Minority Outreach for Grandparents Raising Grandchildren.* Washington, DC: AARP, 2003. Parts I and II available at http://www.aarp.org/research/family/grandparenting/aresearch-import-483.html.

ORGANIZATIONS

Generations United (GU), 1333 H Street, NW, Suite 500 W, Washington, DC, 20005, (202) 289-3979, http://ipath.gu.org.

Grandparents As Parents (GAP), 22048 Sherman Way, Suite 217, Canoga Park, CA, 91303, (818) 264-0880, http://www.grandparentsasparents.com.

National Committee of Grandparents for Children's Rights (NCGCR), http://www.grandparentsforchildren.org.

Granular conjunctivitis *see* Trachoma

Gray oral reading test

Definition

The fourth edition of the Gray Oral Reading Test (GORT-4) is a widely used **assessment** that screens for and diagnoses problems with reading fluency and measures progress in oral reading in children and adolescents aged 6 years to 18 years 11 months.

Purpose

The purposes of the GORT-4 are to:

- identify students who are significantly behind their peers in oral reading proficiency
- identify reading strengths and weaknesses in individual students
- diagnose specific reading problems, such as miscues—including skipping, adding, and substituting words—and mispronunciations
- evaluate and document reading progress resulting from special intervention
- provide an objective measure of progressive oral reading skills from early first grade to college level
- help meet assessment guidelines for Reading First programs
- measure oral reading abilities of children and adolescents for research studies

The GORT-4 evaluates students' ability to read out loud, based on:

- reading rate
- accuracy
- fluency—a combination of rate and accuracy
- comprehension
- overall ability—the combined fluency and comprehension scores

Description

The GORT-4 consists of 14 reading passages of increasing difficulty. Each passage is followed by five comprehension questions. The GORT-4 is most often administered by a **special education** teacher or reading specialist in elementary and secondary schools, clinics, and reading centers. It is administered to students individually. The student reads a text passage aloud, while the teacher times the reading in seconds and monitors the reading for accuracy. The examiner categorizes each type of error, such as word substitutions, additions, deletions, or other deviations from the printed text. These miscues are analyzed for meaning similarity, function similarity, graphic/phonemic similarity, and self-correction. After the reading, the student answers multiple-choice questions relating to the content of the passage, in order to assess reading comprehension. The GORT-4 usually takes 20–30 minutes to administer, depending on how many passages are used. The test is usually continued with text passages of increasing difficulty, until the student reaches a specified number of errors in a passage.

There are two complete and interchangeable forms of the GORT-4, A and B that can be used for retesting students to measure progress over time. The complete GORT-4 consists of:

- an examiner's manual
- a student book
- 25 profile/examiner recording forms for Form A and 25 for Form B

The GORT-4 was published in 2001, replacing the third edition (GORT-3) from 1994. The latter superceded the revised edition of 1986 (GORT-R). The GORT-4 includes a new, easier reading story, increasing the number of text passages from 13 to 14. The GORT-4 also includes all new norms and a new system for adjusting scores that enables the scores on Forms A and B to be interchanged.

Origins

William Scott Gray (1885–1960) is best known as the author of the "Dick and Jane" books, through which generations of children in the United States to learned read. Gray is considered a founding father of reading education in the United States. He earned a bachelor's degree from the University of Chicago and a master's degree from Teachers College of Columbia University. Returning to the University of Chicago for his Ph.D., Gray remained there until his retirement as an emeritus professor in 1950, serving as dean of the college of education from 1917 until 1930.

Literacy education was Gray's passion and his research was devoted to the scientific advancement of reading instruction. He was the author of more than 500 publications on teaching reading and characteristics of readers from early childhood through adulthood. Gray was one of the first to address the diagnosis of reading difficulties and remedial approaches. He developed his first oral reading assessment, Standardized Oral Reading Paragraphs, Grades 1–8, as his 1915 master's thesis. The test went through minor revisions over the years and was published as the Gray Oral Reading Test in 1963.

Gray was a proponent of the sight method of teaching reading. His "Dick and Jane" readers were based on his ideas. Gray believed that the components of a successful reading program included:

- content that is interesting and significant to students
- word study and phonetic analysis to develop independent word-recognition skills, once a student has gained a basic reading vocabulary
- a system of phonics that leads to accurate analysis of longer words encountered after the second grade

Results

The GORT-4 is hand-scored by the examiner, with scoring guidelines provided in the manual:

- The rate is the time in seconds for reading each passage.
- The accuracy is the number of deviations from the printed words of each passage, including incorrect pronunciations.
- The fluency is the combined rate and accuracy scores.
- The oral reading comprehension is the number of correct answers to the comprehension questions.
- The oral reading quotient is obtained by combining the fluency and oral reading comprehension scores.

The rate and accuracy scores for each passage are combined to yield total scores. The raw scores for rate, accuracy, fluency, and comprehension are converted to standard scores, percentile ranks, grade equivalents, and age equivalents. The oral reading quotient is an overall index the student's reading ability.

The GORT-4 has updated and expanded norms, based on a sample of more than 1,600 typical U.S. students between the ages of 6 and 18, stratified to include demographic variables of gender, race, ethnicity, geographic region, and linguistic and socioeconomic backgrounds. Studies have indicated an absence of gender and ethnic bias in the GORT-4. The GORT-4 also has new reliability and validity data. The reliability of the GORT-4 is high for both internal consistency and for testing-retesting of all ages. The test also has extensive validity measures, including studies that demonstrate that the GORT-4 confidently measures oral reading progress over time. GORT-4 scores have been correlated with teacher assessments of student reading ability and with various other standardized reading assessments. The relationship of the GORT-4 to the third edition of the **Wechsler Intelligence Scale for Children** (WISC-III) has also been examined.

KEY TERMS

Age equivalent—A decimal number that indicates the age of a typical child who earns a given score on a standardized test.

Fluency—The ability to speak, read, and write smoothly, easily, and rapidly.

Grade equivalent (GE)—A position on an achievement continuum in terms of beginning grade level and additional months; a decimal number that indicates the grade and month of a typical student who earns that score; most useful for monitoring the development of an individual student over time.

Literacy—The ability to efficiently comprehend and interpret written language and to communicate through written language.

Norm—A standard of achievement, usually derived from the average or median achievement of a large group of a particular age.

Oral reading quotient—A measure of oral reading level relative to age; an overall measure of reading ability.

Percentile—A rank in a population that has been divided into 100 equal groups; thus, test results in the 50th percentile indicate that half of those who took the test scored higher and half scored lower.

Phoneme—A basic unit of sound in a language.

Phonics—Connecting phonemes, or the basic sounds of a language, to graphemes or letters or symbols.

Reading First—A federal program that helps states and school districts implement scientifically based reading programs in kindergarten through the third grade.

Reliability—The extent to which a test or measure yields the same results with repeated trials and different examiners.

Validity—The extent to which a test measures the trait that it is designed to assess.

Parental concerns

Because the time it takes a student to read a passage aloud affects the overall score, the GORT-4 penalizes slower readers who nevertheless read with accuracy and comprehension. The validity of the

GORT-4 comprehension subtest has also been called into question. A 2006 study examined the comprehension subtest to determine the extent to which reading was required to answer the comprehension questions. The study found that when students answered the questions without reading the passages, their accuracy on most of the questions was above the chance level. Furthermore, the study found that under normal GORT administration, the best predictor of answering a question correctly was the passage-independence of the question, rather than how well the child read the passage. These passage-independent questions were not sensitive to reading disabilities, nor did they correlate with performance on other reading comprehension tests.

A 2010 study examined GORT-4 scores for typically developing second- and fourth-grade children who spoke African-American English (AAE). There was a significant correlation between higher AAE usage, as measured by the Diagnostic Evaluation of Language Variation-Screening Test (DELV-ST), and lower scores on the GORT-4 comprehension subtest and lower overall GORT-4 scores. There was also a significant correlation between students's grade levels and their GORT-4 scores, especially on the rate subtest. The study's authors concluded that the GORT-4 should be used cautiously for determining the reading skills of AAE-speaking children.

Because most reading tests have not been standardized with adults who have very low literacy skills, child-standardized tests, including the GORT-4, are often used to assess reading ability in adults. A 2009 study found that the GORT-4 should be interpreted very cautiously when used to assess the reading comprehension skills of adults who read at approximately third- through fifth-grade equivalency levels.

Resources

BOOKS

Bryant, Brian R., Minyi Shih, and Diane Pedrotty Bryant. "The Gray Oral Reading Test, Fourth Edition (GORT-4)." In *Practitioner's Guide to Assessing Intelligence and Achievement,* edited by Jack A. Naglieri and Sam Goldstein. Hoboken, NJ: Wiley, 2009.

Champion, Tempii B., et al. "A Preliminary Investigation of Second- and Fourth-Grade African American Students' Performance on the Gray Oral Reading Test, Fourth Edition." In *Research with Implications for Assessing the Language of African American English Speakers,* edited by Frances A. Burns and Gloria Toliver Weddington. Hagerstown, MD: Lippincott, Williams, & Wilkins, 2010.

Gray, William S. *Gray Oral Reading Test.* Indianapolis, IN: Bobbs-Merrill, 1963.

Wiederholt, J. Lee, and Brian R. Bryant. Gray Oral Reading Test (GORT-4). Austin, TX: Pro-Ed, 2001.

———. Gray Oral Reading Tests, 3rd ed. Austin, TX: Pro-Ed, 1994.

Wiederhold, J. Lee, Brian R. Bryant, and William S. Gray. GORT-R, Gray Oral Reading Tests, rev. ed. Austin, TX: Pro-Ed, 1986.

PERIODICALS

Champion, Tempii B., et al. "A Preliminary Investigation of Second- and Fourth-Grade African American Students' Performance on the Gray Oral Reading Test, Fourth Edition." *Topics in Language Disorders* 30 no. 2 (April–June 2010): 145–153.

Greenberg, Daphne, et al. "Measuring Adult Literacy Students' Reading Skills Using the Gray Oral Reading Test." *Annals of Dyslexia* 59 no. 2 (December 2009): 133–149.

Keenan, Janice M., and Rebecca S. Betjemann. "Comprehending the Gray Oral Reading Test Without Reading It: Why Comprehension Tests Should Not Include Passage-Independent Items." *Scientific Studies of Reading* 10 no. 4 (2006): 363–380.

OTHER

Jorgenson, Gerald W. "Gray, William Scott (1885–1960)." Education.com, http://www.education.com/reference/article/gray-william-scott-1885-1960 (accessed October 8, 2010).

"Reading Assessment Database—Overview." SEDL, http://www.sedl.org/reading/rad (accessed October 8, 2010).

ORGANIZATIONS

Education Resources Information Center, ERIC Program c/o CSC, 655 15th St. NW, Suite 500, Washington, DC, 20005, (800) LET-ERIC (538-3742), http://www.eric.ed.gov.

Learning Point Associates, 1120 East Diehl Rd., Suite 200, Naperville, IL, 60563-1486, (630) 649-6500, (800) 356-2735, (630) 649-6700, http://www.learningpt.org.

Literacy Information and Communication System, info@lincs.ed.gov, http://lincs.ed.gov.

SEDL, 4700 Mueller Blvd., Austin, TX, 78723, (512) 476-6861, (800) 476-6861, (512) 476-2286, info@sedl.org, http://www.sedl.org.

Margaret Alic, PhD

Grieving **see Death and mourning**

Gross motor skills

Definition

Gross motor skills involve the ability to control the large muscles of the body for walking, running, sitting, **crawling**, and other activities.

Gross motor skills

Age	Skill
One month	May hold up head momentarily.
Two months	Lifts head when placed on stomach. Holds up head briefly when held in a seated or standing position.
Three months	Holds head and shoulders up when placed on stomach. Puts weight on forearms.
Four months	Holds head up well in sitting position. Can lift head to a 90-degree angle when placed stomach. May start to roll over.
Five months	Has full head control. When pulled by hands to a sitting position, the head stays in line with body.
Six months	Rolls over (front to back first). Bears a large percentage of body weight when held in a standing position.
Seven months	Can stand with support. May sit without support for short periods. Pushes upper part of body up while on stomach.
Eight months	Stands while holding onto furniture. Sits well unsupported. Gets up on hands and knees; may start to crawl backward.
Nine months	Crawls first by pulling body forward with hands. May move around a room by rolling.
Ten months	Pulls up to standing. Is very steady while sitting; moves from sitting to crawling position and back. Crawls well.
Eleven months	"Cruises," walking while hanging onto furniture. Walks with two hands held.
Twelve months	Walks with one hand held. May walk with hands and feet. Stands unsupported for longer periods of time.
Fifteen months	Walks without help. Crawls up stairs. Gets into a standing position without support.
Eighteen months	Seldom falls while walking. Can walk and pull toy. Runs. Climbs stairs holding railing. May walk backward.
Two years	Kicks a ball. Walks up and down stairs, two feet per step.
Two and a half years	Jumps with both feet. Jumps off step. Can walk on tiptoe.
Three years	Goes upstairs one foot per step. Stands on one foot briefly. Rides tricycle. Runs well.
Four years	Skips on one foot. Throws ball well overhand. Jumps a short distance from standing position.
Five years	Hops and skips. Good balance. Can skate or ride scooter.

SOURCE: *Miller-Keane Encyclopedia and Dictionary of Medicine, Nursing, and Allied Health, 7th ed.*, and Child Development Institute, http://www.childdevelopmentinfo.com.

(Table by PreMediaGlobal. Reproduced by permission of Gale, a part of Cengage Learning.)

Description

Motor skills are deliberate and controlled movements requiring both muscle development and maturation of the central nervous system. In addition, the skeletal system must be strong enough to support the movement and weight involved in any new activity. Once these conditions are met, children learn new physical skills by practicing them until each skill is mastered.

Gross motor skills, like fine motor skills, which involve control of the fingers and hands, develop in an orderly sequence. Although norms for motor development have been charted in detail by researchers and clinicians over the past 50 years, the pace at which these skills develop varies considerably from child to child. The more complex the skill, the greater the possible variation among normal children. For example, the normal age for learning to walk has a range of several months, while the age range for turning the head, a simpler skill that occurs much earlier, is considerably narrower. In addition to variations among children, an individual child's rate of progress varies as well, often including rapid spurts of development and frustrating periods of delay. Although rapid motor development in early childhood is often a good predictor of coordination and athletic ability later in life, there is no proven correlation between a child's rate of motor development and his or her **intelligence**. In most cases, a delay in mastering a specific motor skill is temporary and does not indicate a serious problem. However, medical help should be sought if a child is significantly behind his peers in motor development or if he regresses, losing previously acquired skills.

Infancy and toddlerhood

The sequence of gross motor development is determined by two developmental principles that also govern physical growth. The cephalo-caudal pattern, or head-to-toe development, refers to the way the upper parts of the body, beginning with the head, develop before the lower ones. Thus, infants can lift their heads and shoulders before they can sit up, which in turn precedes standing and walking. The other pattern of both development and maturation is proximo-distal, or from the trunk to extremities. One of the first things an infant achieves is head control. Although babies are born with virtually no head or neck control, most infants can lift their heads to a 45-degree angle by the age of four to six weeks, and they can lift both their heads and chests at an average age of eight weeks. Most infants can turn their heads to both sides within 16 to 20 weeks and lift their heads while lying on their backs within 24 to 28 weeks. By about 36 to 42 weeks, or 9 to 10 months, most infants can sit up unassisted for substantial periods of time with both hands free for playing.

One of the major tasks in gross motor development is locomotion, or the ability to move from one place to another. An infant progresses gradually from rolling (8–10 weeks) to creeping on her stomach and dragging her

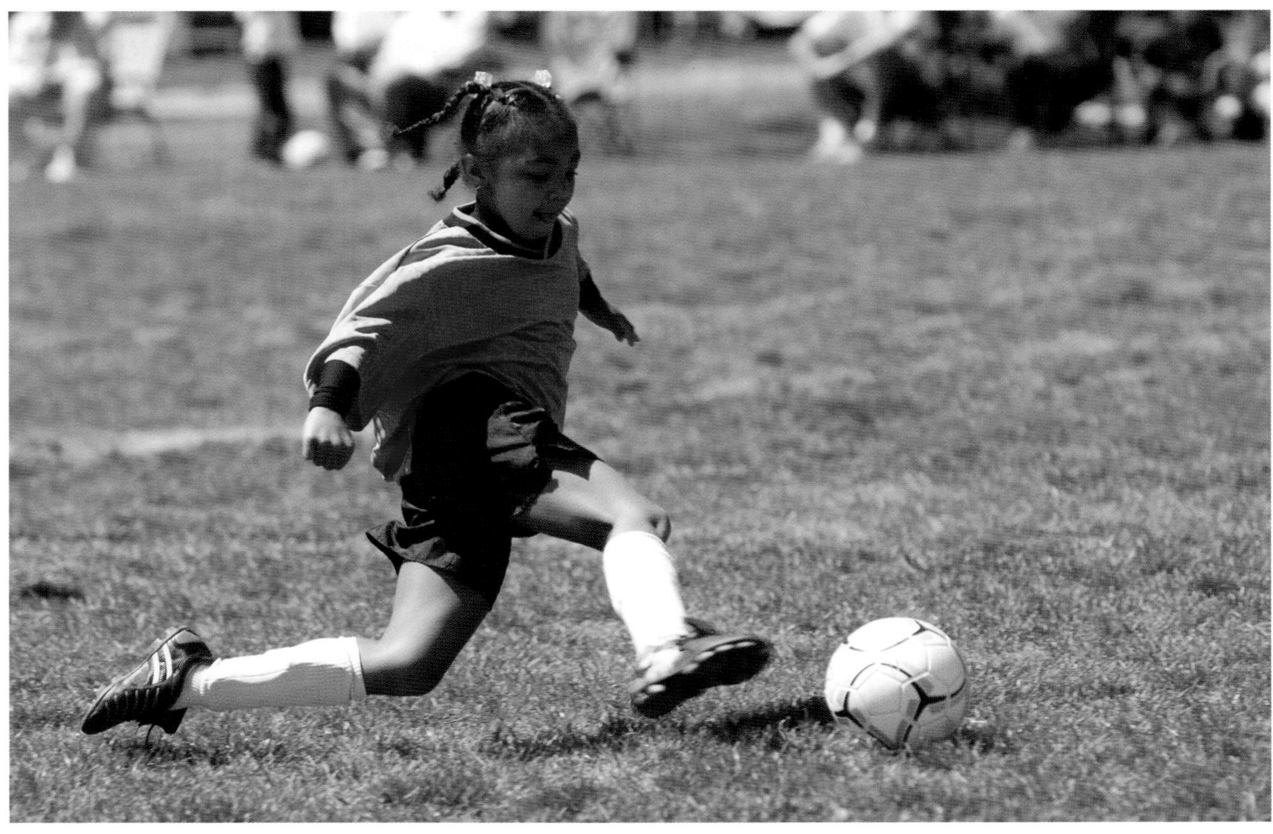

A young girl using her gross motor skills (large muscle movements) to play soccer. *(© iStockPhoto.com/bonnie jacobs.)*

legs behind her (6–9 months) to actual crawling (7–12 months). While the infant is learning these temporary means of locomotion, he or she is gradually becoming able to support increasing amounts of weight while in a standing position. In the second half year of life, babies begin pulling themselves up on furniture and other stationary objects. By the ages of 28–54 weeks, on average, they begin "cruising," or navigating a room in an upright position by holding on to the furniture to keep their balance. Eventually, they are able to walk while holding on to an adult with both hands, and then with only one. They usually take their first uncertain steps alone between the ages of 36 and 64 weeks and are competent walkers by the ages of 52–78 weeks. By the age of two years, children have begun to develop a variety of gross motor skills. They can run fairly well and negotiate stairs holding on to a banister with one hand and putting both feet on each step before going on to the next one. Most infants this age climb (some very actively) and have a rudimentary ability to kick and throw a ball.

Preschool children

During a child's first two years, most parents consider gross motor skills a very high priority; a child's first steps are a universally celebrated developmental milestone. By the time a child is a preschooler, however, many parents shift the majority of their attention to the child's **cognitive development** in preparation for school. In addition, gross motor activity at these ages requires increasing amounts of space, equipment, and supervision. However, gross motor skills remain very important to a child's development, and maintaining a youngster's instinctive love of physical activity can make an important contribution to future fitness and health.

By the age of three, children walk with good posture and without watching their feet. They can also walk backwards and run with enough control for sudden stops or changes of direction. They can hop, stand on one foot, and negotiate the rungs of a jungle gym. They can walk up stairs alternating feet but usually still walk down putting both feet on each step. Other achievements include riding a tricycle and throwing a ball, although children in this age group have trouble catching balls because they hold their arms out in front of their bodies no matter what direction the ball comes from. Four-year-old children typically can balance or hop on one foot, jump forward and backward over objects, and climb and descend stairs alternating feet. They can bounce and

KEY TERMS

Central nervous system (CNS)—Part of the nervous system consisting of the brain, cranial nerves and spinal cord. The brain is the center of higher processes, such as thought and emotion, and is responsible for the coordination and control of bodily activities and the interpretation of information from the senses. The cranial nerves and spinal cord link the brain to the peripheral nervous system, that is, the nerves present in the rest of body.

Fine motor skills—The ability to make smooth, controlled movements using the small muscles in the fingers, hand, and wrist.

catch balls and throw accurately. Some four-year-olds also can skip. Children this age have gained an increased degree of self-consciousness about their motor activities that leads to increased feelings of pride and success when they master a new skill. This self-awareness, however, can also create feelings of inadequacy when they think that they have failed. This concern with success can also lead them to try daring activities beyond their abilities, so they need to be monitored especially carefully.

School-age children

School-age children, who are not going through the rapid, unsettling growth spurts of early childhood or **adolescence**, are quite skilled at controlling their bodies and are generally good at a wide variety of physical activities, although the ability varies based on their level of maturation and their physique. Motor skills are approximately equal in boys and girls at this stage, except that boys have more forearm strength and girls have greater flexibility. Five-year-old children can skip, jump rope, catch a bounced ball, walk on their tiptoes, balance on one foot for over eight seconds, and engage in beginning acrobatics. Some can even ride a small two-wheeler bicycle. Eight- and nine-year-olds typically can ride a bicycle, swim, roller-skate, ice-skate, jump rope, scale fences, use a saw, hammer, and garden tools, and play a variety of **sports**. Many of the sports prized by adults, however, which are often scaled down for play by children, require higher levels of distance judgment and **hand-eye coordination**, as well as quicker reaction times, than are reasonable for middle childhood. Games that are well suited to the motor skills of elementary school-age children include kick ball, dodge ball, and team relay races.

In adolescence, children develop increasing coordination and motor ability. They also gain greater physical strength and prolonged endurance. Adolescents are able to develop better distance judgment and hand-eye coordination than their younger counterparts. With practice, they can master the skills necessary for adult sports.

Difficulties with gross motor skills

Not all children develop gross motor skills in a smooth progression. Several studies of school-aged children indicate that about 6% have significant problems with clumsiness, boys more often than girls. In 1975 a physician named Sasson S. Gubbay coined the term "clumsy child syndrome" to describe problems in gross motor skills severe enough to cause social or academic difficulties in children of normal intelligence without any diagnosable neurological or medical conditions. The American Psychiatric Association's *Diagnostic and Statistical Manual of Mental Disorders*, fourth edition, text revision (DSM-IV-TR), redefined "clumsy child syndrome" as Developmental Coordination Disorder, or DCD. The *DSM-IV-TR* criteria for DCD are as follows:

- "Performance in daily activities that require motor coordination is substantially below the given the person's age and measured intelligence. This change may manifest as marked delays in achieving motor milestones (such as walking, crawling, or sitting) and as dropping things, clumsiness, poor performance in sports, or poor handwriting."
- The poor coordination "significantly interferes with the child's academic achievement and activities of daily living (ADLs)."
- The clumsiness "is not due to a general medical condition (such as cerebral palsy or muscular dystrophy) or a pervasive developmental disorder."
- If the child is mentally retarded, "the difficulties with motor skills are greater than those usually associated with mental retardation."

Relatively little is known about the causes of DCD as of 2010, in part because motor skills are the result of a complex interplay of sensory perception, cognitive interpretation of sensory information, volition (will or intention), motivation, planning a motor activity, muscle tone, and muscular coordination. Other problems that may contribute to DCD are poor posture; poor muscle tone (too loose or too tense); problems with sensory integration; and problems with muscle strength, sequencing, or speed of movements.

Several different pathways are activated in the brain during a single movement, making research on this disorder difficult. For example, consider a child playing baseball who wants to field a batted ball and throw it to first base. The reticular system in the child's brain alerts the child to the activity on the field. Auditory and visual inputs tell him (or her) that the ball has been struck by the batter and the direction and speed that the ball is moving. The child's proprioceptive system tells him the general spatial orientation of his body and arms. Motor planning and the memory of playing in previous games tell him whether he can move fast enough to catch the ball and make the throw to first; they also allow him to correct his movements while he is running to avoid colliding with other players or tripping over the thrown bat. If any of these systems is not functioning adequately, or if the information from the various systems is not integrated rapidly enough, the child may move clumsily and ineffectively rather than smoothly and efficiently.

DCD is thought to occur at the same rate in all races and ethnic groups; however, it does appear to run in families, and it may coexist with attention-deficit/hyperactivity disorder (AD/HD) in about 50% of children diagnosed with DCD. It may be diagnosed at any age during **infancy** or childhood. The child's doctor will typically ask the parents whether the clumsiness represents the loss of skills previously attained, whether it affects only one side of the body, and whether it has gotten worse; if the answer to any of these questions is yes, the child is likely to have a neurological disorder of some kind rather than DCD. DCD is not progressive and tends to affect both sides of the body. The doctor will also need to exclude such other possible causes of clumsiness as traumatic brain injury or orthopedic disorders. After examining the child's eyes and evaluating the child's muscle tone, reflexes, and the functioning of the cranial nerves, the doctor will usually ask the child to perform certain movements (such as standing erect for 15 seconds with arms extended and feet together; hopping in place; or standing with one foot directly in front of the other with eyes closed for 15 seconds) that can be done in the office. There are several other tests of gross motor skills that the doctor may administer.

If the child is diagnosed with DCD, his or her teachers should be informed so that they do not attribute academic difficulties to laziness or sloppiness. In many schools, physical education teachers can arrange for the child to participate in sports or other physical activities that will match his or her motor abilities. **Swimming** is a particularly good activity that offers children with DCD to have some kind of athletic success; horseback riding is another. **Occupational therapy** is useful for children who have suffered from teasing by classmates, and a skilled physical therapist can design a program of exercises tailored to the individual child with DCD. There were, however, no medications or surgical treatments for DCD as of 2010.

Resources

BOOKS

Piek, Jan P. *Infant Motor Development*. Champaign, IL: Human Kinetics, 2006.

OTHER

Floet, Anna M. W., and J. Martin Maldonado-Duran. "Motor Skills Disorder." eMedicine Web site. January 22, 2010, http://emedicine.medscape.com/article/915251-overview (accessed July 15, 2010).

Logsdon, Anne. "Gross Motor Skills." About.com Website, http://learningdisabilities.about.com/od/df/p/finemotorskills.htm (accessed July 15, 2010).

ORGANIZATIONS

American Academy of Family Physicians, P. O. Box 11210, Shawnee Mission, KS, 66207, (913)906-6000, (800) 274-2237, (913) 906-6075, http://familydoctor.org.

American Academy of Pediatrics, 141 Northwest Point Boulevard, Elk Grove Village, IL, 60007-1098, (847) 434-4000, (847) 434-8000, http://www.aap.org.

American Physical Therapy Association, 1111 North Fairfax Street, Alexandria, VA, 22314-1488, (703) 684-APTA (2782), TDD: (703) 683-6748, (800) 999-APTA (2782), (703) 683-6748, http://www.apta.org.

Tish Davidson, AM

Growth ***see*** **Skeletal development**

Growth hormone tests

Definition

Growth hormone (hGH), or somatotropin, is a hormone responsible for normal body growth and development by stimulating protein production in muscle cells and energy release from the breakdown of fats. Tests for growth hormone include the Somatotropin hormone test, Somatomedin C, Growth hormone suppression test (glucose loading test), and Growth hormone stimulation test (Arginine test or Insulin tolerance test).

Purpose

Growth hormone tests are ordered for the following reasons:

- to identify growth deficiencies, including delayed puberty and small stature in adolescents that result from pituitary or thyroid malfunction

- to aid in the diagnosis of hyperpituitarism that is evident in gigantism or acromegaly
- to screen for inadequate or reduced pituitary gland function
- to assist in the diagnosis of pituitary tumors or tumors related to the hypothalamus, an area of the brain
- to evaluate hGH therapy

Precautions

Taking certain drugs such as amphetamines, dopamine, corticosteroids, and phenothiazines may increase and decrease growth hormone secretion, respectively. Other factors influencing hGH secretion include stress, **exercise**, diet, and abnormal glucose levels. These tests should not be done within a week of any radioactive scan.

Description

Several hormones play important roles in human growth. The major human growth hormone (hGH), or somatotropin, is a protein made up of 191 amino acids that is secreted by the anterior pituitary gland and coordinates normal growth and development. Human growth is characterized by two spurts, one at **birth** and the other at **puberty**. hGH plays an important role at both of these times. Normal individuals have measurable levels of hGH throughout life. However, levels of hGH fluctuate during the day and are affected by eating and exercise. Receptors that respond to hGH exist on cells and tissues throughout the body. The most obvious effect of hGH is on linear **skeletal development**. But the metabolic effects of hGH on muscle, the liver, and fat cells are critical to its function. Surprisingly, a 2004 study reported that obese people have lower-than-normal levels of human growth hormone in their bodies. Humans have two forms of hGH, and the functional difference between the two is unclear. They are both formed from the same gene, but one lacks the amino acids in positions 32–46.

hGH is produced in the anterior portion of the pituitary gland by somatotrophs under the control of hormonal signals in the hypothalamus. Two hypothalamic hormones regulate hGH; they are growth hormone-releasing hormone (GHRH) and growth hormone—inhibiting hormone (GHIH). When blood glucose levels fall, GHRH triggers the secretion of stored hGH. As blood glucose levels rise, GHRH release is turned off. Increases in blood protein levels trigger a similar response. As a result of this hypothalamic feedback loop, hGH levels fluctuate throughout the day. Normal plasma hGH levels average 1–3 ng/ML with peaks as high as 60 ng/ML. In addition, plasma glucose and amino acid availability for growth is also regulated by the hormones adrenaline, glucagon, and insulin.

Most hGH is released at night. Peak spikes of hGH release occur around 10 P.M., midnight, and 2 A.M. The logic behind this night-time release is that most of hGH's effects are controlled by other hormones, including the somatomedins, IGH-I and IGH-II. As a result, the effects of hGH are spread out more evenly during the day.

A number of hormonal conditions can lead to excessive or diminished growth. Because of its critical role in producing hGH and other hormones, an abnormal pituitary gland will often yield altered growth. **Dwarfism** (very small stature) can be due to underproduction of hGH, lack of IGH-I, or a flaw in target tissue response to either of these growth hormones. Overproduction of hGH or IGH-I, or an exaggerated response to these hormones can lead to **gigantism** or **acromegaly**, both of which are characterized by a very large stature.

Gigantism is the result of hGH overproduction in early childhood leading to a skeletal height up to 8 feet (2.5m) or more. Acromegaly results when hGH is overproduced after the onset of puberty. In this condition, the epiphyseal plates of the long bone of the body do not close, and they remain responsive to additional stimulated growth by hGH. This disorder is characterized by an enlarged skull, hands and feet, nose, neck, and tongue.

Somatotropin

Somatotropin is used to identify hGH deficiency in adolescents with short stature, delayed sexual maturity, and other growth deficiencies. It also aids in documenting excess hGH production that is responsible for gigantism or acromegaly, and confirms underactivity or overproduction of the pituitary gland (hypopituitarism or hyperpituitarism). However, due to the episodic secretion of hGH, as well as hGH production in response to stress, exercise, or other factors, random assays are not an adequate determination of hGH deficiency. To negate these variables and obtain more accurate readings, a blood sample can be drawn one to 1.5 hours after **sleep** (hGH levels increase during sleep), or strenuous exercise can be performed for 30 minutes before blood is drawn (hGH levels increase after exercise). The hGH levels at the end of an exercise period are expected to be maximal.

Somatomedin C

The somatomedin C test is usually ordered to detect pituitary abnormalities, hGH deficiency, and acromegaly. Also called insulin-like growth factor (IGF-1), somatomedin C is considered a more accurate reflection of the blood concentration of hGH because such variables as time of day, activity levels, or diet do not influence the results. Somatomedin C is part of a group of peptides called somatomedins through which hGH exerts its effects. Because it circulates in the bloodstream bound to long-lasting proteins, it is more stable than hGH. Levels of somatomedin C depend on hGH levels, however. As a result, somatomedin C levels are low when hGH levels are deficient. Abnormally low test results of somatomedin C require an abnormally reduced or absent hGH during an hGH stimulation test in order to diagnose hGH deficiency. Nonpituitary causes of reduced somatomedin C include **malnutrition**, severe chronic illness, severe liver disease, **hypothyroidism**, and Laron's dwarfism.

Growth hormone stimulation test

The hGH stimulation test, also called hGH Provocation test, Insulin Tolerance, or Arginine test, is performed to test the body's ability to produce human growth hormone, and to identify suspected hGH deficiency. A normal patient can have low hGH levels, but if hGH is still low after stimulation, a diagnosis can be more accurately made.

Insulin-induced **hypoglycemia** (via intravenous injection of insulin) stimulates hGH and corticotropin secretion as well. If such stimulation is unsuccessful, then there is a malfunction of the anterior pituitary gland. Blood samples may be obtained following an energetic exercise session lasting 20 minutes.

A substance called hGH-releasing factor has recently been used for hGH stimulation. This approach promises to be more accurate and specific for hGH deficiency caused by the pituitary. Growth hormone deficiency is also suspected when x ray determination of bone age indicates retarded growth in comparison to chronologic age. At present, the best method to identify hGH-deficient patients is a positive stimulation test followed by a positive response to a therapeutic trial of hGH.

Growth hormone suppression test

Also called the glucose loading test, this procedure is used to evaluate excessive baseline levels of human growth hormone, and to confirm diagnosis of gigantism in children and acromegaly in adults. The procedure requires two different blood samples, one drawn before the administration of 100 g of glucose (by mouth), and a second sample two hours after glucose ingestion.

Normally, a glucose load suppresses hGH secretion. In a patient with excessive hGH levels, failure of suppression indicates anterior pituitary dysfunction and confirms a diagnosis of **acromegaly and gigantism**.

Preparation

Somatotropin: This test requires a blood sample. The patient should fast, with nothing to eat or drink from midnight the night before the test. Stress and/or exercise increases hGH levels, so the patient should be at complete rest for 30 minutes before the blood sample is drawn. If the physician has requested two samples, they should be drawn on consecutive days at approximately the same time on both days, preferably between 6 A.M. and 8 A.M.

Somatomedin C: This test requires a blood sample. The patient should have nothing to eat or drink from midnight the night before the test.

Growth hormone stimulation: This test requires intravenous administration of medications and the withdrawal of frequent blood samples, which are obtained at 0, 60, and 90 minutes after injection of arginine and/or insulin. The patient should have nothing to eat or drink after midnight the night before the test.

Growth hormone suppression: This test requires two blood samples, one before the test and another two hours after administration of 100 g of glucose solution by mouth. The patient should have nothing to eat or drink after midnight, and physical activity should be limited for 10–12 hours before the test.

Risks

Growth hormone stimulation: Only minor discomfort is associated with this test, and results from the insertion of the IV line and the low blood sugar (hypoglycemia) induced by the insulin injection. Some patients may experience sleepiness, sweating, and/or nervousness, all of which can be corrected after the test by ingestion of cookies, juice, or a glucose infusion. Severe cases of hypoglycemia may cause ketosis (excessive amounts of fatty acid byproducts in the body), acidosis (a disturbance of the body's acid-base balance), or shock. With the close observation required for the test, these are unlikely.

Growth hormone suppression: Some patients experience nausea after the administration of this amount of glucose. Ice chips can alleviate this symptom.

Normal results

Normal results may vary from laboratory to laboratory but are usually within the following ranges:

Somatotropin:

- men: 5 ng/mL
- women: less than 10 ng/mL
- children: 0–10 ng/mL
- newborn: 10–40 ng/mL

KEY TERMS

Acromegaly—A rare disease resulting from excessive growth hormone caused by a benign tumor. If such a tumor develops within the first 10 years of life, the result is gigantism (in which growth is accelerated) and not acromegaly. Symptoms include coarsening of the facial features, enlargement of the hands, feet, ears, and nose, jutting of the jaw, and a long face.

Dwarfism, pituitary—Short stature. When caused by inadequate amounts of growth hormone (as opposed to late growth spurt or genetics), hGH deficiency results in abnormally slow growth and short stature with normal proportions.

Gigantism—Excessive growth, especially in height, resulting from overproduction during childhood or adolescence of growth hormone by a pituitary tumor. Untreated, the tumor eventually destroys the pituitary gland, resulting in death during early adulthood. If the tumor develops after growth has stopped, the result is acromegaly, not gigantism.

Pituitary gland—The pituitary is the most important of the endocrine glands (glands that release hormones directly into the bloodstream). Sometimes referred to as the "master gland," the pituitary regulates and controls the activities of other endocrine glands and many body processes.

Somatomedin C:

Adult: 42–110 ng/mL

Child:

- 0–8 years: Girls 7–110 ng/mL; Boys 4–87 ng/mL
- 9–10 years: Girls 39–186 ng/mL; Boys 26–98 ng/mL
- 11–13 years: Girls 66–215 ng/mL; Boys 44–207 ng/mL
- 14–16 years: Girls 96–256 ng/mL; Boys 48 255 ng/mL

Growth hormone stimulation: greater than 10 ng/mL.

Growth hormone suppression: Normally, glucose suppresses hGH to levels of undetectable to 3 ng/mL in 30 minutes to two hours. In children, rebound stimulation may occur after two to five hours.

Abnormal results

Somatotropin hormone: Excess hGH is responsible for the syndromes of gigantism and acromegaly. Excess secretion is stimulated by **anorexia nervosa**, stress, hypoglycemia, and exercise. Decreased levels are seen in hGH deficiency, dwarfism, **hyperglycemia**, **failure to thrive**, and delayed sexual maturity.

Somatomedin C: Increased levels contribute to the syndromes of gigantism and acromegaly. Stress, major surgery, hypoglycemia, starvation, and exercise stimulate hGH secretion, which in turn stimulates somatomedin C.

Growth hormone stimulation: Decreased levels are seen in pituitary deficiency and hGH deficiency. Diseases of the pituitary can result in failure of the pituitary to secrete hGH and/or all the pituitary hormones. As a result, the hGH stimulation test will fail to stimulate hGH secretion.

Growth hormone suppression: The acromegaly syndrome elevates base hGH levels to 75 ng/mL, which in turn are not suppressed to less than 5 ng/mL during the test. Excess hGH secretion may cause unchanged or rising hGH levels in response to glucose loading, confirming a diagnosis of acromegaly or gigantism. In such cases, verification of results is required by repeating the test after a one-day rest.

Resources

PERIODICALS

"Weight-loss Hormone." *Better Nutrition* (May 2004): 32.

Janis O. Flores
Teresa G. Odle

Gum disease **see** **Periodontal disease**

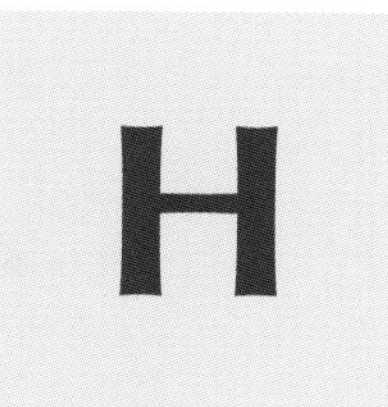

Haemophilus influenzae infections ***see*** **Hemophilus infections**

Haemophilus influenzae type B vaccine ***see*** **Hib vaccine**

Hair loss ***see*** **Alopecia**

Hallucinogens

Substances that cause hallucination-perception of things or feelings that have no foundation in reality-when ingested.

Hallucinogens, or psychedelics, are substances that alter users' thought processes or moods to the extent that they perceive objects or experience sensations that in fact have no basis in reality. Many natural and some synthetic substances have the ability to bring about hallucinations. In fact, because of the ready market for such chemicals, they are manufactured in illegal chemical laboratories for sale as hallucinogens. LSD (lysergic acid diethylamide) and many so-called designer drugs have no useful clinical function.

Hallucinogens have long been a component in the religious rites of various cultures, both in the New and Old Worlds. Among the oldest are substances from mushroom or cactus plants that have been in use in Native American rites since before recorded history. Hallucinogenic mushrooms have been used for centuries in rites of medicine men to foresee the future or

Percentage of high school students who ever used ecstasy or hallucinogenic drugs, by sex, race/ethnicity, and grade, 2009

	Ever used ecstasy*			Ever used hallucinogenic drugs**		
	Female %	Male %	Total %	Female %	Male %	Total %
Race/ethnicity						
White†	5.3	7.4	**6.4**	6.2	11.5	**9.0**
Black†	3.8	6.5	**5.1**	1.4	5.1	**3.3**
Hispanic	7.5	8.9	**8.2**	6.6	9.2	**7.9**
Grade						
9	4.6	5.2	**4.9**	5.0	6.6	**5.9**
10	4.6	5.7	**5.2**	4.5	10.0	**7.4**
11	6.9	10.3	**8.7**	6.9	10.7	**8.9**
12	6.0	9.9	**8.0**	5.6	14.2	**10.0**
Total %	**5.5**	**7.6**	**6.7**	**5.5**	**10.2**	**8.0**

*Used ecstasy (also called MDMA) one or more times during their life
**Used hallucinogenic drugs (e.g., LSD, acid, PCP, angel dust, mescaline, or mushrooms) one or more times during their life
†Non-Hispanic

SOURCE: Centers for Disease Control and Prevention. Youth Risk Behavior Surveillance—United States, 2009. Surveillance Summaries, June 4, 2010. *MMWR* 2010;59(No. SS-5).

(Table by PreMediaGlobal. Reproduced by permission of Gale, a part of Cengage Learning.)

communicate with the gods. The mushroom is consumed by eating it or by drinking a beverage in which the mushroom has been boiled. The effects are similar to those experienced by an LSD user–enhancement of colors and sounds, introspective interludes, perception of nonexistent or absent objects or persons, and sometimes terrifying, threatening visions.

Another ancient, natural hallucinogenic substance is derived from the Mexican peyote cactus. The flowering head of the cactus contains a potent alkaloid called mescaline. Hallucinogenic substances can be found in a number of other plant species.

In the 1960s, hallucinogens were discovered and embraced by the hippie movement, which incorporated drugs into its culture. In addition, artists, poets, and writers of the time believed that the use of hallucinogens enhanced their creative prowess.

Use of LSD, the most widely known hallucinogen, declined after large numbers of users experienced serious, sometimes fatal, effects during the 1960s. In the United States, LSD was classified as a Schedule I drug according to the Controlled Substance Act of 1970. That designation is reserved for drugs considered unsafe, medically useless, and with a high potential for abuse.

LSD made a comeback in the 1990s, becoming the most abused drug of people under 20 years of age. Its low cost at the time ($1 to $5 per "hit"), ready availability, and a renewed interest in 1960s culture were blamed for the resurgence. A 1993 survey reported that 13% of 18- to 25-year-olds had used hallucinogens, in most cases LSD, at least once. By 2003, a national survey showed that use of LSD among 10th through 12th graders had declined almost three fold from 1999 levels, even as use of some drugs remained steady or increased.

Drugs such as LSD are often differentiated from less potent psychedelics, which have the primary effect of inducing euphoria, relaxation, stimulation, relief from **pain**, or relief from **anxiety**. The most popular drug in this group remains **marijuana**, which is available worldwide and constitutes one of the primary money crops in the United States. Opiates such as heroin or morphine, phencyclidine (PCP), and certain tranquilizers such as diazepam (Valium) also belong to this category.

The problem is that teens often begin with one drug and then experiment with another, such as LSD. Many of these drugs are used at parties, dances, and clubs. One drug that has been used more in recent years is MDMA, or ecstasy, which can cause serious side effects as well. Research in 2004 reported that increased use of ecstasy led to greater use of stimulants and hallucinogens.

LSD was first synthesized in 1938 by Dr. Albert Hofmann, a Swiss chemist who was seeking a **headache** remedy. Years later, he accidentally ingested a small, unknown quantity, and shortly afterward he was forced to stop his work and go home. Hofmann lay in a darkened room and later recorded in his diary that he was in a dazed condition and experienced "an uninterrupted stream of fantastic images of extraordinary plasticity and vividness ... accompanied by an intense kaleidoscope-like play of colors."

Three days later, Hofmann purposely took another dose of LSD to verify that his previous experience was the result of taking the drug. He ingested what he thought was a small dose (250 micrograms), but which is actually about five times the amount needed to induce pronounced hallucinations in an adult male. His second hallucinatory experience was even more intense, and his journal describes the symptoms of LSD toxicity: a metallic taste, difficulty in breathing, dry and constricted throat, cramps, paralysis, and visual disturbances.

LSD is one of the most potent hallucinogens known, and no therapeutic benefits have been discovered. The usual dose for an adult is 50-100 micrograms. (A microgram is one millionth of a gram.) Higher doses will produce more intense effects and lower doses will produce milder effects. The so-called "acid trip" can be induced by swallowing the drug, smoking it (usually with marijuana), injecting it, or rubbing it on the skin. Taken by mouth, the drug will take about 30 minutes to have any effect and up to an hour for its full effect to be felt, which will last 2 to 4 hours.

The physiological effects of LSD include blurred vision, dilation of the pupils of the eye, muscle weakness and twitching, and an increase in heart rate, blood pressure, and body temperature. The user may also salivate excessively and shed tears, and the hair on the back of his arms may stand erect. Pregnant women who use LSD or other hallucinogens may have a miscarriage, because these drugs cause the muscles of the uterus to contract. Such a reaction in pregnancy would expel the fetus.

To the observer, the user usually will appear quiet and introspective. Most of the time the user will be unwilling or unable to interact with others, to carry on a conversation, or engage in intimacies. At times even moderate doses of LSD will have profoundly disturbing effects on an individual. Although the physiological effects will seem uniform, the psychological impact of the drug can be terrifying. The distortions in reality, exaggeration of perception and other effects can be horrifying, especially if the user is unaware that he has been given the drug. This constitutes what is called the "bad trip."

Among the psychological effects reported by LSD users is depersonalization, the separation from one's body, yet with the knowledge that the separated mind is observing the passing scene. A confused body image (the user cannot tell where his own body ends and the surroundings begin) also is common. A distorted perception of reality often occurs. For example, the user's perception of colors, distance, shapes, and sizes is inconsistent and unreliable. In addition, the user may perceive absent objects and forms without substance. He may also taste colors or smell sounds, a mixing of the senses called synesthesia. Sounds, colors, and taste are all greatly enhanced, though they may constitute an unrealistic and constantly changing tableau.

The user often talks non-stop on a variety of subjects, often uttering meaningless phrases. But he may also become silent and immobile for long periods of time as he listens to music or contemplates a flower or his thumb. Mood swings are frequent, alternating suddenly between total euphoria and complete despair.

Some users will exhibit symptoms of paranoia. They become suspicious of people around them and tend to withdraw from others. Feelings of anxiety can also surface when the user is removed from a quiet environment and exposed to everyday stimuli. Activities such as standing in line with other people or walking down a city sidewalk may seem impossible to handle. Users have been known to jump off buildings or walk in front of moving trucks.

How LSD and other hallucinogens produce these bizarre effects remains unknown. The drug attaches to certain chemical binding sites widely spread through the brain, but what ensues thereafter has yet to be described. A person who takes LSD steadily with the doses close together can develop a tolerance to the drug. That is, the amount of drug that once produced a pronounced "high" no longer is effective. A larger dose is required to achieve the same effect. However, if the individual keeps increasing his drug intake he will soon pass over the threshold into the area of toxicity.

Discontinuing LSD or the other hallucinogens, especially after having used them for an extended period of time, is not easy. The residual effects of the drugs produce toxic symptoms and "flashbacks," which are similar to an LSD "trip."

Currently, the most common way to use LSD is by licking the back of a stamp torn from a perforated sheet of homemade stamps. The drug is coated on the back of the sheet of stamps or is deposited as a colored dot on the paper. Removing one stamp, the user places it on his tongue and allows the LSD to dissolve in his saliva. Because a tiny amount can produce strong effects, overdoses are common.

Teens often experiment with LSD or other hallucinogens in reaction to poor **family** relationships and psychological problems. Others are prompted by curiosity, **peer pressure**, and the desire to escape from feelings of isolation or despair. Typical physical signs of hallucinogen use include rapid breathing, muscle twitching, chills and shaking, upset stomach, enlarged pupils, confusion, and poor coordination.

Resources

BOOKS

Robbins, Paul R. *Hallucinogens.* Springfield, NJ: Enslow, 1996.

PERIODICALS

Fernandes, B. "The Long, Strange Trip Back." *World Press Review* 40, September 1993, pp. 38-39.

Monroe, Judy. "Designer Drugs: CAT & LSD." *Current Health* 21, September 1994, p. 13.

"The Negative Side of Nostalgia." *Medical Update* 17, July 1993, p. 3.

Perlstein, Steve. "Overall teen Drug Use Falls for Second Year in Row: Inhalant Use in Grade 8 a 'Warning Sign'." *Clinical Psychiatry News* (March 2004): 1-3.

Porush, D. "Finding God in the Three-Pound Universe: The Neuroscience of Transcendence." *Omni* 16, October 1993, pp. 60-62.

"Rave Realities; The Truth About Club Drugs." *Science World* (January 12, 2004): S8.

Scholey, Andrew B., et al. "Increased Intensity of Ecstasy and Polydrug Usage in the More Experienced Recreational Ecstast/MDMA Users: a WWW Study." *Addictive Behaviors* (June 2004):743-752.

Hallucinogens and related disorders

Definition

Hallucinogens are a chemically diverse group of drugs that cause changes in a person's thought processes, perceptions of the physical world, and sense of time passing. Hallucinogens can be found naturally in some plants and can be synthesized in the laboratory. Most hallucinogens are abused as recreational drugs. Hallucinogens are also called psychedelic drugs.

Description

Use of hallucinogens is at least as old as civilization. Many cultures have recorded eating certain plants specifically to induce visions or alter the perception of reality. Often these hallucinations were part of a religious or prophetic experience. Shamans in Siberia were known to eat the hallucinogenic mushroom *Amanita muscaria.* The ancient Greeks and the Vikings also used naturally occurring plant hallucinogens. Peyote, a spineless cactus native to the southwestern United States and Mexico, was used by native peoples, including the Aztecs, to produce visions.

Although several hundred plants are known to contain compounds that cause hallucinations, most hallucinogens are synthesized in illegal laboratories for delivery as street drugs. The best known hallucinogens are lysergic acid diethylamide (LSD), mescaline, psilocybin, and MDMA (ecstasy). Phencyclidine (PCP, angel dust) can produce hallucinations, as can amphetamines and **marijuana**, but these drugs are considered dissociative drugs, rather than hallucinogens, and act by a different pathway from classic hallucinogens. Dextromorphan, the main ingredient in many **cough** medicines, has become popular among some populations because of the PCP-like hallucinations it produces. In addition, new designer drugs that are chemical variants of classic hallucinogens are apt to appear on the street at any time. A drug that only recently was added to Schedule I of the 1970 Controlled Substances Act (the classification for many other "hard" drugs with no known therapeutic value) is 5-methoxy-N, N-diisopropyltryptamine (5-MeO-DIPT), a drug derived from the chemical tryptamine that is more commonly known as Foxy or Foxy Methoxy. A related hallucinogen, dimethyltryptamine, occurs naturally in plants in the Amazon but is now synthesized in labs. This drug, more commonly known as DMT, can be a powerful hallucinogen.

Although the various hallucinogens produce similar physical and psychological effects, they are a diverse group of compounds. However, all hallucinogens appear to affect the brain in similar ways. While the mechanism of action of hallucinogens is not completely understood, researchers have shown that these drugs bind with one type of serotonin receptor ($5\text{-}HT_2$) in the brain.

Serotonin is a neurotransmitter that facilitates transmission of nerve impulses in the brain and is associated with feelings of well-being, as well as many physiological responses. When a hallucinogenic compound binds with serotonin receptors, serotonin is blocked from those receptor sites, and nerve transmission is altered. There is an increase in free (unbound) serotonin in the brain. The result is a distortion of the senses of sight, sound, and touch, disorientation in time and space, and alterations of mood. In the case of hallucinogen intoxication, however, a person is not normally delirious, unconscious, or dissociated. He or she is aware that these changes in perception are caused by the hallucinogen.

LSD

LSD was first synthesized by Alfred Hoffman for a pharmaceutical company in Germany in 1938 while he was searching for a **headache** remedy. Hoffman discovered the hallucinogenic properties of LSD accidentally in 1943. The drug became popular with counterculture "hippies" in the mid-1960s when its sense-altering properties were reputed to offer a window into enhanced **creativity** and self-awareness. LSD also occurs naturally in morning glory seeds.

Pure LSD is a white, odorless, crystalline powder that dissolves easily in water, although contaminants can cause it to range in color from yellow to dark brown. LSD was listed as a Schedule I drug under the Controlled Substance Act of 1970, meaning that it has no medical or legal uses and has a high potential for abuse. LSD is not easy to manufacture in a home laboratory, and some of its ingredients are controlled substances that are difficult to obtain. However, LSD is very potent, and a small amount can produce a large number of doses.

On the street, LSD is sold in several forms. Microdots are tiny pills smaller than a pinhead. Windowpane is liquid LSD applied to thin squares of gelatin. Liquid LSD can also be sprayed on sugar cubes. The most common street form of the drug is liquid LSD sprayed onto blotter paper and dried. The paper, often printed with colorful or psychedelic pictures, is divided into tiny squares, each square being one dose. Liquid LSD can also be sprayed on the back of a postage stamp and licked off. Street names for the drug include acid, yellow sunshine, windowpane, cid, doses, trips, and boomers.

Mescaline

Mescaline is a naturally occurring plant hallucinogen. Its primary source is the cactus *Lophophora williamsii.* This cactus is native to the southwestern United States and Mexico. The light blue-green plant is spineless and has a crown called a peyote button. This button contains mescaline and can be eaten or made into a bitter tea. Mescaline is also the active ingredient of at least ten other cacti of the genus *Trichocereus* that are native to parts of South America.

Mescaline was first isolated in 1897 by the German chemist Arthur Hefftner and first synthesized in the laboratory in 1919. Some experiments were done with the drug to determine if it was medically useful, but no medical uses were found. However, peyote is culturally significant. It has been used for centuries as part of religious celebrations and vision quests of Native Americans. The Native American Church, which fuses elements of Christianity with indigenous practices, has long used peyote as part of its religious practices.

In 1970 mescaline was listed as a Schedule I drug under the Controlled Substances Act. However, that same year the state of Texas legalized peyote for use in Native American religious ceremonies. In 1995, a federal law was passed making peyote legal only for this use in all 50 states.

Psilocybin

Psilocybin is the active ingredient in what are known on the street as magic mushrooms, shrooms, mushies, or Mexican mushrooms. There are several species of mushrooms that contain psilocybin, including *Psilocybe mexicana, P. muscorumi,* and *Stropharia cubensis.* These mushrooms grow in most moderate, moist climates.

Psilocybin-containing mushrooms are usually cooked and eaten (they have a bitter taste), or dried and boiled to make a tea. Although psilocybin can be made synthetically in the laboratory, there is no street market for synthetic psilocybin, and virtually all the drug comes from cultivated mushrooms. In the United States, it is legal to possess psilocybin-containing mushrooms, but it is illegal to traffic in them, and psilocybin and psilocyn (another psychoactive drug found in small quantities in these mushrooms) are both Schedule I drugs.

MDMA

MDMA, short for 3,4-methylenedioxymethamphetamine, and better known as ecstasy, XTC, E, X, or Adam, has become an increasingly popular club drug since the 1980s. The hallucinogenically active portion of the drug is chemically similar to mescaline, while its stimulant portion is similar to methamphetamine. MDMA was first synthesized in 1912 by a German pharmaceutical company looking for a new compound that would stop bleeding. The company patented the drug, but never did anything with it. A closely related drug, methylenedioxyamphetimine or MDA, was tested by a pharmaceutical company as an appetite suppressant in the 1950s, but its use was discontinued when it was discovered to have hallucinogenic properties. In the 1960s, MDA was a popular drug of abuse in some large cities such as San Francisco.

During the early 1980s therapists experimented with MDMA, which was legal at the time, as a way to help patients open up and become more empathetic. Recreational use soon followed, and it was declared an illegal Schedule I drug in 1985. For about a year between 1987 and 1988, the drug was again legal as the result of court challenges, but it permanently joined other Schedule I hallucinogens in March 1988.

MDMA is a popular club drug often associated with all-night raves or dance parties. The drug, sold in tablets, is attractive because it combines stimulant effects that allow ravers to dance for hours with a feeling of empathy, reduced **anxiety**, and reduced inhibitions, and euphoria. Some authorities consider MDA and MDMA stimulant-hallucinogens and do not group them with classic hallucinogens such as LSD, but research indicates that MDA and MDMA affect the brain in the same way as classic hallucinogens. The American Psychiatric Association considers MDMA as a drug that can cause hallucinogen-related disorders.

Causes and symptoms

A cause of hallucinogen use is that hallucinogens are attractive to recreational drug users for a number of reasons, including:

- they are minimally addictive and there are no physical withdrawal symptoms upon stopping use.
- they produce few serious or debilitating physical side effects.
- they do not usually produce a delusional state, excessive stupor, or excessive stimulation.
- they do not cause memory loss with occasional use.
- they are easily and cheaply available.
- they produce a high that gives the illusion of increasing creativity, empathy, or self-awareness.
- deaths from overdoses are rare.

Despite their perceived harmlessness, strong hallucinogens such as LSD can cause frightening and anxiety-evoking emotional experiences, known as bad trips. Flashbacks, where the sensations experienced while under the influence of a drug recur uncontrollably without drug use, can occur for months after a single drug use. During hallucinogen intoxication, reality may be so altered that a person may endanger himself by believing he is capable of feats such as flying off buildings. Hallucinogens also may induce or cause a worsening of latent psychiatric disorders such as anxiety, depression, and psychosis. Hallucinogens can also cause paranoia, long-term memory loss, personality changes (especially if there is a latent psychiatric disorder), and psychological drug dependence.

Psychological symptoms

Hallucinogens work primarily on the perception of reality. They usually do not create true hallucinations, which are imagined visions or sounds (voices heard in the head, for example) in the absence of any corresponding reality. Instead, classic hallucinogens alter the perception of something that is physically present. A face may appear to "melt" or colors may become brighter, move, and change shape. Sounds may be "seen," rather than heard.

More than with other drugs, the mental state of the hallucinogen user and the environment in which the drug is taken influence the user's experience. LSD, especially, is known for symptoms that range from mellowness and psychedelic visions (good trips) to anxiety and panic attacks (bad trips). Previous good experiences with a drug do not guarantee continued good experiences. People with a history of psychiatric disorders are more likely to experience harmful reactions, as are those who are given the drug without their knowledge.

Normally, mescaline and psilocybin produce uniformly milder symptoms than LSD. During a single drug experience, the user can experience a range of symptoms. Mood can shift from happy to sad or pleasant to frightening and back again several times. Some symptoms occur primarily with MDMA, as indicated. Psychological symptoms of hallucinogen intoxication include:

- distortion of sight, sound, and touch
- confusion of the senses—sounds are "seen" or vision is "heard"
- disorientation in time and space
- delusions of physical invulnerability (especially with LSD)
- paranoia
- unreliable judgment and increased risk taking
- anxiety attacks
- flashbacks after the drug has been cleared from the body
- blissful calm or mellowness
- reduced inhibitions
- increased empathy (MDMA)
- elation or euphoria
- impaired concentration and motivation
- long-term memory loss
- personality changes, especially if there is a latent psychiatric disorder
- psychological drug dependence

Physical symptoms

Although the primary effects of hallucinogens are on perceptions, some physical effects do occur. Physical symptoms include:

- increased blood pressure
- increased heart rate
- nausea and vomiting (especially with psilocybin and mescaline)
- blurred vision which can last after the drug has worn off
- poor coordination
- enlarged pupils
- sweating
- diarrhea (plant hallucinogens)
- restlessness
- muscle cramping (especially clenched jaws with MDMA)
- dehydration (MDMA)
- serious increase in body temperature leading to seizures (MDMA)

Demographics

Hallucinogen use, excluding MDMA, peaked in the United States late 1960s as part of the counter-culture movement. Hallucinogen use then gradually declined until the early 1990s, when it again picked up. A recent government survey found that about 33.7 million Americans (13.9%) age 12 or older report having tried a hallucinogen at least once in their lives. About 22.4 million Americans (9.2% of the population) age 12 or older report having used LSD at least once, with 104,000 reporting use within the last month. Among teenagers, use of these drugs has remained fairly stable with some declines in recent years.

A recent U.S. government survey found that about 11.5 million Americans age 12 or older report having tried MDMA at least once. About 0.2% of the population reported having used the drug in the last month. Among adolescents, use of the drug appears to have increased in recent years. A total of 6.5% of twelfth graders reported having tried MDMA in the past month according to a recent survey.

Diagnosis

Although not all experts agree, the diagnosis of mental disorders, recognizes two hallucinogen-related disorders: hallucinogen dependence and hallucinogen abuse. Hallucinogen dependence is the continued use of hallucinogens even when the substances cause the affected individual significant problems, or when the individual knows of adverse effects (memory impairment while intoxicated, anxiety attacks, flashbacks), but continues to use the substances anyway. "Craving" hallucinogens after not using them for a period of time has been reported. Hallucinogen abuse is repeated use of hallucinogens even after they have caused the user impairment that undermines his or her ability to fulfill obligations at work, school, or home, but the use is usually not as frequent as it is among dependent users. In addition to these two disorders, the American Psychiatric Association recognizes eight hallucinogen-induced disorders. These are:

- hallucinogen intoxication
- hallucinogen persistent perception disorder (flashbacks)
- hallucinogen intoxication delirium
- hallucinogen-induced psychotic disorder with delusions
- hallucinogen-induced psychotic disorder with hallucinations
- hallucinogen-induced mood disorder
- hallucinogen-induced anxiety disorder
- hallucinogen-related disorder not otherwise specified

Hallucinogen dependence and abuse are normally diagnosed from reports by the patient or person accompanying the patient of use of a hallucinogenic drug. Active hallucinations and accompanying physical symptoms can confirm the diagnosis, but do not have to be present. Routine drug screening does not detect LSD in the blood or urine, although specialized laboratory methods can detect the drug. Hallucinogen dependence differs from other drug dependence in that there are no withdrawal symptoms when the drug is stopped, and the extent of tolerance, (needing a higher and higher dose to achieve the same effect) appears minimal.

Hallucinogen intoxication is diagnosed based on psychological changes, perceptual changes, and physical symptoms that are typical of hallucinogen use. These changes must not be caused by a general medical condition, other **substance abuse**, or another mental disorder.

Hallucinogen persisting perception disorder, better known as flashbacks, occur after hallucinogen use followed by a period of lucidity. Flashbacks may occur weeks or months after the drug was used, and may occur after a single use or many uses.

To be diagnosed as a psychiatric disorder, flashbacks must cause significant distress or interfere with daily life activities. They can come on suddenly with no warning, or be triggered by specific environments. Flashbacks may include emotional symptoms, seeing colors, geometric forms, or, most commonly, persistence of trails of light across the visual field. They may last for months. Flashbacks are most strongly associated with LSD.

Hallucinogen intoxication delirium is rare unless the hallucinogen is contaminated by another drug or chemical such as strychnine. In hallucinogen intoxication, the patient is still grounded in reality and recognizes that the experiences of altered perception are due to using a hallucinogen. In hallucinogen intoxication delirium, the patient is no longer grounded in reality. Hallucinogen-induced psychotic disorders are similar in that the patient loses touch with reality. Psychotic states can occur immediately after using the drug, or days or months later.

Hallucinogen-induced mood disorder and hallucinogen-induced anxiety disorder are somewhat controversial, as hallucinogen use may uncover latent or preexisting anxiety or **mood disorders** rather than being the cause of them. However, it does appear that MDMA use can cause major depression.

Treatments

Acute treatment is aimed at preventing the patient from harming himself or anyone else. Since most people experiencing hallucinogen intoxication remain in touch with reality, "talking down" or offering reassurance and support that emphasizes that the disturbing sensatinos, anxiety, panic attack, or paranoia will pass as the drug wears off is often helpful. Patients are kept in a calm, pleasant, but lighted environment, and are encouraged to move around while being helped to remain oriented to reality. Occasionally, drugs such as lorazepam are given for anxiety. Complications in treatment occur when the hallucinogen has been contaminated with other street drugs or chemicals. The greatest life-threatening risk is associated with MDMA, in which users may develop dangerously high body temperatures. Reducing the patient's temperature is an essential acute treatment.

Treatment for long-term effects of hallucinogen use involve long-term psychotherapy after drug use has stopped. Many people find 12-step programs or group support helpful. In addition, underlying psychiatric disorders must be addressed.

Prognosis

Because hallucinogens are not physically addictive, many people are able to stop using these drugs successfully. However, users may be haunted by chronic problems such as flashbacks or mood and anxiety disorders either brought about or worsened by use of hallucinogens. It is difficult to predict who will have long-term complications and who will not.

Prevention

Hallucinogen use is difficult to prevent, because these drugs have a reputation for being nonaddictive and "harmless." Drug education and social outlets that provide people with a sense of self-worth are the best ways to prevent hallucinogen and other substance abuse.

Resources

BOOKS

American Psychiatric Association. *Diagnostic and Statistical Manual of Mental Disorders,* 4th ed., Text rev. Washington, D.C.: American Psychiatric Association, 2000.

Galanter, Marc, and Herbert D. Kleber, eds. *Textbook of Substance Abuse Treatment,* 2nd ed. Washington, D.C.: American Psychiatric Press, Inc., 1999.

Giannini, James. *Drug Abuse: A Family Guide to Detection, Treatment and Education.* Los Angeles: Health Information Press, 1999.

Holland, Julie, ed. *Ecstasy: The Complete Guide.* Rochester, Vermont: Park Street Press, 2001.

Sadock, Benjamin J., and Virginia A. Sadock, eds. *Comprehensive Textbook of Psychiatry,* 7th ed., Vol. 1. Philadelphia: Lippincott Williams and Wilkins, 2000.

OTHER

Office of National Drug Control Policy. "Drug Facts: Club Drugs." (2007). Available online at: http://www.whitehousedrugpolicy.gov/drugfact/club/index.html.

Office of National Drug Control Policy. "Drug Facts: Hallucinogens." (2007) Available online at: http://www.whitehousedrugpolicy.gov/drugfact/hallucinogens/index.html.

Substance Abuse and Mental Health Services Administration. (2006). *Results from the 2005 National Survey on Drug Use and Health: National Findings* (Office of Applied Studies, NSDUH Series H-30, DHHS Publication No. SMA 06-4194). Rockville, MD. Available online at: http://www.oas.samhsa.gov/NSDUH/2k5NSDUH/2k5results.htm.

ORGANIZATIONS

National Clearinghouse for Alcohol and Drug Information, P. O. Box 2345, Rockville MD, 20852, (800) 729-6686, http://www.health.org.

National Institute on Drug Abuse, 5600 Fishers Lane, Room 10 A-39, Rockville MD, 20857, (888) 644-6432, http://niad.nih.gov.

Partnership for a Drug-Free America, 405 Lexington Avenue, New York NY, 10174, (212) 922-1560, http://www.drugfreeamerica.org.

Tish Davidson, AM
Emily Jane Willingham, PhD

Hand-eye coordination

Definition

Hand-eye coordination involves the ability of the brain to synchronize vision with **fine motor skills**.

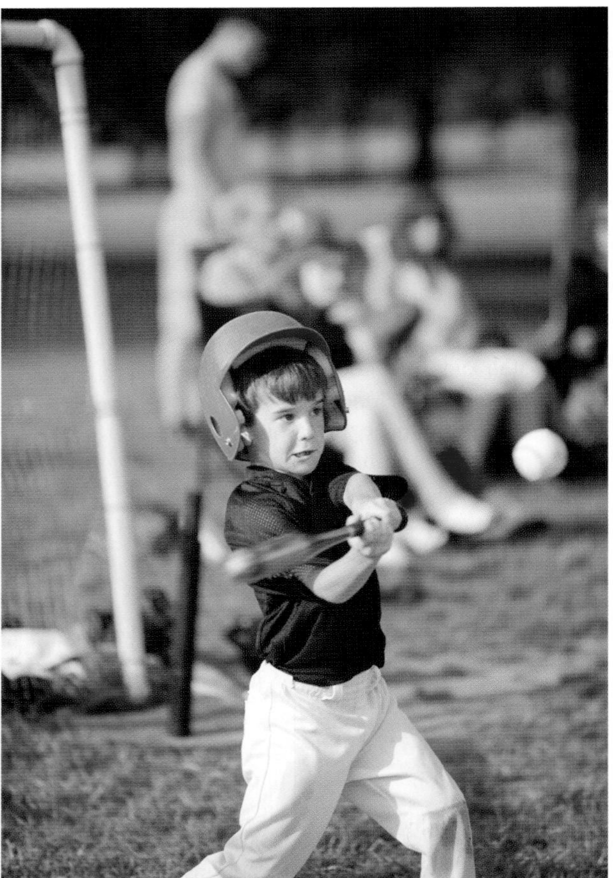

Good hand-eye coordination is needed to play baseball. *(Sonya Etchison/Shutterstock.com.)*

Description

Infancy

Hand-eye coordination begins developing in **infancy**. Although it is an instinctive developmental achievement that cannot be taught, parents can hasten its progress by providing their children with stimulating **toys** and other objects that will encourage them to practice reaching out for things and grasping them.

Until the age of eight weeks, infants are too nearsighted to see objects at distances farther than about eight inches from their faces, and they have not yet discovered their hands, which are held in fists throughout this period. By the age of two to two-and-a-half months, the eyes focus much better, and babies can follow a moving object with their gaze, even turning their heads to keep sight of it longer. However, when children this age drop an object, they will try to find it by feeling rather than looking for it, and although they play with their hands, they do it without looking at them.

By three months, most infants will have made an important hand-eye connection; they can deliberately bring their hands into their field of vision. By now they are watching their hands when they play with them. They also swipe at objects within their view, a repetitive activity that provides practice in estimating distance and controlling the hands. Attempts to grab onto things (which usually fail) consist of a series of tries, with the child looking at the object and then at the hand, moving the hand closer to it, and then re-sighting the object and trying again.

At the age of four or five months, hand-eye coordination is developed sufficiently for an infant to manipulate toys and begin to seek them out. By the age of six months, the infant can focus on objects at a distance and consistently follow them with the eyes. At this point, infants can sight an object and reach for it without repeatedly looking at their hands; they sense where their hands are and can move them straight to the object, keeping their eyes on the object the entire time. By the final months of the first year, infants can shift their gaze between objects held in both hands and compare them to each other.

Toddlerhood

The toddler stage brings further progress in hand-eye coordination, resulting in the control necessary to manipulate objects with increasing sophistication. The ability to sight and grasp objects accurately improves dramatically with the acquisition of the "pincer grasp." This ability to grasp objects between the thumb and forefinger develops between the ages of 12 and 15 months. Around the same time, children begin stacking objects on top of each other. Most children can stack two blocks by the age of 15 months and three by the age of 18 months. At this age they also begin emptying, gathering, and nesting objects, or placing one object inside another. Toddlers also can draw horizontal and vertical pencil lines and circular scribbles, twist dials, push levers, pull strings, pound pegs, string large beads, put a key in a lock, and turn book pages. Eventually, they are able to stack as many as six blocks, unwrap small objects, manipulate snap toys, and play with clay. Between the ages of 15 and 23 months there is significant improvement in feeding skills, such as using a spoon and a cup.

Preschool years

During the **preschool** period, hand-eye coordination progresses to the point of near independence at self-care activities. A four-year-old is learning to handle eating utensils well and button even small buttons. Four-year-old children can also handle a pencil competently, copy geometric shapes and letters, and use scissors. By the age of five, a child's hand-eye coordination appears quite advanced, although it will continue to be fine-tuned for several more years. The child approaches, grasps, and releases objects with precision and accuracy. The five year old may use the same toys as preschoolers, but manipulates them with greater skill and purpose and can complete a familiar jigsaw puzzle with lightning speed. An important milestone in hand-eye progress at this stage is the child's ability to tie his or her own shoelaces.

School-aged children

At the age of six, a child's visual orientation changes somewhat. Children of this age and older shift their gaze more frequently than younger children. They also have a tendency to follow the progress of an object rather than looking directly at it, a fact that has been linked to the practice of some six–year–old children using their fingers to mark their places when they are reading. Even when absorbed in tasks, they look away frequently, although their hands remain active.

Hand-eye coordination improves through middle childhood, with advances in speed, timing, and coordination. By the age of nine, the eyes and hands are well differentiated, that is, each can be used independently of the other, and improved finger differentiation is evident as well. Nine-year-olds can use carpentry and garden tools with reasonable skill and complete simple sewing projects.

KEY TERMS

Fine motor skills—The ability to make smooth, controlled movements using the small muscles in the fingers, hand, and wrist.

Resources

OTHER

Reilly, Peter. "Hand–Eye Test." World of Psychology. January 8 2007, http://www.handeyetest.com (accessed September 26, 2010).

Rosseau, Robert. "How to Improve Hand Eye Coordination." Bodyomics.com, http://www.bodyomics.com/articles/hand_eye_coordination.html (accessed September 26, 2010).

ORGANIZATIONS

American Academy of Family Physicians (AAFP), PO Box 11210, Shawnee Mission KS, 66207 (913) 906–6000, (800) 274–2237, (913) 906–6075, http://familydoctor.org.

American Academy of Neurology (AAN), 1080 Montreal Ave., St. Paul MN, 55116 (651) 695–2717, (800) 879–1960, (651) 695–2791, http://www.aan.com.

American Academy of Pediatrics (AAP), 141 Northwest Point Blvd., Elk Grove Village IL, 60007–1098, (847) 434–4000 (847) 434–8000, http://www.aap.org.

Tish Davidson, AM

Hand-foot-and-mouth disease

Definition

Hand-foot-and-mouth disease is an infection of young children in which characteristic fluid-filled blisters appear on the hands, feet, and inside the mouth.

Demographics

Hand-foot-and-mouth disease is very common among young children and often occurs in clusters of children who are in daycare together.

An outbreak of hand-foot-and-mouth disease occurred in Singapore in 2000, with more than 1,000 diagnosed cases, all in children, resulting in four deaths. A smaller outbreak occurred in Malaysia in 2000. In 1998, a serious outbreak of enterovirus 71 in Taiwan resulted in more than one million cases of hand-foot-and-mouth disease. Of these, there were 405 severe cases and 78 deaths, 71 of which were children younger than five years of age.

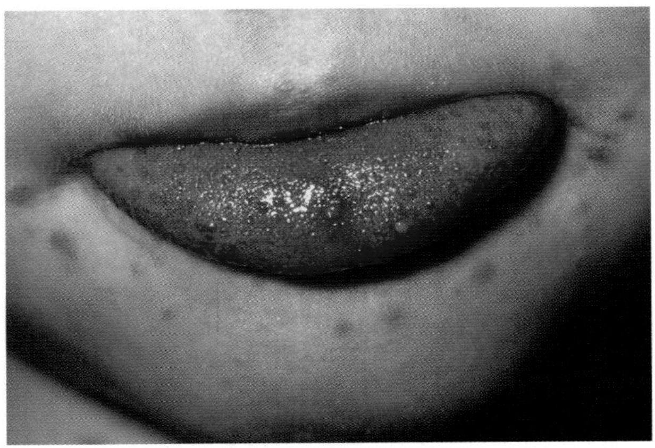

Skin lesions on the tongue and around the mouth of a five-year-old boy due to hand-foot-mouth disease. *(Dr. P. Marazzi/Photo Researchers, Inc.)*

Hand-foot-and-mouth should not be confused with foot and mouth disease, which infects cattle but is extremely rare in humans. An outbreak of foot and mouth disease swept through Great Britain and into other parts of Europe and South America in 2001.

Description

Coxsackie viruses belong to a family of viruses called enteroviruses. These viruses live in the gastrointestinal tract, and are therefore present in feces. They can be spread easily from one person to another when poor hygiene allows the virus within the feces to be passed from person to person. After exposure to the virus, development of symptoms takes only four to six days. Hand-foot-and-mouth disease can occur year-round, although the largest number of cases are in summer and fall months.

Causes and symptoms

Hand-foot-and-mouth disease is very common among young children, and often occurs in clusters of children who are in daycare together. It is spread when poor hand-washing after a diaper change or contact with saliva (drool) allows the virus to be passed from one child to another.

Within about four to six days of acquiring the virus, an infected child may develop a relatively low-grade **fever**, ranging from 99-102°F (37-38.9°C). Other symptoms include fatigue, loss of energy, decreased appetite, and a sore sensation in the mouth that may interfere with feeding. After one to two days, fluid-filled bumps (vesicles) appear on the inside of the mouth, along the surface of the tongue, on the roof of the mouth, and on the insides of the cheeks. These are tiny blisters, about three to seven millimeters in diameter. Eventually, they may appear on the palms of the hands and on the soles of the feet. Occasionally, these vesicles may occur in the diaper region.

The vesicles in the mouth cause the majority of discomfort, and the child may refuse to eat or drink due to **pain**. This phase usually lasts for an average of a week. As long as the bumps have clear fluid within them, the disease is at its most contagious. The fluid within the vesicles contains large quantities of the causative viruses. Extra care should be taken to avoid contact with this fluid.

Diagnosis

Diagnosis is made by most practitioners solely on the basis of the unique appearance of blisters of the mouth, hands, and feet, in a child not appearing very ill.

KEY TERMS

Enteroviruses—Viruses which live in the gastrointestinal tract. Coxsackie viruses, viruses that cause hand–foot–mouth disease, are an enterovirus.

Vesicle—A bump on the skin filled with fluid.

Treatment

There are no treatments available to cure or decrease the duration of the disease. Medications like **acetaminophen** or ibuprofen may be helpful for decreasing pain, and allowing the child to eat and drink. It is important to try to encourage the child to take in adequate amounts of fluids, in the form of ice chips or popsicles if other foods or liquids are too uncomfortable.

Alternative treatment

There are no effective alternative treatments for hand-foot-and-mouth disease.

Prognosis

The prognosis for a child with hand-foot-and-mouth disease is excellent. The child is usually completely better within about a week of the start of the illness.

Prevention

Prevention involves careful attention to hygiene. Thorough, consistent hand-washing practices, and discouraging the sharing of clothes, towels, and stuffed **toys** are all helpful. Virus continues to be passed in the feces for several weeks after infection, so good hygiene should be practiced long after all signs of infection have passed.

Resources

BOOKS

Morag, Abraham, and Pearay L. Ogra. "Viral Infections." In Behrman, Richard, editor. *Nelson Textbook of Pediatrics,* 16th ed. Philadelphia: W.B. Saunders Co., 2000.

PERIODICALS

Lee T.C., et al. "Diseases Caused by Enterovirus 71 Infection." *The Pediatric Infectious Disease Journal.* 28(10) (October 2009): 904–10.

Ooi M.H., et al. "Identification and Validation of Clinical Predictors for the risk of Neurological Involvement in Children with Hand, Foot, and Mouth Disease in Sarawak." *BMC Infectious Diseases.* 9 (January 19 2009): 3.

Rosalyn Carson–DeWitt, MD
Karl Finley

Handedness

Definition

Handedness refers to person's natural preference for using one hand over the other when performing manual tasks.

Demographics

Roughly 90% of humans are right-handed; in the United States, 8–15% of the adult population is thought to be left-handed. Men are three times more likely to be left-handed than women, and homosexuals have a higher rate of left-handedness than heterosexuals.

Description

The term handedness (sometimes called laterality) describes a characteristic form of specialization whereby a person, by preference, uses one hand for such clearly identified activities as writing. For example, a person who uses his or her right hand for activities requiring skill and coordination (e.g., writing, drawing, cutting) is defined as right-handed. Because left-handed children who are forced to write with their right hand sometimes develop the ability to write with both hands, the term ambidexterity is often used in everyday parlance to denote balanced handedness. True ambidexterity, in the sense of being able to perform the same task equally well with both hands, is rare, however; most left-handed people who have learned to write with the right hand prefer using only the left hand for other purposes. For example, both Babe Ruth and Lou Gehrig were forced to learn to write with the right hand when they were children, but they hit and threw only with the left hand as baseball players.

Causes

An often misunderstood phenomenon, handedness is a result of the human brain's unique development. While the human mind is commonly thought of as a single entity, research in brain physiology and anatomy has demonstrated that various areas of the brain control different mental aptitudes and that the physiological structure of the brain affects our mental functions. The brain's fundamental structure is dual (i.e., there are two cerebral hemispheres), and this duality is an essential quality of the human body. Generally speaking, each hemisphere is connected to sensory receptors on the opposite side of the body. In other words, the left hemisphere of the cerebral cortex controls the right hand. When scientists started studying the brain's anatomy, they learned that the two hemispheres are not identical. In fact, the French physician and anthropologist Paul Pierre Broca (1824–1880) and the German neurologist and psychiatrist Carl Wernicke (1848–1905) produced empirical evidence that important language centers were located in the left hemisphere. Since Broca's findings were based on right-handed subjects, and since right-handedness is predominant in humans, psychologists felt prompted to develop the notion of the left hemisphere as the dominant part of the brain.

Furthermore, Broca formulated a general rule stating that the hemisphere that governs language skills is always opposite from a person's preferred side. In other words, the left hemisphere always controls a right-handed person's language abilities. According to Broca's rule, left-handedness would indicate a hemispheric switch. Handedness research, however, uncovered a far more complex situation. While Broca's rule works for right-handers, left-handed people present a rather puzzling picture. Namely, researchers have discovered that only about two out of ten left-handers follow Broca's rule. In other words, most left-handed people violate Broca's rule by having their language center in the left hemisphere. Furthermore, the idea of clearly defined cerebral dominance seems compromised by the fact that some 70% of left-handed people have bilateral hemispheric control of language.

Hemispheric dominance is not the only explanation that has been offered for handedness. Some researchers have proposed that exposure to higher levels of testosterone before **birth** increases the chances of the child's being left-handed. This theory is thought to explain why more boys than girls are left-handed. Another theory associates left-handedness in the child with a high level of emotional stress on the mother during the birth process.

Development of handedness

While hemispheric dominance can be observed in animals, only humans have a clearly defined type of dominance. In other words, while animals may be right- or left-"pawed," only humans are predominantly right-handed. The American developmental psychologist Arnold Gesell (1880–1961), known for his pioneering work in scientific observation of child behavior, noted that infants display signs of handedness as early as the age of four weeks. At that age, according to Gesell, right-handed children assume a "fencing" position, right arm and hand extended; by the age of one, right-handedness is clearly established, the child using the right hand for a variety of operations, and the left for holding and gripping. Predominant right-handedness in humans has led researchers to define right-handedness as genetically coded. This raises the question of if left-handedness also has a genetic basis, is it possible to establish inheritance patterns? Empirical studies, even studies of identical **twins**, have failed to establish left-handedness as a genetic trait. For example, a person with two left-handed parents has only a 35% chance of being left-handed.

Challenges of left-handedness

In the past, left-handedness was associated with emotional and behavioral problems. This association led to the popular belief, strengthened by folklore, that left-handed people are somehow flawed. In addition, left-handedness has also been associated with immunological problems and a shorter life span. While not devoid of any foundation, these ideas are based on inconclusive, and sometimes even deceptive, evidence. For example, a 1991 study that purported to demonstrate that left-handed people died on average 9 years earlier than their right-handed counterparts of the same sex born in the same year has been shown to be seriously flawed. The "case of the disappearing southpaws" is now attributed to the fact that people born before 1940 were under much greater pressure to switch hands as children than people in later generations, which would explain why there is a higher proportion of left-handed people in younger age groups in the United States.

An even greater challenge than right-handed scissors and can openers is what psychologist Stanley Coren calls "handism," the belief that right-handedness is "better" than left-handedness. The idea that left-handers need to conform to a dominant standard has traditionally been translated into punitive educational practices whereby left-handed children were physically forced to write with their right hand. For example, both King George VI (father of the current Queen Elizabeth II of England) and Nelson Rockefeller (a former governor of New York) were both forced in childhood to wear long strings attached to the left wrist. When their fathers saw them using the left hand for any purpose, they would tug the string violently. It is thought that George VI's lifelong stammer resulted from this punitive treatment.

Some historians think that "handism" may have been a by-product of ancient warfare and the development of professional armies by the time of the later Roman Republic (c. 100 BC). A left-handed recruit for the heavy infantry in the Roman army was trained to use the *gladius*, the short sword used in combat, with his right hand by having his left hand tied to his side during the Roman equivalent of basic training. The reason for this practice was that Roman heavy infantrymen stood in continuous lines in battle formation, with each legionary's shield touching the shield of the soldier next to him. A left-handed soldier would have broken the formation, in addition to risking striking the legionary to his immediate left with his sword.

While there is a growing awareness among educators and parents that left-handedness should not be suppressed, the left-handed child is still exposed to a variety of pressures, some subtle, some crude, to conform. These pressures are reinforced by a tradition of maligning left-handed people. Among the Inuit, for example, left-handedness was associated with sorcery. In medieval Japan, a man was allowed to **divorce** his wife if he discovered after the wedding that she was left-handed. Major religious traditions, such as Christianity, Buddhism, and Islam, have described left-handedness in negative terms. In Islam, for example, the left hand is associated with defecation, because a devout Muslim will use only the left hand to clean himself after using the toilet.

Current language is also a rich repository of recorded animosity toward left-handers. For example, the modern English "left" evolved from the Anglo-Saxon *lyft*, which means "weak." The Latin word *sinister*, meaning "unfavorable" as well as denoting the left side, is still used to denote something evil; and *gauche*, the French word for left, generally indicates awkwardness. The German adjective *linkisch*, from *links* (left), means "awkward" or "wrong"; *weit links* means "very much mistaken." The numerous expressions which imply that "left" is the opposite of "good" include such phrases as "a left-handed compliment."

Disadvantages of left-handedness

Being a left-handed child still has many disadvantages, despite the efforts made in recent years to accept left-handedness as a normal human difference. Even children whose parents and teacher tolerate their left-handedness often suffer in school. For example, a left-handed student's paper may be downgraded for being "sloppy" because of the teacher's unconscious reaction to handwriting that just does not seem "right." In addition, art and science projects may receive unfair criticism because the teacher did not realize that the left-handed student was struggling with instruments and equipment designed for the right-handed majority. Scissors designed for right-handed people, for example, are uncomfortable for left-handers to grip. In Japan, left-handed sushi chefs must order knives designed specially for left-handers, because the Japanese knife has its cutting edge ground to slant to one side, unlike the symmetrical cutting edge of European or American knives. Lastly, left-handed surgeons rarely receive help with handedness-related problems during their medical training; of a group of left-handed surgeons in the United States surveyed in 2004, only 10% received training in coping with their left-handedness during their residency years, and only 13% worked in residency programs that provided them with left-handed surgical instruments.

KEY TERMS

Cerebral cortex—Brain region responsible for reasoning, mood, and perception.

Testosterone—A male steroid hormone produced in the testes and responsible for the development of secondary sex characteristics.

Advantages of left-handedness

On the other hand, those who are left-handed have the advantage in some fields. In baseball, left-handed batters have the advantage of being one step closer to first base, thus making it easier to beat a close play. They also have a better angle of vision for seeing balls thrown by right-handed pitchers. Left-handed soldiers have the advantage of a surprise factor in hand-to-hand combat, since most of the opponents will be right-handed; Alexander the Great was an outstanding left-handed swordsman. Left-handedness is not a disadvantage in the fine arts, as such famous painters as Michelangelo, Leonardo da Vinci, and Pablo Picasso were all left-handed.

Resources

BOOKS

Wolman, David. *A Left-hand Turn Around the World: Chasing the Mystery and Meaning of All Things Southpaw.* New York: MJF Books, 2007.

OTHER

Ambidextrous Children at Higher Risk for Learning Problems. MedlinePlus HealthDay.com. January 25, 2010. [accessed July 16, 2010]. file:///C:/DOCUME~1/HP_ADM~1/LOCALS~1/Temp/fullstory_94482.htm

Left-handedness: Does it Mean Anything? PsychologistWorld.com. Undated. [accessed July 16, 2010], http://www.psychologistworld.com/influence_personality/handedness.php

Needleman, Robert. "What is 'Handedness'?" Dr.Spock.com August 26, 2004. [accessed July 16, 2010], http://www.drspock.com/article/0,1510,5812,00.html

ORGANIZATIONS

Handedness Research Institute, 674 E. Cottage Grove, Suite 200, Bloomington IN, 47408, (812) 855-4691, http://www.handedness.org.

Left-Handed Liberation Society, 375 N. Stephanie Street, Suite 1411, Henderson NV, 89014-8909, (888) 30-LEFTY, bsands@adelphia.ne or bsands1@roadrunner.com, http://www.lefthander.com.

Rebecca J. Frey, PhD
Tish Davidson, AM

Happy puppet syndrome **see Angelman syndrome**

Harelip **see Cleft lip and palate**

Hashimoto's thyroiditis **see Hypothyroidism**

Haverhill fever **see Rat-bite fever**

Hay fever **see Allergic rhinitis**

HBF test **see Fetal hemoglobin test**

HBV **see Hepatitis B vaccine**

Head injury

Definition

Injury to the head may damage the scalp, skull, or brain. The most important consequence of head trauma is traumatic brain injury. Head injury may occur either as a closed head injury, such as the head hitting a car's windshield, or as a penetrating head injury, as when a bullet pierces the skull. Both may cause damage that ranges from mild to profound. Very severe injury can be fatal because of profound brain damage.

Description

External trauma to the head is capable of damaging the brain, even if there is no external evidence of damage. More serious injuries can cause skull fracture, blood clots between the skull and the brain, or bruising and tearing of the brain tissue itself.

Injuries to the head can be caused by traffic accidents, **sports injuries**, falls, workplace accidents, assaults, or bullets. Most people have had some type of head injury at least once in their lives, but rarely do they require a hospital visit.

Each year about two million people have a serious head injury, and up to 750,000 of them are severe enough to require hospitalization. Brain injury is most likely to occur in males between ages 15 and 24, usually as a result of car and motorcycle accidents. About 70% of all accidental deaths are due to head injuries, as are most of the disabilities that occur after trauma.

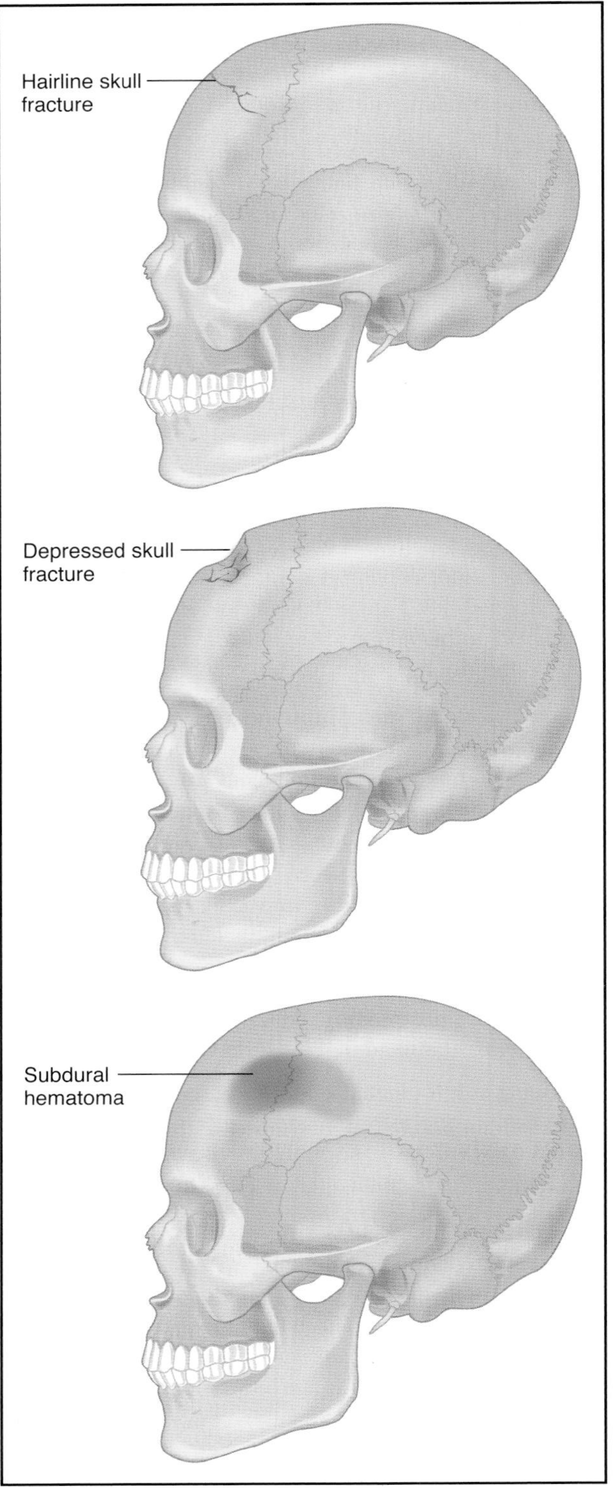

Illustration depicting three types of head injury: hairline fracture, depressed fracture, and subdural hematoma. *(Illustration by Electronic Illustrators Group. Reproduced by permission of Gale, a part of Cengage Learning.)*

A person who has had a head injury and who is experiencing the following symptoms should seek medical care immediately:

- serious bleeding from the head or face
- loss of consciousness, however brief
- confusion and lethargy
- lack of pulse or breathing
- clear fluid drainage from the nose or ear

Causes and symptoms

A head injury may cause damage both from the direct physical injury to the brain and from secondary factors, such as lack of oxygen, brain swelling, and disturbance of blood flow. Both closed and penetrating head injuries can cause swirling movements throughout the brain, tearing nerve fibers and causing widespread bleeding or a blood clot in or around the brain. Swelling may raise pressure within the skull (intracranial pressure) and may block the flow of oxygen to the brain.

Head trauma may cause a **concussion**, in which there is a brief loss of consciousness without visible structural damage to the brain. In addition to loss of consciousness, initial symptoms of brain injury may include:

- memory loss and confusion
- vomiting
- dizziness
- partial paralysis or numbness
- shock
- anxiety

After a head injury, there may be a period of impaired consciousness followed by a period of confusion and impaired memory with disorientation and a breakdown in the ability to store and retrieve new information. Others experience temporary amnesia following head injury that begins with memory loss over a period of weeks, months, or years before the injury (retrograde amnesia). As the patient recovers, memory slowly returns. Post-traumatic amnesia refers to loss of memory for events during and after the accident.

Epilepsy occurs in 2–5% of people who have had a head injury; it is much more common in people who have had severe or penetrating injuries. Most cases of epilepsy appear right after the accident or within the first year, and become less likely with increased time following the accident.

Closed head injury

Closed head injury refers to brain injury without any penetrating injury to the brain. It may be the result of a direct blow to the head; of the moving head being rapidly stopped, such as when a person's head hits a windshield in a car accident; or by the sudden deceleration of the head without its striking another object. The kind of injury the brain receives in a closed head injury is determined by whether or not the head was unrestrained upon impact and the direction, force, and veloçity of the blow. If the head is resting on impact, the maximum damage will be found at the impact site. A moving head will cause a "contrecoup injury" where the brain damage occurs on the side opposite the point of impact, as a result of the brain slamming into that side of the skull. A closed head injury also may occur without the head being struck, such as when a person experiences whiplash. This type of injury occurs because the brain is of a different density than the skull, and can be injured when delicate brain tissues hit against the rough, jagged inner surface of the skull.

Penetrating head injury

If the skull is fractured, bone fragments may be driven into the brain. Any object that penetrates the skull may implant foreign material and dirt into the brain, leading to an infection.

Skull fracture

A skull fracture is a medical emergency that must be treated promptly to prevent possible brain damage. Such an injury may be obvious if blood or bone fragments are visible, but it is possible for a fracture to have occurred without any apparent damage. A skull fracture should be suspected if there is:

- blood or clear fluid leaking from the nose or ears
- unequal pupil size
- bruises or discoloration around the eyes or behind the ears
- swelling or depression of part of the head

Intracranial hemorrhage

Bleeding (hemorrhage) inside the skull may accompany a head injury and cause additional damage to the brain. A blood clot (hematoma) may occur if a blood vessel between the skull and the brain ruptures; when the blood leaks out and forms a clot, it can press against brain tissue, causing symptoms from a few hours to a few weeks after the injury. If the clot is located between the bones of the skull and the covering of the brain (dura), it is called an epidural hematoma. If the clot is between the dura and the brain tissue itself, the condition is called a **subdural hematoma**. In other cases, bleeding may occur deeper inside the brain. This condition is called intracerebral hemorrhage or intracerebral contusion (from the word for bruising).

In any case, if the blood flow is not stopped, it can lead to unconsciousness and **death**. The symptoms of bleeding within the skull include:

- nausea and vomiting
- headache
- loss of consciousness
- unequal pupil size
- lethargy

Post-concussion syndrome

If the head injury is mild, there may be no symptoms other than a slight **headache**. There also may be confusion, **dizziness**, and blurred vision. While the head injury may seem to have been quite mild, in many cases symptoms persist for days or weeks. Up to 60% of patients who sustain a mild brain injury continue to experience a range of symptoms called "post-concussion syndrome," as long as six months or a year after the injury.

The symptoms of **post-concussion syndrome** can result in a puzzling interplay of behavioral, cognitive, and emotional complaints that can be difficult to diagnose, including:

- headache
- dizziness
- mental confusion
- behavior changes
- memory loss
- cognitive deficits
- depression
- emotional outbursts

Diagnosis

The extent of damage in a severe head injury can be assessed with computed tomography (CT) scan, **magnetic resonance imaging** (MRI), positron emission tomography (PET) scans, electroencephalograms (EEG), and routine neurological and neuropsychological evaluations.

Doctors use the Glasgow Coma Scale to evaluate the extent of brain damage based on observing a patient's ability to open his or her eyes, respond verbally, and respond to stimulation by moving (motor response). Patients can score from three to 15 points on this scale. People who score below eight when they are admitted usually have suffered a severe brain injury and will need rehabilitative therapy as they recover. In general, higher scores on the Glasgow Coma Scale indicate less severe brain injury and a better prognosis for recovery.

Patients with a mild head injury who experience symptoms are advised to seek out the care of a specialist; unless a family physician is thoroughly familiar with medical literature in this newly emerging area, experts warn that there is a good chance that patient complaints after a mild head injury will be downplayed or dismissed. In the case of mild head injury or post-concussion syndrome, CT and MRI scans, electroencephalograms (EEG), and routine neurological evaluations all may be normal because the damage is so subtle. In many cases, these tests cannot detect the microscopic damage that occurs when fibers are stretched in a mild, diffuse injury. In this type of injury, the axons lose some of their covering and become less efficient. This mild injury to the white matter reduces the quality of communication between different parts or the brain. A PET scan, which evaluates cerebral blood flow and brain metabolism, may be of help in diagnosing mild head injury.

Patients with continuing symptoms after a mild head injury should call a local chapter of a head-injury foundation that can refer patients to the best nearby expert.

Treatment

If a concussion, bleeding inside the skull, or skull fracture is suspected, the patient should be kept quiet in a darkened room, with head and shoulders raised slightly on a pillow or blanket.

After initial emergency treatment, a team of specialists may be needed to evaluate and treat the problems that result. A penetrating wound may require surgery. Those with severe injuries or with a deteriorating level of consciousness may be kept hospitalized for observation. If there is bleeding inside the skull, the blood may need to be surgically drained; if a clot has formed, it may need to be removed. Severe skull **fractures** also require surgery.

Supportive care and specific treatments may be required if the patient experiences further complications. People who experience seizures, for example, may be given anticonvulsant drugs, and people who develop fluid on the brain (**hydrocephalus**) may have a shunt inserted to drain the fluid.

In the event of long-term disability as a result of head injury, there are a variety of treatment programs available, including long-term rehabilitation, coma treatment centers, transitional living programs, behavior management programs, life-long residential or day treatment programs and independent living programs.

KEY TERMS

Computed tomography scan (CT)—A diagnostic technique in which the combined use of a computer and x rays produce clear cross-sectional images of tissue. It provides clearer, more detailed information than x rays alone.

Electroencephalogram (EEG)—A record of the tiny electrical impulses produced by the brain's activity. By measuring characteristic wave patterns, the EEG can help diagnose certain conditions of the brain.

Magnetic resonance imaging (MRI)—A diagnostic technique that provides high quality cross-sectional images of organs within the body without x rays or other radiation.

Positron emission tomography (PET) scan—A computerized diagnostic technique that uses radioactive substances to examine structures of the body. When used to assess the brain, it produces a three-dimensional image that reflects the metabolic and chemical activity of the brain.

Prognosis

Prompt, proper diagnosis and treatment can help alleviate some of the problems after a head injury. It usually is difficult to predict the outcome of a brain injury in the first few hours or days; a patient's prognosis may not be known for many months or even years.

The outlook for someone with a minor head injury generally is good, although recovery may be delayed and symptoms such as headache, dizziness, and cognitive problems can persist for up to a year or longer after an accident. This can limit a person's ability to work and cause strain in personal relationships.

Serious head injuries can be devastating, producing permanent mental and physical disability. Epileptic seizures may occur after a severe head injury, especially a penetrating brain injury, a severe skull fracture, or a serious brain hemorrhage. Recovery from a severe head injury can be very slow, and it may take five years or longer to heal completely. Risk factors associated with an increased likelihood of memory problems or seizures after head injury include age, length and depth of coma, duration of post-traumatic and retrograde amnesia, presence of focal brain injuries, and initial Glasgow Coma Scale score.

As researchers learn more about the long-term effects of head injuries, they have started to uncover links to later conditions. A 2003 report found that mild brain injury during childhood could speed up expression of **schizophrenia** in those who were already likely to get the disorder because of genetics. Those with a history of a childhood brain injury, even a minor one, were more likely to get familial schizophrenia than a sibling and to have earlier onset. Another study in 2003 found that people who had a history of a severe head injury were four times more likely to develop Parkinson's disease than the average population. Those requiring hospitalization for their head injuries were 11 times as likely. The risk did not increase for people receiving mild head injuries.

Prevention

Many severe head injuries could be prevented by wearing protective helmets during certain **sports**, or when riding a bike or motorcycle. Seat belts and airbags can prevent many head injuries that result from car accidents. Appropriate protective headgear always should be worn on the job where head injuries are a possibility.

Resources

BOOKS

Daisley, Audrey, Rachel Tams, and Udo Kischka. *Head Injury.* New York: Oxford University Press, 2009.

Huff, Eane. *Heads Up: Finding Possibility and Purpose with Head Injury.* Parker, CO: Outskirts Press, 2009.

Mason, Michael Paul. *Head Cases: Stories of Brain Injury and Its Aftermath.* New York: Farrar, Straus and Giroux, 2009.

Smith, Terry. *Surviving Head Trauma: A Guide to Recovery Written by a Traumatic Brain Injury Patient.* Bloomington, IN: iUniverse, 2009.

PERIODICALS

"Childhood Head Injury Tied to Later Schizophrenia." *The Brown University Child and Adolescent Behavior Letter* (June 2003): 5.

"Link to Head Injury Found." *Pain & Central Nervous System Week* (June 9, 2003): 3.

ORGANIZATIONS

American Epilepsy Society, 342 N. Main St., West Hartford CT, 06117-2507, (860) 586-7505, http://www.aesnet.org.

Brain Injury Association of America, 1608 Spring Hill Road, Suite 110, Vienna VA, 22182, (703) 761-0750, http://www.biausa.org.

Brain Injury Resource Center, P.O. Box 84151, Seattle WA, 98124, (206) 621- 8558, http://www.headinjury.com.

Family Caregiver Alliance, 425 Bush St., Ste. 500, San Francisco CA, 94108, (800) 445-8106, http://www.caregiver.org.

Head Trauma Support Project, Inc, 2500 Marconi Ave., Ste. 203, Sacramento CA, 95821, (916) 482-5770

National Head Injury Foundation, 333 Turnpike Rd., Southboro MA, 01722, (617) 485-9950

National Institute of Neurological Disorders and Stroke (NINDS), P.O. Box 5801, Bethesda MD, 20824, (301) 496-5751, (800) 352-9424, http://www.ninds.nih.gov.

Carol A. Turkington
Teresa G. Odle
Laura Jean Cataldo, RN, EdD

Head lice ***see* Lice infestation**

Head Start programs

Definition

Head Start began in 1965 as a **preschool** program for three- to five-year-old children from low-income families in the United States. Its original aim was to prepare children for success in school through an early structured learning program. As of 2010 the program has expanded to include nutritional programs for newborns, services for homeless children and the children of migrant workers, and Native American children.

Canada began a program for First Nations, Inuit, and Métis children in 1995 modeled on the Head Start program in the United States. Called the Aboriginal Head Start (AHS) program, it is under the direction of Health Canada as of 2010.

Demographics

Head Start serves approximately 980,000 children across the United States as of 2010, 57% of whom are four years old or older, and 43% three years old or younger. Most programs are a half-day in length and include lunch. The curriculum is not the same in every program, but in most cases school readiness is stressed. Children may be taught the alphabet and numbers, and to recognize colors and shapes. Health care is an important aspect of the program. Children in Head Start are monitored to keep them up to date on their immunizations and screening is available for hearing and vision.

Many local programs are integrated to include children with such special needs as a physical or mental handicap. Class size is limited to between 17 and 20 children, with two teachers. Parents are encouraged to volunteer their time in the classroom, or to work as teacher aides. Most programs are aimed at four-year-olds, who attend Head Start for one year before starting kindergarten. Some programs are for two years, and others are for infants and toddlers who participate with their parents.

Eligibility for Head Start was originally limited to families at or below the federal poverty level. The 2007 reauthorization of the program, allows as many as 10% of any funded program's enrollment to come from over-income families or families experiencing emergency situations. In addition, the 2007 Head Start Act includes a provision to offer local programs the option of serving children from 100 to 130% of the federal poverty guidelines.

In 2005 (the last year for which financial data are available), Head Start programs had a $6.8 billion budget, which covered 1,604 different programs operating more than 48,000 classrooms scattered across the United States, at an average cost of $7,222 per child. The staff of Head Start programs that year included 212,000 paid personnel and 1.1 million volunteers.

Description

Head Start began in 1965 as part of the War on Poverty program launched by the administration of president Lyndon B. Johnson. Nearly half the nation's poor people were children under age 12, and Head Start was developed to respond to the needs of poor children as early as possible. A few privately funded pre-school programs for poor children in inner cities and rural areas had shown marked success in raising children's intellectual skills. Many low-income children also had unrecognized health problems and had not been immunized. Head Start was envisioned as a comprehensive program that would provide health and nutritional services to poor children, while also developing their cognitive skills. The program aimed to involve parents. Many parents of children in the program were employed as teacher's aides, so that they would understand what their children were learning, and help carry on that learning at home.

Head Start has been moved from one government department to another since it began as an eight-week summer program in 1965 under the auspices of the Office of Economic Opportunity. In 1969 the program was moved to the Office of Child Development within what was then called the Department of Welfare. When Congress passed the Head Start Act in 1981, the program was transferred to the Department of Health and Human Services (HHS). As of 2010, Head Start is under the jurisdiction of the Administration for Children and Families (ACF) within the HHS.

Expansion of Head Start programs

Head Start added a new program in 1994 known as Early Head Start. This program, intended to serve children from **birth** through three years of age, was established in order to meet children's nutritional and emotional needs before they are old enough to enter standard Head Start programs. Early Head Start programs are administered locally, in most cases by a combination of nonprofit agencies and local school systems.

Head Start received reauthorization from Congress in 2007 and was extended to cover previously underserved or unserved groups:

- Migrant and seasonal Head Start. Established to serve the children of migrant and seasonal workers. Because of the nature of the work done by the parents, these programs run for longer hours per day but fewer months per year than standard Head Start programs. Children between the ages of six months and five years are eligible.
- Homeless children. Homeless children are defined by HHS as not only homeless children in a shelter or other outreach program, or those living in motels or cars but also those "sharing the housing of others due to loss of housing, economic hardship, or similar reason."
- American Indian/Alaska Native Head Start. These services are primarily for disadvantaged preschool children as well as infants and toddlers.
- Children with disabilities. As of the 2007 reauthorization, all Head Start programs are required to provide full services to children with disabilities, up to 10% of their total enrollment.

In 2007, Head Start added stipulations about the academic credentials required of Head Start teachers. The 2007 Head Start Act mandates that all teachers must have an associate degree in a related field by 2013, and half must have bachelor's degrees by that date. Head Start teachers are paid an average of $26,000 per year (as of 2009), compared to the $45,000 to $50,000 that public school teachers receive.

Canadian AHS programs

Canadian AHS programs are similar to their counterparts in the United States in their emphasis on parental involvement; meeting children's emotional, social, health, nutritional and psychological needs; and tailoring each program to the specific circumstances of the local community. Most AHS programs as of 2010 are half-day and operate five days a week for children between the ages of three and five. Health Canada provides general oversight; however, there is no standard curriculum imposed on all AHS centers.

The primary difference between AHS programs and Head Start programs in the United States is the emphasis given to preserving the aboriginal cultures and languages of Canada. Children in AHS programs are given instruction in their tribal languages as well as English or French.

KEY TERMS

Aboriginal—A general term for the inhabitants of any country or territory who were there before the arrival of European colonists.

First Nations—The Canadian term for the original inhabitants of Canada; roughly equivalent to the use of "Native Americans" in the United States.

Métis—The Canadian term for people of mixed European and First Nations heritage.

Evaluations of the program

The Head Start program was political from its inception. Head Start was launched with much fanfare by Claudia (Lady Bird) Johnson, Lyndon Johnson's wife, and presidents from Lyndon Johnson to George W. Bush have praised the program and taken credit for its successes. Measuring the program's actual success is not a simple matter. Head Start is said to save taxpayers' money, because children who attend Head Start are more likely to graduate high school and get a job than their peers who do not attend Head Start. However, the precise long-term benefits of Head Start are difficult to gauge, and researchers disagree even about the short-term benefits. Nevertheless, one government publication states that, in the long term, $6 are saved for every $1 invested in the Head Start program. Other studies merely suggest that Head Start graduates are more likely than their peers to stay in the proper grade level for their age in elementary school.

Disagreement about the short-term and long-term benefits of Head Start programs has continued into 2010. Several recent studies have noted that Head Start programs are not effective in reducing obesity, which presently affects about one-third of children enrolled in these programs. This failure is attributed to "parents and staff sometimes shar[ing] cultural beliefs that were inconsistent with preventing obesity, such as the belief that heavier children are healthier." Another ongoing concern is the difficulty of involving minority parents in their children's early education. As of 2010 there are 13 clinical studies evaluating the effectiveness of Head Start programs in helping children with **asthma**; preventing obesity in children; treating depression in the children's mothers; improving children's dental health; and preventing behavior disorders in the children.

Resources

BOOKS

Gillette, Michael J. *Launching the War on Poverty: An Oral History*. New York: Oxford University Press, 2010.

Rose, Elizabeth. *The Promise of Preschool: From Head Start to Universal Pre-kindergarten*. New York: Oxford University Press, 2010.

Zigler, Edward, and Sally J. Styfco. *The Hidden History of Head Start*. New York: Oxford University Press, 2010.

PERIODICALS

de la Cruz, A.M., and P. McCarthy. "Alberta Aboriginal Head Start in Urban and Northern Communities: Longitudinal Study Pilot Phase." *Chronic Diseases in Canada* 30 (March 2010): 40–45.

D'Onise, K., et al. "Can Preschool Improve Child Health Outcomes? A Systematic Review." *Social Science and Medicine* 70 (May 2010): 1423–40.

Hammer, C.S., et al. "The Language and Literacy Development of Head Start Children: A Study Using the Family and Child Experiences Survey Database." *Language, Speech, and Hearing Services in Schools* 41 (January 2010): 70–83.

Hughes, C.C., et al. "Barriers to Obesity Prevention in Head Start." *Health Affairs* 29 (March-April 2010): 454–62.

Mendez, J.L. "How Can Parents Get Involved in Preschool? Barriers and Engagement in Education by Ethnic Minority Parents of Children Attending Head Start." *Cultural Diversity and Ethnic Minority Psychology* 16 (January 2010): 26–36.

Welsh, J.A., et al. "The Development of Cognitive Skills and Gains in Academic School Readiness for Children from Low-Income Families." *Journal of Educational Psychology* 102 (February 2010): 43–53.

Whitaker, R.C., et al. "Reaching Staff, Parents, and Community Partners to Prevent Childhood Obesity in Head Start, 2008." *Preventing Chronic Disease* 7 (May 2010): A54.

OTHER

"Early Head Start (EHS)." Early Childhood Learning and Knowledge Center, Office of Head Start, http://eclkc.ohs.acf.hhs.gov/hslc/Early%20Head%20Start (accessed September 18, 2010).

U.S. Department of Health and Human Services Administration for Children and Families. *Head Start Impact Study, First Year Findings* May 2005, http://www.acf.hhs.gov/programs/opre/hs/impact_study/reports/first_yr_execsum/first_yr_execsum.pdf (accessed September 18, 2010).

Williams, Lylee. *Aboriginal Head Start Program* National Indian and Inuit Community Health Representatives Organization [Canada], http://www.niichro.com/Child/child4.html (accessed September 18, 2010).

ORGANIZATIONS

Aboriginal Head Start, Childhood and Youth Division, Health Promotion and Programs Branch, Health Canada, 3rd Floor, Emerald Plaza, 1547 Merivale Road, Nepean Ontario Canada, K1A 0L3, (613) 946-9744, (613) 952-7733, http://www.hc-sc.gc.ca/fniah-spnia/famil/develop/ahsor-papa_intro-eng.php.

Administration of Children and Families (ACF) Office of Head Start (OHS), 8th Floor Portals Building, Washington DC, 20024, (866) 763-6481, http://eclkc.ohs.acf.hhs.gov/hslc.

National Head Start Association (NHSA), 1651 Prince St., Alexandria VA, 22314, (703) 739-0875, (703) 739-0878, http://www.nhsa.org.

A. Woodward
Rebecca J. Frey, PhD

Headache

Definition

A headache involves **pain** in the head which can arise from many disorders or may be a disorder in and of itself.

Description

There are three types of primary headaches: tension-type (muscular contraction headache), migraine (vascular

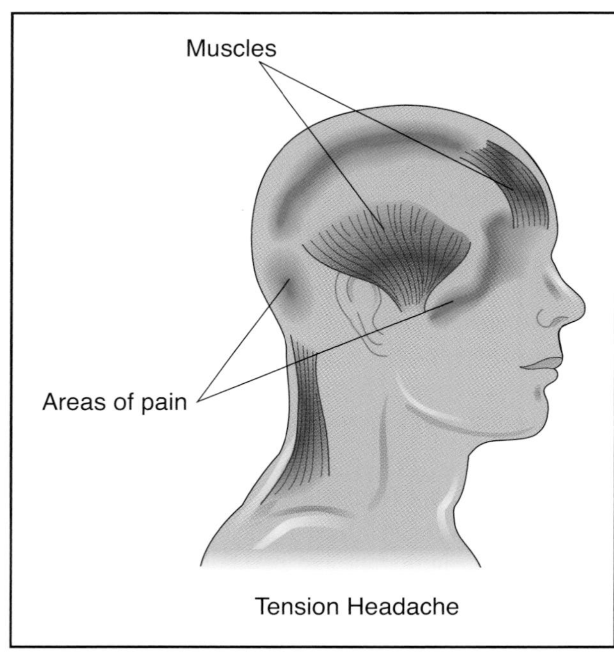

Tension headaches are the most common type of headache and are caused by severe muscle contractions triggered by stress or exertion. Tension headaches usually occur in the front of the head, although they may also appear at the top or the back of the skull. *(Illustration by Electronic Illustrators Group. Reproduced by permission of Gale, a part of Cengage Learning.)*

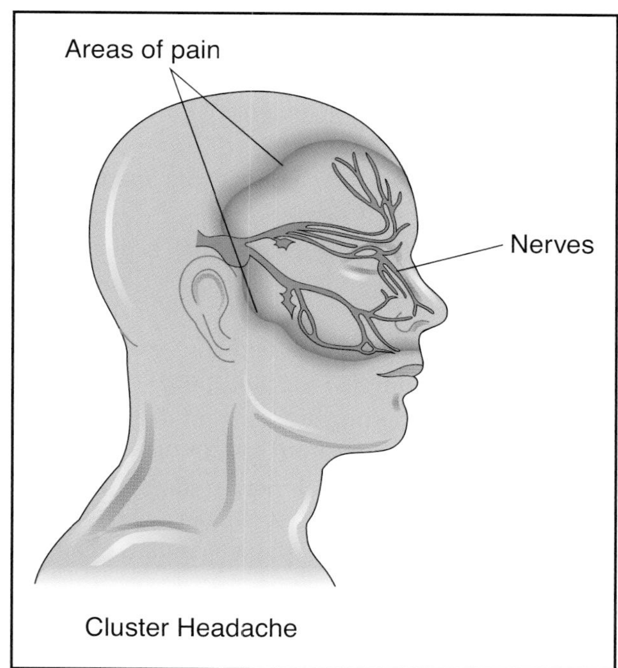

The primary cluster headache symptom is excruciating one-sided head pain located behind an eye or near the temple. Secondary symptoms include eye tearing, nasal congestion, and a runny nose. *(Illustration by Electronic Illustrators Group. Reproduced by permission of Gale, a part of Cengage Learning.)*

headaches), and cluster. Virtually everyone experiences a tension-type headache at some point. An estimated 18% of American women suffer migraines, compared to 6% of men. Cluster headaches affect fewer than 0.5% of the population, and men account for approximately 80% of all cases. Headaches caused by illness are secondary headaches and are not included in these numbers.

Approximately 40–45 million people in the United States suffer chronic headaches. Headaches have an enormous impact on society due to missed workdays and productivity losses.

Causes and symptoms

Traditional theories about headaches link tension-type headaches to muscle contraction, and migraine and cluster headaches to blood vessel dilation (swelling). Pain-sensitive structures in the head include blood vessel walls, membranous coverings of the brain, and scalp and neck muscles. Brain tissue itself has no sensitivity to pain. Therefore, headaches may result from contraction of the muscles of the scalp, face or neck; dilation of the blood vessels in the head; or brain swelling that stretches the brain's coverings. Involvement of specific nerves of the face and head may also cause characteristic headaches. Sinus inflammation is a common cause of headache. Keeping a headache diary may help link headaches to stressful occurrences, menstrual phases, food triggers, or medication.

Tension-type headaches are often brought on by stress, overexertion, loud noise, and other external factors. The typical tension-type headache is described as a tightening around the head and neck, and an accompanying dull ache.

Migraines are intense throbbing headaches occurring on one or both sides of the head, usually on one side. The pain is accompanied by other symptoms such as nausea, **vomiting**, blurred vision, and aversion to light, sound, and movement. Migraines often are triggered by food items, such as red wine, chocolate, and aged cheeses. For women, a hormonal connection is likely, since headaches occur at specific points in the menstrual cycle, with use of **oral contraceptives**, or the use of hormone replacement therapy after menopause. Research shows that a complex interaction of nerves and neurotransmitters in the brain act to cause migraine headaches.

Cluster headaches cause excruciating pain. The severe, stabbing pain centers around one eye, and eye tearing and nasal congestion occur on the same side. The headache lasts from 15 minutes to four hours and may recur several times in a day. Heavy smokers are more likely to suffer cluster headaches, which also are associated with alcohol consumption.

Diagnosis

Since headaches arise from many causes, a physical exam assesses general health and a neurologic exam evaluates the possibility of neurologic disease as a cause for the headache. If the headache is the primary illness, the doctor asks for a thorough history of the headache. Questions revolve around its frequency and duration, when it occurs, pain intensity and location, possible triggers, and any prior symptoms. This information aids in classifying the headache.

Warning signs that should point out the need for prompt medical intervention include:

- "Worst headache of my life." This may indicate subarachnoid hemorrhage from a ruptured aneurysm (swollen blood vessel) in the head or other neurological emergency.
- Headache accompanied by one-sided weakness, numbness, visual loss, speech difficulty, or other signs. This may indicate a stroke. Migraines may include neurological symptoms.
- Headache that becomes worse over a period of 6 months, especially if most prominent in the morning

or if accompanied by neurological symptoms. This may indicate a brain tumor.
- Sudden onset of headache. If accompanied by fever and stiff neck, this can indicate meningitis.

Headache diagnosis may include neurological imaging tests such as computed tomography scan (CT scan) or **magnetic resonance imaging** (MRI).

Treatment

Headache treatment is divided into two forms: abortive and prophylactic. Abortive treatment addresses a headache in progress, and prophylactic treatment prevents headache occurrence.

Tension-type headaches can be treated with aspirin, **acetaminophen**, ibuprofen, or naproxen. In early 1998, the FDA approved extra-strength Excedrin, which includes **caffeine**, for mild migraines. Physicians continue to investigate and monitor the best treatment for migraines and generally prefer a stepped approach, depending on headache severity, frequency and impact on the patient's quality of life. A group of drugs called triptans are usually preferred for abortive treatment. About seven triptans are available in the United States and the pill forms are considered most effective. They should be taken as early as possible during the typical migraine attack. The most common prophylactic therapies include antidepressants, beta blockers, calcium channel blockers and antiseizure medications. Antiseizure medications have proven particularly effective at blocking the actions of neurotransmitters that start migraine attacks. Topiramate (Topamax) was shown effective in several combined clinical trials in 2004 at 50 to 200 mg per day.

In 2004, a new, large study added evidence to show the effectiveness of botulinum toxin type A (Botox) treatment to prevent headache pain for those with frequent, untreatable tension and migraine headaches. Patients were treated every three months, with two to five injections each time. They typically received relief within two to three weeks.

Cluster headaches may also be treated with ergotamine and sumatriptan, as well as by inhaling pure oxygen. Prophylactic treatments include prednisone, calcium channel blockers, and methysergide.

Alternative treatment

Alternative headache treatments include:

- acupuncture or acupressure
- biofeedback
- chiropractic
- herbal remedies using feverfew (*Chrysanthemum parthenium*), valerian (*Valeriana officinalis*), white willow (*Salix alba*), or skullcap (*Scutellaria lateriflora*), among others
- homeopathic remedies chosen specifically for the individual and his/her type of headache
- hydrotherapy
- massage
- magnesium supplements
- regular physical exercise
- relaxation techniques, such as meditation and yoga
- transcutaneous electrical nerve stimulation (TENS) (A procedure that electrically stimulates nerves and blocks the signals of pain transmission.)

KEY TERMS

Abortive—Referring to treatment that relieves symptoms of a disorder.

Analgesics—A class of pain-relieving medicines, including aspirin and Tylenol.

Biofeedback—A technique in which a person is taught to consciously control the body's response to a stimulus.

Chronic—Referring to a condition that occurs frequently or continuously or on a regular basis.

Prophylactic—Referring to treatment that prevents symptoms of a disorder from appearing.

Transcutaneous electrical nerve stimulation—A method that electrically stimulates nerve and blocks the transmission of pain signals, called TENS.

Prognosis

Headaches are typically resolved through the use of **analgesics** and other treatments. Research in 2004 showed that people who have migraine headaches more often than once a month may be at increased risk for **stroke**.

Prevention

Some headaches may be prevented by avoiding triggering substances and situations, or by employing alternative therapies, such as **yoga** and regular **exercise**. Since **food allergies** often are linked with headaches, especially cluster headaches, identification and elimination of the allergy-causing food(s) from the diet can be an important preventive measure.

Parental concerns

It is important for parents to reassure their child that most headaches are not caused by a serious illness. Parents can help their child create and maintain a headache diary to record headache symptoms, triggers, as well as the duration and frequency of the headaches. Parents should make sure their child drinks enough fluids, eats three well-balanced meals each day, gets plenty of sleep, and balances activities to avoid an over-crowded schedule that may cause stress and lead to a headache. When headaches occur, parents should allow the child to take a nap; a dark, quiet room is usually preferred by the child. In addition, parents can help the child learn relaxation techniques to help relieve or prevent headache symptoms. If the headaches are linked to anxiety or depression, the parents should ask the child's doctor for a referral to a counselor who can provide additional assistance.

Resources

PERIODICALS

Kruit, Mark C., et al. "Migraine as a Risk Factor for Subclinical Brain Lesions." *JAMA, Journal of the American Medical Association* January 28, 2004: 427–435.

Norton, Patrice G. W. "Botox Stops Headache Pain in Recalcitrant Cases." *Clinical Psychiatry News* March 2004: 72.

Taylor, Frederick, et al. "Diagnosis and Management of Migraine in Family Practice." *Journal of Family Practice* January 2004: S3–S25.

ORGANIZATIONS

American Council for Headache Education (ACHE), 19 Mantua Road, Mt. Royal NJ, 08061, (800 255-2243, http://www.achenet.org.

National Headache Foundation 428 W. St. James Place, Chicago IL, 60614 (800) 843-2256, http://www.headaches.org.

Julia Barrett
Teresa G. Odle

Hearing development and function

Definition

Hearing development and function involve the formation of structures in the ear and brain that allow vibrations to be converted into meaningful language. Hearing is essential to the understanding and production of spoken language.

Description

Hearing is the transformation of vibrations or sound waves in the air into electrical signals that can be interpreted by the brain. Research has shown that fetuses begin reacting to sound at around 14 weeks of after conception, and they develop the ability to hear sounds between weeks 17 and 20. Pregnant women have reported feeling their fetus move in response to loud noises at 31 weeks (7 weeks before full-term delivery). Some research indicates that babies listen to their mother's voice during the last few months of pregnancy. Babies who were read to by their mothers before **birth** showed early ability to pick out their mother's voice from among other female voices.

Newborns are sensitive to the location, frequency, pitch, and volume of sounds. Loud sounds startle them, while rhythmic, repetitive sounds tend to soothe them. During the second month of life, they become sensitive to a wider range of sounds, reacting to a variety of medium-range sounds that can affect them differently depending on their mood. For example, a child at this age may enjoy the sound of a vacuum cleaner when feeling happy and become upset by it when in an irritable mood. Research shows that infants can hear higher frequencies than adults can, a fact that may be related to the adult instinct to produce "baby talk" at higher pitches than their normal speaking voices. In addition, infants can detect a broad range of pitches and discriminate among different speech sounds At the age of six months, they can tell the difference between sounds that differ as little as 10 decibels in loudness.

Human infants are acutely attuned to the human voice and prefer it above all other sounds. In fact, they prefer the higher pitch ranges characteristic of female voices. They also are attentive to the human face and may stare at it intensely if the face is talking. These preferences are present at birth. By about seven months, a baby should turn his or her head toward voices and by nine months should turn around if a parent calls from behind the child. At the end of the first year, a baby with normal hearing will be trying to repeat sounds that parents make. By age two, a toddler should be able to point to a body part or an object or follow a simple command without seeing the speaker's lips move.

Baring injury or illness, hearing remains stable through most of childhood and early adulthood. However, as individuals age, they often first lose the ability to hear high-frequency sounds, and then gradually lose the ability to hear soft and low-pitched sounds. About 30% of adults over age 60 have significant hearing loss.

How we hear

The ear has three parts: the outer ear, the middle ear, and the inner ear. When something produces a sound, it causes a vibration. The three parts of the ear function together to collect these vibrations, amplify them, and convert them to an electrical signal that will move along a nerve to the brain where it will be processed into meaningful information.

THE OUTER EAR The outer or external ear consists of two parts. The pinna is made of cartilage and is the part of the ear that is visible. The role of the pinna is to collect sound waves and direct them into the ear canal. In humans, the pinnae are firmly attached to the skull and moves very little, thus humans can more easily hear sounds that are produced in front rather than behind them. Some animals such as dogs and horses have pinnae that move easily. Movement of the pinnae helps these animals hear sounds that originate behind or to the side of them.

The ear canal, also called the external auditory meatus, is a twisting tube about 1 inch (2.5 cm) long and about 4 mm wide that connects the pinna to the eardrum. Within the ear canal are glands that produce earwax (cerumen). Earwax provides some protection against bacteria, **foreign objects** and water that enter the ear.

THE MILDDLE EAR The eardrum, also called the tympanic membrane, is located at the end of the ear canal. The eardrum is a thin, taut, concave membrane. When sound waves pass down the ear canal, the eardrum vvibrates like the head of a drum. Behind the inner side of the eardrum are a series of three tiny bones (ossicles). The malleus (sometimes called the "hammer") is attached on one side to the eardrum and on the other side to the incus ("anvil"). The other side of the incus is attached to the stapes ("stirrup"). These three bones relay the sound vibrations to the cochlea.

Unlike the inner ear, which is fluid filled, the middle ear is filled with air. The Eustachian tube, connects the middle ear to the mouth. The purpose of the Eustachian tube is to equalize air pressure on either side of the eardrum. Vibrations are passed along the ossicles most effectively when the pressure is equalized. When changing altitudes, a person may notice that his or her ears "pop." This occurs when there is a temporary inequality in the air pressure on either side of the eardrum.

THE INNER EAR The inner ear is filled with fluid and consists of two parts. The vestibular section of the inner dear helps the body sense acceleration and deceleration as well as rotational motion. This helps maintain balance and allows the body to remain oriented in space. The vestibular section does not play a role in hearing.

The hearing apparatus of the inner ear is called the cochlea. The cochlea contains three fluid-filled, coiled canals. The main canal contains the organ of corti. The organ of corti consists of hundreds of extremely sensitive hair cells. Movement of fluid in the organ of corti causes the hair cells to vibrate. When they vibrate they create an electrochemical signal that is sent along nerve cells to the temporal lobe of the brain. Here the nerve impulses are processed and integrated with other nerve impulses to create meaningful information that we call sound.

Common problems

Congenital hearing loss is one of them most common **birth defects**. An estimated 10 per 1,000 children are born with hearing loss in the United States. Between 2 and 4 per 1,000 have profound hearing loss, and about 4 more per 1,000 have enough hearing loss to affect language acquisition unless the loss is corrected through hearing aids. About 65% of all children with hearing loss are born deaf, and an additional 12% become deaf before the age of 3. A hearing loss delays speech and language acquisition, interferes with **cognitive development**, disrupts socially skill acquisition, and usually delays progress in school.

As of mid-2010, in the United States 43 states plus the District of Columbia have passed laws requiring universal hearing screening of newborns. In other states, newborn hearing screening is voluntary, but is widely performed. Since universal screening was begun the age at which hearing loss is identified has dropped from 2.5 years in 1988 to about 3 months in 2010. Early detection and intervention are crucial in preventing or minimizing developmental and educational delays. Researchers have shown that a child with hearing impairment that goes

KEY TERMS

Congenital—Present at birth.

Eustachian tube—A tube that connects the middle ear to the mouth. The purpose of the Eustachian tube is to equalize air pressure on either side of the eardrum.

Electroencephalogram (EEG)—A recording of the electrical activity of the brain.

undetected beyond 6 months of age will show a delay in understanding speech (receptive speech) and producing speech (expressive speech). When intervention is begun before 6 months of age, children with mild-to-moderate hearing impairment usually progress in language at close to the same speed as their hearing peers.

Parental concerns

Universal hearing screening detects most hearing loss in infants. Parents also can test the hearing of a young child at home by clapping or making some other loud noise and seeing if the sound elicits a startled response. By the age of six months, infants will look around for the source of the noise.

Hearing should be evaluated regularly by a child's **pediatrician**. Infants and children can have their hearing tested by **audiometry**, in which frequency perception is assessed by listening to sounds through earphones in a soundproof room. Alternately, tympanometry, which works by measuring sound waves bouncing off the eardrum with a special probe inserted into the ear. Brainstem auditory-evoked response (BAER) measures brain waves through a test that is similar to an electroencephalogram (EEG). If hearing loss is suspected, these tests can tell the physician something about whether the problem is in transmission of sounds to the inner ear or in transmission of nerve impulses to the brain. For additional information on hearing loss, please see the entry for hearing impairment.

Resources

BOOKS

Moller, Aage R. *Hearing: Anatomy, Physiology, and Disorders of the Auditory System,* 2nd ed. Boston: Academic Press, 2006.

Yost, William A. *Fundamentals of Hearing: An Introduction,* 5th ed. San Diego: Academic Press, 2007.

OTHER

Effects of Hearing Loss on Development. American Speech-Language-Hearing Association. Undated [accessed September 12, 2010], http://www.asha.org/public/hearing/disorders/effects.htm

Hearing, Ear Infections and Deafness. National Institute on Deafness and Other Communication Disorders. August 19, 2010 [accessed September 12, 2010], http://www.nidcd.nih.gov/health/hearing

How We Hear. Audiologists Awareness Campaign. [accessed September 12, 2010], http://www.audiologyawareness.com/hearinfo_howhear.asp

Your Child's Hearing Development Checklist. National Institute on Deafness and Other Communication Disorders. June 7, 2010 [accessed September 12, 2010], http://www.nidcd.nih.gov/health/hearing/silence.htm

ORGANIZATIONS

American Academy of Audiology, 11730 American Plaza Drive, Suite 300, Reston VA, 20190, (800) AAA-2336, (703) 790-8631, http://www.audiology.org.

American Speech-Language-Hearing Association (ASHA), 2200 Research Boulevard, Rockville MD, 20850-3289, (301) 296-5700; TTY (301) 296-5650, (800) 638-8255, (301) 296-8580, actioncenter@asha.org, http://www.asha.org.

National Institute on Deafness and Other Communication Disorders, 31 Center Drive, MSC 2320, Bethesda MD, 20892-2320.nidcdinfo@nidcd.nih.gov, http://www.nidcd.nih.gov.

Tish Davidson, AM

Hearing impairments

Definition

Hearing impairments are conditions that cause hearing loss.

Demographics

Congenital hearing loss is one of them most common **birth defects**. An estimated 10 per 1,000 children are born with hearing loss in the United States. Between 2 and 4 per 1,000 have profound hearing loss, and about 4 more per 1,000 have enough hearing loss to affect language acquisition unless the loss is corrected through hearing aids. About 65% of all children with hearing loss are born deaf, and an additional 12% become deaf before the age of 3. About 30% of adults over age 60 have significant hearing loss. Hearing impairments are more common in adult men than in adult women.

Description

The ear has three parts: the outer ear, the middle ear, and the inner ear. When something produces a sound, it causes a vibration. The three parts of the ear function together to collect these vibrations, amplify them, and convert them to an electrical signal that will move along a nerve to the brain where it will be processed into meaningful information. (For more information on the structure and function of the ear, please see the entry hearing development and function.)

Hearing impairments are most commonly categorized by which parts of the ear are affected. Conductive hearing loss is caused by a problem in the outer or middle or ear that interferes with the conduction of vibrations to the inner ear. Sensorineural hearing loss involves an abnormality of the cochlea of the inner ear or damage to the auditory nerve that carries electrochemical signals generated by sound waves to the brain. Mixed hearing loss indicates a combination of both of these types. Hearing impairments also are classified as prelingual (before a child can learn to speak) or postlingual (after language acquisition has occurred), and genetic or nongenetic (based on whether it is inherited).

Yet another way hearing loss is classified is by severity. Normal hearing is generally defined as the ability to hear sounds of 15 decibels (dB) or less. A person with a mild hearing loss can only hear sounds that are between 15 and 40 or 45 dB or louder. At this level of hearing loss, speech and conversation are unaffected, but there is some difficulty hearing distant sounds. A moderate hearing loss means that only sounds registering 40 to 60 or 70 dB can be heard. At this level, the ability to hear normal conversation and form sounds is affected. With severe hearing loss, a person can only hear sounds that register 60 to 90 dB and needs a hearing aid to be able to discern more than an occasional word of conversation. A profound hearing loss is defined as the inability to hear sounds that are under 90 dB, meaning that only very loud sounds—much louder than those used in conversation—can be heard. A person with profound hearing loss may hear somewhat better with a hearing aid but will still generally be unable to articulate words normally.

Causes and symptoms

The most frequent cause of hearing impairment in children is **otitis media**, or infection of the middle ear, which is very common in children between the ages of 6 months and 2 years and can occur in older and younger children as well. Ordinarily it causes a mild-to-moderate, temporary conductive hearing loss that disappears when the condition clears up. However, persistent or recurrent infections may cause an ongoing moderate hearing loss that can interfere with speech and **language development**.

Certain physical conditions are associated with conductive hearing loss because they increase the likelihood of middle ear infections. **Cleft palate**, which impairs middle ear drainage through the Eustachian tubes, leads to conductive hearing loss in 30% of children with this condition. Other head and facial abnormalities, such as Treacher-Collins syndrome also can cause conductive hearing loss, as can **Down syndrome**, which is characterized by narrow ear canals that are conducive to middle ear infections. About 80% of children with Down syndrome sustain some degree of hearing loss. Trauma to the ear that damages (perforates) the eardrum or the bones of the inner ear also can cause conductive hearing loss.

Another cause of conductive hearing loss is excessive build-up of earwax (cerumen), which can keep sound waves from reaching the eardrum (tympanic membrane). Earwax, which protects the ear from dust and other foreign matter, is produced by glands in the outer ear canal and normally works its way out of the ear naturally. However, sometimes excessive amounts can build up and harden in the outer ear canal, causing a gradual decrease in hearing and, in some cases, irritating the canal. Earwax can usually be removed at home (with a doctor's instructions) by flushing out the ears with water after using special drops to soften the wax. If necessary, the doctor can remove earwax by suction or with a flushing fluid.

Sensorineural hearing loss has a variety of causes including over 70 known genetically inherited conditions, which account for approximately half of all severe sensorineural hearing losses. Problems occurring during **birth** or shortly afterward (e.g., asphyxia, where the baby fails to breathe) can cause inner ear or nerve damage. Hearing loss also may result from intrauterine infections during pregnancy, the best known of which is **rubella** (German measles) contracted during the first trimester of pregnancy. Other viruses known to cause sensorineural hearing loss include **toxoplasmosis**, herpes, and cytomegalovirus (CMV). Bacterial infections in **infancy** (e.g., **meningitis**, measles) are another cause of hearing impairment. It is also thought that the noise from incubators may affect the hearing of premature infants.

Older children and adults may develop hearing loss through damage caused by repeated exposure to loud noise. There is increasing concern that high volume sound played directly into the ears by earbuds used to listen to portable music devices may cause hearing loss. Workplace noise can also cause hearing loss, especially for workers who are exposed to repeated, very loud sounds (e.g., someone who works regularly with a jackhammer). Hearing loss also occurs naturally with aging. About 30% of adults over age 60 have significant hearing loss.

Certain drugs, including some **antibiotics**, diuretics ("water pills"), **analgesics** (e.g., aspirin, ibuprofen, naproxen) and anticancer drugs can all cause hearing loss if used over a long time or at incorrect dosages.

Diagnosis

As of mid-2010, in the United States 43 states plus the District of Columbia have passed laws requiring

KEY TERMS

Down syndrome—The most prevalent of a class of genetic defects known as trisomies, in which cells contain three copies of certain chromosomes rather than the usual two. Down syndrome, or trisomy 21, usually results from three copies of chromosome 21.

Otitis media—Inflammation of the middle ear commonly called an ear infection.

universal hearing screening of newborns. In other states, newborn hearing screening is voluntary, but is widely performed. Since universal screening was begun the age at which hearing loss is identified has dropped from 2.5 years in 1988 to about 3 months in 2010. Early detection and intervention are crucial in preventing or minimizing developmental and educational delays.

Tests

An audiologist is a person trained to evaluate hearing loss. Various methods of testing hearing loss are available including testing by **audiometry**, in which frequency perception is assessed by listening to sounds through earphones in a soundproof room. Alternately, tympanometry, which works by measuring sound waves bouncing off the eardrum with a special probe inserted into the ear. Brainstem auditory-evoked response (BAER) measures brain waves through a test that is similar to an electroencephalogram (EEG). If hearing loss is suspected, these tests can tell the physician something about whether the problem is in transmission of sounds to the inner ear or in transmission of nerve impulses to the brain. Additional tests may be ordered based on initial findings.

Treatment

Common treatment methods for otitis media problem include prolonged low doses of antibiotics and an outpatient procedure called a **myringotomy**, in which a small tube is inserted through the eardrum to drain fluid and equalize the pressure between the middle ear and the ear canal.

A variety of hearing aids are available. The postauricular, or behind-the-ear, hearing aid fits behind the ear and is connected to a plastic earmold, which is custom-fitted to each person. (These must be replaced frequently in rapidly growing young children.) An person with sufficient residual hearing can use the less noticeable in-the-ear or in-the-canal hearing aids, in which the entire apparatus fits inside the ear. In addition to these traditional hearing aids, recent technological advances have made several newer devices available. The transposer changes high-pitched sounds inaudible to many hearing-impaired persons into lower-pitched sounds they can hear. Hearing aids that can be programmed by computer are custom-fitted to an individual's particular type of hearing loss.

The device that has received the greatest degree of attention in hearing-impaired children is the cochlear implant, which, attached directly to the cochlea in a surgical procedure, functionally "replaces" the damaged hair cells of persons with sensorineural hearing loss. The implant itself, consisting of electrodes implanted into the cochlea through a hole drilled in the mastoid bone, works together with two external components: a speech processor, which is commonly worn on the belt or carried in a pocket, and a microphone. Unlike hearing aids, which can only help children who have some residual hearing, **cochlear implants** can help those whose hearing is completely destroyed. While cochlear implants do not restore full normal hearing, they offer potentially substantial improvement in speech recognition and production, as well the ability to hear and identify common sounds such as car horns and doorbells. However, within the deaf community, there is considerable debate about the appropriateness of these devices.

Prognosis

A variety of educational approaches are used to meet the needs of hard of hearing and deaf individuals. A variety of systems, known as oral approaches, use spoken rather than sign language for all communication needs. They may rely on lip reading or on the extension of residual hearing made possible by today's powerful hearing aids and cochlear implants, or on a combination of both methods. One of these, the auditory-verbal approach, relies on enhanced residual hearing, teaching children to speak by having them listen to spoken language. Its ultimate goal is to enable children with hearing loss to attend regular schools and participate fully in the life of the hearing world around them. Another method, Cued Speech, supplements lip reading skills with a set of eight phonetically based hand shapes. Each hand shape represents several combinations of consonant sounds in order to help children learn how words and letters sound. (Vowel sounds are represented by a series of diagrams showing different placements in and around the mouth.) The phonetic mastery made possible by Cued Speech can enable hearing-impaired children to become familiar with a variety of dialects besides their own and learn spoken foreign languages as well.

In contrast to oral methods, the Bilingual-Bicultural (or Bi-Bi) approach treats the hearing impaired as a separate culture with its own language (American Sign Language, or ASL). With this approach, ASL is taught as the primary language and standard English (written only) as a secondary one. In addition, children learn about the history, contributions, and customs of deaf culture, and their parents are encouraged to learn ASL and become active in the Deaf community. A contrasting approach that incorporates signing is called Total Communication, which is based on a philosophy of inclusiveness that embraces all forms of communication that can help a hearing-impaired child communicate and learn, including hearing amplification, signs, gestures, lip reading, and finger spelling. However, unlike the Bilingual-Bicultural approach, Total Communication uses signing systems based on English (collectively referred to as Manually Coded English or MCE) rather than American Sign Language, which is a separate language system distinct from English. Manually Coded English systems include Signed English, Seeing Essential English and its spin-off, Signing Exact English, and Contact Signing (formerly called Pidgin Sign English). Within the Deaf community, there is a great deal of sometimes acrimonious debate about the way to properly educate deaf children, with deaf parents of deaf children often preferring the Bi-Bi approach while hearing parents of deaf children often preferring a spoken English approach.

Prevention

Today, children and adolescents may be creating hearing loss by tuning in to loud technology. A poll conducted in 2006 found that about one-half of high school students have at least one symptom of hearing loss. Many experts believe part of the reason is that so many teens listen to loud headphones. Children start with loud **toys**, **video games** and other technology, and soon crank up the volume on MP3 players, which are designed for children as young as three years old. Adults can help prevent hearing loss by consistently using ear protection when working in noisy environments.

Resources

BOOKS

Carmen, Richard E. *The Consumer Handbook on Hearing Loss and Hearing Aids: A Bridge to Healing,* 3rd ed. Sedona, AZ: Auricle Ink Publishers, 2009.

Luterman, David. *Children with hearing loss: A Family Guide.* Sedona, AZ: Auricle Ink Publishers, 2006.

Moller, Aage R. *Hearing: Anatomy, Physiology, and Disorders of the Auditory System,* 2nd ed. Boston: Academic Press, 2006.

OTHER

Hearing Disorders and Deafness. MedlinePlus. August 20, 2010 [accessed September 12, 2010], http://www.nlm.nih.gov/medlineplus/hearingdisordersanddeafness.html

Hearing, Ear Infections and Deafness. National Institute on Deafness and Other Communication Disorders. August 19, 2010 [accessed September 12, 2010], http://www.nidcd.nih.gov/health/hearing

Noise and Hearing Loss Prevention. National Institute for Occupational Safety and Health. [accessed September 12, 2010], http://www.cdc.gov/niosh/topics/noise/default.html

Your Child's Hearing Development Checklist. National Institute on Deafness and Other Communication Disorders. June 7, 2010 [accessed September 12, 2010], http://www.nidcd.nih.gov/health/hearing/silence.htm

ORGANIZATIONS

American Academy of Audiology, 11730 American Plaza Drive, Suite 300, Reston VA, 20190, (800) AAA-2336, (703) 790-8631, http://www.audiology.org.

American Society for Deaf Children, 800 Florida Ave NE #2047, Washington DC, 20002-3695, (800) 942-2732 or (866) 895-4206, (410) 795-0965, asdc@deafchildren.org, http://www.deafchildren.org.

American Speech-Language-Hearing Association (ASHA), 2200 Research Boulevard, Rockville MD, 20850-3289, (301) 296-5700; TTY (301) 296-5650, (800) 638-8255, (301) 296-8580, actioncenter@asha.org, http://www.asha.org.

National Institute on Deafness and Other Communication Disorders, 31 Center Drive, MSC 2320, Bethesda MD, 20892-2320.nidcdinfo@nidcd.nih.gov, http://www.nidcd.nih.gov.

Tish Davidson, AM

Hearing test with an audiometer **see Audiometry**

Heart disease, congenital **see Congenital heart disease**

Heart murmurs

Definition

A heart murmur is an abnormal extra sound during the heartbeat cycle made by blood moving through the heart and its valves. It is detected by the physician's examination using a stethoscope and may sound like a swishing or whooshing noise. Some heart murmurs are congenital (present at **birth**) while others develop later in life. In adults, most abnormal heart murmurs are caused by infections, other diseases, or aging.

Demographics

Innocent heart murmurs are quite common in the general population. Exact statistics are difficult to obtain; however, one Dutch study reported in the mid-1990s that 41% of schoolchildren between the ages of 5 and 14 years had grade 1 (barely audible) innocent heart murmurs, while 14% had grade 2 or grade 3 murmurs.

Description

A heart which is beating normally makes two sounds, "lubb," which is heard when the valves between the atria and ventricles close; and "dupp," which is heard when when the valves between the ventricles and the major arteries close. The first sound (lubb) is known as S1 in medical shorthand, and the second heart sound (dupp or dub) is known as S2. A heart murmur is a series of vibratory sounds made by turbulent blood flow. The sounds are longer than normal heart sounds and can be heard between the normal sounds of the heart.

Heart murmurs are common in children and can also result from heart or valve defects. Nearly two-thirds of heart murmurs in children are produced by normal hearts and are harmless. This type of heart murmur is usually called an "innocent" heart murmur. It can also be called "functional" or "physiologic." Innocent heart murmurs are usually very faint, intermittent, and occur in a small area of the chest. Pathologic heart murmurs may indicate the presence of a serious heart defect. They are louder, continual, and may be accompanied by a click or gallop.

Some heart murmurs are continually present; others occur only when the heart is working harder than usual, including during **exercise** or certain types of illness. Heart murmurs can be diastolic or systolic. Those that occur during relaxation of the heart between beats are called diastolic murmurs. Those that occur during contraction of the heart muscle are called systolic murmurs. Murmurs that can be heard throughout the heartbeat cycle are called continuous murmurs. The characteristics of the murmur may suggest specific alterations in the heart or its valves.

Heart murmurs are evaluated according to several characteristics:

- Timing. Timing refers to whether the murmur is systolic, diastolic, or continuous.
- Shape. Shape refers to the loudness of the murmur over time. Some grow louder (crescendo); some grow softer (decrescendo); and some grow louder and then softer (crescendo/decrescendo).
- Location. This characteristic refers to the place on the front of the chest where the doctor can best hear the murmur.
- Radiation. Radiation refers to the direction of the movement of the sound of the murmur. In general, heart murmurs radiate in the direction of the blood flow.
- Intensity. Intensity refers to the loudness of the murmur and is graded on a scale of 1 to 6. A grade 1 murmur is difficult to hear at all; grade 3 can be heard all over the portion of the chest over the heart; grade 5 can be heard with the stethoscope partly off the chest; and grade 6 is loud enough to be heard with the stethoscope completely off the chest.
- Pitch. The pitch of a murmur can be low, medium, or high.
- Quality. This characteristic refers to unusual aspects of the murmur's sound. Some murmurs can be described as harsh, rumbling, blowing, or even musical.

Risk factors

Risk factors for heart murmurs in an unborn child include:

- Family history of heart murmurs or heart defects.
- Illnesses during pregnancy, particularly poorly controlled diabetes and rubella (German measles).
- Using alcohol or illegal drugs during pregnancy.

There are no known risk factors for innocent heart murmurs in the general population as of 2010.

Causes and symptoms

Heart murmurs in general are caused by the turbulence of blood flowing through the chambers and valves of the heart or the blood vessels near the heart strongly enough to produce audible sounds. Sometimes **anxiety**, stress, **fever**, **anemia**, an overactive thyroid gland, and pregnancy will cause innocent murmurs that can be heard by a physician using a stethoscope. Pathologic heart murmurs, however, are caused by structural abnormalities of the heart. These include defective heart valves or holes in the walls of the heart. Valve problems are more common. Valves that do not open completely cause blood to flow through a smaller opening than normal, while those that do not close properly may cause blood to go back through the valve.

KEY TERMS

Atria (singular, atrium)—The upper two chambers of the heart.

Auscultation—The medical term for listening to the sounds of the heart or other body organs.

Cardiologist—A doctor who specializes in diagnosing and treating disorders of the heart.

Congenital—Present at birth.

Echocardiogram—A non-invasive ultrasound test that shows an image of the inside of the heart. An echocardiogram can be performed to identify any structural problems which cause a heart murmur.

Electrocardiogram—A test that shows the electrical activity of the heart by placing electronic sensors on the patient. This test can be used to confirm the presence of a heart murmur.

Innocent—The medical term for a harmless heart murmur.

Pathologic—Characterized by disease or the structural and functional changes due to disease. Pathologic heart murmurs may indicate a heart defect.

Ventricles—The lower two chambers of the heart.

A hole in the wall between the left and right sides of the heart, called a septal defect, can cause heart murmurs. Some septal defects close on their own; others require surgery to prevent progressive damage to the heart.

The symptoms of heart murmurs differ depending on the cause of the heart murmur. Innocent heart murmurs and those which do not impair the function of the heart have no symptoms. Murmurs that are due to severe abnormalities of a heart valve may cause shortness of breath, **dizziness**, chest pains, faintness, a bluish discoloration of the skin of the fingertips and lips, swollen veins in the neck, heavy sweating with little exertion, palpitations, and lung congestion.

Diagnosis

The diagnosis of a heart murmur begins with taking a careful patient history. The doctor may ask about a family history of heart murmurs or heart disease. The doctor may also ask about symptoms that may be associated with heart disorders, such as fainting, chest **pain**, a bluish tinge to the complexion, shortness of breath, weight gain, and swelling. The doctor will also check the size of the patient's liver by feeling the abdomen, and look for swollen neck veins.

Examination

Heart murmurs can be heard during an office examination when a **pediatrician** or primary care physician listens to the heart through a stethoscope during a regular checkup. The doctor's listening to heart or other body sounds is called auscultation. After listening to the heart sounds, the doctor will also check for any unusual sounds in the lungs. Very loud heart murmurs and those with clicks or extra heart sounds should be evaluated further. The doctor may ask the patient to stand, squat, hold the breath while bearing down, or squeeze an object in the hand during auscultation. These maneuvers help the doctor to evaluate the location and possible cause of the murmur.

Infants with heart murmurs who do not thrive, eat, or breathe properly, and older children who lose consciousness suddenly or are intolerant of exercise should also be evaluated. If the murmur sounds suspicious, the physician may order a chest x ray, an electrocardiogram, and an echocardiogram. A primary care physician may refer the patient to a cardiologist, who is a doctor who specializes in diagnosing and treating heart disorders.

Tests

An electrocardiogram (ECG) displays the heart's activity and may reveal muscle thickening, damage, or a lack of oxygen. Electrodes covered with conducting jelly are placed on the patient's chest, arms, and legs. They send impulses of the heart's activity through a monitor (oscilloscope) to a recorder which traces them on paper. The test takes about 10 minutes and is commonly performed in a physician's office. An exercise ECG can reveal additional information.

An echocardiogram (cardiac ultrasound), may be ordered to identify a structural problem that is causing the heart murmur. An echocardiogram uses sound waves to create an image of the heart's chambers and valves. The technician applies gel to a hand-held transducer then presses it against the patient's chest. The sound waves are converted into an image that can be displayed on a monitor. Performed in a cardiology outpatient diagnostic laboratory, the test takes 30 minutes to an hour.

In some cases the doctor may administer a drug to further evaluate a murmur. The two compounds used most often for such tests are amyl nitrite, which expands blood vessels and lowers blood pressure; and methoxamine, which has the opposite effect, namely constricting blood vessels and raising blood pressure.

Procedures

In some cases the doctor may recommend cardiac catheterization to evaluate the condition of the patient's heart. This procedure involves the use of x-ray and ultrasound imaging to guide a long thin tube called a catheter through a major blood vessel into the heart. The doctor can inject a dye visible on x-ray through the catheter and trace its flow through the chambers of the heart in order to identify problems in the valves or other structures of the heart.

Treatment

Traditional

Innocent heart murmurs do not affect the patient's health and require no treatment. Treatment when needed is directed toward the cause of the heart murmur. Heart murmurs due to septal defects may require surgery. Those due to valvular defects may require **antibiotics** to prevent infection during certain surgical or dental procedures. Severely damaged or diseased valves can be repaired or replaced through surgery.

Drugs

Some heart murmurs can be managed with various medications. Depending on the specific cause of the murmur, the doctor might prescribe one or more of the following types of drugs:

- Diuretics. Diuretics, sometimes called water pills, are drugs that remove fluid from the blood by increasing urinary output. They can be used to lower blood pressure, as high blood pressure can worsen a heart murmur.
- Angiotensin-converting enzyme (ACE) inhibitors: These are another class of drugs often prescribed to lower high blood pressure.
- Statins. Statins are a group of drugs given to control blood cholesterol levels. High blood cholesterol is a risk factor for making some heart valve problems worse.
- Digoxin (Lanoxin). Also known as digitalis, digoxin is a drug that increases the strength of the heart muscle's contractions, making the heart pump blood more efficiently.
- Aspirin or other anticoagulants. Anticoagulants, sometimes called blood thinners, are drugs that prevent blood clots from forming in the heart, thus lowering the risk of a stroke or heart attack.

Alternative

There are no alternative treatments for heart murmurs that require surgical treatment, although there are alternative therapies that are helpful for pre- and post-surgical support of the patient. If the heart murmur is innocent, heart activity can be supported using the herb hawthorn (*Crataegus laevigata* or *C. oxyacantha*) or coenzyme Q10. These remedies improve heart contractility and the heart's ability to use oxygen. If the murmur is valvular in origin, herbs that act like antibiotics as well as options that build resistance to infection in the valve areas may be considered.

Prognosis

The prognosis of a heart murmur depends on its cause. Most children with innocent heart murmurs grow out of them by the time they reach adulthood. Severe causes of heart murmurs may progress to severe symptoms and **death**.

Prevention

Apart from keeping diabetes under control and avoiding drug or alcohol abuse during pregnancy, there is no known way to prevent heart murmurs as of 2010.

Resources

BOOKS

Auscultation Skills: Breath and Heart Sounds, 4th ed. Philadelphia:Wolters Kluwer/Lippincott Williams and Wilkins Health, 2010.

Driscoll, David J. *Fundamentals of Pediatric Cardiology.* Philadelphia: Lippincott Williams and Wilkins, 2006.

PERIODICALS

Conn, R.D., and J.H. O'Keefe. "Cardiac Physical Diagnosis in the Digital Age: An Important But Increasingly Neglected Skill (from Stethoscopes to Microchips)." *American Journal of Cardiology* 104 (August 15, 2009): 590–95.

Dunn, F.G. "Physical Examination: Include Heart Murmurs." *BMJ* 340 (January 19, 2010): c290.

Federspiel, M.G. "Cardiac Assessment in the Neonatal Population." *Neonatal Network* 29 (May-June 2010): 135–42.

Guntheroth, W.G. "Innocent Murmurs: A Suspect Diagnosis in Non-pregnant Adults." *American Journal of Cardiology* 104 (September 2009): 735–37.

Hanifin, C. "Cardiac Auscultation 101: A Basic Science Approach to Heart Murmurs." *Journal of the American Academy of Physician Assistants* 23 (April 2010): 44–48.

Teixeira, O.H. "Distinguishing Innocent from Pathologic Murmurs in Neonates." *Journal of Pediatrics* 155 (August 2009): 300.

OTHER

American Heart Association (AHA). *Innocent Heart Murmurs*, http://www.americanheart.org/presenter.jhtml?identifier=170

Mayo Clinic. *Heart Murmurs*, http://www.mayoclinic.com/health/heart-murmurs/DS00727

MedlinePlus Medical Encyclopedia. *Heart Murmurs and Other Sounds*, http://www.nlm.nih.gov/medlineplus/ency/article/003266.htm

National Heart, Lung, and Blood Institute (NHLBI). *Heart Murmur*, http://www.nhlbi.nih.gov/health/dci/Diseases/heartmurmur/hmurmur_what.html

National Heart, Lung, and Blood Institute (NHLBI). *How the Heart Works: Heart Contraction and Blood Flow* This is an animation with written text and voiceover illustrating the cycle of the human heartbeat. It takes about 4 minutes to play, http://www.nhlbi.nih.gov/health/dci/Diseases/hhw/hhw_pumping.html

Seattle Children's Hospital. *Heart Murmurs*, http://www.seattlechildrens.org/medical-conditions/heart-blood-conditions/heart-murmurs/

ORGANIZATIONS

American College of Cardiology (ACC), Heart House, 2400 N Street NW, Washington DC, 20037, 202-375-6000, 202-375-7000, http://www.acc.org/.

American Heart Association, 7272 Greenville Avenue, Dallas TX, 75231, 301-592-8573, 800-242-8721, 301-592-8563, www.americanheart.org.

Center for Adults with Congenital Heart Disease, University of Chicago Medical Center, 5841 S. Maryland Avenue, Chicago IL, 60637, 888-UCH-0200, http://www.uchospitals.edu/specialties/heart/services/adult-congenital-heart/.

National Heart, Lung, and Blood Institute (NHLBI), Health Information Center, P.O. Box 30105, Bethesda MD, 20824-0105, 301-592-8573, 240-629-3246, nhlbiinfo@nhlbi.nih.gov, http://www.nhlbi.nih.gov/.

Lori De Milto
Rebecca J. Frey, PhD

Heat disorders

Definition

Heat disorders are a group of physically related illnesses caused by prolonged exposure to hot temperatures, restricted fluid intake, or failure of the body's temperature regulation mechanisms. Disorders of heat exposure include heat cramps, heat exhaustion, and heat **stroke** (also called sunstroke). Hyperthermia is the general name given to heat-related illnesses. The two most common forms of hyperthermia are heat exhaustion and heat stroke, which is especially dangerous and requires immediate medical attention.

Demographics

Anyone can develop hyperthermia. However, seniors and young children are more likely to be affected than young or middle-aged adults. The United States Centers for Disease Control and Prevention (CDC) report that more than 330 individuals die of heat-related causes each year. More deaths occur in years that have significant heat waves, and more individuals die of heat-related illness during the summer months. More than 40% of the individuals who die of heat-related causes each year are over the age of 65.

Description

Heat disorders are harmful to people of all ages, but their severity is likely to increase as people age. Heat cramps in a 16-year-old may be heat exhaustion in a 45-year-old and heat stroke in a 65-year-old.

Regardless of extreme weather conditions, the healthy human body keeps a steady temperature of approximately 98.6°F (37°C). The body's temperature regulating mechanisms rely on the thermal regulating centers in the brain. Through these complex centers, the body tries to adapt to high temperatures by adjusting the amount of salt in the perspiration. Salt helps the cells in body tissues retain water. In hot weather, a healthy body will lose enough water to cool the body while creating the lowest level of chemical imbalance. In hot weather, or during vigorous activity, the body perspires. As perspiration evaporates from the skin, the body is cooled. If the body loses too much salt and fluids, the symptoms of **dehydration** can occur.

Risk factors

The very young, very old, obese individuals and those with cardiovascular problems are at increased risk of experiencing a heat disorder. Alcohol and diseases that impair the ability to sweat are associated with a higher risk of heat-related illness.

Individuals taking certain medications are more likely to be affected because the medications can interfere with the body's normal cooling mechanisms. Individuals taking some blood pressure and heart medications, allergy medications, diet pills, water pills, cold medicines, medicines to prevent seizures, **laxatives**, and thyroid pills are at increased risk for hyperthermia.

Heat cramps

Heat cramps are the least severe of the heat-related illnesses. This heat disorder is often the first signal that the body is having difficulty with increased temperature.

Individuals exposed to excessive heat should think of heat cramps as a warning sign to a potential heat-related emergency.

Heat exhaustion

Heat exhaustion is a more serious and complex condition than heat cramps. Heat exhaustion can result from prolonged exposure to hot temperatures, restricted fluid intake, or failure of temperature regulation mechanisms of the body. It often affects athletes, firefighters, construction workers, factory workers, and anyone who wears heavy clothing in hot humid weather.

Heatstroke

Heat exhaustion can develop rapidly into heatstroke. Heatstroke can be life threatening. Because of its seriousness and its high potential for causing **death**, immediate medical attention is critical when problems first begin. Heat stroke, like heat exhaustion, is also a result of prolonged exposure to hot temperatures, restricted fluid intake, or failure of temperature regulation mechanisms of the body. However, the severity of impact on the body is much greater with heatstroke.

Causes and symptoms

Heat cramps

Heat cramps are painful **muscle spasms** caused by the excessive loss of salts (electrolytes) due to heavy perspiration. The muscle tissue becomes less flexible, causing **pain**, difficult movement, and involuntary tightness. Heavy exertion in extreme heat, restricted fluid intake, or failure of temperature regulation mechanisms of the body may lead to heat cramps. This disorder occurs more often in the legs and abdomen than in other areas of the body. Individuals at higher risk are those working in extreme heat, elderly people, young children, people with health problems, and those who are unable to naturally and properly cool their bodies. Individuals with poor circulation and who take medications to reduce excess body fluids (diuretics) can be at risk when conditions are hot and humid.

Heat exhaustion

Heat exhaustion is caused by exposure to high heat and humidity for many hours, resulting in excessive loss of fluids and salts through heavy perspiration. The skin may appear cool, moist, and pale. The individual may complain of **headache** and nausea with a feeling of overall weakness and exhaustion. **Dizziness**, faintness, and mental confusion are often present, as is rapid and weak pulse. Breathing becomes fast and shallow. Fluid loss reduces blood volume and lowers blood pressure. Yellow or orange urine often is a result of inadequate fluid intake, along with associated intense thirst. Insufficient water and salt intake or a deficiency in the production of sweat place an individual at high risk for heat exhaustion.

Heatstroke

Heatstroke is caused by overexposure to extreme heat, resulting in a breakdown in the body's heat regulating mechanisms. The body's temperature reaches a dangerous level, as high as 106°F (41.1°C). An individual with heat stroke has a body temperature higher than 104°F (40°C). Other symptoms include mental confusion with possible combativeness and bizarre behavior, staggering, and faintness.

The pulse becomes strong and rapid (160–180 beats per minute) with the skin taking on a dry and flushed appearance. There is often very little perspiration. The individual can quickly lose consciousness or have convulsions. Before heat stroke, an individual experiences heat exhaustion and the associated symptoms. When the body can no longer maintain a normal temperature, heat exhaustion becomes heatstroke. Heatstroke is a life-threatening medical emergency that requires immediate initiation of life-saving measures.

Diagnosis

The diagnosis of heat cramps usually involves observation of symptoms such as muscle cramping and thirst. Diagnosis of heat exhaustion or heatstroke, however, may require a physician to review the medical

KEY TERMS

Convulsions—Also termed seizures; a sudden violent contraction of a group of muscles.

Electrolyte—ions in the body that participate in metabolic reactions. The major human electrolytes are sodium (Na+), potassium (K+), calcium (Ca 2+), magnesium (Mg2+), chloride (Cl-), phosphate (HPO4 2-), bicarbonate (HCO3-), and sulfate (SO4 2-). Careful and regular monitoring of electrolytes and intravenous replacement of fluid and electrolytes are part of the acute care in many illnesses.

Intravenous (iv)—The process of giving a liquid through a vein.

Rehydration—The restoration of water or fluid to a body that has become dehydrated.

history, document symptoms, and obtain a blood pressure and temperature reading. The physician also may take blood and urine samples for further laboratory testing. A test to measure the body's electrolytes also can give valuable information about chemical imbalances caused by the heat-related illness.

Treatment

Heat cramps

The care of heat cramps includes placing the individual at rest in a cool environment, while giving cool water with one teaspoon of salt per quart of water or giving a commercial **sports** drink (e.g., Gatorade). Usually rest and liquids are all that is needed for the patient to recover. Mild stretching and massaging of the muscle area follows once the condition improves. The individual should not take salt tablets since this may actually worsen the condition. When the cramps stop, the person usually can start activity again if there are no other signs of illness. The individual needs to continue drinking fluids and should be watched carefully for further signs of heat-related illnesses.

Heat exhaustion

An individual who shows signs of heat exhaustion should stop all physical activity and immediately be moved to a cool place out of the sun, preferably a cool, air-conditioned location. She or he should then lay down with feet slightly elevated, remove or loosen clothing, and drink cold (but not iced), slightly salty water or a commercial sports drink. Rest and replacement of fluids and salt is usually all the treatment that is needed, and hospitalization is rarely required. Following rehydration, the person usually recovers rapidly.

Heatstroke

Simply moving the individual afflicted with heatstroke to a cooler place is not enough to reverse internal overheating. Emergency medical assistance should be called immediately. While waiting for help to arrive, quick action to lower body temperature must take place. Treatment involves getting the victim to a cool place, loosening clothes or undressing the heat stroke victim, and allowing air to circulate around the body. The next important step is wrapping the individual in wet towels or clothing, and placing ice packs in areas with the greatest blood supply. These areas include the neck, under the arm and knees, and in the groin. The individual can even be placed into a bathtub full of cool water to help speed cooling. A fan can be used to circulate air over dampened skin to simulate sweating and help the cooling process. Once the patient is under medical care, cooling treatments may continue as appropriate. The individual's body temperature will be monitored constantly to guard against overcooling. Breathing and heart rate will be monitored closely, and fluids and electrolytes will be replaced intravenously. Anticonvulsant drugs may be given to help reduce shivering, which warms the body up. After severe heat stroke, bed rest may be recommended for several days.

Prognosis

Prompt treatment for heat cramps is usually very effective with the individual returning to activity thereafter. Treatment of heat exhaustion usually brings full recovery in one to two days. Heatstroke is a very serious condition and its outcome depends upon general health and age. Due to the high internal temperature of heatstroke, permanent damage to internal organs is possible.

Prevention

Because heat cramps, heat exhaustion, and heatstroke are all essentially different levels of severity of the same disorder, the prevention of the onset of all heat disorders is similar. Strenuous **exercise** should be avoided when it is very hot or humid. Individuals exposed to extreme heat conditions should drink plenty of fluids. Wearing light and loose-fitting clothing in hot weather is important, regardless of the activity. It is important to consume water often and not to wait until thirst develops. If perspiration is excessive, fluid intake should be increased. When urine output decreases, fluid intake should also increase. Eating lightly salted foods can help replace salts lost through perspiration. Ventilation in any working areas in warm weather must be adequate. This can be achieved as simply as opening a window or using an electric fan. Proper ventilation will promote adequate sweat evaporation to cool the skin.

Resources

BOOKS

Barton, Bob. *Safety, Risk, and Adventure in Outdoor Activities.* Thousand Oaks, CA: Paul Chapman, 2007.

Spengler, Daniel P., Andrew Connaughton, and Andrew T. Pittman. *Risk Management in Sport and Recreation.* Champaign, IL: Human Kinetics, 2006.

PERIODICALS

Holcomb, Susan Simmons. "Pediatric Heatstroke" *Nursing* (September 2009) 39(9):64.

"What Can Be Done to Avoid Or At Least Recognize Heatstroke Before It's Too Late For Help?" *Mayo Clinic Health Letter* (July 2009) 27(7): 8.

"When Does Heat Stroke Occur, and What Are the Signs? *Johns Hopkins Medical Letter* (August 2000) 21(6): 8.

OTHER

Medline Plus. Heat Illness. December 5, 2009, http://www.nlm.nih.gov/medlineplus/heatillness.html

University of Maryland Medical Center. Dehydration and Heat Stroke. January 25, 2008, http://www.umm.edu/non_trauma/dehyrat.htm

Jeffrey P. Larson, RPT
Tish Davidson, A.M.

Heavy metal poisoning

Definition

Heavy metal **poisoning** is the toxic accumulation of heavy metals in the soft tissues of the body.

Description

Heavy metals are chemical elements that have a specific gravity (a measure of density) at least five times that of water. The heavy metals most often implicated in accidental human poisoning are lead, mercury, arsenic, and cadmium. More recently, thallium has gained some attention in the media as the poison used in several murder cases in the 1990s. Some heavy metals, such as zinc, copper, chromium, iron, and manganese, are required by the body in small amounts, but these same elements can be toxic in larger quantities.

Heavy metals may enter the body in food, water, or air, or by absorption through the skin. Once in the body, they compete with and displace essential **minerals** such as zinc, copper, magnesium, and calcium, and interfere with organ system function. People may come in contact with heavy metals in industrial work, pharmaceutical manufacturing, and agriculture. Children may be poisoned as a result of playing in contaminated soil. **Lead poisoning** in adults has been traced to the use of lead-based glazes on pottery vessels intended for use with food, and contamination of Ayurvedic and other imported herbal remedies. Arsenic and thallium have been mixed with food or beverages to attempt **suicide** or poison others.

Another form of **mercury poisoning** that is seen more and more frequently in the United States is self-injected mercury under the skin. Some boxers inject themselves with mercury in the belief that it adds muscle bulk. Metallic mercury is also used in folk medicine or religious rituals in various cultures. These practices increase the risk of mercury poisoning of children in these ethnic groups or subcultures.

Causes and symptoms

Symptoms will vary, depending on the nature and the quantity of the heavy metal ingested. Patients may complain of nausea, **vomiting**, **diarrhea**, stomach **pain**, **headache**, sweating, and a metallic taste in the mouth. Depending on the metal, there may be blue-black lines in the gum tissues. In severe cases, patients exhibit obvious impairment of cognitive, motor, and language skills. The expression “mad as a hatter” comes from the mercury poisoning prevalent in 17th-century France among hatmakers who soaked animal hides in a solution of mercuric nitrate to soften the hair.

Diagnosis

Heavy metal poisoning may be detected using blood and urine tests, hair and tissue analysis, or x ray. The diagnosis is often overlooked, however, because many of the early symptoms of heavy metal poisoning are nonspecific. The doctor should take a thorough patient history with particular emphasis on the patient’s occupation.

In childhood, blood lead levels above 80 ug/dL generally indicate lead poisoning, however, significantly lower levels (>30 ug/dL) can cause **mental retardation** and other cognitive and behavioral problems in affected children. The Centers for Disease Control and Prevention considers a blood lead level of 10 ug/dL or higher in children a cause for concern. In adults, symptoms of lead poisoning are usually seen when blood lead levels exceed 80 ug/dL for a number of weeks.

Blood levels of mercury should not exceed 3.6 ug/dL, while urine levels should not exceed 15 ug/dL. Symptoms of mercury poisoning may be seen when mercury levels exceed 20 ug/dL in blood and 60 ug/dL in urine. Mercury levels in hair may be used to gauge the severity of chronic mercury exposure.

Since arsenic is rapidly cleared from the blood, blood arsenic levels may not be very useful in diagnosis. Arsenic in the urine (measured in a 24-hour collection following 48 hours without eating seafood) may exceed 50 ug/dL in people with arsenic poisoning. If acute arsenic or thallium poisoning is suspected, an x ray may reveal these substances in the abdomen (since both metals are opaque to **x rays**). Arsenic may also be detected in the hair and nails for months following exposure.

Cadmium toxicity is generally indicated when urine levels exceed 10 ug/dL of creatinine and blood levels exceed 5 ug/dL.

Thallium poisoning often causes hair loss (**alopecia**), **numbness**, and a burning sensation in the skin as well as nausea, vomiting, and **dizziness**. As little as 15–

20 mg of thallium per kilogram of body weight is fatal in humans; however, smaller amounts can cause severe damage to the nervous system.

Treatment

When heavy metal poisoning is suspected, it is important to begin treatment as soon as possible to minimize long-term damage to the patient's nervous system and digestive tract. Heavy metal poisoning is considered a medical emergency, and the patient should be taken to a hospital emergency room.

The treatment for most heavy metal poisoning is chelation therapy. A chelating agent specific to the metal involved is given either orally, intramuscularly, or intravenously. The three most common chelating agents are calcium disodium edetate, dimercaprol (BAL), and penicillamine. The chelating agent encircles and binds to the metal in the body's tissues, forming a complex; that complex is then released from the tissue to travel in the bloodstream. The complex is filtered out of the blood by the kidneys and excreted in the urine. This process may be lengthy and painful, and typically requires hospitalization. Chelation therapy is effective in treating lead, mercury, and arsenic poisoning, but is not useful in treating cadmium poisoning. To date, no treatment has been proven effective for cadmium poisoning. Thallium poisoning is treated with a combination of Prussian blue (potassium ferric hexacyanoferrate) and a diuretic, because about 35% of it is excreted in the urine; however, if treatment is not started within 72 hours of ingesting the poisoning, damage to the patient's nervous system may be permanent.

In cases of acute mercury, arsenic, or thallium ingestion, vomiting may be induced. Activated charcoal may be given in cases of thallium poisoning. Washing out the stomach (gastric lavage) may also be useful. The patient may also require treatment such as intravenous fluids for such complications of poisoning as shock, **anemia**, and kidney failure.

Patients who have taken arsenic, thallium, or mercury in a suicide attempt will be seen by a psychiatrist as part of emergency treatment.

Prognosis

The chelation process can only halt further effects of the poisoning; it cannot reverse neurological damage already sustained.

Prevention

Because arsenic and thallium were commonly used in rat and insect poisons at one time, many countries have tried to lower the rate of accidental poisonings by banning the use of heavy metals in pest control products. Thallium was banned in the United States as a rodent poison in 1984. As a result, almost all recent cases of arsenic and thallium poisoning in the United States were deliberate rather than accidental.

Because exposure to heavy metals is often an occupational hazard, protective clothing and respirators should be provided and worn on the job. Protective clothing should then be left at the work site and not worn home, where it could carry toxic dust to family members. Industries are urged to reduce or replace the heavy metals in their processes wherever possible. Exposure to environmental sources of lead, including lead-based paints, plumbing fixtures, vehicle exhaust, and contaminated soil, should be reduced or eliminated.

People who use Ayurvedic or traditional Chinese herbal preparations as alternative treatments for various illnesses should purchase them only from reliable manufacturers.

KEY TERMS

Alopecia—Loss of hair.

Chelation—The process by which a molecule encircles and binds to a metal and removes it from tissue.

Heavy metal—One of 23 chemical elements that has a specific gravity (a measure of density) at least five times that of water.

Prussian blue—The common name of potassium ferric hexacyanoferrate, a compound approved in the United States for treatment of thallium poisoning. Prussian blue gets its name from the fact that it was first used by artists in 1704 as a dark blue pigment for oil paints. It has also been used in laundry bluing and fabric printing.

Resources

BOOKS

Beers, Mark H., MD, and Robert Berkow, MD., editors. "Poisoning." In *The Merck Manual of Diagnosis and Therapy.* 18th ed., Whitehouse Station, NJ: Merck Research Laboratories, 2006.

Beers, Mark H., MD, and Robert Berkow, MD., editors. "Psychiatric Emergencies." In *The Merck Manual of Diagnosis and Therapy.* 18th ed., Whitehouse Station, NJ: Merck Research Laboratories, 2006.

Wilson, Billie A., Margaret T. Shannon, and Carolyn L. Stang. *Nurses Drug Guide 2000.* Stamford, CT: Appleton & Lange, 2000.

PERIODICALS

Boyarsky, Igor, DO, and Adrain D. Crisan, MD. "Toxicity, Thallium." *eMedicine* August 3, 2004, http://www.emedicine.com/emerg/topic926.htm.

Centers for Disease Control and Prevention (CDC). "Adult Blood Lead Epidemiology and Surveillance—United States, 2002." *Morbidity and Mortality Weekly Report* 53 (July 9, 2004): 578–582.

Counter, S. A., and L. H. Buchanan. "Mercury Exposure in Children: A Review." *Toxicology and Applied Pharmacology* 198 (July 15, 2004): 209–230.

Ferner, David J., MD. "Toxicity, Heavy Metals." *eMedicine* May 25, 2001, *http://www.emedicine.com/EMERG/topic237.htm.*

Prasad, V. L. "Subcutaneous Injection of Mercury: 'Warding Off Evil.'" *Environmental Health Perspectives* 111 (September 2004): 1326–1328.

Schilling, U., R. Muck, and E. Heidemann. "Lead Poisoning after Ingestion of Ayurvedic Drugs." [in German] *Medizinische Klinik* 99 (August 15, 2004): 476–480.

Thompson, D. F., and E. D. Callen. "Soluble or Insoluble Prussian Blue for Radiocesium and Thallium Poisoning?" *Annals of Pharmacotherapy* 38 (September 2004): 1509–1514.

ORGANIZATIONS

American Society of Health-System Pharmacists (ASHP), 7272 Wisconsin Avenue, Bethesda MD, 20814, (301) 657-3000, http://www.ashp.org.

Centers for Disease Control and Prevention (CDC), 1600 Clifton Road, Atlanta GA, 30333, (404) 498-1515, (800) 311-3435, http://www.cdc.gov.

Food and Drug Administration, Office of Inquiry and Consumer Information, 5600 Fisher Lane, Room 12-A-40, Rockville MD, 20857, (301) 827-4420, http://www.fda.gov/fdahomepage.html.

National Institute of Environmental Health Sciences (NIEHS), P.O. Box 12233, MD K3-16, Research Triangle Park, NC, 27713 (919) 361-9408, http://tools.niehs.nih.gov.

Bethany Thivierge
Rebecca J. Frey, PhD

Heimlich maneuver

Definition

The Heimlich maneuver is an emergency procedure for removing a foreign object lodged in the airway that is preventing a person from breathing. It is also known as abdominal thrusts.

Purpose

Each year, between 2,800 and 4,000 adults die in the United States because they accidentally inhale rather than swallow food. The food gets stuck and blocks their trachea (windpipe), making breathing impossible. **Death** follows rapidly unless the food or other foreign material

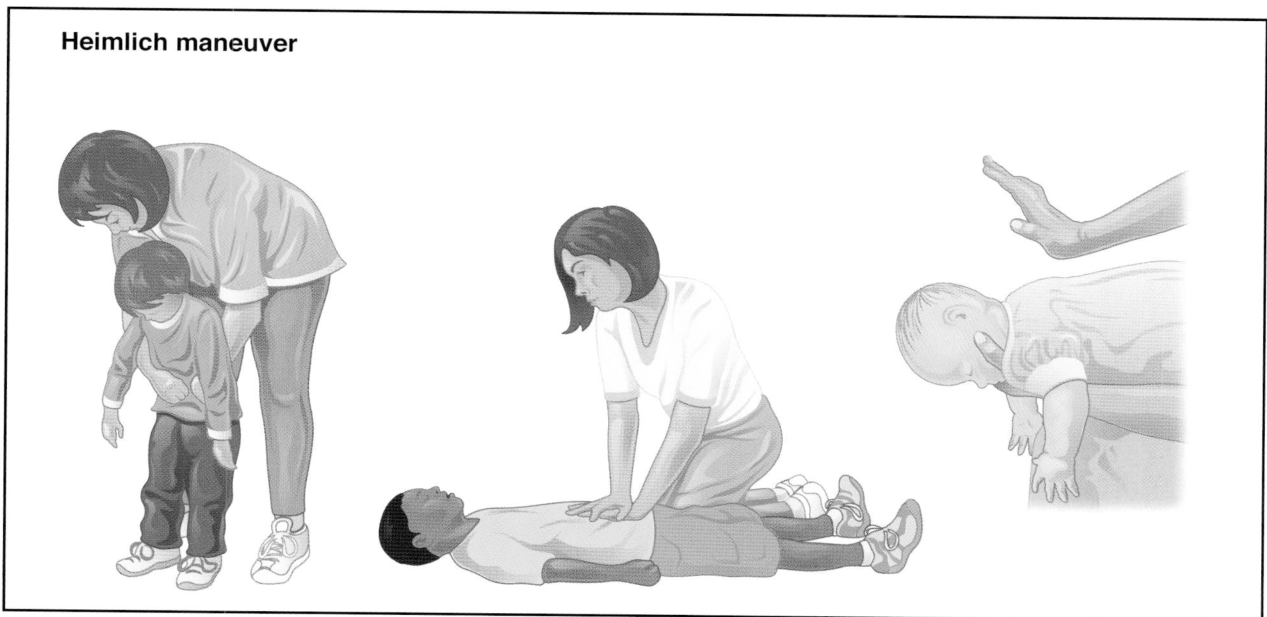

Illustration showing the three ways to perform the Heimlich maneuver: with choking victim standing, with victim lying down, and on an infant. *(Illustration by Electronic Illustrators Group. Reproduced by permission of Gale, a part of Cengage Learning.)*

can be displaced from the airway. This condition is so common it has been nicknamed the "café coronary."

In 1974, Dr. Henry Heimlich first described an emergency technique for expelling foreign material blocking the trachea. This technique, now called the Heimlich maneuver or abdominal thrust, is simple enough that it can be performed immediately by anyone trained in the maneuver. The Heimlich maneuver is a standard part of all **first aid** courses.

The theory behind the Heimlich maneuver is that by compressing the abdomen below the level of the diaphragm, air is forced out of the lungs under pressure. This air dislodges the obstruction in the trachea and brings the foreign material back up into the mouth.

The Heimlich maneuver is used mainly when such solid materials as food, coins, vomit, or small **toys** are blocking the airway. There has been some controversy about whether the Heimlich maneuver is appropriate to use routinely on **near-drowning** victims. After several studies of the effectiveness of the Heimlich maneuver on reestablishing breathing in near-drowning victims, the American Red Cross and the American Heart Association both recommend that the Heimlich maneuver be used only as a last resort after traditional airway clearance techniques and **cardiopulmonary resuscitation** (CPR) have been tried repeatedly and failed; or if it is clear that a solid foreign object is blocking the airway.

Demographics

There are no exact statistics on the number of times the Heimlich maneuver is performed in an average year, or the circumstances or age groups of the persons treated, although one study done in California stated that 4% of 513 patients treated for a foreign body in the airway died and that the average age of patients treated was 65. The Heimlich maneuver was the most commonly used intervention, with an 86% success rate.

Description

The Heimlich maneuver can be performed on all people. Modifications are necessary if the person **choking** is very obese, pregnant, a child, or an infant. Indications that a person's airway is blocked include:

- inability to speak or cry out
- face turning blue from lack of oxygen
- desperate grabbing at the throat
- weak cough with labored breathing producing a high-pitched noise
- all of the above, followed by unconsciousness

Performing the Heimlich maneuver on adults

To perform the Heimlich maneuver on a conscious adult, the rescuer stands behind the affected person, who may be either sitting or standing. The rescuer makes a fist with one hand and places it, thumb toward the person choking, below the rib cage and above the waist. The rescuer encircles the other person's waist, placing the other hand on top of the fist.

In a series of six to 10 sharp and distinct thrusts upward and inward, the rescuer attempts to develop enough pressure to force the foreign object back up the trachea. If the maneuver fails, it is repeated. It is important not to give up if the first attempt fails. As the choking person is deprived of oxygen, the muscles of the trachea relax slightly. Because of this loosening, it is possible that a foreign object may be expelled on a second or third attempt.

If the individual choking is unconscious, the rescuer should place the person supine on the floor; bend the chin forward; make sure the tongue is not blocking the airway; and feel in the mouth for any **foreign objects**, being careful not to push them further into the airway. The rescuer kneels astride the choking person's thighs and places the fists between the bottom of the choking person's breastbone and navel. The rescuer then executes a series of six to 10 sharp compressions by pushing inward and upward.

After the abdominal thrusts, the rescuer repeats the process of lifting the chin, moving the tongue, feeling for and possibly removing any foreign material. If the airway is not clear, the rescuer repeats the abdominal thrusts as often as necessary. If the foreign object has been removed, but the victim is not breathing, the rescuer starts CPR.

Performing the Heimlich maneuver under special circumstances

OBVIOUSLY PREGNANT OR VERY OBESE PEOPLE The main difference in performing the Heimlich maneuver on this group of people is in the placement of the fists. Instead of using abdominal thrusts, chest thrusts are used. The rescuer's fists are placed against the middle of the breastbone (sternum), and the motion of the chest thrust is in and downward, rather than upward. If the person choking is unconscious, the chest thrusts are similar to those used in CPR.

CHILDREN The technique in children over one year of age is the same as in adults, except that the amount of force used is less than that used with adults, in order to avoid damaging a child's ribs, breastbone, and internal organs.

INFANTS UNDER ONE YEAR OLD The rescuer sits down and positions the infant along the rescuer's forearm with the infant's face pointed toward the floor and at a lower level than the infant's chest. The rescuer's hand supports the infant's head. The forearm rests on the rescuer's own thigh for additional support. Using the heel of the other hand, the rescuer administers four or five rapid blows to the infant's back between the shoulder blades.

After administering the back blows, the rescuer sandwiches the infant between both arms. The infant is turned over so that it lies face up, supported by the rescuer's opposite arm. Using the free hand, the rescuer places the index and middle finger on the center of the breastbone and makes four sharp chest thrusts. This series of back blows and chest thrusts is alternated until the foreign object is expelled.

SELF-ADMINISTRATION OF THE HEIMLICH MANEUVER To apply the Heimlich maneuver to oneself, a choking person should make a fist with one hand and place it in the middle of the body at a spot above the navel and below the breastbone, then grasp the fist with the other hand and push sharply inward and upward. If this fails, the choking person should press the upper abdomen over the back of a chair, edge of a table, porch railing or something similar, and thrust up and inward until the object is dislodged.

Benefits

The Heimlich maneuver usually results in the expulsion and removal of an obstruction in the throat; in many situations, the person's life is saved. The choking person suffers no permanent effects from the episode.

Precautions

If possible, have someone nearby call 911 while the rescuer performs the Heimlich maneuver.

It is important to have training and practice in the correct use of the maneuver. Incorrect application of the Heimlich maneuver can damage the chest, ribs, heart, or internal organs of the person on whom it is performed. People may also vomit after being treated with the Heimlich maneuver. It is important to prevent aspiration of the vomitus.

Preparation

Any adult, adolescent, or responsible older child can be trained to perform the Heimlich maneuver. Knowing how to perform it may save someone's life. Before doing the maneuver, it is important to determine whether the airway is completely blocked. If the choking person can talk or cry, the Heimlich maneuver is not appropriate. If the airway is not completely blocked, the choking person should be allowed to try to **cough** up the foreign object without assistance.

Aftercare

Once the obstruction is removed, most persons who experience an episode of choking recover without any further care. Persons who have an obstruction that cannot be dislodged but are able to breathe should be taken to an emergency room for treatment.

Risks

Many people vomit after being treated with the Heimlich maneuver. Depending on the length and severity of the choking episode, the person may need to be taken to a hospital emergency room. In addition, even when the maneuver is performed correctly, the person being treated often suffers **bruises** in the abdominal area. Occasionally, one or more ribs of the choking person may be broken during administration of the Heimlich maneuver. The elderly are more likely to suffer bruises or broken ribs during the maneuver than younger adults.

Applying the Heimlich maneuver too vigorously may result in an injury to the internal organs of the choking person. There may be some local **pain** and tenderness at the point where the rescuer's fist was placed. In infants, a rescuer should never attempt to sweep the baby's mouth without looking to remove

KEY TERMS

Aspiration—The entry of body secretions or foreign material into the trachea and lungs.

Diaphragm—The thin layer of muscle that separates the chest cavity, which contains the lungs and heart, from the abdominal cavity, which contains the intestines and digestive organs.

Sternum—The breastbone. The sternum is located over the heart, is the point of attachment for ribs at the front of the body and provides protection to the heart beneath it.

Trachea—The windpipe. A tube extending from below the voice box into the chest where it splits into two branches, the bronchi, that lead to each lung.

foreign material. This is likely to push the material farther down the trachea. If the foreign material is not removed, the person choking will die from lack of oxygen.

Health care team roles

Anyone can be trained to successfully apply the Heimlich maneuver. Most of the applications each year are provided by trained volunteers. Health professionals may become involved. Paramedics may apply the Heimlich maneuver to a choking person. Physicians, physician assistants and nurses may provide additional treatment in a hospital emergency room. Nurses may provide some follow-up care.

Research and general acceptance

There is some debate as of 2010 over the benefit of slapping the person's upper back to help dislodge the material in the windpipe. Dr. Heimlich has long maintained that back slaps should not be done because they drive the material deeper into the windpipe. However, the American Red Cross and the American Heart Association presently recommend the use of hard blows with the heel of the rescuer's hand on the upper back of the victim. The number to be used varies by training organization, but is usually between five and 20. The back slap is designed to create pressure behind the blockage, assisting the patient in dislodging the article in the airway. The Mayo Clinic article listed below recommends five back slaps before beginning the abdominal thrusts of the Heimlich maneuver, and alternating between five back blows and five abdominal thrusts until the food or other object is dislodged.

Resources

BOOKS

American Academy of Orthopaedic Surgeons. *First Aid, CPR, and AED Standard*. Sudbury, MA: Jones and Bartlett Publishers, 2010.

Dvorchak, George E., Jr. *The Pocket First Aid Field Guide: Treatment of Outdoor Emergencies*. New York: Skyhorse Publishing, 2010.

National Safety Council. *Basic Pediatric First Aid, CPR, and AED*. Boston: McGraw-Hill Higher Education, 2008.

PERIODICALS

Chillag, S., et al. "The Heimlich Maneuver: Breaking Down the Complications." *Southern Medical Journal* 103 (February 2010): 147–150.

Drinka, P. "Broken Ribs Following CPR or the Heimlich Maneuver." *Journal of the American Medical Directors Association* 10 (May 2009): 283–84.

Lee, S.L., et al. "Complications as a Result of the Heimlich Maneuver." *Journal of Trauma* 66 (March 2009): E34–E35.

Soroudi, A., et al. "Adult Foreign Body Airway Obstruction in the Prehospital Setting." *Prehospital Emergency Care* 11 (January-March 2007): 25–29.

OTHER

American Heart Association. *Heimlich Maneuver*, http://www.americanheart.org/presenter.jhtml?identifier=4605

Broomfield, James, MD. "Heimlich Maneuver on Self." *Discovery Health*, January 4, 2007, http://health.discovery.com/encyclopedias/illnesses.html?article=671

Heimlich Institute. *How to Do the Heimlich Maneuver*, http://www.heimlichinstitute.org/page.php?id=34

Howcast. *How to Perform the Heimlich Maneuver* This is a video demonstration of the maneuver that takes about 2-1/2 minutes to watch, http://www.youtube.com/watch?v=tEIiEAn7b-U

Mayo Clinic. *Choking: First Aid*, http://www.mayoclinic.com/health/first-aid-choking/FA00025

MedlinePlus Medical Encyclopedia. *Heimlich Maneuver*, http://www.nlm.nih.gov/medlineplus/ency/article/000047.htm

Nathan, Joan. "A Heimlich in Every Pot." *New York Times*, February 3, 2009. This is a first-person account by a cookbook author who was saved from choking by a celebrity chef at a dinner party, http://www.nytimes.com/2009/02/04/opinion/04nathan.html?ref=opinion

ORGANIZATIONS

American Heart Association National Center, 7272 Greenville Avenue, Dallas TX, 75231, 800-AHA-USA-1, http://www.americanheart.org/presenter.jhtml?identifier=1200000.

American Red Cross National Headquarters, 2025 E Street, NW, Washington DC, 20006, 202-303-5000, http://www.redcross.org/.

Heimlich Institute, 311 Straight Street, Cincinnati OH, 45219, 513-559-2100, http://www.heimlichinstitute.org/default.php.

L. Fleming Fallon, Jr., MD, PhD, DrPH
Rebecca J. Frey, PhD

Hemangiomas *see* **Birthmarks**

Hemoglobin F test *see* **Fetal hemoglobin test**

Hemophilia

Definition

Hemophilia is a coagulation disorder arising from a genetic defect of the X chromosome; the defect can either be inherited or result from spontaneous gene mutation. In each type of hemophilia (hemophilias A, B, and C), a critical coagulation protein is missing, causing individuals to bleed

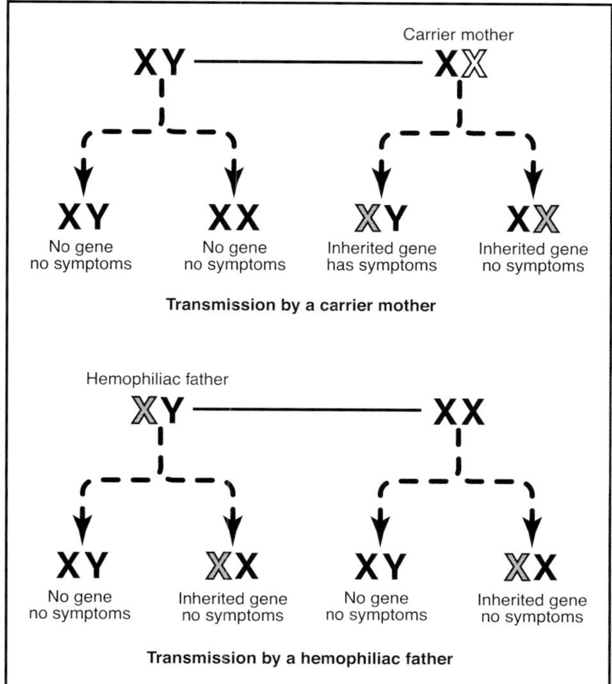

Chart showing how hemophilia is transmitted on the X chromosome. However, some 30 percent of hemophilia cases are caused by random genetic mutation. *(Illustration by Electronic Illustrators Group. Reproduced by permission of Gale, a part of Cengage Learning.)*

for long periods of time before clotting occurs. Depending on the degree of the disorder in the affected individual, uncontrolled bleeding may occur spontaneously with no known initiating event, or occur after specific events such as surgery, dental procedures, immunizations, or injury.

Demographics

According to the National Heart, Lung, and Blood Institute (NHLBI), hemophilia affects about 18,000 people in the United States, and each year, about 400 babies are born with the disorder, which usually occurs only in males with very rare exceptions. Worldwide, hemophilia A is the most common type of the disorder with about 1 in 4,000 males born with the disorder. As for hemophilia B, it occurs approximately in 1 of 20,000 newborn males. In 2008, an Orphanet report estimated the European prevalence of hemophilia at 7.7 per 100,000 persons. The mortality rate for patients with hemophilia is twice that of the healthy male population. For severe hemophilia, the rate is increased 4–6 times.

Hemophilia A and B are observed in all ethnic and racial groups, with some prevalence reported in Chinese populations.

Description

The normal mechanism for blood clotting is a complex series of events (coagulation cascade) involving interaction between the injured blood vessel, blood cells called platelets, 13 specific coagulation factors (designated by Roman numerals I through XIII), and other substances that circulate in the blood.

When a blood vessel is injured in a way that causes bleeding, platelets collect over the injured area, and form a temporary plug to prevent further bleeding. This temporary plug, however, is too disorganized to serve as a long–term solution, so a series of chemical events occur, resulting in the formation of a more reliable plug. The final plug involves tightly woven fibers of a material called fibrin. The production of fibrin requires the interaction of several chemicals, in particular a series of proteins called clotting factors. At least thirteen different clotting factors have been identified.

The clotting cascade, as it is usually called, is the series of events required to form the final fibrin clot. The cascade uses a technique called amplification to rapidly produce the proper sized fibrin clot from the small number of molecules initially activated by the injury.

In hemophilia, certain clotting factors are either decreased in quantity, absent, or improperly formed. Because the clotting cascade uses amplification to rapidly plug up a bleeding area, absence or inactivity of just one clotting factor can greatly increase bleeding time.

Hemophilia A is the most common type of bleeding disorder and involves decreased activity of factor VIII. There are three levels of factor VIII deficiency: severe, moderate, and mild. This classification is based on the percentage of normal factor VIII activity present:

- Individuals with less than 1% of normal factor VIII activity level have severe hemophilia. Half of all people with hemophilia A fall into this category. Such individuals frequently experience spontaneous bleeding, most frequently into their joints, skin, and muscles. Surgery or trauma can result in life–threatening hemorrhage, and must be carefully managed.
- Individuals with 1–5% of normal factor VIII activity level have moderate hemophilia, and are at risk for heavy bleeding after seemingly minor traumatic injury.
- Individuals with 5–40% of normal factor VIII activity level have mild hemophilia, and must prepare carefully for any surgery or dental procedures.

Individuals with hemophilia B have symptoms very similar to those of hemophilia A, but the deficient factor is factor IX. This type of hemophilia is also known as Christmas disease.

Hemophilia C is very rare, and much more mild than hemophilia A or B; it involves factor XI.

Risk factors

Hemophilia is a genetic disorder, which is usually inherited. The hemophilia gene is passed down from a parent to a child. Individuals with a family history of the condition are accordingly at higher risk for haemophilia,

Causes and symptoms

Hemophilia A and B are both caused by a genetic defect present on the X chromosome. (Hemophilia C is inherited in a different fashion.) About 70% of all people with hemophilia A or B inherited the disease. The other 30% develop from a spontaneous genetic mutation.

The following concepts are important to understanding the inheritance of these diseases. All humans have two chromosomes determining their gender: females have XX, males have XY. Because the trait is carried only on the X chromosome, it is called "sex–linked." The chromosome's flawed unit is referred to as the gene.

Both factors VIII and IX are produced by a genetic defect of the X chromosome, so hemophilia A and B are both sex–linked diseases. Because a female child always receives two X chromosomes, she nearly always will receive at least one normal X chromosome. Therefore, even if she receives one flawed X chromosome, she will still be capable of producing a sufficient quantity of factors VIII and IX to avoid the symptoms of hemophilia. Such a person who has one flawed chromosome, but does not actually suffer from the disease, is called a carrier. She carries the flaw that causes hemophilia and can pass it on to her offspring. If, however, she has a son who receives her flawed X chromosome, he will be unable to produce the right quantity of factors VIII or IX, and he will suffer some degree of hemophilia. (Males inherit one X and one Y chromosome, and therefore have only one X chromosome.)

In rare cases, a hemophiliac father and a carrier mother can pass on the right combination of parental chromosomes to result in a hemophiliac female child. This situation, however, is rare. The vast majority of people with either hemophilia A or B are male.

About 30% of all people with hemophilia A or B are the first member of their family to ever have the disease. These individuals have had the unfortunate occurrence of a spontaneous mutation; meaning that in their early development, some random genetic accident befell their X chromosome, resulting in the defect causing hemophilia A or B. Once such a spontaneous genetic mutation takes place, offspring of the affected person can inherit the newly–created, flawed chromosome.

In the case of severe hemophilia, the first bleeding event usually occurs prior to eighteen months of age. In some babies, hemophilia is suspected immediately, when a routine **circumcision** (removal of the foreskin of the penis) results in unusually heavy bleeding. Toddlers are at particular risk, because they fall frequently, and may bleed into the soft tissue of their arms and legs. These small bleeds result in bruising and noticeable lumps, but don't usually need treatment. As a child becomes more active, bleeding may occur into the muscles; a much more painful and debilitating problem. These muscle bleeds result in **pain** and pressure on the nerves in the area of the bleed. Damage to nerves can cause **numbness** and decreased ability to use the injured limb.

Some of the most problematic and frequent bleeds occur into the joints, particularly into the knees and elbows. Repeated bleeding into joints can result in scarring within the joints and permanent deformities. Individuals may develop arthritis in joints that have suffered continued irritation from the presence of blood. Mouth injuries can result in compression of the airway, and, therefore, can be life–threatening. A blow to the head, which might be totally insignificant in a normal individual, can result in bleeding into the skull and brain. Because the skull has no room for expansion, the hemophiliac individual is at risk for brain damage due to blood taking up space and exerting pressure on the delicate brain tissue.

People with hemophilia are at very high risk of hemorrhage (severe, heavy, uncontrollable bleeding) from injuries such as motor vehicle accidents and also from surgery.

Some other rare clotting disorders such as **Von Willebrand disease** present similar symptoms but are not usually called hemophilia.

Diagnosis

Examination

If hemophilia is suspected, or if a person has a bleeding problem, a physician typically takes personal and family medical histories to establish whether the family has a history of frequent or heavy bleeding and bruising.

Tests

Various tests are available to measure, under very carefully controlled conditions, the length of time it takes to produce certain components of the final fibrin clot. The activated partial thromboplastin time (APTT) is performed and will typically be prolonged while a prothrombin time (PT) will likely be normal. Factor assays, measurement

KEY TERMS

Amplification—A process by which something is made larger. In clotting, only a very few chemicals are released by the initial injury; they result in a cascade of chemical reactions which produces increasingly larger quantities of different chemicals, resulting in an appropriately–sized, strong fibrin clot.

Coagulation—Blood clotting.

Coagulation factors—Specific coagulation proteins in the blood required for clotting. Coagulation proteins are designated with roman numerals I through XIII.

Factors—Coagulation factors are substances in the blood, such as proteins and minerals, that are necessary for clotting. Each clotting substance is designated with roman numerals I through XIII.

Fibrin—The final substance created through the clotting cascade, which provides a strong, reliable plug to prevent further bleeding from the initial injury.

Hemorrhage—Very severe, massive bleeding that is difficult to control. Hemorrhage can occur in hemophiliacs after what would be a relatively minor injury to a person with normal clotting factors.

Mutation—A permanent change in the genetic material that may alter a trait or characteristic of an individual, or manifest as disease, and can be transmitted to offspring.

Platelets—Small disc–shaped structures that circulate in the blood stream and participate in blood clotting.

Trauma—Injury.

methods performed by the clinical laboratory, can determine the percentage of factors VIII and IX present compared to normal percentages. This information helps to confirm a diagnosis of hemophilia and identifies the type and severity of hemophilia present.

Hemophilia A and B are classified as mild, moderate, or severe, depending on the amount of clotting factor VIII or IX in the blood. Mild hemophilia is diagnosed if 5–30% of the normal clotting factors are present. With 1–5% of the normal clotting factors present, the haemophilia is diagnosed as moderate, and as severe when less than 1% of the normal clotting factors are present.

Procedures

Individuals with a family history of hemophilia may benefit from genetic counseling before deciding to have a baby. Families with a positive history of hemophilia can also have tests done during a pregnancy to determine whether the fetus is a hemophiliac. The test called chorionic villius sampling examines proteins for the defects that lead to hemophilia. This test, which is associated with a 1% risk of miscarriage, can be performed at 10–12 weeks. The test called **amniocentesis** examines the DNA of fetal cells shed into the amniotic fluid for genetic mutations. Amniocentesis, which is associated with a one in 200 risk of miscarriage, is performed at 16–18 weeks gestation.

Treatment

Traditional

The most important thing that individuals with hemophilia can do to prevent complications of his disease is to avoid injury. This is accomplished with replacement therapy to replace the clotting factor that is missing or present in low amounts. Hemophiliacs are also typically vaccinated against hepatitis.

In replacement therapy, various types of factors VIII and IX are available to replace a patient's missing factors. These are administered intravenously (directly into the patient's veins by needle). Cryoprecipitate, for example, is a single–or multiple–donor human plasma preparation rich in coagulation factors; it is made available as a frozen concentrate. Fresh frozen plasma is a single–donor preparation of factor–rich plasma; it is used primarily for replacing factor XI in individuals with hemophilia C. Concentrated factor preparations may be obtained from a single donor, by pooling the donations of as many as thousands of donors, or by laboratory creation through highly advanced genetic techniques. These preparations are administered directly into the individual's veins (intravenous administration). In 2008, the United States Food and Drug Administration (FDA) approved a new formulation of the genetically engineered version of Factor VIIa that can be stored at room temperature for up to two years.

The frequency of treatment with factors depends on the severity of the individual patient's disease. Patients with relatively mild disease will only require treatment in the event of injury, or to prepare for scheduled surgical or dental procedures. Patients with more severe disease will require regular treatment to avoid spontaneous bleeding.

While appropriate treatment of hemophilia can both decrease suffering and be life–saving, complications associated with treatment can also be quite serious. About

20% of all patients with hemophilia A begin to produce chemicals in their bodies which rapidly destroy infused factor VIII. The presence of such a chemical may greatly hamper efforts to prevent or stop a major hemorrhage.

Individuals who receive factor prepared from pooled donor blood are at risk for serious infections that may be passed through blood. Hepatitis, a severe and potentially fatal viral liver infection, may be contracted from pooled factor preparations. Recently, a good deal of concern has been raised about the possibility of hemophiliacs contracting a fatal slow virus infection of the brain (Creutzfeldt–Jakob disease) from blood products. Unfortunately, pooled factor preparations in the early 1980s were contaminated with human **immunodeficiency** virus (HIV), the virus which causes **AIDS**. A large number of hemophiliacs were infected with HIV and some statistics show that HIV is still the leading cause of **death** among hemophiliacs. Currently, careful methods of donor testing, as well as methods of inactivating viruses present in donated blood, have greatly lowered this risk.

Drugs

Desmopressin (DDAVP) is a synthetic hormone used in the treatment of mild to moderate hemophilia A. DDAVP is not used to treat hemophilia B or severe hemophilia A. DDAVP usually is given by injection or as nasal spray. Since it wears off when used often, DDAVP is given only in specific situations. For example, before dental work or before certain physical activities to prevent or reduce bleeding. Antifibrinolytic medicines, such as tranexamic acid and aminocaproic acid, may also be used with replacement therapy. These medications are typically used before dental work or to treat bleeding from the mouth or nose or mild intestinal bleeding.

Medications or drugs that promote bleeding, such as aspirin, should be avoided.

Alternative

The most exciting new treatments currently being researched involve efforts to transfer new genes to hemophiliacs. These new genes would have the ability to produce the missing factors. As yet, these techniques are not being performed on humans, but there is great hope that eventually this type of gene therapy will be available.

Clinical trials for the treatment of hemophilia are currently sponsored by the National Institutes of Health (NIH) and other agencies. In 2009, NIH reported 196 on–going or recently completed studies. Some examples include the following:

- The evaluation of the safety of gene transfer for the treatment of severe hemophilia B. (NCT00076557)
- The study of musculoskeletal function in people with hemophilia in developing countries. (NCT00324493)
- The study of allergic reactions to factor IX in patients with hemophilia B. (NCT00195221)
- A study evaluating inhibitor specificity in hemophilia A. (NCT00151385)

Clinical trial information is constantly updated by NIH and the most recent information on hemophilia trials can be found at: http://clinicaltrials.gov/ct2/results?term=hemophilia

Home remedies

At home, certain steps can help avoid excessive bleeding. They include regular **exercise** to build up muscles and protect joints, avoiding aspirin and nonsteroidal anti–inflammatory drugs (Advil, Motrin, others) that can aggravate bleeding, practising good dental hygiene to avoid having teeth pulled out, and using protective equipment in **sports** and physical activities to minimize injuries.

Prognosis

Prognosis is very difficult to generalize. Because there are so many variations in the severity of hemophilia, and because much of what befalls a hemophiliac patient will depend on issues such as physical activity level and accidental injuries, statistics on prognosis are not generally available.

Prevention

Because of its genetic origins, hemophilia cannot be prevented in those born with the inherited defects or factor deficiencies. However, individuals who have a family history of hemophilia may benefit from **genetic testing** and counseling before deciding to have a baby. The most important way for individuals with hemophilia to prevent complications of the disease is to avoid activities that may lead to injury. Those individuals who require dental work or any type of surgery may need to be pre–treated with an infusion of factor VIII to avoid hemorrhage. Hemophiliacs should also avoid medications or drugs that promote bleeding; aspirin is one such medication and many prescription drugs have anticoagulant properties.

Resources

BOOKS

Freedman, Jeri. *Hemophilia (Genetic Diseases)*. New York, NY: Rosen Publishing Group, 2006.

Gray, Laura, and Christine Chamberlain. *The Gift of Experience: Conversations About Hemophilia.* Brunswick, ME: Camden Writers, 2008.

Lee, Christine A., et al., editors. *Textbook of Hemophilia.* Boston, MA: Blackwell Publishing, 2010.

Parker, Philip M. *Hemophilia—A Bibliography and Dictionary for Physicians, Patients, and Genome Researchers.* San Diego, CA: Icon Health Publications, 2007.

Raabe, Michelle. *Hemophilia (Genes and Disease).* New York, NY: Chelsea House Publishers, 2008.

PERIODICALS

Douma–van Riet, D. C., et al. "Physical fitness in children with haemophilia and the effect of overweight." *Haemophilia* 15, no. 2 (March 2009): 519–527.

Ghosh, K., and S. Shetty. "Immune response to FVIII in hemophilia A: an overview of risk factors." *Clinical Reviews in Allergy & Immunology* 37, no. 2 (October 2009): 58–66.

Kessler, C. M. "Advances in the treatment of hemophilia." *Clinical Advances in Hematology & Oncology* 6, no. 3 (March 2008): 184–187.

Oldenburg, J., et al. "Haemophilia care then, now and in the future." *Haemophilia* 15, suppl. 1 (January 2009): 2–7.

Petrini, P., and A. Seuser. "Haemophilia care in adolescents—compliance and lifestyle issues." *British Journal of Haematology* 15, suppl. 1 (January 2009): 15–19.

Rodriguez, N. I., and W. K. Hoots. "Advances in hemophilia: experimental aspects and therapy." *Pediatric Clinics of North America* 55, no. 2 (April 2008): 357–376.

Sherry, D. D. "Avoiding the impact of musculoskeletal pain on quality of life in children with hemophilia." *Orthopaedic Nursing* 27, no. 2 (March–April 2008): 103–108.

Stine, K. C., and D. L. Becton. "Bleeding disorders: when is normal bleeding not normal?" *Journal of the Arkansas Medical Society* 106, no. 2 (August 2009): 40–42.

Viiala, N. O., et al. "Gene therapy for hemophilia: clinical trials and technical tribulations." *Seminars in Thrombosis and Hemostasis* 35, no. 1 (February 2009): 81–92.

Zhang, B. "Recent developments in the understanding of the combined deficiency of FV and FVIII." *British Journal of Haematology* 145, no. 1 (April 2009): 15–23.

OTHER

"Frequently Asked Questions About Hemophilia." *World Federation of Hemophilia* Information Page, http://www.wfh.org/index.asp?lang=EN&url=2/1/1_1_1_FAQ.htm (accessed December 17, 2009).

"Hemophilia." *Genetics Home Reference* Information Page, http://ghr.nlm.nih.gov/condition=hemophilia (accessed December 17, 2009)

"Hemophilia." *Medline Plus* Health Topic, http://www.nlm.nih.gov/medlineplus/hemophilia.html (accessed December 17, 2009)

"Hemophilia." *NHLBI* Information Page, http://www.nhlbi.nih.gov/health/dci/Diseases/hemophilia/hemophilia_what.html (accessed December 17, 2009)

ORGANIZATIONS

American Society of Pediatric Hematology and Oncology (ASPHO), 4700 W. Lake Ave., Glenview IL, 60025, (847) 375-4716, info@aspho.org, http://www.aspho.org.

National Heart, Lung, and Blood Institute (NHLBI), P.O. Box 30105, Bethesda MD, 20824-0105, (301) 592-8573, (240) 629-3246, nhlbiinfo@nhlbi.nih.gov, http://www.nhlbi.nih.gov.

National Hemophilia Foundation, 116 West 32nd St., 11th Floor, New York NY, 10001, (212) 328-3700, (212) 328-3777, handi@hemophilia.org, http://www.hemophilia.org.

World Federation of Hemophilia, 1425 René Lévesque Blvd. W., Suite 1010, Montréal QC Canada, H3G 1T7, (514) 875-7944, (514) 875-8916, wfh@wfh.org, http://www.wfh.org.

Jennifer F. Wilson, MS
Culvert L. Lee, MS
Monique Laberge, PhD

Hemophilus infections

Definition

Hemophilus infections, most of which are due to *Haemophilus influenzae* infections, are a group of contagious diseases that are caused by a gram-negative bacterium, and affect only humans. Some hemophilus infections are potentially fatal.

Description

H. influenzae is a common organism worldwide; it has been found in the nasal secretions of as many as 90% of healthy individuals in the general population. Hemophilus infections are characterized by acute inflammation with a discharge (exudate). They may affect almost any organ system, but are most common in the respiratory tract. The organism can be transmitted by person-to-person contact, or by contact with nasal discharges and other body fluids. Hemophilus infections in the United States are most likely to spread in the late winter or early spring.

The primary factor influencing the rate of infection is age; children between the ages of six months and four years are most vulnerable to *H. influenzae*. In previous years, about 50% of children would acquire a hemophilus infection before reaching one year of age; almost all children would develop one before age three. These figures are declining, however, as a result of the increasing use of hemophilus vaccines for children.

Adults are also susceptible to hemophilus diseases. *H. influenzae* pneumonia is a common nosocomial infection (illnesses contracted in hospitals). The rate of hemophilus infections in the adult population has increased over the past 40 years. The reasons for this change are unclear, but some researchers speculate that the overuse of **antibiotics** has led to the development of drug-resistant strains of *H. influenzae*. The risk factors for hemophilus infections among adults include:

- smoking
- alcoholism
- chronic lung disease
- old age
- living in a city or institutional housing with a large group of people
- poor nutrition and hygiene
- HIV infection, or other immune system disorder

Causes and symptoms

Hemophilus infections are primarily caused by *Haemophilus influenzae*, a gram-negative bacterium that is capable of spreading from the nasal tissues and upper airway, where it is usually found, to the chest, throat, or middle ear. The organism sometimes invades localized areas of tissue, producing **meningitis**, infectious arthritis, **conjunctivitis**, cellulitis, **epiglottitis**, or inflammation of the membrane surrounding the heart. The most serious infections are caused by a strain called *H. influenzae* b (Hib). Before routine **vaccination**, Hib was the most common cause of bacterial meningitis, and responsible for most of the cases of acquired **mental retardation** in the United States.

Hemophilus infections in children

BACTERIAL SEPSIS IN THE NEWBORN Bacterial sepsis (sepsis is the presence of illness-causing microorganisms, or their poisons, in the blood) is a potentially fatal illness in newborn infants. The child may acquire the disease organism as it passes through the mother's **birth** canal, or from the hospital environment. *H. influenzae* can also produce inflammations of the eye (conjunctivitis) in newborn children. The signs of sepsis may include **fever**, crankiness, feeding problems, breathing difficulties, pale or mottled skin, or drowsiness. Premature birth is the most significant risk factor for hemophilus infections in newborns.

EPIGLOTTITIS Epiglottitis is a potentially fatal hemophilus infection. Although children are more likely to develop epiglottitis, it can occur in adults as well. When the epiglottis (a piece of cartilage behind the tongue which protects the opening to the windpipe by opening and closing) is infected, it can swell to the point where it blocks the windpipe. The symptoms of epiglottitis include a sudden high fever, drooling, the feeling of an object stuck in the throat, and **stridor**. The epiglottis will look swollen and bright red if the doctor examines the patient's throat with a laryngoscope (a viewing device).

MENINGITIS Meningitis caused by Hib is most common in children between nine months and four years of age. The child usually develops upper respiratory symptoms followed by fever, loss of appetite, **vomiting**, **headache**, and a stiff or sore neck or back. In severe cases, the child may have convulsions or go into shock or coma.

OTHER INFECTIONS Hib is the second most common cause of middle ear infection and **sinusitis** in children. The symptoms of sinusitis include fever, **pain**, bad breath, and coughing. Children may also develop infectious arthritis from Hib. The joints most frequently affected are the large weight-bearing joints.

Hemophilus infections in adults

PNEUMONIA Hib **pneumonia** is the most common hemophilus infection in adults. The symptoms include empyema (sputum containing pus), and fever. The hemophilus organism can usually be identified from sputum samples. Hib pneumonia is increasingly common in the elderly.

MENINGITIS Meningitis caused by Hib can develop in adults as a complication of an ear infection or sinusitis. The symptoms are similar to those in children but are usually less severe in adults.

Diagnosis

The diagnosis is usually based on a combination of the patient's symptoms and the results of blood counts, cultures, or antigen detection tests.

Laboratory tests

Laboratory tests can be used to confirm the diagnosis of hemophilus infections. The bacterium can be grown on chocolate agar, or identified by blood cultures or Gram stain of body fluids. Antigen detection tests can be used to identify hemophilus infections in children. These tests include latex agglutination and electrophoresis.

Other laboratory findings that are associated with hemophilus infections include **anemia** (low red blood cell count), and a drop in the number of white blood cells in children with severe infections. Adults often show an abnormally high level of white blood cells; cell counts of 15,000–30,000/mm^3 are not unusual.

Treatment

Because some hemophilus infections are potentially fatal, treatment is started without waiting for the results of laboratory tests.

Medications

Hemophilus infections are treated with antibiotics. Patients who are severely ill are given ampicillin or a third-generation cephalosporin, such as cefotaxime or ceftriaxone, intravenously. Patients with milder infections are given oral antibiotics, including amoxicillin, cefaclor, erythromycin, or trimethoprim-sulfamethoxazole. Patients who are allergic to penicillin are usually given cefaclor or trimethoprim-sulfamethoxazole.

Patients with Hib strains that are resistant to ampicillin may be given chloramphenicol. Chloramphenicol is not a first-choice drug because of its side effects, including interference with bone marrow production of blood cells.

The duration of antibiotic treatment depends on the location and severity of the hemophilus infection. Adults with respiratory tract infections, or Hib pneumonia, are usually given a 10–14 day course of antibiotics. Meningitis is usually treated for 10–14 days, but a seven-day course of treatment with ceftriaxone appears to be sufficient for infants and children. Ear infections are treated for seven to 10 days.

Supportive care

Patients with serious hemophilus infections require bed rest and a humidified environment (such as a **croup** tent) if the respiratory tract is affected. Patients with epiglottitis frequently require intubation (insertion of a breathing tube) or a tracheotomy to keep the airway open. Patients with inflammation of the heart membrane, pneumonia, or arthritis may need surgical treatment to drain infected fluid from the chest cavity or inflamed joints.

Supportive care also includes monitoring of blood cell counts for patients using chloramphenicol, ampicillin, or other drugs that may affect production of blood cells by the bone marrow.

Prognosis

The most important factors in the prognosis are the severity of the infection and promptness of treatment. Untreated hemophilus infections—particularly meningitis, sepsis, and epiglottitis—have a high mortality rate. Bacterial sepsis of the newborn has a mortality rate between 13–50%. The prognosis is usually good for patients with mild infections who are treated without delay. Children who develop Hib arthritis sometimes have lasting problems with joint function.

KEY TERMS

Bacterium—A microscopic one-celled organism. *Haemophilus influenzae* is a specific bacterium.

Epiglottitis—Inflammation of the epiglottis. The epiglottis is a piece of cartilage behind the tongue that closes the opening to the windpipe when a person swallows. An inflamed epiglottis can swell and close off the windpipe, thus causing the patient to suffocate.

Exudate—A discharge produced by the body. Some exudates are caused by infections.

Gram-negative—A term that means that a bacterium will not retain the violet color when stained with Gram's dye. *Haemophilus influenzae* is a gram-negative bacterium.

Intubation—The insertion of a tube into the patient's airway to protect the airway from collapsing. Intubation is sometimes done as an emergency procedure for patients with epiglottitis.

Nosocomial—Contracted in a hospital. Pneumonia caused by *H. influenzae* is an example of a nosocomial infection.

Sepsis—Invasion of body tissues by disease organisms or their toxins. Sepsis may be either localized or generalized. *Haemophilus influenzae* can cause bacterial sepsis in newborns.

Stridor—A harsh or crowing breath sound caused by partial blockage of the patient's upper airway.

Tracheotomy—An emergency procedure in which the surgeon cuts directly through the patient's neck into the windpipe in order to keep the airway open.

Prevention

Hemophilus vaccines

There are three different vaccines for hemophilus infections used to immunize children in the United States: PRP-D, HBOC, and PRP-OMP. PRP-D is used only in children older than 15 months. HBOC is administered to infants at two, four, and six months after birth, with a booster dose at 15–18 months. PRP-OMP is administered to infants at two and four months, with the third dose at the child's first birthday. All three vaccines are given by intramuscular injection. About 5% of children may develop fever or soreness in the area of the injection.

Other measures

Other preventive measures include isolating patients with respiratory hemophilus infections; treating appropriate contacts of infected patients with rifampin; maintaining careful standards of cleanliness in hospitals, including proper disposal of soiled tissues; and washing hands properly.

Resources

BOOKS

Chambers, Henry F. "Infectious Diseases: Bacterial & Chlamydial." In *Current Medical Diagnosis and Treatment, 1998*, edited by Stephen McPhee, et al., 37th ed. Stamford: Appleton & Lange, 1997.

Rebecca J. Frey, PhD

Henoch-Schonlein purpura ***see*** **Allergic purpura**

Hepatitis A

Definition

Hepatitis A is an infectious disease of the liver caused by the HAV virus. The disease is usually transmitted by food or water contaminated by human wastes containing the virus or by close human contact. As far as is known, only humans can get hepatitis A; it is not carried by other animals.

Hepatitis A was previously known as infectious hepatitis because it spread relatively easily from those infected to close household contacts.

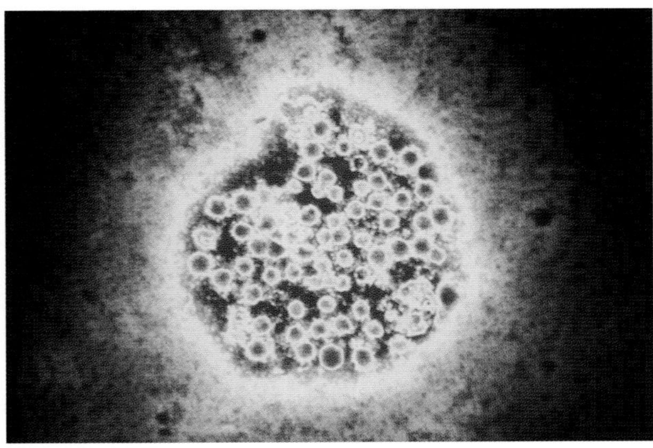

Hepatitis A virus magnified 225,000 times. *(Custom Medical Stock Photo, Inc. Reproduced by permission.)*

Demographics

Hepatitis A is much more common in Africa, Asia, and South America than in the United States. The rates of hepatitis A in North America have been steadily dropping since the 1980s due to improvements in public health policies and sanitation; on the other hand, the rates of hepatitis A among frequent travelers have been rising during the same time period.

In 1988 the Centers for Disease Control and Prevention (CDC) reported 32,000 cases in the United States; in 2003, 7653 cases were reported. The CDC estimates that nearly 25,000 people contracted hepatitis A in the United States in 2007, although the number of reported cases is much lower because many people do not show symptoms of the disease. In developing countries, children below the age of 2 account for most new cases of hepatitis A; in the United States, the age group most often affected is children between the ages of 5 and 14.

The states with the highest incidence of hepatitis A account for 50 percent of the reported cases. According to the **American Academy of Pediatrics**, 11 states have a rate of HAV infection that is at least twice the national average, or 20 cases per every 100,000 people. The states are: Arizona, Alaska, California, Idaho, Nevada, New Mexico, Oklahoma, Oregon, South Dakota, Utah, and Washington.

Males and females are equally likely to get hepatitis A, as are people from all races and ethnic groups in the United States.

Description

Hepatitis A is an inflammation of the liver caused by the HAV virus, also called enterovirus 72, which was first identified in 1973. It differs from **hepatitis B** and hepatitis C in that it does not cause long-term liver damage. Even though people can take several weeks or months to recover completely from hepatitis A, they have lifelong immunity afterward. Complications from hepatitis A are rare and usually limited to people with chronic liver disease or those who have received a liver transplant.

Hepatitis A varies in severity, running an acute course, generally starting within two to six weeks after contact with the virus, and lasting no longer than two or three months. Children and younger adults may have no symptoms at all, although they can still spread the disease. In general, adults are more likely to have noticeable symptoms than children or teenagers. The most common symptom is loss of energy and overall tiredness.

Some people develop a mild flu-like illness with **diarrhea**, low-grade **fever**, nausea, **vomiting**, and

muscle cramps. People with more severe symptoms may have **pain** in the abdomen in the area of the liver (below the rib cage on the right side of the body); they may notice that their urine has turned dark brown or that they have jaundice—yellowing of the skin and the whites of the eyes. Some have an itchy skin rash.

HAV may occur in single cases after contact with an infected relative or sex partner. Alternately, epidemics may develop when food or drinking water is contaminated by the feces of an infected person. In the public's mind, outbreaks of hepatitis A usually are linked with the eating of contaminated food at a restaurant. It is true that food-handlers, who may themselves have no symptoms, can start an alarming, widespread epidemic. Many types of food can be infected by sewage containing HAV, but such shellfish as clams and oysters are common culprits.

Most people diagnosed with hepatitis A feel better within four to six weeks after the symptoms begin, although about 15 percent of patients may take up to 9 months to regain their energy and feel normal again.

Risk factors

Some people are at increased risk of hepatitis A;

- People who travel to parts of the world with high rates of the disease and poor sanitation, including the Middle East, South America, Eastern Europe, Mexico and Central America, Africa, Southeast Asia, and the Caribbean.
- Male homosexuals.
- People who use illicit drugs, whether injected or taken by mouth.
- Medical researchers and laboratory workers who may be exposed to HAV.
- Child care workers and children in day care centers. Children at day care centers make up an estimated 14–40% of all cases of HAV infection in the United States. Changing diapers transmits infection through fecal-oral contact. Toys and other objects may remain contaminated for some time. Often a child without symptoms brings the infection home to siblings and parents.
- Troops living under crowded conditions at military camps or in the field.
- Homeless people.

Causes and symptoms

Causes

Hepatitis A is caused by a virus that is transmitted by close personal contact with an infected person, by needle sharing, and by eating food or drinking water contaminated by fecal matter. After the virus enters the body, it multiplies in the cells of the liver, causing inflammation of the liver and a general response from the **immune system** that leads to most of the symptoms of the illness.

The HAV virus is shed from the liver into the bile (a digestive fluid secreted by the liver) and then into the person's stools between 15 and 45 days before symptoms appear. That means that people can spread the virus through their feces before they know that they are sick. In the United States, hepatitis A is most commonly spread by food handlers who do not wash their hands properly after using the bathroom; by childcare workers who do not wash their hands after changing a baby's diaper; by anal sex; and by eating raw shellfish harvested from sewage-polluted waters. In very rare cases the virus can be transmitted through blood transfusions.

Symptoms

Often the first symptoms to appear are fatigue and general achiness. Those who like to drink coffee or smoke cigarettes may lose their taste for them. The liver often enlarges, causing pain or tenderness in the right upper part of the abdomen. As many as three out of four children have no symptoms of HAV infection, but about 85% of adults will have symptoms.

In addition to fatigue, the most common symptoms of hepatitis A include:

- Low-grade fever (101°F).
- Nausea, vomiting, and diarrhea.
- Loss of appetite and weight loss.
- Swelling of the liver and pain in the area of the abdomen over the liver.
- Tea- or coffee-colored urine.
- Jaundice.
- An itchy rash or a generalized sensation of itching.
- Pale or clay-colored stools.
- Muscle pains.

Diagnosis

Diagnosis of hepatitis A is made on the basis of the patient's history, findings during an office examination, and a blood test for HAV.

Examination

The doctor may suspect that a patient has hepatitis A during a physical examination in the office by feeling the area over the liver for signs of swelling and pain; taking

KEY TERMS

Antibody—A substance made by the body in response to a foreign body, such as a virus, which is able to attack and destroy the invading virus.

Antiemetic—A type of drug given to control nausea and vomiting.

Contamination—The process by which an object or body part becomes exposed to an infectious agent such as a virus.

Bile—A yellow-green fluid secreted by the liver that aids in the digestion of fats.

Epidemic—A situation where a large number of infections by a particular agent, such as a virus, develops in a short time. The agent is rapidly transmitted to many individuals.

Hepatitis—The medical term for inflammation of the liver. It can be caused by toxic substances or alcohol as well as infections.

Immune globulin—A preparation of antibodies that can be given before exposure for short-term protection against hepatitis A and for persons who have already been exposed to hepatitis A virus. Immune globulin must be given within two weeks after exposure to hepatitis A virus for maximum protection.

Incubation period—The interval from initial exposure to an infectious agent, such as a virus, and the first symptoms of illness.

Jaundice—A yellowish discoloration of the skin and whites of the eyes caused by increased levels of bile pigments from the liver in the patient's blood.

Relapse—A temporary recurrence of the symptoms of a disease.

Vaccine—A substance prepared from a weakened or killed microorganism which, when injected, helps the body to form antibodies that will prevent infection by the natural microorganism.

the patient's temperature; and checking the skin and eyes for signs of **jaundice**.

Tests

A definite diagnosis is provided by a blood test for antibodies to the HAV virus. There is a specific antibody called hepatitis A IgM antibody that develops when HAV is present in the body. This test always registers positive when a patient has symptoms, and should continue to register positive for four to six months. However, hepatitis A IgM antibody will persist lifelong in the blood and is protective against reinfection.

In some cases the doctor may also have the sample of blood checked for abnormally high levels of liver enzymes.

Treatment

Traditional

There is no specific drug treatment for hepatitis A, as **antibiotics** cannot be used to treat virus infections. Most people can care for themselves at home by making sure they get plenty of fluids and adequate **nutrition**. People whose appetite has been affected may benefit from eating small snacks throughout the day rather than three main meals, and eating soft and easily digested foods.

Patients with hepatitis A should avoid drinking alcohol, which makes it harder for the liver to recover from inflammation. Patients should also tell their doctor about any other over-the-counter or prescription drugs they are taking, because the drugs may need to be stopped temporarily or have the dosages changed.

Drugs

Patients with hepatitis A may take **acetaminophen** to reduce fever and relieve pain. Patients with mild vomiting may be prescribed antiemetics (drugs to control nausea); the drug most commonly prescribed for hepatitis patients is metoclopramide (Reglan). Those with severe vomiting may need to be hospitalized in order to receive intravenous fluids.

Prognosis

Most people recover fully from hepatitis A within a few weeks or months. Between 3 and 20 percent have relapses (temporary recurrences of symptoms) for as long as 6 to 9 months after infection. In the United States, serious complications are infrequent and deaths are very rare. As many as 75% of adults over 50 years of age in North America will have blood test evidence of previous hepatitis A.

About 1 percent of patients develop liver failure following HAV infection, mostly those over 60 or those with chronic liver disease. In these cases liver transplantation may be necessary for the patient's survival. There are about 100 deaths from hepatitis A reported each year in the United States.

Prevention

Hepatitis A can be prevented by a vaccine called Havrix that is given before exposure to the HAV virus.

The vaccine is given in 2 shots, the second given between 6 and 18 months after the first. It confers immunity against hepatitis A for at least 20 years. Those who should receive the vaccine include people in the military and those who travel abroad frequently; men who have sex with other men; people who use intravenous drugs; people with **hemophilia** who must receive human blood products; and people who have chronic hepatitis B or C infection.

People who have been exposed to the HAV virus should be given immune globulin to protect them against getting sick, because Havrix is not effective in people who have already been exposed to HAV. Children under the age of 2 should be given immune globulin or a newer vaccine (described below) rather than Havrix to protect them against HAV.

A vaccine against hepatitis A introduced in 2007 is called Epaxal; there is a version for children called Epaxal Junior that appears to be a good choice for mass **vaccination** programs. Unlike Havrix, Epaxal Junior can be given to children above the age of one year.

Everyone can reduce their risk of hepatitis A by observing the following precautions:

- Practice good personal hygiene; wash hands frequently, especially after using the toilet or changing a child's diaper.
- When traveling, drink only bottled water; avoid raw or undercooked meat or shellfish; and avoid eating fresh fruits or vegetables unless you have washed and peeled them yourself.
- Avoid sharing drinking glasses and eating utensils. If someone in the family has hepatitis A, wash their glasses and utensils separately in hot, soapy water.
- Avoid sexual contact with anyone who has hepatitis A.

Resources

BOOKS

Dworkin, Mark S. *Outbreak Investigations around the World: Case Studies in Infectious Disease Field Epidemiology*. Sudbury, MA: Jones and Bartlett, Publishers, 2010.

Feigin, Ralph D., et al, eds. *Feigin and Cherry's Textbook of Pediatric Infectious Diseases*, 6th ed. Philadelphia, PA: Saunders/Elsevier, 2009.

Richman, Douglas D., Richard J. Whitley, and Frederick G. Hayden, eds. *Clinical Virology*, 3rd ed. Washington, DC: ASM Press, 2009.

Younossi, Zobair M., ed. *Practical Management of Liver Diseases*. New York: Cambridge University Press, 2008.

PERIODICALS

Ackerman, L.K. "Update on Immunizations in Children and Adolescents." *American Family Physician* 77 (June 1, 2008): 1561–68.

Bovier, P.A. "Epaxal: A Virosomal Vaccine to Prevent Hepatitis A Infection." *Expert Review of Vaccines* 7 (October 2008): 1141–1150.

Costas, L., et al. "Vaccination Strategies against Hepatitis A in Travelers Older Than 40 Years: An Economic Evaluation." *Journal of Travel Medicine* 16 (September-October 2009): 344–48.

Degertekin, B., and A.S. Lok. "Update on Viral Hepatitis: 2008." *Current Opinion in Gastroenterology* 25 (May 2009): 180–85.

Dentinger, C.M. "Emerging Infections: Hepatitis A." *American Journal of Nursing* 109 (August 2009): 29–33.

Gitto, S., et al. "Alcohol and Viral Hepatitis: A Mini-Review." *Digestive and Liver Disease* 41 (January 2009): 67–70.

Lugoboni, F., et al. "Bloodborne Viral Hepatitis Infections among Drug Users: The Role of Vaccination." *International Journal of Environmental Research and Public Health* 6 (January 2009): 400–413.

Todd, E.C., et al. "Outbreaks Where Food Workers Have Been Implicated in the Spread of Foodborne Disease. Part 4. Infective Doses and Pathogen Carriage." *Journal of Food Protection* 71 (November 2008): 2339–2373.

OTHER

American Liver Foundation. *Hepatitis A*, http://www.liverfoundation.org/education/info/hepatitisa/

Centers for Disease Control and Prevention (CDC). *Hepatitis A Vaccination*, http://www.cdc.gov/vaccines/vpd-vac/hepa/default.htm

Gilroy, Richard A., and Sandeep Mukherjee. "Hepatitis A." *eMedicine*, August 26, 2008, http://emedicine.medscape.com/article/177484-overview

Mayo Clinic. *Hepatitis A*, http://www.mayoclinic.com/health/hepatitis-a/DS00397

National Institute of Allergy and Infectious Diseases (NIAID). *Hepatitis A*, http://www3.niaid.nih.gov/topics/hepatitis/hepatitisA/

ORGANIZATIONS

American College of Gastroenterology (ACG), P.O. Box 342260, Bethesda MD, 20827-2260, 301-263-9000, http://www.acg.gi.org/.

American Liver Foundation (ALF), 75 Maiden Lane, Suite 603, New York NY, 10038, 212-668-1000, 212-483-8179, http://www.liverfoundation.org/.

Centers for Disease Control and Prevention (CDC), 1600 Clifton Road, Atlanta GA, 30333, 800-232-4636, cdcinfo@cdc.gov, http://www.cdc.gov.

National Institute of Allergy and Infectious Diseases (NIAID), 6610 Rockledge Drive, MSC 6612, Bethesda MD, 20892-6612, 301-496-5717, 866-284-4107, 301-402-3573, http://www3.niaid.nih.gov.

World Health Organization (WHO), Avenue Appia 20, 1211 Geneva 27 Switzerland, + 41 22 791 21 11, + 41 22 791 31 11, info@who.int, http://www.who.int/en/.

Larry I. Lutwick, MD
Monique Laberge, PhD
Rebecca J. Frey, PhD

Hepatitis B

Definition

Hepatitis B is a viral infection of the liver transmitted through the blood or body fluids of someone who is infected. It is also called serum hepatitis because it can be transmitted through blood serum, the liquid portion of blood.

Hepatitis B is the most common serious liver infection worldwide. The disease has two forms: an acute form that lasts a few weeks, and a chronic form that can last for years, leading to cirrhosis, liver failure, liver **cancer**, and even **death**. Acute hepatitis B has a 5 percent chance of leading to the chronic form of the infection in adults; however, infants infected during the mother's pregnancy have a 90 percent chance of developing chronic hepatitis B, and children have a 25–50 percent chance.

Demographics

There are about 100,000 new cases of hepatitis B in the United States each year; it is estimated that 1–1.4 million people carry the disease and that 12 million Americans (1 in 20) have been infected by the disease. Hepatitis B causes about 5100 deaths in the United States each year; on average, one American health care worker dies each day from hepatitis B. In the rest of the world, as many as a third of the population (2 billion people) are chronic carriers of the disease. Chronic hepatitis B affects approximately 400 million people around the world as of 2009 and contributes to an estimated 1 million deaths worldwide each year.

The age group most commonly affected by hepatitis B in the United States is adults between the ages of 20 and 50. The routine immunization of children against the disease since 1990 has led to a decline in the rate of acute hepatitis in North America for the past two decades. African Americans are more likely to be infected than either Hispanics or Caucasians; however, Alaskan Eskimos and Pacific Islanders have higher rates of carrier status than members of other racial groups. Asian Americans are at increased risk of severe liver damage from hepatitis B compared to members of other racial groups. More males than females are infected with hepatitis B in all races and age groups.

Description

Hepatitis B has an incubation period of 1–6 months. About 50 percent of people with the acute form of the disease have no symptoms at all; the others experience

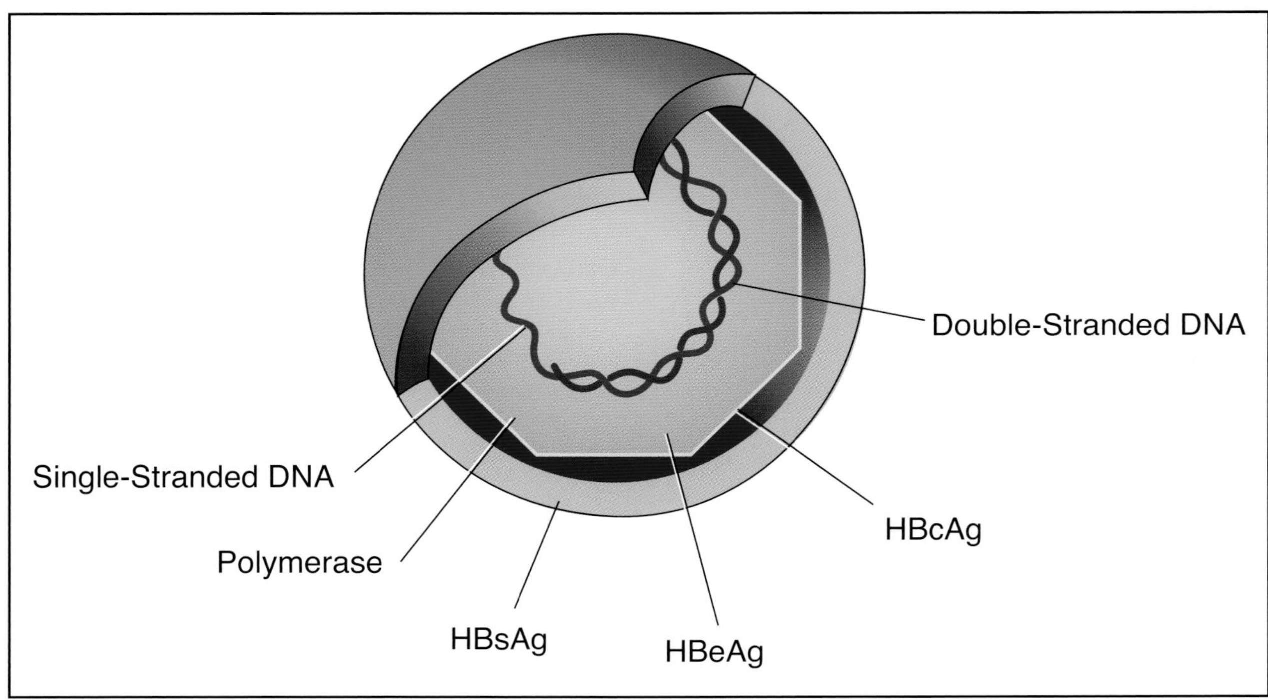

Hepatitis B virus (HBV) is composed of an inner protein core and an outer protein capsule. The outer capsule contains the hepatitis B surface antigen (HBsAg). The inner core contains HBV core antigen (HBcAg) and hepatitis B e-antigen (HBeAg). This cell also contains polymerase, which catalyzes the formation of the cell's DNA. HBV is the only hepatitis-causing virus that has DNA, instead of RNA. *(Illustration by Electronic Illustrators Group. Reproduced by permission of Gale, a part of Cengage Learning.)*

loss of appetite, nausea and **vomiting**, and **jaundice** around 12 weeks after getting infected. Some patients may also have joint **pain**, itchy skin, or abdominal pain. Many of these patients assume that they have **influenza**.

Patients with chronic hepatitis may have no symptoms at all. The one-third who do eventually fall ill have the same symptoms as patients with the acute form of the disease. About two-thirds of people with chronic HBV are carriers of the virus. They may never get sick themselves but they can transmit the infection to others. The remaining one-third of people with chronic hepatitis B develop liver disease that can lead to permanent scarring of the liver. Between 15 and 25 percent of people with chronic hepatitis B eventually die of liver disease.

Although there are many ways of passing on HBV, the virus is not very easily transmitted by indirect contact because it is a bloodborne pathogen. There is no need to worry that such casual contact as shaking hands will expose one to hepatitis B, and there is no reason not to share a workplace or even a restroom with an infected person. On the other hand, hepatitis B virus is a durable virus that can survive outside the body for at least 7 days. During that time, the virus can still cause disease if it enters the body of a person who is not infected. For that reason it is necessary to clean any surface contaminated by blood spills (including those that have dried) carefully with a mixture of chlorine bleach and water. Medical or dental instruments must be sterilized with particular care.

People who have been infected by HBV and have recovered from the infection are protected against hepatitis B for the rest of their lives. People can also be protected by receiving a vaccine against the disease but must have a repeat **vaccination** every 5–10 years.

Risk factors

Risk factors for hepatitis B include:

- Having unprotected sex with a partner regardless of sexual orientation.
- Having a large number of sexual partners.
- Being infected with another sexually transmitted disease (STD), particularly gonorrhea or chlamydia.
- Sharing needles with other intravenous drug users.
- Having a family member with chronic HBV infection.
- Having had a blood transfusion or use of blood products before 1972.
- Needing hemodialysis for kidney disease.
- Frequent travels to parts of the world with high rates of hepatitis B. These include the Middle East, southern Africa, China, Southeast Asia, Brazil, and the Pacific Islands.
- Emigrating from or adopting a child from any of the countries listed above.
- Working in a hospital, clinic, or other facility requiring frequent exposure to blood, open wounds, or other body secretions. Health care workers at risk include dentists and dental hygienists as well as physicians, nurses, and laboratory technicians.
- Working as a police officer, firefighter, or other emergency first responder.
- Being a prison inmate.
- Living or working in a facility for the developmentally disabled.

Causes and symptoms

Causes

Hepatitis B is caused by a virus known as HBV. With the exception of HBV, all the common viruses that cause hepatitis are known as RNA viruses because they contain ribonucleic acid or RNA as their genetic material. HBV is the only deoxyribonucleic acid or DNA virus that is a major cause of hepatitis. HBV is made up of several fragments called antigens that stimulate the body's **immune system** to produce the antibodies that can neutralize or even destroy the infecting virus. It is in fact the immune reaction, not the virus, that seems to cause the liver inflammation associated with hepatitis B.

Hepatitis B is primarily a bloodborne infection but can also be transmitted through contact with the semen, vaginal secretions, or saliva of an infected person. The virus enters the body through injection, a break in the skin, or contact with the mucous membranes that line the mouth, genitals, and rectum. People cannot get hepatitis B from food or from shaking hands, sneezing or coughing, **breastfeeding**, or casual contact with an infected person.

Symptoms

ACUTE HEPATITIS B In the United States, a majority of acute HBV infections occur in teenagers and young adults. Half of these youth never develop symptoms, and only about 20%—or one in five infected patients—develop severe symptoms and yellowing of the skin (jaundice). Jaundice occurs when the infected liver is unable to get rid of certain colored substances, or pigments, as it normally does. The remaining 30% of patients have only "flu-like" symptoms and will probably not even be diagnosed as having hepatitis unless certain blood tests are performed.

The most commom symptoms of acute hepatitis B are loss of appetite, nausea, generally feeling poorly, and pain or tenderness in the right upper part of the abdomen (where the liver is located). Compared to patients with **hepatitis A** or C, those with HBV infection are less able to continue their usual activities and require more time resting in bed.

Occasionally patients with HBV infection will develop joint swelling and pain (arthritis) as well as **hives** or a skin rash before jaundice appears. The joint symptoms usually last no longer than three to seven days.

Typically the symptoms of acute hepatitis B do not persist longer than two or three months. If they continue for four months, the patient has an abnormally long-lasting acute infection. In a small number of patients—probably fewer than 3%—the infection keeps getting worse as the liver cells die off. Jaundice deepens, and patients may bleed easily when the levels of coagulation factors (normally made by the liver) decrease. Large amounts of fluid collect in the abdomen and beneath the skin (edema).

A few people (less than 1% of patients) develop a severe form of hepatitis B known as fulminant hepatitis. This form of the disease appears rapidly and can cause death if not treated at once. Its symptoms include:

- Sudden collapse.
- Mental confusion, hallucinations, or extreme sleepiness.
- Jaundice.
- Noticeable swelling of the abdomen.

CHRONIC HEPATITIS B HBV infection lasting longer than six months is said to be chronic. After this time it is much less likely that the infection will disappear. Most infants infected with HBV at **birth** and many children infected between 1 and 5 years of age become chronically infected. Not all carriers of the virus develop chronic liver disease; in fact, a majority of carriers have no symptoms. About one in every four HBV carriers, however, develops liver disease that gets worse over time as the liver becomes more and more scarred and less able to carry out its normal functions. The hepatitis B virus accounts for 5–10% of cases of chronic end-stage liver disease in the United States. A badly scarred liver is called cirrhosis. Patients are likely to have an enlarged liver and spleen, as well as tiny clusters of abnormal blood vessels in the skin that resemble spiders.

The most serious complication of chronic HBV infection is liver cancer. Worldwide this is the most common cancer to occur in men. Nevertheless, the overall chance that liver cancer will develop at any time in a patient's life is probably much lower than 10%. Patients with chronic hepatitis B who drink or smoke are more likely to develop liver cancer. It is not unusual for a person to simultaneously have both HBV infection and infection by HIV (human **immunodeficiency** virus, the cause of **AIDS**). One study reported that men infected with both HIV and HBV were more likely to die from liver disease than people infected with just one of the diseases.

KEY TERMS

Antibody—A substance formed in the body in response to a foreign body, such as a virus, which can then attack and destroy the invading virus.

Antigen—Part of an invading microorganism, such as a virus, that causes tissue damage (in hepatitis, to the liver), and that also stimulates the body's immune system to produce antibodies.

Carrier—A person who is infected with a virus or other disease organism but does not develop the symptoms of the disease.

Chronic—Long-term or recurrent.

Cirrhosis—Disruption of normal liver function by the formation of scar tissue and nodules in the liver.

Fulminant—Referring to a disease that comes on suddenly with great severity.

Hepatitis—A general term for inflammation of the liver. It can be caused by toxic substances or alcohol as well as infections.

Jaundice—A yellowish discoloration of the skin and whites of the eyes caused by increased levels of bile pigments from the liver in the patient's blood.

Pathogen—Any biological agent that causes illness or disease in its host. A pathogen may be a virus, bacterium, fungus, or prion.

Vaccine—A substance prepared from a weakened or killed virus which, when injected, helps the body to form antibodies that will attack an invading virus and may prevent infection altogether.

Diagnosis

Hepatitis B is diagnosed by one or more blood tests, since patients may not have any apparent symptoms. In a number of cases, the person is diagnosed following a routine blood test given as part of an annual health checkup. The most common clue is abnormal **liver function** results.

Examination

Many patients infected with hepatitis B will not have any visible symptoms during a routine office examination. In some cases, however, the doctor may observe swelling or tenderness in the right upper quadrant of the patient's abdomen; enlargement of the spleen; a low-grade **fever**; reddening of the palms of the hands; and signs of jaundice. If the disease has progressed to cirrhosis, the doctor may be able to detect the presence of fluid in the abdomen.

Tests

To confirm the diagnosis of hepatitis B, the doctor will take one or more blood samples for testing:

- A test of the patient's liver function, if this has not already been done.
- Tests for antibodies to the hepatitis B virus. A positive result means that the person has either been effectively vaccinated against HBV or has been infected at some point in the past and has recovered.
- Tests for the surface antigen of the hepatitis B virus (HBsAg). The surface antigen is the outer coating of the virus. A positive HBsAg test means that the patient is currently infected and can pass on the virus to others.
- Hepatitis B DNA test. This blood test measures the levels of virus in the patient's blood.

Procedures

Patients with chronic active hepatitis B may be given a computed tomography (CT) scan or ultrasound imaging of the liver to see whether the liver has been damaged by the infection. The doctor may also perform a liver biopsy. This test involves inserting a long hollow needle into the patient's liver through the abdomen and withdrawing a small amount of tissue for examination under a microscope.

Treatment

Traditional

There are few treatment options for chronic hepatitis B. If the patient has no symptoms and little sign of liver damage, the doctor may suggest monitoring the levels of HBV in the patient's blood periodically rather than starting drug treatment right away.

If the patient develops fulminant hepatitis B or their liver is otherwise severely damaged by HBV, the only option is a liver transplant. This is a serious operation with a lengthy recovery period; its success also depends on finding a suitable donor liver.

Drugs

Patients who know that they have been exposed to the hepatitis B virus can be treated by administering three shots of the HBV vaccine to prevent them from developing an active infection. Those who have already developed symptoms of the acute form of the disease may be given intravenous fluids to prevent **dehydration** or antinausea medications to stop vomiting. There is no medication as of late 2009 that can prevent acute hepatitis B from becoming chronic once the symptoms begin.

There are seven different drugs approved in the United States to treat chronic hepatitis B in adults as of 2009, but they do not work in all patients and may produce severe side effects. These drugs include adefovir dipivoxil (Hepsera), alpha interferon (Intron A), pegylated interferon (Pegasys), entecavir (Baraclude), telbivudine (Telzeka), tenofovir (Viread), and lamivudine (Zeffix or Epivir-HBV). The two interferons are given by injection; the other five drugs are taken by mouth in pill form once a day. Most doctors will wait until the patient's liver function begins to worsen before administering these drugs. The drugs do not cure the infection; what they do is lower the patient's risk of severe liver damage by slowing or preventing the hepatitis B virus from reproducing further.

The only drugs approved as of 2009 for treating chronic hepatitis B in children are alpha interferon (Intron A) and lamivudine (Zeffix or Epivir-HBV).

Alternative

There are no alternative or complementary therapies that are definitely known to be useful in treating or preventing hepatitis B. One herbal remedy, milk thistle (*Silybum marianum*), has been recommended by some alternative practitioners as beneficial to liver function and as a treatment for cirrhosis and viral hepatitis. The seeds of the plant are used to make capsules, extracts, and herbal teas to be taken by mouth.

Several studies have been done on the benefits of milk thistle; however, the studies are of uneven quality and the findings inconclusive as of 2009. The only major side effects of milk thistle are headaches and mild gastrointestinal upset (**diarrhea**, laxative effect, and nausea). While milk thistle is not known to be harmful, patients diagnosed with hepatitis B who wish to try this herb should consult their doctor first.

Prognosis

Each year an estimated 150,000 persons in the United States get hepatitis B. More than 10,000 will require hospital care, and as many as 5,000 will eventually die from complications of the infection. About 90% of all those infected will have acute disease only. It is the remaining 10% with chronic infection who account for most serious complications and deaths from HBV infection. Even when no symptoms of liver disease develop, chronic carriers remain a threat to others by serving as a source of infection.

Patients with acute hepatitis B usually recover; the symptoms go away in 2–3 weeks, and the liver itself returns to normal in about 4 months. Other patients have a longer period of illness with very slow improvement. The course of chronic HBV infection in any particular patient is unpredictable. Some patients who do well at first may later develop serious complications. Chronic hepatitis leads to an increased risk of cirrhosis and liver cancer, and eventual death in about 1 percent of cases.

Prevention

Hepatitis B can be prevented by vaccination with a vaccine called Engerix-B. An adult patient is given the first two doses of the vaccine a month apart and the third dose 6 months later. The vaccine is recommended for all persons under the age of 20; it can be given to newborns and infants as part of their regular vaccination series. Children usually receive the first vaccine between birth and two months of age, the second shot at one to four months, and the third at six to 18 months. The vaccine is generally required for all children born on or after January 1, 1992, before they enter school. The vaccine is available for older children who may have not been immunized before 1992 and is recommended to be given before age 11 or 12.

Others who should be vaccinated include health care workers, military personnel, firefighters and police, people who travel frequently to countries with high rates of hepatitis B, people with **hemophilia**, people who must be treated for kidney disease, people who inject illegal drugs, and men who have sex with men. A study published in 2009 reported that the immunity conferred by the vaccine lasts for at least 22 years.

Other preventive measures include:

- Practicing safe sex.
- Not sharing needles, razors, toothbrushes, or any other personal item that might have blood on it.
- Avoiding getting a tattoo or body piercing, as some people who perform these procedures do not sterilize their needles and other equipment properly.
- Getting tested for HBV infection if pregnant, as the virus can be transmitted from a mother to her unborn baby.
- Consulting a doctor before taking an extended trip to any country with high rates of hepatitis B.
- As noted above, carefully disinfecting any blood-stained surface or material with a mixture of chlorine bleach and water.

Resources

BOOKS

Feigin, Ralph D., et al, eds. *Feigin and Cherry's Textbook of Pediatric Infectious Diseases*, 6th ed. Philadelphia, PA: Saunders/Elsevier, 2009.

Freedman, Jeri. *Hepatitis B.* New York: Rosen Publishing, 2009.

Mathet, Veronica B. *Genetic Diversity and Variability of Hepatitis B virus (HBV).* New York: Nova Science Publishers, 2009.

Richman, Douglas D., Richard J. Whitley, and Frederick G. Hayden, eds. *Clinical Virology*, 3rd ed. Washington, DC: ASM Press, 2009.

Wilt, Timothy J., et al. *Management of Chronic Hepatitis B.* Rockville, MD: U.S. Department of Health and Human Services, Agency for Healthcare Research and Quality, 2008.

Younossi, Zobair M., ed. *Practical Management of Liver Diseases.* New York: Cambridge University Press, 2008.

PERIODICALS

Bertoletti, A., and A. Gehring. "Therapeutic Vaccination and Novel Strategies to Treat Chronic HBV Infection." *Expert Review of Gastroenterology and Hepatology* 3 (October 2009): 561–69.

Carey, I., and P.M. Harrison. "Monotherapy Versus Combination Therapy for the Treatment of Chronic Hepatitis B." *Expert Opinion on Investigational Drugs* 18 (November 2009): 1655–66.

Degertekin, B., and A.S. Lok. "Update on Viral Hepatitis: 2008." *Current Opinion in Gastroenterology* 25 (May 2009): 180–85.

Jones, J., et al. "Adefovir Dipivoxil and Pegylated Interferon-alpha for the Treatment of Chronic Hepatitis B: An Updated Systematic Review and Economic Evaluation." *Health Technology Assessment* 13 (July 2009): 1–172.

Kim, H.N., et al. "Hepatitis B Vaccination in HIV-infected Adults: Current evidence, Recommendations and Practical Considerations." *International Journal of STD and AIDS* 20 (September 2009): 595–600.

Lim, S.G., et al. "Prevention of Hepatocellular Carcinoma in Hepatitis B Virus Infection." *Journal of Gastroenterology and Hepatology* 24 (August 2009): 1352–57.

Lugoboni, F., et al. "Bloodborne Viral Hepatitis Infections among Drug Users: The Role of Vaccination." *International Journal of Environmental Research and Public Health* 6 (January 2009): 400–413.

McMahon, B.J., et al. "Antibody Levels and Protection after Hepatitis B Vaccine: Results of a 22-year Follow-up Study and Response to a Booster Dose." *Journal of Infectious Diseases* 200 (November 1, 2009): 1390–96.

Poynard, T., et al. "Impact of Interferon-alpha Treatment on Liver Fibrosis in Patients with Chronic Hepatitis B: An Overview of Published Trials." *Gastroentérologie clinique et biologique* 33 (October-November 2009): 916–22.

Wong, V.W., and H.L. Chan. "Severe Acute Exacerbation of Chronic Hepatitis B: A Unique Presentation of a Common Disease." *Journal of Gastroenterology and Hepatology* 24 (July 2009): 1179–86.

OTHER

American Liver Foundation. *Hepatitis B, http://www.liver-foundation.org/education/info/hepatitisb/*

Centers for Disease Control and Prevention (CDC). *Hepatitis B, http://www.cdc.gov/hepatitis/HepatitisB.htm*

Mayo Clinic. *Hepatitis B, http://www.mayoclinic.com/health/hepatitis-b/DS00398*

National Center for Complementary and Alternative Medicine (NCCAM). *Herbs at a Glance: Milk Thistle, http://nccam.nih.gov/health/milkthistle/ataglance.htm*

National Library of Medicine (NLM). *Hepatitis B* This is an online tutorial with voiceover; viewers have the option of a self-playing version, an interactive version with questions, or a text version, *http://www.nlm.nih.gov/medlineplus/tutorials/hepatitisb/htm/index.htm*

Pyrsopoulos, Nikolaos T., and K. Rajender Reddy. "Hepatitis B." *eMedicine*, June 19, 2009, *http://emedicine.medscape.com/article/177632-overview*

ORGANIZATIONS

American College of Gastroenterology (ACG), P.O. Box 342260, Bethesda MD, 20827-2260, 301-263-9000, http://www.acg.gi.org/.

American Liver Foundation (ALF), 75 Maiden Lane, Suite 603, New York NY, 10038, 212-668-1000, 212-483-8179, http://www.liverfoundation.org/.

Centers for Disease Control and Prevention (CDC), 1600 Clifton Road, Atlanta GA, 30333, 800-232-4636, cdcinfo@cdc.gov, http://www.cdc.gov.

Hepatitis B Foundation, 3805 Old Easton Road, Doylestown PA, 18902, 215-489-4900, 215-489-4313, info@hepb.org, http://www.hepb.org/.

National Institute of Allergy and Infectious Diseases (NIAID), 6610 Rockledge Drive, MSC 6612, Bethesda MD, 20892-6612, 301-496-5717, 866-284-4107, 301-402-3573, http://www3.niaid.nih.gov.

World Health Organization (WHO), Avenue Appia 20, 1211 Geneva 27 Switzerland, + 41 22 791 21 11, + 41 22 791 31 11, info@who.int, http://www.who.int/en/.

David A. Cramer, MD
Monique Laberge, PhD
Rebecca J. Frey, PhD

Hepatitis B vaccine

Definition

The **hepatitis B** vaccine (HBV or HepB) is an injection that protects individuals from contracting hepatitis B, a serious disease caused by the hepatitis B virus.

Purpose

The purpose of hepatitis B **vaccination** is to prevent hepatitis B infection. Hepatitis B infection can lead to both acute illness and serious, chronic, often fatal conditions such as liver **cancer** and cirrhosis.

Description

The hepatitis B vaccine consists of a small protein from the surface of the hepatitis B virus called the hepatitis B surface antigen (HBsAg). The vaccine cannot cause Hepatitis B infection. After vaccination with HBV, the person's **immune system** recognizes HBsAg as foreign and produces antibodies that attach to the protein (anti-HBs). These specific antibodies remain in the blood for many years, possibly for a lifetime. Later, if the individual becomes infected with the hepatitis B virus, the antibodies recognize the protein and stimulate the immune system to produce large quantities of specific antibodies that attach to and destroy the virus and prevent the disease.

Universal childhood vaccination has been practiced in the United States since 1991. HBV usually is the first vaccine a child receives, most often while still in the hospital within 24 hours after **birth**. The second and third HBV immunizations are administered by the age of 18 months in conjunction with other routine childhood vaccinations.

Vaccine formulations

The HBsAg in HBVs is referred to as recombinant because it is genetically engineered. The gene encoding the DNA for HBsAg is introduced into common baker's yeast. The yeast is grown in vats in which large amounts of HBsAg are produced. The yeast cells are broken, and the HBsAg is isolated and purified. It is adsorbed into aluminum hydroxide.

Two HBVs are approved for use in the United States. Recombivax HB, manufactured by Merck & Company, is as of 2010 available as a pediatric/adolescent formulation (orange cap) and as an adult formulation (green cap). Engerix-B, made by SmithKline Beecham Biologicals, is as of 2010 available as a pediatric formulation (blue cap) and as an adult formulation (orange cap). In general these HBVs are interchangeable and either or both can be used in an individual immunization series. An HBV derived from the blood serum of people with hepatitis B was as of 2004 no longer produced in the United States.

Packaged hepatitis B vaccine contains the following:

- up to 95% HBsAg, with 10 to 40 micrograms of HBsAg per milliliter of vaccine
- no more than 5% yeast protein
- a small amount of aluminum hydroxide (0.5 mg/mL)
- very small amounts of other additives to stabilize and preserve the vaccine

Hepatitis B in children

The U.S. Centers for Disease Control and Prevention (CDC) estimates that before the launch of the infant HBV immunization program, about 33,000 American children of non-infected mothers acquired hepatitis B by the age of ten. This number has substantially decreased. In 2007, 4,519 cases of acute Hepatitis B in the United States were reported, the lowest ever recorded. However, this number is thought to be about a ten-fold underestimate because many new cases do not cause symptoms and are not reported. With universal vaccination of newborns, the pattern of infection has shifted, and the highest rates are among adults, particularly males aged 25–44 years.

Hepatitis B is a potentially serious disease caused by the hepatitis B virus. It may result in inflammation and damage to the liver. Hepatitis B infection may be without symptoms or with acute or short-lived symptoms that can include:

- jaundice (a yellowing of the skin and whites of the eyes)
- joint pain
- stomach pain
- itchy red hives on the skin

The hepatitis B virus is eventually cleared from the bodies of most infected adolescents and adults. Only about 2–6% of infected older children and adults develop chronic hepatitis B and can continue to transmit the virus to other people. By contrast 90% of infants and 30% of young children infected with hepatitis B develop chronic disease: the younger the child, the more likely that a hepatitis B infection will become chronic. The consequences of chronic hepatitis B infection may include:

- chronic liver disease
- cirrhosis
- liver cancer
- liver failure

There is no cure for hepatitis B and approximately one-fourth of chronic hepatitis B victims die of cirrhosis or liver cancer, including children who do not survive to young adulthood. Of the approximately 1.25 million Americans with chronic hepatitis B, 20–30% were infected as infants or children.

Risk of childhood infection

Those with the highest risk for infection are older adolescents and adults engaging in high-risk behaviors such as drug use and unprotected sex with multiple partners. Health care workers are also at higher risk because of the increased chance of needle stick and contact with blood of infected patients.

Far less common sources of childhood hepatitis B infection include:

- breast milk from an infected mother
- contact with blood, saliva, tears, or urine from an infected household member
- cuts
- blood transfusions

However, the following children are at particular risk for hepatitis B infection:

- children of immigrants and refugees or children adopted from regions where hepatitis B is endemic, including Asia, Sub-Saharan Africa, the Amazon Basin, Eastern Europe, and the Middle East
- Alaskan natives and Pacific Islanders
- children living in households with a chronically hepatitis-B-infected person
- children living in institutions
- children receiving hemodialysis
- children receiving certain blood products

Children born to infected mothers

Children of hepatitis B-infected mothers are at a 10–85% risk of becoming infected during birth. The CDC estimates that in 2007 about 22,000 American infants were born to mothers infected with hepatitis B, making infant vaccination critical for these children. In addition, children of hepatitis B-infected mothers are at high risk of becoming infected before the age of five unless they are vaccinated early. Mothers who have emigrated from countries with high rates of endemic hepatitis B are more likely to be infected.

Children under the age of five who become infected with hepatitis B are at high risk for chronic infection and severe liver damage and disease later in life, even though initially they may have no symptoms. These infected children have a 90% risk of chronic hepatitis B infection and as many as 25% of them will die of chronic liver disease as adults.

Mothers with acute or chronic infectious hepatitis B can be identified by a blood test for HBsAg. Children born to mothers who have hepatitis B or whose hepatitis B status is unknown should receive their first HBV dose within 12 hours of birth. The second and third doses are given at two and six months of age. HBV can safely be given to pregnant and **breastfeeding** women. In many parts of the world, vaccine intervention before birth is required to prevent hepatitis B infection and its consequences in newborns.

It is recommended that newborns whose mothers are HBsAg-positive receive hepatitis B immune globulin (HBIG)—a preparation of serum containing high levels of antibodies to hepatitis B—as well as HBV within 12 hours of birth. About 70% of these newborns will be protected from chronic hepatitis B. A child's immune response to either hepatitis B infection or to HBV can be measured by a blood test for antibodies to HBsAg (anti-HBs). If a vaccinated child is exposed to hepatitis B, a measure of the anti-HBs in the blood will indicate whether another dose of HBV is required. Infants born to mothers who are HBsAg-positive should be tested for anti-HBs three to nine months following their last dose of vaccine. Their anti-HB levels should be at least 10 milli-international units per milliliter (mIU/mL), indicating that they are immune due to vaccination.

Recommended dosage

The immune response to HBV varies among individuals. Therefore, the HBV dose should be determined by a medical professional. In general, the following immunization schedule is recommended:

- Newborns: first dose injected into the anterolateral thigh muscle within 24 hours after birth and one month and six months after the first dose, for a total of three doses.
- Older child or adolescent: three-dose series for individuals not previously vaccinated. Otherwise, two doses of adult formulation HBV separated by at least four months.
- High-risk adults (e.g., health care workers, intravenous drug users, individuals with multiple sexual partners): in consultation with a physician and depending on previous immunization, a three-dose series.

Precautions

Individuals should not receive HBV if they are allergic to baker's yeast or to any other components in a combination vaccine or have had a previous allergic reaction to HBV.

HBV is highly effective in protecting against hepatitis B. HBV also protects against the related hepatitis D virus, which occurs as a co-infection with hepatitis B and usually results in more severe disease symptoms. However, the immune response to HBV varies among individuals, apparently due to genetic variations in the immune systems. In addition, the following medical conditions may cause individuals to benefit less from HBV:

- stomach pain
- cirrhosis (scarring) of the liver
- immune system impairment
- medical conditions requiring kidney dialysis

The duration of hepatitis B immunity following infant vaccination is not known As of 2008, immunity was found to last at least 20 years for individuals who

KEY TERMS

Antibody—A special protein made by the body's immune system as a defense against foreign material (bacteria, viruses, etc.) that enters the body. It is uniquely designed to attack and neutralize the specific antigen that triggered the immune response.

Antigen—A substance (usually a protein) identified as foreign by the body's immune system, triggering the release of antibodies as part of the body's immune response.

Booster immunization—An additional dose of a vaccine to maintain immunity to the disease.

Cirrhosis—A chronic degenerative disease of the liver, in which normal cells are replaced by fibrous tissue and normal liver function is disrupted. The most common symptoms are mild jaundice, fluid collection in the tissues, mental confusion, and vomiting of blood. Cirrhosis is associated with portal hypertension and is a major risk factor for the later development of liver cancer. If left untreated, cirrhosis leads to liver failure.

Hepatitis B immune globulin—HBIG, a blood serum preparation containing anti-hepatitis-B antibodies (anti-HBs) that is administered along with HBV to children born to hepatitis-B-infected mothers.

Immunity—Ability to resist the effects of agents, such as bacteria and viruses, that cause disease.

had received a complete series of injections beginning at birth. Duration studies are ongoing.

HBV is safe for pregnant and breastfeeding women. It may safely be given at the same time as other vaccines.

Side effects

Pediatric

Although most children experience no side effects from HBV, the most common side effects are as follows:

- fatigue or irritability in up to 20% of children
- soreness at the point of the injection, lasting one to two days, in about one out of eleven children and adolescents
- a mild to moderate fever in one out of 14 children and adolescents

Other less common side effects of HBV include:

- a purple spot, hard lump, redness, swelling, pain, or itching at the point of injection
- unusual tiredness or weakness
- dizziness
- fever of 100°F (37.7°C) or higher
- headache

Other rare reactions to HBV include:

- general feeling of discomfort or illness
- aches or pain in joints or muscles
- skin rash or welts that may occur days or weeks after receiving the vaccine
- blurred vision or other vision changes
- muscle weakness or numbness or tingling in the arms and legs
- back pain or stiffness or pain in the neck or shoulder
- chills
- diarrhea or stomach cramps
- nausea or vomiting
- increased sweating
- sore throat or runny nose
- itching
- decreased or lost appetite
- sudden redness of the skin
- swelling of glands in the armpit or neck
- difficulty sleeping

Although allergic reactions to HBV are rare, if they occur emergency medical help should be sought immediately. Symptoms of an allergic reaction include:

- reddening of the skin, especially around the ears
- swelling of the eyes, face, or inside of the nose
- hives
- itching, especially of the feet or hands
- sudden and severe tiredness or weakness
- difficulty breathing or swallowing

Parental concerns

Preparing a child for an injection

Most children are afraid of injections; however, there are simple methods for easing a child's **fear**. Prior to the vaccination parents should take the following steps:

- Tell children that they will be getting a shot and that it will feel like a prick; however, it will only sting for a few seconds.
- Explain to children that the shot will prevent them from becoming sick.
- Have older siblings comfort and reassure a younger child.
- Bring along the child's favorite toy or blanket.
- Never threaten children by telling them they will get a shot.
- Read the vaccination information statement and ask questions of the medical practitioner.

During the vaccination parents should take the following steps:

- Hold the child.
- Make eye contact with the child and smile.
- Talk softly and comfort the child.
- Distract the child by pointing out pictures or objects or using a hand puppet.
- Sing or tell the child a story.
- Have the child tell a story.
- Teach the child to focus on something other than the shot.
- Help the child take deep breaths.
- Allow the child to cry.
- Stay calm.

Comforting restraint

Parents may choose to use a comforting restraint method while their child is receiving an injection. These methods enable the parent to control and steady the child's arm while not holding the child down. With infants and toddlers, the following holds may be effective:

- The child is held on the parent's lap.
- The child's arm is behind the parent's back, held under the parent's arm.

- The parent's arm and hand control the child's other arm.
- The child's feet are held between the parent's thighs and steadied with the parent's other arm.

With older children, the following positions may be effective:

- The child is held on the parent's lap or stands in front of the seated parent.
- The parent's arms embrace the child.
- The child's legs are between the parent's legs.

After the injection

Following an injection parents should help in the following ways:

- Hold and caress a child or breastfeed an infant.
- Talk soothingly and reassuringly.
- Hug and praise the child for doing well.
- Review the information for possible side effects.
- Use a cool, wet cloth to reduce soreness or swelling at the injection site.
- Check the child for rashes over the following few days.
- In addition, parents should remember the following:
- The child may eat less during the first 24 hours following a vaccination.
- The child should drink plenty of fluids.
- The medical practitioner may suggest a non-aspirin pain reliever for the child.

Interactions

There are no known drug interactions.

Resources

BOOKS

Sears, Robert, MD. *The Vaccine Book: Making The Right Decision for Your Child.* New York: Little, Brown, 2007.

OTHER

Hepatitis B Information for Health Professionals. United States Centers for Disease Control and Prevention. March 12, 2009, http://www.cdc.gov/hepatitis/HBV/index.htm

Hepatitis B. World Health Organization. October 10, 2008, http://www.who.int/immunization/topics/hepatitis_b/en/index.html

Sharma, Poonam, et al. Hepatitis B. eMedicine.com. May 1, 2008, http://emedicine.medscape.com/article/964662-overview

Vaccines. United States Centers for Disease Control and Prevention (CDC). March 30, 2010, http://www.cdc.gov/vaccines

ORGANIZATIONS

American Academy of Family Physicians, P. O. Box 11210, Shawnee Mission KS, 66207, (913)906-6000, (800) 274-2237, (913) 906-6075, http://familydoctor.org.

American Academy of Pediatrics, 141 Northwest Point Boulevard, Elk Grove Village IL, 60007-1098, (847) 434-4000, (847) 434-8000, http://www.aap.org.

United States Centers for Disease Control and Prevention (CDC), 1600 Clifton Road, Atlanta GA, 30333, (404) 639-3534, 800-CDC-INFO (800-232-4636). TTY: (888) 232-6348, inquiry@cdc.gov, http://www.cdc.gov.

World Health Organization, Avenue Appia 20, 1211 Geneva 27 Switzerland, +22 41 791 21 11, +22 41 791 31 11, info@who.int, http://www.who.int.

Margaret Alic, PhD
Tish Davidson, AM

Hepatoblastoma

Definition

Hepatoblastoma is a rare type of liver **cancer** that affects infants and children.

Demographics

Incidence of hepatoblastoma is uncommon when compared to the incidence rates of other types of solid tumors which can affect infants and children. About 100 new cases are diagnosed annually in the United States. In the U.S., the incidence of hepatoblastoma is rising especially in premature infants who were born with low **birth** weights or with very low birth weights. Hepatoblastoma is the most commonly diagnosed histologic type of pediatric liver cancer accounting for approximately 70% of all primary liver cancers in children.

In Japan, **vaccination** has lead to a decrease in the incidence of hepatoblastoma. Rates of this type of childhood cancer are higher in developing nations and is thought to be a result of increased exposure to carcinogens.

This type of cancer is more likely to affect white children, although black children with hepatoblastoma often have poorer outcomes. Males are affected more often than female children. Hepatoblastomas are typically diagnosed prior to age three years. Children diagnosed with this type of liver cancer after age three usually have a worse prognosis. Although this type of cancer can be diagnosed in adolescents and in adults, incidence in these age groups is extremely rare.

Description

Hepatoblastomas originate from undifferentiated liver precursor cells. Most hepatoblastomas are encapsulated. Tumors are typically confined to one lobe of the liver, usually the right lobe. Hepatoblastomas have the capacity to spread beyond the liver. The most common sites for metastases are the lungs and the central nervous system.

Risk factors

Hepatoblastomas are associated with several types of familial or hereditary cancer syndromes and cancer predisposition syndromes including:

- Beckwith-Wiedemann syndrome
- Li-Fraumeni syndrome
- Simpson-Golabi-Behmel syndrome
- trisomy 18
- glycogen storage disorders
- neurofibromatosis type 1
- familial adenomatous polyposis (FAP) (estimates are that as many as 1 in every 20 cases of hepatoblastoma may be associated with this disorder)

Other risk factors associated with the development of hepatoblastoma include maternal use of **oral contraceptives**, **fetal alcohol syndrome**, and **prematurity** especially in premature infants born with low or very low birth rates. Individuals diagnosed with dysplastic kidney or Meckel diverticulum are at higher risk for the development of hepatoblastoma. Premature infants, especially those born at low or very low birth rates, who were given the drug erythropoietin in the neonatal intensive care unit may be at higher risk. Exposure to the carcinogen bromochloroacetic acid has been linked to the development of hepatoblastoma.

There are six subtypes or variants of hepatoblastoma. Identifying the subtype is critical to appropriate staging of the tumor and in determining optimal treatment strategies.

The six subtypes of hepatoblastoma are:

- epithelial type fetal pattern
- epithelial type embryonal and fetal pattern
- epithelial type macrotrabecular pattern
- epithelial type small cell undifferentiated pattern
- mixed epithelial and mesenchymal type with teratoid features
- mixed epithelial and mesenchymal type without teratoid features

KEY TERMS

Carcinogen—A cancer-causing agent.

Encapsulated—Enclosed, such as in a capsule.

Vascularity—Characterized by a large number of vessels such as blood vessels and/or lymph vessels.

Causes and symptoms

The cause of hepatoblastoma is unknown. Developing hepatoblastoma cells appear to look very much like cells of normally developing liver tissue. A disturbance involving liver cell development in the embryo may result in hepatoblastoma formation. An alteration in the signaling pathway is being investigated for its role in hepatoblastoma development.

Most children with hepatoblastoma have no symptoms at the time of diagnosis other than a painless abdominal mass. Therefore, disease may be advanced by the time a diagnosis is confirmed. As the disease progresses children may experience anorexia, pathologic **fractures**, severe **anemia** and rarely, rupture of the tumor with hemorrhage if the tumor is left untreated.

Children with a family history of a familial or hereditary cancer syndrome or cancer predisposition syndrome associated with the development of hepatoblastoma, such as FAP, should be screened regularly for rising alpha-feta protein (AFP) levels as AFP is considered a tumor marker for hepatoblastoma. The goal is to diagnose liver cancer prior to the onset of symptoms.

Diagnosis

Tests

Tests used to establish the diagnosis of hepatoblastoma include a complete blood count (CBC) with differential, liver enzyme studies, and measurement of alpha-protein (AFP).

Anemia and thrombocytosis may be present at the time of diagnosis. The AFP level is typically elevated in children with hepatoblastoma. AFP levels often drop once successful treatment is initiated. Therefore, AFP levels are monitored frequently during treatment to assess response to treatment and after completion of treatment to determine evidence of recurrence of disease.

Radiographic and imaging tests used in the diagnosis of hepatoblastoma include abdominal **x rays**, abdominal ultrasound, CT scans, **magnetic resonance imaging** (MRI), and positron emission (PET) scanning. An echocardiogram will be performed to determine baseline cardiac function prior to the start of anthracyline **chemotherapy**. Additional echocardiograms will be repeated periodically once chemotherapy has started to assess for toxicity to the heart.

Other tests which may be ordered in preparation for treatment with chemotherapy include tests to measure **kidney function** such as glomerular filtration rate and/or creatinine clearance. A baseline hearing test will also be ordered prior to the start of chemotherapy since some of the drugs used to treat hepatoblastoma may cause hearing loss.

Procedures

Prior to the start of therapy, a surgical diagnosis is confirmed. The goal of the surgery is complete removal or resection of the tumor when possible. Tumor removed during surgical resection is sent for pathologic evaluation. If the entire tumor cannot be removed during the resection, then an open biopsy is conducted. Needle biopsy of hepatoblastoma is contraindication due to the high vascularity of the tumor and of the liver.

Treatment

Chemotherapy is often very effective in treating hepatoblastoma. The chemotherapy drugs cisplatin, 5-fluorouracil (5FU), vincristine (VCR) doxorubicin have shown the most antitumor activity against hepatoblastoma. Other chemotherapy agents including carboplatin, paclitaxel and etoposide may be used to treat patients with advanced or metastatic disease.

The current standard chemotherapy treatment regimen is cisplatin/5-FU/VCR which may be started 2–4 weeks after surgery. Treatment generally consists of six cycles administered every 2–4 weeks. Testing of AFP levels is conducted at intervals to determine response to therapy.

Results of some international clinical trials have indicated that preoperative chemotherapy may significantly improve outcomes. Some clinicians are advocating that all patients diagnosed with hepatoblastoma receive preoperative chemotherapy.

Children diagnosed with hepatoblastoma that cannot be completely resected and those with metastatic disease should be referred for evaluation of a liver transplant in centers which specialize in these types of complex procedures.

Radiation therapy may be used to treat hepatoblastoma. However, radiation doses are limited by the amount of radiation exposure the liver can tolerate.

Prognosis

Prognosis after treatment for hepatoblastoma is dependent upon stage at diagnosis and favorable histology. Patients with favorable histology and whose tumors are able to be completely resected followed by chemotherapy have a survival rate of 100%.

Prevention

The cause of many cases of hepatoblastoma is unknown. Some cases of this type of rare tumor are more likely to occur in patients with a family history of some types of familial or hereditary cancer syndromes and some types of cancer predisposition syndromes. Patients with a family history of FAP, hemihypertrophy, or Beckwith-Wiedemann syndrome should participate in screening of AFP levels every 3 months until the child is at least 4 years old. Children diagnosed with hepatoblastoma should be evaluated for FAP as they may be at increased risk for the early development of colon polyps which are often the precursors of adenocarcinoma of the colon.

Resources

PERIODICALS

Ang, J.P., Heath, J.A., Donath, S., Khurana, & Auldist, A."Treatment Outcomes for Hepatoblastoma: An Institution's Experience over Two Decades."*Pediatr Surg Int.* (Feb 2007); 23(2): 103–9.

D'Antiga, L., Vallortigara, F., Cillo, U., et al."Features Predicting Unresectability in Hepatoblastoma."*Cancer.* (Sep 1, 2007); 110(5): 1050–8.

Horton, J.D., Lee, S., Brown, S.R., Bder, J., Meier, D. E."Survival Trends in Children with Hepatoblastoma." *Pediatr Surg Int.*(May 2009); 25(5): 407–12.

Perilongo, G., Maibach, R., Shafford, E., et al."Cisplatin versus Cisplatin Plus Doxorubicin for Standard-Risk Hepatoblastoma." *N Engl J Med.*(Oct 22, 2009); 361(17): 1662–70.

OTHER

"Childhood Liver Cancer Treatment (PDQ)." July 2, 2010 [cited August 21, 2010], http://www.cancer.gov/cancertopics/pdq/treatment/childliver/Patient

Willert, J.R., & Dahl, G."Hepatoblastoma."eMedicine. January 4, 2010 [cited August 21, 2010], http://www.emedicine.medscape.com

Melinda Granger Oberleitner,
RN, DNS, APRN, CNS

Hereditary fructose intolerance

Definition

Hereditary fructose intolerance is an inherited condition where the body does not produce the chemical needed to break down fructose (fruit sugar).

Description

Fructose is a sugar found naturally in fruits, vegetables, honey, and table sugar. Fructose intolerance is a disorder caused by the body's inability to produce an enzyme called aldolase B (also called fructose 1-phosphate aldolase) that is necessary for absorption of fructose. The undigested fructose collects in the liver and kidneys, eventually causing liver and kidney failure. One person in about 20,000 is born with this disorder. It is reported more frequently in the United States and Northern European countries than in other parts of the world. It occurs with equal frequency in males and females.

Causes and symptoms

Fructose intolerance is an inherited disorder passed on to children through their parents' genes. Both the mother and father have the gene that causes the condition, but may not have symptoms of fructose intolerance themselves. (This is called an autosomal recessive pattern of inheritance.) The disorder will not be apparent until the infant is fed formula, juice, fruits, or baby foods that contain fructose. Initial symptoms include **vomiting**, **dehydration**, and unexplained **fever**. Other symptoms include extreme thirst and excessive urination and sweating. There will also be a loss of appetite and a failure to grow. Tremors and seizures caused by low blood sugar can occur. The liver becomes swollen and the patient becomes jaundiced with yellowing of the eyes and skin. Left untreated, this condition can lead to coma and **death**.

Diagnosis

Urine tests can be used to detect fructose sugar in the urine. Blood tests can also be used to detect *hyperbilirubinemia* and high levels of liver enzymes in the blood. A liver biopsy may be performed to test for levels of enzymes present and to evaluate the extent of damage to the liver. A fructose-loading test where a dose of fructose is given to the patient in a well-controlled hospital or clinical setting may also be used to confirm fructose intolerance. Both the biopsy and the loading test can be very risky, particularly in infants that are already sick.

KEY TERMS

Aldolase B—Also called fructose 1-phosphate aldolase, this chemical is produced in the liver, kidneys, and brain. It is needed for the breakdown of fructose, a sugar found in fruits, vegetables, honey, and other sweeteners.

Hyperbilirubinemia—A condition where there is a high level of bilirubin in the blood. Bilirubin is a natural by-product of the breakdown of red blood cells, however, a high level of bilirubin may indicate a problem with the liver.

Liver biopsy—A surgical procedure where a small piece of the liver is cut out for examination. A needle or narrow tube may be inserted either directly through the skin and muscle or through a small incision and passed into the liver for collection of a sample of liver tissue.

Treatment

Once diagnosed, fructose intolerance can be successfully treated by eliminating fructose from the diet. Patients usually respond within three to four weeks and can make a complete recovery if fructose-containing foods are avoided. Early recognition and treatment of the disease is important to avoid damage to the liver, kidneys, and small intestine.

Prognosis

If the condition is not recognized and the diet is not well controlled, death can occur in infants or young children. With a well-controlled diet, the child can develop normally.

Prevention

Carriers of the gene for hereditary fructose intolerance can be identified through DNA analysis. Anyone who is known to carry the disease or who has the disease in his or her **family** can benefit from genetic counseling. Since this is a hereditary disorder, there is currently no known way to prevent it other than assisting at-risk individuals with family planning and reproductive decisions.

Resources

OTHER

"What Is Hereditary Fructose Intolerance?" Hereditary Fructose Intolerance & Aldolase Homepage, http://www.bu.edu/aldolase

ORGANIZATIONS

National Institute of Diabetes, Digestive and Kidney Diseases (NIDDK), 31 Center Drive, MSC 2560, Bldg 31, Rm 9A06, Bethesda MD, 20892-2560, (301) 496-3583, http://www2.niddk.nih.gov/.

Altha Roberts Edgren

KEY TERMS

Autosomal dominant—A pattern of inheritance in which the dominant gene on any non-sex chromosome carries the defect.

Chromosome—A threadlike structure in the cell which transmits genetic information.

Hereditary hemorrhagic telangiectasia

Definition

Hereditary hemorrhagic telangiectasia is an inherited condition characterized by abnormal blood vessels which are delicate and prone to bleeding. Hereditary hemorrhagic telangiectasia is also known as Rendu-Osler-Weber disease.

Description

The term telangiectasia refers to a spot formed, usually on the skin, by a dilated capillary or terminal artery. In hereditary hemorrhagic telangiectasia these spots occur because the blood vessel is fragile and bleeds easily. The bleeding may appear as small, red or reddish-violet spots on the face, lips, inside the mouth and nose or the tips of the fingers and toes. Other small telangiectasias may occur in the digestive tract.

Unlike **hemophilia**, where bleeding is caused by an ineffective clotting mechanism in the blood, bleeding in hereditary hemorrhagic telangiectasia is caused by fragile blood vessels. However, like hemophilia, bleeding may be extensive and can occur without warning.

Causes and symptoms

Hereditary hemorrhagic telangiectasia, an autosomal dominant inherited disorder, occurs in one in 50,000 people.

Recurrent nosebleeds are a nearly universal symptom in this condition. Usually the nosebleeds begin in childhood and become worse with age. The skin changes begin at **puberty**, and the condition becomes progressively worse until about 40 years of age, when it stabilizes.

Diagnosis

The physician will look for red spots on all areas of the skin, but especially on the upper half of the body, and in the mouth and nose and under the tongue.

Treatment

There is no specific treatment for hereditary hemorrhagic telangiectasia. The bleeding resulting from the condition can be stopped by applying compresses or direct pressure to the area. If necessary, a laser can be used to destroy the vessel. In severe cases, the leaking artery can be plugged or covered with a graft from normal tissue.

Prognosis

In most people, recurrent bleeding results in an iron deficiency. It is usually necessary to take iron supplements.

Prevention

Hereditary hemorrhagic telangiectasia is an inherited disorder and cannot be prevented.

ORGANIZATIONS

American Medical Association, 515 N. State St., Chicago IL, 60612, (312) 464-5000, http://www.ama-assn.org.

Association of Birth Defect Children, 3526 Emerywood Lane, Orlando FL, 32806, (305) 859-2821

Dorothy Elinor Stonely

Hermaphroditism

Definition

Hermaphroditism is a rare condition in which ovarian and testicular tissue exist in the same person. The testicular tissue contains seminiferous tubules or spermatozoa. The ovarian tissue contains follicles or corpora albicantia. The condition is the result of a chromosome anomaly.

Description

Among human beings, hermaphroditism is an extremely rare anomaly in which gonads for both sexes are present. External genitalia may show traits of both sexes, and in which the chromosomes show male-female mosaicism (where one individual possesses both the male XY and female XX chromosome pairs). There are two different variants of hermaphroditism: true hermaphroditism and pseudohermaphroditism. There are female and male pseudohermaphrodites. True hermaphroditism refers to the presence of both testicular and ovarian tissue in the same individual. The external genitalia in these individuals may range from normal male to normal female. However, most phenotypic males have **hypospadias**. Pseudohermaphroditism refers to gonadal dysgenesis.

Genetic profile

The most common karyotype for a true hermaphrodite is 46XX. DNA from the Y chromosome is translocated to one of the X-chromosomes. The karyotype for male pseudohermaphrodites is 46XY. Female pseudohermaphroditism is more complicated. The condition is caused by deficiencies in the activity of enzymes. The genetic basis for three enzyme deficiencies have been identified. Deficiency of 3B hydroxysteroid dehydrogenase - Type 2 is due to an abnormality on chromosome 1p13.1. Deficiency of 21-Hydroxylase is due to an abnormality on chromosome 6p21.3. Deficiency of 11B-Hydroxylase - Type 1 is due to an abnormality on chromosome 8q21.

Demographics

True hermaphrodites are extremely rare. Approximately 500 individuals have been identified in the world to date. Because of the ambiguity of genitalia and difficulties in making an accurate diagnosis, the incidence of pseudohermaphroditism is not well established. The incidence of male pseudohermaphroditism has been estimated at between 3 and 15 per 100,000 people. The incidence of female pseudohermaphroditism has been estimated at between one and eight per 100,000 people.

Signs and symptoms

True hermaphroditism is characterized by ambiguous internal and external genitalia. On internal examination (most often using laparoscopy), there is microscopic evidence of both ovaries and testes. Male pseudohermaphroditism is also characterized by ambiguous internal and external genitalia. However, gonads are often (but not always) recognizable as testes. These are frequently softer than normal. An affected person is often incompletely masculinized. Female pseudohermaphroditism is characterized by female internal genitals. External genitals tend to appear as masculine. This is most commonly characterized by clitoral hypertrophy. Most hermaphrodites are infertile although a small number of pregnancies have been reported.

Diagnosis

True hermaphroditism is often diagnosed after laparoscopic investigation. An initial suspicion of male pseudohermaphroditism is often made by inspection of external genitals. This is confirmed by chromosomal analysis and assays of hormones such as testosterone. Initial suspicion of female pseudohermaphroditism is also made by inspection of external genitals. This is confirmed by analysis of chromosomes and hormonal assay. Laparoscopic examination usually reveals nearly normal female internal genitals.

Treatment and management

Early assignment of gender is important for the emotional well being of any person with ambiguous genitalia. A decision to select a gender of rearing is based on the corrective potential of the ambiguous genitalia, rather than using chromosome analysis. Once the decision is made regarding gender, there should be no question in the family's mind regarding the gender of the child from that point on.

Corrective surgery is used to reconstruct the external genitalia. In general, it is easier to reconstruct female genitalia than male genitalia, and the ease of reconstruction will play a role in selecting the gender of rearing. Treating professionals must be alert for stress in persons with any form of hermaphroditism and their families.

Prognosis

With appropriate corrective surgery, the appearance of external genitalia may appear normal. However, other problems such as virilization may appear later in life. As of 2010, there is some interest among persons with ambiguous genitalia at **birth** to reverse their gender of rearing.

Resources

BOOKS

Rappaport, Robert. "Female Pseudohermaphroditism." *Nelson Textbook of Pediatrics.* Edited by Richard E. Behrman et al. 16th ed. Philadelphia, W.B. Saunders, 2000, p. 1760.

Rappaport, Robert. "Male Pseudohermaphroditism." *Nelson Textbook of Pediatrics.* Edited by Richard E. Behrman et al. 16th ed. Philadelphia, W.B. Saunders, 2000, pp. 1761-1764.

Rappaport, Robert. "True Hermaphroditism." *Nelson Textbook of Pediatrics.* Edited by Richard E. Behrman et al. 16th ed. Philadelphia, W.B. Saunders, 2000, pp. 1765-1766.

KEY TERMS

Corpora albicantia—Plural of corpus albicans. A corpus albicans is the scar tissue that remains on an ovarian follicle after ovulation.

Dysgenesis—Defective or abnormal formation of an organ or part usually occurring during embryonic development.

Follicle—A pouch-like depression.

Mosaicism—A genetic condition resulting from a mutation, crossing over, or nondisjunction of chromosomes during cell division, causing a variation in the number of chromosomes in the cells.

Semineferous tubules—Long, threadlike tubes that are packed in areolar tissue in the lobes of the testes.

Spermatozoa—Mature male germ cells that develop in the seminiferous tubules of the testes.

Wilson, Jean D., and James E. Griffin. "Disorders of Sexual Differentiation." *Harrison's Principles of Internal Medicine.* Edited by Anthony S. Fauci, et al. 14th ed. New York: McGraw-Hill, 1998, pp. 2119-2131.

PERIODICALS

Denes F. T., B. B. Mendonca, and S. Arap. "Laparoscopic Management of Intersexual States." *Urology Clinics of North America* 28, no. 1 (2001): 31-42.

Krstic Z. D., et al. "True Hermaphroditism: 10 Years' Experience." *Pediatric Surgery International* 16, no. 8 (2000): 580-583.

Wiersma, R. "Management of the African Child With True Hermaphroditism." *Journal of Pediatric Surgery* 36, no. 2 (2001): 397-399.

Zucker, K. J. "Intersexuality and Gender Identity Differentiation." *Annual Review of Sexual Research* 10 (1999): 1-69.

ORGANIZATIONS

Genetic Alliance, 4301 Connecticut Ave. NW, #404, Washington DC, 20008-2304, (202 966-5557, (888) 394-3937 (800) 336-GENE, info@geneticalliance.org, http://www.geneticalliance.org.

Hermaphrodite Education and Listening Post, PO Box 26292, Jacksonville NY, 32226.help@jaxnet.com, http://users.fdn.com/~help/hermaph.html.

Intersex Society of North America, PO Box 301, Petaluma CA, 94953-0301, http://www.isna.org.

March of Dimes Birth Defects Foundation, 1275 Mamaroneck Ave., White Plains NY, 10605, (888) 663-4637, resourcecenter@modimes.org, http://www.modimes.org.

L. Fleming Fallon, Jr., MD, DrPH

Hernia

Definition

Hernia is a general term used to describe a bulge or protrusion of an organ through the structure or muscle that normally contains it.

Demographics

The frequency of hernias varies greatly depending on the type of hernia. Hernias tend to be more common in the elderly than in younger individuals. Hernias also are more common in infants and children, often caused by the abdominal wall not closing completely after **birth**.

Hiatal hernias are very common, although most do not produce serious symptoms and many individuals never even know they have one. About 10% of individuals under the age of 40 have hiatal hernias. This number increases with age, with about 70% of individuals over age 70 having this type of hernia.

Abdominal hernias are more common in males than in females. About 25% of men have an inguinal hernia at some time in their lives, and only about 2% of women ever have one. Over 1 million surgeries are performed each year to repair abdominal hernias.

Description

There are many different types of hernias. The most familiar type is that which occur in the abdomen when part of the intestine protrudes through the abdominal wall. This may occur in different areas and, depending on the location, the hernia is given a different name.

An inguinal hernia appears as a bulge in the groin and may come and go depending on the position of the person or their level of physical activity. It can occur with or without **pain**. In men, the protrusion may descend into the scrotum. Inguinal hernias account for 80% of all hernias and are more common in men.

Femoral hernias are similar to inguinal hernias but appear as a bulge slightly lower. They are more common in women and are often caused by the strain that pregnancy puts on the abdominal area.

A ventral hernia is also called an incision hernia because it generally occurs as a bulge in the abdomen at the site of an old surgical scar. It is caused by thinning or stretching of scar tissue. It occurs more frequently in people who are obese or pregnant.

An umbilical hernia appears as a soft bulge at the navel (umbilicus). It is caused by a weakening of the area or an imperfect closure of the area in infants. This type of

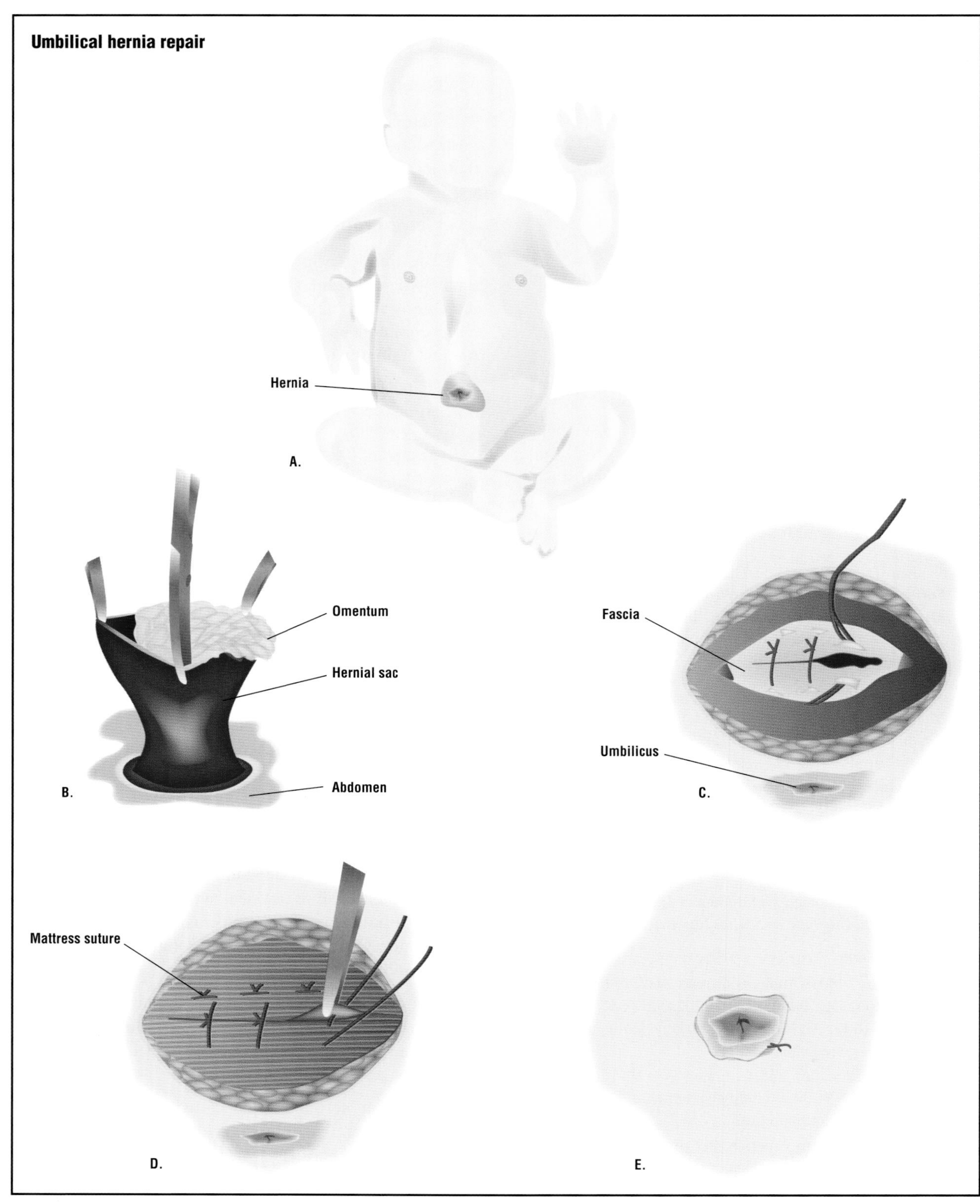

Baby with an umbilical hernia (A). To repair, the hernia is cut open (B), and the contents replaced in the abdomen. Connecting tissues, or fascia, are sutured closed (C), and the skin is repaired (D). *(Illustration by PreMediaGlobal. Reproduced by permission of Gale, a part of Cengage Learning.)*

hernia is more common in women due to pregnancy, and in Chinese and African American infants. Some umbilical hernias in infants disappear without treatment within the first year.

A hiatal or diaphragmatic hernia is different from abdominal hernias in that it is not visible on the outside of the body. With a hiatal hernia, the stomach bulges upward through the muscle that separates the chest from the abdomen (the diaphragm). This type of hernia occurs more often in women than in men, and it is treated differently from other types of hernias.

Causes and symptoms

Most hernias result from a weakness in the abdominal wall. In many cases an infant is born with this weakness(congenital), and in other cases weakness can develop later in life. Any increase in pressure in the abdomen, such as recurring coughing, straining, heavy lifting, or pregnancy, can be a considered a causative factor in developing an abdominal hernia. Obesity or recent excessive weight loss, as well as aging and previous surgery, are also risk factors.

Most abdominal hernias appear suddenly when the abdominal muscles are strained. The individual may feel tenderness, a slight burning sensation, or a feeling of heaviness in the bulge. It may be possible for the individual to push the hernia back into place with gentle pressure, or the hernia may disappear by itself when the person reclines. Being able to push the hernia back is called reducing it. On the other hand, some hernias cannot be pushed back into place, and are termed incarcerated or irreducible.

A hiatal hernia may also be caused by obesity, pregnancy, aging, or previous surgery. About 50% of all people with hiatal hernias do not have any symptoms. If symptoms exist they usually include heartburn, usually 30–60 minutes following a meal. There may be some mid chest pain due to gastric acid from the stomach being pushed up into the esophagus (gastric reflux). The pain and heartburn usually are worse when lying down. Frequent belching and feelings of abdominal fullness may also be present.

Diagnosis

Generally, abdominal hernias need to be seen and felt to be diagnosed. Usually the hernia will increase in size with an increase in abdominal pressure, so the doctor may ask the person to **cough** while he or she feels the area. Once a diagnosis of an abdominal hernia is made, the doctor usually will refer the individual to a surgeon for a consultation. Surgery provides the only cure for a hernia through the abdominal wall.

With a hiatal hernia, the preliminary diagnosis is based on the symptoms reported by the person. The doctor may then order tests to confirm the diagnosis. One possible test is called a barium swallow test. During this procedure, the individual drinks a chalky white barium solution and then undergoes an abdominal x ray. The barium causes any protrusion through the diaphragm show up more clearly on the x ray. Hiatal hernias often are diagnosed using endoscopy. This procedure is done by a gastroenterologist (a specialist in digestive diseases). During an endoscopy the person is given an intravenous sedative and a small tube is inserted through the mouth, then into the esophagus and stomach where the doctor can look at the hernia using a small tube or camera. The procedure takes about 30 minutes and usually causes no discomfort. It is done on an outpatient basis.

Treatment

Once an abdominal hernia occurs it tends to increase in size. Some patients with abdominal hernias take a watch and wait approach before deciding on surgery. In these cases, they must avoid strenuous physical activity such as heavy lifting or straining with **constipation**. They may also wear a truss, which is a support worn like a belt to keep a small hernia from protruding. People can

KEY TERMS

Endoscopy—A diagnostic procedure in which a tube is inserted through the mouth, into the esophagus and stomach. It is used to visualize various digestive disorders, including hiatal hernias.

Herniorrhaphy—Surgical repair of a hernia.

Incarcerated hernia—A hernia that cannot be reduced, or pushed back into place inside the abdominal wall.

Reducible hernia—A hernia that can be gently pushed back into place or that disappears when the person lies down.

Laparoscopic surgery—A minimally invasive surgery in which a camera and surgical instruments are inserted through a small incision.

Strangulated hernia—A hernia that is so tightly incarcerated outside the abdominal wall that the intestine is blocked and the blood supply to that part of the intestine is cut off.

tell if their hernia is getting worse if they develop severe constant pain, nausea and **vomiting**, or if the bulge does not return to normal when lying down or when they try to gently push it back in place. In these cases they, should consult their doctor immediately. In most cases, surgery is eventually required to correct the hernia.

Surgery

There are risks to not surgically repairing a hernia. Left untreated, a hernia may become incarcerated, which means it can no longer be reduced or pushed back into place. With an incarcerated hernia, the intestine become trapped, or strangulated, outside the abdomen. This can lead to a blockage in the intestine. If strangulation is severe, it may cut off the blood supply to the intestine and part of the intestine will die. Because of the risk of tissue death (necrosis) and gangrene, and because the hernia can block food from moving through the bowel, a strangulated hernia is a medical emergency requiring immediate surgery. Repairing a hernia before it becomes incarcerated or strangulated is much safer than waiting until complications develop.

Surgical repair of a hernia is called a herniorrhaphy. The surgeon will push the bulging part of the intestine back into place and sew the overlying muscle back together. When the muscle is not strong enough, the surgeon may reinforce it with a synthetic mesh.

Surgery can be done on an outpatient basis. It usually takes 30 minutes in children and 60 minutes in adults. It can be done under either local or general anesthesia and is frequently done laparoscopically. In this type of surgery, a tube that allows visualization of the abdominal cavity is inserted through a small puncture wound. Several small punctures are made to allow surgical instruments to be inserted. This type of surgery avoids a larger incision and significantly reduces the time required for recovery.

Hiatal hernias normally are treated without surgery. The focus of the treatment is to reduce the symptoms associated with **gastroesophageal reflux disease** (GERD) associated with the hernia. Treatments include:

- avoiding reclining after meals
- avoiding spicy foods, acidic foods, alcohol, and tobacco
- eating small, frequent, bland meals
- eating a high-fiber diet.

Several types of medications can help manage the symptoms of gastric reflux and heartburn a hiatal hernia. Antacids are used to neutralize gastric acid and decrease heartburn. Drugs that reduce the amount of acid produced in the stomach (H2 blockers) are also used. This class of drugs includes famotidine (Pepcid), cimetidine (Tagamet), and ranitidine (Zantac). Omeprazole (Prilosec) is a proton pump inhibitor (PPI) drug, which is another class of drugs that suppress gastric acid secretion and are used for symptoms associated with hiatal hernias. Another option may be metoclopramide (Reglan), a drug that increases the tone of the muscle around the esophagus and causes the stomach to empty more quickly. This drug, however, can have serious side effects.

Alternative treatment

Visceral manipulation, done by a trained therapist, can help replace the stomach to its proper positioning. An alternative to H2 blocker and PPI drugs is deglycyrrhizinated licorice (DGL). This helps balance stomach acid by improving the protective substances that line the stomach and intestines and by improving blood supply to these tissues. DGL does not interrupt the normal function of stomach acid.

As with traditional therapy, dietary modifications are important. Small, frequent meals will keep pressure down on the esophageal sphincter. Also, raising the head of the bed several inches with blocks or books can help with both the quality and quantity of **sleep**.

Prognosis

Abdominal hernias generally do not recur in children but can recur in up to 10% of adult patients. Surgery is considered the only cure, and the prognosis is excellent if the hernia is corrected before it becomes strangulated.

Hiatal hernias are treated successfully with medication and diet modifications 85% of the time.

Prevention

Some hernias can be prevented by maintaining a reasonable weight, not **smoking**, avoiding heavy lifting, preventing constipation, and following a moderate **exercise** program to maintain good abdominal muscle tone.

Resources

PERIODICALS

Goran, Augustin, et al. "Abdominal Hernias in Pregnancy." *Journal of Obstetrics and Gynecology Research* (April 2009) 35(2): 203–211.

Kingsnorth, Andrew N. "Hernia Surgery: From Guidelines to Clinical Practice." *Annals of the Royal College of Surgeons of England* (May 2009) 91(4): 273–279.

OTHER

Hernia Resource Center. All About Hernias. 2007, http://www.herniainfo.com/content/about.aspx

Medline Plus. Hernia. February 8, 2010, http://www.nlm.nih.gov/medlineplus/hernia.html

ORGANIZATIONS

The British Hernia Centre, 87 Watford Way, London England United Kingdom, NW4 4RS, + 44-20 8201 7000, +44 20 8202 6714, experts@hernia.org, http://www.hernia.org/.

Joyce S. Siok, RN
Tish Davidson, AM

Herpes simplex

Definition

Herpes simplex is a virus that causes blister-like open sores, usually on the mouth or genitals of the infected person.

Demographics

There are two distinct types: herpes simplex virus type 1 (HSV-1) and herpes simplex virus type 2 (HSV-2). Both types of HSV are common worldwide. HSV-1 is transmitted from person to person by close contact, such as kissing. In the United States, by age 30, half of all individuals of high socioeconomic status are infected with HSV-1, and 80% of all individuals of low socioeconomic status carry the virus, although many of those infected do not show symptoms.

HSV-2 is transmitted through sexual contact, thus its distribution is related to the age at which sexual activity begins and the extent of sexual activity within a population. Infection is more common in women than men, and in the United States infection is more common among blacks than whites. As many as 90% of people infected with HSV-2 are unaware that they carry the virus because they have either no symptoms or very mild symptoms. The number of people infected with HSV-2 has been increasing worldwide since the mid-1990s.

Description

HSV-1 usually is associated with infections of the lips, mouth, and face. HSV-1 sores are referred to as oral herpes, **cold sores**, or **fever** blisters. HSV-2, or **genital herpes**, is a sexually transmitted disease (STD) and usually is associated with genital ulcers or sores. The first symptoms often occur within 2–20 days after contact with an infected person, although individuals may be infected with HSV-1 and/or HSV-2 and not develop any symptoms or the development of symptoms may be delayed.

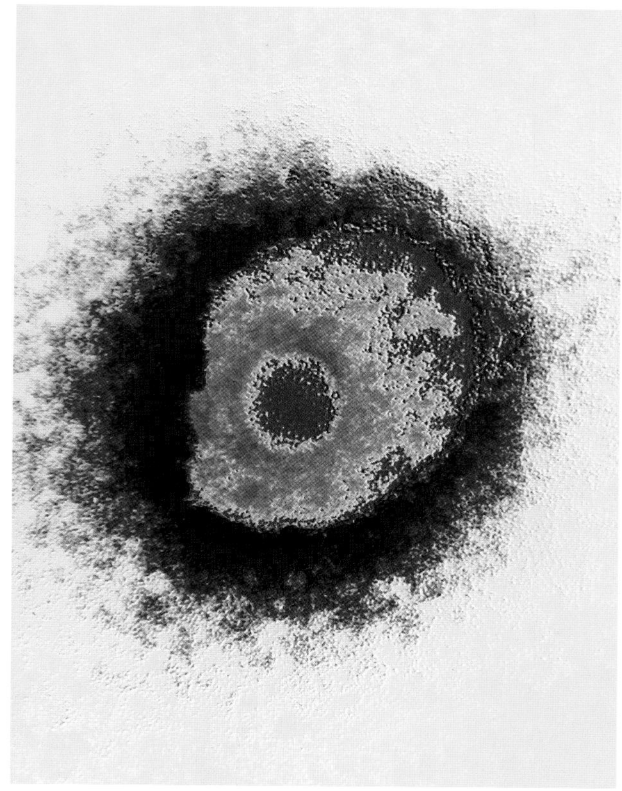

A false-color transmission electron microscopy (TEM) image of a herpes simplex virus. *(Custom Medical Stock Photo, Inc. Reproduced by permission.)*

Risk factors

Risk factors for HSV-2 infection include having many sexual partners and having unprotected sex. HSV-2 can also be transmitted by oral sex and cause sores on the lips. **Cancer** patients, especially those who are undergoing **chemotherapy** or radiation treatments, are at greater risk of primary (first) and secondary (recurrent) herpes infections, as are individuals with HIV/AIDS or other conditions in which the **immune system** is weakened.

Causes and symptoms

HSV virus causes sores on mucous membranes, most often in the mouth and in the genital region. Once HSV enters the body it spreads to nearby mucosal areas through nerve cells. Typically, 50–80% of people with oral herpes experience a prodrome (symptoms of oncoming disease) of **pain**, burning, **itching**, or **tingling** at the site where blisters will form. This prodrome stage may last anywhere from a few hours to one to two days. The herpes infection prodrome occurs in both the primary infection and recurrent infections.

Symptoms of the primary infection usually are more severe than those of recurrent infections. The primary infection can cause symptoms similar to those experienced in other viral infections, including lack of energy, **headache**, fever, and swollen lymph nodes in the neck. The first sign of infection is formation of fluid-filled blisters that may last up to two weeks. However, the pain in the area may last much longer.

Once an individual becomes infected with HSV, the virus remains in the body for the life of that individual. During periods of latency there are no symptoms. At times the infected person may shed the virus, even in the absence of visible symptoms, and infect others. Individuals infected with the virus can have recurrent infections or flare-ups; however, recurrent infections usually have milder and shorter symptoms. Nevertheless, cancer patients and others with compromised immune systems can have severe recurrences and serious complications.

Women who develop their first (primary) HSV-2 infection during pregnancy are at greater risk of delivering babies with **birth defects**. An active genital herpes sore at the time of **birth** can cause extremely serious results, including blindness, birth defects, and even **death**. **Cesarean section** may be advisable for mothers with active herpes sores at the time of delivery.

Diagnosis

Often, herpes infection is diagnosed from symptoms and by visually examining the sores.

Tests

Testing for neonatal herpes infections may include special smears and/or viral cultures, blood antibody levels, and polymerase chain reaction (PCR) testing of spinal fluid. Cultures are usually obtained from skin vesicles, eyes, mouth, rectum, urine, stool, and blood. For older children and adults, if there is a question as to the cause of a sore, a tissue sample or culture can be taken to determine what type of virus or other microorganism is responsible. For herpes, it is preferable to have this test done within the first 48 hours after symptoms first show up for a more accurate result.

Treatment

Drugs

There is no cure for HSV infection, although **antiviral drugs** have some effect in lessening the symptoms, decreasing the length of herpes outbreaks, and preventing complications in immunocompromised individuals. There is evidence that some of these drugs also may prevent future outbreaks. For the best results drug treatment should begin during the prodrome stage before blisters are visible. Depending upon the length of the outbreak, drug treatment could continue up to 10 days.

Acyclovir (Zovirax) is often the drug of choice for herpes infection and can be given intravenously or taken by mouth. It can be applied directly to sores as an ointment but is not very useful in this form. A liquid form for children is also available. Acyclovir is effective in treating both the primary infection and recurrent outbreaks. When taken by mouth to prevent an outbreak, acyclovir reduces the frequency of herpes outbreaks. Other antiviral drugs used to treat HSV infection include penciclovir (Denavir), valacyclovir (Valtrex), and famciclovir (Famvir).

Alternative and complementary therapies

A number of steps may relieve the symptoms of herpes infections. It is important to keep the blisters or sores clean and dry with an agent such as cornstarch. One should avoid touching the sores, and wash hands frequently. Local application of ice may relieve the pain. Over-the-counter medication for fever, pain, and inflammation, such as aspirin, **acetaminophen**, or ibuprofen, may help. Children should never be given aspirin because of the possible development of **Reye's syndrome**.

Sexual intercourse should be avoided during both the active stage and the prodrome stages. During an outbreak of cold sores salty foods, citrus foods (oranges etc.), and other foods that irritate the sores should be avoided. Over-the-counter lip products that contain the chemical "phenol" (such as Blistex Medicated Lip Ointment) and numbing ointments (such as Anbesol) help to relieve the pain of cold sores. A bandage may be placed over the sores to protect them and prevent spreading the virus to other sites on the lips or face.

A diet rich in the amino acid lysine may help prevent recurrences of cold sores. Foods that contain high levels of lysine include most vegetables, legumes, fish, turkey, and chicken. Oral lysine supplements in the amount of 1000 mg per day may help sores heal faster. There is a belief that foods with high lysine-to-arginine ratio will help prevent outbreaks of herpes simplex. That has not

KEY TERMS

Reye's syndrome—A rare but often fatal disease that involves the brain, liver, and kidneys. It may broungt on by giving salicylates to children (but not adults) who have a viral infection.

been proven, and it is important to include foods that have a low lysine-to-arginine ratio also, such as nuts, onion, garlic, and green vegetables. It is also suggested that the amount of arginine in the diet be limited as there is a belief that arginine is needed for herpes virus growth. This amino acid is found in peanuts, beer, chocolate, gelatin, and raisins.

Prognosis

Infection is permanent. Although symptom-free periods are common, during these times individuals may still shed the virus into their saliva and genital secretions and infect others. Life-threatening neurological complications may occur in individuals who are immunocompromised, and HSV-2 infection during pregnancy and delivery can cause birth defects or serious harm to the infant.

Prevention

It is almost impossible to prevent HSV-1 infection. Limiting the number of sexual partners reduces the likelihood of becoming with HSV-2. Using a condom may help discourage infection, but does not fully protect against spread of the virus.

Resources

BOOKS

Ebel, Charles and Anna Wald. *Managing Herpes: Living and Loving With HSV.* Research Triangle Park, NC: American Social Health Association, 2007.

Warren, Terri. *The Good News About the Bad News: Herpes, Everything You Need to Know.* Oakland, CA: New Harbinger Publications, 2009.

OTHER

"Genital Herpes." United States Center for Disease Control and Prevention. February 26, 2009 [August 29, 2009], http://www.cdc.gov/std/Herpes

"Herpes simplex." MedlinePlus. August 14, 2009 [August 29, 2009], http://www.nlm.nih.gov/medlineplus/herpessimplex.html

ORGANIZATIONS

American Social Health Association, PO Box 13827, Research Triangle Park NC, 27709, (919) 361-8400, (800) 227-8922, (919) 361-8425, http://www.ashastd.org.

National Institute of Allergy and Infectious Diseases Office of Communications and Government Relations, 6610 Rockledge Drive, MSC 6612, Bethesda MD, 20892-6612, (301) 496-5717, (866) 284-4107 or TDD: (800)877-8339 (for hearing impaired), (301) 402-3573, http://www3.niaid.nih.gov.

Belinda M. Rowland, Ph. D.
Tish Davidson, A.M.

Hib vaccine

Definition

The Hib vaccine is an injection that helps protect children from contracting infections due to *Haemophilus influenzae* type B (Hib), a bacterium that is capable of causing serious illness and potential **death** in children under age five.

Purpose

Hib vaccine provides protection against *Haemophilus influenzae* type b infection.

Description

H. influenzae type B (Hib) is a common organism worldwide; it is found in most healthy individuals in the general population. Small children can pick up the bacteria from people who are not aware that they are carriers. When the bacteria spread to the lungs and bloodstream, serious illness, including **pneumonia** and **meningitis**, can result. Another serious disease stemming from this pathogen is **epiglottitis**, an infection of the epiglottis that cause swelling of the airways and potential death.

About 80% of people who develop Hib infections are children under age 5, with children age 6–12 months at

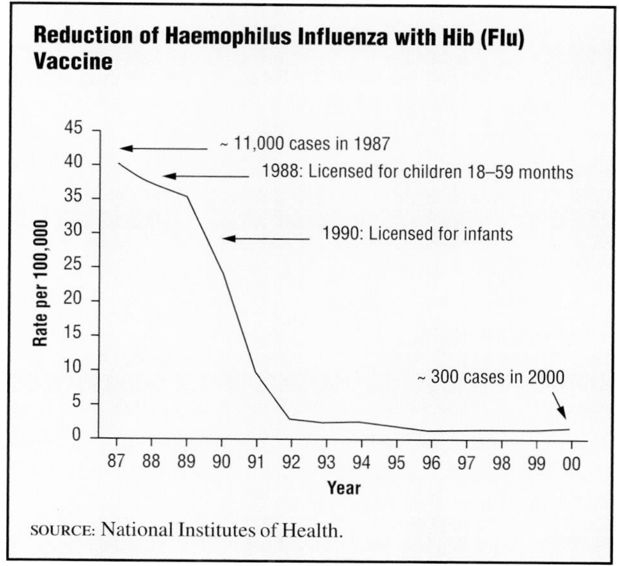

After the introduction of the Hib vaccine, instances of Haemophilus influenzae infection declined dramatically and have remained steady into the twenty-first century. *(Graph by PreMediaGlobal. Reproduced by permission of Gale, a part of Cengage Learning.)*

greatest risk for developing meningitis, and children over age 2 years at greatest risk for developing epiglottitis. In the United States before the introduction of a vaccine against Hib in the mid-1980s, each year about 20,000 cases of invasive (serious) Hib infection occurred in children and resulted in 1,000 deaths. Since **vaccination** against Hib has become standard in developed countries, the rate of infection has declined by about 95%.

In other countries where Hib immunization is common, a similar decrease has been seen. However, in the developing world vaccination rates are quite low, and Hib infection remains a significant cause of pediatric death. The World Health Organization (WHO) estimates that vaccination coverage is as low as 8% of children in the poorest countries, such as those in sub-Saharan Africa, and is less than 50% in many developing countries. WHO estimated that in the mid-2000s, Hib was responsible for 3 million serious illnesses and 386,000 deaths annually, primarily in countries where vaccination coverage is low.

United States Centers for Disease Control (CDC) and the World Health Organization (WHO) recommend that all infants be vaccinated against Hib disease. In general, the vaccine is considered highly effective, with few side effects. Failure to fully vaccinate and an age of under 5 years are the greatest risk factors for developing Hib infection.

Recommended dosage

According to the **American Academy of Pediatrics** and the United States Centers for Disease Control (CDC), immunization should consist of a series of shots given at age 2 months, 4 months, 6 months and between 12 and 15 months of age. Children older than five years and adults do not need vaccination, unless they have serious health problem that lowers immunity, such as HIV infection, **sickle cell disease**, or are being treated for **cancer**.

Precautions

Infants less than six weeks of age should not receive the Hib vaccine. Those children with moderate to severe illness should wait for vaccination until they are well. If a child has had a severe reaction to Hib vaccine, another dose should not be administered.

Side effects

Like any vaccine or medication, Hib vaccine is capable of causing a serious allergic reaction; however, this is extremely rare. Most children show no side effects from the vaccine. Of those that do, the most common side effects include inflammation at the injection site and slight **fever**, which can usually occur within 24 hours of the injection and can last two or three days. Any low-grade fever or soreness can be treated with ibuprofen or **acetaminophen** as recommended by the **pediatrician**. Serious reactions, including high fever, difficulty breathing, and fast heartbeat should receive immediate medical treatment.

KEY TERMS

Epiglottitis—Inflammation and swelling of the epiglottis, a flap of tissue in the throat that prevents food from entering the airways leading to the lungs. A swollen epiglottis can lead to difficulty breathing.

Meningitis—A serious, sometimes fatal, bacterial or viral disease in which the membranes lining the brain and spinal cord (the meninges) become infected.

Interactions

Interactions between Hib vaccine and other drugs, food, or herbs have not been reported. The Hib vaccine can be safely given at the same time as other childhood vaccines.

Resources

BOOKS

Sears, Robert, MD. *The Vaccine Book: Making The Right Decision for Your Child.* New York: Little, Brown, 2007.

OTHER

Devarajan, Vidya R. Haemophilus Influenzae Infection. EMedicine.com, December 17, 2009, http://emedicine.medscape.com/article/218271-overview

United States Centers for Disease Control. Haemophilus Influenzae Type b (Hib) Vaccine: What You Need to Know. Undated [accessed April 9, 2010], http://www.cdc.gov/vaccines/pubs/vis/downloads/vis-hib.pdf

Vaccines. United States Centers for Disease Control and Prevention (CDC). March 30, 2010, http://www.cdc.gov/vaccines

World Health Organization. Haemophilus Influenzae Type B (HiB). 2010, http://www.who.int/mediacentre/factsheets/fs294/en

ORGANIZATIONS

American Academy of Family Physicians, P. O. Box 11210, Shawnee Mission KS, 66207, (913)906-6000, (800) 274-2237, (913) 906-6075, http://familydoctor.org.

American Academy of Pediatrics, 141 Northwest Point Boulevard, Elk Grove Village IL, 60007-1098, (847) 434-4000, (847) 434-8000, http://www.aap.org.

United States Centers for Disease Control and Prevention (CDC), 1600 Clifton Road, Atlanta GA, 30333, (404) 639-3534, 800-CDC-INFO (800-232-4636). TTY: (888) 232-6348, inquiry@cdc.gov, http://www.cdc.gov.

World Health Organization, Avenue Appia 20, 1211 Geneva 27 Switzerland, +22 41 791 21 11, +22 41 791 31 11, info@who.int, http://www.who.int.

Kristine Krapp
Tish Davidson, AM

Hiccups

Definition

Hiccups are the result of an involuntary, spasmodic contraction of the diaphragm followed by the closing of the throat.

Demographics

A hiccup bout is an episode lasting more than a few minutes. If hiccups last longer than 48 hours, they are considered persistent or protracted. Hiccups lasting longer than one month are termed intractable. The longest recorded attack is 6 decades.

Hiccups can occur at any age and in utero. Pre-term infants spend up to 2.5% of their time hiccupping. Although hiccups occur less frequently with age, intractable hiccups are more common in adult life. Females develop hiccups more frequently during early adulthood than males of the same age.

Hiccups are one of the most common, but thankfully mildest, disorders to which humans are prey. Virtually everyone experiences them at some point, but they rarely last long or require a doctor's care. Occasionally, a bout of hiccups will last longer than two days, earning it the name "persistent hiccups." Very few people will experience intractable hiccups, in which hiccups last longer than one month.

Description

A hiccup involves the coordinated action of the diaphragm and the muscles that close off the windpipe (trachea). The diaphragm is a dome-shaped muscle separating the chest and abdomen, normally responsible for expanding the chest cavity for inhalation. Sensation from the diaphragm travels to the spinal cord through the phrenic nerve and the vagus nerve, which pass through the chest cavity and the neck. Within the spinal cord, nerve fibers from the brain monitor sensory information and adjust the outgoing messages that control contraction. These messages travel along the phrenic nerve.

Irritation of any of the nerves involved in this loop can cause the diaphragm to undergo involuntary contraction, or spasm, pulling air into the lungs. When this occurs, it triggers a reflex in the throat muscles. Less than a tenth of a second afterward, the trachea is closed off, making the characteristic "hic" sound.

Causes and symptoms

Hiccups can be caused by central nervous system disorders, injury or irritation to the phrenic and vagus nerves, and toxic or metabolic disorders affecting the central or peripheral nervous systems. They may be of unknown cause or may be a symptom of psychological stress. Hiccups often occur after drinking carbonated beverages or alcohol. They may also follow overeating or rapid temperature changes. Persistent or intractable hiccups may be caused by any condition which irritates or damages the relevant nerves, including:

- overstretching of the neck
- laryngitis
- heartburn (gastroesophageal reflux)
- irritation of the eardrum (which is innervated by the vagus nerve)
- general anesthesia
- surgery
- bloating
- tumor
- infection
- diabetes

Diagnosis

Hiccups are diagnosed by observation, and by hearing the characteristic sound. Diagnosing the cause of intractable hiccups may require imaging studies, blood tests, pH monitoring in the esophagus, and other tests.

Treatment

Most cases of hiccups will disappear on their own. Home remedies which interrupt or override the spasmodic nerve circuitry are often effective. Such remedies include:

- holding one's breath for as long as possible
- breathing into a paper bag

- swallowing a spoonful of sugar
- bending forward from the waist and drinking water from the wrong side of a glass

Treating any underlying disorder will usually cure the associated hiccups. Chlorpromazine (Thorazine) relieves intractable hiccups in 80% of cases. Metoclopramide (Reglan), carbamazepam, valproic acid (Depakene), and phenobarbital are also used. As a last resort, surgery to block the phrenic nerve may be performed, although it may lead to significant impairment of respiration.

Prognosis

Most cases of hiccups last no longer than several hours, with or without treatment.

Prevention

Some cases of hiccups can be avoided by drinking in moderation, avoiding very hot or very cold food, and avoiding cold showers. Carbonated beverages when drunk through a straw deliver more gas to the stomach than when sipped from a container; therefore, avoid using straws.

Resources

PERIODICALS

Krysiak W, Szabowski S, Stepien M, Krzywkowska K, Krzywkowski A, Marciniak P. Hiccups as a Myocardial Ischemia Symptom. *Pol Arch Med Wewn.* Mar 2008;118 (3):148-51.

Suh WM, Krishnan SC. Violent hiccups: An Infrequent Cause of Bradyarrhythmias. *West J Emerg Med.* Aug 2009;10 (3):176-7.

Richard Robinson
Karl Finley

High-risk pregnancy

Definition

A pregnancy that has maternal or fetal complications requiring special medical attention or bed rest is considered high-risk. Complications, as used here, mean that the risk of illness or **death** before or after delivery is greater than normal for the mother or baby.

Demographics

According to the U.S. Centers for Disease Control and Prevention (CDC) there were 13.1 maternal deaths for every 100,000 live births in the United States in 2004. There was a large racial disparity in maternal deaths, with African American women experiencing 36.1 deaths per 100,00 live births in 2004 and white women experiencing 9.8 deaths per 100,000 live births the same year. The rate for Hispanic women was 8.5 per 100,000 live births. Over the past 100 years deaths due to pregnancy and **childbirth** have declined hugely. In the early 1900s, giving **birth** was one of the most dangerous things a woman could do, with more than 600 women dying for every 100,000 live births in the year 1915.

Other statistics provide maternal mortality information by total female population, instead of per number of live births. In 2006, there were 115 deaths per 100,000 population due to pregnancy and childbirth among African American women, 70 deaths per 100,000 population among Hispanic and Latino women, 113 deaths per 100,000 population among white women, and 20 deaths per 100,000 population among Asian women. Common causes of death in women of childbearing age are problems related to pregnancy and delivery, including blood clots that travel to the lungs, anesthesia complications, bleeding, infection, and high blood pressure complications (pre-eclampsia and eclampsia).

A baby dies before, during, or shortly after birth in 16 out of 1,000 deliveries in the United States. Almost 50% of these deaths are stillbirths, which are sometimes unexplained. In 2005 there were 4.54 deaths in newborns before age 28 days per 1,000 live births, a total of 18,782 neonatal deaths. Risk factors for stillbirth and neonatal can be present before pregnancy occurs or develop during the course of the pregnancy.

Description

Risk factors in pregnancy are those findings discovered during prenatal assessment that are known to have a potentially negative effect on the outcome of the pregnancy, either for the woman or the fetus. This evaluation determines whether the mother has characteristics or conditions that make her or her baby more likely to become sick or die during the pregnancy.

The pregnant woman's interview at her first visit to the health care provider is conducted by the nurse, who obtains the data necessary to begin the high-risk screening. The physician or midwife caring for the pregnant woman will review the prenatal assessment sheet, order lab data, and obtain ultrasounds to determine if any risk factors are present. If it is determined that a woman has a high-risk pregnancy, she should be referred to a perinatologist for advanced care. This is the specialist who establishes and implements the medical regimen needed for the particular maternal/fetal complications likely to occur and the interdisciplinary team associated with the perinatal center works in its management. The perinatal team usually comprises a nutritionist, social worker, nurse educators, geneticists, ultrasonographers, and additional nursing staff who are responsible for the monitoring and supervising of ongoing team care of the patient.

Causes and symptoms

All risk factors do not threaten pregnancy to the same extent. The risk of complications is increased by **smoking**, poor nutritional habits, drug and alcohol abuse, domestic violence, prepregnancy maternal health status, psychosocial factors, prior health care, the presence of chronic medical problems in the mother, past history of repeated preterm delivery, multiple gestation, and abnormalities of the fetus or placenta. A woman with a high-risk pregnancy may have an earlier labor and delivery depending upon the fetal or maternal complication present and, likewise, present with symptoms dependent on the condition. Since the placenta supplies the baby with its nutrients and oxygen, any condition that threatens the blood supply to it threatens fetal development.

The threat of a preterm delivery is the most common reason for a referral to a perinatal center, which is linked to obstetric and newborn services that provide the highest level of care for a pregnant woman and her baby. A preterm delivery may occur because of a premature rupture of membranes (the bag of water surrounding the baby breaks) or preterm labor. There is a strong correlation of vaginal or uterine infection with the pregnant woman's water breaking, and there are laboratory tests that are predictive of a woman's risk of experiencing preterm labor.

Diagnosis

A risk-scoring sheet is used by many health care agencies during the prenatal assessment to establish if a woman may be at risk for complications during her pregnancy. This score sheet is implemented at the first prenatal visit, becomes a part of the woman's record, and is updated throughout the pregnancy as necessary. A woman's age affects pregnancy risk, as girls 15 years old and under are more likely to develop high blood pressure, protein in the urine and fluid accumulation, or seizures. They also are more likely to have underweight or undernourished babies. A woman 35 or older has a greater risk of developing high blood pressure or diabetes, as well as a much higher risk of having a chromosomal abnormality such as **Down syndrome**. A woman shorter than five feet or a woman weighing less than 100 pounds before pregnancy has a greater risk of having a small or preterm baby.

Laboratory data and ultrasound also are used to determine high-risk pregnancies by specific blood tests and imaging of the baby. A pregnancy may begin classified as low risk but be changed to a classification of high risk secondary to complications determined from the ongoing assessment of the pregnant woman. Since many of these complications can be managed with proper treatment, it is essential that a pregnant woman make and keep regular obstetric appointments.

Treatment

Treatment will vary, depending upon the maternal or fetal complication present. Generally, a woman with severe high-risk factors in pregnancy should be referred to a perinatal center to obtain the highest level of care for herself and her baby. Interventions to improve health status might include nutritional assessment; physical examination; teaching modalities for smoking cessation, drug and alcohol programs; prescribing medications related to the condition or changing pre-pregnancy medications (known to cause problems in the fetus); serial ultrasounds to learn fetal status; **amniocentesis**; fetal transfusions; fetal surgery; **antepartum testing**; bed rest; home health care; hospitalization; and early delivery. In a post-term pregnancy (greater than 42 weeks), the death of a baby is three times more likely than that of a normal term pregnancy (37–40 weeks). The treatment in this case would be to induce labor or perform a **cesarean section** before problems start to occur.

Prognosis

Advances in the management of complications in high-risk pregnancies have provided women with a means of controlling their risks, which substantially increases the potential for a successful outcome. Since it is impossible to guarantee a good outcome in a normal pregnancy, it is even more difficult to ensure that a high-risk pregnancy will result in a healthy infant and mother. A woman who strictly adheres to the medical regimen established for her, however, will greatly increase her chances of a positive result.

Prevention

The early weeks of pregnancy are the most crucial ones for the fetus. Many women do not know they are pregnant until several weeks after conception, so education about the need for preconceptional care is essential. Preconception counseling guides a woman in planning a healthy pregnancy. These are some of the factors to which attention must be paid:

- family history
- medical history
- past pregnancies
- current medications

KEY TERMS

Amniocentesis—A procedure that uses ultrasound to guide a needle into the amniotic sac (bag of waters) surrounding the baby and obtain fluid to analyze for genetic abnormalities.

Antepartum—This refers to the time period of the woman's pregnancy from conception and onset of labor.

Down syndrome—The most prevalent of a class of genetic defects known as trisomies, in which cells contain three copies of certain chromosomes rather than the usual two. Down syndrome, or trisomy 21, usually results from three copies of chromosome 21.

Perinatal—Refers to the period shortly before and after birth, generally from around the 20th week of pregnancy to one to four weeks after birth.

Perinatologist—A specialist in the branch of obstetrics that deals with the high-risk pregnant woman and her fetus.

Preconceptional—This refers to the time period before pregnancy, i.e., conception, occurs.

Ultrasonographer—The person who performs the radiologic technique of ultrasound in which deep structures of the body are visualized.

- lifestyle
- environment
- infections

The number one preventable cause of **mental retardation** in infants is the alcohol use during pregnancy. Alcohol can cause problems ranging from miscarriage to severe behavioral problems in the baby or developing child even if no obvious physical **birth defects** are apparent. **Fetal alcohol syndrome** is seen in about two out of 1,000 live births.

Cigarette smoking is the most common **addiction** among pregnant women in the United States, and despite the health hazards of smoking being well known, only about 20% of these women actually quit during pregnancy. One risk of smoking during pregnancy is having a baby who may die from **sudden infant death syndrome** (SIDS).

Drugs known to cause birth defects when taken during pregnancy include: alcohol, dilantin (phenytoin), any drug that interferes with the actions of **folic acid**, lithium, streptomycin, tetracycline, thalidomide, warfarin (Coumadin), and isotretinoin (Accutane), which is prescribed for **acne**.

Infections that may cause birth defects include: **herpes simplex**, viral hepatitis, the flu, **mumps**, German measles (**rubella**), **chickenpox** (**varicella**), syphilis, **toxoplasmosis** (occurs from eating undercooked meat and handling kitty litter), **listeriosis**, and infections from the coxsackievirus or cytomegalovirus (CMV). Many adults have been exposed to coxsackievirus and CMV when they were younger, but many have not. Those who have not been exposed should pay careful attention to any illnesses they have early in their pregnancy, noting the onset, presence of **fever**, muscle aches and pains, and duration of illness to report to their physician.

Hemolytic disease of the newborn (destruction of the red blood cells) can occur when Rh incompatibility exists between child and mother. The most common cause of incompatible blood types is Rh incompatibility, such as when the mother has Rh-negative blood and the father has Rh-positive blood. The baby may have Rh-positive blood, in which case the mother's body produces antibodies against the baby's blood. Fortunately, the mother can be treated with Rhogham [Rh0(D)immune globulin], which can be given to the mother in the first 72 hours after delivery and at the twenty-eighth week of pregnancy; it will destroy any antibodies produced by her blood and significantly decrease the risk associated with pregnancies with Rh-factor incompatibilities.

There are, however, other incompatible blood factors during the prenatal assessment period that can cause **anemia** in the fetus and require ongoing monitoring. The greatest gift a woman can give to herself and her baby is to plan her pregnancy with preconceptional counseling. Many women are frequently deficient in folic acid, a B vitamin used in the synthesis of ribonucleic acid (RNA) and essential, in large quantities, for optimal protein synthesis in the fetus. This is especially true in the early weeks of pregnancy, when all cell division and organ development is occurring. Thus, the best prevention for a high risk pregnancy is good planning.

Resources

BOOKS

Gilbert, Elizabeth S. *Manual of High Risk Pregnancy and Delivery*, 5th ed. Maryland Heights, MO: Mosby Elsevier, 2011.

James, David K., ed. *High Risk Pregnancy: Management Options*, 5th ed. Philadelphia, PA: Saunders/Elsevier, 2011.

Platt, Elizabeth S. *100 Questions and Answers about Your High-Risk Pregnancy*. Sudbury, MA: Jones & Bartlett Publishers, 2008.

Raab, Diana with Errol Norwitz. *Your High-Risk Pregnancy: A Practical and Supportive Guide*. Alameda, CA: Hunter House, 2009.

PERIODICALS

Holland, Marium G., et al. "Late Preterm Birth: How Often is it Avoidable?" *American Journal of Obstetrics and Gynecology,* (October 2009), 104(4), 404.e1-4.

Vidaeff, Alex C., and Susan M. Ramin. "Management Strategies for the Prevention of Preterm Birth."*Current Opinion in Obstetrics and Gynecology,* (December 2009), 21(6), 480-484.

ORGANIZATIONS

American Academy of Pediatrics, 141 Northwest Point Boulevard, Elk Grove Village IL, 60007-1098, (847) 434-4000, (847) 434-8000, http://www.aap.org.

American College of Obstetricians and Gynecologists, P.O. Box 96920, Washington DC, 20090-6920, (202)638-5577, http://www.acog.org.

American Pregnancy Association, 431 Greenway Drive, Suite 800, Irving TX, 75038, (972) 550-0140, (972) 550-0800, Questions@AmericanPregnancy.org, http://www.americanpregnancy.org.

Linda K. Bennington, R.N.C., M.S.N., C.N.S.
Tish Davidson, A.M.

High blood pressure ***see* Hypertension**

High cholesterol ***see* Cholesterol, high**

Hip dysplasia, congenital ***see* Congenital hip dysplasia**

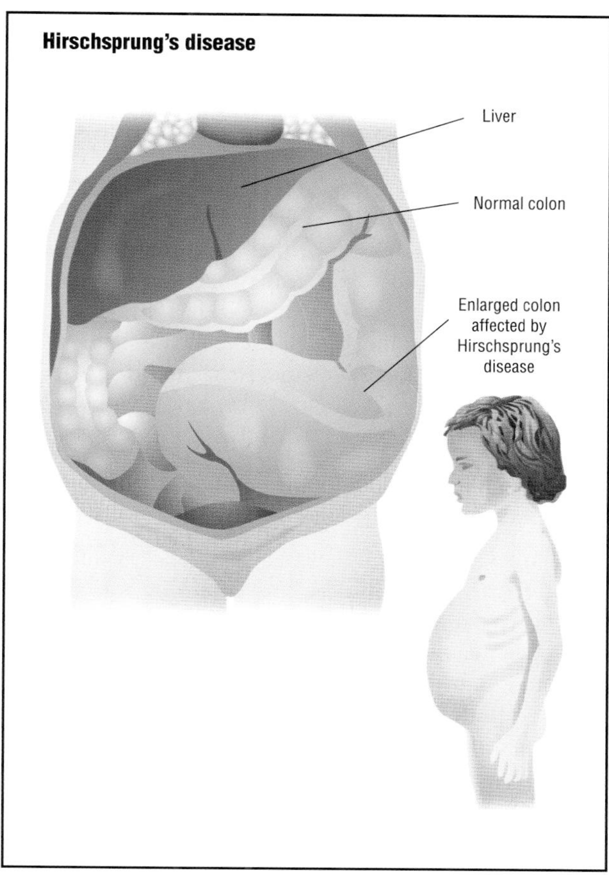

In Hirschsprung's disease, the flow of contents through the large intestine is halted, causing some areas to enlarge greatly. This causes many symptoms in the patient, including a distended abdomen. *(Illustration by PreMediaGlobal. Reproduced by permission of Gale, a part of Cengage Learning.)*

Hirschsprung's disease

Definition

Hirschsprung's disease, also known as congenital megacolon or aganglionic megacolon, is an abnormality in which certain nerve fibers are absent in segments of the bowel, resulting in severe bowel obstruction. It was first identified in 1886 by a physician named Harold Hirschsprung.

Description

Hirschsprung's disease is caused when certain nerve cells (called parasympathetic ganglion cells) in the wall of the large intestine (colon) do not develop before **birth**. Without these nerves, the affected segment of the colon lacks the ability to relax and move bowel contents along. This causes a constriction and as a result, the bowel above the constricted area dilates due to stool becoming trapped, producing megacolon (dilation of the colon). The disease can affect varying lengths of bowel segment, most often involving the region around the rectum. In up to 10% of children, however, the entire colon and part of the small intestine are involved. This condition is known as total colonic aganglionosis, or TCA.

Hirschprung's disease occurs once in every 5,000 live births, and it is about four times more common in males than females. Between 4% and 50% of siblings are also afflicted. The wide range for recurrence is due to the fact that the recurrence risk depends on the gender of the affected individual in the **family** (i.e., if a female is affected, the recurrence risk is higher) and the length of the aganglionic segment of the colon (i.e., the longer the segment that is affected, the higher the recurrence risk).

Causes and symptoms

Hirschsprung's disease occurs early in fetal development when, for unknown reasons, there is either failure of nerve cell development, failure of nerve cell migration, or arrest in nerve cell development in a segment of the bowel. The absence of these nerve fibers, which help control the movement of bowel contents, is what results in intestinal obstruction accompanied by other symptoms.

There is a genetic basis to Hirschsprung's disease, and it is believed that it may be caused by different genetic factors in different subsets of families. Proof that genetic factors contribute to Hirschprung's disease is that it is known to run in families, and it has been seen in association with some chromosome abnormalities. For example, about 10% of children with the disease have **Down syndrome** (the most common chromosomal abnormality). Molecular diagnostic techniques have identified many genes that cause susceptibility to Hirschprung's disease. As of the early 2000s, a total of six genes have been identified: the RET gene, the glial cell line-derived neurotrophic factor gene, the endothelin-B receptor gene, endothelin converting enzyme, the endothelin-3 gene, and the Sry-related transcription factor SOX10. Mutations that inactivate the RET gene are the most frequent, occurring in 50% of familial cases (cases which run in families) and 15–20% of sporadic (non-familial) cases. Mutations in these genes do not cause the disease, but they make the chance of developing it more likely. Mutations in other genes or environmental factors are required to develop the disease, and these other factors are not understood. As of 2004, at least three chromosomes are known to be involved: 13q22, 21q22, and 10q. Hirschsprung's disease has also been reported in association with abnormal forms of chromosome 18.

For persons with a ganglion growth beyond the sigmoid segment of the colon, the inheritance pattern is autosomal dominant with reduced penetrance (risk closer to 50%). For persons with smaller segments involved, the inheritance pattern is multifactorial (caused by an interaction of more than one gene and environmental factors, risk lower than 50%) or autosomal recessive (one disease gene inherited from each parent, risk closer to 25%) with low penetrance.

The initial symptom is usually severe, continuous **constipation**. A newborn may fail to pass meconium (the first stool) within 24 hours of birth, may repeatedly vomit yellow- or green-colored bile and may have a distended (swollen, uncomfortable) abdomen. Occasionally, infants may have only mild or intermittent constipation, often with **diarrhea**.

While two-thirds of cases are diagnosed in the first three months of life, Hirschsprung's disease may also be diagnosed later in **infancy** or childhood. Occasionally, even adults are diagnosed with a variation of the disease. In older infants, symptoms and signs may include anorexia (lack of appetite or inability to eat), lack of the urge to move the bowels or empty the rectum on physical examination, distended abdomen, and a mass in the colon that can be felt by the physician during examination. It should be suspected in older children with abnormal bowel habits, especially a history of constipation dating back to infancy and ribbon-like stools.

Occasionally, the presenting symptom may be a severe intestinal infection called enterocolitis, which is life-threatening. The symptoms are usually explosive, watery stools and **fever** in a very ill-appearing infant. It is important to diagnose the condition before the intestinal obstruction causes an overgrowth of bacteria that evolves into a medical emergency. Enterocolitis can lead to severe diarrhea and massive fluid loss, which can cause **death** from **dehydration** unless surgery is done immediately to relieve the obstruction.

Hirschsprung's disease sometimes occurs in children with other disorders of the autonomic nervous system, such as congenital central hypoventilation syndrome, a breathing disorder. Other syndromes associated with Hirschsprung disease include congenital deafness and Waardenburg syndrome, a genetic disorder characterized by facial abnormalities and the loss of normal pigmentation in the hair, skin, and the iris of the eye.

Diagnosis

Hirschsprung's disease in the newborn must be distinguished from other causes of intestinal obstruction. The diagnosis is suspected by the child's medical history and physical examination, especially the rectal exam. The diagnosis is confirmed by a barium enema x ray, which shows a picture of the bowel. The x ray will indicate if a segment of bowel is constricted, causing dilation and obstruction. A biopsy of rectal tissue will reveal the absence of the nerve fibers. Adults may also undergo manometry, a balloon study (device used to enlarge the anus for the procedure) of internal anal sphincter pressure and relaxation.

Treatment

Hirschsprung's disease is treated surgically. The goal is to remove the diseased, nonfunctioning segment of the bowel and restore bowel function. This is often done in two stages. The first stage relieves the intestinal obstruction by performing a colostomy. This is the creation of an opening in the abdomen (stoma) through which bowel contents can be discharged into a waste bag. When the child's weight, age, or condition is deemed appropriate, surgeons close the stoma, remove the diseased portion of bowel, and perform a "pull-through" procedure, which repairs the colon by connecting functional bowel to the anus. The pull-through operation usually establishes fairly normal bowel function.

Children with total colonic aganglionosis occasionally fail to benefit from a pull-through procedure. One option in treating these patients is the construction of an ileoanal S-pouch.

The surgeon may recommend a permanent ostomy if the child has Down syndrome in addition to Hirschsprung disease, as these children usually have more difficulty with bowel control.

Prognosis

Overall, prognosis is very good. Most infants with Hirschsprung's disease achieve good bowel control after surgery, but a small percentage of children may have lingering problems with soilage or constipation. These infants are also at higher risk for an overgrowth of bacteria in the intestines, including subsequent episodes of enterocolitis, and should be closely followed by a physician. Mortality from enterocolitis or surgical complications in infancy is 25–30%.

Prevention

Hirschsprung's disease is a congenital abnormality that has no known means of prevention. It is important to diagnose the condition early in order to prevent the development of enterocolitis. Genetic counseling can be offered to a couple with a previous child with the disease or to an affected individual considering pregnancy to discuss recurrence risks and treatment options. Prenatal diagnosis is not available as of the late 2000s.

Resources

BOOKS

Beers, Mark H., MD, and Robert Berkow, MD., editors. "Congenital Anomalies." In *The Merck Manual of Diagnosis and Therapy*. 18th ed., Whitehouse Station, NJ: Merck Research Laboratories, 2006.

PERIODICALS

Chen, M. L., and T. G. Keens. "Congenital Central Hypoventilation Syndrome: Not Just Another Rare Disorder." *Paediatric Respiratory Reviews* 5 (September 2004): 182–189.

Lal, D. R., P. F. Nichol, B. A. Harms, et al. "Ileo-Anal S-Pouch Reconstruction in Patients with Total Colonic Aganglionosis after Failed Pull-Through Procedure." *Journal of Pediatric Surgery* 39 (July 2004): e7–e9.

Martucciello, G., et al. "Pathogenesis of Hirschprung's Disease." *Journal of Pediatric Surgery* 35 (2000): 1017–1025.

Munnes, M., et al. "Familial Form of Hirschprung Disease: Nucleotide Sequence Studies Reveal Point Mutations in the RET Proto-oncogene in Two of Six Families But Not in Other Candidate Genes." *American Journal of Medical Genetics* 94 (2000): 19–27.

Neville, Holly, MD, and Charles S. Cox, Jr., MD. "Hirschsprung Disease." *eMedicine* July15, 2003, *http://www.emedicine.com/ped/topic1010.htm.*

Prabhakara, K., H. E. Wyandt, X. L. Huang, et al. "Recurrent Proximal 18p Monosomy and 18q Trisomy in a Family with a Maternal Pericentric Inversion of Chromosome 18." *Annales de génétique* 47 (July-September 2004): 297–303.

ORGANIZATIONS

American Pseudo-Obstruction & Hirschsprung's Society, 158 Pleasant St., North Andover MA, 01845, (978) 685-4477

National Organization for Rare Disorders (NORD), 55 Kenosia Avenue, P. O. Box 1968, Danbury CT, 06813-1968 (203) 744-0100, (800) 999-6673, http://www.rarediseases.org.

Pull-thru Network, 316 Thomas St., Bessemer AL, 35020, (205) 428-5953

Amy Vance, MS, CGC
Rebecca J. Frey, PhD

Histiocytosis X

Definition

Histiocytosis X is a generic term that refers to an increase in the number of histiocytes, a type of white blood cell, that act as scavengers to remove foreign material from the blood and tissues. Since recent research demonstrated Langerhan cell involvement as well as histiocytes, this led to a proposal that the term Langerhans Cell Histiocytosis (LCH) be used in place of histiocytosis X. Either term refers to three separate illnesses (listed in order of increasing severity): eosinophilic granuloma, Hand-Schuller-Christian disease and Letterer-Siwe disease.

Description

Epidermal (skin) Langerhans cells (a form of dendritic cell) accumulate with other immune cells in various parts of the body and cause damage by the release of chemicals. Normally, Langerhans cells recognize foreign material, including bacteria, and stimulate the **immune system** to react to them. Langerhans cells are usually found in skin, lymph nodes, lungs, and the gastrointestinal tract. Under abnormal conditions these cells affect skin, bone, and the pituitary gland as well as the lungs, intestines, liver, spleen, bone marrow, and brain. Therefore, the disease is not confined to areas where Langerhans cells are normally found. The disease is more common in children than adults and tends to be most severe in very young children.

Histiocytosis X or LCH is a family of related conditions characterized by a distinct inflammatory and proliferative process but differs from each other in which parts of the body are involved. The least severe of the histiocytosis X/LCH family is eosinophilic granuloma. Approximately 60–80% of all diagnosed cases are in this classification, which usually occurs in children aged 5–10 years. The bones are involved 50–75% of the time, which includes the skull or mandible, and the long bones. If the bone marrow is involved, **anemia** can result. With skull involvement, growths can occur behind the eyes, bulging them forward. One recent case study involved swelling of the eyes caused by histiocytosis in a three-year-old girl. The lungs are involved less than 10% of the time, and this involvement signals the worst prognosis.

Next in severity is Hand-Schuller-Christian disease, a chronic, scattered form of histiocytosis. It occurs most commonly from the age of one to three years and is a slowly progressive disease that affects the softened areas of the skull, other flat bones, the eyes, and skin. Letterer-Siwe disease is the acute form of this series of diseases. It is generally found from the time of **birth** to one year of age. It causes an enlarged liver, bruising and skin lesions, anemia, enlarged lymph glands, other organ involvement, and extensive skull lesions.

Causes and symptoms

This is a rare disorder affecting approximately 1 in 200,000 children or adults each year. The International Histiocyte Society formed a registry in 2000 that has registered a total of 274 adults from 13 countries as of 2003. Because histiocytic disorders are so rare, little research has been done to determine their cause. Over time, histiocytosis may lessen in its assault on the body but there are still problems from damage to the tissues. There are no apparent inheritance patterns in these diseases with the exception of a form involving the lymphatic system; of the 274 adults in the international registry, only one came from a family with a history of the disease.

The symptoms of histiocytosis are caused by substances called cytokines and prostaglandins, which are normally produced by histiocytes and act as messengers between cells. When these chemicals are produced in excess amounts and in the wrong places, they cause tissue swelling and abnormal growth. Thus, symptoms may include painful lumps in the skull and limbs as well as **rashes** on the skin. General symptoms may include: poor appetite, failure to gain weight, recurrent **fever**, and irritability. Symptoms from other possible sites of involvement include:

- gums: swelling, usually without significant discomfort
- ear: chronic discharge
- liver or spleen: abdominal discomfort or swelling
- pituitary: This gland at the base of the brain is affected at some stage in approximately 20%–30% of children causing a disturbance in water balance to produce thirst and frequent urination.
- eyes: Due to the bony disease, behind-the-eye bulging may occur (exophthalmos)
- lungs: breathing problems

Diagnosis

The diagnosis can be made only by performing a biopsy, that is, taking a tissue sample under anesthesia from a site in the patient thought to be involved. Blood and urine tests, chest and other **x rays**, **magnetic resonance imaging** (MRI) and **computed tomography scans** (**CAT** scans) (to check the extent of involvement), and possibly bone marrow or breathing tests may be required to confirm the diagnosis.

Treatment

Although this disease is not **cancer**, most patients diagnosed with it are treated in cancer clinics. There are two reasons for this:

- Historically, cancer specialists treated it before the cause was known.
- The treatment requires the use of drugs typically required to treat cancer.

Any cancer drugs utilized are usually given in smaller doses, which diminishes the severity of their side effects. Radiation therapy is rarely used, and special drugs may be prescribed for skin symptoms. If there is only one organ affected, **steroids** may be injected locally, or a drug called indomethacin may be used. Indomethacin is an anti-inflammatory medication that may achieve a similar response with less severe side effects.

Prognosis

The disease fluctuates markedly. If only one system is involved, the disease often resolves by itself. Multisystem disease usually needs treatment although it may disappear spontaneously. The disease is not normally fatal unless organs vital to life are damaged. In general, the younger the child at diagnosis and the more organs involved, the poorer the outlook. If the condition resolves, there could still be long-term complications because of the damage done while the disease was active.

Resources

BOOKS

Beers, Mark H., MD, and Robert Berkow, MD., editors. "Histiocytic Syndromes." In *The Merck Manual of Diagnosis and Therapy.* 18th ed., Whitehouse Station, NJ: Merck Research Laboratories, 2006.

Behrman, Richard E., Robert Kliegman, and Hal B. Jenson, editors.*Nelson Textbook of Pediatrics.* Philadelphia: W. B. Saunders, 2000.

PERIODICALS

Arico, M., M. Girschikofsky, T. Genereau, et al. "Langerhans Cell Histiocytosis in Adults. Report from the International Registry of the Histiocyte Society." *European Journal of Cancer* 39 (November 2003): 2341–2348.

Eckhardt, A., and A. Schulze. "Maxillofacial Manifestations of Langerhans Cell Histiocytosis: A Clinical and Therapeutic Analysis of 10 Patients." *Oral Oncology* 39 (October 2003): 687–694.

Kobyahsi, M., O. Yamamoto, Y. Suenaga, and M. Asahi. "Electron Microscopic Study of Langerhans Cell Histiocytosis." *Journal ofDermatology* July 27, 2000: 453–7.

Levy, J., T. Monos, J.Kapelushnik, et al. "Langerhans Cell Histiocytosis with Periorbital Cellulitis." *American Journal of Ophthalmology* 136 (November 2003): 939–942.

OTHER

"Immunity Disorders." *NurseMinerva.* June 26, 2001, http://nurseminerva.co.uk/immunity.htm.

ORGANIZATIONS

Histiocytosis Association of America, 302 North Broadway, Pitman NJ, 08071, (800) 548-2758, http://www.histio.org.

Linda K. Bennington, CNS
Rebecca J. Frey, PhD

Hitting **see** Acting out

HIV **see** AIDS

Hives

Definition

Hives are due to an allergic skin reaction and cause localized redness, swelling, and **itching**.

Description

Hives are a reaction of the body's **immune system** that causes areasof the skin to swell, itch, and become reddened (wheals). When the reaction islimited to small areas of the skin, it is called "urticaria."Involvement of

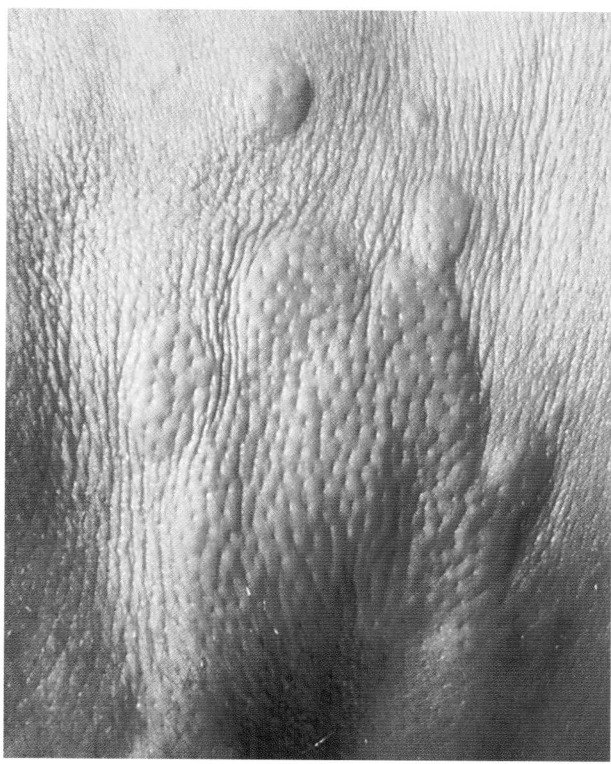

Hives on the back of a young woman's legs. Hives is an allergic reaction that ranges in size from small spots to patches measuring several inches across. *(Custom Medical Stock Photo, Inc. Reproduced by permission.)*

larger areas, such as whole sections of a limb, is called "angioedema." Hives can be round or they can form rings or largepatches. Hives can also form wheals or welts, which are red lesions with a red flare at the borders.

Demographics

It is estimated that five percent of all people will develop urticaria at some pointin their lives. Hives are more common in women than in men. Of those with chronic hives, lasting six weeks or more, about 80% are idiopathic, meaning no cause, allergic, or otherwise, can be found.

Causes and symptoms

Causes

Hives occur due to an allergic reaction. The body's immune system is normally responsible for protection from foreign invaders. When it becomes sensitized to normally harmless substances, the resulting reaction is called an allergy. An attack of hives is set off when such a substance, called an allergen, is ingested, inhaled, or otherwise contacted. The allergen interacts with immunecells called mast cells, which reside in the skin, airways, and digestive system. When mast cells encounter an allergen, they release histamine and other chemicals, both locally and into the blood stream. These chemicals cause blood vessels to become more porous, allowing fluid to accumulate in tissue and leading to the swollen and reddish appearance of hives. Some of the chemicals released sensitize **pain** nerve endings, causing the affected area to become itchy and sensitive.

A wide variety of substances may cause hives in sensitive people, including foods, drugs, and insect **bites** or **stings**. Common culprits include:

- nuts, especially peanuts, walnuts, and Brazil nuts
- fish, mollusks, and shellfish
- eggs
- wheat
- milk
- strawberries
- food additives and preservatives
- penicillin or other antibiotics
- flu vaccines
- tetanus toxoid vaccine
- gamma globulin
- bee, wasp, and hornet stings
- bites of mosquitoes, fleas, and scabies

Symptoms

Urticaria is characterized by redness, swelling, and itching of small areas of the skin. These patches usually grow and recede in less than a day, but may be replaced by hives in other locations. Angioedema is characterized by more diffuse swelling. Swelling of the airways may cause wheezing and respiratory distress. In severe cases, airway obstruction may occur.

Diagnosis

Hives are easily diagnosed by visual inspection. The cause of hives is usually apparent, but may require a careful medical history in some cases.

Treatment

Mild cases of hives are treated with **antihistamines**, such as diphenhydramine (Benadryl) or desloratadine (Clarinex). Clarinex is non–sedating, meaning it will not make patients drowsy. More severe cases may require oral corticosteroids, such as prednisone. Topical corticosteroids are not effective. Airway swelling may require emergency injection of epinephrine (adrenaline).

Alternative treatment

An alternative practitioner will try to determine what allergic substance is causing the reaction and help the patient eliminate or minimize its effects. To deal with the symptoms of hives, an oatmeal bath may help to relieve itching. Chickweed (*Stellaria media*), applied as a poultice (crushed or chopped herbs applied directly to the skin) or added to bath water, may also help relieve itching. Several homeopathic remedies, including *Urtica urens* and *Apis* (*Apis mellifica*), may help relieve the itch, redness, or swelling associated with hives.

Prognosis

Most cases of hives clear up within one to seven days without treatment, providing the cause (allergen) is found and avoided.

Prevention

Preventing hives depends on avoiding the allergen causing them. Analysis of new items in the diet or new drugs taken may reveal the likely source of the reaction. Chronic hives may be aggravated by stress, **caffeine**, alcohol, or tobacco; avoiding these may reduce the frequency of reactions.

Resources

PERIODICALS

Kirn, F. Timothy. "Desloratadine Improves Urticaria inClinical Setting." *Skin & Allergy News* September 2004:41.

ORGANIZATIONS

American Academy of Dermatology (AAD), 930 E. Woodfield Rd., Schaumburg IL, 60173, http://www.aad.org.

American Podiatric Medical Association (APMA), 9312 Old Georgetown Rd., Bethesda MD, 20814–1698, (301) 571–9200, http://www.apma.org.

Richard Robinson
Teresa G. Odle
Karl Finley

Home birth

Definition

A home birth occurs when a mother gives birth at her home instead of in a hospital or birthing center.

Purpose

Proponents of home birth suggest that giving birth at home provides a special, intimate birthing experience unlike any that can be achieved at the hospital. They suggest that it provides a variety of benefits to the mother and baby and allows for greater involvement of other **family** members and friends. Home birth allows mothers to make more choices for themselves during labor and delivery. The purpose of any birthing method is to provide the best, safest, birthing experience possible for both the mother and the baby.

Demographics

Until around 1900 all births were home births. In the beginning of the twentieth century, women started moving towards giving birth in hospitals. The availability of emergency care for the woman and child in the hospital setting led to decreases in maternal and **infant mortality**, as well as a decrease in the number of stillbirths. In many places in the world today, the majority of births still occur inside the home.

The number of hospital births continued to increase in the United States until 1969 when it reached about 99% of all births. The percentage of hospital births remains at around 99% as of 2010.

According to the United States Centers for Disease Control and Prevention (CDC) there were 38,568 out-of-hospital births in 2006, of which 24,970 were home births. White women were the most likely to choose to give birth at home, as were women who had previously had several children, women over age 25, and women who were married. Home births were highest for women over age 45 and those who previously had given birth to 8 or more live children. Home births were more common in rural counties with fewer than 100,000 residents.

In 2006 approximately 61% of home births were attended by midwives, of which a little more than one-fourth were attended by certified nurse-midwives.

Description

A home birth is a birth that occurs in the woman's home instead of at a hospital or birthing center. Home births are generally attended by a doctor, nurse, or in most cases by a professional midwife. Other professionals may also attend, such as masseurs, chiropractors, or doctors of naturopathic medicine. A home birth can be attended by any friends and family members the parents would like have present.

Like every mother, every home birth is different. Home births generally are tailored to the mothers's wishes about **pain** medication, medical intervention, location, and other aspects. At a home birth, the delivery can occur anywhere the mother desires, including in bed, on the floor, or on a special mat. Some home births are also water births, in which the woman sits in a tub of warm water during labor and delivery.

Women who give birth at home can eat and drink as much or as little as they wish during labor. Medical guidelines generally strongly discourage the mother from eating or drinking anything during labor, although as of 2010 the necessity of not allowing the mother to drink any fluids at all was beginning to be questioned.

Other aspects of a home birth vary from woman to woman and from midwife to midwife. Some midwives provide intravenous fluids to women if needed, whereas others are not qualified to provide this service. The amount and type of medical care that midwives are qualified to and comfortable with providing differs. Women considering home birth should be sure to talk to the midwife who will be attending them about these issues well before labor begins.

A significant number of women who begin giving birth at home are transferred to the hospital. Transfer is generally due to complications or because the woman no longer desires or feels able to complete giving birth at home. In many cases transfer is required because labor stops progressing.

Benefits

Proponents of home birth point to a wide range of benefits for women with low-risk pregnancies. First, there is the opportunity to give birth in a familiar place with as many family members and friends gathered around as the woman desires. Additionally, women who give birth at home can exercise more control over their labor and delivery. They can take a shower, walk around, and eat or drink as desired without being limited by the hospital's guidelines or rules.

Other potential benefits of home birth include the reduced likelihood of infection of the mother or newborn, and the reduced likelihood of **cesarean section**. Many proponents of home birth point to the reduction in medical interventions during home birth as one of the primary benefits of choosing to give birth at home.

Giving birth at home may be a better emotional experience for the mother. The setting is familiar, which may reduce **anxiety**. Reduced anxiety is believed to lead to a less painful labor and delivery, as well as a faster labor in some cases. Some people believe that giving birth at home is a more holistic, calmer experience for both the mother and the newborn baby.

KEY TERMS

Certified nurse-midwife—A nurse-midwife who has been certified by the American College of Nurse-Midwives.

Certified professional midwife—A midwife certified by the North American Registry of Midwives.

Lay midwife—A midwife who has not completed any official certification or training.

Licensed midwife—A midwife licensed by the state or locality in which she practices.

Preeclampsia—A pregnancy-related condition that causes high blood pressure and swelling.

Precautions

Women with high-risk pregnancies should not give birth at home. High-risk pregnancies are highly likely to require specialized medical intervention to protect the health of the baby, the mother, or often both. Women with diabetes, high blood-pressure or toxemia (preeclampsia), a baby in an unusual birth position, a baby with an irregular heartbeat or who are pregnant with multiple fetuses should not give birth at home. Any time that there is a suspicion there is something unusual about or wrong with the pregnancy the woman should not choose home birth. Women who are giving birth preterm should also not give birth at home.

Preparation

Preparation for a home birth takes special care and planning. In addition to usual preparations for birth, such as parenting or birthing classes, accumulation of everything the baby will need in its first days, and the emotional preparation of the mother, father, and other family members, preparing for home birth requires some additional care.

A midwife or other professional who will attend the birth should be carefully researched and selected. It is important to find a birthing professional who shares the parents' views about birth and with whom the mother is comfortable.

The mother and midwife should work together to develop a plan for what will happen if there are unexpected complications during labor and delivery. Some midwives have doctors or hospitals they work with who agree in advance to provide care for the midwive's patients in case of an emergency.

Mothers and other family members should prepare for a transfer in case it is necessary. Even if transfer is not expected to occur, it pays to be prepared with insurance cards, a bag or suitcase full of clothes for the mother and the new baby, and other supplies.

Aftercare

Care after a home birth is similar to care after a hospital bed birth. The baby is cleaned, the umbilical cord is cut, and the mother is treated as needed. After a home birth the mother often chooses to feed the baby right away. Breast feeding the baby shortly after birth can help clear out the baby's nose, mouth, and throat.

After a home birth the baby should be taken to a **pediatrician** within the first 24 hours after birth. Numerous screenings, tests, and a **hepatitis B vaccine** usually are given at birth. Practitioners assisting in home births are often not set up to do all these things in the home. However, this care can successfully administered at a doctor's office within next day.

Risks

The main risk of a home birth is not any specific complication or emergency, but instead it is the risk due to delay of care if a complication or emergency develops. A home is not equipped to provide the complex medical care needed to treat complications that occur during birth. Even the seemingly least complicated and healthiest pregnancy can become an emergency in only a few seconds. When there is an emergency during labor or delivery even a few minutes can make the difference between life and **death** or permanent disability.

When considering home birth women should consider how far the home is from a hospital, and how long transfer would take if an emergency were to occur. Women who live far from a hospital are at much higher risk for serious negative outcomes if problems occur during labor or delivery in the home. Not only physical distance but also expected total travel time, from calling an ambulance to arriving at the hospital door, should be taken into account factors such as the likely amount of traffic and the average speed of emergency response in the area.

Research and general acceptance

Home birth is an extremely controversial topic. On one side are advocates who believe that home birth is an experience that has benefits not reproducible in a hospital or birthing center and that restricting a woman's right to give birth at home is restricting her right to choose what happens to her body and her baby. On the other side are people who believe that home birth adds unnecessary danger to the birthing process, a process that is always highly variable and that can develop life-threatening complications at any time. People against home birth often argue that women who choose home birth are putting the birthing "experience" ahead of what is healthiest and safest for themselves and their babies.

The American Medical Association and the American Congress of Obstetricians and Gynecologists passed statements against home birth. Midwives associations are for home birth as a safe and more personal alternative to hospital birth.

There is one thing that everyone in the home birth debate agrees on. If a woman has a **high-risk pregnancy** or is giving birth preterm, she should not have a home birth. Even the most devoted practitioners and supporters of home birth openly acknowledge that there are some situations that a hospital is much better equipped to handle than anything that could be set up in a home.

There are no clear statistics providing evidence of the benefits of home birth, although there are many anecdotal stories by women who have done so and by career midwives. One issue that complicates the picture is the high incidence of transfer birth to the hospital of women who start home birth. There is wide disparity in the percentage of transfers reported by different sources. Most agree that more than 1 in 10 women who begin home birth will be transferred to the hospital. Some reports suggest that in the United States about one in four women giving birth for the first time will be transferred.

The high rate of transfer makes the interpretation of statistics about home birth difficult. Many statistics showing the benefits of home birth count only those babies delivered at home, which removes all the women transferred to the hospital from consideration. In general, it seems that there is evidence for a decreased incidence of caesarian section and somewhat fewer medical interventions for women who choose home birth.

Statistics about the **safety** of home birth are thrown around by both sides of the debate. It is often hard to determine what the real facts are without reading the original journal articles, which are often written in very technical medical language. There are a few things to consider, however, when assessing statistics given by either side of the debate.

- Who is providing the statistics?
- What source are they citing? Is it a well-known, reputable source?
- Are the statistics for women who started giving birth at home, or only for those who completed giving birth at home? Transfer rates are very high, so this difference can be very important.
- Are the statistics for long term outcomes, or did the study only look at outcomes right after birth?
- Do the statistics provide information on who attended the births?
- Are all the births used in the statistics intended home births? Unintended home births are quite different, as they usually involve an unprepared mother and only unskilled and untrained individuals attending the birth.
- Are the statistics really for just home births? Sometimes statistics for births occurring outside the hospital include births that occur in cars, subways, and other unintended and less than ideal locations.

Training and certification

A variety of different people may be involved in a home birth. Some doctors with medical degrees and special training and experience in home births provide their services to women who choose to give birth at home. Registered nurses, and nurse-midwives also offer their services. The most common professionals who attend home births are midwives, but the variety of certifications of midwives can be confusing.

Registered nurse-midwives are individuals who have both achieved the status of registered nurse, and who have received special training or experience in midwifery. A certified nurse-midwife is a nurse-midwife who has been certified by the American College of Nurse-Midwives. A certified professional midwife is an individual who does not necessarily have the credentials to be a nurse, but who has significant training and experience in the art of providing midwife care and who is certified by North American Registry of Midwives.

A lay midwife is a midwife who has not completed any official certification or training. She has usually become a midwife through experience assisting another midwife with births and/or through self-study. A lay midwife is not certified by an professional organization.

A licensed midwife is a midwife who is legally licensed to provide midwife care in a specific state or locality. Some states do not license any midwives, although many people are working to change this situation. In some state a midwife must have an agreement with a doctor or hospital to provide back-up care if any unforeseen complications arise when the mother is under the midwife's care.

Resources

BOOKS

Buckley, Sarah J. *Gentle Birth, Gentle Mothering: A Doctor's Guide to Natural Childbirth and Gentle Early Parenting Choices.* Berkeley: Celestial Arts, 2009.

Chapman, Vicky, and Cathy Charles, eds. *The Midwife's Labour and Birth Handbook,* 2nd ed. Malden, MA: Wily-Blackwell, 2009.

Cook, Kalena, and Margaret Christensen. *Birthing a Better Way: 12 Secrets of Natural Childbirth.* Denton, TX: University of North Texas Press, 2010.

Gabriel, Cynthia. *Natural Hospital Birth: The Best of Both Worlds.* Boston, MA: Harvard Common Press, 2011.

Spatafora, Denise. *Better Birth: The Ultimate Guide to Childbirth From Home Birth To Hospitals.* Hoboken, NJ: Wiley, 2009.

PERIODICALS

Doyle, Michelle K. "Choosing Where to Have Your Baby." *Journal of Midwifery & Women's Health* (March-April 2010), 55(2), 195.

Lieberman, Linda. "Are We Ready to Standardize Homebirth?" *Midwifery Today with International Midwife,* (2010), 93, 68-9.

Vedam, Saraswathi, Jessica Aaker, and Kathrin Stoll. "Assessing Certified Nurse-Midwives's Attitudes Towards Planned Home Birth." *Journal of Midwifery & Women's Health,* (March-April 2010), 55(2), 133-42.

ORGANIZATIONS

American College of Nurse-Midwives, 8403 Colesville Rd, Suite 1550, Silver Spring MD, 20919, (240) 485-1800, (240) 485-1818, http://www.midwife.org.

American College of Obstetricians and Gynecologists, P.O. Box 96920, Washington DC, 20090-6920, (202)638-5577, http://www.acog.org.

Association of Women's Health, Obstetric, and Neonatal Nurses, 2000 L St., NW, Suite. 740, Washington DC, 20036, (202) 261-2400, (800) 673-8499. Toll free in Canada (800) 245-0231, (202) 728-0575, customerservice@awhonn.org, http://www.awhonn.org.

Tish Davidson, A.M.

Home schooling

Definition

Home schooling is the education of children at home rather than in a public or private school setting. Teaching the children is often done by a parent or guardian however, the use of tutors is also sometimes employed.

Demographics

Home schooling is perhaps the fastest growing trend in education in the United States, as well as in Canada, Australia, New Zealand, and the United Kingdom. According to the U.S. Department of Education, about 500,000 students, or about 1 percent of the total school age population, were taught at home in 1996. By 1999 the official figure had reached 850,000, or 1.7 percent of the student population, and by 2003, 1.1 million or 2.2 percent. The Department of Education's figures jumped 30 percent over one five-year period, and some researchers say the number of home-schooled children is growing at about 25 percent annually. As of 2010, there is an estimated number of two million home-schoolers in the U.S.

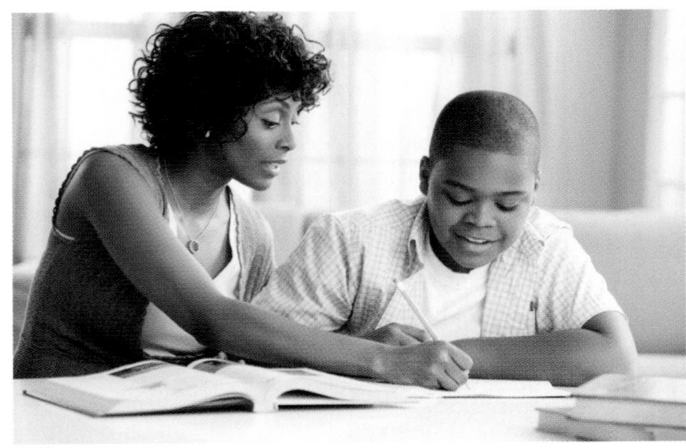

A mother home schooling her son. *(© Blend Images/Alamy.)*

Racial or ethnic ratios have remained fairly consistent since the mid-1990s: 2.7 percent of Caucasian students are home-schooled, 1.3 percent of African American students, and 0.7 percent of Hispanic students. Home schooling is now legal in every state, though requirements vary. Some states require parents who teach their children at home to have teacher's certificates or college degrees; some require extensive monitoring by public school officials. Some states have specific curriculum and testing requirements, while others ask only that parents notify the school district that they plan to teach their children at home.

Description

Home schooling involves a tremendous commitment from parents. At least one parent must be willing to work closely with the child, plan lessons, keep abreast of requirements, and perhaps negotiate issues with the school district. The most common home school arrangement is for the mother to teach while the father works outside the home. There are a variety of educational materials geared for the home school published by dozens of suppliers. Some are correspondence courses that grade students' work; some are full curricula; and some are single topic workbooks or drill materials in such areas as math or phonics. Many of the curriculum providers are identifiably Christian, including several major home school publishers such as Bob Jones University Press, Alpha Omega Publications, and Home Study International. A major nonreligious provider of home school materials is the Calvert School in Baltimore.

Other philosophies and models of education represented in home schooling include:

- The classical model. This rigorous and systematic approach to education began in the universities of the medieval West and was ultimately derived from the ancient Greek notion of education as *paideia*, or bringing the student into the full excellence of human thought and culture. The "Great Books" tradition, which began at the University of Chicago in the 1950s, is a modern version of this educational ideal. The Great Books Foundation, which is still based in Chicago, recently added a Junior Great Books program to its offerings.
- Waldorf (Steiner) education. Waldorf or Steiner education is a worldwide system of schooling based on the ideas of Rudolf Steiner (1861-1925), an anthroposophist who believed that children's cognitive, emotional, and physical growth take place in three stages representing the gradual embodiment of an immortal soul in a human body. Waldorf education emphasizes the development of the child's oral rather than written language (foreign languages are taught as early as first grade); an unusual amount of time devoted to arts and crafts; freedom to explore the outdoors; and a movement art called eurhythmy.
- Montessori method. This approach to education focuses on the individuality of each child, the natural joy of learning, the child's freedom to explore subjects that interest him or her within appropriate limits, and guidance in practical life skills that include kind and gracious interactions with other people.
- Individual tutoring. This tradition of education goes back as far as the philosopher Aristotle, who was the private tutor of Alexander the Great. More recently, bright middle-class children in the United Kingdom sometimes went to live with the tutor in his or her family home for several months to a year as part of intensive preparation for university entrance.
- Accelerated or college-level online courses for gifted students. Stanford and other leading universities have set up online courses that home-schooled students with particular interests in mathematics, physics, English literature, or the arts can take for college credit while still living at home. This type of challenging online program is particularly helpful for students with exceptional talent or interest in one particular field.

Background and history of home schooling

Before the mid-nineteenth century, home schooling was common in North America and Europe. Public schools became widespread in the United States in the 1830s, though many rural families found it inconvenient for their children to travel long distances to school. The first compulsory education law was passed in 1852; by the turn of the twentieth century, children in most communities were required to attend school, usually through eighth grade. Home schooling became for the most part obsolete. But dissatisfaction with public education led some parents and educators back to the home school option in the 1970s. The writings of Raymond and Dorothy Moore, two former U.S. Department of Education officials, and John Holt, author of several books on education, gave credence and national presence to a growing home school movement. The number of families schooling at home grew tremendously in the 1980s, with the majority of such families being fundamentalist Protestants. The rise in home schooling led to numerous legal confrontations; through changes in state laws and precedent-setting legal cases, however, many barriers to home schooling dropped away by the early 1990s. Simultaneously, many studies of home-schooled children demonstrated that they scored consistently better than or equal to their peers from traditional schools on academic achievement tests.

Reasons for home schooling

Reasons for schooling children at home differ from **family** to family. The majority of families in the United States choose home schooling for religious reasons. About 80 percent of families who home school identify themselves as Christian, with many coming from fundamentalist or evangelical sects, although Roman Catholics now also have religiously oriented home–schooling materials. Many Christian families, as well as some Jewish families, prefer to home-school because they **fear** public schools foster a moral environment at odds with their own. Furthermore, they may disagree with the curriculum or fear the influence of non-Christian students on their children. Muslim families are also interested in home schooling; according to one Canadian report, Muslims represent the fastest-growing segment of families choosing home schooling for religious reasons.

On the other hand, a growing number of families home-school for nonreligious reasons. Some parents believe that children should be allowed to learn at their own pace. Raymond Moore claims that children are not ready for formal academic learning until age eight or ten, or even older. Home-schooled children need not follow a regular school curriculum, which teaches reading in first grade, for example, and multiplication in the third grade. The home-schooling parent and child might determine together when the child is ready to read or multiply. Other parents choose to home-school because their children are gifted in one field or another and bored in school. Parents of children with physical handicaps or other special needs often prefer to home-school, as do military families and others that must move frequently due to one or both parents' occupation. It is significant that 85 percent of home–schooling parents mention concern for the child's physical **safety** as one reason for their decision to educate the child at home, according to the National Center for Education Statistics (NCES). Home-schooling is most popular in the primary grades; about one-third of all home-schooled students eventually return to conventional schools, usually for high school.

Curriculum

Figures vary as to how many home schools use published curricula or correspondence courses, but the Department of Education estimated in 1996 that it was between 25 and 50 percent; the rest used a curriculum that the parents and/or child had devised. The most recent (2003) figures from NCES indicate that home-schooling parents use the following resources for books, curricula, and other educational materials:

- public library: 78 percent
- home–schooling catalog or publisher: 77 percent
- retail bookstore: 68 percent
- education publisher not affiliated with home–schooling: 60 percent
- Internet or correspondence distance learning: 41 percent
- church, synagogue, or other religious institution: 37 percent
- local public school or district: 23 percent

The education writer John Holt, a champion of home schooling, suggested that no particular area of study was essential. He recommended what he called "unschooling," advising parents to use such real-life activities as work in a family business, writing letters, bookkeeping, observing nature, and talking with old people as meaningful academic lessons. Home schools might fall anywhere on this spectrum between the tightly planned study of a formal curriculum to Holt's free-form approach to experiential learning.

Considerations

Some legal obstacles still remain for parents who home school. For instance, some parents who teach their children at home have sued school districts for denying access to school equipment or **extracurricular activities**. While some public and private schools have accommodated home-schooled children with access to science labs and participation in **sports** teams, others have resisted. Many parents who have opted to home-school vilify public schools, while educators often stress that home-schooled children are not fully socialized because they are not exposed to children from different backgrounds and levels of ability. Though there is some remaining social stigma attached to children who have been home-schooled, a recent University of Michigan study of home-schooled children found them to be well-adjusted socially.

Parents interested in teaching their children at home must find out what laws apply to their state and school district. Many resources are available through the organizations listed below.

KEY TERMS

Home Schooling—Teaching children at home rather than sending them to a public or private school.

Research and evaluation

Home-schooling does not appear to hinder children's later adjustment to the adult world but rather fosters it. A study commissioned by the Home School Legal Defense Association (HSLDA) reported in 2003 that adults who were home-schooled as children are more satisfied with their education as well as more involved in their communities than those who attended conventional public or private schools: 71 percent participate in community activities (church or synagogue-related groups, sports teams, neighborhood associations, etc.) compared to 37 percent of American adults in the same age groups who went to public schools. Seventy-six percent of home-school "graduates" voted within the last five years, compared to 29 percent of the general adult population; and 59 percent of those who were home–schooled reported that they were "very happy" with their education, compared to 27 percent of the general population.

Resources

BOOKS

Cousins, Ruth. *College Admission 101: A Guide for Homeschooling Families.* Bloomington, IN: CrossBooks Publishing, 2010.

Haskins, Sonya. *Homeschooling for the Rest of Us: How Your One-of-a-Kind Family Can Make Homeschooling and Real Life Work.* Ada, MI: Bethany House, 2010.

Kunzman, Robert. *Write These Laws on Your Children: Inside the World of Conservative Christian Homeschooling.* Boston, MA: Beacon Press, 2010.

LearningExpress Editors. *Homeschooling FAQs: 101 Questions Every Homeschooling Parent Should Ask.* New York, NY: LearningExpress, LLC., 2010.

Linsenbach, Sherri. *The Everything Homeschooling Book: All you need to create the best curriculum and learning environment for your child,* 2nd ed. Avon, MA: Adams Media, 2010.

McGrath, Sara. *Unschooling: A Lifestyle of Learning.* Raleigh, NC: lulu.com, 2010.

Weldon, Laura Grace. *Free Range Learning: How Homeschooling Changes Everything.* . PRESCOTT, AZ: Hohm Press, 2010.

PERIODICALS

Gordon, Amy. "Catholic Homeschooling." *Catholic Insight* 13 (July-August 2005): 41.

"Homeschoolers Support a Range of Businesses." *Colorado Springs Business Journal,* March 31, 2006.

Pride, Mary. "It's Never Too Soon." *Practical Homeschooling* 70 (May-June 2006): 1-2.

Smith, Catherine Arnott, Ph.D. "In a Class of Their Own: Homeschoolers and Public Libraries Are a Perfect Combination." *School Library Journal* 51 (October 2005): 13.

OTHER

National Center for Education Statistics (NCES). *Homeschooling in the United States: 2003* Washington, DC: NCES, 2006. Available online at, http://nces.ed.gov/pubs2006/homeschool/index.asp.

ORGANIZATIONS

Great Books Foundation
Junior Great Books
Address:35 East Wacker Drive, Suite 2300
Chicago, IL 60601-2205
Telephone: Toll-free (800) 222-5870
Website: www.greatbooks.org

Home School Legal Defense Association (HSLDA)
Address: P.O. Box 3000
Purcellville, VA 20134
Telephone: (540) 338-5600
Website: www.hslda.org

National Home Education Network (NHEN)
Address: P.O. Box 1652
Hobe Sound, FL 33475
Fax (no telephone): (413) 581-1463
Website: http://www.homeschool-curriculum-and-support.com/index.html

Stanford University Education Program for Gifted Youth (EPGY)
Address: Ventura Hall, 220 Panama Street
Stanford, CA 94305-4101
Telephone: (800) 372-EPGY
Website: http://epgy.stanford.edu

Laura Jean Cataldo, RN, Ed.D.

Homosexuality

Definition

Homosexuality is the enduring emotional, romantic, or sexual attraction to individuals of one's own gender.

Description

For most of history, open discussions about homosexuality-sexual attraction to people of one's own gender-have been taboo. Men and women with a homosexual orientation are referred to as gay, while the term lesbian refers to women only. **Bisexuality** refers to persons who are attracted to members of either sex. Homosexuality and bisexuality were classified as a mental disorder until 1973, when the American Psychiatric Association removed them from the ***Diagnostic and Statistical Manual of Mental Disorders.*** Some decades later, bias and discrimination against gay people and bisexuals still exist, but sexual orientation is discussed more openly. Much more, however, is known about gay men than about gay women or bisexuals, who have not been studied as extensively.

There are no reliable statistics on the number of people who are homosexual, whether in the United States or in other countries. The American researcher Alfred C. Kinsey conducted extensive surveys on sexual behavior in the 1950s, and estimated that about 4 percent of men and 3 percent of women were exclusively homosexual; however, his research found that 37 percent of men and 28 percent of women had had some sexual experience with a person of their own gender. Most researchers in the 1990s estimate the percentage of the population with homosexual orientation at 2 to 5 percent, while recognizing that the estimate is based on projections rather than hard statistics.

The four components of human sexuality are biological sex, **gender identity** (the psychological sense of being male or female), sexual orientation, and social sex role (adherence to cultural norms for feminine and masculine behavior). Sexual orientation refers to emotional, romantic, sexual, or affectionate feelings of attraction to individuals of a particular gender. Sexual orientation may or may not be reflected by the individual in his or her behavior, because feelings of attraction may be repressed or ignored for any number of reasons. It is also important to distinguish between homosexuality and transsexuality; a homosexual is a person who is attracted to and aroused by members of his or her own sex; a transsexual is a person who believes that his or her innate gender is different from his or her biologically determined gender. In addition, homosexuality should be distinguished from transvestism (cross-dressing), which refers to the practice of dressing in the clothing of the opposite sex. Cross-dressing, which is much more common in men than in women, is often independent of a person's sexual orientation.

Through history, various theories have been proposed regarding the source and development of sexual orientation. Many scientists believe that sexual orientation is shaped for most people at an early age through complex interactions among biological, psychological, and social factors. With regard to biological factors, there is no consensus as of the early 2000s as to the role of genetics, hormonal influences on the brain prior to **birth**, neurochemical differences in the brain after birth, or structural differences in the brain in determining sexual orientation; research in these areas is ongoing.

One outline of the developmental process involved in one's sexual orientation identifies four stages (age ranges given are generalizations):

- Sensitization (early and middle childhood): a period of vague awareness of being different, but the feelings are nonspecific and nonsexual in nature.
- Identity confusion (early teens): the person may be aware of feelings toward others of the same sex, may deny such feelings, or may be experimenting with sex. Use of Internet chat rooms at this age may serve to explore feelings, but also makes younger teenagers vulnerable to online predators.
- Identity assumption (18-21 years): the person now identifies as gay, lesbian, or bisexual (GLB) to him- or herself. He or she may or may not disclose his or her identity to friends, or may have several different sets of friends, some of whom know and others who do not. The person may or may not join adult gay support groups or social groups. Males in this age group are more likely to engage in unsafe sexual practices; they are at increased risk of anal cancer, eating disorders, and drug abuse. They should receive regular health screening and preventive health services.
- Commitment (after 21): the person openly acknowledges a GLB orientation to parents and other relatives. Males should continue to receive regular health screening.

The process of identity development for lesbians and gay men, usually called "coming out," has been found to be strongly related to psychological adjustment. Being able to discuss one's sexual orientation is a sign of positive mental health and strong **self-esteem** for a gay man or lesbian. But even for those gays and lesbians who have adjusted psychologically to their sexual orientation, false stereotypes and prejudice make the process of "coming out" challenging. Lesbian and gay people must risk rejection by **family**, friends, co-workers, and religious institutions when they share their sexual orientation. For this reason it is unethical for a **pediatrician** or other medical professional to disclose a teenager's homosexuality to his or her parents without the patient's permission.

In addition, violence and discrimination are still real threats. Legal protection from discrimination and violence for gay and lesbian people is important. Some states categorize violence against an individual on the basis of her or his sexual orientation as a "hate crime" with more stringent punishment. Most U.S. states have laws against educational, employment, or housing discrimination on the basis of sexual orientation as of the early 2000s.

Some well-meaning parents have sought therapy to help their child change his or her sexual orientation, especially when the admission of homosexuality seems to be causing the child great emotional pain. In 1990, the American Psychological Association stated that scientific evidence does not support conversion therapy; in fact, the evidence reveals that it can actually be psychologically damaging to attempt conversion. Sexual orientation is a complex component of one's personality not limited to sexual behavior. Altering sexual orientation is to attempt to alter a key aspect of the individual's identity.

Like people of other sexual orientations, a percentage of gays and lesbians seek counseling. They may see a therapist for any of the reasons many people seek help–coping with grief, **anxiety**, or other mental health or relationship difficulties; they are, however, at increased risk of depression and **substance abuse** disorders. In addition, they may seek psychological help in adjusting to their sexual orientation and in dealing with prejudice, discrimination, and rejection. Families who are adjusting to the news that one of their members is homosexual may also seek counseling to help with the complex feelings and prejudices that such news may elicit.

Since sexual orientation usually (though not always) emerges in adolescence—already a stage of challenging emotional, social, and physical development—families of adolescent gays and lesbians should learn as much as they can about sexual orientation. Educational materials and support and discussion groups exist for both adolescents and their family members.

Resources

BOOKS

American Psychiatric Association. *Diagnostic and Statistical Manual of Mental Disorders*, fourth edition, text revision. Washington, DC: American Psychiatric Association, 2000.

Bamberg-Smith, Barbara A. *The Psychology of Sex and Gender*. Boston: Pearson/Allyn and Bacon, 2007.

Diamant, Louis, and Richard D. McAnulty, eds. *The Psychology of Sexual Orientation, Behavior, and Identity: A Handbook*. Westport, CT: Greenwood Press, 1995.

Garnets, L. D. and D. C. Kimmel. *Psychological Perspectives on Lesbian, Gay, and Bisexual Experiences*, 2nd ed. New York: Columbia University Press, 2003.

Perrin, Ellen C. *Sexual Orientation in Child and Adolescent Health Care*. New York: Kluwer Academic/Plenum Publishers, 2002.

PERIODICALS

Eisenberg, M. E., and D. Resnick. "Suicidality among Gay, Lesbian, and Bisexual Youth: The Role of Protective Factors." *Journal of Adolescent Health* 39 (November 2006): 662-668.

Knight, Daniel, MD. "Health Care Screening for Men Who Have Sex with Men." *American Family Physician* 69 (May 1, 2004): 2149-2156.

Reitman, David S., MD. "Sexuality: Sexual Orientation." *eMedicine*, June 12, 2006. Available online at, *http://www.emedicine.com/ped/topic2773.htm*.

OTHER

American Academy of Child and Adolescent Psychiatry (AACAP). Facts for Families #63. *Gay, Lesbian and Bisexual Adolescents* Washington, DC: AACAP, 2006.

ORGANIZATIONS

American Academy of Child and Adolescent Psychiatry (AACAP), 3615 Wisconsin Ave. NW, Washington DC, 20016, (202) 966-7300, http://www.aacap.org.

Gay Men's Health Crisis (GMHC), The Tisch Building, 119 West 24th Street, New York NY, 10011, (212) 367-1000, (800) AIDS-NYC (800-243-7692), http://www.gmhc.org.

National Gay and Lesbian Task Force, 1325 Massachusetts Avenue, NW, Suite 600, Washington DC, 20005, (202 393-5177, http://www.thetaskforce.org.

Parents and Friends of Lesbians and Gays (PFLAG), 1726 M Street, NW, Suite 400, Washington DC, 20036, 202-467-8180, http://www.pflag.org.

Society for Adolescent Medicine (SAM), 1916 Copper Oaks Circle, Blue Springs MO, 64015, (816) 224-8010, http://www.adolescenthealth.org.

HPV *see* Human papillomavirus

HPV vaccination

Definition

HPV **vaccination** refers to the administration of a vaccine to protect against human papillovirus (HPV) infection.

Purpose

Human papillomavirus (HPV) is the most common sexually-transmitted virus in the United States. Most HPV infections do not cause any symptoms, and disappear on their own. But it is now known that HPV can cause cervical **cancer** in women. Every year in the United States, approximately 11,000 women are diagnosed with cervical cancer and 4,000 die from it. Cervical cancer is the second leading cause of cancer deaths among women around the world. It is estimated that as much as two-thirds of the cervical cancer deaths around the world could be eliminated if all women were immunized with the HPV vaccine prior to infection with HPV.

There are approximately 40 types of genital HPV. In the United States, about 20 million people are infected, with about 6.2 million new cases of genital HPV infection reported each year. Some HPV types can cause cervical cancer in women and can also cause other kinds of cancer in both men and women. HPV infection has been linked to oropharyngeal cancer and cancers of the anus, vulva, vagina, and penis. Other types of HPV can cause **genital warts** in both males and females or **warts** in the upper respiratory tract. The HPV vaccines work by preventing the most common types of HPV that cause cervical cancer and genital warts.

Description

In June 2006, the Advisory Committee on Immunization Practices (ACIP) voted to recommend the first vaccine developed to prevent cervical cancer and other diseases in females caused by certain types of genital human papillomavirus (HPV). This vaccine, Gardasil, manufactured by the pharmaceutical company Merck, is a quadrivalent vaccine that protects against four HPV types (types 6, 11, 16, and 18), which together cause 70% of cervical cancers and 90% of genital warts. The Food and Drug Administration (FDA) licensed this vaccine for use in girls and women, between the ages of 9–26 years. Gardasil has also been approved by the FDA for use in males ages 9 to 26 years to prevent genital warts caused by HPV types 6 and 11.

In 2009 drug manufacturer GlaxoSmithKline released a second HPV vaccine, Cervarix. Cervarix is a bivalent vaccine, meaning it protects against HPV infection from two HPV types (types 16 and 18) which can cause precancerous and cancerous tumors of the cervix. Cervarix does not protect against genital warts (caused by HPV types 6 and 11). Cervarix has been approved by the FDA for use in females ages 10 to 25 years for the prevention of cervical cancer caused by HPV types 16 and 18.

KEY TERMS

Cervical cancer—Cancer of the entrance to the womb (uterus). The cervix is the lower, narrow part of the uterus (womb).

Cervical cancer screening—Use of the Papanicolaou (Pap) smear test to detect cervical cancer in the early curable stage.

Intramuscularly—A medication given by needle into a muscle.

Pathogen—A disease–causing microorganism.

Quadrivalent vaccine—A vaccine that protects against four pathogens.

Virus—A microorganism smaller than a bacteria, which cannot grow or reproduce apart from a living cell. Viruses cause many common human infections, and are also responsible for many rare diseases.

Wart—A raised growth on the surface of the skin or other organ.

Recommended dosage

The HPV vaccine is routinely administered to girls 11 and 12 years of age and is given in a series of three injections over a six-month period. The second and third doses are given one and six months after the first dose. Each dose of quadrivalent HPV vaccine is 0.5 mL, administered intramuscularly. It is important for girls to get vaccinated before their first sexual contact, i.e., before they can be exposed to HPV. For immunized girls, the vaccine can prevent almost 100% of the diseases caused by the types of HPVs targeted by the vaccine. Girls as young as 9 years old can receive the vaccine. The vaccine is also recommended for girls and women 13 through 26 years of age who did not receive it when they were younger. Additional (booster) doses are not recommended at this time. Studies are underway to determine whether booster vaccinations are necessary. HPV vaccine may be given at the same time as other vaccines.

Precautions

Vaccines can cause severe allergic reactions, like all medications. The risk of a vaccine causing serious harm, or **death**, is extremely small. Overwhelmingly, health practitioners recommend vaccination over the risk of suffering the disease against which it protects. However, some girls should not get the HPV vaccine. They include:

- Any girl who has ever had a life-threatening allergic reaction to yeast, to any other component of HPV vaccine, or to a previous dose of HPV vaccine.
- Pregnant women should not get vaccinated since no data is yet available on its safety in mothers and the unborn baby. Women who are breast feeding may safely get the vaccine.
- Girls with moderate or severe illnesses should wait until they recover.

Protection from HPV vaccine is expected to be long-lasting. However, vaccinated women still need cervical cancer screening because the vaccine does not protect against all HPV types that cause cervical cancer.

Side effects

According to the CDC, the following problems may follow HPV vaccination:

- Pain at the injection site (8 people in 10)
- Redness or swelling at the injection site (1 person in 4)
- Mild fever (100°F/37.8°C) (1 person in 10)
- Itching at the injection site (1 person in 30)
- Moderate fever (102°F/38.9°C) (1 person in 65)

A small number of patients receiving the HPV vaccine have experienced syncope (fainting) or seizures. Patients receiving the vaccine should be observed for 15 minutes after receiving each dose.

Interactions

The FDA has licensed the HPV vaccine as safe and effective. This vaccine has been tested in thousands of females (9 to 26 years of age) around the world no serious interactions or side effects.

Some medicines may interact with HPV vaccine. Alkylating agents (eg, cyclophosphamide), antimetabolites (eg, fluorouracil, methotrexate), cytotoxics (eg, cisplatin), or corticosteroids (eg, prednisone) may decrease the HPV vaccine's effectiveness.

Resources

BOOKS

Nardo, Don. *Human Papillomavirus (HPV).* Farmington Hills: Lucent Books (Gale), 2007.

PERIODICALS

Ault, K. A. "Long–term efficacy of human papillomavirus vaccination." *Gynecologic Oncology* 107, no. 2 (November 2007): S27–S30.

Brisson, M., Van de Velde, N., De Wals, P., Boily, M. C. "Estimating the number needed to vaccinate to prevent diseases and death related to human papillomavirus infection." *Canadian Medical Association Journal* 177, no. 5 (August 2007): 464–468.

Bryan, J. T. "Developing an HPV vaccine to prevent cervical cancer and genital warts." *Vaccine* 25, no. 16 (2007): 3001–3006.

Garcia, F. A., Saslow, D. "Prophylactic human papillomavirus vaccination: a breakthrough in primary cervical cancer prevention." *Obstetrics and Gynecology Clinics of North America* 34, no. 4 (December 2007): 761–781.

Giuliano, A. R. "Human papillomavirus vaccination in males." *Gynecology and Oncolgy* 107, suppl. 2 (November 2007): S24–S26.

Hairon, N. "HPV vaccination of girls to help prevent cervical cancer." *Nursing Times* 103, no. 45 (2007): 23–24.

Hutchinson, D.J., Klein, C.K."Human Papillomavirus disease and vaccines."*American Journal of Health-System Pharmacy*65, no. 22 (2009):2105–2112.

Nour, N.M."Cervical cancer: A preventable death."*Reviews in Obstetrics and Gynecology*2, no. 4 (2009):240–244.

OTHER

HPV Vaccination Webpage, CDC (February 4, 2010), http://www.cdc.gov/vaccines/vpd-vac/hpv/default.htm

HPV Vaccine Questions and Answers Webpage, CDC (June 26, 2008), http://www.cdc.gov/std/hpv/STDFact-HPV-vaccine-young-women-htm

Human Papillomavirus (HPV) Prevention and HPV Vaccine: Questions and Answers Webpage, Public Health Agency of Canada (June 18, 2007), http://www.phac-aspc.gc.ca/std-mts/hpv-vph/hpv-vph-vaccine_e.html

Human Papillomavirus (HPV) Vaccines: Questions and Answers Webpage, National Cancer Institute (October 22, 2009), http://www.cancer.gov/cancertopics/factsheet/Prevention/HPV-vaccine

Vaccine Information: Human papillomavirus (HPV) Webpage, National Network for Immunization Information (March 23, 2010), http://www.immunizationinfo.org/vaccines/human-papillomavirus-hpv

ORGANIZATIONS

Centers for Disease Control and Prevention (CDC), 1600 Clifton Road, Atlanta GA, 30333, (404) 498-1515, (800) 311-3435, http://www.cdc.gov.

National Institute of Allergy and Infectious Disease, 31 Center Drive MSC 2520, Building 31, Room 7A-50, Bethesda MD, 20892-2520, (301) 496-5717, (800) 877-8339 (TTY), http://www.niaid.nih.gov/default.htm.

National Network for Immunization Information, 301 University Blvd, Galveston TX, 77555-0350, (409) 772-0199, nnii@i4ph.org, http://www.immunizationinfo.org/.

National Vaccine Program Office, U.S. Department of Health & Human Services, 200 Independence Avenue, SW, Washington D.C., 20201, (877) 696-6775, http://www.hhs.gov/nvpo/.

Monique Laberge, PhD
Melinda Granger Oberleitner, RN, DNS, APRN, CNS

Huffing **see Inhalants and related disorders**

Human bite infections

Definition

Human bite infections are potentially serious infections caused by rapid growth of bacteria in broken skin.

Description

Bites—animal and human—are responsible for about 1% of visits to emergency rooms. Bite injuries are more common during the summer months.

Closed–fist injury

In adults, the most common form of human bite is the closed–fist injury, sometimes called the "fight bite." These injuries result from the breaking of the skin over the knuckle joint when a person's fist strikes someone's teeth during a fight.

Causes and symptoms

In children, bite infections result either from accidents during play or from fighting. Most infected **bites** in adults result from fighting.

The infection itself can be caused by a number of bacteria that live in the human mouth. These include streptococci, staphylococci, anaerobic organisms, and *Eikenella corrodens*. Infections that begin less than 24 hours after the injury are usually produced by a mixture of organisms and can cause a necrotizing infection (causing the **death** of a specific area of tissue), in which tissue is rapidly destroyed. If a bite is infected, the skin will be sore, red, swollen, and warm to the touch.

Diagnosis

In most cases the diagnosis is made by an emergency room physician on the basis of the patient's history.

Because the human mouth contains a variety of bacteria, the physician will order a laboratory culture to choose the most effective antibiotic.

Treatment

Treatment involves surgical attention as well as medications. Because bites cause puncturing and tearing of skin rather than clean-edged cuts, they must be

KEY TERMS

Antibiotic—A drug used to treat infections caused by bacteria and other microorganisms.

Bacteria—Single-celled microorganisms that can be seen only through a microscope. Many bacteria cause disease.

carefully cleansed. The doctor will wash the wound with water under high pressure and debride it. Debridement is the removal of dead tissue and **foreign objects** from a wound to prevent infection. If the bite is a closed-fist injury, the doctor will look for torn tendons or damage to the spaces between the joints. Examination includes **x rays** to check for bone **fractures** or foreign objects in the wound.

Doctors do not usually suture a bite wound because the connective tissues and other structures in the hand form many small closed spaces that make it easy for infection to spread. Emergency room doctors often consult surgical specialists if a patient has a deep closed-fist injury or one that appears already infected.

The doctor will make sure that the patient is immunized against **tetanus**, which is routine procedure for any open wound. A study released in June 2004 showed that routine use of **antibiotics** for human bites may not be necessary, as physicians try to minimize overuse of antibiotics. Superficial **wounds** in low-risk areas may no longer need antibiotic treatment, but more serious human bites to high-risk areas such as the hands should be treated with antibiotics to prevent serious infection. Patients with closed-fist injuries may need inpatient treatment in addition to an intravenous antibiotic.

Prognosis

The prognosis depends on the location of the bite and whether it was caused by a child or an adult. Bites caused by children rarely become infected because they are usually shallow. Between 15–30% of bites caused by adults become infected, with a higher rate for closed-fist injuries.

Prevention

Prevention of human bite infections depends upon prompt treatment of any bite caused by a human being, particularly a closed-fist injury.

Resources

PERIODICALS

"Do All Human Bite Wounds Need Antibiotics?" *Emergency Medicine Alert* June 2004: 3.

ORGANIZATIONS

Centers for Disease Control and Prevention (CDC), 1600 Clifton Road, Atlanta GA, 30333, (404) 498-1515, (800) 311-3435, http://www.cdc.gov.

National Institute of Allergy and Infectious Disease 31 Center Drive MSC 2520, Building 31, Room 7A-50, Bethesda MD, 20892-2520 (301) 496-5717, (800) 877-8339 (TTY), http://www.niaid.nih.gov/default.htm.

ORGANIZATIONS

Centers for Disease Control and Prevention (CDC), 1600 Clifton Rd., Atlanta GA, 30333, 800-311-3435, http://www.cdc.gov.

National Institutes of Health (NIH), 9000 Rockville Pike, Bethesda MD, 20892, 301-496-4000, http://www.nih.gov/index.html.

Rebecca J. Frey, Ph.D.
Teresa G. Odle
Laura Jean Cataldo, RN, Ed.D.

Human papilloma virus

Definition

HPV infection is a sexually transmitted disease (STD) caused by 30-40 of the 130 or so known strains of human papillomavirus, the name of a group of viruses that infect the skin and mucous membranes of humans and some animals. In humans these sexually transmitted strains can cause **genital warts**, precancerous changes in the tissues of the female vagina, or cervical **cancer**. Other strains of HPV are responsible for **warts** on the soles of the feet (plantar warts), common warts on the hands, and flat warts on the face or legs.

Demographics

In recent years HPV infection has become the most common STD in the United States. Approximately 20 million Americans are infected with HPV as of 2009, and another 6.2 million people become newly infected each year. According to one study, 27 percent of women between the ages of 14 and 59 are infected with one or more types of HPV, and 35% of homosexual men. The Centers for Disease Control and Prevention (CDC) estimates that more than 80 percent of American women will contract at least one strain of genital HPV by age 50. About 75-80 percent of sexually active Americans of either sex will be infected with HPV at some point in their lifetime.

As far as is known, men and women are at equal risk of being infected with HPV, as are members of all races and ethnic groups.

In terms of specific illnesses associated with HPV, 11,000 women are diagnosed with cervical cancer each year in the United States and 3,900 women die of the disease. Another 5,800 women are diagnosed with cancers of the vagina and the external female genitals, while 3,300 men are diagnosed with cancer of the penis or the anal area. The risk of anal cancer is 17 to 31 times higher among gay and bisexual men than among heterosexual men.

Description

The family of human papilloma viruses includes a large number of genetically related viruses. Many of these cause warts, including the warts commonly found on the skin. Another group of HPV preferentially infect the mucosal surfaces of the genitals, including the penis, vagina, vulva, and cervix. These are spread among adults by sexual contact. One group of HPV that infect the genitals causes soft warts, often designated condylomata acuminata. These genital warts are quite common and rarely if ever become cancerous. The most common of these low-risk HPV types are designated HPV 6 and 11.

The second group of viruses, termed high-risk HPV types, is associated with the development of cervical cancer. Individuals infected with these viruses are at higher risk for the development of precancerous lesions. Typically, infection with these viruses is common in adolescents and women in their twenties, and usually do not result in cancerous growth. The most common high-risk HPV is type 16. The appearance of abnormal cells containing high-risk HPV types is seen most frequently in women over the age of 30 who have abnormal Pap smears.

It is possible that other viruses work together with human papilloma viruses to produce precancerous changes in tissue. Cases of tongue cancer have been reported in which HPV was found together with Epstein-Barr virus, or EBV. **Smoking**, the use of **oral contraceptives** for birth control for longer than 5 years, and suppression of the **immune system** are also thought to be factors that combine with HPV infection to lead to precancerous lesions in tissue.

Risk factors

Some people are at greater risk of sexually transmitted HPV than others:

- Gay and bisexual men.
- People with HIV or other diseases that weaken the immune system.
- Males or females below age 25. Younger people appear to be more biologically vulnerable to the HPV virus.
- People who have large numbers of sexual partners.
- People in relationships with partners who have sex with many other people.
- People who must take drugs that suppress the immune system.

Causes and symptoms

Causes

The cause of sexually transmitted HPV infection is one or more strains of the human papillomavirus. The virus enters the body through small breaks in the skin surface or in the mucous membranes lining the genitals. In most cases the body fights off the virus within a few weeks. In some people, however, HPV remains dormant for a period ranging from a few weeks to three years in one of the lower layers of skin cells. The virus then begins to replicate (copy itself) when these cells mature and move upward to the surface of the skin. The virus affects the shape of the cells, leading to the formation of noticeable warts, precancerous changes in skin cells, or cervical cancer. About 1 percent of sexually active adults in the United States have genital warts at any one time; about 10 percent of women with high-risk HPV in the tissues of their cervix will develop long-lasting HPV infections that put them at risk for cervical cancer.

The percentages of cancers caused by high-risk types of HPV are as follows:

- Cervical cancer: 100%.
- Anal cancer: 90%.
- Cancer of the vulva: 40%.
- Vaginal cancer: 40%.
- Oropharyngeal cancer: 12%.
- Oral cancer: 3%.

Symptoms in adults

Symptoms of sexually transmitted HPV infection may include:

- Genital warts. These appear as bumps or clusters of fleshy outgrowths around the anus or on the genitals. Some may grow into large cauliflower-shaped masses. Genital warts usually appear within weeks or months after sexual contact with an infected person. If left untreated, genital warts may go away, remain unchanged, or increase in size or number but will not turn into cancers. It is possible, however, for a person to be infected with a high-risk strain of HPV as well as one of the strains that cause genital warts; therefore the appearance of genital warts does not necessarily mean that the person is not at risk of cancer.

- Precancerous changes in the tissues of the female cervix. These are flat growths on the cervix that cannot be seen or felt by the infected woman.
- Cancer. High-risk strains of HPV can cause cancers of the mouth and throat as well as cancers of the anal area and the male and female genitals. These typically take years to develop after infection. In men, symptoms of anal cancer may include bleeding, pain, or a discharge from the anus, or changes in bowel habits. Early signs of cancer of the penis may include thickening of the skin, tissue growths, or sores.

It is not fully understood as of 2010 why most infections with high-risk HPV are of short duration, while a small percentage persist and eventually transform cervical cells to a state of cancerous growth.

Symptoms in children

In addition to producing precancerous lesions in some patients, HPV infections in women are a health concern because they can be transmitted to the respiratory tract of a baby during **childbirth**. This type of HPV infection may lead to a rare disorder known as juvenile-onset recurrent respiratory papillomatosis (JO-RRP) or laryngeal papillomatosis, in which papillomas or warts form in the child's airway, producing hoarseness or partial blockage of the windpipe. Although laryngeal papillomatosis can occur in HPV-infected adults, 60–80% of cases occur in children, most of them younger than three years.

Laryngeal papillomatosis is usually diagnosed by laryngoscopy. Surgery, whether traditional or laser surgery, is the usual treatment for JO-RRP, but the warts often recur and require additional surgery to remove them. In extreme cases, the patient may be given a tracheotomy, a procedure in which a hole is cut through the throat into the windpipe and a tube is inserted to keep the breathing hole open. A newer treatment for the disorder is photodynamic therapy or PDT. In PDT, a special light-sensitive dye is injected into the patient's blood. The dye collects in the tumors rather than in healthy tissue. When bright light of a specific wavelength is shined on the throat, it destroys the tumors containing the dye.

Cidofovir and interferon are often given as adjuvant treatments for this disease as of the early 2000s. JO-RRP is a serious illness, leading to **death** in a significant number of affected children. In a very few cases, respiratory papillomatosis can lead to cancer as well as breathing difficulties.

KEY TERMS

Ablative—Also known as "ablation" and referring to the surgical removal of lesions associated with HPV.

Biopsy—The removal of a small bit of tissue for diagnostic examination

Cervical intra-epithelial neoplasia (CIN)—A pre-cancerous condition in which a group of cells grow abnormally on the cervix but do not extend into the deeper layers of this tissue.

Cervix—The narrow neck or outlet of a woman's uterus.

Colposcopy—Procedure in which the cervix is examined using a special microscope.

Condylomata acuminata (singular, condyloma acuminatum)—The medical term for infectious warts on the genitals caused by HPV.

Cryotherapy—The use of liquid nitrogen or other forms of extreme cold to destroy tissue.

Epithelial—Referring to the epithelium, the layer of cells forming the epidermis of the skin and the surface layer of mucous membranes.

High-risk HPV type—A member of the HPV family of viruses that is associated with the development of cervical cancer and precancerous growths.

Pap test—A screening test for cervical cancer devised by Giorgios Papanikolaou (1883–1962) in the 1940s.

Photodynamic therapy (PDT)—A treatment for tumors in which a light-sensitive dye is injected into the blood (or skin) to be taken up selectively by the tumors. Light of a specific wavelength is then applied to the affected area to kill the tumors.

Topical—Referring to a type of medication applied directly to the skin or outside of the body.

Tracheotomy—A surgical procedure in which a hole is cut through the neck to open a direct airway through an incision in the trachea (windpipe).

Diagnosis

There is no general blood, urine, or imaging test for HPV infection. The diagnosis of genital warts is obvious based on their location and appearance. The doctor may, however, use a vinegar solution to identify HPV-infected areas on the skin of the genitals. The vinegar solution will turn white if HPV is present. Since genital warts are caused by low-risk strains of HPV, the doctor does not need to identify the specific strain of the virus that is present.

Sexually active women should be screened periodically for the presence of changes in the tissues of the cervix. The most common test is the Papanikolaou test or Pap smear, invented by a Greek physician in the 1940s. To perform a Pap smear, the doctor takes a small spatula to obtain cells from the outer surface of the cervix and smears the collected cells on a slide that is then examined in a laboratory for signs of any abnormal cells. If abnormal or questionable cells are found, the doctor may order an HPV DNA test, which can identify the DNA of 13 high-risk types of HPV in cells taken from the cervix.

There are no HPV screening tests for men as of 2009; however, some doctors are suggesting that anal Pap smears for men who have sex with men would be useful in early detection of anal cancer.

Tests

The relationship among HPV, precancerous cellular changes, and cervical cancer have led to the suggestion that testing for the presence of HPV can be a useful addition to Pap smears. Pap smears involve microscopic analysis of cells removed from the cervix. The results of these tests are generally reported as either normal or consistent with the presence of cancer or a precancerous condition. Patients receiving the latter diagnosis usually are treated either by excisional or ablative therapy surgery or some other means in order to remove the tumor or precancerous lesion.

In some cases the cytologist or pathologist examining a Pap smear reports a "borderline" result when abnormal cells are observed, but it is not possible to distinguish whether the changes seen are due to early precancerous changes or to inflammation caused by some infectious agent or irritant. In these cases, some physicians and scientists believe that testing for the presence of HPV can help to identify those women who should be closely followed for the development of early cancerous lesions, or who should undergo colposcopy, a procedure to examine the cervix for precancerous lesions. These cancer precursors, termed cervical intraepithelial neoplasia (CIN) when identified early, before they have become invasive, can almost always be completely removed by minor surgery, essentially curing the patient before the cancer has had a chance to develop. The cervical tissue removed, which includes the precancerous tissue, is examined as part of a biopsy to confirm the diagnosis, and if requested by a doctor, can be tested for the presence of high-risk HPV types.

Treatment

Traditional

Patients with genital warts should *never* use over-the counter-preparations designed to remove common or flat warts from the hands or face. Doctors can treat genital warts with various medical or surgical techniques:

- Cryotherapy. Cryotherapy uses liquid nitrogen to freeze the warts. The dead tissue in the wart falls away from the skin beneath in about a week.
- Imiquimod. Imiquimod (Aldara) is a topical cream that gets rid of genital warts by stimulating the body's immune system to fight the virus that causes the warts.
- Podofilox. Podofilox (Condylox) is a topical medication available in liquid or gel form that destroys the wart tissue.
- Surgery. The doctor can remove the wart by drying it out with an electric needle and then scraping the tissue with a sharp instrument called a curette. Lasers can also be used to remove genital warts.

Low-grade precancerous changes in the tissue of the female cervix are not usually treated directly because most of them will eventually go away on their own without developing into cancer. The patient should, however, see the doctor for follow-up Pap smears to make sure that the tissues are returning to normal. High-risk precancerous lesions are removed, usually by surgery, cryotherapy, electrocauterization, or laser surgery.

Since the incidence of latent and recurrent infections is high, the eradication of HPV is not always 100% effective. It is essential to be aware that HPV is a sexually transmitted disease and women must engage in safe sex practices to decrease the risk of spreading the virus or becoming reinfected. A vaccine effective against four of the HPV types most likely to cause genital warts or cervical cancer was approved for use in 2006; it is described more fully under Prevention below. As of 2009, researchers are working on developing vaccines that protect against additional types of the HPV virus.

Prognosis

The prognosis of sexually transmitted HPV infections depends on the patient's age, number of sexual partners, gender, and the condition of their immune system. Women are significantly more likely than men to develop cancers following HPV infection. However, most people of either sex with normally functioning immune systems who are infected with HPV will clear the infection from their bodies within two years.

Prevention

Preventive measures that people can take to lower their risk of HPV infection include:

- Abstaining from sex, or having sex only with an uninfected partner who is faithful.
- Reducing the number of sexual partners.

- Using condoms regularly during sexual intercourse.
- For women, using a new vaccine called Gardasil. Approved by the Food and Drug Administration (FDA) in 2006, Gardasil is a vaccine that protects against the four types of HPV that cause most cervical cancers and genital warts. The vaccine is recommended for 11- and 12-year-old girls. It is also recommended for girls and women age 13 through 26 who have not yet been vaccinated or completed the vaccine series. Gardasil works best in girls who have not yet been sexually active. It is given as a series of three shots over a six-month period.

A second human papillomavirus vaccine, Cervarix, was approved in Europe, Australia, and the Philippines in 2007. It is awaiting FDA approval for use in the United States as of September 2009.

In addition to giving the available preventive vaccines to women, some doctors think it might be a useful preventive measure to vaccinate men as well to protect their female partners against infection. As of 2009, however, male **vaccination** for HPV is still under discussion rather than being put into clinical practice.

Resources

BOOKS

Gonzales, Lissette. *Frequently Asked Questions about Human Papillomavirus*. New York: Rosen, 2009.

Krueger, Hans, et al. *HPV and Other Infectious Agents in Cancer: Opportunities for Prevention and Public Health*. New York: Oxford University Press, 2010.

Marr, Lisa. *Sexually Transmitted Diseases: A Physician Tells You What You Need to Know*, 2nd ed. Baltimore: Johns Hopkins University Press, 2007.

Nardo, Don. *Human Papillomavirus (HPV)*. Detroit, MI: Lucent Books, 2007.

Rosenblatt, Alberto. *Human Papillomavirus*. New York: Springer, 2009.

PERIODICALS

Burki, T. "Should Males Be Vaccinated against HPV?" *Lancet Oncology* 10 (September 2009): 845.

Haug, C. "The Risks and Benefits of HPV Vaccination." *Journal of the American Medical Association* 302 (August 19, 2009): 795–95.

Hershey, J.H., and L.F. Velez. "Public Health Issues Related to HPV Vaccination." *Journal of Public Health Management and Practice* 15 (September-October 2009): 384–92.

Lindsey, K., et al. "Anal Pap Smears: Should We Be Doing Them?" *Journal of the American Academy of Nurse Practitioners* 21 (August 2009): 437–43.

O'Connor, M. B., and C. O'Connor. "The HPV Vaccine for Men." *International Journal of STD and AIDS* 20 (April 2009): 290–91.

Printz, C. "HPV Status Predicts Survival of Oropharyngeal Cancer Patients." *Cancer* 115 (September 15, 2009): 4045.

Samara, R. N., and S. N. Khleif. "HPV as a Model for the Development of Prophylactic and Therapeutic Cancer Vaccines." *Current Molecular Medicine* 9 (August 2009): 766–73.

Wang, Z., et al. "Detection of Human Papilloma Virus Subtypes 16 and P16(ink4a) in Invasive Squamous Cell Carcinoma of the Fallopian Tube and Concomitant Squamous Cell Carcinoma in Situ of the Cervix." *Journal of Obstetrics and Gynaecology Research* 35 (April 2009): 385–89.

OTHER

Centers for Disease Control and Prevention (CDC) Fact Sheet. *HPV and Men*, http://www.cdc.gov/std/hpv/STDFact-HPV-and-men.htm

Centers for Disease Control and Prevention (CDC). *Human Papillomavirus (HPV) Infection*, http://www.cdc.gov/std/hpv/default.htm

Gearhart, Peter A., and Thomas C. Randall. "Human Papillomavirus." *eMedicine*, August 4, 2009, http://emedicine.medscape.com/article/219110-overview

Mayo Clinic. *HPV Infection*, http://www.mayoclinic.com/health/hpv-infection/DS00906

National Cancer Institute (NCI), http://www.cancer.gov/cancertopics/factsheet/Risk/HPV

National Institute of Allergy and Infectious Diseases (NIAID). *Human Papillomavirus and Genital Warts*, http://www3.niaid.nih.gov/topics/genitalWarts

National Institute on Deafness and Other Communication Disorders (NIDCD). *Laryngeal Papillomatosis*, http://www.nidcd.nih.gov/health/voice/laryngeal.htm

ORGANIZATIONS

American College of Obstetricians and Gynecologists (ACOG), 409 12th St., S.W., P.O. Box 96920, Washington DC, 20090-6920, 202-638-5577, resources@acog.org, http://www.acog.org/.

American Social Health Association (ASHA), P.O. Box 13827, Research Triangle Park NC, 27709, 919-361-8400, 800-227-8922, 919-361-8425, http://www.ashastd.org/index.cfm.

Centers for Disease Control and Prevention (CDC), 1600 Clifton Road, Atlanta GA, 30333, 800-232-4636, cdcinfo@cdc.gov, http://www.cdc.gov.

National Cancer Institute, 6116 Executive Blvd., Room 3036A, Bethesda MD, 20892-8322, 800-422-6237, cancergovstaff@mail.nih.gov, http://www.cancer.gov.

National Institute of Allergy and Infectious Diseases (NIAID), 6610 Rockledge Drive, MSC 6612, Bethesda MD, 20892-6612, 301-496-5717, 866-284-4107, 301-402-3573, http://www3.niaid.nih.gov.

National Institute on Deafness and Other Communication Disorders (NIDCD), 31 Center Drive, MSC 2320, Bethesda MD, 20892-2320, (800) 241-1044, (301) 770-8977, nidcdinfo@nidcd.nih.gov, http://www.nidcd.nih.gov/index.asp.

Warren Maltzman, PhD
Rebecca J. Frey, PhD

Hunter's syndrome *see* **Mucopolysaccharidoses**

Huntington disease

Definition

Huntington disease (HD) is an inherited, progressive, neurodegenerative disease causing uncontrolled physical movements and mental deterioration. The disease was discovered by George Huntington of Pomeroy, Ohio, who first described a hereditary movement disorder.

Demographics

HD is estimated to occur in the United States at a rate of 4.1-8.4 cases per 100,000 people. In most European countries, prevalence ranges from 1.63-9.95 per 100,000 people. It is lower in Finland and Japan (less than 1 case per 100,000 people). Pockets of isolated populations with western European ancestors exist where the prevalence is higher. For example, these include the region of lake Maracaibo in Venezuela (700 per 100,000 people), the island of Mauritius (46 per 100,000 people), and Tasmania (17.4 per 100,000 people). HD is a disease that affects males and females equally.

The mean age at HD onset ranges from 35-44 years. HD onset in patients younger than 10 years and older than 70 years is rare. Modifying genes and environmental factors are thought to influence the age of onset. Fpr example, the Venezuelan age of onset (34.35 y) is on average higher than that of Americans (37.47 y) and Canadians (40.36 y).

Description

Huntington disease is also called Huntington chorea, from the Greek word for "dance," referring to the involuntary movements that develop as the disease progresses. It is occasionally referred to as "Woody Guthrie disease" for the American folk singer who died from it. Huntington disease causes progressive loss of cells in areas of the brain responsible for some aspects of movement control and mental abilities. A person with HD gradually develops abnormal movements and changes in cognition (thinking), behavior and personality.

Risk factors

Children of a parent who carries the gene responsible for HD have a 50% chance of inheriting the abnormal gene.

Causes and symptoms

Mutations in the HTT gene cause Huntington disease. This gene provides instructions for making a protein called huntingtin, a protein that is believed to play an important role in the development of brain neurons. The HTT mutation involves lengthening a DNA segment known as a CAG trinucleotide repeat. The extra building blocks in the huntingtin gene cause the protein that is made from it to contain an extra section. It is currently thought that this extra protein section interacts with other proteins in brain cells where it occurs, and that this interaction ultimately leads to cell **death**.

The HD gene is a dominant gene, meaning that only one copy of it is needed to develop the disease. HD affects both males and females. The gene may be inherited from either parent, who will also be affected by the disease. A parent with the HD gene has a 50% chance of passing it on to each offspring. The chances of passing on the HD gene are not affected by the results of previous pregnancies.

The symptoms of HD fall into three categories: motor or movement symptoms, personality and behavioral changes, and cognitive decline. The severity and rate of progression of each type of symptom can vary from person to person.

Early motor symptoms include restlessness, twitching and a desire to move about. Handwriting may become less controlled, and coordination may decline. Later symptoms include:

- Dystonia, or sustained abnormal postures, including facial grimaces, a twisted neck, or an arched back.
- Chorea, in which involuntary jerking, twisting or writhing motions become pronounced.
- Slowness of voluntary movements, inability to regulate the speed or force of movements, inability to initiate movement, and slowed reactions.
- Difficulty speaking and swallowing due to involvement of the throat muscles.
- Localized or generalized weakness and impaired balance ability.
- Rigidity, especially in late-stage disease.

Personality and behavioral changes include depression, irritability, **anxiety** and apathy. The person with HD may become impulsive, aggressive, or socially withdrawn.

Cognitive changes include loss of ability to plan and execute routine tasks, slowed thought, and impaired or inappropriate judgment. Short-term memory loss usually occurs, although long-term memory is usually not

KEY TERMS

Chorea—Involuntary writhing movements.

Cognition—The mental activities associated with thinking, learning, and memory.

Computed tomography (CT) scan—An imaging procedure that produces a three–dimensional picture of organs or structures inside the body, such as the brain.

Deoxyribonucleic acid (DNA)—The genetic material in cells that holds the inherited instructions for growth, development, and cellular functioning.

Heimlich maneuver—An action designed to expel an obstructing piece of food from the throat. It is performed by placing the fist on the abdomen, underneath the breastbone, grasping the fist with the other hand (from behind), and thrusting it inward and upward.

Neurodegenerative—Relating to degeneration of nerve tissues.

Neuron—A cell that is specialized to conduct nerve impulses.

affected. The person with late-stage HD usually retains knowledge of his environment and recognizes family members or other loved ones, despite severe cognitive decline.

Diagnosis

Examination

Diagnosis of HD begins with a detailed medical history, and a thorough physical and **neurological exam**. Family medical history is very important as HD is inherited.

Tests

Magnetic resonance imaging (MRI) or computed tomography scan (CT scan) imaging may be performed to look for degeneration in the basal ganglia and cortex, the brain regions most affected in HD.

A genetic test is available for confirmation of the clinical diagnosis. In this test, a small blood sample is taken, and DNA from it is analyzed to determine the CAG repeat number. A person with a repeat number of 30 or below will not develop HD. A person with a repeat number between 35 and 40 may not develop the disease within their normal life span. A person with a very high number of repeats (70 or above) is likely to develop the juvenile-onset form. An important component of **genetic testing** is extensive genetic counseling

Prenatal testing is also available. A person at risk for HD may obtain fetal testing without determining whether she herself carries the gene. This test, also called a linkage test, examines the pattern of DNA near the gene in both parent and fetus, but does not analyze for the triple nucleotide repeat (CAG). If the DNA patterns do not match, the fetus can be assumed not to have inherited the HD gene, even if present in the parent. A pattern match indicates the fetus probably has the same genetic makeup of the at-risk parent.

Treatment

Traditional

There is no cure for HD, nor any treatment that can slow the rate of progression. Treatment is aimed at reducing the disability caused by the motor impairments, and treating behavioral and emotional symptoms.

Physical therapy is used to maintain strength and compensate for lost strength and balance. Stretching and range of motion exercises help minimize contracture, or muscle shortening, a result of weakness and disuse. The physical therapist also advises on the use of mobility aids such as walkers or wheelchairs.

Occupational therapy is used to design compensatory strategies for lost abilities in the activities of daily living, such as eating, dressing, and grooming. The occupational therapist advises on modifications to the home that improve **safety**, accessibility, and comfort.

Difficulty swallowing may be lessened by preparation of softer foods, blending food in an electric blender, and taking care to eat slowly and carefully. Use of a straw for all liquids can help. The potential for **choking** on food is a concern, especially late in the disease progression. Caregivers should learn the use of the **Heimlich maneuver**. In addition, passage of food into the airways increases the risk for **pneumonia**. A gastric feeding tube may be needed, if swallowing becomes too difficult or dangerous.

Speech difficulties may be partially compensated by using picture boards or other augmentative communication devices. Loss of cognitive ability affects both speech production and understanding. A speech-language pathologist can work with the family to develop simplified and more directed communication strategies, including speaking slowly, using simple words, and repeating sentences exactly.

Drugs

Motor symptoms may be treated with drugs, although some studies suggest that anti-chorea treatment rarely improves function. Chorea (movements caused by abnormal muscle contractions) can be suppressed with drugs that deplete dopamine, an important brain chemical regulating movement. As HD progresses, natural dopamine levels fall, leading to loss of chorea and an increase in rigidity and movement slowness. Treatment with L-dopa (which resupplies dopamine) may be of some value. Frequent reassessment of the effectiveness and appropriateness of any drug therapy is necessary. In August 2008 the Food and Drug Administration (FDA) approved tetrabenazine to treat Huntington's chorea, making it the first drug approved for use in the United States to treat HD.

Early behavioral changes, including depression and anxiety, may respond to drug therapy. Maintaining a calm, familiar, and secure environment is useful as the disease progresses. Support groups for both patients and caregivers form an important part of treatment.

Alternative

As of 2009, 548 clinical trials for the treatment of Huntington's disease were being sponsored by the National Institutes of Health (NIH) and other agencies. A few examples include:

- The study of early brain and behavioral changes in people who have the gene expansion for HD, but are currently healthy and have no symptoms. (NCT00051324)
- The evaluation of the effect of atomoxetine on daily activities such as attention and focus, thinking ability and muscle movements in subjects with early HD. (NCT00368849)
- The collection of prospective data from individuals who are part of HD family to learn more about HD, develop potential treatments for HD, and to plan for future research studies of experimental drugs aimed at slowing or postponing the onset and progression of HD. (NCT00313495)
- The evaluation of the safety of the drug ursodiol in people with HD and the study of how the compound is processed by the body. (NCT00514774)
- The evaluation of the safety and tolerability of dimebon in people with HD. (NCT00387270)
- The effectiveness of a music therapy program to improve holistically the psychological, somatic, and social symptoms of patients with HD. (NCT00178360)
- The assessment of the impact of minocycline on the progression of symptoms of HD. (NCT00277355)

Clinical trial information is constantly updated by NIH and the most recent information on Huntington's disease trials can be found at: http://clinicaltrials.gov/search/term=Huntington%27s%20Disease

Prognosis

The person with Huntington disease may be able to maintain a job for several years after diagnosis, despite the increase in disability. Loss of cognitive functions and increase in motor and behavioral symptoms eventually prevent the person with HD from continuing employment. Ultimately, severe motor symptoms prevent mobility. Death usually occurs 15-20 years after disease onset. Progressive weakness of respiratory and swallowing muscles leads to increased risk of respiratory infection and choking, the most common causes of death. Future research in this area is currently focusing on nerve cell transplantation.

Prevention

Genetic testing is available for HD and should be considered if there is a family history of the disease. The Huntington's Disease Society of America has reputable pre-test and post-test counseling information.

Resources

BOOKS

Knowles, Johanna. *Huntington's Disease.* New York, NY: Rosen Publishing Group, 2006.

Lawrence, David, M. *Huntington's Disease.* New York, NY: Chelsea House Publications, 2009.

Lo, Donald C., and Robert E. Hughes. *The Neurobiology of Huntington's Disease.* Boca Raton, FL: CRC Press, 2009.

Quarrell, Oliver W. J. *Huntington's Disease (The Facts).* Oxford, UK: Oxford University Press, 2008.

Sulaiman, Sandy. *Learning to Live With Huntington's Disease: One Family's Story.* London, UK: Jessica Kingsley Publishers, 2007.

Wexler, Alice. *The Woman Who Walked into the Sea: Huntington's and the Making of a Genetic Disease.* Ann Harbor, MI: Sheridan Books, 2008.

PERIODICALS

Aubeeluck, A., and E. Wilson. "Huntington's disease. Part 1: essential background and management." *British Journal of Nursing* 17, no. 3 (February 2008): 146–151.

Blekher, T., et al. "Visual scanning and cognitive performance in prediagnostic and early–stage Huntington's disease. Part 2: treatment and management issues in juvenile HD." *Movement Disorders* 24, no. 4 (March 2009): 533–540.

Busse, M. E., et al. "Mobility and falls in people with Huntington's disease." *Journal of Neurology, Neurosurgery, and Psychiatry* 80, no. 1 (January 2009): 88–90.

Harper, S. Q. "Progress and challenges in RNA interference therapy for Huntington disease." *Archives of Neurology* 66, no. 8, (August 2009): 933–938.

Kim, M., et al. "Stem cell–based cell therapy for Huntington disease: a review." *Neuropathology* 28, no. 1 (February 2008): 1–9.

Lahiri, N., and S. J. Tabrizi. "Huntington's disease: a tale of two genes." *Neurology* 73, no. 16 (October 2009): 1254–1255.

Videnovic, A., et al. "Daytime somnolence and nocturnal sleep disturbances in Huntington disease." *Parkinsonism & related disorders* 15, no. 6 (July 2009): 471–474.

Williams, J. K., et al. "Caregiving by teens for family members with Huntington disease." *Journal of Family Nursing* 15, no. 3 (August 2009): 273–294.

OTHER

"Genetic Testing for Huntington's Disease." *HDSA* Referral List, http://www.hdsa.org/living-with-huntingtons/family-care/living-at-risk/genetic-testing-centers.html (accessed December 12, 2009)

"Huntington's Disease." *Genetics Home Reference* Information Page, http://ghr.nlm.nih.gov/condition=huntingtondisease (accessed December 12, 2009)

"Huntington's Disease." *Madisons Foundation* Information Page, http://www.madisonsfoundation.org/index.php/component/option,com_mpower/diseaseID,190 (accessed December 12, 2009)

"Huntington's Disease." *Medline Plus* Health Topic, http://www.nlm.nih.gov/medlineplus/huntingtonsdisease.html (accessed December 12, 2009)

"Huntington's Disease." *NINDS* Information Page, http://www.ninds.nih.gov/disorders/huntington/huntington.htm (accessed December 12, 2009)

ORGANIZATIONS

Hereditary Disease Foundation., 3960 Broadway, 6th Floor, New York NY, 10032, (212) 928-2121, (212) 928-2172, cures@hdfoundation.org, http://www.hdfoundation.org.

Huntington's Disease Society of America (HDSA), 505 Eighth Avenue, Suite 902, New York NY, 10018, (212) 242-1968, (800) 345-4372, (212) 239-3430, hdsainfo@hdsa.org, http://www.hdsa.org.

Huntington Society of Canada, 151 Frederick Street, Suite 400, Kitchener ON Canada, NH2 2M2, (519) 749-7063, (800) 998-7398, (519) 749-8965, info@huntingtonsociety.ca, http://www.huntingtonsociety.ca.

International Huntington Association (IHA), Callunahof 8, St Harfsen The Netherlands, 7217, + 31-573-431595, + 31-573-431719, iha@huntington-assoc.com, http://www.huntington-assoc.com.

National Institute of Neurological Disorders and Stroke (NINDS), PO Box 5801, Bethesda MD, 20824, (301) 496-5751, (800) 352-9424, http://www.ninds.nih.gov.

Laith Gulli, MD
Monique Laberge, PhD

Hurler's syndrome

Definition

A severe genetic disorder that causes skeletal deformity and **mental retardation**.

Description

Hurler's syndrome belongs to the broader category of mucopolysaccharidosis (MPS), a type of disease caused by an excess accumulation of certain substances (mucopolysaccharides) found in connective tissue. There are six major types of mucopolysaccharidosis, all produced by various enzyme deficiencies that cause mucopolysaccharides to be stored in cells. It is possible to screen for these conditions because the stored mucopolysaccharides leak into the urine. MPS occurs in an estimated 1 in 25,000 live births.

Hurler's syndrome, named for Gertrud Hurler (1889-1965), the German **pediatrician** who first identified the condition in 1919, is one of the more common forms of mucopolysaccharidosis. Like most other types of MPS, it is an autosomal recessive trait. Caused by a deficiency in the enzyme alpha-L-iduronidase, it is characterized by mental and growth retardation, short, broad bones, a humpback, joint stiffness, and limited joint function. Children with Hurler's syndrome have slow growth during the second six months of life and generally stop growing altogether by the age of two. The corneas become clouded, and facial deformities develop, including a prominent forehead, coarse features, thick earlobes, a sunken nasal bridge, excessively full lips, and upturned nostrils. The spine becomes shortened, the liver and spleen enlarged, the chest deformed, and the abdomen protruding. After the age of three, the mouth is usually held open. Children afflicted by Hurler's syndrome usually die by the age of 10 from heart failure or **pneumonia**. Recently, physicians have had some success in treating the condition with bone marrow transplants. Prenatal screening for Hurler's syndrome may be done through either **amniocentesis** or chorionic villus sampling by testing for levels of the associated enzyme in cultured fetal cells.

Hyaline membrane disease **see Respiratory distress syndrome**

Hydrocephalus

Definition

Hydrocephalus is an abnormal expansion of cavities (ventricles) within the brain that is caused by the accumulation of cerebrospinal fluid. Hydrocephalus comes from two Greek words: *hydros* means water and *cephalus* means head.

There are two main varieties of hydrocephalus: congenital and acquired. An obstruction of the cerebral

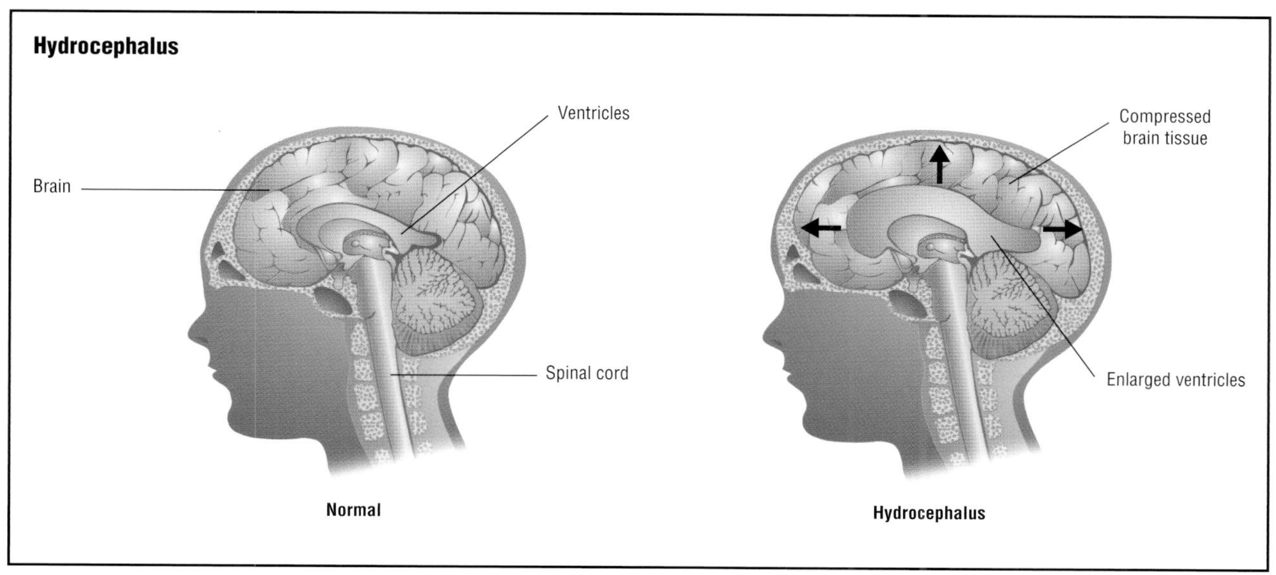

A normal brain (left) and one showing the enlarged ventricles of hydrocephalus. The additional fluid in the ventricles causes increased pressure on the brain. *(Illustration by PreMediaGlobal. Reproduced by permission of Gale, a part of Cengage Learning.)*

aqueduct (aqueductal stenosis) is the most frequent cause of congenital hydrocephalus. Acquired hydrocephalus may result from **spina bifida**, intraventricular hemorrhage, **meningitis**, head trauma, tumors, and cysts.

Description

Hydrocephalus is the result of an imbalance between the formation and drainage of cerebrospinal fluid (CSF). Approximately 500 milliliters (about a pint) of CSF is formed within the brain each day, by epidermal cells in structures collectively called the choroid plexus. These cells line chambers called ventricles that are located within the brain. There are four ventricles in a human brain. Once formed, CSF usually circulates among all the ventricles before it is absorbed and returned to the circulatory system. The normal adult volume of circulating CSF is 150 mL. The CSF turn-over rate is more than three times per day. Because production is independent of absorption, reduced absorption causes CSF to accumulate within the ventricles.

There are three different types of hydrocephalus. In the most common variety, reduced absorption occurs when one or more passages connecting the ventricles become blocked. This prevents the movement of CSF to its drainage sites in the subarachnoid space just inside the skull. This type of hydrocephalus is called "noncommunicating." In a second type, a reduction in the absorption rate is caused by damage to the absorptive tissue. This variety is called "communicating hydrocephalus."

Both of these types lead to an elevation of the CSF pressure within the brain. This increased pressure pushes aside the soft tissues of the brain. This squeezes and distorts them. This process also results in damage to these tissues. In infants whose skull bones have not yet fused, the intracranial pressure is partly relieved by expansion of the skull, so that symptoms may not be as dramatic. Both types of elevated-pressure hydrocephalus may occur from **infancy** to adulthood.

A third type of hydrocephalus, called "normal pressure hydrocephalus," is marked by ventricle enlargement without an apparent increase in CSF pressure. This type affects mainly the elderly.

Hydrocephalus has a variety of causes including:

- congenital brain defects
- hemorrhage, either into the ventricles or the subarachnoid space
- infection of the central nervous system (syphilis, herpes, meningitis, encephalitis, or mumps)
- tumor

Hydrocephalus is believed to occur in approximately one to two of every 1,000 live births. The incidence of adult onset hydrocephalus is not known. There is no known way to prevent hydrocephalus.

Causes and symptoms

Hydrocephalus that is congenital (present at **birth**) is thought to be caused by a complex interaction of genetic and environmental factors. Aqueductal stenosis, an obstruction of the cerebral aqueduct, is the most frequent cause of congenital hydrocephalus. As of 2001, the genetic factors are not well understood. According to the British Association for Spina Bifida and Hydrocephalus, in very rare circumstances, hydrocephalus is due to hereditary factors, which might affect future generations.

Signs and symptoms of elevated-pressure hydrocephalus include:

- headache
- nausea and vomiting, especially in the morning
- lethargy
- disturbances in walking (gait)
- double vision
- subtle difficulties in learning and memory
- delay in children achieving developmental milestones

Irritability is the most common sign of hydrocephalus in infants. If this is not treated, it may lead to lethargy. Bulging of the fontanelles, or the soft spots between the skull bones, may also be an early sign. When hydrocephalus occurs in infants, fusion of the skull bones is prevented. This leads to abnormal expansion of the skull.

Symptoms of normal pressure hydrocephalus include dementia, gait abnormalities, and incontinence (involuntary urination or bowel movements).

Diagnosis

Imaging studies—x ray, computed tomography scan (CT scan), ultrasound, and especially **magnetic resonance imaging** (MRI)—are used to assess the presence and location of obstructions, as well as changes in brain tissue that have occurred as a result of the hydrocephalus. Lumbar puncture (spinal tap) may be performed to aid in determining the cause when infection is suspected.

Treatment

The primary method of treatment for both elevated and normal pressure hydrocephalus is surgical installation of a shunt. A shunt is a tube connecting the ventricles of the brain to an alternative drainage site, usually the abdominal cavity. A shunt contains a one-way valve to prevent reverse flow of fluid. In some cases of non-communicating hydrocephalus, a direct connection can be made between one of the ventricles and the subarachnoid space, allowing drainage without a shunt.

Installation of a shunt requires lifelong monitoring by the recipient or family members for signs of recurring hydrocephalus due to obstruction or failure of the shunt. Other than monitoring, no other management activity is usually required.

Some drugs may postpone the need for surgery by inhibiting the production of CSF. These include acetazolamide and furosemide. Other drugs that are used to delay surgery include glycerol, digoxin, and isosorbide.

Some cases of elevated pressure hydrocephalus may be avoided by preventing or treating the infectious diseases which precede them. Prenatal diagnosis of congenital brain malformation is often possible, offering the option of family planning.

Prognosis

The prognosis for elevated-pressure hydrocephalus depends on a wide variety of factors, including the cause, age of onset, and the timing of surgery. Studies indicate that about half of all children who receive appropriate treatment and follow-up will develop IQs greater than 85. Those with hydrocephalus at birth do better than those with later onset due to meningitis. For individuals with normal pressure hydrocephalus, approximately half will benefit by the installation of a shunt.

Resources

BOOKS

Toporek, Chuck, and Kellie Robinson. *Hydrocephalus: A Guide for Patients, Families & Friends.* Cambridge, Mass.: O'Reilly &Associates, 1999.

PERIODICALS

"Hydrocephalus." *Review of Optometry* 137, no. 8 (August 15, 2000): 56A.

OTHER

"Hydrocephalus." *American Association of Neurological Surgeons/Congress of Neurological Surgeons*, http://www.neurosurgery.org/pubpages/patres/hydrobroch.html

"Hydrocephalus." *Institute for Neurology and Neurosurgery.* Beth Israel Medical Center, New York, NY, http://nyneurosurgery.org/child/hydrocephalus/hydrocephalus.htm.

"Hydrocephalus." National Library of Medicine. *MEDLINEplus*, http://www.nlm.nih.gov/medlineplus/hydrocephalus.html

ORGANIZATIONS

Association for Spina Bifida and Hydrocephalus, 42 Park Rd, PeterboroughPE1 2UQ UK, 0173 355 5988, 017 3355 5985, postmaster@asbah.org, http://www.asbah.demon.co.uk.

Hydrocephalus Foundation, Inc. (HyFI), 910 Rear Broadway, Saugus MA, 01906, (781) 942-1161, HyFI1@netscape.net, http://www.hydrocephalus.org.

L. Fleming Fallon, MD, PhD, DrPH

Hyper-IgM syndrome

Definition

Hyper-IgM syndrome (also known as hypogammaglobulinemia with hyper IgM) is a group of primary **immunodeficiency** disorders in which the child's body fails to produce certain specific types of antibodies. The term *primary* means that the disorder is present from **birth**, in contrast to secondary immunodeficiencies (such as **AIDS**), which are acquired later in life by previously healthy persons. The five subtypes of hyper-IgM syndrome identified as of 2010 are caused by mutations in three genes that govern the body's T and B cells, which are types of white blood cells or lymphocytes. T cells assist in the maturation of B cells and regulate the production of antibodies, which are protein molecules produced as the first line of the immune system's defense against disease-causing organisms. B cells actually make the antibodies.

There are two patterns of inheritance in these syndromes. The more common of the two, known as X-linked hyper-IgM syndrome (XHIM or HIGM1), is caused by an abnormal gene on the X chromosome and affects only boys. Between 65% and 70% of all known cases of hyper-IgM syndrome are XHIM (HIGM1). The less common forms are autosomal recessive and occur in children who have inherited an abnormal gene from both parents. The less common forms affect girls as well as boys.

The five subtypes of hyper-IgM syndrome known as of 2010 are as follows:

- Hyper-IgM syndrome type 1 (XHIM or HIGM1). This is the X-linked form of the syndrome. It is caused by a mutation of the *CD40LG* gene on the long arm of the X chromosome at locus Xq26. The mutation affects the ability of T cells to direct the antibody production of B cells.
- Hyper-IgM syndrome type 2 (HIGM2). This form is caused by a mutation of the *AICDA* gene on the short arm of chromosome 12 at 12p13. In this form, B cells cannot recombine genetic material, which they must do in order to switch from producing one type of antibody to another. Children with HIGM2 suffer recurrent bacterial, respiratory, and gastrointestinal infections, but rarely have the opportunistic infections found in boys with XHIM.
- Hyper-IgM syndrome type 3 (HIGM3). This subtype of the syndrome is caused by a mutation in the *CD40* gene. In this form, B cells are unable to receive chemical signals from T cells. Children with HIGM3 have the same clinical symptoms as those with XHIM.
- Hyper-IgM syndrome type 4 (HIGM4). This subtype is also characterized by the inability of B cells to recombine genetic material. It was discovered only in 2005 and little is known about it as of 2010.
- Hyper-IgM syndrome type 5 (HIGM5). Identified in only three patients as of 2010, this subtype is caused by a mutation in the *UNG* gene on chromosome 12. Children with HIGM5 have the same clinical symptoms as those with HIGM2.

Demographics

All forms of hyper-IgM syndrome are very rare disorders. One group of researchers at Johns Hopkins University estimates the incidence of XHIM in the general North American population as one in 1,030,000 males, while the National Institutes of Health (NIH) estimates that XHIM affects one baby boy in every 2 million. The incidence of the four non-X-linked subtypes has not been established as of 2010, but they are known to be much less common than XHIM; as noted above, only three cases of subtype 5 (HIGM5) have been reported as of 2010. Only 15 cases of subtype 4 (HIGM4) are known as of 2010.

Researchers are not certain as of 2010 whether these disorders are more common in some racial or ethnic groups than others or whether they are equally common in all parts of the world; as of 2010, cases of XHIM have been reported in Asian and African families as well as in families of European descent. The only registries of patients diagnosed with hyper-IgM syndrome are located in Europe and the United States. The registry that was established in the United States in 1997 contains the records of 79 patients from 60 unrelated families, while the European database contains the records of XHIM patients from 130 unrelated families. The U.S. registry has data on the racial background of 75 of its patients: 52 were Caucasian, 12 were African American, 9 were Asian American, one was both African and Asian American, and one was both Caucasian and Asian American.

Description

Hyper-IgM syndrome appears during the first year of life when the child develops recurrent infections of the respiratory tract that do not respond to standard antibiotic treatment, along with chronic **diarrhea**. Other early symptoms may include enlarged tonsils; swelling of the liver and spleen; enlarged lymph nodes; or opportunistic infections. Children with XHIM are more likely to develop enlarged lymph nodes than children with other primary immunodeficiency disorders. Opportunistic infections are caused by organisms that do not usually cause disease in people with normally functioning immune systems. The most common opportunistic infection in children with XHIM is a lung disease known as *Pneumocystis jirovecii* (formerly known as *Pneumocystis carinii*) pneumonia. Children with either XHIM or the four non-X-linked subtypes of the syndrome who are not diagnosed early may show delays in growth and normal weight gain.

Hyper-IgM syndrome is a disorder with a high degree of morbidity, which means that patients diagnosed with it often develop or suffer from other diseases or disorders. The most common comorbid conditions associated with XHIM and HIGM3 include the following:

- Recurrent and chronic infections of the lungs and sinuses leading to chronic dilation of the bronchi (the larger air passageways) in the lungs. This condition, called bronchiectasis, is marked by frequent attacks of coughing that bring up pus-streaked mucus.
- Chronic diarrhea leading to weight loss and malnutrition. The diarrhea is usually caused by opportunistic infections of the digestive tract; the most common disease agents are *Cryptosporidium parvum*, *Giardia lamblia*, *Campylobacter*, or rotaviruses.
- Frequent mouth ulcers, skin infections, and inflammation of the area around the rectum (proctitis). These complications are associated with neutropenia, a condition in which the blood has an abnormally low number of neutrophils. Neutrophils are a special type of white blood cell that ingest bacteria and other foreign substances. The connection between hyper-IgM syndrome and neutropenia is not fully understood.
- Infections of the bones and joints leading to arthritis or osteomyelitis.
- Disorders of the nervous system caused by meningoencephalitis, or inflammation of the brain and its overlying layers of protective tissue. Patients with these disorders may have problems with thinking clearly, have difficulty walking normally, or develop paralysis on one side of the body (hemiplegia).
- Liver disease. About 70 percent of patients with XHIM develop liver disease by age 30, usually as a result of recurrent *Cryptosporidium* infections.
- Malignant tumors, most commonly non-Hodgkin's lymphoma or cancers of the gall bladder and liver.

Causes and symptoms

Causes

X-linked hyper-IgM syndrome is caused by a mutation in a gene on the X chromosome that affects the patient's T cells. The gene has been identified at locus Xq26. Normal T cells produce a ligand (a small molecule that links to larger molecules) known as CD40. CD40 is a protein found on the surface of T cells that signals B cells to stop producing IgM, which is the antibody that is first produced in response to invading organisms and switch to producing IgG, IgA, and IgE, which are more specialized antibodies. As a result, boys with XHIM have abnormally low levels of IgG and IgA in their blood, with normal or higher than normal levels of IgM. Because they lack these so-called second line of defense antibodies, they are more vulnerable to infections.

About 70 percent of patients diagnosed with XHIM have inherited the disorder through their mother; about 30 percent of cases, however, are caused by new mutations. Females who carry the defective gene have a 50 percent chance of passing it on to their sons but are not affected themselves by the disorder. The daughters of carriers have a 50 percent risk of carrying the defective gene to the next generation.

Symptoms

The symptoms of hyper-IgM syndrome usually become noticeable after the affected baby is six months to a year old. Over 50% of males with XHIM develop symptoms by age one year, and more than 90% are symptomatic by age four years. At this point the antibodies received from the mother during pregnancy are no longer present in the baby's blood. The child develops a series of severe ear, throat, or chest infections that do not clear up with standard antibiotic treatment. Another early warning sign is recurrent or chronic diarrhea. In addition, the child may have more than one infection at the same time. The most common telltale symptom, however, is PCP; in fact, the frequency of *Pneumocystis jirovecii* pneumonia in children with hyper-IgM syndrome was a useful clue to geneticists searching for the mutation that causes the disorder.

The Jeffrey Modell Foundation (JMF) and the American Red Cross have drawn up a list of 10 warning signs of hyper-IgM syndrome and other primary immunodeficiency disorders:

- The child has eight or more ear infections within one year.
- The child has two or more serious sinus infections within one year.
- The child has been treated with antibiotics for two months or longer with little effect.
- The child has been diagnosed with pneumonia more than twice within the past year.

KEY TERMS

Antibody—A special protein made by the body's immune system as a defense against foreign material (bacteria, viruses, etc.) that enters the body. Each antibody is uniquely designed to attack and neutralize the specific antigen that triggered the immune response.

B cell—A type of white blood cell derived from bone marrow. B cells are sometimes called B lymphocytes. They secrete antibodies and have a number of other complex functions within the human immune system.

Bronchiectasis—A disorder of the bronchial tubes marked by abnormal stretching, enlargement, or destruction of the walls. Bronchiectasis is usually caused by recurrent inflammation of the airway.

Human leukocyte antigen (HLA)—A group of protein molecules located on bone marrow cells that can provoke an immune response. A donor's and a recipient's HLA types should match as closely as possible to prevent the recipient's immune system from attacking the donor's marrow as a foreign material that does not belong in the body.

Immunoglobulin G (IgG)—Immunoglobulin type gamma, the most common type found in human blood and tissue fluids.

Ligand—Any type of small molecule that binds to a larger molecule. Hyper-IgM syndrome is caused by a lack of a ligand known as CD40 on the surfaces of the T cells in the child's blood.

Lymphocyte—A type of white blood cell that participates in the immune response. The two main groups of lymphocytes are the B cells that have antibody molecules on their surface and T cells that destroy antigens.

Morbidity—A disease or abnormality. In statistics it also refers to the rate at which a disease or abnormality occurs.

Neutropenia—A condition in which the number of neutrophils, a type of white blood cell (leukocyte) is abnormally low.

Opportunistic infection—An infection that is normally mild in a healthy individual, but which takes advantage of an ill person's weakened immune system to move into the body, grow, spread, and cause serious illness.

Osteomyelitis—An infection of the bone and bone marrow, usually caused by bacteria.

Primary immunodeficiency disease (PIDD)—A group of approximately 150 hereditary or genetic conditions that affect the normal functioning of the human immune system.

Prophylactic—Referring to a drug or practice intended to prevent the spread or occurrence of disease or infection.

Stem cell—An undifferentiated cell that retains the ability to develop into any one of a variety of cell types.

T cell—A type of white blood cell that is produced in the bone marrow and matured in the thymus gland. It helps to regulate the immune system's response to infections or malignancy.

Thrush—An infection of the mouth caused by a yeast and characterized by a whitish growth and ulcers.

- If an infant, the child is not growing or gaining weight normally.
- The child has repeatedly developed deep skin abscesses.
- If older than 12 months, the child has persistent thrush (fungal infection of the mouth).
- The child needs intravenous antibiotics to clear infections.
- The child has two or more deep-seated infections (meningitis, osteomyelitis, sepsis, or cellulitis).
- Other family members have been diagnosed with a primary immunodeficiency disorder.

Diagnosis

Most children with hyper-IgM syndrome are diagnosed before they are a year old; about 40 percent have PCP at the time of diagnosis. If the doctor has seen the child on a regular basis since birth, there will be a record of the number of infections the child has had, the length of time the child has had each infection, and the child's response to treatment. If the doctor suspects a primary immunodeficiency disorder, he or she will ask the parents about a family history of such disorders.

Examination

The next step in diagnosis is a thorough physical examination. Children with primary immunodefiencies are often underweight or small for their age and may look pale or generally unwell. The doctor will listen for unusual sounds in the lungs when the child breathes in and out and will check the child's skin and the inside of the mouth for **rashes**, ulcers, or sores. As the doctor palpates (feels) the child's abdomen, he or she will pay particular attention to the size of the spleen and liver. The doctor will also examine the child's joints and the lymph nodes in the neck for signs of swelling.

Tests

The doctor will order a blood test to screen the child for an immunodeficiency disorder. The most common tests performed to screen for hyper-IgM syndrome are a complete blood count (CBC) and a quantitative immunoglobulin test. The CBC will help to determine whether the child has neutropenia. The quantitative test measures the levels of the different types of immunoglobulins in the blood as well as the total level of all immunoglobulins. A child with hyper-IgM syndrome will be found to have abnormally low levels of IgA and IgG antibodies and a normal or elevated level of IgM.

The doctor may also order x-ray studies of the child's chest or sinuses in order to determine whether lung damage has already occurred or to make a baseline evaluation of the child's lungs.

Procedures

The diagnosis of hyper-IgM syndrome can be confirmed by two tests: a measurement of CD40 ligand protein expression performed after stimulating some T cells from the patient's blood in the laboratory; or by molecular genetics testing for the defective CD40 gene. If a child has XHIM, the T cells in the sample will not show an increase in CD 40 ligand protein after stimulation. The genetics test involves DNA sequencing and has been available since the early 2000s. As of 2010 the test can successfully identify mutations in 99% of affected males.

Treatment

Traditional

Intravenous immunoglubulin (IVIG) has been the mainstay of treatment for a number of primary immunodeficiencies since it was first approved by the Food and Drug Administration (FDA) in the early 1980s. IVIG involves the infusion of immunoglobulins derived from donated blood plasma directly into the patient's bloodstream as a protection against infection. In the case of children with XHIM, IVIG is given to replace the missing IgG antibodies and to reduce or normalize the IgM level. IVIG infusions are usually given every three to four weeks for the remainder of the patient's life. They can be given in an outpatient clinic or in the patient's home. Patients with neutropenia may be treated with G-CSF (Neupogen), a protein given by injection that stimulates the body to produce more neutrophils.

IVIG therapy is the most effective treatment for the non-X-linked subtypes of the syndrome as of the early 2000s.

IVIG does have potentially severe side effects, including nausea, **vomiting**, difficulty breathing, and an increased risk of kidney dysfunction or failure. An alternative is subcutaneous (beneath the skin) immune globulin (SCIG) therapy, given weekly. The only product of this type as of 2010 approved by the FDA is Vivaglobin, approved in 2006 for treatment of primary immunodeficiency disorders. Patients can administer Vivaglobin to themselves at home after being trained by their doctor; it takes about 1 hour to infuse the weekly dose under the skin. SCIG therapy has been well received by patients for its effectiveness as well as its convenience compared to IVIG.

Drugs

Boys diagnosed with XHIM are given **antibiotics** as a prophylactic (preventive) treatment to protect them against *Pneumocystis jirovecii* pneumonia. They are usually started on a regimen of trimethoprim-sulfamethoxazole (Bactrim or Septra) as soon as they are diagnosed.

An experimental treatment for XHIM is recombinant human CD40 ligand (rhuCD40L), an artificial form of the protein needed for proper antibody production. Researchers have found that giving artificial CD40 ligand to specially bred immunodeficient mice improves their ability to make IgA and IgG antibodies. The National Institutes of Health (NIH) completed a study to evaluate the effectiveness of this treatment in humans in 2008 but no reports of its effectiveness in XHIM patients specifically have been published as of summer 2010.

Transplantation

Bone marrow transplantation (BMT), which is also referred to as hematopoietic stem cell transplantation (HSCT), is considered to be curative for primary immunodeficiency disorders. Although BMT has been performed on children with severe immunodeficiency disorders since the 1980s, it was usually restricted to those with limited life expectancy because of complications associated with transplantation. Several advances since the late 1990s, however, have made this form of treatment more feasible for boys with XHIM. These advances include better matching of potential donors and recipients through more accurate tissue typing and improved surgical techniques. As of 2010, however, doctors recommended that boys with XHIM be given BMT before they develop significant infections or organ damage. This form of treatment is not recommended for patients who already have signs of liver damage.

The best source of bone marrow for transplantation is the affected child's siblings. They will be tissue-typed to determine whether their bone marrow has the same human leukocyte antigens (HLA) as the affected child. Human leukocyte antigens are genetically determined proteins that allow the body to distinguish between its own cells and those from an outside source. The closer the HLA match between a bone marrow donor and recipient, the lower the chances that the recipient's body will reject the transplanted tissue. In addition to siblings, another choice is bone marrow from one of the parents, who shares half the affected child's HLA antigens. With the expansion of bone marrow registries since the early 2000s, it is also possible to use bone marrow from an unrelated donor whose tissues closely match those of the affected child. These are called matched unrelated donor (MUD) transplants. The most successful bone marrow transplants in hyper-IgM children, however, have used marrow donated by HLA-identical siblings.

Another approach to transplantation as a cure for hyper-IgM syndrome is the use of stem cells from cord blood. This technique was first used for immunodeficiency disorders in 1988. Stem cells are undifferentiated precursor cells whose daughter cells can differentiate into more specialized cells. The stem cells used for transplantation are taken from blood collected from a baby's umbilical cord or the placenta (afterbirth) immediately following delivery. Cord blood from healthy siblings can be used for transplantation to treat XHIM patients. Stem cell transplants from cord blood have two advantages over bone marrow transplants: they have a lower rate of rejection in recipients, and they can be stored ahead of time. Families with a history of primary immunodeficiency disorders can save cord blood in private storage facilities for later use if needed.

Diet and nutrition

Nutritional concerns for children with XHIM are related to infections of the digestive tract resulting in chronic diarrhea. The primary risks with chronic diarrhea are **dehydration** and **malnutrition**. To prevent dehydration, the doctor may recommend a clear liquid diet for infants and toddlers during episodes of diarrhea. If the child is able to keep the clear liquids down, milk or diluted formula can be given. The child's rectal area should be coated with petroleum jelly to reduce irritation.

If the diarrhea is caused by *Cryptosporidium* or another infectious organism, the child's diapers and bed linens should be washed separately from the rest of the family's laundry, and the bathroom should be cleaned regularly with a disinfectant.

Parental concerns

Hyper-IgM syndrome has a major impact on the family of a child diagnosed with the disease. The following are some of the important concerns for parents:

- High financial costs. Children diagnosed with hyper-IgM syndrome require careful monitoring for liver function, lung function, nutritional status, oral hygiene, and normal growth patterns as well as blood antibody levels. In most cases the child will be seen every three to six months by a clinical immunologist as well as his primary care doctor. Such procedures as bone marrow transplantation, IVIG, or subcutaneous immune globulin are also costly.
- Emotional wear and tear on the family. In addition to the extra time and attention required for the affected child, parents are likely to confront emotional problems in the family, ranging from resentment on the part of siblings to anxiety about the affected child's survival and decisions about future pregnancies. Support groups and/or family therapy may be helpful.
- Genetic testing. Genetic counselors recommend having the affected child's siblings tested to see whether they are carriers of the defective gene.
- Education and future employment. Children who are receiving IVIG treatment can attend a regular school and participate in most sports provided that minor injuries are treated promptly. Adults with hyper-IgM syndrome can attend college or graduate school and work in most fields of employment.
- Peer pressure in adolescence. It is important for parents to warn children with hyper-IgM syndrome that smoking, alcohol consumption, and the use of recreational drugs are far more dangerous for them than for adolescents with normal immune systems.

Prognosis

The prognosis for children diagnosed with XHIM is still generally poor as of 2010; morbidity and mortality for this disorder are significantly higher than for other primary immunodeficiency disorders. A study done in 2000 indicated that only 20 percent of patients with hyper-IgM syndrome survived to the age of 25. The most common causes of early **death** are pneumonia, **encephalitis**, **cancer**, and liver failure.

However, researchers expect the outlook to improve for children in treatment as of 2010, particularly those patients who are good candidates for bone marrow transplantation. In one Japanese study, five out of seven patients who received BMT survived, with four of the five producing T cells with normal CD40 ligand without supplementary IVIG therapy. As of 2010, boys with XHIM who receive allogeneic HCT are reported to have a 70%–75% long-term survival rate. In general, children who are treated with IVIG and/or BMT as infants have a better prognosis than those who are diagnosed after the age of two years.

Prevention

As all known subtypes of hyper-IgM syndrome are caused by genetic mutations, there is no way to prevent the disorders after the child is born. Parents who already have a child with hyper-IgM syndrome or who come from families with a history of primary immunodeficiency disorders may wish to consider genetic counseling and prenatal **genetic testing** with future pregnancies.

There are, however, some preventive measures that families can take to lower the risk of opportunistic infections and other complications in children with hyper-IgM syndrome. These precautions include the following:

- Practicing good hygiene, including careful washing of the hands before and after meals and after using the toilet. Antibacterial hand wipes can be packed with school lunches.
- Careful cleansing of even small cuts or scrapes with an antiseptic liquid or cream.
- Proper dental care. Children with primary immunodeficiency syndromes are at increased risk of tooth decay and gum disorders as well as thrush and mouth ulcers.
- Avoiding the use of vaccines made from live viruses (measles, poliovirus, mumps, rubella). Vaccines made with killed viruses should be given regularly.
- Having the home water supply tested for possible contamination by *Cryptosporidium parvum*.
- Avoiding crowded stores, theaters, or athletic events during flu season.
- Giving the affected child his or her own room if possible.
- Having other family members take primary responsibility for the care of household pets. Children with hyper-IgM syndrome are highly susceptible to infection from animal bites.
- Making sure the affected child has a yearly pulmonary (lung) function test to catch any lung infections and loss of breathing capacity early.

Resources

BOOKS

Immune Deficiency Foundation (IDF). *IDF Patient and Family Handbook for Primary Immune Deficiency Diseases*, 4th ed. Towson, MD: IDF, 2007.

Rezaei, Nima, Asghar Aghamohammadi, and Luigi Notarangelo, eds. *Primary Immunodeficiency Diseases: Definition, Diagnosis, and Management*. New York: Springer, 2008.

Strober, Warren. *Immunology: Clinical Case Studies and Disease Pathophysiology*. Hoboken, NJ: Wiley-Blackwell, 2009.

PERIODICALS

Aghamohammadi, A., et al. "Clinical and Laboratory Findings in Hyper-IgM Syndrome with Novel CD40L and AICDA Mutations." *Journal of Clinical Immunology* 29 (November 2009): 769–76.

Bishu, S., et al. "CD40 Ligand Deficiency: Neurologic Sequelae with Radiographic Correlation." *Pediatric Neurology* 41 (December 2009): 419–27.

Davies, E.G., and A.J. Thrasher. "Update on the Hyper Immunoglobulin M Syndromes." *British Journal of Haematology* 149 (April 2010): 167–80.

Gardulf, A., et al. "Prognostic Factors for Health-related Quality of Life in Adults and Children with Primary Antibody Deficiencies Receiving SCIG Home Therapy." *Clinical Immunology* 126 (January 2008): 81–88.

Hsu, A.P., et al. "Mutation Analysis in Primary Immunodeficiency Diseases: Case Studies." *Current Opinion in Allergy and Clinical Immunology* 9 (December 2009): 517–24.

Rangel-Santos, A., et al. "Molecular Characterization of Patients with X-linked Hyper-IgM Syndrome: Description of Two Novel CD40L Mutations." *Scandinavian Journal of Immunology* 69 (February 2009): 169–73.

Vale, A.M., and H.W. Schroeder, Jr. "Clinical Consequences of Defects in B-cell Development." *Journal of Allergy and Clinical Immunology* 125 (April 2010): 778–87.

OTHER

Genetics Home Reference. *X-linked Hyper IgM Syndrome*, http://ghr.nlm.nih.gov/condition/x-linked-hyper-igm-syndrome

Immune Deficiency Foundation (IDF). *Hyper IgM Syndrome*, http://www.primaryimmune.org/publications/book_pats/e_ch08.pdf

Immune Deficiency Foundation (IDF). *What Is a Primary Immunodeficiency Disease?* http://www.primaryimmune.org/about_pi/about_pi.htm

Jeffrey Modell Foundation (JMF). *10 Warning Signs of Primary Immunodeficiency*, http://www.info4pi.org/

aboutPI/index.cfm?section=aboutPI&content=warningsigns&TrkId=24&CFID=39029460&CFTOKEN=77999062

Johnson, Judith, and Alexandra H. Filipovich. *X-Linked Hyper-IgM Syndrome* This is a highly technical discussion of XHIM from the National Library of Medicine's *GeneReviews*, http://www.ncbi.nlm.nih.gov/bookshelf/br.fcgi?book=gene∂=xlhi

National Institute of Child Health and Human Development (NICHD). *Primary Immunodeficiency*, http://www.nichd.nih.gov/health/topics/Primary_Immunodeficiency.cfm

National Organization for Rare Disorders (NORD). *Hyper IgM Syndrome*, http://www.rarediseases.org/search/rdbdetail_abstract.html?disname=Hyper%20IgM%20Syndrome

Park, C. Lucy. "X-Linked Immunodeficiency with Hyper IgM." *eMedicine*, February 20, 2009, http://emedicine.medscape.com/article/889104-overview

ORGANIZATIONS

American Academy of Allergy, Asthma, and Immunology (AAAAI), 555 East Wells Street, Suite 1100, Milwaukee WI, 53202, 414-272-6071, info@aaaai.org, http://www.aaaai.org/.

Immune Deficiency Foundation (IDF), 40 West Chesapeake Avenue, Suite 308, Towson MD, 21204, 800-296-4433, idf@primaryimmune.org, http://www.primaryimmune.org/.

Jeffrey Modell Foundation (JMF), 747 Third Avenue, New York NY, 10017, 212-819-0200, 212-764-4180, info@jmfworld.org, http://www.info4pi.org/index.cfm.

National Institute of Child Health and Human Development (NICHD)., Bldg 31, Room 2A32, MSC 2425, 31 Center Drive, Bethesda MD, 20892, 800-370-2943, 866-760-5947, NICHDInformationResourceCenter@mail.nih.gov, http://www.nichd.nih.gov/.

National Organization for Rare Disorders (NORD), 55 Kenosia Avenue, P.O. Box 1968, Danbury CT, 06813, 203-744-0100, 800-999-6673, 203-798-2291, http://www.rarediseases.org/.

U.S. Immunodeficiency Network (USIDNET), 40 West Chesapeake Avenue, Suite 308, Towson MD, 21204, 410-321-6647, 800-296-4433, 410-321-9165, info@usidnet.org, http://www.usidnet.org/index.cfm.

Rebecca J. Frey, PhD

Hyperbilirubinemia **see** Jaundice

Hyperglycemia

Definition

Hyperglycemia is an abnormally high level of glucose (sugar) in the blood, which occurs when the body has too little insulin or cannot utilize insulin properly. Hyperglycemia is usually associated with **diabetes mellitus**, but transient hyperglycemia can be also caused by pregnancy, illness, injury, or other stresses. Prolonged hyperglycemia can damage multiple organ systems.

Demographics

Reported cases of diabetes, which is the primary cause of hyperglycemia, have increased at least two-fold over the past two decades in most parts of the world. However the incidence of diabetes varies greatly, both in neighboring regions with differing lifestyles and in countries with genetically similar populations. The annual incidence ranges from 0.61 cases per 100,000 people in China to 41.4 cases per 100,000 in Finland. The incidence of diabetes appears to increase with distance from the equator.

As of 2007 it was estimated that 7.8% of Americans have diabetes, of which approximately 24% are undiagnosed, and the incidence continues to rise. In addition three to eight percent of American women develop gestational diabetes during pregnancy.

The majority of new diabetes cases in children are type 1, formerly known as juvenile–onset diabetes. Although type 1 can develop at any age, its incidence increases with age until mid-puberty and then declines. Caucasians have the highest rate of type 1 diabetes and Chinese have the lowest rate. Type 1 diabetes is 1.5 times as likely to develop in American whites as in American blacks or Hispanics. However evidence suggests that when immigrants move to an area with a higher incidence of type 1 diabetes, their rates of diagnosis increase. Furthermore children are increasingly being diagnosed with type 2 diabetes, formerly known as adult-onset. This trend is particularly true for children from ethnic and racial minorities. Diabetic adolescents are especially susceptible to hyperglycemia, both because of fluctuating hormone levels and because many adolescents have erratic eating and sleeping patterns.

Hyperglycemia often goes untreated. A recent study from Detroit reported that 41% of people with sustained hyperglycemia failed to get appropriate treatment within six months. Another 25% went one year without treatment and 11% failed to get appropriate care for up to two years.

Description

Insulin, a hormone produced by the pancreas, is required for the processing of carbohydrates, fats, and proteins. Insulin reduces blood glucose levels by:

- enabling glucose to enter muscle cells
- stimulating glycogenesis—the conversion of glucose to glycogen for storage

- inhibiting glycogenolysis—the release of stored glucose from liver glycogen
- inhibiting gluconeogenesis—the breakdown of protein and fat for glucose in the liver and kidneys
- slowing the breakdown of fat to triglycerides, free fatty acids, and ketones
- stimulating fat storage

Deficiencies in the production or utilization of insulin cause hyperglycemia because circulating glucose is not used or stored and gluconeogenesis continues unabated. The excess glucose overwhelms the kidneys, causing increased urination (osmotic diuresis), excess sugar in the urine (glycosuria), thirst, and **dehydration**. Because the body cannot utilize glucose, fats and proteins are broken down for energy, producing ketones as waste products that are excreted in the urine. In the absence of insulin, ketone build-up in the blood leads to diabetic ketoacidosis (DKA) and potentially to a life-threatening diabetic coma. Children with type 1 diabetes who develop DKA can waste away and die.

All diabetics have occasional episodes of hyperglycemia—which is usually detected by regularly checking their blood sugar levels—and hyperglycemia is a major cause of diabetes-related complications. Hyperglycemia impairs immunity and can make patients susceptible to recurrent infections, particularly infections of the skin and urinary and respiratory tracts. Serious, long–term consequences of prolonged hyperglycemia depend on a variety of factors and usually develop later in life. These complications include nerve damage and diabetic neuropathy, **stroke**, blindness, and the need for amputations.

Persistent hyperglycemia during pregnancy can lead to fetal **gigantism**, premature delivery, and increased infant morbidity and mortality. DKA during pregnancy may result in fetal **death**. Sick infants often have low amounts or poorly functioning insulin, which can lead to hyperglycemia.

Risk factors

Type 1 diabetes is usually due to inherited factors that affect insulin production. Diabetes in newborns is usually related to an inherited defect in a potassium channel in the cells that secrete insulin. Risk factors for type 2 diabetes include gestational diabetes during pregnancy, advancing age, obesity, and a sedentary lifestyle.

Risk factors for untreated or delayed treatment of hyperglycemia in diabetics include:

- poor control of blood glucose over time
- lower income levels or poverty
- poor adherence to medication
- absence of regular physician visits
- higher prescription drug co-payments

Causes and symptoms

Hyperglycemia is usually caused by:

- insufficient insulin administration by type 1 diabetics
- insulin ineffectiveness in type 2 diabetics
- diabetics who eat more or exercise less than they planned
- stress from illness, even a minor infection such as a cold or flu
- acute stress from trauma, heart attack, or stroke
- emotional stresses from family, school, work, or relationship problems

Hyperglycemia is sometimes caused other factors, conditions, or diseases including:

- excessive food intake
- metabolic syndrome
- pregnancy
- drugs, including corticosteroids, tricyclic antidepressants, diuretics, epinephrine, estrogens in birth control pills or hormone replacement therapies, lithium, phenytoin (Dilantin), salicylates, beta–blockers such as metoprolol
- liver problems
- hyperthyroidism
- acromegaly—growth hormone overproduction
- Cushing's syndrome
- chronic renal failure
- pancreatitis
- pancreatic cancer

Hyperglycemia in newborns can result from glucose infusions given to low-birth-weight infants or from physiological stress associated with surgery, **respiratory distress syndrome**, or sepsis.

Although some diabetics never experience symptoms of hyperglycemia, most experience hyperglycemic symptoms even before they are diagnosed with diabetes. It is important to recognize the symptoms of hyperglycemia so that it can be treated quickly:

- frequent urination
- severe thirst
- frequent hunger
- hunger even after eating
- weakness
- fatigue

- blurred vision
- rapid weight loss
- nausea
- vomiting
- dry mouth
- itchy skin
- impotence
- hyperventilation—breathing faster and deeper
- abnormal heart rate
- confusion
- coma
- recurrent infections or poor wound healing with chronic hyperglycemia

The primary symptoms of hyperglycemia in children are usually increased frequency of urination and increased urine volume. This can lead to nighttime urination and incontinence, but may be overlooked in infants due to their high fluid intake and diaper use. Babies often have no noticeable symptoms. Some children with hyperglycemia become irritable or ill-tempered and experience general malaise, **headache**, and weakness.

Diabetics can develop DKA at lower blood sugar levels when they are ill; thus DKA is most often triggered by infection. In children with type 1 diabetes, DKA usually develops gradually over a few days as blood sugar levels rise. However DKA can develop in less than 24 hours. Frequent urination and increased thirst are the first signs of DKA. Other symptoms include:

- flushed face
- headache
- shortness of breath
- deep, labored breathing
- fruity smelling breath from ketones
- abdominal pain, especially in children
- nausea and vomiting
- dry skin
- very dry mouth
- severe dehydration
- blurred vision
- rapid heartbeat
- drowsiness and lethargy
- coma

Hyperglycemic hyperosmolar syndrome (HHS) is a life-threatening complication of type 2 diabetes, characterized by extremely high blood glucose levels without ketone production, severe dehydration, and reduced consciousness. The blood becomes thick with glucose, salts, and other substances (hyperosmolarity). It may be brought on by infection or other illness or medications.

KEY TERMS

Diabetic hyperglycemic hyperosmolar syndrome; HHS—A life–threatening complication of type 2 diabetes in which blood sugar levels are extremely high.

Diabetic ketoacidosis; DKA—A serious complication of diabetes in which organic compounds called ketones reach very high levels in the blood.

Glycogen—A polysaccharide that is the principal source of stored glucose in humans.

Glycosuria—Abnormal amounts of sugar in the urine.

Insulin—A protein hormone synthesized in the pancreas and secreted by beta cells of the islets of Langerhans. Insulin is required for the metabolism of carbohydrates, lipids, and proteins, and regulates blood sugar levels by facilitating the uptake of glucose into tissues, converting sugars to glycogen, fatty acids, and triglycerides, and preventing the release of glucose from the liver.

Ketones—Organic compounds that build up in the blood and urine from the breakdown of fat and which are poisonous at high levels.

Osmotic diuresis—Increased urination caused by sugar or other substances in the urine.

Diagnosis

Tests

Hyperglycemia is diagnosed by measuring blood glucose levels. In non-pregnant adults the normal range for blood glucose before a meal (fasting) is 70–130 milligrams (mg) per deciliter (dL) of blood. A normal non–fasting blood glucose level is less than 180 mg/dL or 9 nanomoles (nm) per liter (L). A non-fasting blood glucose concentration above 200 mg/dL or 11 nm/L is diagnostic of diabetes. Glycosuria occurs at blood glucose levels above 180 mg/dL. However physicians often individualize blood glucose goals for each patient.

The A1C test measures average blood-glucose levels over two to three months. Non-diabetics score at about five percent on the A1C test. The American Diabetes Association (ADA) recommends that most people with diabetes keep their A1C levels at or below seven percent.

Routine urinalysis includes a measure of glucose in the urine. With normal **kidney function**, glucose is found in the urine only when it is abnormally high in the blood. Ketones in the urine are measured when blood glucose is over 240 mg/dL.

Treatment

Traditional

The standard treatment for hyperglycemia is injection of insulin, usually in combination with intravenous fluids and salts (electrolytes). DKA is treated with insulin, electrolytes, and fluids. In children and adolescents these components must be carefully adjusted for the patient's weight and administered with great precision. HHS is treated with fluids, potassium, and insulin. DKA and HHS usually require hospitalization.

Home remedies

Diabetics can often lower their blood sugar by exercising and/or eating less food. However if ketones are present in the urine, **exercise** can increase blood sugar.

Prognosis

The long-term consequences of prolonged hyperglycemia can include:

- intellectual impairment in children under four years of age
- increased susceptibility to infection
- retinopathy or blindness
- cataracts
- progressive kidney failure
- high blood pressure
- peripheral vascular disease
- early coronary artery disease
- nerve damage including peripheral and autonomic neuropathy

Age-specific mortality from diabetic hyperglycemia is probably twice that of the general population. Most deaths result from delayed diagnosis or from neglected treatment. The overall mortality rate from DKA is 1.2–9%. Children aged one to four years and adolescents are at particularly high risk for cerebral edema (swelling) from DKA. Of the one percent of children with DKA who develop cerebral edema, 57% recover completely, 21% have some type of neurological damage, and 21% die. The mortality rate from HHS may be as high as 40%.

Prevention

Prevention requires good diabetes management, careful monitoring of blood sugar levels, and early detection and correction of hyperglycemia. Hyperglycemia with type 1 diabetes can be prevented by carefully balancing dietary intake, physical activity, and insulin administration. Women are usually screened for gestational diabetes between the 24th and 28th week of pregnancy.

Parental concerns

Parents of a diabetic child may live with the uncertainty of possible hyperglycemic episodes but can be reassured by knowing that continuous glucose monitoring, a proper diet as advised by the pediatrician, insulin therapy if prescribed, and appropriate exercise can control the disease and help avoid extremes that lead to hyperglycemia. It is important to maintain close contact with the child's diabetes team of professionals and to learn as much as possible about the disease and the symptoms to watch for in the child that may signal hyperglycemia. The parents of school-age children should make sure that teachers also understand the warning signs of hyperglycemia so that immediate medical attention can be given when needed.

Resources

BOOKS

Galmer, Andrew. *Diabetes.* Westport, CT: Greenwood Press, 2008.

Magic Foods for Better Blood Sugar. London: Reader's Digest, 2008.

PERIODICALS

Bunker, Katie. "30 Things You Should Know About Managing Diabetes." *Diabetes Forecast* 61(4) (April 2008): 54–6.

Dungan, Kathleen M., Susan S. Braithwaite, and Jean–Charles Preiser. "Stress Hyperglycaemia." *Lancet* 373(9677) (May 23–29, 2009): 1798–1807.

Pagán, Camille Noe. "'I Beat Sugar with Food.'" *Prevention* 61(4) (April 2009): 102–12.

OTHER

American Diabetes Association. "Hyperglycemia (High Blood Glucose)." Living With Diabetes, http://www.diabetes.org/living–with–diabetes/treatment–and–care/blood–glucose–control/hyperglycemia.html (accessed September 26, 2010).

"Glucose." Lab Tests Online, http://www.labtestsonline.org/understanding/analytes/glucose/test.html (accessed September 26, 2010).

"Hyperglycemia—Infants." MedlinePlus, http://www.nlm.nih.gov/medlineplus/ency/article/007228.htm (accessed September 26, 2010).

Lamb, William H. "Diabetes Mellitus, Type 1." eMedicine, http://emedicine.medscape.com/article/919999–overview (accessed September 26, 2010).

National Diabetes Information Clearinghouse. "Your Guide to Diabetes: Type 1 and Type 2." http://diabetes.niddk.nih.gov/dm/pubs/type1and2/index.htm (accessed September 26, 2010).

ORGANIZATIONS

American Diabetes Association (ADA), 1701 North Beauregard St., Alexandria VA, 22311, (800) 342–2383 (DIABETES), AskADA@diabetes.org, http://www.diabetes.org.

Juvenile Diabetes Research Foundation International (JDRFI), 26 Broadway, 14th Floor, New York NY, 10004, (800) 533–CURE (2873), (212) 785–9595, info@jdrf.org, http://www.jdf.org.

National Institute of Diabetes and Digestive and Kidney Diseases (NIDDK), Building 31, Room 9A06, 31 Center Dr., MSC 2560, Bethesda MD, 20892–2560, (301) 496–3583, http://www2.niddk.nih.gov.

Margaret Alic, PhD

Hyperhidrosis

Definition

Hyperhidrosis is a disorder marked by excessive sweating. It usually begins at **puberty** and affects the palms, soles, and armpits.

Description

Sweating is the body's way of cooling itself and is a normal response to a hot environment or intense **exercise**. Excessive sweating unrelated to these conditions can be a problem for some people. Those with constantly moist hands may feel uncomfortable shaking hands or touching, while others with sweaty armpits and feet may have to contend with the unpleasant odor that results from the bacterial breakdown of sweat and cellular debris (bromhidrosis). People with hyperhidrosis often must change their clothes at least once a day, and their shoes can be ruined by the excess moisture. Hyperhidrosis may contribute to such skin diseases as athlete's foot (tinea pedis) and **contact dermatitis**.

In addition to excessive sweat production, the texture and color of the skin itself may be affected by hyperhidrosis. The skin may turn pink or bluish white. Severe hyperhidrosis of the soles of the feet may produce cracks, fissures, and scaling of the skin.

Hyperhidrosis in general and axillary hyperhidrosis (excessive sweating in the armpits) in particular are more common in the general population than was previously thought. A group of dermatologists in Virginia reported in 2004 that 2.8% of the United States population, or about 7.8 million persons, have hyperhidrosis. Of this group, slightly more than half (4 million persons) have axillary hyperhidrosis. One-third of the latter group, or about 1.3 million persons, find that the condition significantly interferes with daily activities and is barely tolerable. Only 38% had ever discussed their excessive sweating with their doctor.

Causes and symptoms

There are three basic forms of hyperhidrosis: emotionally induced; localized; and generalized. Emotionally induced hyperhidrosis typically affects the palms of the hands, soles of the feet, and the armpits. Localized hyperhidrosis typically affects the palms, armpits, groin, face, and the area below the breasts in women, while generalized hyperhidrosis may affect the entire body.

Hyperhidrosis may be either idiopathic (of unknown cause) or secondary to **fever**, metabolic disorders, **alcoholism**, menopause, Hodgkin lymphoma, **tuberculosis**, various types of **cancer**, or the use of certain medications. The medications most commonly associated with hyperhidrosis are propranolol, venlafaxine, **tricyclic antidepressants**, pilocarpine, and physostigmine.

Most cases of hyperhidrosis begin during childhood or **adolescence**. Hyperhidrosis that begins in adult life should prompt the doctor to look for a systemic illness, medication side effect, or metabolic disorder.

Hyperhidrosis affects both sexes equally and may occur in any age group. People of any race may be affected; however, for some unknown reason, Japanese are affected 20 times more frequently than members of other ethnic groups.

Diagnosis

Hyperhidrosis is diagnosed by patient report and a physical examination. In many cases the physician can directly observe the excessive sweating.

Tests

The doctor may perform an iodine starch test, which involves spraying the affected areas of the patient's body with a mixture of 500 g of water-soluble starch and 1 g iodine crystals. Areas of the skin producing sweat turn black.

The doctor will order other laboratory or imaging tests if he or she suspects that the sweating is associated with another disease or disorder.

KEY TERMS

Dermatitis—A skin condition characterized by a red, itchy rash. It may occur when the skin comes in contact with something to which it is sensitive.

Treatment

Most over-the-counter antiperspirants are not strong enough to effectively prevent hyperhidrosis. To treat the disorder, doctors prescribe 20% aluminum chloride hexahydrate solution (Drysol). It is applied at night to the affected areas and then wrapped in a plastic film until morning. Drysol works by blocking the sweat pores. Formaldehyde and glutaraldehyde-based solutions can also be prescribed; however, formaldehyde may trigger an allergic reaction and glutaraldehyde can stain the skin (for this reason it is primarily applied to the soles).

Drugs

Anticholinergic drugs may be given. These drugs include such medications as propantheline, oxybutynin, and benztropine.

Injections of botulinum toxin (Botox) given under the skin work well for some patients. Botox works to stop the excessive sweating by preventing the transmission of nerve impulses to the sweat glands. These injections must be repeated every 4-12 months.

Alternative

An electrical device that emits low-voltage current can be held against the skin to reduce sweating. These treatments are usually conducted in a doctor's office on a daily basis for several weeks, followed by weekly visits. Dermatologists recommend that patients wear clothing made of natural or absorbent fabrics, avoid high-buttoned collars, use talc or cornstarch, and keep underarms shaved.

The only permanent cure for hyperhidrosis of the palms is a surgical procedure known as a sympathectomy. To treat severe excessive sweating, a surgeon can remove a portion of the nerve near the top of the spine that controls palm sweat. Few neurosurgeons in the United States will perform the procedure because it often results in compensatory sweating in other regions of the body. Alternatively, it is possible to surgically remove the sweat gland-bearing skin of the armpits, but this is a major procedure that may require skin grafts.

More recently, liposuction under the armpits has been successfully used to treat hyperhidrosis in this region of the body. The liposuction removes some of the excess sweat glands responsible for axillary hyperhidrosis. The procedure also has the advantage of leaving smaller scars and being less disruptive to the overlying skin.

Prognosis

Hyperhidrosis is not associated with increased mortality; it primarily affects the patient's quality of life rather than longevity. While the condition cannot be cured without radical surgery, it can usually be controlled effectively.

Resources

BOOKS

Mooney, Jean. *Illustrated Dictionary of Podiatry and Foot Science.* St Louis: Churchill Livingstone Elsevier, 2009.

Willoughby, William Franklin. *Regulation of the Sweating System.* New York: Nabu Press, 2010.

PERIODICALS

Licht, P.B., and H.K. Pilegaard. "Severity of Compensatory Sweating after Thoracoscopic Sympathectomy." *Annals of Thoracic Surgery* 78 (August 2004): 427–431.

Strutton, D.R., J.W. Kowalski, D.A. Glaser, and P.E. Stang. "U.S. Prevalence of Hyperhidrosis and Impact on Individuals with Axillary Hyperhidrosis: Results from a National Survey." *Journal of the American Academy of Dermatology* 51 (August 2004): 241–248.

OTHER

Altman, Rachel, and Robert Schwartz. "Hyperhidrosis." *eMedicine* March 12, 2010, http://emedicine.medscape.com/article/1073359-overview (accessed October 10, 2010).

ORGANIZATIONS

American Academy of Dermatology (AAD), P.O. Box 4014, Schaumburg IL, 60168-4014, (847) 330-0230, http://www.aad.org.

Carol A. Turkington
Rebecca J. Frey, PhD
Laura Jean Cataldo, RN, EdD

Hypertension

Definition

Hypertension is high blood pressure. Blood pressure is the force of blood pushing against the walls of arteries as it flows through them. Arteries are the blood vessels that carry oxygenated blood from the heart to the body's tissues.

Normal blood pressure ranges* in children, by age, gender, and height percentile

Boys

Age	Percentile of height						
	5th	10th	25th	50th	75th	90th	95th
1	80–105/34–61	81–106/35–62	83–108/36–63	85–110/37–64	87–112/38–65	88–113/39–66	89–114/39–66
2	84–109/39–66	85–110/40–67	87–111/41–68	88–113/42–69	90–115/43–70	92–117/44–71	92–117/44–71
3	86–111/47–71	87–112/44–71	89–114/45–72	91–116/46–73	93–118/47–74	94–119/48–75	95–120/48–75
4	88–113/47–74	89–114/48–75	91–116/49–76	93–118/50–77	95–120/51–78	96–121/51–78	97–122/52–79
5	90–115/50–77	91–116/51–78	93–118/52–79	95–120/53–80	96–121/54–81	98–123/55–81	98–123/55–82
6	91–116/53–80	92–117/53–80	94–119/54–81	96–121/55–82	98–123/56–83	99–124/57–84	100–125/57–84
7	92–117/55–82	94–118/55–82	95–120/56–83	97–122/57–84	99–124/58–85	100–125/59–86	101–126/59–86
8	94–119/56–83	95–120/57–84	97–122/58–85	99–123/59–86	100–125/60–87	102–127/60–87	102–127/61–88
9	95–120/57–84	96–121/58–85	98–123/59–86	100–125/57–87	102–127/61–88	103–128/61–88	104–129/62–89
10	97–122/58–85	98–123/59–86	100–125/60–86	102–127/61–88	103–128/61–88	105–130/62–89	106–130/63–90
11	99–124/59–86	100–125/59–86	102–127/60–87	104–129/61–88	105–130/62–89	107–132/63–90	107–132/63–90
12	101–126/59–86	102–127/60–87	104–129/61–88	106–131/62–89	108–133/63–90	109–134/63–90	110–135/64–91
13	104–128/60–87	105–130/60–87	106–131/61–88	108–133/62–89	110–135/63–90	111–136/64–91	112–137/64–91
14	106–131/60–87	107–132/61–88	109–134/62–89	111–136/63–90	113–138/64–91	114–139/65–92	115–140/65–92
15	109–134/61–88	110–135/62–89	112–136/63–90	113–138/64–91	115–140/65–92	117–142/66–93	117–142/66–93
16	111–136/63–90	113–137/63–90	114–139/64–91	116–141/65–92	118–143/66–93	119–144/67–94	120–145/67–94
17	114–139/65–92	115–140/66–93	116–141/66–93	118–143/67–94	120–145/68–95	121–146/69–96	122–147/70–97

Girls

Age	Percentile of height						
	5th	10th	25th	50th	75th	90th	95th
1	83–108/38–64	84–108/39–64	85–109/39–65	86–111/40–65	88–112/41–66	89–113/41–67	90–114/42–67
2	85–109/41–69	85–110/44–69	87–111/44–70	88–112/45–70	89–114/46–71	91–115/46–72	91–116/47–62
3	86–111/47–73	87–111/48–73	88–113/48–74	89–114/49–75	91–115/50–75	92–116/50–76	93–117/51–76
4	88–112/50–76	88–113/50–76	90–114/51–76	91–115/52–77	92–117/52–78	94–118/53–79	94–119/54–79
5	89–114/52–78	90–114/53–78	91–116/53–79	93–117/54–79	94–118/55–80	95–120/55–81	96–120/56–81
6	91–115/54–80	92–116/54–80	93–117/55–80	94–119/56–81	96–120/56–82	97–121/57–83	98–122/58–83
7	93–117/55–81	93–118/56–81	95–119/56–82	96–120/57–82	97–122/58–83	99–123/58–84	99–124/59–84
8	95–119/57–82	95–120/57–82	96–121/57–83	98–122/58–83	99–123/59–84	100–125/60–85	101–125/60–86
9	96–121/58–83	97–121/58–83	98–123/58–84	100–124/59–84	101–125/60–85	102–127/61–86	103–127/61–87
10	98–123/59–84	99–123/59–84	100–125/59–85	102–126/60–86	103–127/61–86	104–129/62–87	105–129/62–88
11	100–125/60–85	101–125/60–85	102–126/60–86	103–128/61–87	105–129/62–87	106–130/63–88	107–131 /63–89
12	102–127/61–86	103–127/61–86	104–128/61–87	105–130/62–88	107–131/63–88	108–132/64–89	109–133/64–90
13	104–128/62–87	105–129/62–87	106–130/62–88	107–132/63–89	109–133/64–89	110–134/65–90	110–135/65–91
14	106–130/63–88	106–131/63–88	107–132/63–89	109–133/64–90	110–135/65–90	111–136/66–91	112–136/66–92
15	107–131/64–89	108–132/64–89	109–133/64–90	110–134/64–91	111–136/66–91	113–137/67–92	113–138/67–93
16	108–132/64–90	108–133/64–90	110–134/64–90	111–135/66–91	112–137/66–92	114–138/67–93	114–139/68–93
17	108–133/64–90	109–133/65–90	110–134/65–91	111–136/66–91	113–137/67–92	114–138/67–93	115–139/68–93

*Ranges are given as systolic blood pressure (mmHg)/diastolic blood pressure (mmHg).

SOURCE: *The Fourth Report on the Diagnosis, Evaluation, and Treatment of High Blood Pressure in Children and Adolescents.* National Heart, Lung, and Blood Institute, National Institutes of Health, Department of Health and Human Services, May 2005. Available online at: http://www.nhlbi.nih.gov/health/prof/heart/hbp/hbp_ped.pdf (accessed September 24, 2010).

(Table by PreMediaGlobal. Reproduced by permission of Gale, a part of Cengage Learning.)

Demographics

Hypertension is a major health problem, especially because it has no symptoms. Many people have hypertension without knowing it. In the United States, about 50 million people age six and older have high blood pressure. Hypertension is more common in men than women and in people over the age of 65 than in younger persons. More than half of all Americans over the age of 65 have hypertension. It also is more common in African-Americans than in white Americans.

Description

As blood flows through arteries it pushes against the inside of the artery walls. The more pressure the blood exerts on the artery walls, the higher the blood pressure will be. The size of small arteries also affects the blood pressure. When the muscular walls of arteries are relaxed, or dilated, the pressure of the blood flowing through them is lower than when the artery walls narrow, or constrict.

Blood pressure is highest when the heart beats to push blood out into the arteries. When the heart relaxes to fill with blood again, the pressure is at its lowest point. Blood pressure when the heart beats is called systolic pressure. Blood pressure when the heart is at rest is called diastolic pressure. When blood pressure is measured, the systolic pressure is stated first and the diastolic pressure second. Blood pressure is measured in millimeters of mercury (mm Hg). For example, if a person's systolic pressure is 120 and diastolic pressure is 80, it is written as 120/80 mm Hg. The American Heart Association has long considered blood pressure less than 140 over 90 normal for adults. However, the National Heart, Lung, and Blood Institute in Bethesda, Maryland released new clinical guidelines for blood pressure in 2003, lowering the standard normal readings. A normal reading was lowered to less than 120 over less than 80.

Hypertension is serious because people with the condition have a higher risk for heart disease and other medical problems than people with normal blood pressure. Serious complications can be avoided by getting regular blood pressure checks and treating hypertension as soon as it is diagnosed.

If left untreated, hypertension can lead to the following medical conditions:

- arteriosclerosis, also called atherosclerosis
- heart attack
- stroke
- enlarged heart
- kidney damage

Arteriosclerosis is hardening of the arteries. The walls of arteries have a layer of muscle and elastic tissue that makes them flexible and able to dilate and constrict as blood flows through them. High blood pressure can make the artery walls thicken and harden. When artery walls thicken, the inside of the blood vessel narrows. **Cholesterol** and fats are more likely to build up on the walls of damaged arteries, making them even narrower. Blood clots also can get trapped in narrowed arteries, blocking the flow of blood.

Arteries narrowed by arteriosclerosis may not deliver enough blood to organs and other tissues. Reduced or blocked blood flow to the heart can cause a heart attack. If an artery to the brain is blocked, a **stroke** can result.

Hypertension makes the heart work harder to pump blood through the body. The extra workload can make the heart muscle thicken and stretch. When the heart becomes too enlarged it cannot pump enough blood. If the hypertension is not treated, the heart may fail.

The kidneys remove the body's wastes from the blood. If hypertension thickens the arteries to the kidneys, less waste can be filtered from the blood. As the condition worsens, the kidneys fail and wastes build up in the blood. Dialysis or a kidney transplant are needed when the kidneys fail. About 25% of people who receive kidney dialysis have kidney failure caused by hypertension.

Risk factors

Even though the cause of most hypertension is not known, some people have risk factors that increase their chance of developing hypertension. Many of these risk factors can be avoided to lower the chance of developing hypertension or as part of a treatment program to lower blood pressure.

Risk factors for hypertension include:

- age over 60
- male sex
- race
- heredity
- salt sensitivity
- obesity
- inactive lifestyle
- heavy alcohol consumption
- use of oral contraceptives

Some people inherit a tendency to get hypertension. People with family members who have hypertension are more likely to develop it than those whose relatives are not hypertensive. People with these risk factors can avoid or eliminate other risk factors to lower their chance of developing hypertension. A 2003 report found that the rise in incidence of high blood pressure among children is most likely due to an increase in the number of overweight and obese children and adolescents.

Causes and symptoms

Many different actions or situations can normally raise blood pressure. Physical activity can temporarily raise blood pressure. Stressful situations can make blood pressure go up; when the stress goes away, blood pressure usually returns to normal. These temporary increases in blood pressure are not considered hypertension. A diagnosis of hypertension is made only when a person has multiple high blood pressure readings over a period of time.

The cause of hypertension is not known in 90–95% of the people who have it. Hypertension without a known cause is called primary or essential hypertension.

When a person has hypertension caused by another medical condition, it is called secondary hypertension. Secondary hypertension can be caused by a number of different illnesses. Many people with kidney disorders have secondary hypertension. The kidneys regulate the balance of salt and water in the body. If the kidneys cannot rid the body of excess salt and water, blood pressure goes up. Kidney infections, a narrowing of the arteries that carry blood to the kidneys, called renal artery stenosis, and other kidney disorders can disturb the salt and water balance.

Cushing's syndrome and tumors of the pituitary and adrenal glands often increase levels of the adrenal gland hormones cortisol, adrenalin, and aldosterone, which can cause hypertension. Other conditions that can cause hypertension are blood vessel diseases, thyroid gland disorders, some prescribed drugs, **alcoholism**, and pregnancy.

One of the most dangerous features of hypertension is the fact that it does not usually cause any symptoms. Individuals may not be aware that they have the condition, or they may mistakenly downplay its importance, simply because it is not causing any discernible problems. Without treatment, the deleterious effects of hypertension progress unchecked.

When blood pressure becomes extremely high, for example over 180/110 mmHg (termed malignant hypertension), symptoms such as **headache**, visual disturbances, **anxiety**, and shortness of breath may occur. If left untreated, stroke may supervene or a hypertensive crisis, in which organs cannot receive an adequate blood supply and begin to fail.

Diagnosis

Examination

Because hypertension does not cause symptoms, it is important to have blood pressure checked regularly. Blood pressure is measured with an instrument called a sphygmomanometer. A cloth-covered rubber cuff is wrapped around the upper arm and inflated. When the cuff is inflated, an artery in the arm is squeezed to momentarily stop the flow of blood. Then, the air is let out of the cuff while a stethoscope placed over the artery is used to detect the sound of the blood spurting back through the artery. This first sound is the systolic pressure, the pressure when the heart beats. The last sound heard as the rest of the air is released is the diastolic pressure, the pressure between heart beats. Both sounds are recorded on the mercury gauge on the sphygmomanometer.

A typical physical examination to evaluate hypertension includes:

- medical and family history
- physical examination
- ophthalmoscopy: Examination of the blood vessels in the eye
- chest x ray
- electrocardiograph (ECG)
- blood and urine tests

The medical and family history help the physician determine if the patient has any conditions or disorders that might contribute to or cause the hypertension. A family history of hypertension might suggest a genetic predisposition for hypertension.

The physical exam may include several blood pressure readings at different times and in different positions. The physician uses a stethoscope to listen to sounds made by the heart and blood flowing through the arteries. The pulse, reflexes, and height and weight are checked and recorded. Internal organs are palpated, or felt, to determine if they are enlarged.

Because hypertension can cause damage to the blood vessels in the eyes, the eyes may be checked with a instrument called an ophthalmoscope. The physician will look for thickening, narrowing, or hemorrhages in the blood vessels.

Tests

A chest x ray can detect an enlarged heart or other vascular (heart) abnormalities.

An electrocardiogram (ECG) measures the electrical activity of the heart. It can detect if the heart muscle is enlarged and if there is damage to the heart muscle from blocked arteries.

Urine and blood tests may be done to evaluate health and to detect the presence of disorders that might cause hypertension.

Treatment

Depending on the results of diagnostic tests, childhood hypertension is generally treated with such lifestyle changes as:

- reducing salt and fat intake
- losing weight

- getting regular exercise
- quitting smoking
- reducing alcohol consumption

Dietary guidelines are individualized, based on the child's blood pressure levels and specific needs. In children older than two years of age, the following low-fat dietary guidelines are recommended:

- Total fat intake should comprise 30 percent or less of total calories consumed per day.
- Calories consumed as saturated fat should equal no more than 8 to 10 percent of total calories consumed per day.
- Total cholesterol intake should be less than 300 mg/dl per day.

Elevated blood pressure can be reduced by an eating plan that emphasizes fruits, vegetables, and low-fat dairy foods, and which is low in saturated fat, total fat, and cholesterol. The DASH diet is recommended for patients with hypertension and includes whole grains, poultry, fish, and nuts. Fats, red meats, sodium, sweets, and sugar-sweetened beverages are limited. Sodium should also be reduced to no more than 1,500 milligrams per day.

A gradual transition to a heart-healthy diet can help decrease a child's risk of coronary artery disease and other health conditions in adulthood. Parents can replace foods high in fat with grains, vegetables, fruits, lean meat, and other foods low in fat and high in complex carbohydrates and protein. They can resist adding salt to foods while cooking and avoid highly processed foods that are usually high in sodium, such as fast foods, canned foods, boxed mixes, and frozen meals.

Prognosis

There is no cure for hypertension. However, it can be well controlled with proper treatment. Therapy with a combination of lifestyle changes and antihypertensive medicines can keep blood pressure at levels that will not cause damage to the heart or other organs. The key to avoiding serious complications of hypertension is to detect and treat it before damage occurs. Because antihypertensive medicines control blood pressure, but do not cure it, patients must continue taking the medications to maintain reduced blood pressure levels and avoid complications.

Prevention

Prevention of hypertension centers on avoiding or eliminating known risk factors.

Parental concerns

Parents should reinforce with the child that hypertension is a serious condition that can cause more health problems later in life. Parents should work with their child to make dietary changes and increase their activity level to manage hypertension and prevent it from getting worse. Everyone can benefit when a heart-healthy lifestyle is followed, so the dietary and activity changes made for the hypertensive child will benefit the entire family.

Resources

BOOKS

Goldman, Lee and Dennis Ausiello., eds. *Cecil Textbook of Medicine.*, 23rd ed. Philadelphia: Saunders Elsevier, 2008.

Libby, P., et al. *Braunwald's Heart Disease*, 8th ed. Philadelphia: Saunders, 2007.

PERIODICALS

McNamara, Damian. "Obesity Behind Rise in Incidence of Primary Hypertension." *Family Practice News* April 1, 2003: 45-51.

McNamara, Damian. "Trial Shows Efficacy of Lifestyle Changes for BP: More Intensive Than Typical Office Visit." *Family Practice News* July 1, 2003: 1-2.

"New BP Guidelines Establish Diagnosis of Pre-hypertension: Level Seeks to Identify At-risk Individuals Early." *Case Management Advisor* July 2003: S1.

"New Hypertension Guidelines: JNC-7." *Clinical Cardiology Alert* July 2003: 54-63.

ORGANIZATIONS

American Heart Association, 7272 Greenville Avenue, Dallas TX, 75231, (800) 242-8721, http://www.americanheart.org.

National Heart, Lung and Blood Institute, P.O. Box 30105, Bethesda MD, 20824-0105, (301) 592-8573, (240) 629-3246, nhlbiinfo@nhlbi.nih.gov, http://www.nhlbi.nih.gov.

Texas Heart Institute, P.O. Box 20345, Houston TX, 77225-0345, (800) 292-2221, hic@heart.thi.tmc.edu, http://www.texasheart.org.

Toni Rizzo
Teresa G. Odle

Hyperthyroidism

Definition

Hyperthyroidism is the overproduction of thyroid hormones by an overactive thyroid gland. More

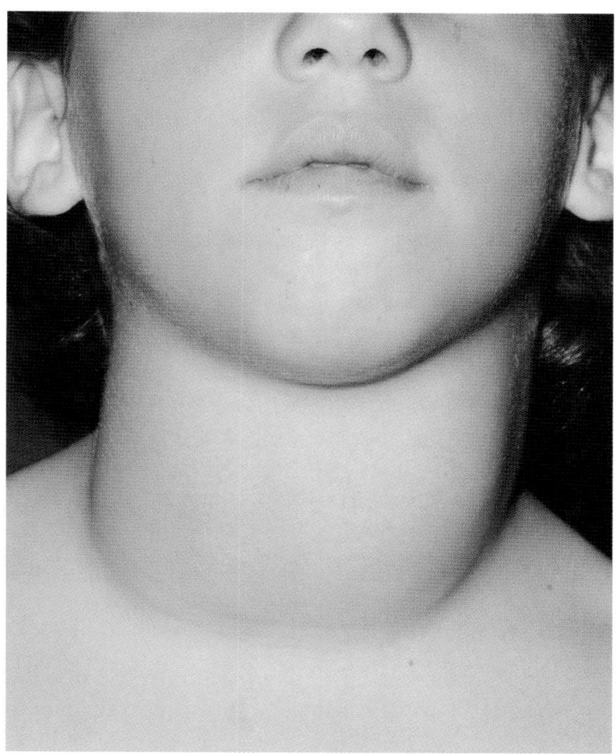

A symptom of hyperthyroidism is the enlargement of the thyroid gland, as seen in this child's neck. *(© Lester V. Bergman/Corbis.)*

specifically, the thyroid gland produces too much of a hormone called thyroxine.

The term *hyperthyroidism* covers any disease which results in overabundance of thyroid hormone. Other names for hyperthyroidism, or specific diseases within the category, include Graves' disease, diffuse toxic goiter, Basedow's disease, Parry's disease, and thyrotoxicosis.

Demographics

Hyperthyroidism is a fairly common disorder; the National Institute of Diabetes and Digestive and Kidney Diseases (NIDDK) estimates that about 1% of the population of the United States and Canada has some form of hyperthyroidism. It is primarily a disease of adults; most patients are 35 or older at the time of diagnosis. Only about 5% of patients are younger than 15 years of age. The peak age for hyperthyroidism caused by Graves' disease is 35 to 40 years; hyperthyroidism caused by multinodular goiter is more common in adults over 50 than in younger adults.

The disease is 10 times more common in women than in men, and the annual incidence of hyperthyroidism in the United States is about one per 1,000 women. About 7% of women of childbearing age develop postpartum thyroiditis in the year after they give **birth**. Between 3% and 7% of American adults develop thyroid nodules. Occult hyperthyroidism may occur in patients over 65 and is characterized by a distinct lack of typical symptoms. Diffuse toxic goiter occurs in as many as 80% of patients with hyperthyroidism.

Among children, about five times as many girls as boys develop hyperthyroidism. Almost all cases of pediatric hyperthyroidism are the form called Graves' disease. There is a form of hyperthyroidism called neonatal Graves' disease, which occurs in infants born of mothers with Graves' disease. Children with such other conditions as trisomy 21 (**Down syndrome**), Addison's disease, diabetes, systemic lupus erythematosus, rheumatoid arthritis, myasthenia gravis, vitiligo, pernicious **anemia**, and immune thrombocytopenic purpura are more likely to develop Graves' disease.

Hyperthyroidism is equally common among Caucasians, Asians, and Hispanics in the United States but is less common among African Americans. The reason for this difference is not known as of 2009.

Description

Located in the front of the neck, the thyroid gland is a butterfly-shaped structure lying between the Adam's apple and the collarbone. It takes its name from a Greek word meaning "shield." It consists of two lobes about 2 inches in length (in adults) connected by a thin strip of tissue called the isthmus. The thyroid gland weighs about a tenth of an ounce in newborns and 0.6–1.5 ounces in adults. One of the largest endocrine glands in the body, the thyroid controls the rate at which the body **burns** energy, its sensitivity to other hormones, and its manufacture of proteins.

The thyroid gland produces two hormones: thyroxine (T_4) and triiodothyronine (T_3, which regulate the body's metabolic rate by helping to form protein ribonucleic acid (RNA) and increasing oxygen absorption in every cell. In turn, the production of these hormones is controlled by thyroid-stimulating hormone (TSH), which is produced by the pituitary gland. Hyperthyroidism occurs when production of the thyroid hormones increases despite the level of TSH being produced. The excessive amount of thyroid hormones in the blood increases the body's metabolism, producing both mental and physical symptoms.

Risk factors

Risk factors for hyperthyroidism include:

- Female sex.
- Age over 60.

- Family history of thyroid disorders. Some genes have been identified as of 2009 that increase a person's susceptibility to autoimmune thyroid disease.
- Personal history of thyroid surgery or goiter.
- Having type 1 diabetes, pernicious anemia, or primary adrenal insufficiency.
- Pregnancy.
- Giving birth within the past 6 months.
- Eating large amounts of iodine-containing foods.
- Use of medications containing iodine, particularly amiodarone (Cordarone), a drug given to treat irregular heart rhythms.

Causes and symptoms

Causes

Hyperthyroidism is often associated with the body's production of autoantibodies in the blood that cause the thyroid to grow and secrete excess thyroid hormone. This condition, as well as other forms of hyperthyroidism, may be inherited. It accounts for 70–75% of cases of hyperthyroidism.

Other causes of hyperthyroidism include multinodular goiter or Plummer's disease (about 15–20% of cases of hyperthyroidism), a condition in which adenomas (nodules or lumps) form within the thyroid gland and cause it to secrete a larger than normal amount of thyroid hormone; and thyroiditis, a condition in which a malfunction of the **immune system** or a viral infection causes the thyroid gland to leak thyroid hormone. Last, hyperthyroidism can be caused by taking too much thyroid hormone in tablet form. In a few very rare cases, hyperthyroidism can be caused by a malignant (cancerous) tumor in the thyroid gland.

Symptoms

Regardless of the cause or age of the patient, hyperthyroidism produces the same symptoms, including sudden weight loss with increased appetite, shortness of breath and fatigue, intolerance of heat, heart palpitations, increased frequency of bowel movements, warm and smooth skin, weak muscles, tremors, **anxiety**, and difficulty sleeping. Women of childbearing age may also notice decreased menstrual flow and irregular menstrual cycles.

The symptoms of hyperthyroidism are often less noticeable in older adults, and may consist mainly of an increased heart rate, heat intolerance, and a tendency to become tired during ordinary activities. In addition, beta blockers (a type of heart medication) can mask the symptoms of hyperthyroidism in seniors.

Patients with Graves' disease often have a goiter (visible enlargement of the thyroid gland), although as many as 10 percent do not. These patients may also have bulging eyes. Thyroid storm, a serious form of hyperthyroidism, may show up as sudden and acute symptoms, some of which mimic typical hyperthyroidism, as well as the addition of **fever** (104°F or higher), substantial weakness, extreme restlessness, confusion, emotional swings or psychosis, or coma. Fortunately, such a fulminant course of Graves' disease is rare in children and adolescents.

Babies with neonatal Graves' disease may suffer from **prematurity**, airway obstruction, and heart failure. **Death** occurs in as many as 16 percent of these babies, and other complications from which survivors may suffer include **craniosynostosis** (early closure of the sutures of the skull, which can result in compression of the growing brain), and **developmental delay**.

Diagnosis

The diagnosis of hyperthyroidism is based on a combination of patient history, a physical examination, and the results of laboratory and imaging tests. In most cases, patients are evaluated and treated by an endocrinologist rather than a family doctor.

Examination

Patients concerned that they may have nodules in their thyroid or an enlarged thyroid can conduct a "neck check" at home by examining their neck below the Adam's apple and above the collarbone while swallowing water and looking in a handheld mirror. Detailed instructions for the neck check can be found at the AACE link under the "Other" resources listed below.

An endocrinologist will look for physical signs and symptoms indicated by the patient's history during an office examination. The patient will typically be asked to lift the head and swallow several times while the doctor feels the part of the neck containing the thyroid gland. On inspection, the physician may note such symptoms as a goiter, warm, smooth, and moist skin, eye bulging or a staring gaze, high blood pressure, irregular heart rhythm, hyperactivity, overactive reflexes, tremor, and muscle weakness. Pregnancy or recent **childbirth**, or a family history of thyroid disorders may also be clues to a diagnosis of hyperthyroidism.

Tests

A simple blood test can be performed to determine the amount of thyroid hormone in the patient's blood. The American Thyroid Association recommends that adults,

KEY TERMS

Adenoma—The medical term for a benign (noncancerous) tumor that originates in a gland. Thyroid nodules are one type of adenoma.

Endocrine gland—Any gland that makes hormones and secretes them directly into the bloodstream.

Endocrinologist—A doctor who specializes in diagnosing and treating disorders of the endocrine glands and the hormones they secrete.

Fulminant—Referring to a disease process that is explosive in onset, severe, and potentially deadly.

Goiter—Chronic enlargement of the thyroid gland.

Gonads—Organs that produce gametes (eggs or sperm), i.e. the ovaries and testes.

Graves' disease—An autoimmune disorder of the thyroid gland, in which the gland swells to twice its normal size and secretes too much thyroid hormone. Graves' disease accounts for 70–75% of cases of hyperthyroidism. It is named for an Irish doctor named Robert James Graves, who described a case of the disorder in 1835.

Hormone—A chemical released by specialized cells that affects cells in other parts of the body. Hormones regulate such body processes as growth, metabolism, the immune system, reproduction, hunger, and mood.

Multinodular goiter—A condition in which benign lumps of tissue (nodules) form within the thyroid gland and cause it to secrete too much thyroid hormone. It is also called Plummer's disease.

Palpitations—Rapid and forceful heartbeat.

Postpartum—After childbirth.

Radioisotope—One of two or more atoms with the same number of protons but a different number of neutrons with a nuclear composition. In nuclear scanning, radioactive isotopes are used as a diagnostic agent.

Thyroid storm—A rare but potentially life-threatening complication of hyperthyroidism, characterized by fever over 104°F, irregular heart rhythm, vomiting, diarrhea, dehydration, coma, and death.

Thyroidectomy—Surgical removal of the thyroid gland.

Thyroiditis—Inflammation of the thyroid gland. It can be caused by a viral infection, a malfunction of the immune system, or certain medications.

Thyrotoxicosis—Another term for hyperthyroidism.

Vitiligo—A chronic skin disorder that causes loss of pigmentation (color) from patches of skin, most often on the face, hands, and wrists.

particularly women, have this blood test to detect thyroid problems every 5 years starting at age 35. The diagnosis is usually straightforward with this combination of clinical history, physical examination, and routine blood hormone tests. Radioimmunoassay, or a test to show concentrations of thyroid hormones with the use of a radioisotope mixed with fluid samples, helps confirm the diagnosis.

A thyroid scan is a nuclear medicine procedure involving injection of a radioisotope dye that will tag the thyroid and help produce a clear image of inflammation or involvement of the entire thyroid. Other tests can determine thyroid function and thyroid-stimulating hormone levels. Ultrasonography, **computed tomography scans** (CT scan), and **magnetic resonance imaging** (MRI) may provide visual confirmation of a diagnosis or help to determine the extent of involvement.

Procedures

The doctor may also order a fine needle aspiration biopsy (FNAB), a procedure in which the doctor inserts a thin needle into a suspected thyroid nodule to extract a sample of cells for examination under a microscope. The doctor usually uses an ultrasound monitor to guide the needle. A FNAB can be performed in an outpatient clinic or a doctor's office; it is safer and less invasive than an open surgical biopsy.

Treatment

Traditional

Treatment of hyperthyroidism will depend on the specific disease and individual circumstances such as age, severity of disease, and other conditions affecting a patient's health. No single approach to treatment works for all patients.

Drugs

Hyperthyroidism is usually treated with medications whenever possible. The two types of drugs most often prescribed are antithyroid drugs and radioactive iodine.

ANTITHYROID DRUGS Antithyroid drugs are often administered to help the patient's body cease overproduction of thyroid hormones. The antithyroid drugs most commonly prescribed are methimazole (Tapazole) and propylthiouracil (PTU). About 20% to 30% of patients with Graves' disease will have long-term remission of hyperthyroidism after treatment with antithyroid drugs for a period of 12-18 months. It takes several weeks or months for antithyroid drugs to bring the patient's level of thyroid hormone into the normal range. Patients may be given beta blockers for symptom relief during this period.

Antithyroid drugs are also used in preparation for either radioiodine treatment or surgery in patients diagnosed with multinodular goiter. These medications may work for young adults, pregnant women, and others. Women who are pregnant should be treated with the lowest dose required to maintain thyroid function in order to minimize the risk of **hypothyroidism** in the infant.

Antithyroid drugs can have unpleasant side effects, such as **rashes**, **itching**, or increased susceptibility to infection due to a decreased level of white blood cells. In rare cases these medications can lead to liver failure.

RADIOACTIVE IODINE Radioactive iodine (iodine-131) is often prescribed to damage cells that make thyroid hormone. The cells need iodine to make the hormone, so they will absorb any iodine found in the body. The patient may take an iodine capsule daily for several weeks, resulting in the eventual shrinkage of the thyroid in size, reduced hormone production and a return to normal blood levels. Some patients may receive a single larger oral dose of radioactive iodine to treat the disease more quickly. This should only be done for patients who are not of reproductive age or are not planning to have children, since a large amount can concentrate in the reproductive organs (gonads). The risk of long-term side effects is low, however, as radioactive iodine has been used for over 60 years to treat patients with hyperthyroidism and doctors have followed these patients carefully.

Most patients who are given iodone-131 eventually develop hypothyroidism, which is an abnormally low level of thyroid hormone. Most endocrinologists do not consider this side effect of iodine-131 to be a major problem, however, because hypothyroidism is easier to treat and has fewer long-term complications than hyperthyroidism.

BETA BLOCKERS Beta blockers may be used in the treatment of patients with hyperthyroidism even though they do not suppress the activity of the thyroid gland. They are useful in regulating the patient's heart rhythm and reducing such symptoms as palpitations, tremor, and nervousness until antithyroid medications can begin to take effect. The beta blockers most often prescribed for hyperthyroidism are the longer-acting drugs like atenolol (Tenormin), metoprolol (Lopressor), and nadolol (Corgard).

Surgery

Some patients may undergo surgery to treat hyperthyroidism. Surgery is usually recommended when the results of a FNAB indicate that the patient has a malignancy in the thyroid, or when the thyroid gland is so enlarged that it is putting pressure on the patient's windpipe or esophagus.

Most commonly, patients treated with thyroidectomy in the form of partial or total removal of the thyroid suffer from large goiter and have suffered relapses, even after repeated attempts to address the disease through drug therapy. Some patients may be candidates for surgery because they were not good candidates for iodine therapy, or refused iodine administration. Patients receiving thyroidectomy or iodine therapy must be carefully monitored for years to watch for signs of hypothyroidism, or insufficient production of thyroid hormones, which can occur as a complication of thyroid production suppression.

Alternative

Consumption of such foods as broccoli, Brussels sprouts, cabbage, cauliflower, kale, rutabagas, spinach, turnips, peaches, and pears can help naturally suppress thyroid hormone production. Caffeinated drinks and dairy products should be avoided. Under the supervision of a trained physician, high dosages of certain vitamin/mineral combinations can help to alleviate hyperthyroidism.

Prognosis

Hyperthyroidism is generally treatable and carries a good prognosis. Most patients lead normal lives with proper treatment. Thyroid storm, however, can be life-threatening and can lead to heart, liver, or kidney failure. Luckily, this form of fulminant hyperthyroidism is rare in children and adolescents.

Hyperthyroidism is associated with an increased risk of Alzheimer's disease in later life even when the thyroid dysfunction has been successfully treated. The reason for this association is not fully understood as of 2009.

Prevention

Although a periodic neck check at home cannot prevent hyperthyroidism in the strict sense of prevention, it can help in detecting the condition earlier rather than later.

There are no known prevention methods for hyperthyroidism, since its causes are either inherited or not completely understood as of 2010. The best prevention tactic is knowledge of family history and close attention to symptoms and signs of the disease. Careful attention to prescribed therapy can prevent complications of the disease.

Resources

BOOKS

Cooper, David S. *Medical Management of Thyroid Disease*, 2nd ed. New York: Informa Healthcare, 2009.

Mertens, Lionel, and Jeremy Bogaert, eds. *Handbook of Hyperthyroidism: Etiology, Diagnosis, and Treatment*. Hauppauge, NY: Nova Science, 2009.

Shannon, Joyce Brennfleck. *Endocrine and Metabolic Disorders Sourcebook*, 2nd ed. Detroit, MI: Omnigraphics, 2007.

PERIODICALS

Baloch, Z.W., and V.A. LiVolsi. "Fine-needle Aspiration of the Thyroid: Today and Tomorrow." *Best Practice and Research: Clinical Endocrinology and Metabolism* 22 (December 2008): 929–39.

Brown, R.S. "Autoimmune Thyroid Disease: Unlocking a Complex Puzzle." *Current Opinion in Pediatrics* 21 (August 2009): 523–28.

Hegedüs, L. "Treatment of Graves' Hyperthyroidism: Evidence-based and Emerging Modalities." *Endocrinology and Metabolism Clinics of North America* 38 (June 2009): 355–71.

Kaguelidou, F., et al. "Graves' Disease in Childhood: Advances in Management with Antithyroid Drug Therapy." *Hormone Research* 71 (June 2009): 310–317.

Kharlip, J., and D.S. Cooper. "Recent Developments in Hyperthyroidism." *Lancet* 373 (June 6, 2009): 1930–32.

Kohl, B.A., and S. Schwartz. "Surgery in the Patient with Endocrine Dysfunction." *Medical Clinics of North America* 93 (September 2009): 1031–47.

Mistry, N., et al. "When to Consider Thyroid Dysfunction in the Neurology Clinic." *Practical Neurology* 9 (June 2009): 145–56.

Tan, Z.S., and R.S. Vasan. "Thyroid Function and Alzheimer's Disease." *Journal of Alzheimer's Disease* 16 (March 2009): 503–07.

Yildizhan, R., et al. "Fetal Death Due to Upper Airway Compromise Complicated by Thyroid Storm in a Mother with Uncontrolled Graves' Disease: A Case Report." *Journal of Medical Case Reports* 28 (May 2009): 7297.

OTHER

American Association of Clinical Endocrinologists (AACE). "How to Take the Thyroid 'Neck Check'." http://www.aace.com/public/awareness/tam/2006/pdfs/NeckCheckCard.pdf

American Thyroid Association (ATA). *Hyperthyroidism*, http://www.thyroid.org/patients/patient_brochures/hyperthyroidism.html

Hormone Foundation. *Hyperthyroidism*, http://www.hormone.org/Thyroid/hyperthyroidism.cfm

Lee, Stephanie L., and Sonia Ananthakrishnan. "Hyperthyroidism." *eMedicine*, June 8, 2009, http://emedicine.medscape.com/article/121865-overview

Mayo Clinic. *Hyperthyroidism*, http://www.mayoclinic.com/health/hyperthyroidism/DS00344

National Institute of Diabetes and Digestive and Kidney Diseases (NIDDK). *Hyperthyroidism*, http://endocrine.niddk.nih.gov/pubs/Hyperthyroidism/index.htm

Reid, Jeri R., and Stephen F. Wheeler. "Hyperthyroidism: Diagnosis and Treatment." *American Family Physician* 72 (August 15, 2005): 623–36, http://www.aafp.org/afp/20050815/623.html

ORGANIZATIONS

American Academy of Otolaryngology—Head and Neck Surgery, 1650 Diagonal Road, Alexandria VA, 22314, 703-836-4444, http://www.entnet.org/.

American Association of Clinical Endocrinologists (AACE), 245 Riverside Ave., Suite 200, Jacksonville FL, 32202, 904-353-7878, http://www.aace.com/.

American Thyroid Association (ATA), 6066 Leesburg Pike, Suite 550, Falls Church VA, 22041, 703-998-8890, 703-998-8893, thyroid@thyroid.org, http://www.thyroid.org/.

Hormone Foundation, 8401 Connecticut Avenue, Suite 900, Chevy Chase MD, 20815, 800–HORMONE, 301-941-0259, hormone@endo-society.org, http://www.hormone.org/.

National Institute of Diabetes and Digestive and Kidney Diseases (NIDDK), Building 31, Rm 9A06, 31 Center Drive, MSC 2560, Bethesda MD, 20892-2560, 301-496-3583, http://www2.niddk.nih.gov/Footer/ContactNIDDK.htm, http://www2.niddk.nih.gov/.

Teresa G. Odle
Rosalyn Carson-DeWitt, MD
Rebecca J. Frey, PhD

Hypertonia **see** Spasticity

Hypoglycemia

Definition

The condition called hypoglycemia is literally translated as low blood sugar. Hypoglycemia occurs when blood sugar (or blood glucose) concentrations fall below a level necessary to properly support the body's need for energy and stability throughout its cells.

Demographics

Attempts at quantifying the incidence of hypoglycemia is challenging, as many individuals do not regularly record, nor report the occurrence of this condition to their healthcare provider. It is thought to affect as many as 1 out of 1,000 people and can occur for a variety of reasons. Episodes of hypoglycemia occurring at night (nocturnal hypoglycemia) are commonly undetected by patients and it is believed that about 6% of all deaths in diabetes are due to unrecognized nocturnal hypoglycemia.

Description

Carbohydrates are the main dietary source of the glucose that is manufactured in the liver and absorbed into the bloodstream to fuel the body's cells and organs. Glucose concentration is controlled by hormones, primarily insulin and glucagon. Glucose concentration also is controlled by epinephrine (adrenalin) and norepinephrine, as well as growth hormone. If these regulators are not working properly, levels of blood sugar can become either excessive (as in **hyperglycemia**) or inadequate (as in hypoglycemia). If a person has a blood sugar level of 50 mg/dl or less, he or she is considered hypoglycemic, although glucose levels vary widely from one person to another.

Hypoglycemia can occur in several ways:

Drug-induced hypoglycemia

Drug-induced hypoglycemia, a complication of diabetes, is the most commonly seen and most dangerous form of hypoglycemia.

Hypoglycemia occurs most often in diabetics who must inject insulin periodically to lower their blood sugar. While other diabetics also are vulnerable to low blood sugar episodes, they have a lower risk of a serious outcome than insulin-dependent diabetics. Unless recognized and treated immediately, severe hypoglycemia in the insulin-dependent diabetic can lead to generalized convulsions followed by amnesia and unconsciousness. **Death**, though rare, is a possible outcome.

In insulin-dependent diabetics, hypoglycemia known as an insulin reaction or insulin shock can be caused by several factors. These include overmedicating with manufactured insulin, missing or delaying a meal, eating too little food for the amount of insulin taken, exercising too strenuously, drinking too much alcohol, or any combination of these factors.

Reactive hypoglycemia

Reactive hypoglycemia (also called postprandial hypoglycemia) occurs about 2–4 hours after eating a meal. A number of reasons for this reaction have been proposed, but no single cause has been identified.

In some cases, this form of hypoglycemia appears to be associated with malfunctions or diseases of the liver, pituitary, adrenals, liver, or pancreas. These conditions are unrelated to diabetes. Children intolerant of a natural sugar (fructose) or who have inherited defects that affect digestion also may experience hypoglycemic attacks. Some children with a negative reaction to aspirin also experience reactive hypoglycemia. It sometimes occurs among people with an intolerance to the sugar found in milk (galactose), and it also often begins before diabetes strikes later on.

Fasting hypoglycemia

Fasting hypoglycemia sometimes occurs after long periods without food, but it also happens occasionally following strenuous **exercise**, such as running in a marathon.

Other factors sometimes associated with hypoglycemia include:

- pregnancy
- a weakened immune system
- a poor diet high in simple carbohydrates
- prolonged use of drugs, including antibiotics
- chronic physical or mental stress
- heartbeat irregularities (arrhythmias)
- allergies
- breast cancer
- high blood pressure treated with beta-blocker medications (after strenuous exercise)
- upper gastrointestinal tract surgery

Causes and symptoms

When carbohydrates are eaten, they are converted to glucose that goes into the bloodstream and is distributed throughout the body. Simultaneously, a combination of chemicals that regulate how our body's cells absorb that sugar is released from the liver, pancreas, and adrenal glands. These chemical regulators include insulin, glucagon, epinephrine (adrenalin), and norepinephrine. The mixture of these regulators released following digestion of carbohydrates is never the same, since the amount of carbohydrates that are eaten is never the same.

Interactions among the regulators are complicated. Any abnormalities in the effectiveness of any one of the regulators can reduce or increase the body's absorption of glucose. Gastrointestinal enzymes such as amylase and lactase that break down carbohydrates may not be functioning properly. These abnormalities may produce hyperglycemia or hypoglycemia, and can be detected when the level of glucose in the blood is measured.

Cell sensitivity to these regulators can be changed in many ways. Over time, a person's stress level, exercise patterns, advancing age, and dietary habits influence cellular sensitivity. For example, a diet consistently overly rich in carbohydrates increases insulin requirements over time. Eventually, cells can become less receptive to the effects of the regulating chemicals, which can lead to glucose intolerance.

Diet is both a major factor in producing hypoglycemia as well as the primary method for controlling it. Diets typical of western cultures contain excess carbohydrates, especially in the form of simple carbohydrates such as sweeteners, which are more easily converted to sugar. In poorer parts of the world, the typical diet contains even higher levels of carbohydrates. Fewer dairy products and meats are eaten, and grains, vegetables, and fruits are consumed. This dietary trend is balanced, however, since people in these cultures eat smaller meals and usually use carbohydrates more efficiently through physical labor.

Early symptoms of severe hypoglycemia, particularly in the drug-induced type of hypoglycemia, resemble an extreme shock reaction. Symptoms include:

- cold and pale skin
- numbness around the mouth
- apprehension
- heart palpitations
- emotional outbursts
- hand tremors
- mental cloudiness
- dilated pupils
- sweating
- fainting

Mild attacks, however, are more common in reactive hypoglycemia and are characterized by extreme tiredness. Patients first lose their alertness, then their muscle strength and coordination. Thinking grows fuzzy, and finally the patient becomes so tired that he or she becomes "zombie-like," awake but not functioning. Sometimes the patient will actually fall asleep. Unplanned naps are typical of the chronic hypoglycemic patient, particularly following meals.

Additional symptoms of reactive hypoglycemia include headaches, double vision, staggering or inability to walk, a craving for salt and/or sweets, abdominal distress, premenstrual tension, chronic colitis, **allergies**, ringing in the ears, unusual patterns in the frequency of urination, skin eruptions and inflammations, **pain** in the neck and shoulder muscles, memory problems, and sudden and excessive sweating.

Unfortunately, a number of these symptoms mimic those of other conditions. For example, the depression, insomnia, irritability, lack of concentration, crying spells, **phobias**, forgetfulness, confusion, unsocial behavior, and suicidal tendencies commonly seen in nervous system and psychiatric disorders also may be hypoglycemic symptoms. It is very important that anyone with symptoms that may suggest reactive hypoglycemia see a doctor.

Because all of its possible symptoms are not likely to be seen in any one person at a specific time, diagnosing hypoglycemia can be difficult. One or more of its many symptoms may be due to another illness. Symptoms may persist in a variety of forms for long periods of time. Symptoms also can change over time within the same person. Some of the factors that can influence symptoms include physical or mental activities, physical or mental state, the amount of time passed since the last meal, the amount and quality of **sleep**, and exercise patterns.

Diagnosis

Drug-induced hypoglycemia

Once diabetes is diagnosed, the patient then monitors his or her blood sugar level with a portable machine called a glucometer. The diabetic places a small blood sample on a test strip that the machine can read. If the test reveals that the blood sugar level is too low, the diabetic can make a correction by eating or drinking an additional carbohydrate.

Reactive hypoglycemia

Reactive hypoglycemia only can be diagnosed by a doctor. Symptoms usually improve after the patient has gone on an appropriate diet. Reactive hypoglycemia was diagnosed more frequently 10–20 years ago than today. Studies have shown that most people suffering from its symptoms test normal for blood sugar, leading many doctors to suggest that actual cases of reactive hypoglycemia are quite rare. Some doctors think that people with hypoglycemic symptoms may be particularly sensitive to the body's normal postmeal release of the hormone epinephrine, or are actually suffering from some other physical or mental problem. Other doctors believe reactive hypoglycemia actually is the early onset of diabetes that occurs after a number of years. There continues to be disagreement about the cause of reactive hypoglycemia.

A common test to diagnose hypoglycemia is the extended oral glucose tolerance test. Following an overnight fast, a concentrated solution of glucose is drunk and blood samples are taken hourly for five to six hours. Though this test remains helpful in early identification of diabetes, its use in diagnosing chronic reactive hypoglycemia has lost favor because it can trigger hypoglycemic symptoms in people with otherwise normal glucose readings. Some doctors now recommend that blood sugar be tested at the actual time a person experiences hypoglycemic symptoms.

Treatment

Treatment of the immediate symptoms of hypoglycemia can include eating sugar. For example, a patient can eat a piece of candy, drink milk, or drink fruit juice. Glucose tablets can be used by patients, especially those who are diabetic. Effective treatment of hypoglycemia over time requires the patient to follow a modified diet. Patients usually are encouraged to eat small, but frequent, meals throughout the day, avoiding excess simple sugars (including alcohol), fats, and fruit drinks. Those patients with severe hypoglycemia may require fast-acting glucagon injections that can stabilize their blood sugar within approximately 15 minutes.

Alternative treatment

A holistic approach to reactive hypoglycemia is based on the belief that a number of factors may create the condition. Among them are heredity, the effects of other illnesses, emotional stress, too much or too little exercise, bad lighting, poor diet, and environmental pollution. Therefore, a number of alternative methods have been proposed as useful in treating the condition. Homeopathy, acupuncture, and applied kinesiology, for example, have been used, as have herbal remedies. One of the herbal remedies commonly suggested for hypoglycemia is a decoction (an extract made by boiling) of gentian (*Gentiana lutea*). It should be drunk warm 15–30 minutes before a meal. Gentian is believed to help stimulate the endocrine (hormone-producing) glands.

In addition to the dietary modifications recommended above, people with hypoglycemia may benefit from supplementing their diet with chromium, which is believed to help improve blood sugar levels. Chromium is found in whole grain breads and cereals, cheese, molasses, lean meats, and brewer's yeast. Hypoglycemics should avoid alcohol, **caffeine**, and cigarette smoke, since these substances can cause significant swings in blood sugar levels.

Prevention

Drug-induced hypoglycemia

Preventing hypoglycemic insulin reactions in diabetics requires taking glucose readings through frequent blood sampling. Insulin then can be regulated based on those readings. Continuous glucose monitoring sensors have been developed to help diabetics remain more aware of possible hypoglycemic episodes. These monitors even can check for episodes while the patient sleeps, when many will experience severe hypoglycemia but not know it. Those who don't pay attention to severe hypoglycemia events or who have had previous severe hypoglycemia are the most likely to have future severe hypoglycemia. An audible alert can let the patient know immediately that he or she needs to take care of his or her blood sugar level. Continuous monitoring has proved particularly helpful in pediatric patients with Type 1 diabetes.

Maintaining proper diet also is a factor. Programmable insulin pumps implanted under the skin have proven useful in reducing the incidence of hypoglycemic episodes for insulin-dependent diabetics. As of late 1997, clinical studies continue to seek additional ways to control diabetes and drug-induced hypoglycemia. Tests of a substance called pramlintide indicate that it may help improve glycemic control in diabetics.

Reactive hypoglycemia

The onset of reactive hypoglycemia can be avoided or at least delayed by following the same kind of diet used to control it. While not as restrictive as the diet diabetics must follow to keep tight control over their disease, it is quite similar.

There are a variety of diet recommendations for the reactive hypoglycemic. Patients should:

- avoiding overeating
- never skipping breakfast
- including protein in all meals and snacks, preferably from sources low in fat, such as the white meat of chicken or turkey, most fish, soy products, or skim milk
- restricting intake of fats (particularly saturated fats, such as animal fats), and avoiding refined sugars and processed foods
- being aware of the differences between some vegetables, such as potatoes and carrots. These vegetables have a higher sugar content than others (like squash and broccoli). Patients should be aware of these differences and note any reactions they have to them.
- being aware of differences found in grain products. White flour is a carbohydrate that is rapidly absorbed into the bloodstream, while oats take much longer to break down in the body.
- keeping a "food diary." Until the diet is stabilized, a patient should note what and how much he/she eats and drinks at every meal. If symptoms appear following a meal or snack, patients should note them and look for patterns.

- eat fresh fruits, but restrict the amount they eat at one time. Patients should remember to eat a source of protein whenever they eat high sources of carbohydrate like fruit. Apples make particularly good snacks because, of all fruits, the carbohydrate in apples is digested most slowly.
- following a diet that is high in fiber. Fruit is a good source of fiber, as are oatmeal and oat bran. Fiber slows the buildup of sugar in the blood during digestion.

A doctor can recommend a proper diet, and there are many cookbooks available for diabetics. Recipes found in such books are equally effective in helping to control hypoglycemia.

Prognosis

Like diabetes, there is no cure for reactive hypoglycemia, only ways to control it. While some chronic cases will continue through life (rarely is there complete remission of the condition), others will develop into type II (age onset) diabetes. Hypoglycemia appears to have a higher-than-average incidence in families where there has been a history of hypoglycemia or diabetes among their members, but whether hypoglycemia is a controllable warning of oncoming diabetes has not yet been determined by clinical research.

A condition known as hypoglycemia unawareness can develop in those who do not control their blood glucose, particularly in people with Type 1 diabetes. These people may lose notice of the automatic warning symptoms of hypoglycemia that normally occur as their bodies become so used to frequent periods of hypoglycemia. It is not a permanent event, but can be treated by careful avoidance of hypoglycemia for about two weeks.

Resources

BOOKS

Colbert, Don, M.D. *The New Bible Cure for Diabetes.* Lake Mary, FL: Siloam Press, 2009.

Kenrose, Stephanie. *The Reactive Hypoglycemia Cookbook.* Charleston, SC: CreateSpace, 2010.

Kenrose, Stephanie. *The Reactive Hypoglycemia Sourcebook.* Raleigh, NC: Lulu, 2009.

Pierce, Dino Paul, CFT, CPT, RD, CDE. *The Diabetes Handbook: Create Awareness and a New You.* Charleston, SC: CreateSpace, 2009.

Vaughn, Richard, A. *Beating The Odds: 64 Years of Diabetes Health.* Charleston, SC: CreateSpace, 2010.

PERIODICALS

Brauker, James, et al. "Use of Continuous Glucose Monitoring Alerts to Better Predict, Prevent and Treat Postprandial Hyperglycemia." *Diabetes* June 2003: 90-91.

Gertzman, Jerilyn, et al. "Severity of Hypoglycemia and Hypoglycemia Unawareness Are Associated with the Extent of Unsuspected Nocturnal Hypoglycemia." *Diabetes* June 2003:146-151.

Kumar, Rajeev, and Miles Fisher. "Impaired Hypoglycemia Awareness: Are we Aware?" *Diabetes and Primary Care* Summer 2004: 33–38.

Ludvigsson, Johnny, and Ragnar Hanas. "Continuous Subcutaneous Glucose Monitoring Improved Metabolic Control in Pediatric Patients With Type 1 Diabetes: A Controlled Crossover Study." *Pediatrics* May 2003: 933-936.

ORGANIZATIONS

American Diabetes Association, 1701 North Beauregard Street, Alexandria VA, 22311, (800) 342-2383, http://www.diabetes.org.

Hypoglycemia Association, Inc, 18008 New Hampshire Ave., PO Box 165, Ashton MD, 20861-0165

National Hypoglycemia Association, Inc., PO Box 120, Ridgewood NJ 07451, (201) 670-1189

The Hypoglycemia Support Foundation, Inc, http://www.hypoglycemia.org/default.asp.

Martin W. Dodge, Ph.D.
Teresa G. Odle
Ken R. Wells
Laura Jean Cataldo, RN, Ed.D.

Hypogonadism

Definition

Hypogonadism is the condition more prevalent in males in which the production of sex hormones and germ cells are inadequate.

Description

Gonads are the organs of sexual differentiation—in the female, they are ovaries; in the male, the testes. Along with producing eggs and sperm, they produce sex hormones that generate all the differences between men and women. If they produce too little sex hormone, then either the growth of the sexual organs or their function is impaired.

The gonads are not independent in their function, however. They are closely controlled by the pituitary gland. The pituitary hormones are the same for males and females, but the gonadal hormones are different. Men produce mostly androgens, and women produce mostly estrogens. These two hormones regulate the development of the embryo, determining whether it is a male or a female. They also direct the adolescent maturation of sex organs into their adult form. Further, they sustain those organs and their function throughout the reproductive years. The effects of estrogen reach beyond that to sustain bone strength and protect the cardiovascular system from degenerative disease.

Hormones can be inadequate during or after each stage of development—embryonic and adolescent. During each stage, inadequate hormone stimulation will prevent normal development. After each stage, a decrease in hormone stimulation will result in failed function and perhaps some shrinkage. The organs affected principally by sex hormones are the male and female genitals, both internal and external, and the female breasts. Body hair, fat deposition, bone and muscle growth, and some brain functions are also influenced.

Causes and symptoms

Sex is determined at the moment of conception by sex chromosomes. Females have two X chromosomes, while males have one X and one Y chromosome. If the male sperm with the Y chromosome fertilizes an egg, the baby will be male. This is true throughout the animal kingdom. Genetic defects sometimes result in changes in the chromosomes. If sex chromosomes are involved, there is a change in the development of sexual characteristics.

Female is the default sex of the embryo, so most of the sex organ deficits at **birth** occur in boys. Some, but not all, are due to inadequate androgen stimulation. The penis may be small, the testicles undescended (cryptorchidism) or various degrees of "feminization" of the genitals may be present.

After birth, sexual development does not occur until **puberty**. Hypogonadism most often shows up as an abnormality in boys during puberty. Again, not every defect is due to inadequate hormones. Some are due to too much of the wrong ones. Kallmann's syndrome is a birth defect in the brain that prevents release of hormones and appears as failure of male puberty. Some boys have adequate amounts of androgen in their system but fail to respond to them, a condition known as androgen resistance.

Female problems in puberty are not caused by too little estrogen. Even female reproductive problems are rarely related to a simple lack of hormones, but rather to complex cycling rhythms gone wrong. All the problems with too little hormone happen during menopause, which is a normal hypogonadism.

A number of adverse events can damage the gonads and result in decreased hormone levels. The childhood disease **mumps**, if acquired after puberty, can infect and destroy the testicles—a disease called viral orchitis. Ionizing radiation and **chemotherapy**, trauma, several drugs (spironolactone, a diuretic and ketoconazole, an antifungal agent), alcohol, **marijuana**, heroin, methadone, and environmental toxins can all damage testicles and decrease their hormone production. Severe diseases in the liver or kidneys, certain infections, sickle cell **anemia**, and some cancers also affect gonads. To treat some male cancers, it is necessary to remove the testicles, thereby preventing the androgens from stimulating **cancer** growth. This procedure, still called castration or *orchiectomy*, removes androgen stimulation from the whole body.

For several reasons the pituitary can fail. It happens rarely after pregnancy. It used to be removed to treat advanced breast or prostate cancer. Sometimes the pituitary develops a tumor that destroys it. Failure of the pituitary is called hypopituitarism and, of course, leaves the gonads with no stimulation to produce hormones.

Besides the tissue changes generated by hormone stimulation, the only other symptoms relate to sexual desire and function. Libido is enhanced by testosterone, and male sexual performance requires androgens. The role of female hormones in female sexual activity is less clear, although hormones strengthen tissues and promote healthy secretions, facilitating sexual activity.

Diagnosis

Presently, there are accurate blood tests for most of the hormones in the body, including those from the pituitary and even some from the hypothalamus. Chromosomes can be analyzed, and gonads can, but rarely are, biopsied.

Treatment

Replacement of missing body chemicals is much easier than suppressing excesses. Estrogen replacement is recommended for nearly all women after menopause for its many beneficial effects. Estrogen can be taken by mouth, injection, or skin patch. It is strongly recommended that the other female hormone, progesterone, be taken as well, because it prevents overgrowth of uterine lining and uterine cancer. Testosterone replacement is available for males who are deficient.

Resources

BOOKS

Carr, Bruce R., and Karen D. Bradshaw. "Disorders of the Ovary and Female Reproductive Tract." In *Harrison's Principles of Internal Medicine*, edited by Anthony S. Fauci, et al. New York: McGraw-Hill, 1998.

J. Ricker Polsdorfer, MD

Hypopigmentation *see* Albinism

Hypospadias and epispadias

Definition

Hypospadias is a congenital defect, primarily of males, in which the urethra opens on the underside (ventrum) of the penis. It is one of the most common congenital abnormalities in the United States, occurring in about one of every 125 live male births. The corresponding defect in females is an opening of the urethra into the vagina and is rare.

Epispadias (also called bladder exstrophy) is a congenital defect of males in which the urethra opens on the upper surface (dorsum) of the penis. The corresponding defect in females is a fissure in the upper wall of the urethra and is quite rare.

Description

In a male, the external opening of the urinary tract (external meatus) is normally located at the tip of the penis. In a female, it is normally located between the clitoris and the vagina.

In males with hypospadias, the urethra opens on the inferior surface or underside of the penis. In females with hypospadias, the urethra opens into the cavity of the vagina.

In males with epispadias, the urethra opens on the superior surface or upper side of the penis. In females with epispadias, there is a crack or fissure in the wall of the urethra and out of the body through an opening in the skin above the clitoris.

During the embryological development of males, a groove of tissue folds inward and then fuses to form a tube that becomes the urethra. Hypospadias occurs when the tube does not form or does not fuse completely. Epispadias is due to a defect in the tissue that folds inward to form the urethra.

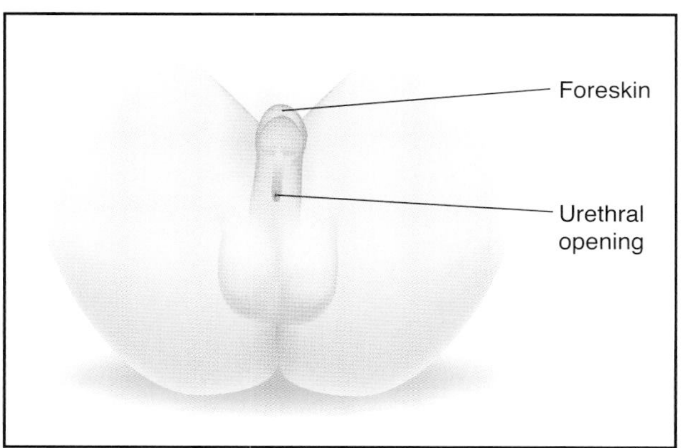

Hypospadias, a condition in which the urethral opening is not at the tip of the penis, but rather along the penile shaft. *(Illustration by Argosy, Inc. Reproduced by permission of Gale, a part of Cengage Learning.)*

During the development of a female, similar processes occur to form the urethra. The problem usually is insufficient length of the tube that becomes the urethra. As a result, the urethra opens in an abnormal location, resulting in a hypospadias. Occasionally, fissures form in the bladder. These may extend to the surface of the abdomen and fuse with the adjacent skin. This condition is most commonly identified as a defect in the bladder although it is technically an epispadias.

Hypospadias in males generally occur alone. Female hypospadias may be associated with abnormalities of the genital tract, since the urinary and genital tracts are formed in the same embryonic process.

Because it represents incomplete development of the penis, some experts think that insufficient male hormone may be responsible for hypospadias.

In males, the incidence of hypospadias is approximately one per 250 to 300 live births. Epispadias is much less common, having an incidence of about one per 100,000 live male births.

In females, hypospadias is much less common than in males. It appears about once in every 500,000 live female births. Epispadias is even rarer. Reliable estimates of the prevalence of epispadias in females are not available. Epispadias in females is often diagnosed and recorded as a bladder anomaly.

Causes and symptoms

Hypospadias and epispadias are congenital defects of the urinary tract. This means they occur during intrauterine development. There is no genetic basis for the defects. Specific causes for hypospadias are not known. This means that blood relatives do not have increased chances of developing them. Reports have shown some rise in prevalence of hypospadias among offspring of mothers who work in certain occupations where they may be exposed to chemicals that disrupt the endocrine system. However, a large trial ending in 2003 showed that aside from a slight increased risk among women who were hairdressers from 1992–1996, there is no evidence that maternal occupation or certain chemical exposure increases risk of hypospadias. The role of chemicals in the development of the defect remains uncertain.

Concern was once raised that use of the antihistamine loratadine (Claritin) early in pregnancy might cause hypospadias. However, a national clinical trial revealed in 2004 that there was no link between the drug and risk of second or third-degree hypospadias.

KEY TERMS

Continence—Control of urination or bowel movement.

Urethra—The tube through which urine passes from the bladder to the outside of the body.

Hypospadias usually is not associated with other defects of the penis or urethra. In males, it can occur at any site along the underside of the penis. In females, the urethra exits the body in an abnormal location. This usually is due to inadequate length of the urethra.

Epispadias is associated with bladder abnormalities. In females, the front wall of the bladder does not fuse or close. The bladder fissure may extend to the external abdominal wall. In such a rare case, the front of the pelvis also is widely separated. In males, the bladder fissure extends into the urethra and simply becomes an opening somewhere along the upper surface of the penis.

Hypospadias is associated with difficulty in assigning gender to babies. This occurs when gender is not obvious at **birth** because of deformities in the sex organs.

Diagnosis

Male external urinary tract defects are discovered at birth during the first detailed examination of the newborn. Female urethral defects may not be discovered for some time due to the difficulty in viewing the infant vagina.

Treatment

Surgery is the treatment of choice for both hypospadias and epispadias. All surgical repairs should be undertaken early and completed without delay. This minimizes psychological trauma.

In males with hypospadias, one surgery usually is sufficient to repair the defect. With more complicated hypospadias (more than one abnormally situated urethral opening), multiple surgeries may be required. In females with hypospadias, surgical repair technically is more complicated but can usually be completed in a brief interval of time.

Repairing an epispadias is more difficult. In males, this may involve other structures in the penis. Males should not be circumcised since the foreskin often is needed for the repair. Unfortunately, choices may be required that affect the ability to inseminate a female partner. Reproduction requires that the urethral meatus be close to the tip of the penis. Cosmetic appearance and ability to urinate (urinary continence) usually are the primary goals. Surgery for these defects is successful 70 to 80% of the time. Modern treatment of complete male epispadias allows for an excellent genital appearance and achievement of urinary continence.

In females, repair of epispadias may require multiple surgical procedures. Urinary continence and cosmetic appearance are the usual primary considerations. Urinary continence usually is achieved although cosmetic appearance may be somewhat compromised. Fertility is not usually affected. Repair rates that are similar or better than those for males usually can be achieved for females.

Hypospadias in both males and females is more of a nuisance and hindrance to reproduction than a threat to health. If surgery is not an option, the condition may be allowed to persist. This usually leads to an increased risk of infections in the lower urinary tract.

Prognosis

With adequate surgical repair, most males with simple hypospadias can lead normal lives with a penis that appears and functions in a normal manner. This includes fathering children. Females with simple hypospadias also have normal lives, including conceiving and bearing children.

The prognosis for epispadias depends on the extent of the defect. Most males with relatively minor epispadias lead normal lives, including fathering children. As the extent of the defect increases, surgical reconstruction generally is acceptable. However, many of these men are unable to conceive children. Most epispadias in females can be surgically repaired. The chances of residual disfigurement increase as the extent of the epispadias increases. Fertility in females is not generally affected by epispadias.

Resources

BOOKS

Dhar, Panchali. *Before the Scalpel: What Everyone Should Know About Anesthesia.* New Haven, CT: Tell Me Press, LLC, 2010.

Liebmann–Smith, Joan., and Jacqueline Egan. *Baby Body Signs: The Head–to–Toe Guide to Your Child's Health, from Birth Through the Toddler Years.* New York, NY: Bantam, 2010.

PERIODICALS

Kubetin, Sally Koch. "Hypospadias, Loratadine Use in Pregnancy: No Link." *Pediatric News* July 2004.

"Molecular Epidemiology of Hypospadias: Genetic and Environmental Risk Factors." *Health & Medicine Week* December 15, 2003: 424.

Vrijheid, M., et al. "Risk of Hypospadias in Relation to Maternal Occupational Exposure to Potential Endocrine

Disrupting Chemicals." *Occupational and Environmental Medicine* August 2003: 543–548.

OTHER

Hatch, David A. "Abnormal Development of the Penis and Male Urethra." Genitourinary Development, http://www.meddean.luc.edu/lumen/MedEd/urology/abnpendv.htm (accessed September 11, 2010).

The Penis.com, http://www.the–penis. com/hypospadias.html (accessed September 11, 2010).

Society for Pediatric Urology, http://www.spuonline.org (accessed September 11, 2010).

ORGANIZATIONS

Association for the Bladder Exstrophy Community, 3075 First St., La Salle MI, 48145, (866) 300–2222, http://www.bladderexstrophy.com.

Hypospadias and Epispadias Association, 240 W. 44th St., Suite 2, New York NY, 10036, (212) 382–3471, http://heainfo.org.

L. Fleming Fallon, Jr., MD, PhD.
Teresa G. Odle
Laura Jean Cataldo, RN, Ed.D.

Hypothyroidism

Definition

Hypothyroidism is a condition in which a person's thyroid gland is not producing enough hormone. It may be caused by an autoimmune disorder, a genetic defect in a newborn, certain medications, surgical removal of the thyroid gland, radiation therapy for **cancer**, and other reasons.

There are three main types of hypothyroidism. The most common is primary hypothyroidism, in which the thyroid doesn't produce an adequate amount of T_4. Secondary hypothyroidism develops when the pituitary gland does not release enough of the thyroid-stimulating hormone (TSH) that prompts the thyroid to manufacture T_4. Tertiary hypothyroidism results from a malfunction of the hypothalamus, the part of the brain that controls the endocrine system. Drug-induced hypothyroidism, an adverse reaction to medication, occurs in two of every 10,000 people, but rarely causes severe hypothyroidism.

Demographics

According to the National Institute of Diabetes and Digestive and Kidney Diseases (NIDDK), between 3 and 5 percent of the general population in the United States and Canada has some form of hypothyroidism. Apart from cretinism, which affects one child in every 3,000–4,000, hypothyroidism is largely a disease of adults. The most common form of primary hypothyroidism in North America is Hashimoto's disease, an autoimmune disorder that is diagnosed in about 14 women out of every 1000 and 1 man in every 2000.

Caucasians and Hispanics (particularly Mexican Americans) in North America have higher rates of hypothyroidism than African Americans. The reason for this difference is not known as of 2009.

Internationally, however, the most common cause of hypothyroidism is a lack of iodine in the diet. The prevalence of hypothyroidism caused by iodine deficiency in developing countries is 2–5%, increasing to 15% by age 75.

Description

Hypothyroidism is an endocrine disorder; that is, it is caused by underfunctioning of a gland that is part of the endocrine system—a group of small organs located throughout the body that regulate growth, metabolism, tissue function, and emotional mood. The thyroid gland itself is a butterfly-shaped organ weighing between half an ounce and 1.5 ounces in adults that lies at the base of the throat below the Adam's apple and above the collarbone. It takes its name from a Greek word meaning "shield." The thyroid consists of two lobes about 2 inches in length (in adults) connected by a thin strip of tissue called the isthmus.

Hypothyroidism develops when the thyroid gland fails to produce or secrete as much thyroxine (T_4) as the body needs. Because T_4 regulates such essential functions as heart rate, digestion, physical growth, and mental development, an insufficient supply of this hormone can slow life-sustaining processes, damage organs and tissues in every part of the body, and lead to life-threatening complications.

Hypothyroidism is not easy to diagnose because its symptoms are found in a number of other diseases; it often comes on slowly; and it may produce few or no symptoms in younger adults. In general, hypothyroidism is characterized by a slowing down of both physical and mental activities.

Risk factors

Risk factors for hypothyroidism include:

- Sex. Women are at greater risk of hypothyroidism than men. The female/male ratio among adults is between 2:1 and 8:1, depending on the age group being studied.

- Age over 50. In one Massachusetts study, 6 percent of women over 60 and 2.5 percent of men over 60 were found to be hypothyroid.
- Race. According to the National Institutes of Health (NIH), the rates of hypothyroidism in the United States are highest among Caucasians (5.1 percent) and Hispanics (4.1 percent) and lowest among African Americans (1.7 percent).
- Obesity.
- Having a small body size at birth and low body mass index during childhood.
- Family history of autoimmune disease.
- Having Turner syndrome, a genetic disorder in which a girl is born with only one X chromosome instead of the normal two. Turner syndrome affects 1 in every 2500 girls.

Causes and symptoms

Causes

The most common causes of hypothyroidism are:

- Hashimoto's disease. This is an autoimmune disorder in which the patient's immune system attacks the thyroid gland, leading to tissue destruction.
- Treatment for hyperthyroidism. People who have been treated for an oversupply of thyroid hormone (hyperthyroidism) with radioactive iodine (iodine-131) may lose their ability to produce enough thyroid hormone.
- Surgery on the thyroid gland.
- Radiation therapy for the treatment of head or neck cancer.
- Medications. Lithium, given to treat some psychiatric disorders, and certain heart medications may affect the functioning of the thyroid gland. Other drugs known to suppress thyroid function include amiodarone, a heart medication; interferon alpha, given to treat cancer; and stavudine, a drug used to treat HIV infection.
- Pregnancy. As many as 10 percent of women may become hypothyroid in the first year after childbirth, particularly if they have diabetes.
- Viral infections. These can cause a short-term inflammation of the thyroid gland known as thyroiditis in some people.
- A tumor in the pituitary gland. The pituitary gland produces a hormone called thyroid-stimulating hormone or TSH. Low levels of TSH can lead to secondary hypothyroidism.
- Congenital. About one baby in every 3,000–4,000 is born with a defective thyroid gland or no gland at all.
- Too little iodine in the diet. This cause of hypothyroidism is most common in developing countries; it is rare in North America and Europe.

Symptoms

Not every patient with an underactive thyroid has the same symptoms or has them with the same severity. Common symptoms of hypothyroidism, however, include the following:

- Increased sensitivity to cold weather.
- Dry, itchy skin and a pale or yellowish complexion.
- Dry brittle hair that falls out easily and nails that break or split.
- Constipation.
- Goiter (swelling in the front of the neck caused by thyroid enlargement).
- Hoarse voice and puffy facial skin.
- Unexplained weight gain of 10–20 pounds, most of which is fluid.
- Sore and aching muscles, most commonly in the shoulders and hips.
- In women, extra-long menstrual periods or unusually heavy bleeding.
- Weak leg muscles.
- Decreased sweating.
- Arthritis.
- Memory loss or difficulty concentrating.
- Slowed heart rate (less than 60 beats per minute) and lowered blood pressure.
- Depression.

Diagnosis

Adults

Hypothyroidism in adults can be difficult to diagnose because many of its early symptoms are not unique to it. In addition, the symptoms typically come on gradually; the person may simply feel tired or less energetic than usual, or develop dry, itchy skin and brittle hair that falls out easily. Hypothyroidism is sometimes referred to as a "silent" disease precisely because the early symptoms may be so mild that no one realizes anything is wrong. The classic symptoms of hypothyroidism—sensitivity to cold, puffy complexion, decreased sweating, and coarse skin—may occur in only 60 percent of patients. In addition, the patient's loss of energy and low mood may be misdiagnosed as a psychiatric disorder, most commonly major depression. It may take months to years before the person or their doctor begins to suspect a problem with the thyroid gland.

KEY TERMS

Congenital—Present at birth.

Cretinism—A form of hypothyroidism found in some newborns.

Endocrine system—A system of small organs located throughout the body that regulate metabolism, growth and puberty, tissue function, and mood. The thyroid gland is part of the endocrine system.

Endocrinologist—A doctor who specializes in diagnosing and treating disorders of the endocrine glands and the hormones they secrete.

Goiter—A swelling in the neck caused by an enlarged thyroid gland.

Hashimoto's disease—An autoimmune disorder that is the most common cause of primary hypothyroidism. It was the first disease to be recognized as an autoimmune disorder. It is named for a Japanese doctor, Hakaru Hashimoto, who first described it in 1912.

Hormone—A chemical released by specialized cells that affects cells in other parts of the body. Hormones regulate such body processes as growth, metabolism, the immune system, reproduction, hunger, and mood.

Hyperthyroidism—A disease condition in which the thyroid gland produces too much thyroid hormone.

Hypothyroidism—A disease condition in which the thyroid gland does not produce enough thyroid hormone.

Metabolism—The chemical changes in living cells in which new materials are taken in and energy is provided for vital processes,

Myxedema—A synonym for hypothyroidism. Myxedema coma is a condition in which a person with untreated hypothyroidism loses consciousness. It is potentially fatal.

Thyroid-stimulating hormone (TSH)—A hormone produced by the pituitary gland that stimulates the thyroid gland to produce the hormones that regulate metabolism. Also called thyrotropin.

Thyroiditis—Inflammation of the thyroid gland. It can be caused by a viral infection, a malfunction of the immune system, or certain medications.

Thyroxine (T_4)—The thyroid hormone that regulates many essential body processes.

Triiodothyronine (T_3)—A thyroid hormone similar to thyroxine but more powerful. Preparations of triiodothyronine are used in treating hypothyroidism.

It's important to see a doctor if any of these symptoms appear unexpectedly. People whose hypothyroidism remains undiagnosed and untreated may eventually develop myxedema. Symptoms of this rare but potentially deadly complication include enlarged tongue, swollen facial features, hoarseness, and physical and mental sluggishness.

Myxedema coma can cause unresponsiveness; irregular, shallow breathing; and a drop in blood pressure and body temperature. The onset of this medical emergency can be sudden in people who are elderly or have been ill, injured, or exposed to very cold temperatures; have recently had surgery; or use sedatives or antidepressants. Without immediate medical attention, myxedema coma can be fatal.

Children

In the United States, newborn infants between 24 and 72 hours old are tested for congenital thyroid deficiency (cretinism) using a test that measures the levels of thyroxine in the infant's blood. If the levels are low, the physician will likely repeat the blood test to confirm the diagnosis. The physician may take an x ray of the infant's legs. In an infant with hypothyroidism, the ends of the bones have an immature appearance. Treatment within the first few months of life can prevent **mental retardation** and physical abnormalities.

Older children who develop hypothyroidism may suddenly stop growing. If the child was above average height before the disease occurred, he or she may now be short compared to other children of the same age. Therefore, the most important feature of hypothyroidism in a child is a decrease in the rate of growth in height. If the disease is recognized early and adequately treated, the child will grow at an accelerated rate until reaching the same growth percentile where the child measured before the onset of hypothyroidism. Diagnosis of hypothyroidism in school-age children is based on the patient's observations, medical history, physical examination, and thyroid function tests.

Examination

The doctor may notice such signs of hypothyroidism during an office examination as dry skin, facial puffiness, a goiter in the neck, thin or brittle hair, poor muscle tone, pale complexion, and a slower than normal heart rate. As previously mentioned, however, it is possible for a person with hypothyroidism not to have these symptoms.

Tests

The diagnosis of hypothyroidism is usually made by tests of the patient's thyroid function following a careful history of the patient's symptoms. The first test is a blood test for thyroid-stimulating hormone, or TSH. TSH is a hormone produced by the pituitary gland in the brain that stimulates the thyroid gland to produce thyroid hormone. When the thyroid gland is not producing enough hormone, the pituitary gland secretes more TSH; thus a high level of TSH in the blood indicates that the thyroid gland is not as active as it should be.

The TSH test, however, does not always detect borderline cases of hypothyroidism. The doctor may order additional tests to measure the levels of thyroid hormone as well as TSH in the patient's blood. If the doctor thinks that the patient may have Hashimoto's disease, he or she may test for the presence of abnormal antibodies in the blood. Because Hashimoto's disease is an autoimmune disorder, there will be two or three types of anti-thyroid antibodies in the patient's blood in about 90 percent of cases.

A woman being tested for hypothyroidism should let her doctor know if she is pregnant or **breastfeeding** and all patients should be sure their doctors are aware of any recent procedures involving radioactive materials or contrast media.

Procedures

In some cases, the doctor may also order an ultrasound study of the patient's neck in order to evaluate the size of the thyroid gland or take a small sample of thyroid tissue in order to make sure that the gland is not cancerous. The usual procedure for obtaining the tissue sample is a fine-needle aspiration biopsy or FNAB. To perform a FNAB, the doctor inserts a thin needle into the thyroid to extract a sample of cells for examination under a microscope. The doctor usually uses an ultrasound monitor to guide the needle. A FNAB can be performed in an outpatient clinic or a doctor's office; it is safer and less invasive than an open surgical biopsy.

Treatment

Traditional

Medications are the treatment of choice for hypothyroidism.

Drugs

Treatment for hypothyroidism consists of a daily dose of a synthetic form of thyroid hormone sold under the trade names of Synthroid, Levothroid, or Levoxyl. The patient is told that the drug must be taken as directed for the rest of his or her life.

In the early weeks of treatment, the patient will need to see the doctor every four to six weeks to have their TSH level checked and the dose of medication adjusted. After the doctor is satisfied with the dosage level and the patient's overall health, checkups are done every six to 12 months. The reason for this careful measurement of the medication is that too much of the synthetic hormone increases the risk of osteoporosis in later life or abnormal heart rhythms in the present. Aging, other medications, and changes in weight and general health can also affect how much replacement hormone a patient needs, and regular TSH tests are used to monitor hormone levels. Patients should not switch from one brand of thyroid hormone to another without a doctor's permission.

Medications and over-the-counter preparations that can affect the body's absorption of synthetic thyroid hormone include cholestyramine (Questran), antacids that contain aluminum hydroxide, calcium supplements, and iron supplements. A high intake of soy products or a diet high in fiber can also affect the body's absorption of the hormone, and the patient's doctor may need to adjust the dosage.

Congenital hypothyroidism or cretinism is also treated with synthetic thyroid hormone. Most hospitals now screen newborns for thyroid problems, because untreated cretinism can lead to lifelong physical and mental developmental disorders.

Regular **exercise** and a high-fiber diet can help maintain thyroid function and prevent **constipation**.

Alternative

Alternative treatments are primarily aimed at strengthening the thyroid and will not eliminate the need for thyroid hormone medications. Herbal remedies to improve thyroid function and relieve symptoms of hypothyroidism include bladder wrack (*Fucus vesiculosus*), which can be taken in capsule form or as a tea. Some foods, including cabbage, peaches, radishes, soybeans, peanuts, and spinach, can interfere with the production of thyroid hormones. Anyone with hypothyroidism may want to avoid these foods.

The Shoulder Stand **yoga** position (at least once daily for 20 minutes) is believed to improve thyroid function.

One alternative treatment for hypothyroidism that should *not* be used is coconut oil. There is no evidence that coconut oil stimulates the thyroid gland, and a few studies suggest that it may actually lower thyroid function.

Prognosis

The prognosis for patients with hypothyroidism is very good, provided they take their medication as directed. They can usually live a normal life with a normal life expectancy. Children with cretinism have a good prognosis if the disorder is caught and treated early; some develop **learning disorders**, however, in spite of early treatment.

The chief risks to health are related to lack of treatment for hypothyroidism. If low levels of thyroid hormone are not diagnosed and treated, patients are at increased risk of goiter, an enlarged heart, and severe depression. In addition, women with untreated hypothyroidism have a higher risk of giving **birth** to babies with **cleft palate** and other **birth defects**.

One rare but potentially life-threatening complication of long-term untreated hypothyroidism is myxedema coma. In this condition, which is usually triggered by stress or illness, the person becomes extremely sensitive to cold, may be unusually drowsy, or lose consciousness. Heart rate, blood pressure, and breathing may all be abnormally low. Myxedema coma requires emergency treatment in a hospital with intravenous thyroid hormone and intensive care nursing.

Prevention

There are no proven ways to prevent hypothyroidism as of 2010 because the disorder has so many possible causes.

Resources

BOOKS

Cooper, David S. *Medical Management of Thyroid Disease*, 2nd ed. New York: Informa Healthcare, 2009.

Pratt, Maureen. *The First Year—Hypothyroidism: An Essential Guide for the Newly Diagnosed*, 2nd ed., revised and updated. New York: Marlowe and Co., 2007.

Rone, James K. *The Thyroid Paradox: How to Get the Best Care for Hypothyroidism*. Laguna Beach, CA: Basic Health Publications, 2007.

Shannon, Joyce Brennfleck. *Endocrine and Metabolic Disorders Sourcebook*, 2nd ed. Detroit, MI: Omnigraphics, 2007.

Skugor, Mario. *Thyroid Disorders: A Cleveland Clinic Guide*. Cleveland, OH: Cleveland Clinic Press, 2006.

PERIODICALS

Alexander, E.K. "Thyroid Function: The Complexity of Maternal Hypothyroidism During Pregnancy." *Nature Reviews: Endocrinology* 5 (September 2009): 480–81.

Baloch, Z.W., and V.A. LiVolsi. "Fine-needle Aspiration of the Thyroid: Today and Tomorrow." *Best Practice and Research: Clinical Endocrinology and Metabolism* 22 (December 2008): 929–39.

Brown, R.S. "Autoimmune Thyroid Disease: Unlocking a Complex Puzzle." *Current Opinion in Pediatrics* 21 (August 2009): 523–28.

Carson, M. "Assessment and Management of Patients with Hypothyroidism." *Nursing Standard* 23 (January 7–13, 2009): 48–56.

Counts, D., and S.K. Varma. "Hypothyroidism in Children." *Pediatrics in Review* 30 (July 2009): 251–58.

Miller, M.C., and A. Agrawal. "Hypothyroidism in Postradiation Head and Neck Cancer Patients: Incidence, Complications, and Management." *Current Opinion in Otolaryngology and Head and Neck Surgery* 17 (April 2009): 111–115.

Mistry, N., et al. "When to Consider Thyroid Dysfunction in the Neurology Clinic." *Practical Neurology* 9 (June 2009): 145–56.

Wirsing, N., and A. Hamilton. "How Often Should You Follow Up on a Patient with Newly Diagnosed Hypothyroidism?" *Journal of Family Practice* 58 (January 2009): 40–41.

OTHER

American Thyroid Association. *Hypothyroidism*, http://www.thyroid.org/patients/brochures/Hypo_brochure.pdf

Bharaktiya, Shikha, et al. "Hypothyroidism." *eMedicine*, July 23, 2009, http://emedicine.medscape.com/article/122393-overview

Mayo Clinic. *Hypothyroidism (Underactive Thyroid)*, http://www.mayoclinic.com/health/hypothyroidism/DS00353

National Institute of Diabetes and Digestive and Kidney Diseases (NIDDK). *Hypothyroidism*, http://endocrine.niddk.nih.gov/pubs/Hypothyroidism/index.htm

ORGANIZATIONS

American Academy of Otolaryngology—Head and Neck Surgery, 1650 Diagonal Road, Alexandria VA, 22314, 703-836-4444, http://www.entnet.org/.

American Association of Clinical Endocrinologists (AACE), 245 Riverside Ave., Suite 200, Jacksonville FL, 32202, 904-353-7878, http://www.aace.com/.

American Thyroid Association (ATA), 6066 Leesburg Pike, Suite 550, Falls Church VA, 22041, 703-998-8890, 703-998-8893, thyroid@thyroid.org, http://www.thyroid.org/.

Hormone Foundation, 8401 Connecticut Avenue, Suite 900, Chevy Chase MD, 20815, 800–HORMONE, 301-941-0259, hormone@endo-society.org, http://www.hormone.org/.

National Institute of Diabetes and Digestive and Kidney Diseases (NIDDK), Building 31. Rm 9A06, 31 Center Drive, MSC 2560, Bethesda MD, 20892-2560, 301-496-3583, http://www2.niddk.nih.gov/Footer/ContactNIDDK.htm, http://www2.niddk.nih.gov/.

Judith Sims, M.S.
Rebecca J. Frey, PhD

Hypotonia

Definition

Hypotonia means "low tone," and refers to a physiological state in which a muscle has decreased tone, or tension. A muscle's tone is a measure of its ability to resist passive elongation or stretching. Hypotonia usually involves reduced muscle strength as well as lowered tone.

Demographics

Hypotonia is the most common muscular abnormality seen in neonatal (newborn) neurological disorders. It affects males and females equally, and shows no preponderance in any particular ethnic group or race. An increase in the occurrence of hypotonia in recent years is correlated with increased survival rates of infants born significantly premature, since these children are at increased risk for neurological problems.

Description

Hypotonia is better understood as a sign or symptom than a diagnosis. It is most often seen in newborns (congenital) and infants, but it may persist through **adolescence** into adulthood. Another name for infantile hypotonia is floppy baby syndrome. This refers to the tendency of a hypotonic infant's arms, legs, and head to flop or dangle loosely when they are picked up or moved. In the past, the term "benign congenital hypotonia" was used for many cases in which no obvious cause for the hypotonia could be detected. Better diagnostic techniques and increased knowledge of neuromuscular disorders,

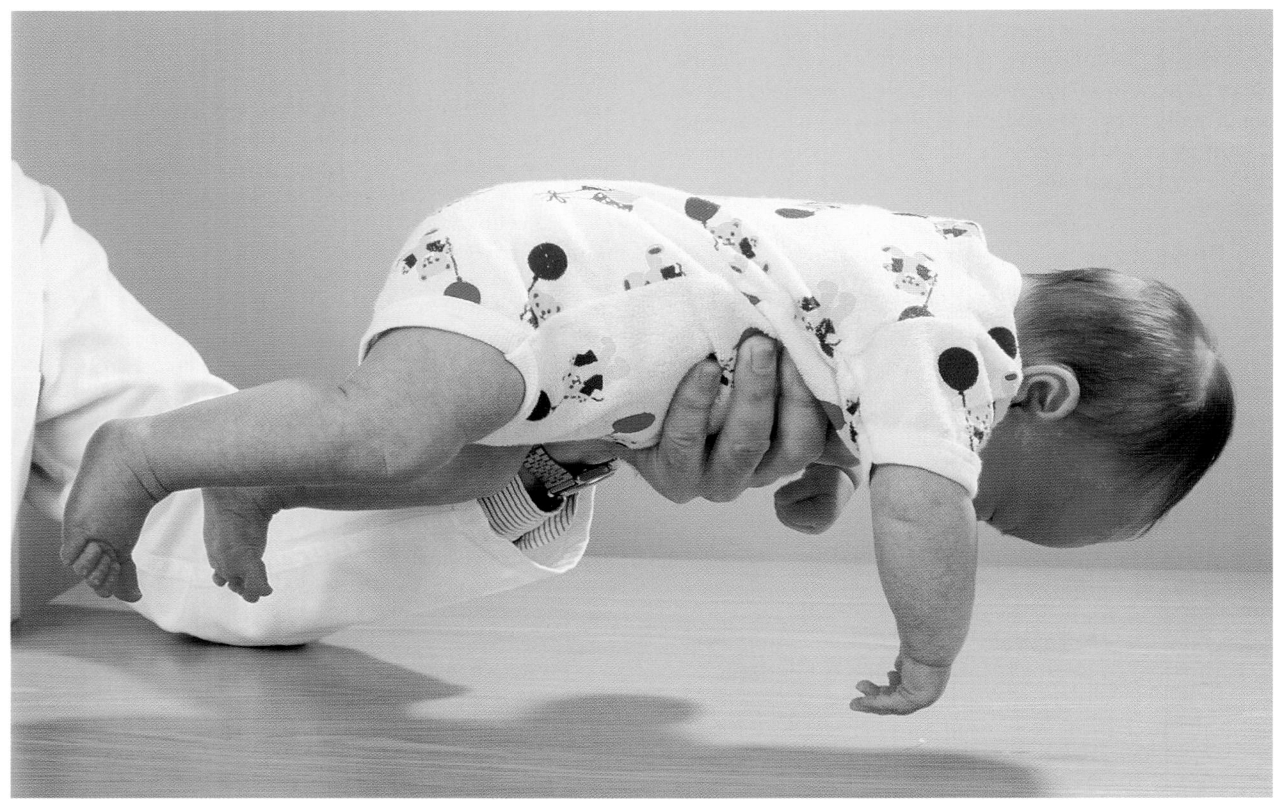

A six-week-old baby girl is held horizontally by the trunk in a test for hypotonia, sometimes called "floppy infant syndrome." The girl is normal. *(Saturn Stills/Photo Researchers, Inc.)*

however, have resulted in much less frequent use of this term.

Hypotonia is of concern to parents and pediatricians because it is often associated with or leads to other problems. In addition to low muscle tone, infants with hypotonia may also exhibit excessive flexibility of the joints (hypermobility), decreased deep tendon reflexes (e. g., tapping the knee joint produces little or no muscle jerk), and difficulties with sucking and swallowing. Children in whom hypotonia persists often show delays in such **gross motor skills** as sitting up, **crawling**, and walking. They may also have difficulties with coordination and exhibit speech delays. In some cases, symptoms may persist into adulthood. Hypotonia itself is not associated with decreased intellectual development, but the underlying cause may pose significant risks for **developmental delay** and **mental retardation**.

Risk factors

Risk factors for hypotonia include:

- Premature birth.
- Traumatic injury to the central nervous system.
- Family history of inherited disorders that affect the nerves and muscles.

Causes and symptoms

The causes of hypotonia are varied and numerous. Some involve trauma to, or diseases of, the brain or spinal cord (CNS), while others affect the peripheral nerves, neuromuscular junction, or the muscles themselves. A disorder of the nervous system is a neuropathy, while a muscle disease is a myopathy. A neuromuscular condition is one in which a neurological disorder results in associated muscular symptoms.

CNS trauma and infection are perhaps the most common cause of hypotonia, both in infants and in children. Insult to the brain may occur prenatally (before **birth**), perinatally (around the time of birth), or postnatally (after birth).

Prenatal CNS damage may be caused by certain maternal/fetal infections, maternal diseases, problems with the placenta or umbilical cord, or maternal use of harmful substances such as alcohol or certain drugs. Most congenital brain malformations, however, have no discernible cause and are likely due to chance maldevelopment of a very complex organ. Perinatal asphyxia/hypoxia (lack of oxygen to the baby's brain) occurs less frequently than is commonly believed, but does present a risk for CNS damage that can result in hypotonia. The greatest risk for asphyxia/hypoxia is from complicated and/or premature deliveries. Infants who are born healthy may sustain postnatal brain injury if they suffer from breathing difficulties, develop an infection in the lining of the brain (see **Meningitis**), or suffer some other type of physical trauma or abuse.

A number of different **genetic disorders** are associated with hypotonia, and may affect the nerves (and by extension the muscles), or the muscles only. Most genetic conditions are generalized (affecting multiple muscle groups) and progressive. Some genetic conditions are hereditary (autosomal recessive or X-linked recessive) and some are sporadic (chromosomal disorders). Hereditary conditions would typically imply a 25% recurrence risk for siblings on the affected child, while the chance for another child with the same chromosomal abnormality is usually about 2–3%.

While it is less common, hypotonia may develop in an adult. This is again most often the result of CNS trauma or disease, usually affecting the cerebellum. The primary function of the cerebellum is control of balance and coordination, including maintaining passive tension/tone of the muscles, such as muscular control required for standing.

Diagnosis

Determining which diagnostic tests to administer depends on the clinician's judgment of what is most likely to be the underlying cause of the hypotonia. This in turn is based upon the history and physical findings. In some cases, different doctors will order different tests based upon their area of expertise. There is always a possibility that a diagnosis will not be determined. The term for hypotonia without a diagnosis is idiopathic, which literally means "of unknown cause."

Examination

Tests

Diagnosis of the cause of hypotonia may involve a number of different medical methods, procedures, and tests. These include:

- A complete prenatal (before birth) and perinatal (around the time of birth) history. Along with this a complete family medical history should be obtained
- A physical examination to determine the degree of hypotonia and the muscles affected
- An electromyelogram (EMG) measures muscle response to electrical stimulation
- A nerve conduction velocity (NCV) test, which measures a nerve's ability to transmit electrical impulses to and from the muscle

KEY TERMS

Congenital—Present at birth.

Hydrocephalus—A condition in which there is an abnormal buildup of cerebrospinal fluid in the ventricles (internal cavities) of the brain.

Idiopathic—Of spontaneous origin or unknown cause.

Muscle tone—Also termed tonus; the normal state of balanced tension in the tissues of the body, especially the muscles.

Myopathy—Any abnormal condition or disease of muscle tissue, characterized by muscle weakness and wasting.

Neuromuscular—Involving both the muscles and the nerves that control them.

Neuropathy—A disease or abnormality of the peripheral nerves (the nerves outside the brain and spinal cord). Major symptoms include weakness, numbness, paralysis, or pain in the affected area.

Sporadic—Rare and scattered or random in occurrence.

Tone—A readiness to contract that makes resting muscle resistant to stretching.

- Electroencephalogram (EEG), a test that measures the electrical activity in the brain
- A muscle biopsy to analyze the microscopic structure of affected muscle
- Biochemical tests of muscle tissue and blood
- Genetic tests to look for possible sporadic (chance occurrence) or hereditary genetic errors affecting the brain, nerves, and/or muscles
- Imaging studies (CT scan or MRI) of the brain and spinal cord

Treatment

Treatment team

Along with normal pediatric care, specialists who may be involved in the care of a child with hypotonia include developmental pediatricians (specialists in child development), neurologists, neonatologists (specialists in the care of newborns), geneticists, occupational therapists, physical therapists, speech therapists, orthopedists, pathologists (conduct and interpret biochemical tests and tissue analysis), and specialized nursing care. Depending on the cause and progression of hypotonia, treatment and evaluation may be needed throughout life.

Traditional

Unlike the wide array of potential causes of hypotonia, treatment options for low muscle tone are somewhat limited. In very severe cases, treatment may be primarily supportive, such as mechanical assistance with basic life functions like breathing and feeding, physical therapy to prevent muscle atrophy and maintain joint mobility, and measures to try and prevent such opportunistic infections as **pneumonia**. Therapy for infants and young children may also include sensory stimulation programs. Treatments to improve neurological status might involve such approaches as medication for a **seizure disorder**, medicines or supplements to stabilize a metabolic disorder, or surgery to help relieve the pressure from **hydrocephalus** (increased fluid in the brain). If the neurologic condition is untreatable, physical and **occupational therapy** may help to improve muscle tone, strength, and coordination.

In all cases, frequent or periodic monitoring of muscle tone and performance, along with neurological status, should be done to determine if the hypotonia is worsening, static, or improving. Effective recovery and rehabilitation can only be achieved if an accurate status of the condition is known. Since muscle weakness often accompanies hypotonia, efforts to improve muscle strength may also improve low muscle tone. Some individuals with persistent symptoms may need assistance with mobility, such as a walker or wheelchair. Occupational and physical therapy can assist individuals in developing alternative methods for accomplishing some everyday tasks they may find difficult. **Speech therapy** is primarily directed at young children to help them develop language skills early, but can be beneficial at any age if the muscles of the face and throat are hypotonic.

Prognosis

Determining a prognosis depends on determining a diagnosis for hypotonia. Some genetic conditions are fatal in **infancy**, while others result in permanent disability and mental retardation. For those few genetic metabolic disorders that are treatable, improvement may be dramatic, or minimal. Outcomes for hypotonia caused by CNS trauma or infection depend on the severity of neurologic damage. Mild trauma obviously has the best chance for improvement and recovery, but even significant neurologic deficits may improve over time.

Most individuals with a nongenetic form of hypotonia will improve to some degree. From a broad perspective, some individuals with hypotonia will respond very little or not at all to any treatment method attempted, while in others the condition will resolve on its own; each case is unique.

Prevention

Some genetic disorders associated with hypotonia can be detected during prenatal testing, and some risk factors for preterm birth (infections, **malnutrition**, heavy **smoking** and alcohol consumption) can be avoided. On the other hand, some causes of hypotonia cannot be avoided, and idiopathic hypotonia cannot be predicted.

Resources

BOOKS

Berger, Itai, and Michael S. Schimmel, eds. *Hot Topics in Neonatal Neurology*. New York: Nova Science Publishers, 2008.

Rowland, Lewis P., and Timothy A. Pedley, eds. *Merritt's Neurology*, 12th ed. Philadelphia: Lippincott Williams and Wilkins, 2010.

PERIODICALS

Harris, S.R. "Congenital Hypotonia: Clinical and Developmental Assessment." *Developmental Medicine and Child Neurology* 50 (December 2008): 889–92.

Martin, K., et al. "Clinical Characteristics of Hypotonia: A Survey of Pediatric Physical and Occupational Therapists." *Pediatric Physical Therapy* 19 (Fall 2007): 217–26.

van Adel, B.A., and M.A. Tamopolsky. "Metabolic Myopathies: Update 2009." *Journal of Clinical Neuromuscular Disease* 10 (March 2009): 97–121.

OTHER

Colorado Springs Down Syndrome Association. *Exercises and Stimulation Therapy for Hypotonia*, http://www.csdsa.org/artthera.asp

MedlinePlus Medical Encyclopedia. *Hypotonia*, http://www.nlm.nih.gov/medlineplus/ency/article/003298.htm

Muscular Dystrophy Association (MDA). *Facts about Myopathies*, http://www.mda.org/publications/PDFs/FactsAboutMyopathies.pdf

National Institute of Neurological Disorders and Stroke (NINDS). *Hypotonia Information Page*, http://www.ninds.nih.gov/disorders/hypotonia/hypotonia.htm

National Organization for Rare Disorders (NORD). *Hypotonia, Benign Congenital*, http://www.rarediseases.org/search/rdbdetail_abstract.html?disname=Hypotonia%2C%20Benign%20Congenital

ORGANIZATIONS

American Academy of Pediatrics (AAP), 141 Northwest Point Boulevard, Elk Grove Village IL, 60007, 847-434-4000, 847-434-8000, http://www.aap.org/.

Muscular Dystrophy Association (MDA), 3300 East Sunrise Drive, Tucson AZ, 85718, 800-572-1717, http://www.mda.org/.

National Institute of Child Health and Human Development (NICHD)., Bldg 31, Room 2A32, MSC 2425, 31 Center Drive, Bethesda MD, 20892, 800-370-2943, 866-760-5947, NICHDInformationResourceCenter@mail.nih.gov, http://www.nichd.nih.gov/.

National Institute of Neurological Disorders and Stroke (NINDS), P.O. Box 5801, Bethesda MD, 20824, 800-352-9424 301-496-5751, http://www.ninds.nih.gov/index.htm.

National Organization for Rare Disorders (NORD), 55 Kenosia Avenue, P.O. Box 1968, Danbury CT, 06813, 203-744-0100, 800-999-6673, 203-798-2291, http://www.rarediseases.org/.

Scott J. Polzin, MS, CGC
Rebecca J. Frey, PhD

Hypoxia

Definition

Hypoxia refers to a lack of oxygen in any part of the body. In a neurological context it refers to a reduction of oxygen to the brain despite adequate amounts of blood.

Description

A decrease in oxygen supply to the brain can occur because of **choking**, strangling, suffocation, head trauma, **carbon monoxide poisoning**, cardiac arrest, and as a complication of general anesthesia. A failure to deliver oxygen and glucose to the brain causes a cascade of abnormal events. The extent of damage is directly proportional to the severity of the injury. The severity of cerebral ischemia, a low-oxygen state caused by arterial obstruction or lack of blood supply, and the duration of blood-flow loss in the brain determine the extent of brain damage. The neurons can suffer temporary dysfunction, or they can be irreversibly damaged because nerve cells are highly sensitive to minute changes in oxygen levels. Severe damage involving extensive areas can occur (cerebral infarction). Cerebral hypoxia/ischemia can be caused by a broad spectrum of diseases that affect the cardiovascular pumping system or the respiratory system. There are four types of disorders to consider: focal cerebral ischemia, global cerebral ischemia, diffuse cerebral hypoxia, and cerebral infarction.

Focal cerebral ischemia

Focal cerebral ischemia (FCI) often results from a blood clot in the brain. The blood flow in the affected area is reduced. The reduction may be severe or mild, but usually FCI causes irreversible injury to sensitive neurons. The clinical signs and symptoms last approximately 15–30 minutes.

Global cerebral ischemia

Global cerebral ischemia (GCI) is a serious condition caused by ventricular fibrillation or cardiac asystole, which stops all blood flow to the brain. If the GCI lasts more than five to ten minutes, then it is likely the person will have suffered a loss of consciousness that makes recovery doubtful.

Diffuse cerebral hypoxia

Diffuse cerebral hypoxia (DCH) is limited to conditions that cause mild to moderate hypoxemia, or low arterial-oxygen content due to deficient blood oxygenation. Pure cerebral hypoxia causes cerebral dysfunction but not irreversible brain damage. Pure cerebral hypoxia can occur due to pulmonary disease, altitude sickness, or severe **anemia**.

Cerebral infarction

Cerebral infarction (CI) is a severe condition caused by a focal vascular occlusion in an area of the brain. This causes an area of destruction resulting from a lack of oxygen delivery.

Pathology of cerebral ischemia

Lack of oxygen causes neurons in the brain to die in several ways. Autolysis can occur, which results from the digestion of nerve tissues by enzymes. Cerebral infarction causes the **death** of neurons; transient cessation of the cerebral circulation for a few minutes causes selective areas of ischemic necrosis. This type of necrosis is especially evident in highly vulnerable neurons that are sensitive to abrupt oxygen deprivation. More prolonged periods of moderate-to-severe hypoxemia or carbon monoxide **poisoning** can cause a loss of the outer sheath of neurons.

Molecular mechanisms of cerebral hypoxia

In cases of severe ischemia to brain tissue, the tissue loses structural integrity within a few seconds or a few minutes. Soon after there is an abnormal exchange of ions in neurons through a process called depolarization; this is characterized by an influx of sodium and calcium ions inside the neuron, and a simultaneous efflux of potassium ions outside the neuron.

KEY TERMS

Depolarization—Occurs when a neuron exchanges ions, causing an influx of sodium and calcium inside the cell and an efflux of potassium out of the cell.

Cerebral edema

Cerebral edema refers to abnormal increases in water content in the brain and occurs with all types of cerebral ischemia and hemorrhagic **stroke**. Increased water retention in the brain causes an increase in intracranial pressure. This pressure causes the brain to be pushed against the skull, resulting in neurologic deterioration and death due to herniation. Cerebral edema and herniation of the brain is the cause of death for approximately 75% of all fatal-stroke victims and 33% of fatalities for all ischemic events to the brain.

Symptoms

Symptoms vary depending on the severity of damage. Symptoms of mild cerebral hypoxia can include poor judgment, memory loss, inattentiveness, and a decrease in motor coordination. In more severe cases, there can be permanent neurologic deficits, coma, seizures, or death.

Treatment

Treatment depends on the cause and availability of equipment. Treatment is urgent and includes basic and advanced life-support measures. It is important to maintain breathing, dispense intravenous fluids and medications, and maintain stability with blood products and medications that control blood pressure and seizures. The outlook depends on the extent of cerebral ischemia.

Resources

BOOKS

Goldman, Lee, et al. *Cecil's Textbook of Medicine*, 21st ed. Philadelphia: W. B. Saunders Company, 2000.

ORGANIZATIONS

Brain Injury Association of America, 105 North Alfred St., Alexandria VA, 22314, (800) 444-6443, http://www.biausa.org.

National Rehabilitation Information Center (NARIC), 4200 Forbes Boulevard, Suite 202, Lanham MD, 20706-4829, (301) 562-2400, (301) 562-2401 (800) 346-2742, naricinfo@heitechservices.com, http://www.naric.com.

Laith Farid Gulli, MD

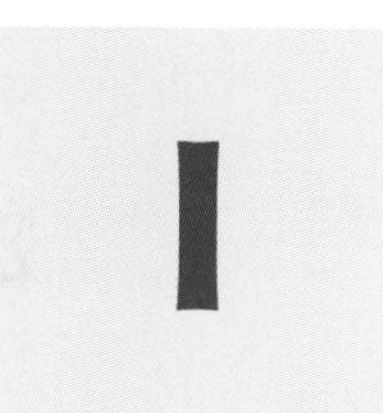

IBS *see* **Irritable bowel syndrome**

Ibuprofen *see* **Nonsteroidal anti-inflammatory drugs**

Idiopathic thrombocytopenic purpura

Definition

Idiopathic thrombocytopenic purpura, or ITP, is a bleeding disorder caused by an abnormally low level of platelets in the patient's blood. Platelets are small plate-shaped bodies in the blood that combine to form a plug when a blood vessel is injured. The platelet plug then binds certain proteins in the blood to form a clot that stops bleeding. ITP's name describes its cause and two symptoms. Idiopathic means that the disorder has no apparent cause. ITP is now often called immune thrombocytopenic purpura rather than idiopathic because of recent findings that ITP patients have autoimmune antibodies in their blood. Thrombocytopenia is another word for a decreased number of blood platelets. Purpura refers to a purplish or reddish-brown skin rash caused by the leakage of blood from broken capillaries into the skin. Other names for ITP include purpura hemorrhagica and essential thrombocytopenia.

Demographics

ITP may be either acute or chronic. The acute form is most common in children between the ages of one and six years; the chronic form is most common in adult females between 30 and 40. ITP is uncommon in adults older than age 60. Between 10% and 20% of children with ITP have the chronic form. ITP does not appear to be related to race, lifestyle, climate, or environmental factors.

In the United States, annual incidence of ITP is difficult to determine because it is thought that most cases of ITP are so mild that medical attention is not needed. Estimates are that ITP affects 5 in every 100,000 children and 2 in every 100,000 adults in the U.S. every year.

Description

ITP is a disorder that affects the overall *number* of blood platelets rather than their function. The normal platelet level in adults is between 150,000 and 450,000/mm^3. Platelet counts below 50,000 mm^3 increase the risk of dangerous bleeding from trauma; counts below 20,000/mm^3 increase the risk of spontaneous bleeding.

Causes and symptoms

In adults, ITP is considered an autoimmune disorder, which means that the body produces antibodies that damage some of its own products—in this case, blood platelets. Some adults with chronic ITP also have other **immune system** disorders, such as systemic lupus erythematosus (SLE) or acute or chronic leukemia. ITP is usually triggered by a viral infection such as infection with **rubella**, **chickenpox**, **measles**, cytomegalovirus, Epstein-Barr virus, or hepatitis virus (A, B, C). It usually begins about two or three weeks after the infection. ITP may also occur as a result of infection with the human **immunodeficiency** virus (HIV). However, most commonly, ITP follows a viral upper respiratory infection or **gastroenteritis**.

Some medications are also linked to the development of ITP. These medications include:

- quinidine or quinine medications
- heparin
- antibiotics such as cephalosporin drugs and rifampicin
- analgesics
- diuretics
- antihypertensives

ITP is also associated with acute and chronic alcohol ingestion and is also seen in individuals with chronic liver disease.

KEY TERMS

Autoimmune disorder—A disorder in which the patient's immune system produces antibodies that destroy some of the body's own products. ITP in adults is thought to be an autoimmune disorder.

Idiopathic—Of unknown cause. Idiopathic refers to a disease that is not preceded or caused by any known dysfunction or disorder in the body.

Petechiae—Small pinpoint hemorrhages in skin or mucous membranes caused by the rupture of capillaries.

Platelet—A blood component that helps to prevent blood from leaking from broken blood vessels. ITP is a bleeding disorder caused by an abnormally low level of platelets in the blood.

Prednisone—A corticosteroid medication that is used to treat ITP. Prednisone works by decreasing the effects of antibody on blood platelets. Long-term treatment with prednisone is thought to decrease antibody production.

Purpura—A skin discoloration of purplish or brownish red spots caused by bleeding from broken capillaries.

Splenectomy—Surgical removal of the spleen.

Thrombocytopenia—An abnormal decline in the number of platelets in the blood.

In children, most cases of ITP are acute while in adults, most cases are chronic.

Acute ITP

Acute ITP is characterized by bleeding into the skin or from the nose, mouth, digestive tract, or urinary tract. The onset is usually sudden. Bleeding into the skin takes the form of purpura or petechiae. Purpura is a purplish or reddish-brown rash or discoloration of the skin; petechiae are small round pinpoint hemorrhages. Both are caused by the leakage of blood from tiny capillaries under the skin surface. In addition to purpura and petechiae, the patient may notice that he or she **bruises** more easily than usual. In extreme cases, patients with ITP may bleed into the lungs, brain, or other vital organs.

Chronic ITP

Chronic ITP has a gradual onset and may have minimal or no external symptoms. The low **platelet count** may be discovered in the course of a routine blood test. Most patients with chronic ITP, however, will consult their primary care doctor because of the purpuric skin rash, nosebleeds, or bleeding from the digestive or urinary tract. Women sometimes go to their gynecologist for unusually heavy or lengthy menstrual periods.

Diagnosis

ITP is usually considered a diagnosis of exclusion, which means that the doctor arrives at the diagnosis by a process of ruling out other possible causes. If the patient belongs to one or more of the risk groups for chronic ITP, the doctor may order a blood test for autoantibodies in the blood early in the diagnostic process.

Physical examination

If the doctor suspects ITP, he or she will examine the patient's skin for bruises, purpuric areas, or petechiae. If the patient has had nosebleeds or bleeding from the mouth or other parts of the body, the doctor will examine these areas for other possible causes of bleeding. Patients with ITP usually look and feel healthy except for the bleeding.

The most important features that the doctor will be looking for during the physical examination are the condition of the patient's spleen and the presence of **fever**. Patients with ITP do not have fever, whereas patients with lupus and some other types of thrombocytopenia are usually feverish. The doctor will have the patient lie flat on the examining table in order to feel the size of the spleen. If the spleen is noticeably enlarged, ITP is usually excluded as the diagnosis.

Laboratory testing

The doctor will order a complete blood count (CBC), a test of clotting time, a bone marrow test, and a test for antiplatelet antibodies if it is available in the hospital laboratory. Patients with ITP usually have platelet counts below 20,000/mm^3 and prolonged bleeding time. The size and appearance of the platelets may be abnormal. The red blood cell count (RBC) and white blood cell count (WBC) are usually normal, although about 10% of patients with ITP are also anemic. The blood marrow test yields normal results. Detection of antiplatelet antibodies in the blood is considered to confirm the diagnosis of ITP.

In most children, examination of the bone marrow is not required to diagnose acute ITP.

Treatment

General care and monitoring

There is no specific treatment for ITP. In most cases, the disorder will resolve without medications or surgery within two to six weeks. Nosebleeds can be treated with ice packs when necessary.

General care includes explaining ITP to the patient and advising him or her to watch for bruising, petechiae, or other signs of recurrence. Children should be discouraged from rough contact **sports** or other activities that increase the risk of trauma. Patients are also advised to avoid using aspirin or ibuprofen (Advil, Motrin) as pain relievers because these drugs lengthen the clotting time of blood.

Treatment with corticosteroids such as oral prednisone or IV methylprednisone are the initial drugs of choice for the treatment of ITP.

Emergency treatment

Patients with acute ITP who are losing large amounts of blood or bleeding into their central nervous system require emergency treatment. This includes transfusions of platelets, intravenous immunoglobulins, or treatment with corticosteroids such as methylprednisone. Prednisone is a steroid medication that decreases the effects of antibody on platelets and eventually lowers antibody production. If the patient has a history of ITP that has not responded to prednisone or immunoglobulins, the surgeon may remove the patient's spleen. This operation is called a splenectomy. The reason for removing the spleen when ITP does not respond to other forms of treatment is that the spleen sometimes keeps platelets out of the general blood circulation.

Medications and transfusions

Patients with chronic ITP can be treated with prednisone, immune globulin, or large doses of intravenous gamma globulin. Although 90% of patients respond to immunoglobulin treatment, it is very expensive. About 80% of patients respond to prednisone therapy. Platelet transfusions are not recommended for routine treatment of ITP. If the patient's platelet level does not improve within one to four months, or requires high doses of prednisone, the doctor may recommend splenectomy. All medications for ITP are given either orally or intravenously; intramuscular injection is avoided because of the possibility of causing bleeding into the skin.

Newer medications which may be used in the treatment of ITP include the monoclonal antibody rituximab (Rituxan) which can be combined with the corticosteroid dexamethasone to treat chronic ITP and thrombopoietin-receptor agonists romiplostim (Nplate) and eltrombopag (Promacta) which work by directly stimulating the bone marrow to increase platelet production.

Surgery

Between 80% and 85% of adults with ITP have a remission of the disorder after the spleen is removed. Splenectomy is usually avoided in children younger than five years because of the increased risk of a severe infection after the operation. However, in older children splenectomy is recommended if the child has been treated for 12 months without improvement; if the ITP is very severe or the patient is getting worse; if the patient begins to bleed into the head or brain; and if the patient is an adolescent female with extremely heavy periods. Relapse of ITP is more common after splenectomy in patients with chronic ITP as compared to those with acute ITP.

Prognosis

The prognosis for recovery from acute ITP is good; 80% of patients recover without special treatment. The prognosis for chronic ITP is also good; most patients experience long-term remissions. In rare instances, however, ITP can cause life-threatening hemorrhage or bleeding into the central nervous system.

Prevention

In most individuals, ITP occurs as a manifestation of another disease or as a consequence of a viral infection. Therefore, at this time ITP cannot be entirely prevented.

Resources

PERIODICALS

Danese, M.D., Lindquist, K., Gleeson, M., Deuson, R., & Mikhael, J. "Cost and Mortality Associated with Hospitalizations in Patients with Immune Thrombocytopenic Purpera." *Am J Hematol.* (Jul 16, 2009).

Fogarty, P.F. & Segal, J.B. "The Epidemiology of Thrombocytopenia Purpera." *Curr Opin Hematol.* (Sep 2007); 14(5): 515–9.

Stasi, R., Evangelista, M.L., Stipa, E., et al. "Idiopathic Thrombocytopenia Purpura: Current Concepts in Pathophysiology and Management." *Thromb Haemost.* (Jan 2008); 99(1): 4–13.

OTHER

Sandler, S.G. & Bhanji, R. "Immune Thrombocytopenia Purpera."eMedicine. May 10, 2010 [cited July 24, 2010], http://www.emedicine.medscape.com/article/202158.

Rebecca J. Frey, PhD
Melinda Granger Oberleitner, RN, DNS

IgA deficiency *see* Immunoglobulin deficiency syndromes

IgG subclasss deficiencies *see* Immunoglobulin deficiency syndromes

Ileus

Definition

Ileus is a partial or complete non-mechanical blockage of the small and/or large intestine. When this blockage occurs the bowel becomes full of gases and fluids. Consequently, patients often report mild abdominal **pain** and bloating. They may also experience poor appetite, nausea, and, sometimes, **vomiting**. The term "ileus" comes from the Latin word for **colic**. Ileus is sometimes also called bowel obstruction, intestinal volvulus, and colonic ileus.

Demographics

The blockage of the intestines from the condition called ileus can occur at any age. In infants and children, it is the major cause of bowel obstruction. In adults, abdominal surgery can often bring about ileus. It occurs throughout the human population, regardless of one's ethnic background or other factors.

Description

There are two types of **intestinal obstructions** (when the bowel does not work correctly), mechanical and non-mechanical. Mechanical obstructions occur because the bowel is physically (structurally) blocked and its contents cannot pass the point of the obstruction. This happens when the bowel twists on itself (volvulus) or as the result of hernias, impacted feces, abnormal tissue growth, or the presence of foreign bodies in the intestines.

Unlike mechanical obstruction, non-mechanical obstruction, called ileus or paralytic ileus, occurs when there is not a structural problem within the bowel but, instead, because peristalsis stops. Peristalsis is the rhythmic contraction that moves material through the bowel. Thus, ileus occurs when the muscles of the bowel wall have failed and they are unable to transport contents through the intestinal tract. Ileus is most often associated with an infection of the peritoneum (the membrane lining the abdomen). It is one of the major causes of bowel obstruction in infants and children.

Another common cause of ileus is a disruption or reduction of the blood supply to the abdomen. Handling the bowel during abdominal surgery can also cause peristalsis to stop so people who have had abdominal surgery are more likely to experience ileus. When ileus results from abdominal surgery, the condition known as postoperative ileus, the condition is often temporary and usually lasts from 48 to 72 hours.

Ileus sometimes occurs as a complication of surgery on other parts of the body, including joint replacement or chest surgery.

Ileus can also be caused by kidney diseases especially when potassium levels decrease. Ileus can also be caused by heart disease and certain **chemotherapy** drugs such as vinblastine (Velban, Velsar) and vincristine (Oncovin, Vincasar PES, Vincrex). Infants with **cystic fibrosis** are more likely to experience meconium ileus (a dark green material in the intestine). Over all, the total rate of bowel obstruction due both to mechanical and non-mechanical causes is one in one thousand people (1/1,000).

Causes and symptoms

The major cause of ileus is operations occurring within and about the intestines. However, normal activity of the intestines usually returns within hours to days after such operations. Other causes of ileus include:

- drugs, such as antacids, chlorpromazine, opioids, warfarin, and amitriptline
- metabolic changes, such as thoe caused by low levels of iron, potassium magnesium, or sodium
- pneumonia
- heart attack (myocardial infarction)
- trauma, such as injuries to the head and spinal column
- pneumonia

When the bowel stops functioning, the following symptoms can occur:

- abdominal cramping
- abdominal distension, discomfort, and tenderness
- poor appetite
- nausea and vomiting, especially after eating
- excessive belching
- constipation
- failure to pass gas (flatulence) or to have a bowel movement (defecation)
- absence of abdominal cramping

Diagnosis

When a doctor listens with a stethoscope to the abdomen, there will be few or no bowel sounds, indicating that the intestine has stopped functioning. Ileus can be confirmed by **x rays** of the abdomen, **computed tomography scans** (CT scans), or ultrasound. It may be necessary to do more invasive tests, such as a barium enema or upper gastrointestinal (GI) series, if the obstruction is mechanical. Blood tests also are useful in diagnosing paralytic ileus.

Barium studies are used in cases of mechanical obstruction, but may cause problems by increasing pressure or intestinal contents if used in ileus. Also, in

KEY TERMS

Bowel—The part of the intestines that is connected to the anus.

Computed tomography scan (or CT scan)—A computer enhanced x-ray study performed to detect abnormalities that do not show up on normal x rays.

Meconium—A greenish fecal material that forms the first bowel movement of an infant.

Peritoneum—The transparent membrane lining the abdominal cavity that holds internal organs in place.

cases of suspected mechanical obstruction involving the gastrointestinal tract (from the small intestine downward) use of barium x rays are contraindicated since they may contribute to the obstruction. In such cases a barium enema should always be performed first.

Treatment

Patients may be treated with supervised bed rest in a hospital and bowel rest. Bowel rest means that nothing is taken by mouth and patients are fed intravenously or through the use of a nasogastric tube. (A nasogastric tube provides relief for patients with vomiting and distension; however, it has not been found helpful with treating ileus itself.) A nasogastric tube is a tube inserted through the nose, down the throat, and into the stomach. A similar tube can be inserted in the intestine. The contents are then suctioned out. In some cases, especially where there is a mechanical obstruction, surgery may be necessary.

Narcotics are often used after surgery for pain relief but can be replaced over time with nonsteroidal anti–inflammatory drugs (NSAIDs), which also help with reducing inflammation. Drug therapies that promote intestinal motility (ability of the intestine to move spontaneously), such as cisapride (Prepulsid, Propulsid) and vasopressin (Pitressin), are sometimes prescribed.

Alternative treatment

Alternative practitioners offer few treatment suggestions, but focus on prevention by keeping the bowels healthy through eating a good diet that is high in fiber and low in fat. If the case is not a medical emergency, homeopathic treatment and traditional Chinese medicine can recommend therapies that may help to reinstate peristalsis.

Prognosis

The outcome of ileus varies depending on its cause. Complications may occur, including infection, **jaundice** (yellow skin discoloration), perforation (hole) in the intestine, or electrolyte imbalances (any of a number of free-ion substances in the body that are not in normal concentrations).

Prevention

Most cases of ileus are not preventable. Surgery to remove a tumor or other mechanical obstruction will help prevent a recurrence.

Some measures that have been recommended to minimize the severity of postoperative ileus or shorten its duration include making sure that any electrolyte imbalances are corrected, and using nonopioid medications to relieve pain, as opioid drugs (including morphine, oxycodone, and codeine) tend to cause **constipation**. One group of drugs that shows promise for treating abdominal pain is a class of medications known as kappa-opioid agonists. As of 2008, however, these drugs are still under investigation for controlling visceral pain in humans. Further clinical studies are needed to determine their ability to treat such pain.

Resources

BOOKS

Beers, Mark H., et al., editors. *The Merck Manual of Diagnosis and Therapy,* 18th ed. Whitehouse Station, NJ: Merck Research Laboratories, 2006.

Feldman, Mark., et al., editors. *Sleisenger and Fordtran's Gastrointestinal and Liver Disease: Pathophysiology/Diagnosis/Management.* Philadelphia: Saunders/Elsevier, 2006.

Townsend, C. M, et al. editors. *Sabiston Textbook of Surgery: The Biological Basis of Modern Surgical Practice,* 18th ed. Philadelphia: Saunders/Elsevier, 2008.

PERIODICALS

Chang, Howard Y., and Anthony J. Lembo. "Opioid–induced Bowel Dysfunction." *Current Treatment Options in Gastroenterology.* 11, no. 1 (February 2008): 11–18.

OTHER

Heller, Jacob L. "Intestinal Obstruction." Medline Plus, U.S. National Library of Medicine and National Institutes of Health. July 23, 2008. [Accessed September 4, 2010], http://www.nlm.nih.gov/medlineplus/ency/article/000260.htm.

Mukherjee, Sandeep, et al. "Ileus." eMedicine, WebMD. December 28, 2009. [Accessed September 4, 2010], http://emedicine.medscape.com/article/178948-overview.

ORGANIZATIONS

ITP Foundation, 40 West Chesapeake Ave., Suite 308, Towson MD, 21204, (203) 655–6954, itpf@itpfoundation.org, http://www.itpfoundation.org/.

Tish Davidson, A. M.
Rebecca J. Frey, PhD

Immobilization

Definition

Immobilization refers to the process of holding a joint or bone in place with a splint, cast, or brace. This is done to prevent an injured area from moving while it heals.

Purpose

Splints, casts, and braces support and protect broken bones, dislocated joints, and such injured soft tissue as tendons and ligaments. Immobilization restricts motion to allow the injured area to heal. It can help reduce **pain**, swelling, and muscle spasm. In some cases, splints and casts are applied after surgical procedures that repair bones, tendons, or ligaments. This allows for protection and proper alignment early in the healing phase.

Precautions

There are no special precautions for immobilization.

Description

When an arm, hand, leg, or foot requires immobilization, the cast, splint, or brace will generally extend from the joint above the injury to the joint below the injury. For example, an injury to the mid-calf requires immobilization from the knee to the ankle and foot. Injuries of the hip and upper thigh or shoulder and upper arm require a cast that encircles the body and extends down the injured leg or arm.

Casts and splints

Casts are generally used for immobilization of a broken bone. Once the doctor makes sure the two broken ends of the bone are aligned, a cast is put on to keep them in place until they are rejoined through natural healing. Casts are applied by a physician, a nurse, or an assistant. They are custom-made to fit each person and are usually made of plaster or fiberglass. Fiberglass weighs less than plaster, is more durable, and allows the skin more adequate airflow than plaster. A layer of cotton or synthetic padding is first wrapped around the skin to cover the injured area and protect the skin. The plaster or fiberglass is then applied over this.

Most casts should not be gotten wet. However, some types of fiberglass casts use Gore-tex padding that is waterproof and allows the person to completely immerse the cast in water when taking a shower or bath. There are some circumstances when this type of cast material can not be used.

A splint is often used to immobilize a dislocated joint while it heals. Splints are also often used for finger injuries, such as **fractures** or baseball finger. Baseball finger is an injury in which the tendon at the end of the finger is separated from the bone as a result of trauma. Splinting also is used to immobilize an injured arm or leg immediately after an injury. Before moving a person who has injured an arm or leg some type of temporary splint

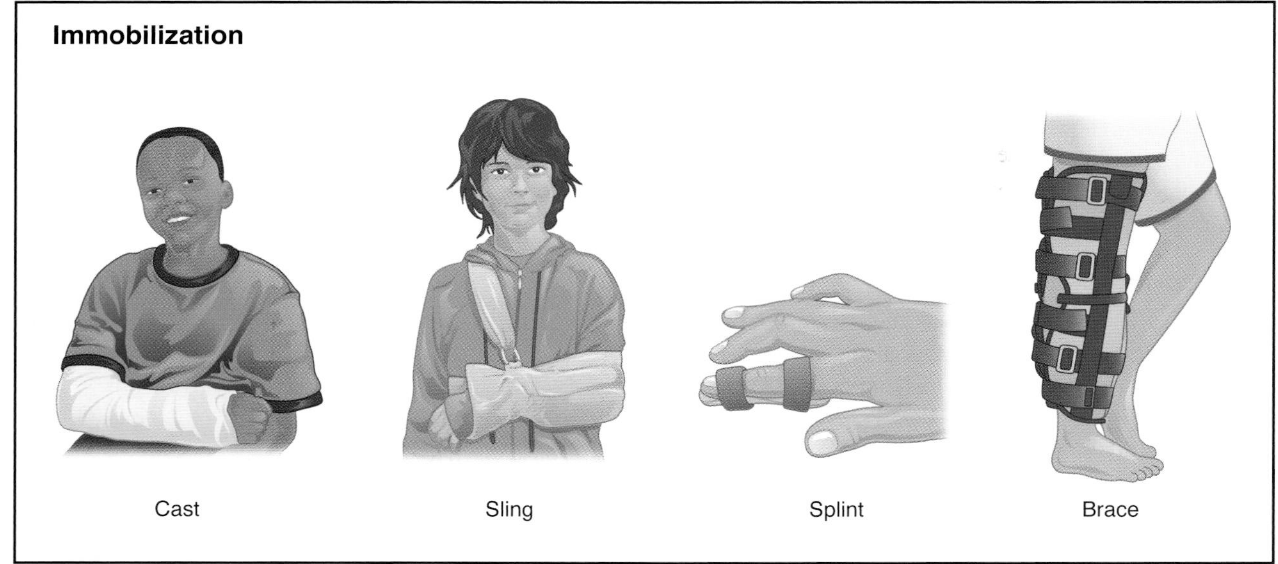

These illustrations feature several types of immobilization techniques, including slings and splints. *(Illustration by Electronic Illustrators Group. Reproduced by permission of Gale, a part of Cengage Learning.)*

should be applied to prevent further injury to the area. Splints may be made of acrylic, polyethylene foam, plaster of paris, or aluminum. In an emergency, a splint can be made from a piece of wood or rolled magazine.

Slings

Slings are often used to support the arm after a fracture or other injury. They are generally used along with a cast or splint but sometimes are used alone as a means of immobilization. They can be used in an emergency to immobilize the arm until the person can be seen by a doctor. A triangular bandage is placed under the injured arm and then tied around the neck.

Braces

Braces are used to support, align, or hold a body part in the correct position. Braces are sometimes used after a surgical procedure is performed on an arm or leg. They can also be used for an injury. Since some braces can be easily taken off and put back on, they are often used when the person must have physical therapy or **exercise** the limb during the healing process. Many braces can also be adjusted to allow for a certain amount of movement.

Braces can be custom-made or a ready-made brace can be used. The off-the-shelf braces are made in a variety of shapes and sizes. They generally have Velcro straps that make the brace easy to adjust, put on, and take off. Both braces and splints offer less support and protection than a cast and may not be a treatment option in all circumstances.

Collars

A collar is generally used for neck injuries. A soft collar can relieve pain by restricting movement of the head and neck. They also transfer some of the weight of the head from the neck to the chest. Stiff collars are generally used to support the neck when there has been a fracture in one of the bones of the neck. Cervical collars are widely used by emergency personnel at the scene of injuries when there is a potential neck or **head injury**.

Traction

Immobilization may also be secured by traction. Traction involves using a method for applying tension to correct the alignment of two structures (such as two bones) and hold them in the correct position. For example, if the bone in the thigh breaks, the broken ends may have a tendency to overlap. Use of traction will hold them in the correct position for healing to occur. The strongest form of traction involves inserting a stainless steel pin through a bony prominence attached by a horseshoe-shaped bow and rope to a pulley and weights suspended over the end of the patient's bed.

Traction must be balanced by countertraction. This is obtained by tilting the bed and allowing the patient's body to act as a counterweight. Another technique involves applying weights pulling in the opposite direction.

Traction for neck injuries may be in the form of a leather or cotton cloth halter placed around the chin and lower back of the head. For very severe neck injuries that require maximum traction, tongs that resemble ice tongs are inserted into small holes drilled in the outer skull.

All traction requires careful observation and adjustment by doctors and nurses to maintain proper balance and alignment of the traction with free suspension of the weights.

Immobilization can also be secured by a form of traction called skin traction. This is a combination of a splint and traction that is applied to the arms or legs by strips of adhesive tape placed over the skin of the arm or leg. Adhesive strips, moleskin, or foam rubber traction strips are applied on the skin. This method is effective only if a moderate amount of traction is required.

Preparation

There are many reasons for immobilization using splints, casts, and braces. Each person should understand his or her diagnosis clearly.

Aftercare

After a cast or splint has been put on, the injured arm or leg should be elevated for 24 to 72 hours. It is recommended that the person lie or sit with the injured arm or leg raised above the level of the heart. Rest combined with elevation will reduce pain and speed the healing process by minimizing swelling.

Fingers or toes can be exercised as much as can be tolerated after casting. This has been found to decrease swelling and prevent stiffness. If excessive swelling is noted, the application of ice to the splint or cast may be helpful.

After the cast, splint, or brace is removed, gradual exercise is usually performed to regain muscle strength and motion. The doctor may also recommend hydrotherapy, heat treatments, and other forms of physical therapy.

Risks

For some people, such as those in traction, immobilization will require long periods of bedrest. Lying in one position in bed for an extended period of time can result in sores on the skin (decubitus ulcers) and skin infection. Long periods of bedrest can also cause a

KEY TERMS

Decubitus ulcers—A pressure sore resulting from ulceration of the skin occurring in persons confined to bed for long periods of time

Ligament—Ligaments are structures that hold bones together and prevent excessive movement of the joint. They are tough, fibrous bands of tissue.

Pneumonia—An acute or chronic disease characterized by inflammation of the lungs and caused by viruses, bacteria, or other microorganisms.

Tendon—Tendons are structures that attach bones to muscles and muscles to other muscles.

buildup of fluid in the lungs or an infection in the lungs (**pneumonia**). Urinary infection can also be a result of extended bedrest.

People who have casts, splints, or braces on their arms or legs will generally spend several weeks not using the injured arm or leg. This lack of use can result in decreased muscle tone and shrinkage of the muscle (atrophy). Much of this loss can usually be regained, however, through rehabilitation after the injury has healed.

Immobility can also cause psychological stress. An individual restricted to a bed with a traction device may become frustrated and bored, and perhaps even depressed, irritable, and withdrawn.

There is the possibility of decreased circulation if the cast, splint, or brace fits too tightly. Excessive pressure over a nerve can cause irritation or possible damage if not corrected. If the cast, splint, or brace breaks or malfunctions, the healing process of the bone or soft tissue can be disrupted and lead to deformity.

Normal results

Normally, the surgical or injured area heals appropriately with the help of immobilization. The form of immobilization can be discontinued, which is followed by an appropriate rehabilitation program under the supervision of a physical therapist to regain range of motion and strength.

Resources

OTHER

"Casts & Splints." *The Center for Orthopaedics and Sports Medicine.* [Accessed December 6, 2010], http://www.arthroscopy.com.

Jeffrey P. Larson, RPT

Immune system

Definition

The immune system is the mechanism that protects the body from foreign substances, foreign cells, and disease-causing microorganism (pathogens). The thymus, spleen, lymph nodes, white blood cells, including the B-cells and T-cells, and antibodies are involved in the immune response, which aims to destroy these foreign bodies.

Description

The body is constantly bombarded with microorganisms, including viruses (such as those that cause colds and **influenza**), bacteria (such as those that cause **pneumonia** and **food poisoning**), parasites, and fungi. The immune system efficiently wages a daily battle to rid the body of most harmful organisms. When the immune system is unable to function because of injury or damage, the consequences can be severe. For instance, acquired immune deficiency syndrome (**AIDS**) is caused by a virus called human **immunodeficiency** virus (HIV) that attacks a key immune system cell, the helper T–cell lymphocyte. Without these cells, the immune system cannot fight off the harmful microorganisms. Without treatment, the person succumbs to infections that a healthy immune system would effortlessly neutralize.

Traditionally scientists have viewed the immune system as a defensive network that protects the "self" from harmful "non-self" invaders. In the mid-1990s, some immunologists modified this view of the immune system, creating a new model of the body's immune system that is able to discriminate between beneficial "non-self" invaders (food or helpful bacteria) and threatening invaders. One of the leading scientists investigating the functioning of the immune system in the 1990s was Polly Matzinger of the National Institute of Allergy and Infectious Diseases in Bethesda, Maryland. Matzinger proposed a model of the immune system that responds to invaders only when cells of the body are injured or damaged. As of 2010, specific parts of this theory were still being challenged by immunology researchers. Some researchers have gone so far as to claim that the "immune system" is not a single system at all but is a combination of independent evolutionary adaptations; thus, no single theory can describe how it works. In the tradition of good scientific research, ideas of how the immune system works are constantly being suggested, challenged, tested, refined, and modified.

No matter what model is used, immunologists generally agree that the immune system consists of three lines of defense. The first line is made up of the physical barriers to foreign material—the skin and mucous membranes—that prevent microorganisms from entering the body. The next line of defense, innate or nonspecific immunity, features responses from cells that surround and digest invaders and from chemicals such as histamine and serum proteins that help to destroy bacteria. The final defense is slower acting but more specific to the invader. This specific immunity calls into action the production of antibodies by lymphocytes or white blood cells produced by the thymus gland and the bone marrow.

Organs of the immune system

The organs of the immune system either make the cells that participate in the immune response or act as sites for immune function. These organs include the lymphatic vessels, lymph nodes, the tonsils, the thymus, Peyer's patches, and spleen. Lymphatic fluid (or lymph) circulates through lymph nodes via the lymphatic vessels. The lymph nodes are small aggregations of tissues located throughout the lymphatic system. Many people are familiar with the lymph nodes below the ear at the angle of the jaw that cause "swollen glands" when one has an infection. Other lymph nodes are located in the armpit and groin. White blood cells (lymphocytes) that function in the immune response are concentrated in the lymph nodes where foreign cells of microorganisms are detected and overpowered.

The tonsils and Peyer's patches contain large numbers of lymphocytes. Located at the back of the throat and under the tongue (tonsils) and in the small intestine and appendix (Peyer's patches), these organs filter out potentially harmful bacteria that may enter the body via the nose, mouth, and digestive system.

The thymus, located within the upper chest region, weighs about 15 grams or one-half ounce at **birth**. It continues to grow until it has roughly doubled in size by the time the child has reached age 12. During childhood, the thymus makes large numbers of the lymphocytes known as T-lymphocytes or T-cells. Around **puberty**, T-cell production is taken over by the lymph nodes and spleen, and the thymus begins to shrink. By adulthood, it is sometimes impossible to detect on **x rays**. If the thymus is removed due to disease or injury before puberty, removal may have a negative effect on both physical growth and the development of immunity to certain organisms.

Bone marrow, found within the hollow interior of bones, also produces lymphocytes that migrate out of the bone marrow to other sites in the body. Because bone marrow is an integral part of the immune system, certain bone **cancer** treatments that require the destruction of bone marrow are high risk because without bone marrow, a person cannot make lymphocytes and thus loses a

KEY TERMS

Antibodies—Proteins that are produced normally by specialized white blood cells after stimulation by a foreign substance (antigen) and that act specifically against the antigen in an immune response.

Antigen—Any foreign substance, usually a protein, that stimulates the body's immune system to produce antibodies.

B-cells (B-lymphocytes)—A type of white blood cell that produce antibodies.

Cytokines—Communication substances secreted by immune system cells that regulate immune system response.

Histamine—A chemical produced by the immune system in response to an allergen.

Immunoglobulin (Ig)—A substance made by B cells that neutralizes specific disease-causing substances and organisms. Also called "antibody." Immunoglobulins are divided into five classes: IgA, IgD, IgE, IgG, and IgM.

Lymph nodes—Small, bean-shaped masses of tissue scattered along the lymphatic system that act as filters and immune monitors, removing fluids, bacteria, or cancer cells that travel through the lymph system. Cancer cells in the lymph nodes are a sign that the cancer has spread and that it might recur.

Lymphocytes—White blood cells that are important in the formation of antibodies. They include B-cells, T-cells, and natural killer cells.

Peyer's patches—A collection of lymphoid tissue found in the small intestine that participates in the immune response.

Spleen—A large lymphatic organ, located just under the left rib cage, that filters the blood.

T-cells (T-lymphocytes)—White blood cells that originate in the thymus gland. T cells regulate the immune system's response to infections, including HIV. CD4 lymphocytes are a subset of T-lymphocytes.

Thymus—An organ that is part of the lymphatic system and in which T-lymphocytes grow and multiply. It is located in the chest behind the breastbone.

Trachea—Commonly called the windpipe, it is the air pathway that connects the nose and mouth to the lungs.

critical part of the immune system. People undergoing bone marrow replacement must be kept in strict isolation to prevent exposure to viruses or bacteria until the new bone marrow begins to function.

The spleen destroys worn-out red blood cells and acts as a reservoir for blood. Any rupture to the spleen can cause dangerous internal bleeding, a potentially fatal condition. The spleen also contains lymphatic tissue and produces lymphocytes.

Overview of immune function

For the immune system to work properly, two things must happen: first, the body must recognize that it is being threatened by a foreign pathogen. Second, the immune response must be quickly activated before many cells are destroyed by the invaders.

BARRIERS: SKIN AND MUCOUS MEMBRANES The skin and mucous membranes act as effective barriers against harmful invaders. The surface of the skin is slightly acidic, which makes it difficult for many microorganisms to survive. In addition, the enzyme lysozyme, which is present in sweat, tears, and saliva, kills many bacteria. Mucous membranes line many of the body's entrances, such as those that open into the respiratory, digestive, and urogenital tract. Microorganisms become trapped in the thick layers of mucus produced by these membranes and are thus prevented from entering the body.

In the upper respiratory tract, the hairs that line the nose also trap bacteria. In addition, many bacteria that are inhaled deeper into the respiratory tract are swept back out again by the cilia—tiny hairs that line the trachea and the bronchi. One reason why smokers are more susceptible to respiratory infections is that cigarette smoke disables the cilia, slowing the movement of mucus and bacteria out of the respiratory tract.

NONSPECIFIC IMMUNE DEFENSES Nonspecific lymphocytes carry out "search and destroy" missions within the body. If these cells encounter a foreign microorganism, they either engulf the foreign invader or destroy the invader with enzymes. The following are nonspecific lymphocytes:

Macrophages are large lymphocytes that engulf foreign cells. Because macrophages ingest other cells, they are also called phagocytes (from two Greek words, *phagein*, to eat and *kytos*, cell).

Neutrophils are cells that migrate to areas where bacteria have invaded, such as entrances created by cuts in the skin. Neutrophils digest microorganisms and release microorganism-killing enzymes. Neutrophils die quickly; the pus that sometimes collects in skin **wounds** contains an accumulation of dead neutrophils.

Natural killer (NK) cells kill body cells infected with viruses by punching a hole in the cell membrane, causing the cell to lyse or break apart.

Fever is a nonspecific response to bacterial or viral invasion. The body responds by increasing its internal temperature, creating conditions that are hostile to the growth of the virus or bacteria.

The inflammatory response is an immune response confined to a small area. When a finger is cut, for example, the area becomes red, swollen, and warm. These signs are evidence of the inflammatory response. Injured tissues send out signals to immune system cells, which quickly migrate to the injured area. These immune cells perform different functions: some engulf bacteria, while others release bacteria-killing chemicals. Other immune cells release a substance called histamine, which causes blood vessels to become wider (dilate), thus increasing blood flow to the area. All of these activities promote healing in the injured tissue.

When the body's immune system reacts to pollen (a harmless substance) as if it were a bacterium, an immune response is prompted in what is known as an allergic reaction. Histamine is released, which dilates blood vessels, causes large amounts of mucus to be produced, and stimulates the release of tears. To combat these reactions, many people who are allergic to pollen take **antihistamines**, drugs that deactivate histamine.

Specific immune defenses

The specific immune response is activated when microorganisms survive or get past the nonspecific defenses. Two types of specific defenses destroy microorganisms in the human body: the cell-mediated response and the antibody response. The cell-mediated response attacks cells that have been infected by viruses. The antibody response attacks both bacteria and "free" viruses that have not yet penetrated cells. Most bacteria do not infect cells, although some do (e.g. the mycobacteria that cause tuberculosis.) The specific immune response depends on the ability of the immune lymphocytes to identify the invader and create immune cells that specifically mark the invader for destruction. Bone marrow produces an amazing array of lymphocytes, each of which is capable of recognizing one specific molecular shape called an antigen.

Two kinds of lymphocytes operate in the specific immune response: T-lymphocytes and B-lymphocytes. T-lymphocytes are made in the thymus gland, while B-lymphocytes are made in bone marrow. B- and T-lymphocytes are individually configured to attack a specific antigen. For example, the blood and lymph of humans have T-cell lymphocytes that specifically target the **chickenpox** virus, T-cell lymphocytes that target the

diphtheria virus, and so on. When T-cell lymphocytes specific for the chickenpox virus encounter a cell infected with this virus, the T-cell multiplies rapidly and destroys the invading virus.

After the invader has been neutralized, some T-cells remain behind. These cells, called memory cells, impart immunity to future attacks by the virus. Once a person has had chickenpox, memory cells quickly stave off subsequent infections. This secondary immune response, involving memory cells, is much faster than the primary immune response. When a human is immunized against a disease, the **vaccination** injects whole or parts of killed viruses or bacteria into the bloodstream, prompting memory cells to be made without a person's developing the disease.

Helper T-cells are a subset of T-cell lymphocytes present in large numbers in the blood and lymphatic system, lymph nodes, and Peyer's patches. When one of the body's macrophage cells ingests a foreign invader, it displays the antigen on its membrane surface. These antigen-displaying-macrophages, or APCs, are the immune system's distress signal. When a helper T-cell encounters an APC, it immediately binds to the antigen on the macrophage. This binding unleashes several powerful chemicals called cytokines. Some cytokines stimulate the growth and division of T-cells, while others play a role in the fever response. Still another cytokine, called interleukin II, stimulates the division of cytotoxic T-cells, key components of the cell-mediated response. The binding also "turns on" the antibody response. Any disease, such as HIV, that destroys helper T-cells destroys the immune system.

Antibodies are made when a B-cell specific for the invading antigen is stimulated to divide. The dividing B-cells, called plasma cells, secrete antibodies composed of a special type of protein called an immunoglobulin (Ig).

T-CELLS T-cell lymphocytes are the primary players in the cell-mediated response. When an antigen-specific helper T-cell is activated, the cell multiplies. The cells produced from this division are called cytotoxic T-cells. Cytotoxic T-cells target and kill cells that have been infected with a specific microorganism. After the infection has subsided, a few memory T-cells persist, so conferring immunity.

Chemical signals activate the immune response; likewise, chemical signals must turn it off. When all the invading microorganisms have been neutralized, special T-cells called suppressor T-cells release cytokines that deactivate the cytotoxic T-cells and the plasma cells, and the cells of the body return to normal functioning.

Immune system disorders

There are three major categories of immune system disorders: immunodeficiencies, autoimmune syndromes, and hypersensitivity. Immunodeficiencies occur when the immune system is inhibited from carrying out its function. **Malnutrition** is the largest single cause of immunodeficiency around the world, as the immune system needs protein to maintain the proper concentration of antibodies in the blood, to produce cytokines, and to support the function of phagocytes. Deficiencies of such single nutrients as iron, copper, selenium, zinc, **vitamins** A, C, E, and B_6, as well as **folic acid**, can also impair the body's immune response. Aging is another factor in immunodeficiency; the body's response to immunizations begins to decline in people older than age 50. Alcohol and drug abuse, obesity, and **smoking** may also contribute to poor immune function. Some diseases associated with immunodeficiency are inherited, such as congenital granulomatous disease, a disorder in which phagocytes have difficulty destroying pathogens.

Autoimmune syndromes are disorders in which the person has a hyperactive immune system that fails to distinguish between the self and the non-self, and attacks a part of the host. Autoimmune diseases include such disorders as Graves' disease, systemic lupus erythematosus (SLE), rheumatoid arthritis (RA), Hashimoto's thyroiditis, ankylosing spondylitis, and type 1 diabetes. Some people are more susceptible than others to developing autoimmune diseases because of genetic factors. Another significant fact about these diseases is that ankylosing spondylitis is the only one more likely to develop in men; all the others show a female preponderance.

Hypersensitivity is an immune response to a pathogen or foreign substance that damages the body's own tissues. Hypersensitivity reactions are divided into four categories according to the time sequence involved and the mechanisms of the body's reaction:

- Type I: Type I hypersensitivity reactions include most allergies; they are immediate, and are mediated by immunoglobulin E (IgE) released from specialized white blood cells known as mast cells and basophils. The symptoms of Type I reactions can range from mild discomfort to death.
- Type II: This type of hypersensitivity reaction occurs when antibodies bind to antigens on the individual's own cells, marking them for destruction by other cells. It is mediated by IgG and IgM antibodies.
- Type III: Type III hypersensitivity reactions are caused by the deposition of immune complexes in various body tissues. Immune complexes are collections of antigens, complement proteins, and IgG and IgM antibodies.
- Type IV: Type IV reactions are sometimes called cell-mediated or delayed type hypersensitivity reactions.

They take several days to develop. Most forms of contact dermatitis (e.g. poison ivy, allergies to jewelry containing nickel, and similar skin rashes) are Type IV reactions. This type is mediated by T-cells, monocytes, and macrophages.

Resources

BOOKS

Parham, Peter. *The Immune System,* 3rd ed. New York: Garland Science, 2009.

Sompayrac, Lauren M. *How the Immune System Works,* 3rd ed. Malden, MA: Blackwell, 2008.

OTHER

"Immune System and Disorders." April 16, 2010. [Accessed September 4, 2010], http://www.nlm.nih.gov/medlineplus/immunesystemanddisorders.html.

National Institute of Allergy and Infectious Diseases (NIAID). "Immune System." October 5, 2008. [Accessed September 4, 2010], http://www.niaid.nih.gov/topics/immuneSystem/pages/whatisimmunesystem.aspx.

ORGANIZATIONS

Allergy and Asthma Network: Mothers of Asthmatics (AANMA), 8201 Greensboro Dr., Suite 300, McLean VA, 22102, (800) 878-4403, (703) 288-5217, http://www.aanma.org.

American Academy of Allergy, Asthma, and Immunology (AAAAI), 555 East Wells St., Suite 1100, Milwaukee WI, 53202-3823, (414) 272-6071, http://www.aaaai.org.

American Autoimmune Related Diseases Association, 22100 Gratiot Ave., East Detroit MI, 48021, (586) 776-3900, (800) 598-4668, (586) 776-3903, http://www.aarda.org.

American College of Allergy, Asthma, and Immunology, 85 West Algonquin Rd., Suite 550, Arlington Heights IL, 60005, (847) 427-1200, (847) 427-1294, info@acaai.org, http://www.acaai.org.

National Institute of Allergy and Infectious Diseases Office of Communications and Government Relations, 6610 Rockledge Dr., MSC 6612, Bethesda MD, 20892-6612, (301) 496-5717, (866) 284-4107 or TDD: (800) 877-8339, (301) 402-3573, http://www3.niaid.nih.gov.

Tish Davidson, AM

Immunization **see Vaccination**

Immunodeficiency

Definition

Immunodeficiency disorders are a group of disorders in which part of the **immune system** is missing or defective. Therefore, the body's ability to fight infections is impaired. As a result, the person with an immunodeficiency disorder has frequent infections—thus, are at greater susceptibility to infection—that are generally more severe and last longer than usual. The infections involving immunodeficiency disorders commonly reside in the skin, throat, ears, sinuses, lungs, brain, spinal cord, urinary tract, and intestines.

Demographics

These disorders are caused by genetic or hereditary defects and can happen to anyone regardless of age or gender. While some immunodeficiency disorders are commonly scattered within the human population, other types are only infrequently found. Even though numerous types of such disorders exist they all have one feature in common: each involves a defect of a specific function of body's overall immune system.

Description

The immune system is the body's main method for fighting infections. Any defect in the immune system decreases a person's ability to fight infections. A person with an immunodeficiency disorder may get more frequent infections, heal more slowly, and have a higher incidence of some cancers.

The normal immune system involves a complex interaction of certain types of cells that can recognize and attack "foreign" invaders (called antigens), such as bacteria, viruses, toxins, fungi, and blood or tissues from other humans or species. It also plays a role in fighting **cancer**. The immune system has both innate and adaptive components. Innate immunity is made up of immune protections people are born with. Adaptive immunity develops throughout life. It adapts to fight off specific invading organisms. Adaptive immunity is divided into two components: humoral immunity and cellular immunity.

The innate immune system is made up of the skin (which acts as a barrier to prevent organisms from entering the body), white blood cells called phagocytes, a system of proteins called the complement system, and chemicals called interferons. When phagocytes encounter an invading organism, they surround and engulf it to destroy it. The complement system also attacks bacteria. The elements in the complement system create a hole in the outer layer of the target cell, which leads to the **death** of the cell.

The adaptive component of the immune system is extremely complex, and is still not entirely understood. It has the ability to recognize an organism or tumor cell as not being a normal part of the body, and to develop a response to attempt to eliminate it.

The humoral response of adaptive immunity involves a type of cell called B-lymphocytes. B-lymphocytes manufacture proteins called antibodies (which are also called immunoglobulins). Antibodies attach themselves to the invading foreign substance. This allows the phagocytes to begin engulfing and destroying the organism. The action of antibodies also activates the complement system. The humoral response is particularly useful for attacking bacteria.

The cellular response of adaptive immunity is useful for attacking viruses, some parasites, and possibly cancer cells. The main type of cell in the cellular response is T-lymphocytes. There are helper T-lymphocytes and killer T-lymphocytes. The helper T-lymphocytes play a role in recognizing invading organisms and they also help killer T-lymphocytes to multiply. As the name suggests, killer T-lymphocytes act to destroy the target organism.

Defects can occur in any component of the immune system or in more than one component (combined immunodeficiency). Different immunodeficiency diseases involve different components of the immune system. The defects can be inherited and/or present at **birth** (congenital) or acquired.

Congenital immunodeficiency disorders

Congenital immunodeficiency is present at the time of birth and is the result of genetic defects. These immunodeficiency disorders are also called primary immunodeficiencies. The disorders are generally classified according to the part of the immune system that is improperly functioning. The World Health Organization (WHO) estimates that over 70 primary immunodeficiency disorders are present around the world. In the United States, the National Institute of Child Health and Human Development estimates about 400 children are born annually with a primary immunodeficiency disorder. It also states that roughly 25,000 to 50,000 people are living in any given year with such a disorder. The number of new cases is rising in the United Sates as new laboratory tests become more commonly available. Congenital immunodeficiencies may occur because of defects in B-lymphocytes, T-lymphocytes, or both. They also can occur in the innate immune system.

HUMORAL IMMUNITY DISORDERS Bruton's agammaglobulinemia, also known as X-linked agammaglobulinemia, a congenital immunodeficiency disorder. The defect results in a decrease or absence of B-lymphocytes, and therefore a decreased ability to make antibodies. People with this disorder are particularly susceptible to infections of the throat, skin, middle ear, and lungs. It is seen only in males because it is caused by a genetic defect on the X chromosome. Since males have only one X chromosome, they always have the defect if the gene is present. Females can have the defective gene but since they have two X chromosomes, there will be a normal gene on the other X chromosome to counter it. Women may pass the defective gene on to their male children.

B LYMPHOCYTE DEFICIENCES If there is an abnormality in either the development or function of B-lymphocytes, the ability to make antibodies will be impaired. This allows the body to be susceptible to recurrent infections.

A type of B-lymphocyte deficiency involves a group of disorders called selective immunoglobulin deficiency syndromes. Immunoglobulin is another name for antibody and there are five different types of immunoglobulins (called IgA, IgG, IgM, IgD, and IgE). The most common type of immunoglobulin deficiency is selective IgA deficiency, which occurs in about one in every 500 white (Caucasian) persons. The amounts of the other antibody types are normal. Some patients with selective IgA deficiency experience no symptoms, while others have occasional lung infections and **diarrhea**. In another immunoglobulin disorder, IgG and IgA antibodies are deficient and there is increased IgM. People with this disorder tend to get severe bacterial infections.

Common variable immunodeficiency is another type of B-lymphocyte deficiency. In this disorder, the production of one or more of the immunoglobulin types is decreased and the antibody response to infections is impaired. It generally develops around the age of 10 to 20 years. The symptoms vary among affected people. Most people with this disorder have frequent infections and some of them also experience **anemia** and rheumatoid arthritis. Many people with common variable immunodeficiency develop cancer.

T-LYMPHOCYTE DEFICIENCIES Severe defects in the ability of T-lymphocytes to mature results in impaired immune responses to infections with antigens, such as viruses, fungi, and certain types of bacteria. These infections are usually severe and can be fatal.

DiGeorge syndrome is a T-lymphocyte deficiency that starts during fetal development and is the result of a deletion in a particular chromosome. Children with DiGeorge syndrome either do not have a thymus or have an underdeveloped thymus. Since the thymus is a major organ that directs the production of T-lymphocytes, these patients have very low numbers of T-lymphocytes. They are susceptible to recurrent infections and usually have physical abnormalities as well. For example, they may have low-set ears, a small receding jawbone, and wide–spaced eyes. People with DiGeorge syndrome are particularly susceptible to viral and fungal infections.

In some cases, no treatment is required for DiGeorge syndrome because T-lymphocyte production improves.

Either an underdeveloped thymus begins to produce more T-lymphocytes or organ sites other than the thymus compensate by producing more T-lymphocytes.

COMBINED IMMUNODEFICIENCIES Some types of immunodeficiency disorders affect both B-lymphocytes and T-lymphocytes. For example, **severe combined immunodeficiency** disease (SCID), sometimes commonly called Bubble Boy Syndrome, is caused by the defective development or function of these two types of lymphocytes. It results in impaired humoral and cellular immune responses. SCID usually is recognized during the first year of life. It tends to cause a fungal infection of the mouth (**thrush**), diarrhea, **failure to thrive**, and serious infections. If not treated with a bone marrow transplant, a person with SCID will generally die from infections before age two. It is reported that the prevalence of SCID is one in 100,000 births, although that figure is regularly considered an underestimate. In some local populations, this figure is much greater. For instance, in the Navajo population within the United States, it is reported that one in 2,000 babies inherit SCID.

DISORDERS OF INNATE IMMUNITY Disorders of innate immunity affect phagocytes or the complement system. These disorders also result in recurrent infections.

Acquired immunodeficiency disorders

Acquired (secondary) immunodeficiency is more common than congenital immunodeficiency. It is frequently the result of an infectious process or other disease, **malnutrition**, medications/drugs, or aging. For example, the human immunodeficiency virus (HIV) is the virus that causes acquired immunodeficiency syndrome (**AIDS**). However, this is not the most common cause of acquired immunodeficiency.

Acquired immunodeficiency often occurs as a complication of other conditions and diseases. For example, the most common causes of acquired immunodeficiency are malnutrition, some types of cancer, and infections. People who weigh less than 70% of the average weight of persons of the same age and gender are considered to be malnourished. Examples of types of infections that can lead to immunodeficiency are **chickenpox**, cytomegalovirus, German **measles**, measles, **tuberculosis**, **infectious mononucleosis** (Epstein–Barr virus), chronic hepatitis, lupus, and bacterial and fungal infections.

In 2003, a new infection emerged that produces immunodeficiency. Severe acute respiratory syndrome (SARS) mysteriously appeared in a hospital in China. It eventually affected 8,000 people in Asia and Canada, killing 800 altogether. **Fever**, lower respiratory tract symptoms, and abnormal chest **x rays** characterize the virus. However, it also produces immunodeficiency. No cases of the disease were reported from July 2003 through December 2003 but scientists feared it would reappear. Thus, the World Health Organization (WHO) set up a network of medical and research professionals to deal with SARS. As of May 2006, the SARS infection has been completely contained. However, it is not considered eradicated so it could return to infect the human population.

Sometimes, acquired immunodeficiency is brought on by drugs used to treat another condition. For example, patients who have an organ transplant are given drugs to suppress the immune system so the body will not reject the organ. Also, some **chemotherapy** drugs, which are given to treat cancer, have the side effect of killing cells of the immune system. During the period of time that these drugs are being taken, the risk of infection increases. It usually returns to normal after the person stops taking the drugs.

Causes and symptoms

Congenital immunodeficiency is caused by genetic defects, which generally occur while the fetus is developing in the womb. These defects affect the development and/or function of one or more of the components of the immune system, such as lymphoid tissue within bone marrow, thymus, lymph nodes, tonsils, spleen, and gastrointestinal tract. Acquired immunodeficiency is the result of a disease process and it occurs later in life. The causes, as described above, can be diseases, infections, or the side effects of drugs given to treat other conditions.

People with an immunodeficiency disorder tend to become infected by organisms that do not usually cause disease in healthy persons. The major symptoms of most immunodeficiency disorders are repeated infections that heal slowly. These chronic infections cause symptoms that persist for long periods of time. People with chronic infection tend to be pale and thin and they may have skin **rashes**. Their lymph nodes tend to be larger than normal and their liver and spleen may also be enlarged. The lymph nodes are small organs that house antibodies and lymphocytes. Broken blood vessels, especially near the surface of the skin, may be seen. This can result in black-and-blue marks in the skin. The person may lose hair from their head. Sometimes, a red inflammation of the lining of the eye (**conjunctivitis**) is present. They may have a crusty appearance in and on the nose from chronic nasal dripping.

Diagnosis

Usually, the first sign that a person might have an immunodeficiency disorder is that they do not improve rapidly when given **antibiotics** to treat an infection. Strong indicators that an immunodeficiency disorder may be present are when rare diseases occur or the patient gets ill from organisms that do not normally cause diseases, especially if the patient repeatedly is infected. If this happens in very young children, it is an indication that a genetic defect may be causing an immunodeficiency disorder. When this situation occurs in older children or young adults, their medical history will be reviewed to determine if childhood diseases may have caused an immunodeficiency disorder. Other possibilities will then be considered, such as recently acquired infections—for example, HIV, hepatitis, tuberculosis, etc.

Laboratory tests are used to determine the exact nature of the immunodeficiency. Most tests are performed on blood samples. Blood contains antibodies, lymphocytes, phagocytes, and complement components—all of the major immune components that might cause immunodeficiency. A blood cell count will determine if the number of phagocytic cells or lymphocytes is below normal. Lower than normal counts of either of these two cell types correlates with immunodeficiencies. The blood cells also are checked for their appearance. Sometimes a person may have normal cell counts but the cells are structurally defective. If the lymphocyte cell count is low, further testing is usually done to determine whether any particular type of lymphocyte is lower than normal. A lymphocyte proliferation test is done to determine if the lymphocytes can respond to stimuli. The failure to respond to stimulants correlates with immunodeficiency. A process called electrophoresis can measure antibody levels. Complement levels can be determined by immunodiagnostic tests.

Treatment

There is no cure for immunodeficiency disorders. Therapy is aimed at controlling infections and, for some disorders, replacing defective or absent components.

Patients with Bruton's agammaglobulinemia must be given periodic injections of a substance called gamma globulin throughout their lives to make up for their decreased ability to make antibodies. The gamma globulin preparation contains antibodies against common invading bacteria. If left untreated, the disease usually is fatal.

Common variable immunodeficiency also is treated with periodic injections of gamma globulin throughout life. Additionally, antibiotics are given when necessary to treat infections.

Patients with selective IgA deficiency usually do not require any treatment. Antibiotics can be given for frequent infections.

In some cases, treatment is not required for DiGeorge syndrome because T-lymphocyte production improves on its own. Either an underdeveloped thymus begins to produce more T-lymphocytes or organ sites other than the thymus compensate by producing more T-lymphocytes. In some severe cases, a bone marrow transplant or thymus transplant can be done to correct the problem.

For patients with SCID, bone marrow transplantation is necessary. In this procedure, healthy bone marrow from a donor who has a similar type of tissue (usually a relative, such as a brother or sister) is removed. The bone marrow is a substance that resides in the cavity of bones. Such marrow produces blood including some of the white blood cells that make up the immune system. The bone marrow of the person receiving the transplant is destroyed and is then replaced with marrow from the donor.

Treatment of the HIV infection that causes AIDS consists of drugs called antiretrovirals. These drugs attempt to inhibit the process that the virus goes through to kill T-lymphocytes. Several of these drugs used in various combinations with one another can prolong the time period before the disease becomes apparent. However, this treatment is not a cure. Other treatments for people with AIDS are aimed at the particular infections and conditions that arise because of the impaired immune system. SARS is a relatively new acquired disease. Treatment to date involves combination therapy with **steroids** and interferon and supplemental oxygen for breathing difficulties. In 2004, the U.S. Food and Drug Administration approved the drug octagam 5% (Immune Globulin Intravenous (Human) 5%), an intravenous immunoglobulin product from the company Octapharma AG, to treat primary immunodeficiency diseases. At that time, the drug had been used in Europe for over ten years for the same purpose.

In most cases, immunodeficiency caused by malnutrition is reversible. The health of the immune system is directly linked to the nutritional status of the patient. Among the essential nutrients required by the immune system are proteins, **vitamins**, iron, and zinc.

For people being treated for cancer, periodic relief from chemotherapy drugs can restore the function of the immune system.

In general, people with immunodeficiency disorders should maintain a healthy diet because malnutrition can aggravate immunodeficiencies. They also should avoid being near people who have colds or are sick because they can easily acquire new infections. For the same reason, they should practice good personal hygiene, especially dental care. People with immunodeficiency

KEY TERMS

Agammaglobulinemia—The lack of gamma globulins in the blood. Antibodies are the main gamma globulins of interest, so this term means a lack of antibodies.

disorders also should avoid eating undercooked food because it might contain bacteria that could cause infection. This food would not cause infection in persons with healthy immune systems but in someone with an immunodeficiency, food is a potential source of infectious organisms. People with immunodeficiency should be given antibiotics at the first indication of an infection.

Prognosis

The prognosis depends on the type of immunodeficiency disorder. People with Bruton's agammaglobulinemia who are given injections of gamma globulin generally live into their 30s or 40s. They often die from chronic infections, usually of the lung. People with selective IgA deficiency generally live normal lives. They may experience problems if given a blood transfusion, and therefore they should wear a Medic Alert bracelet or have some other way of alerting any physician who treats them that they have this disorder.

SCID is the most serious of the immunodeficiency disorders. If a bone marrow transplant is not successfully performed, the child usually will not live beyond two years old.

People with HIV/AIDS are living longer than in the past because of antiretroviral drugs that became available in the mid 1990s. However, AIDS still is a fatal disease. People with AIDS usually die of opportunistic infections, which are infections that occur because the impaired immune system is unable to fight them.

Some complications that can occur include frequent or persistent illnesses and the increased risk from certain cancers. Infections are also much more likely with people having immunodeficiency disorders.

Prevention

There is no way to prevent a congenital immunodeficiency disorder. However, individuals with a congenital immunodeficiency disorder might want to consider getting genetic counseling before having children to find out if there is a chance they will pass the defect on to their children.

Some of the infections associated with acquired immunodeficiency can be prevented or treated before they cause problems. For example, there are effective treatments for tuberculosis and most bacterial and fungal infections. HIV infection can be prevented by practicing "safer sex" and not using illegal intravenous drugs. These are the primary routes of transmitting the virus. For people who do not know the HIV status of the person with whom they are having sex, safer sex involves using a condom.

Malnutrition can be prevented by getting adequate nutrition. Malnutrition tends to be more of a problem in developing countries.

Resources

BOOKS

Abbas, Abul K., and Andrew H. Lichtman. *Basic Immunology: Functions and Disorders of the Immune System.* Philadelphia: Saunders/Elsevier, 2009.

Beers, Mark H., et al., editors. *The Merck Manual of Diagnosis and Therapy,* 18th ed. Whitehouse Station, NJ: Merck Research Laboratories, 2006.

Elgert, Klaus D. *Immunology: Understanding the Immune System,* 2nd ed. Hoboken, NJ: Wiley-Blackwell, 2009.

OTHER

Buckley, Rebecca H. "Immunodeficiency Disorders." Merck Manuals Online Medical Library. September 2008. [Accessed September 4, 2010], http://www.merck.com/mmhe/sec16/ch184/ch184a.html.

Dugdale, David C., III, and Stuart I. Henochowicz. "Immunodeficiency disorders." Medline Plus, U.S. National Library of Medicine and National Institutes of Health. May 2, 2008. [Accessed September 4, 2010], http://www.nlm.nih.gov/medlineplus/ency/article/000818.htm.

Fonseca, Felicia. "A Rare and Once–baffling Disease Forces Navajo Parents to Cope." Indian Country News. December 2007. [Accessed September 4, 2010], http://indiancountrynews.net/index.php?option=com_content&task=view&id=2109&Itemid=1.

"Primary Immunodeficiency." National Institute of Child Health and Human Development. April 7, 2008. [Accessed September 4, 2010], http://www.nichd.nih.gov/publications/pubs/primary_immuno.cfm.

ORGANIZATIONS

Immune Deficiency Foundation, 30 Old Kings Hwy. South, Suite 275, Darien CT, 06820, (800) 296-4433, idf@primaryimmune.org, http://www.primaryimmune.org.

John T. Lohr, PhD
Teresa G. Odle

Immunoglobulin deficiency syndromes

Definition

Immunoglobulin deficiency syndromes are a group of **immunodeficiency** disorders in which the patient has a reduced number of or lack of antibodies.

Demographics

The disorders can appear in anyone, from newborn babies to the elderly.

Description

Immunoglobulins (Ig), also commonly known as antibodies, are gamma globulin proteins. That is, they are a type of protein found in the blood and other fluids of humans and other vertebrates. Immunoglobulins are used to neutralize bacteria, viruses, and other invading foreign substances. There are five major classes of antibodies: IgG, IgM, IgA, IgD, and IgE. Each differs in its functional location, physical properties, and ability to counter foreign substances within the body.

- IgG is the most abundant of the classes of immunoglobulins. It is the antibody for viruses, bacteria, and antitoxins. In addition, it is found in most tissues and plasma. It is also the only Ig that is able to help provide immunity to a mother's fetus.
- IgM is the first antibody present in an immune response.
- IgA is an early antibody for bacteria and viruses. It is found in saliva, tears, and all other mucous secretions such as within respiratory and urogenital tracts.
- IgD activity is not well understood. However, research has shown that it functions primarily as a receptor on B-cells that have yet to be subjected to antigens.
- IgE is present in respiratory secretions. It is an antibody for parasitic diseases (such as those caused by parasitic worms), Hodgkin's disease, hay fever, atopic dermatitis, and allergic asthma.

All antibodies are made by B-lymphocytes (B-cells). Any disease that harms the development or function of B-cells causes a decrease in the amount of antibodies produced. Since antibodies are essential in fighting infectious diseases, people with immunoglobulin deficiency syndromes become ill more often than those without the disorder. However, the cellular **immune system** is still functional so these patients are more prone to infection caused by organisms usually controlled by antibodies. Most of these invading germs (microbes) make capsules, a mechanism used to confuse the immune system. In a healthy body, antibodies can bind to the capsule and overcome the bacteria's defenses. The bacteria that make capsules include the streptococci, meningococci, and *Haemophilus influenzae*. These organisms cause such diseases as otitis, **sinusitis**, **pneumonia**, **meningitis**, osteomyelitis, septic arthritis, and sepsis. Patients with immunoglobulin deficiencies are also prone to some viral infections, including echovirus, enterovirus, and **hepatitis B**. They may also have a bad reaction to the attenuated version of the **polio** virus vaccine.

There are two types of immunodeficiency diseases: secondary and primary. Secondary disorders occur in normally healthy bodies that are suffering from an underlying disease. Once the disease is treated, the immunodeficiency is reversed.

Primary immunodeficiency diseases occur because of defective B-cells or antibodies. They account for approximately 50% of all immunodeficiencies and they are, therefore, the most prevalent type of immunodeficiency disorders. These disorders include:

- X-linked agammaglobulinemia is an inherited disease. The defect is on the X chromosome and, consequently, this disease is seen more frequently in males than females. The defect results in a failure of B-cells to mature. Mature B-cells are capable of making antibodies and developing "memory," a feature in which the B-cell rapidly recognizes and responds to an infectious agent the next time it is encountered. Thus, patients with x-linked agammaglobulinemia do not generate mature B-cells. All classes of antibodies are decreased in agammaglobulinemia. It occurs in about one in 100,000 newborn males, without a predisposition to ethnic origin.
- Selective IgA deficiency, a mild but very common deficiency, is an inherited disease resulting from a failure of B-cells to switch from making IgM, the early antibody, to IgA. Although the number of B-cell is normal, and the B-cells are otherwise normal (they can still make all other classes of antibodies), the amount of IgA produced is limited. This results in more infections of mucosal surfaces, such as the nose, mouth, throat, lungs, digestive tract, and intestines. Roughly no more than one in 333 people are inflicted by the deficiency; however its frequency is dependent on various populations.
- Transient hypogammaglobulinemia of infancy is a temporary disease of unknown cause. Normally, it appears after birth of a child with increased infections but, sometimes, without any symptoms. It is believed to be caused by a defect in the development of T-helper cells (cells that recognize foreign antigens and activate T- and B-cells in an immune response). As the child ages, the number and condition of T-helper cells normally improves and this situation usually corrects

itself. Hypogammaglobulinemia is characterized by low levels of gammaglobulin (antibodies) in the blood. During the disease period, patients have decreased levels of IgG antibodies, and sometimes of IgA and IgM antibodies. In laboratory tests, the antibodies that are present do not react well with infectious bacteria. The incidence of the disease varies widely in infants.

- Common variable immunodeficiency, which includes a group of primary immunodeficiencies, is a defect in both B-cells and T-lymphocytes. The differences of its members are the result of the underlying causes. Most causes are unknown. However, all result in a near complete lack of antibodies in the blood and all occur very frequently with respect to other such related diseases.
- Ig heavy chain deletions is a genetic disease in which part of the antibody molecule is not produced. It results in the loss of several antibody classes and subclasses, including most IgG antibodies and all IgA and IgE antibodies. The disease occurs because part of the gene for the heavy chain has been lost.
- Selective IgG subclass deficiencies is a group of genetic diseases in which some of the subclasses of IgG are not made. There are four subclasses in the IgG class of antibodies. As the B-cell matures, it can switch from one subclass to another. In these diseases there is a defect in the maturation of the B-cells that results in a lack of switching.
- IgG deficiency with hyper-IgM is a disease that results when the B-cell fails to switch from making IgM to IgG. This produces an increase in the amount of IgM antibodies present and a decrease in the amount of IgG antibodies. This disease is the result of a genetic mutation.
- Severe combined immunodeficiency (SCID) is not strictly a deficiency of immunoglobulin, although it is often categorized within this group. It occurs due to the absence or dysfunction of important immune cells called T-cells, or of both T- and B-cells. The condition can be X-linked, in which case more males than females are affected or it can be inherited in an autosomal fashion (in which case males and females can be equally affected). In SCID, the thymus gland (which produces T-cell) may be abnormal.

Causes and symptoms

Immunoglobulin deficiencies are the result of congenital defects affecting the development and function of B lymphocytes (B-cells). There are two main points in the development of B-cells when defects can occur. First, B-cells can fail to develop into antibody-producing cells. X-linked agammaglobulinemia is an example of this disease. Secondly, B-cells can fail to make a particular type of antibody or fail to switch classes during maturation. Initially, when B-cells start making antibodies for the first time, they make IgM. As they mature and develop memory, they switch to one of the other four classes of antibodies. Failures in switching or failure to make a subclass of antibody leads to immunoglobulin deficiency diseases. Another mechanism that results in decreased antibody production is a defect in T-helper cells. Generally, defects in T-helper cells are listed as severe combined immunodeficiencies.

Symptoms are persistent and frequent infections, **diarrhea**, **failure to thrive**, and malabsorption (of nutrients).

Diagnosis

An immunodeficiency disease is suspected when children become ill frequently, especially from the same organisms or from organisms that do not usually cause infection. Standard treatments may also fail. The profile of organisms that cause infection in patients with immunoglobulin deficiency syndrome is unique and is preliminary evidence for this disease. When laboratory tests are performed to verify the diagnosis, blood is collected and analyzed for the content and types of antibodies present. Depending on the type of immunoglobulin deficiency, the laboratory tests will show a decrease or absence of antibodies or specific antibody subclasses.

Treatment

Immunodeficiency diseases cannot be cured. Intravenous administration of immunoglobulin may temporarily boost immunity but these treatments may need to be repeated at regular intervals. Acute or chronic bacterial infections are treated with **antibiotics**; antifungal drugs are also available. Very few drugs are effective against viral diseases. In severe cases, bone marrow transplantation may be considered and can cure some cases of immunodeficiency.

Bone marrow transplantation can, in most cases, completely correct the immunodefiency.

KEY TERMS

Antibody—Another term for immunoglobulin. A protein molecule that specifically recognizes and attaches to infectious agents.

T-helper cell—A type of cell that recognizes foreign antigens and activates T- and B-cells in an immune response.

Prognosis

Patients with immunoglobulin deficiency syndromes must practice impeccable health maintenance and care, paying particular attention to optimal dental care, in order to stay in good health.

Prevention

There is not a known way to prevent immunoglobulin deficiency syndromes.

Resources

BOOKS

Abbas, Abul K. et al. *Basic Immunology: Functions and Disorders of the Immune System.* Philadelphia: Saunders/Elsevier, 2011.

Berkow, Robert, editor. *The Merck Manual of Medical Information: Home Edition.* 2nd ed., Whitehouse Station, NJ: Merck & Co., Inc., 2004.

Coico, Richard. *Immunology: A Short Course.* Hoboken, NJ: Wiley-Blackwell, 2009.

Massoud, Mahmoudi. *Allergy and Asthma: Practical Diagnosis and Management.* New York: McGraw-Hill Medical, 2008.

OTHER

Bascom, Rebecca, and Marina Y Dolina. "Immunoglobulin A Deficiency." eMedicine, WebMD. September 29, 2009. [Accessed September 5, 2010], http://emedic ine.medscape. com/article/136580–overview.

Buckley, Rebecca H. "IgA Deficiency." Merck Manuals Online Medical Library. September 2008. [Accessed September 5, 2010], http://www.merck. com/mmpe/sec13/ch164/ ch164k.html.

Buckley, Rebecca H. "Selective Immunoglobulin Deficiency." Merck Manuals Online Medical Library. September 2008. [Accessed September 5, 2010], http://www.merck.com/ mmhe/sec16/ch184/ch184h.html?qt=Immunoglobulin deficiency&alt=sh.

Dibbern, Donald A., and John M. Routes. "Immunoglobulin D Deficiency." eMedicine, WebMD. December 2, 2009. [Accessed September 5, 2010], http://emedicine.meds-cape.com/article/136803–overview.

Hussain, Iftikhar, and Srividya Sridhara. "Immunoglobulin M Deficiency." eMedicine, WebMD. July 21, 2009. [Accessed September 5, 2010], http://emedic ine.meds-cape.com/article/137693–overview.

Lin, Robert Y., and Robert A. Schwartz. "Immunoglobulin G Deficiency." eMedicine, WebMD. July 9, 2009, http:// emedic ine.medscape.com/article/136897–overview (accessed September 5, 2010).

"Merck Manuals Online Medical Library." Merck. [Accessed September 5, 2010], http://www.merck.com/mmhe/index. html.

Jacqueline L. Longe

Immunotherapy *see* **Allergy shots**

Impetigo

Definition

Impetigo refers to a very localized bacterial infection of the skin. There are two types, bullous and epidemic.

Description

Impetigo is a skin infection that tends primarily to afflict children. Impetigo caused by the bacterium *Staphylococcus aureus* (also known as staph) affects children of all ages. Impetigo caused by the bacteria called group A streptococci (also know as strep) are most common in children ages two to five.

The bacteria that cause impetigo are very contagious. They can be spread by a child from one part of his or her body to another by scratching, or contact with a towel, clothing, or stuffed animal. These same methods can pass the bacteria on from one person to another.

Impetigo tends to develop in areas of the skin that have already been damaged through some other mechanism (a cut or scrape, burn, insect bite, or vesicle from **chickenpox**).

Causes and symptoms

The first sign of bullous impetigo is a large bump on the skin with a clear, fluid-filled top (called a vesicle). The bump develops a scab-like, honey-colored crust. There is usually no redness or **pain**, although the area may be quite itchy. Ultimately, the skin in this area will become dry and flake away. Bullous impetigo is usually caused by staph bacteria.

Epidemic impetigo can be caused by staph or strep bacteria and (as the name implies) is very easily passed

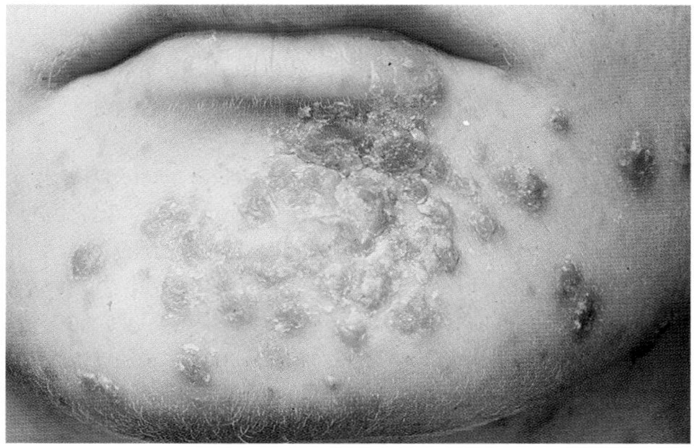

Impetigo is a contagious bacterial skin infection that has affected the area around this patient's nose and mouth. *(Custom Medical Stock Photo, Inc. Reproduced by permission.)*

KEY TERMS

Systemic—Involving the whole body; the opposite of localized.

Ulcer—An irritated pit in the surface of a tissue.

Vesicle—A bump on the skin filled with fluid.

among children. Certain factors, such as heat and humidity, crowded conditions, and poor hygiene increase the chance that this type of impetigo will spread rapidly among large groups of children. This type of impetigo involves the formation of a small vesicle surrounded by a circle of reddened skin. The vesicles appear first on the face and legs. When a child has several of these vesicles close together, they may spread to one another. The skin surface may become eaten away (ulcerated), leaving irritated pits. When there are many of these deep, pitting ulcers, with pus in the center and brownish-black scabs, the condition is called ecthyma. If left untreated, the type of bacteria causing this type of impetigo has the potential to cause a serious kidney disease called glomerulonephritis. Even when impetigo is initially caused by strep bacteria, the vesicles are frequently secondarily infected with staph bacteria.

Impetigo is usually an uncomplicated skin condition. Left untreated, however, it may develop into a serious disease, including osteomyelitis (bone infection), septic arthritis (joint infection), or **pneumonia**. If large quantities of bacteria are present and begin circulating in the bloodstream, the child is in danger of developing an overwhelming systemic infection known as sepsis.

Diagnosis

Characteristic appearance of the skin is the usual method of diagnosis, although fluid from the vesicles can be cultured and then examined in an attempt to identify the causative bacteria.

Treatment

Uncomplicated impetigo is usually treated with a topical antibiotic cream called mupirocin. In more serious, widespread cases of impetigo, or when the child has a **fever** or **swollen glands**, **antibiotics** may be given by mouth or even through a needle placed in a vein (intravenously).

Prognosis

Prognosis for a child with impetigo is excellent. The vast majority of children recover quickly, completely, and uneventfully.

Prevention

Prevention involves good hygiene. This involves handwashing and never sharing towels, clothing, or stuffed animals. Keeping fingernails well-trimmed is another easy precaution to take to avoid spreading the infection from one person to another.

Resources

OTHER

"Impetigo." Medline Plus. [Accessed December 7, 2010], http://www.nlm.nih.gov/medlineplus/ency/article/000860.htm.

PERIODICALS

"Bullous Impetigo." *Archives of Pediatrics and Adolescent Medicine* 151, no. 11 (November 1997): 1168+.

Rosalyn Carson-DeWitt, MD

Impulse control disorders

Definition

Impulse control disorders are a group of psychological disorders characterized by the repeated inability to refrain from performing a particular action that is harmful either to oneself or others.

There is controversy as of 2010 regarding the current classification of impulse control disorders. The most recent (2000) edition of the *Diagnostic and Statistical Manual of Mental Disorders-IV, Text Revision* (also known as the DSM-IV-TR) classifies **trichotillomania**, pathological gambling, **kleptomania** (compulsive **stealing**), **intermittent explosive disorder** (IED), **pyromania** (fire setting), and impulse control disorder not otherwise specified as disorders of impulse control. The differential diagnosis of pyromania and the other five disorders listed under the heading of impulse-control problems includes **antisocial personality disorder** (ASPD), **mood disorders**, conduct disorders (among younger patients), and temporal lobe **epilepsy**. It is not clear whether the impulse-control disorders derive from the same set of causes as ASPD and mood disorders or whether "impulse-control disorder" is simply a catchall category for disorders that are difficult to classify otherwise. In particular, DSM-IV's classification of IED is not universally accepted. Many psychiatrists do not place intermittent explosive disorder into a separate clinical category but consider it a symptom of other psychiatric and mental disorders.

Some American researchers would prefer to categorize pyromania and the other disorders of impulsivity as belonging to the spectrum of obsessive-compulsive disorders. In addition, some researchers include compulsive shopping, compulsive sexual behavior, hoarding, **self-mutilation**, skin picking, and **body dysmorphic disorder** within the category of impulse control disorders. It is likely that the forthcoming fifth edition of DSM (DSM-5), scheduled for publication in May 2013, will reclassify some or all of these disorders.

Demographics

Impulse control disorders as a group are not uncommon in the general population in North America. Some representative demographic statistics:

- Body dysmorphic disorder (BDD): This disorder is thought to affect between 1% and 2% of people in Canada and the United States, although some doctors think that it is underdiagnosed. The average age of patients diagnosed with the disorder is 17. BDD has a high rate of comorbidity, which means that people diagnosed with the disorder are highly likely to have been diagnosed with another psychiatric disorder—most commonly major depression, social phobia, or obsessive-compulsive disorder (OCD). About 29% of patients with BDD eventually try to commit suicide.
- Gambling: Researchers estimate that 1.1% of the adult population in the United States and Canada has had severe problems with gambling in the past year, while another 2.2% has had at least some problems with gambling in the past year. These combined estimates represent 7 million people in the United States alone. Pathological gambling often begins in adolescence or even childhood, particularly in males. It usually begins later in females, however. One study reported that as many as 40% of men begin gambling before age 18, but that women typically begin gambling after age 40.
- Hoarding: The International OCD Foundation notes that one in 50 adults in North America is a hoarder, although some researchers think the figure is closer to one in 20. Hoarders typically begin in their teens, but the average age at diagnosis is 50.
- Intermittent explosive disorder: Although DSM-IV maintains that IED is a rare disorder, other researchers think that it is underdiagnosed. They estimate that 1.4 million persons in the United States currently meet the criteria for IED, with a total of 10 million meeting the lifetime criteria for the disorder.
- Kleptomania: Kleptomania is less common than pathological gambling; the incidence in the general population is estimated to be 0.6%. Kleptomania can begin at any age, although its onset is typically associated with puberty and is reported to be more common among females. The average age of patients in Canada and the United States diagnosed with the disorder as of 2010 is 35 and the average duration of the disorder is 16 years.
- Pyromania: The true incidence of pyromania in adults in the general North American population remains unknown but is thought to be below 1%. Adults diagnosed with pyromania are most likely to be Caucasian males 18 to 35 years old, born in the United States, and living west of the Mississippi. Repeated firesetting appears to be more common in children and adolescents than in adult males. In addition, the incidence appears to be rising in these younger age groups: in 1992, males 18 and younger accounted for 40% of arrests for firesetting; in 2001, they accounted for 55%.
- Self-mutilation/self-cutting: Self-harm is most common in adolescents and young adults between the ages of 14 and 24 with females at greater risk than males. It is commonly associated with such mental health disorders as borderline personality disorder, depression, anxiety disorders, substance abuse disorders, post-traumatic stress disorder and eating disorders. It can occur at any age, however; elderly self-cutters are the most likely to end by committing suicide.
- Trichotillomania: Trichotillomania is probably an underreported impulse control disorder. Various studies give estimates ranging from a lifetime prevalence of 1.5% for males and 3.4% for females to anywhere from 0.6% to 6% in college students. Another estimate gives a figure of 2.5 million people in the United States as having trichotillomania at some time during their lifetimes.

Description

DSM-IV impulse control disorders

GAMBLING Pathological or problem gambling is classified as a disorder of impulse control by the *Diagnostic and Statistical Manual of Mental Disorders*, fourth edition (DSM-IV), published by the American Psychiatric Association (APA). Pathological gambling is defined by DSM-IV as persistent gambling behavior "that disrupts personal, **family**, or vocational pursuits." It is sometimes called compulsive gambling.

Problem gambling has sometimes been termed a process **addiction**, meaning that although it is an activity rather than a substance, it has a mood-altering effect similar to those of alcohol or other addictive substances. Many problem gamblers have a ritualistic pattern to their behavior, such as placing bets at a certain time of day or day of the week, placing bets on "lucky" numbers or horses with "lucky" names, wearing a certain outfit when going to the racetrack or casino, or carrying a "lucky" object of some kind. This patterned behavior begins the process of mood alteration.

There is no single pattern of gambling that leads to problem gambling. Some problem gamblers gamble on a regular basis while others are episodic or "binge" gamblers who gamble only when they are under emotional stress of some kind. The important feature that distinguishes problem gambling from social gambling is its impact on the person's life, not how often they gamble.

INTERMITTENT EXPLOSIVE DISORDER Intermittent explosive disorder (IED) is a mental disturbance that is characterized by specific episodes of violent and aggressive behavior that may involve harm to others or destruction of property. People diagnosed with IED sometimes describe strong impulses to act aggressively prior to the specific incidents reported to the doctor and/or the police. They may experience racing thoughts or a heightened energy level during the aggressive episode, with fatigue and depression developing shortly afterward. Some report various physical sensations, including tightness in the chest, **tingling** sensations, tremor, hearing echoes, or a feeling of pressure inside the head.

Many people diagnosed with IED appear to have general problems with anger or other impulsive behaviors between explosive episodes. Some are able to control aggressive impulses without acting on them while others act out in less destructive ways, such as screaming at someone rather than attacking them physically.

KLEPTOMANIA Persons with kleptomania experience a recurring and irresistible urge to steal. They do not, however, steal for the value of the item, for its use, or because they cannot afford the purchase. Stolen items are often thrown or given away, returned, or hidden. Kleptomania is distinguished from deliberate theft or shoplifting in which the individual is motivated by a desire to acquire the item, to seek revenge, or to fulfill a dare from peers. Shoplifting is more common than kleptomania; it is estimated that less than 5% of individuals who shoplift exhibit symptoms of kleptomania.

PYROMANIA Pyromania is defined as a pattern of deliberate setting of fires for pleasure or satisfaction derived from the relief of tension experienced before the fire-setting, as distinct from organized planning to set fires as an arsonist or terrorist might do. As of 2010, however, the relationship between pyromania in adults and firesetting among children and adolescents is not well defined. Although pyromania is considered to be a rare disorder in adults, repeated firesetting at the adolescent level is a growing social and economic problem that poses major risks to the health and **safety** of other people and the protection of their property. In the United States, fires set by children and adolescents are more likely to result in someone's **death** than any other type of household disaster.

Pyromania in adults resembles kleptomania and other disorders of impulse control in having a high rate of comorbidity with other disorders, including **substance abuse** disorders and mood disorders. As of 2010, however, few rigorously controlled studies using strict diagnostic criteria have been done on adult patients diagnosed with pyromania or other impulse-control disorders.

TRICHOTILLOMANIA Trichotillomania (TTM) is a disorder characterized by the patient's repetitive pulling of his or her own hair, most commonly scalp hair, but sometimes eyelashes, eyebrows, nose hair, pubic hair, axillary (armpit) hair, or other body hair. It commonly results in noticeable hair loss (**alopecia**), emotional distress, and social or functional impairment. It has been identified in three major age groups: young children, adolescents, and adults. A few cases of trichotillomania beginning in **infancy** have been recorded but are rare. The disorder has a very different course in the different age groups. In children younger than five years, the disorder is usually self-limiting (the child outgrows it), and medical or psychiatric intervention is not required. Young children generally pull their hair in what is termed an unfocused or automatic manner; that is, they pull on the hair without thinking about it and typically do not recall pulling the hair afterward. Some young children will also pull on the hair of other people or pets.

Older adolescents and adults, however, are more likely to manifest focused hair-pulling; that is, they are consciously paying attention to the act of hair-pulling. Some have rituals associated with the TTM, such as pulling the hair in a certain direction, pulling the hair until a particular sensation is felt, pulling the hair on a specific portion of the scalp or body, or pulling their hair in response to a specific trigger or stressor. Adults typically pull their hair as a way of controlling uncomfortable emotions, most often **anxiety** or anger.

After a period of time, TTM results in hair loss, although this loss is not the purpose or goal of the hair pulling. Hair loss occurs because the pulling may cause the hair shaft to break or the hair follicle to prematurely enter a part of its growth cycle known as the catagen phase. In this phase the hair in the follicle stops growing and regresses or falls out. The patient may consider the hair loss to be the result of a scalp disease rather than the result of repeated mild trauma to the hair shaft and hair follicles. Hair-pulling, however, is often accompanied by other actions, including chewing on or swallowing the pulled hair, called trichophagia. Trichophagia can lead to the formation of trichobezoars, or hairballs, in the child's digestive tract. Trichobezoars can cause serious health problems, among them **anemia**, chronic **pain** in the abdomen, nausea and **vomiting**, bowel obstruction, pancreatitis, and bleeding from the digestive tract. In some cases the child may have to undergo surgery to remove the mass of hair that has collected in the digestive tract.

Other disorders categorized as impulse control disorders

BODY DYSMORPHIC DISORDER DSM-IV defines body dysmorphic disorder (BDD) as a condition marked by excessive preoccupation with an imaginary or minor defect in a facial feature or localized part of the body. The diagnostic criteria specify that the condition must be sufficiently severe to cause a decline in the patient's social, occupational, or educational functioning. The current edition of DSM assigns BDD to the larger category of somatoform disorders, which are disorders characterized by physical complaints that appear to be medical in origin but that cannot be explained in terms of a physical disease, the results of substance abuse, or by another mental disorder.

Following the publication of DSM-IV in 1994, some psychiatrists suggested that there is a subtype of BDD, namely muscle dysmorphia. Muscle dysmorphia is marked by excessive concern with one's muscularity and/or fitness. Persons with muscle dysmorphia spend unusual amounts of time working out in gyms or exercising rather than dieting obsessively or seeking plastic surgery. DSM-IV-TR added references to concern about body build and excessive weight lifting to DSM-IV's description of BDD in order to cover muscle dysmorphia.

BDD and muscle dysmorphia can both be described as disorders resulting from the patient's distorted body image. Body image refers to a person's mental picture of his or her outward appearance, including size, shape, and form. It has two major components: how the person perceives their physical appearance and how they feel about their body. Significant distortions in self-perception can lead to intense dissatisfaction with one's body and dysfunctional behaviors aimed at improving one's appearance. Some patients with BDD are aware that their concerns are excessive, but others do not have this degree of insight; about 50 percent of patients diagnosed with BDD also meet the criteria for a delusional disorder.

COMPULSIVE HOARDING Compulsive hoarding was not included as an impulse control disorder in DSM-IV but has become increasingly recognized as a disorder since the mid-1990s. Researchers do not yet agree as to whether hoarding is a distinctive disorder or a symptom of another disorder such as OCD. The International OCD Foundation (IOCDF) defines compulsive hoarding as a disorder in which the person "collects and keeps a lot of items, even things that appear useless or of little value to most people; these items clutter the living spaces and keep the person from using their rooms as they were intended; and these items cause distress or problems in day-to-day activities." The most common inanimate objects collected by hoarders are books, mail, newspapers and magazines, clothing, and containers of various sorts (boxes, string, paper bags, bottles, and plastic bags or deli containers).

Animal hoarding is considered a distinctive form of hoarding because of its potential for real (though unintentional) cruelty to animals and major public health problems. The Hoarding of Animals Research Consortium (HARC) at Tufts University defines animal hoarding as "Having more than the typical number of companion animals; failing to provide even minimal standards of nutrition, sanitation, shelter, and veterinary care, with this neglect often resulting in illness and death from starvation, spread of infectious disease, and untreated injury or medical condition; denial of the inability to provide this minimum care and the impact of that failure on the animals, the household, and human occupants of the dwelling; and persistence, despite this failure, in accumulating and controlling animals." Domestic animals (cats, dogs, rabbits, ferrets, birds, gerbils, and guinea pigs) are the species most commonly hoarded, although there are cases of people hoarding farm animals and even potentially dangerous wild animals.

HARC maintains that animal hoarders differ from people who hoard objects in that they are more seriously mentally impaired and often delusional. The HARC researchers also state that as of 2010, hoarding is increasingly recognized as having more differences from than similarities to OCD and that it is likely to be classified as a distinct disorder in DSM-5.

SELF-CUTTING A condition not listed as an impulse control disorder in DSM-IV that some experts consider to be such a disorder is repetitive self-mutilation, in which people intentionally harm themselves by cutting, burning, or scratching their bodies. Other forms of repetitive self-mutilation include sticking oneself with needles, punching or slapping the face, and swallowing harmful substances. Self-mutilation tends to occur in persons who have suffered traumas early in life, such as **sexual abuse** or the death of a parent, and often has its onset at times of unusual stress. In many cases, the triggering event is a perceived rejection by a parent or romantic interest. Characteristics commonly seen in persons with this disorder include perfectionism, dissatisfaction with one's physical appearance, and difficulty controlling and expressing emotions.

People who practice self-mutilation often claim that it is accompanied by excitement and that it reduces or relieves such negative feelings as tension, anger, anxiety, depression, and loneliness. They also describe it as addictive. Self-mutilating behavior may occur in episodes, with periods of remission, or may be continuous over a number of years. Repetitive self-mutilation often worsens over time, resulting in increasingly serious forms of injury that may culminate in **suicide**.

Risk factors

Risk factors for body dysmorphic disorder and self-cutting include a history of childhood abuse and/or having parents who are obsessed with their own looks or highly critical of the child's appearance.

Risk factors for pathological gambling include:

- A history of depression or anxiety disorders. This risk factor applies to adolescents as well as adults.
- A recent crisis in a person's life, such as retirement or job loss.
- The type of game involved. Some studies indicate that a rapid rate of play (as in roulette or slot machines) makes some types of gambling more addictive than others that have a time lapse between placing a bet and the outcome of the bet.
- A history of attention deficit-hyperactivity disorder (ADHD) in childhood.
- A family history of problem gambling.
- A coexisting substance abuse disorder.
- A personality profile that includes a high level of competitiveness, restlessness, and being easily bored.
- Male sex. In most subcultures in North America, about two-thirds of problem gamblers are men.
- Cultural factors. In some subcultures, such as some Asian and Hispanic cultures, gambling is considered a mark of masculinity and maturity.
- Race and ethnicity. A survey conducted according to DSM-IV criteria for disordered gambling reported in 2009 that the prevalence of disordered gambling is twice as high among Native Americans, African Americans, and Asian Americans as among whites,
- Age. According to DSM-IV, adolescents and college-age young adults are 2–3 times more likely to have problems with gambling than older adults.

Risk factors for hoarding include living alone, being over 40 years of age, and having family members who are hoarders. Race, sex, or income level do not appear to be risk factors for this disorder. The most significant risk factor for animal hoarding is a history of trauma, loss, and/or an attachment disorder in childhood.

The only known risk factors for kleptomania as of 2010 are substance abuse; a diagnosis of paranoid, schizoid, or borderline personality disorder; and a family history of kleptomania, mood disorders, or substance abuse. There are a few isolated cases reported of kleptomania being triggered by traumatic brain injury or exposure to high levels of carbon monoxide.

Risk factors in children and adolescents that contribute to firesetting include:

- Antisocial behaviors and attitudes. Adolescent firesetters have often committed other crimes, including forcible rape (11%), nonviolent sexual offenses (18%), and vandalism of property (19%).
- Sensation seeking. Some youths are attracted to firesetting out of boredom and a lack of other forms of recreation.
- Need for attention. Firesetting becomes a way of provoking reactions from parents and other authorities.
- Lack of social skills. Many youths arrested for firesetting are described by others as "loners" and rarely have significant friendships.
- Lack of fire-safety skills and ignorance of the dangers associated with firesetting.
- Poor supervision on the part of parents and other significant adults.
- Early learning experiences of watching adults use fire carelessly or inapproriately.
- Parental neglect or emotional uninvolvement.
- Parental psychopathology. Firesetters are significantly more likely to have been physically or sexually abused than children of similar economic or geographic backgrounds. They are also more likely to have witnessed their parents abusing drugs or acting violently.
- Peer pressure. Having peers who smoke or play with fire is a risk factor for a child's setting fires himself.
- Stressful life events. Some children and adolescents resort to firesetting as a way of coping with crises in their lives and/or limited family support for dealing with crises.

Risk factors for trichotillomania are still a matter of discussion rather than full agreement among specialists. Some factors that have been mentioned as possibly increasing a person's risk of TTM include:

- In young children, divorce or family breakup.
- In adolescents and older adults, a history or current diagnosis of post-traumatic stress disorder.
- A history or current diagnosis of anxiety, depression, or obsessive-compulsive disorder.

KEY TERMS

Arson—A legal term used in the United States to define the willful burning of any real property (whether an inhabited dwelling or unoccupied building) without consent or with unlawful intent.

Body image—A term that refers to a person's inner picture of his or her outward appearance. It has two components: perceptions of the appearance of one's body, and emotional responses to those perceptions.

Comorbidity—The presence of one or more additional diseases or disorders in a patient diagnosed with a primary disorder.

Delusion—A false belief that is resistant to reason or contrary to actual fact.

Mental status examination (MSE)—A structured way of observing a patient's state of mind in the course of an office interview that takes into account such factors as mood, insight, judgment, ability to reason, as well as general appearance and tone of voice.

Muscle dysmorphia—A subtype of body dysmorphic disorder, described as excessive preoccupation with muscularity and body building to the point of interference with social, educational, or occupational functioning.

Neurotransmitter—Any of several chemicals secreted in the brain that serve to transmit nerve impulses from one neuron to another.

Serotonin—A chemical produced by the brain that functions as a neurotransmitter. Low serotonin levels are associated with mood disorders, particularly depression.

Somatoform disorders—A group of psychiatric disorders in the DSM-IV-TR classification that are characterized by external physical symptoms or complaints. BDD is classified as a somatoform disorder.

Trichobezoar—A mass of hair trapped in the stomach or digestive tract. Trichobezoars in humans are a common complication of trichotillomania,

Trichophagia—The compulsive eating and swallowing of one's hair, sometimes while it is still attached to the head.

Causes and symptoms

The causes of impulse control disorders have not been determined as of 2010. Researchers disagree as to whether these disorders result from learned behavior, the result of biochemical or neurological abnormalities, childhood trauma, genetic factors, or a combination of these. Some scientists have reported abnormally low levels of serotonin, a neurotransmitter that affects mood, in the cerebrospinal fluid of some persons with impulse control disorders. One piece of evidence for the theory that impulse control disorders are linked in some way to neurotransmitter imbalances is that many patients with these disorders are helped by treatment with the selective serotonin reuptake inhibitors or SSRIs (Prozac, Paxil, Luvox, Celexa, Zoloft).

The symptoms of the impulse control disorders are included in the descriptions of each disorder.

Diagnosis

The diagnosis of an impulse control disorder is usually based on a combination of the patient's medical history; legal history if he or she has been involved with the criminal justice system; and an office physical examination in the case of suspected self-cutting, trichotillomania, or body dysmorphic disorder. The doctor may also administer a mental status examination or refer the patient to a neurologist to rule out brain damage, epilepsy, or other abnormalities of the brain and spinal cord, or to a clinical psychologist or psychiatrist for further evaluation. There are a number of questionnaires and inventories that can be administered in the examiner's office to determine whether the patient meets the criteria for a specific impulse control disorder. There are, however, no laboratory tests as of 2010 that can be used to diagnose these disorders.

Treatment

Traditional

The standard course of treatment for impulse control disorders is a combination of medications and psychotherapy. The most successful forms of psychotherapy in treating these disorders are cognitive **behavioral therapy** and psychodynamic psychotherapy; classical psychoanalysis is not helpful in treating these patients. Patients with a severe case of self-cutting thought to be at risk of suicide may be hospitalized.

Drugs

The medications most often given to treat impulse control disorders are the selective serotonin reuptake inhibitors, which work by increasing the level of serotonin in the spaces (synapses) between nerve cells in the central nervous system. The SSRIs include fluoxetine (Prozac), citalopram (Celexa), paroxetine (Paxil), fluvoxamine (Luvox), and sertraline (Zoloft). Nalmefene (Revex), a drug developed to treat alcohol abuse, is undergoing trials as a possible treatment for pathological gambling.

Prognosis

The prognosis varies according to the disorder. Patients with BDD do best with a combination of medical and psychological treatment; however, DSM-IV-TR notes that the disorder "has a fairly continuous course, with few symptom-free intervals, although the intensity of symptoms may wax and wane over time." The prognosis for recovery from pathological gambling is highly variable. In general, individuals without co-occurring substance abuse and mental health disorders have the best prognosis for sustained recovery. Recovery from hoarding depends on the person's age and availability of family support; in general, animal hoarders have a poorer prognosis than those who hoard objects.

Intermittent explosive disorder has a poor prognosis because few persons diagnosed with IED are motivated to get better; one study found that only 13% of those diagnosed with IED sought treatment for it. Kleptomania is also particularly difficult to treat; relapses are common and the disorder can last for years. The prognosis for adults diagnosed with pyromania is generally poor. There are some cases of spontaneous remission among adults, but the rate of spontaneous recovery is not known as of 2010. Recovery from trichotillomania depends in part on the patient's age; while young children typically recover without specialized therapy, adolescents have only a guarded prognosis, and adults generally have a poor prognosis; the average duration of the disorder in adults is 21 years.

Prevention

There is no known way to prevent impulse control disorders as of 2010 because their causes are not yet fully understood.

Resources

BOOKS

Aboujaoude, Elias, and Lorrin M. Koran. *Impulse Control Disorders*. New York: Cambridge University Press, 2010.

Abramowitz, Jonathan S., Dean McKay, and Steven Taylor, eds. *Clinical Handbook of Obsessive-Compulsive Disorder and Related Problems*. Baltimore, MD: Johns Hopkins University Press, 2008.

Adamec, Christine. *Impulse Control Disorders*. New York: Chelsea House, 2008.

American Psychiatric Association. *Diagnostic and Statistical Manual of Mental Disorders*. 4th ed., Text rev. Washington, D.C.: American Psychiatric Association, 2000.

Black, Donald W., and Nancy C. Andreasen. *Introductory Textbook of Psychiatry*, 5th ed. Arlington, VA: American Psychiatric Publishing, 2011.

PERIODICALS

Bohne, A. "Impulse-control Disorders in College Students." *Psychiatry Research* 176 (March 30, 2010): 91-92.

Castrodale, L., et al. "General Public Health Considerations for Responding to Animal Hoarding Cases." *Journal of Environmental Health* 72 (March 2010): 14-18.

Grant, J.E., et al. "Nalmefene in the Treatment of Pathological Gambling: Multicentre, Double-blind, Placebo-controlled Study." *British Journal of Psychiatry* 197 (October 2010): 330-31.

Hintikka, J., et al. "Mental Disorders in Self-Cutting Adolescents." *Journal of Adolescent Health* 44 (May 2009): 464-67.

McCloskey, M.S., et al. "Unhealthy Aggression: Intermittent Explosive Disorder and Adverse Physical Health Outcomes." *Health Psychology* 29 (May 2010): 324-32.

Murray, S.B., et al. "Muscle Dysmorphia and the DSM-V Conundrum: Where Does It Belong? A Review Paper." *International Journal of Eating Disorders* 43 (September 2010): 483-91.

Pertusa, A., et al. "When Hoarding Is a Symptom of OCD: A Case Series and Implications for DSM-V." *Behaviour Research and Therapy* 48 (October 2010): 1012-20.

Stein, D.J., et al. "Trichotillomania (Hair Pulling Disorder), Skin Picking Disorder, and Stereotypic Movement Disorder: Toward DSM-V." *Depression and Anxiety* 27 (June 2010): 611-26.

Wetterneck, C.T., et al. "Current Issues in the Treatment of OC-Spectrum Conditions." *Bulletin of the Menninger Clinic* 74 (Spring 2010): 141-66.

OTHER

American Society for the Prevention of Cruelty to Animals (ASPCA). *Animal Hoarding*. [Accessed December 7, 2010], http://www.aspca.org/fight-animal-cruelty/animal-hoarding.aspx.

Feng, Sing-Yi, and Jagvir Singh. "Body Dysmorphic Disorder." *eMedicine*, May 6, 2010. [Accessed December 7, 2010], http://emedicine.medscape.com/article/914976-overview

Hoarding of Animals Research Consortium (HARC). *Common Questions about Animal Hoarding*. [Accessed December 7, 2010], http://www.tufts.edu/vet/hoarding/abthoard.htm.

International OCD Foundation (IOCDF). *Hoarding Fact Sheet*. [Accessed December 7, 2010], http://www.ocfoundation.org/uploadedFiles/Hoarding%20Fact%20Sheet.pdf?n=3557.

Massachusetts Council on Compulsive Gambling. *Your First Step to Change* [Accessed December 7, 2010], http://s96539219.onlinehome.us/toolkits/FirstStepSite/main.htm.

Mayo Clinic. *Kleptomania* [Accessed December 7, 2010], http://www.mayoclinic.com/health/kleptomania/DS01034.

Mayo Clinic. *Self-injury/Cutting* [Accessed December 7, 2010], http://www.mayoclinic.com/health/self-injury/DS00775.

Menaster, Michael. "Psychiatric Illness Associated with Criminality." *eMedicine*, May 18, 2010. [Accessed December 7, 2010], http://emedicine.medscape.com/article/294626-overview.

University of Minnesota Impulse Control Disorders Clinic. *Principles of Treatment: Pathological Gambling Disorder* [Accessed December 7, 2010], http://www.impulsecontrol-disorders.org/html/treatment.html.

University of Minnesota Impulse Control Disorders Clinic. *What Is Craving?* [Accessed December 7, 2010], http://www.impulsecontroldisorders.org/html/cravings.html.

ORGANIZATIONS

American Psychiatric Association, 1000 Wilson Boulevard, Suite 1825, Arlington VA, 22209-3901, (703) 907-7300, apa@psych.org, http://www.psych.org/.

Hoarding of Animals Research Consortium, [affiliated with Tufts University School of Veterinary Medicine but does not maintain a separate office], http://www.tufts.edu/vet/hoarding/index.html.

Institute for Research on Gambling Disorders, 100 Cummings Center, Suite 207P, Beverly MA, 01915, (978) 299-3040, (978) 524-4162, http://www.gamblingdisorders.org/.

National Alliance on Mental Illness (NAMI), 2107 Wilson Blvd., Suite 300, Arlington VA, 22201-3042, (703) 524-7600, Hotline: (800) 950-NAMI (6264), (703) 524-9094, http://www.nami.org/Hometemplate.cfm.

National Institute of Mental Health (NIMH), 6001 Executive Boulevard, Room 8184, MSC 9663, Bethesda MD, 20892-9663, (301) 443-4513, (866) 615-6464, (301) 443-4279, nimhinfo@nih.gov, http://www.nimh.nih.gov/index.shtml.

Trichotillomania Learning Center (TLC), 207 McPherson Street, Suite H, Santa Cruz CA, 95060, (831) 457-1004, (831) 426-4383, info@trich.org, http://www.trich.org/.

University of Minnesota Impulse Control Disorders Clinic, University of Minnesota Medical Center, 2450 Riverside Avenue South, Minneapolis MN, 55454, (612) 273-8700, http://www.impulsecontroldisorders.org/.

International OCD Foundation (IOCDF), 112 Water Street, Suite 501, Boston MA United States, 02109, (617) 973-5801, (617) 973-5803, info@ocfoundation.org, http://www.ocfoundation.org/.

Rebecca J. Frey, PhD

Inclusion conjunctivitis

Definition

Inclusion **conjunctivitis** is an inflammation of the conjunctiva (the membrane that lines the eyelids and covers the white part, or sclera, of the eyeball) by the bacterium *Chlamydia trachomatis*. Chlamydia is a sexually transmitted organism. Chlamydia was originally called "chlamydozoa" by Polish dermatologist Ludwig Halberstaedter and Czech zoologist Stanislaus von Prowazek in 1907 when they discovered *Chlamydia trachomatis*. Chlamydozoa is the Greek word for "mantle."

Demographics

The disease usually affects teenagers and young adults who are sexually active. In fact, persons with the disease often times also have genital Chlamydia (an infection of the genitals). The disease also occurs in newborn infants. Women are usually more susceptible to the disease than are men and people in urban areas frequently acquire it more than people in rural areas.

Description

Inclusion conjunctivitis is known as neonatal inclusion conjunctivitis in the newborn and as adult inclusion conjunctivitis in the adult; it is also called inclusion blennorrhea, chlamydial conjunctivitis, or **swimming** pool conjunctivitis. It usually occurs from poor personal hygiene, specifically from the transmission of contaminated genital secretions to the eye. This disease affects four of 1,000 (0.4%) live births. Approximately half of the infants born to untreated infected mothers will develop the disease.

Causes and symptoms

Inclusion conjunctivitis in the newborn, called neonatal conjunctivitis, results from passage through an infected **birth** canal and develops from 5 to 12 days after birth. Both eyelids and conjunctivae are swollen and red in color. There may be a discharge of pus from the eyes, swelling of the eyelids, and redness around the eye. Irritation, infection, or blocked tear ducts are three primary causes of inclusion conjunctivitis. In infants, the disease can become very serious.

Most instances of adult inclusion conjunctivitis result from exposure to infected genital secretions. It is transmitted to the eye by fingers and occasionally by the water in swimming pools, poorly chlorinated hot tubs, or by sharing makeup. In adult inclusion conjunctivitis, one eye is usually involved, with a stringy discharge of mucus and pus. There may be little bumps called follicles inside the lower eyelid and the eye is red. Occasionally, the condition damages the cornea, causing cloudy areas and a growth of new blood vessels (neovascularization). Women sometimes report genitourinary symptoms.

Diagnosis

Inclusion conjunctivitis is usually considered when the patient has a follicular conjunctivitis that will not go away, even after using **topical antibiotics**. Diagnosis depends upon tests performed on the discharge from the eye. Gram stains determine the type of microorganism, while culture and sensitivity tests determine which antibiotic will kill the harmful microorganism. Conjunctival scraping determines whether chlamydia is present in cells taken from the conjunctiva.

Treatment

Treatment in the newborn consists of administration of tetracycline ointment to the conjunctiva and erythromycin orally or through intravenous therapy for 14 days. Infants can also be given erythromycin ophthalmic ointment for one week and erythromycin or azithromycin elixir for 2 to 3 weeks. The mother should be treated for cervicitis (inflammation of the uterine cervix) and the father for urethritis (inflammation of the urethra), even if they do not have symptoms of these diseases.

In adults, tetracycline ointment or drops should be applied to the conjunctiva and oral tetracycline, amoxacillin, or erythromycin should be taken for up to three weeks, or doxycycline for one week. A single oral dose of azithromycin helps to control redness in and around the eye, along with mucous discharge. In severe cases, intravenous **antibiotics** may also be used together with topical antibiotics. If a blocked tear duct is to blame, warm and gently massages are given between the nasal area and the eye. They help to reduce swelling and irritation. If the blocked tear duct does not heal within one year, surgery may be necessary.

Patients should have weekly checkups so the doctor can monitor the healing.

Oral tetracycline should not be administered to children whose permanent teeth have not erupted. It should also not be given to nursing or pregnant women.

Prognosis

Untreated inclusion conjunctivitis in the newborn persists for 3 to 12 months and usually heals; however, there may be scarring or neovascularization. The occurrence of it in infants has decreased over the past few decades as more women are screened and treated before they become pregnant. In the adult, if left untreated, the disease may continue for months and cause corneal neovascularization. Even if treated, antibiotics usually do not reverse damage that may have occurred but they may help prevent it if given early enough. The infection can spread to the nasopharynx and the lower respiratory tract. **Pneumonia** can result if left untreated.

KEY TERMS

Cervicitis—Cervicitis is an inflammation of the cervix or neck of the uterus.

Conjunctiva—The conjunctiva is the membrane that lines the eyelids and covers the white part of the eyeball (sclera).

Cornea—The clear dome-shaped structure that covers the colored part of the eye (iris).

Neovascularization—Neovascularization is the growth of new blood vessels.

Urethritis—Urethritis is an inflammation of the urethra, the canal for the discharge of urine that extends from the bladder to the outside of the body.

Prevention

The neonatal infection may be prevented by instilling erythromycin drops or ointment into the eye's conjunctival cul-de-sac at the baby's birth. Many state laws require medical professionals perform such preventative measures to babies born in hospitals. However, it is not prevented by silver nitrate, which was a treatment in the past. Instead, antibiotic eye drops are used.

Chlamydia is a contagious, sexually transmitted disease. Some systemic symptoms include a history of vaginitis, **pelvic inflammatory disease**, or urethritis. Patients with symptoms of these diseases should be treated by a physician.

Resources

BOOKS

Reinhard, Thomas, and Frank Larkin, editors. *Cornea and External Eye Disease.* Berlin: Springer, 2008.

Yanoff, Myron, and Jay J. Kuker. *Ophthalmology.* 3rd ed. Edinburgh, Scotland: Mosby Elsevier, 2009.

OTHER

"Conjunctivitis (Pink Eye) in Newborns" Centers for Disease Control and Prevention. June 4, 2010. [Accessed July 1, 2010], http://www.cdc.gov/conjunctivitis/newborns.html.

"The Many Faces of Chlamydial Infection" Review of Ophthalmology. April 1, 2008. [Accessed July 1, 2010], http://www.revophth.com/index.asp?page=1_13785.htm.

ORGANIZATIONS

American Academy of Ophthalmology (AAO), P. O. Box 7424, San Francisco CA, 94120-7424, (415) 561-8500, (415) 561-8533, http://www.aao.org.

American Optometric Association, 243 North Lindbergh Blvd, St. Louis MO, 63141, (314) 991-4100, http://www.aoanet.org.

Lorraine Steefel, RN

Infancy

Definition

Infancy is the earliest stage of human development. It begins at **birth** and extending to no more than 24 months of age.

Description

Infancy begins at birth; infants during the first 28 days of life are referred to as newborns or neonates. Infancy is the time of most rapid growth and development in an individual's life. Deficits in **nutrition**, medical care, physical and emotional care that occur during infancy can affect an individual for a lifetime.

During infancy, knowledge is gained primarily through sensory impressions and motor activity. Through these two modes of learning, experienced both separately and in combination, infants gradually learn to control their own bodies and objects in the external world.

Fine motor development

Fine motor skills involve deliberate and controlled movements requiring both muscle development and maturation of the central nervous system. Although newborns can move their hands and arms, these motions are reflexes that an infant cannot consciously start or stop.

Infants begin flailing at objects that interest them by two weeks of age but cannot grasp them. By eight weeks, they begin to discover and play with their hands, at first solely by touch, and then, at about three months, by sight as well. At this age, however, deliberate grasp remains largely undeveloped. **Hand-eye coordination** begins to develop between the ages of two and four months, initiating a period of trial-and-error practice at sighting objects and grabbing at them. At four or five months, most infants can grasp an object that is within reach, looking only at the object and not at their hands.

One of the most significant fine motor accomplishments is the pincer grip, which typically appears between the ages of 12 and 15 months. The pincer grip is defined as the ability to hold objects between the thumb and index finger. This gives the infant a more sophisticated ability to grasp and manipulate objects and also to deliberately drop them. By about the age of one year, an infant can drop an object into a receptacle, compare objects held in both hands, stack objects, and nest them within each other.

During the second year of life, children develop the ability to manipulate objects with increasing sophistication, including using their fingers to twist dials, pull strings, push levers, turn book pages, and use crayons to produce crude scribbles. **Handedness**, the dominance of either the right or left hand, usually emerges during this period as well.

Gross motor development

Gross motor skills involve the ability to control the large muscles of the body for walking, running, sitting, **crawling**, and other activities. These skills require both muscle development and maturation of the central nervous system. In addition, the skeletal system must be strong enough to support the movement and weight involved in any new activity. Once these conditions are met, children learn new physical skills by practicing them until each skill is mastered.

One of the first things an infant achieves is head control. Although babies are born with virtually no head or neck control, most infants can lift their heads to a 45-degree angle by the age of four to six weeks, and they can lift both their heads and chests at an average age of eight weeks. Most infants can turn their heads to both sides within 16–20 weeks and lift their heads while lying on their backs within 24–28 weeks. By about 9 months, most infants can sit up unassisted for substantial periods with both hands free for playing.

One of the major tasks in gross motor development is acquiring the ability to move from one place to another. Infants progress gradually from rolling (8–10 weeks) to creeping on their stomachs and dragging their legs behind them (6–9 months) to crawling (7–12 months). While infants are learning these temporary means of locomotion, they are gradually becoming able to support increasing amounts of weight while in a standing position. Around seven or eight months of age, infants begin pulling themselves up on furniture and other stationary objects. By the ages of 28–54 weeks, they begin "cruising," or navigating a room in an upright position by holding on to the furniture to keep their balance. Eventually, they are able to walk while holding on to an adult with both hands and then with only one. They usually take their first uncertain steps alone between the ages of 36–64 weeks and are competent walkers by the ages of 52–78 weeks.

By the age of two years, children have begun to develop a variety of gross motor skills. They can run fairly well and negotiate stairs holding on to a banister with one hand and putting both feet on each step before going on to the next one. Most infants this age climb (some very actively) and have a rudimentary ability to kick and throw a ball, although they cannot control its direction.

Speech and understanding language

Many parents put a high priority on their child beginning to speak. Children understand language before they begin speaking. Many children fit the classic **language development** pattern of first speaking one word "sentences," such as "truck," then joining two words "truck fall," and then three, "my truck fall." This is called a referential style because it also correlates with attention to names for objects and event descriptions. Other children speak in long unintelligible babbles that mimic adult speech cadence and rhythm, so that listeners feel as if they are just unable to quite understand the way the child is pronouncing his words. This style of early speech, with less clearly demarked sentence parts, is called expressive style. Such a child is quite imitative, has a good rote memory, and often engages in language for social purposes—songs, routines, greetings, and so forth. The expressive child seems to be slightly slower at cracking the linguistic code than the referential child but the long term differences between the two styles are not significant.

Emotional development

Emotional development refers to the process by which infants and children begin developing the capacity to experience, express, interpret, and understand emotions. The study of the emotional development of infants and young children is relatively new, having been studied systematically only since the mid-twentieth century. To formulate theories about the development of human emotions, researchers focus on observable display of emotion, such as facial expressions and public behavior. An infant's feelings and experiences cannot be studied by researchers so interpretation of emotion must be limited to signs that can be observed.

Between six and ten weeks, a social smile emerges, usually accompanied by other pleasure-indicative actions and sounds, including cooing and mouthing. This social smile occurs in response to adult smiles and interactions. As infants become more aware of their environment, smiling occurs in response to a wider variety of contexts, for example, they may smile when they see a toy they have previously enjoyed. Laughter begins at around three or four months. It requires a level of **cognitive development** because it demonstrates that the child can recognize incongruity. That is, laughter is usually elicited by actions that deviate from the norm, such as being kissed on the abdomen or a **caregiver** playing peek-a-boo.

During the last half of the first year, infants begin expressing **fear**, disgust, and anger. Unfamiliar situations or objects often elicit fear responses. One of the most common is the presence of an adult stranger, a fear that begins to appear at about seven months. **Separation anxiety**, that is crying when separated from a caregiver, also begins to occur between 7–12 months. Symptoms of fear may include stiffening and crying in a young infant or crying and avoidance of a feared person or object in toddlers. Fear also emerges during this stage as children become able to compare an unfamiliar event with what they know. Anger often is expressed by crying. It serves an adaptive function, signaling to caregivers of the infant's discomfort or displeasure, letting them know that something needs to be changed or altered.

During the second year, infants and toddlers begin express culturally dependent emotions of shame, embarrassment, and pride. They also begin to acquire language and to verbally express their feelings in very rudimentary ways. Being able to express emotions through speech is the first step to developing emotional regulation. A rudimentary capacity for empathy also often appears by age two. The development of empathy requires that children read the emotional cues of other people, understand that other people are distinct from themselves, and have a basic recognition of what the other person is feeling.

Social development

Socialization begins in infancy. Toward the end of the first year, infants begin to recognize the emotions of others, and use this information when reacting to novel situations and people. For example, they may rely on the emotional expressions of their caregivers to determine the **safety** or appropriateness of a particular situation.

By the end of the first year, most infants who are cared for in families develop an attachment relationship, usually with the primary caretaker. This relationship is central to the child's development. Researchers suggest that the quality of the infant's attachment may be predictive of aspects of later development. Youngsters who emerge from infancy with a secure attachment stand a better chance of developing happy, competent relationships with others. The attachment relationship not only forms the emotional basis for the continued development of the parent-child relationship, it can also serve as a foundation upon which subsequent social relationships are built.

Sometime around 18 months of age, children usually begin to assert their desire for autonomy by challenging their caregivers. This behavior is normal for the toddler,

KEY TERMS

Congenital—Present at birth.

Immune system—The mechanism that protects the body from foreign substances, foreign cells, and pathogens. The thymus, spleen, lymph nodes, white blood cells, including the B-cells and T-cells, and antibodies are involved in the immune response, which aims to destroy these foreign bodies.

and a healthy development of independence is facilitated by a caregiver-child relationship that provides support and structure for the child's developing sense of autonomy. In many regards, the security of the initial attachment between infant and parent provides the child with the emotional support to begin exploring the world outside the parent-child relationship.

Common problems

Birth (congenital) defects can range from mild and symptom-free to life-threatening. **Birth defects** can manifest as structural abnormalities or metabolic disorders. They can either be genetic (inherited), be caused by maternal illness during pregnancy, or simply be accidents of development. Some can be permanently corrected through surgery; others will require treatment throughout life, and some will cause disability and **death**. Early intervention generally provides the best prognosis.

Infants have immature immune systems leaving them susceptible to many illnesses. They are subject to the most widespread respiratory disorder, the upper respiratory tract infection known as the **common cold**. Young children can get as many as nine colds a year, each lasting about a week. It is not uncommon for a cold to lead to **bronchitis**, a lower respiratory inflammation of the trachea and bronchial tubes. Acute bronchitis, usually caused by a cold virus, is especially common in children under the age of four years. Other common illnesses cause **vomiting** and **diarrhea**, which can rapidly lead to **dehydration** in infants. Parents need to develop a comfortable relationship with their **pediatrician** who can advise them on how to recognize serious illness, recommend appropriate treatment for mild common illnesses in infancy, and who will monitor their child's growth and development through well baby check ups.

Parental concerns

Every parent's biggest concern is whether their child is healthy and is developing normally. Babies generally progress through certain stages of development in the same order. However, every child is unique and there is a reasonable amount of variation in the timing of these stages in normal, healthy children. In addition, babies do not gain developmental milestones in a steady, linear fashion. They may spurt ahead in one area, for example, learning to walk, while lagging behind in another area such as learning to talk. Parents who are concerned that their child is not reaching developmental milestones in a timely way should consult their pediatrician or other health care professional.

Fine motor skills and gross motor skills develop in an orderly progression but at an uneven pace characterized by both rapid spurts and, at times, frustrating but harmless delays. The more complex the skill, the greater the possible variation among the time it takes normal children to acquire the skill. For example, the normal age for learning to walk has a range of several months, while the age range for turning the head, a simpler skill that occurs much earlier, is considerably narrower. In most cases, difficulty with certain motor skills is temporary and does not indicate a serious problem. Medical help should be sought, however, if a child is significantly behind his peers in multiple aspects of fine motor development or if he regresses, losing previously acquired skills.

Although milestones are discussed for the development of communication skills, many normal, healthy children begin speaking significantly earlier or later than the milestone date. For example, children raised in bilingual families where they regularly hear two languages spoken are, on average, slower to reach these milestones, as they are simultaneously attaining competency in two languages. Parents should refrain from attaching too much significance to either deviation from the average; however, when a child's deviation from the average milestones of development cause the parents concern, a pediatrician should be contacted for advice.

Resources

BOOKS

American Academy of Pediatrics. *Caring for Your Baby and Young Child: Birth to Age 5,* 5th ed. New York: Bantam, 2009.

Sears, William et al. *The Baby Book: Everything You Need to Know About Your Baby From Birth To Age Two,*2nd ed. Boston: Little, Brown, 2003.

OTHER

"Infant and Newborn Care." MedlinePlus. May 17, 2010. [Accessed September 15, 2001], http://www.nlm.nih.gov/medlineplus/infantandnewborncare.html

"Infants & Toddlers—Raising Health Children." United States Centers for Disease Control and Prevention. August 24,

2009. [Accessed September 15, 2010], http://www.cdc.gov/parents/infants/healthy_children.html.

Medical Care for Your 1–2 Year Old. Kids Health/Nemours January 2010. [Accessed September 15, 2010], http://kidshealth.org/parent/growth/medical/med12yr.html.

Medical Care for Your 2–3 Year Old. Kids Health/Nemours October 2008. [Accessed September 15, 2010], http://kidshealth.org/parent/system/doctor/medical_care_2_3.html.

Toddler Health. MedlinePlus. May 17, 2010, [Accessed September 15, 2010]. http://www.nlm.nih.gov/medlineplus/toddlerhealth.html.

ORGANIZATIONS

American Academy of Family Physicians, P. O. Box 11210, Shawnee Mission KS, 66207, (913)906-6000, (800) 274-2237, (913) 906-6075, http://familydoctor.org.

American Academy of Pediatrics, 141 Northwest Point Boulevard, Elk Grove Village IL, 60007-1098, (847) 434-4000, (847) 434-8000, http://www.aap.org.

March of Dimes Foundation, 1275 Mamaroneck Avenue, White Plains NY, 10605, (914) 997-4488, askus@marchofdimes.com, http://www.marchofdimes.com.

National Institute of Child Health and Human Development (NICHD), P.O. Box 3006, Rockville MD, 20847, (800) 370-2943 (800) 320-6942, (866) 760-5947, NICHDInformationResourceCenter@mail.nih.gov, http://www.nichd.nih.gov/publications/pubs/endometriosis.

Tish Davidson, AM

Infant massage

Definition

Infant massage refers to **massage therapy** as specifically applied to infants. In most cases, oil or lotion is used as it would be on an adult subject by a trained and licensed massage therapist. Medical professionals caring for infants might also use massage techniques on infants born prematurely, on those with

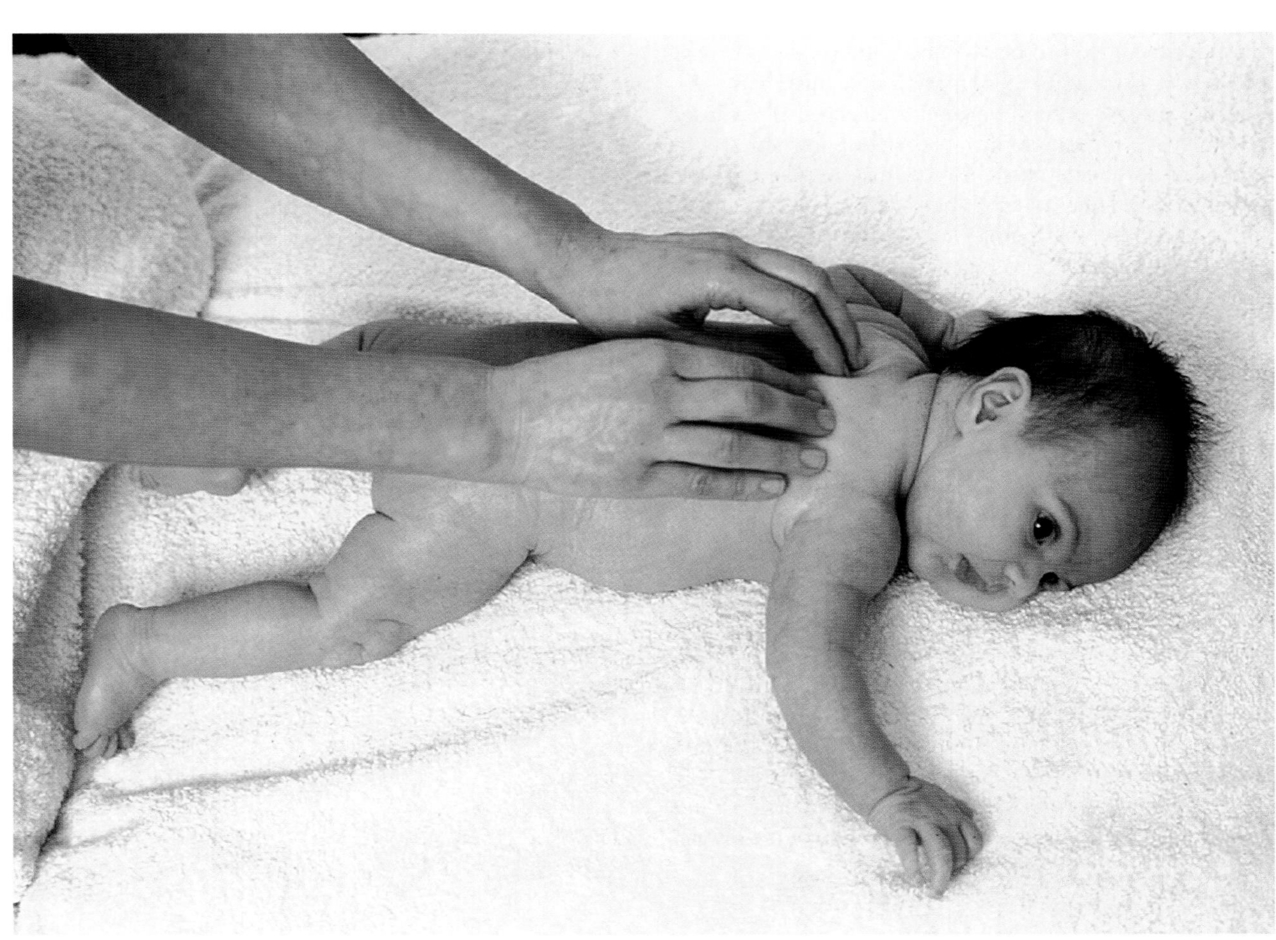

Infant receiving a massage. *(Faye Norman/Photo Researchers, Inc.)*

motor or gastrointestinal problems, or on those who have been exposed to cocaine in utero.

Origins

The practice of massaging infants dates back to ancient times, particularly in Asian and Pacific Island cultures; that is, massage was a component of the baby's regular bath routine among the Maoris and Hawaiians. Touch in these cultures is considered healthful both physically and spiritually. In the West, however, infant massage has received more attention in recent years in conjunction with the popularity of natural **childbirth** and midwife-assisted births. Dr. Frédéric Leboyer, a French physician who was one of the leaders of the natural childbirth movement, helped to popularize infant massage through his photojournalistic book on the Indian art of baby massage.

Infant massage was introduced formally into the United States in 1978 when Vimala Schneider McClure, a **yoga** practitioner who served in an orphanage in Northern India, developed a training program for instructors at the request of childbirth educators. An early research study by R. Rice in 1976 showed that premature babies who were massaged surged ahead in weight gain and neurological development over those who were not massaged. From McClure's training in India, her knowledge of Swedish massage and reflexology, along with her knowledge of yoga postures that she had already adapted for babies, she became the foremost authority on infant massage. In 1986 she founded the International Association of Infant Massage (IAIM), which has 27 chapters worldwide as of 2000.

Benefits

Research from experiments conducted at the Touch Research Institutes at the University of Miami School of Medicine and Nova Southeastern University has been cited for the clinical benefits massage has on infants and children. Tiffany Field, Ph. D., director, noted that the research "... suggests that touch is as important to infants and children as eating and sleeping. Touch therapy triggers many physiological changes that help infants and children grow and develop. For example, massage can stimulate nerves in the brain which facilitate food absorption, resulting in faster weight gain. It also lowers level of stress hormones, resulting in improved immune function."

The benefits of infant massage include:

- relaxation
- relief from stress
- interaction with adults
- stimulation of the nervous system

The results of several studies showed that infant massage alleviates the stress that newborns experience as a result of the enormous change that **birth** brings about in their lives after the 6–9 months they have spent in the womb. Both premature infants and full-term babies need the relaxation that comes from massaging and moving their limbs and muscles. In infants with **colic**, massage provides the relief necessary to disperse gas, ease **muscle spasms**, tone the digestive system and help it work efficiently. Some techniques even help bring relief from **teething** and emotional stress. The stimulation an infant receives from massage can aid circulation, strengthen muscles, help digestion, and relieve **constipation**. The **bonding** that occurs with massage between a parent and child enhances the entire process of bonding that comes with contact through all of the senses, including touch, voice, and sight. It affords a physical experience of quality time between the parents and the child as well as with any significant others in a baby's life.

Description

Various techniques are used in infant massage, with the different strokes specific to a particular therapy. Special handling is used for treating a baby with gas and colic. Some of the strokes are known as "Indian milking," which is a gentle stroking of the child's legs; and the "twist and squeeze" stroke, a gentle squeeze of the muscles in the thigh and calf. The light "feather" strokes often employed in regular Swedish massage are applied at the end of a massage. The procedure is not unlike certain forms of adult massage but extra care must be taken for the fragility of the infant.

There are also specific Chinese techniques of pediatric massage, including massage of children with special needs. In China, these forms of massage can be given by medical professionals but parents are often taught how to do the simpler forms for home treatment of their children.

Preparations

If lotions or oils are used, care is taken to ensure their **safety** on a baby's delicate skin. The most important consideration is to use vegetable oils rather than mineral oils, which can clog the pores in the skin. The oil that is used should be warmed in the caregiver's hands before applying it to the baby's skin. The environment in which the massage is given to an infant should be comfortably warm and as calm and nonthreatening as possible.

Precautions

Extreme caution is necessary when performing infant massage. Strokes are made with the greatest delicacy in order not to harm the infant in any way. Proper techniques are taught by licensed massage therapists ensuring that the infant is treated with appropriate physical touch. Anyone who is unfamiliar with handling a baby should receive appropriate instruction before beginning infant massage.

Side effects

No adverse side effects have been reported when infant massage is done properly after careful instruction, or by a licensed massage therapist who specializes in infant care.

Research & general acceptance

In addition to the study already noted regarding touch therapy, a website devoted to infant massage lists research published as early as 1969 and cites hundreds of individual projects that have been conducted throughout the world focusing on infant massage. Many of the studies are related to the benefits of massage and touch for premature infants and others born with such risk factors as drug dependence. Conclusions regarding the benefits are overwhelmingly positive. The proliferation of therapists licensed in infant massage across the United States and worldwide indicates that infant massage is increasingly recognized as a legitimate health care treatment.

Training & certification

The International Association of Infant Massage (IAIM) has developed a basic course for licensing infant massage therapists. The pioneer in the field, Vimala McClure, began to prepare a course of instruction in the 1970s. The course is introduced in four-day sessions around the United States. Licensing is obtained by those who complete the course, pass a take-home examination, and complete a teaching practicum with five families over a three-month period. IAIM listed its course in 2000 as costing $550 if paid in full two weeks prior to training and $595 after that. It includes a $100 nonrefundable deposit due one month before training. The cities where the basic course was offered in 2000 included Augusta, GA; Gaithersburg, MD; Chicago, IL; Boston, MA; Washington, DC; Charlottesville, VA; Minneapolis, MN; and Albuquerque, NM. In 2000, the International Institute of Infant Massage in Albuquerque also offered an Infant Massage Instructor Certification Course specifically geared to men, entitled "Men Teaching Fathers," and scheduled to last four days.

The licensing of massage therapists varies from state to state, as infant massage qualifies for consideration as medical treatment. Infant massage is becoming an increasingly popular discipline within the field. Numerous websites provide listings for infant massage specialists throughout the United States. The IAIM course is recognized as the official course for infant massage.

Resources

BOOKS

Auckett, Amelia. *Baby Massage: Parent-Child Bonding through Touching.* New York: Newmarket Press, 1982.

Cline, Kyle. *Chinese Massage for Infants and Children: Traditional Techniques for Alleviating Colic, Teething Pain, Earache, and Other Common Childhood Conditions.* Rochester: Inner Traditions International, Limited, 1999.

Fan, Ya-Li. *Chinese Pediatric Massage Therapy: Traditional Techniques for Alleviating Colic, Colds, Earaches, and Other Common Childhood Conditions,* ed. Bob Flaws. Boulder: Blue Poppy Enterprises, 1999.

Gordon, Jay, and Brenda Adderly. *Brighter Baby: Boosting Your Child's Intelligence, Health and Happiness through Infant Therapeutic Massage.* New York: Regnery Publishing, Inc. 1999.

Heinl, Tina. *The Baby Massage Book: Shared Growth through the Hands.* Boston: Sigo Press, 1991.

Leboyer, Frédéric. *Loving Hands: The Traditional Indian Art of Baby Massage.* New York: Knopf, 1976.

McClure, Vimala Schneider. *Infant Massage: A Handbook for Loving Parents.* New York: Bantam Books, 1989.

Walker, Peter. *Baby Massage: A Practical Guide to Massage and Movement for Babies and Infants.* New York: St. Martin's Press, 1996.

OTHER

Gentle Touch Infant Massage Video. Gentle Touch, Inc. 1996.

ORGANIZATIONS

International Association of Infant Massage, PO Box 1045, Oak View CA, 93022

International Institute of Infant Massage, 605 Bledsoe Rd. NW, Albuquerque NM, 87107, (505) 341-9381, (505) 341-9386, http://www.infantmassage.com.

Jane Spehar

Infant mortality

Definition

Infant mortality refers to the statistical rate of infant **death** up to the age of one year, expressed as the number of such deaths per 1,000 live births for a specific geographical area over a given time period, normally one year.

Number of infant (less than one year of age) and neonatal deaths and mortality rates by race and by sex for the United States, 2007

	Infant deaths						Neonatal deaths					
	All races[1]		White		Black		All races[1]		White		Black	
	Number	Rate	Number	Rate	Number	Rate	Number	Rate	Number	Rate	Number	Rate
United States[2]	29,138	6.75	18,807	5.64	8,944	13.24	19,058	4.42	12,333	3.70	5,842	8.65
Male	16,293	7.38	10,540	6.17	4,975	14.49	10,587	4.79	6,845	4.01	3,256	9.48
Female	12,845	6.09	8,267	5.08	3,969	11.94	8,471	4.02	5,488	3.37	2,586	7.78

Note: Rates are infant deaths (less than one year of age) per 1,000 live births in specified group. Infant deaths are based on race of decedent; live births are based on race of mother.
[1]Includes races other than white and black.
[2]Excludes data for Puerto Rico, Virgin Islands, Guam, American Samoa, and Northern Marianas.

SOURCE: Centers for Disease Control and Prevention, National Center for Health Statistics, National Vital Statistics System, "Deaths: Final Data for 2007," *National Vital Statistics Reports* 58, no 19 (May 2010).

(Table by PreMediaGlobal. Reproduced by permission of Gale, a part of Cengage Learning.)

Demographics

According to the Central **Intelligence** Agency (CIA) Fact Book, the highest rate of infant mortality occurs in Angola with an estimated 2010 rate of 178 deaths per 1,000 live births. Angola is followed by Afghanistan (151 per 1,000), then Niger and Mali, both at approximately 114 deaths per 1,000 live births. With the exception of Afghanistan, the 20 countries with the highest rate of infant mortality are all in Africa. The five countries with the lowest projected rate of infant mortality in 2010 are Japan, Sweden, Bermuda, Singapore, and Monaco, with death rates ranging from 2.79 per 1,000 live births (Japan) to 1.78 per thousand (Monaco). The United States ranks at 180 among 224 countries with a rate of 6.14 per 1,000, down from 6.75 in 2003. The relatively high rate of infant deaths in the United States is largely accounted for by high infant mortality rates among low-income minority populations.

Description

Infant mortality is the incidence of death that occurs in the first year after **birth** expressed in relation to every 1,000 live births. Infant mortality is commonly divided into two categories: neonatal deaths (occurring during the first 27 days after birth) and postneonatal deaths (occurring from the age of 28 days to one year). Infant mortality is considered an important indicator of the general level of health for a given population.

Toward the end of the 19th century, before the widespread recognition that bacteria were a major cause of illness, rates of infant mortality throughout the world were much higher than they are today. It was common for 20% or more of all infants in many populations to die before reaching their first birthday and often mortality rates were even higher for children between the ages of one and five years. In the last years of the 19th century, large areas of Russia had an infant mortality rate of nearly 28%. In 1901, the infant mortality rate in England, birthplace of the industrial revolution and capital of a global empire, was 16%. By 1930 the number of infant deaths had declined dramatically in many countries as the causes of infection came to be understood.

Causes and symptoms

Most progress up to this point was due to precautions such as hand washing and sterilization of milk rather than to actual medical advances, since **antibiotics** and sulfa drugs—the first medications that were really effective in fighting infection—were not developed until the late 1930s and were not readily available until the 1940s. Although data on infant mortality in the developing nations is much less complete than the figures for the developed world, it is clear that some of the world's poorer countries made dramatic progress in lowering infant mortality in the 20th century, due in large part to public health programs especially those that have combated malaria through mosquito control. Availability of medication and immunization have also played a major role in improving infant health in developing nations.

Worldwide, common causes of infant mortality are **dehydration** due to **diarrhea**, **pneumonia**, infection, **malnutrition**, malaria, and **birth defects**. In the United States, according to the Centers for Disease Control and Prevention (CDC), in 2005, the 10 leading causes of

KEY TERMS

Congenital—Present at birth.

Dehydration—Excessive water loss by the body.

Malaria—Disease caused by the presence of sporozoan parasites of the genus Plasmodium in the red blood cells, transmitted by the bite of anopheline mosquitoes, and characterized by severe and recurring attacks of chills and fever).

Pneumonia—A disease that causes inflammation of the lungs. It can be caused by a bacterium or a virus.

infant mortality were: (1) birth defects; (2) disorders associated with premature and low birth weight; (3) **sudden infant death syndrome** (SIDS); (4) newborn affected by maternal complications of pregnancy; (5) newborn affected by complications of the placenta, cord and membranes; (6) accidental injury; (7) respiratory distress; (8) infections present during the period of birth; (9) uncontrolled bleeding (hemorrhage) in newborns; and (10) **necrotizing enterocolitis** (an infection of the intestine). The first four causes collectively accounted for more than half of all infant deaths.

Worldwide, infant mortality is linked to income, with poor people and poor countries experiencing higher rates of infant mortality than wealthier individuals and wealthier countries. A cluster of interrelated environmental factors is associated with infant mortality in the United States. These include poverty, inadequate prenatal care, a high rate of teenage pregnancies, and use of drugs, alcohol, and tobacco during pregnancy. The factor most often cited as responsible for the lower rates of infant mortality in other developed nations is the universal availability of free prenatal and maternal health care. Even when free care is available in the United States, low-income women often face significant barriers in obtaining it. They may be unable to take time off work for the lengthy waits that clinic visits often require.

The principal way environmental factors, such as poor prenatal care, affect infant health is through birth weight. Low birth weight percentage defined as weight under 5.5 pounds is responsible for a significant number of neonatal and postneonatal deaths in the United States each year. In addition to being considered a leading cause of infant mortality in its own right, low birth weight is also associated with other causes of infant death including birth defects (congenital abnormalities), sudden infant death syndrome (SIDS), and **respiratory distress syndrome**. Known risk factors for low birth weight are **smoking**, drug and alcohol consumption during pregnancy, teen pregnancy, and multiple fetuses. Other factors thought to be associated with the relatively high levels of low birth weight among infants born in the United States include lower levels of social support, including marital and other emotional support.

Resources

BOOKS

Garrett, Eilidh, et al. editors. *Infant Mortality: A Continuing Social Problem.* Burlington, VT: Ashgate, 2006.

OTHER

CDC Office of Minority Health and Healthy Disparities. "Eliminate Disparities in Infant Mortality." [Accessed September 5, 2010], http://www.cdc.gov/omhd/amh/factsheets/infant.htm.

Central Intelligence Agency. "World Fact Book: Infant Mortality. 2010." [Accessed September 5, 2010], https://www.cia.gov/library/publications/the-world-factbook/rankorder/2091rank.html.

ORGANIZATIONS

National Women's Health Network, 1413 K St., NW, 4th floor, Washington DC, 20005, (202) 682-2640, (202) 682-2646, healthquestions@whn.org, http://www.nwhn.org.

World Health Organization, Avenue Appia 20, 1211 Geneva 27 Switzerland, +22 41 791 21 11, +22 41 791 31 11, info@who.int, http://www.who.int.

Tish Davidson, AM

Infant nutrition

Definition

Children between the ages of **birth** and one year are considered infants. Infants grow very rapidly and have special nutritional requirements that are different from other age groups.

Purpose

Infant nutrition is designed to meet the special needs of very young children and give them a healthy start in life. Children under one year old do not have fully mature organ systems. They need nutrition that is easy to digest and contains enough calories, **vitamins**, **minerals**, and other nutrients to grow and develop normally. Infants also need the proper amount of fluids for their immature kidney's to process. In addition, infant nutrition involves avoiding exposing infants to substances that are harmful to their growth and development.

Description

Infancy is a time of incredibly rapid growth and development. Getting the right kinds of nutrients in the right quantities and avoiding the wrong kinds of substances gives infants the best chance at a healthy start to life. Parents are responsible for seeing that their infant's nutritional needs are met. Infant nutrition is so important that the United States Department of Agriculture has developed the Women, Infants, and Children (WIC) program. This program provides free health and social service referrals, nutrition counseling, and vouchers for healthy foods to supplement the diet of pregnant and **breastfeeding** women, infants, and children up to age 5 who are low-income and nutritionally at risk. In 2004, WIC served about 7.9 million people, including 2 million infants and 1.9 million pregnant and nursing women.

Breastfeeding

Human milk is uniquely suited to the nutrition needs of newborns. Many health organizations, including the **American Academy of Pediatrics** (AAP), the American Medical Association (AMA), the American Dietetic Association (ADA), and the World Health Organization (WHO) support the position that breast milk is the best and most complete form of nutrition for infants. The AAP recommends that infants should be exclusively breastfed for the first 6 months of life and that breastfeeding should continue for at least 12 months.

Breastfeeding in the United States slowly increased in acceptance in the last decade of the twentieth century. In 1998, 64% of American mothers breastfed their babies for a short time after birth. Only 29% were still breastfeeding by the time their baby was 6 months old. The United States Department of Health and Human Services developed a set of health goals for the nation to aim for by the year 2000. One of these goals involved breastfeeding. The Healthy People 2000 goal was for 75% of American women to breastfeed their babies for a period immediately after birth and 50% to breastfeed for the first 6 months of their infant's life. Although there is significant variation in support for breastfeeding among different racial and ethnic groups in the United States, no racial group met this target. In 2000, the Department of Health and Human Services estimated that:

- 45% of African American mothers breastfed their infants for a short time after birth; 19% were breastfeeding at 6 months; 9% at 12 months.
- 66% of Hispanic mothers breastfed their infants for a short time after birth; 28% were breastfeeding at 6 months; 19% at 12 months.
- 68% of white mothers breastfed their infants for a short time after birth; 31% were breastfeeding at 6 months; 17% at 12 months.

Healthy People 2010, the health goals set for Americans during the first decade of the twenty-first century, include eliminating the differences among racial groups in the rate of breastfeeding. The goal for 2010 is for 75% of all women to be breastfeeding shortly after birth, 50% to be breastfeeding at 6 months, and 25% to breastfeed for a full year.

ADVANTAGES OF BREASTFEEDING Research comparing formula-fed and breastfed babies convincingly shows that both full-term and premature breastfed infants have certain advantages over formula fed infants. One of the most important advantages conferred by breast milk is an increased resistance to infection.

An infant is born with an immature **immune system** that does not become fully functional for about two years. Since immune system cells make antibodies to fight infection, an incompletely developed immune system leaves the infant vulnerable to many bacterial and viral infections. However, the nursing mother has a fully developed immune system and many of the antibodies and other components of her immune system pass into her breast milk. Nursing infants take in their mother's antibodies along with the other nutrients in breast milk. These antibodies survive passage through the infant's digestive system and are absorbed into the infant's blood, where they help protect against infection. Well-designed studies have repeatedly documented the fact that breastfed babies have fewer ear infections, bouts of **diarrhea**, respiratory infections, and cases of **meningitis** than formula-fed babies. Overall, the **death** rate of breastfeed babies during the first year of life is lower than the death rate of formula-fed babies.

Another way that breastfeeding protects against infection is by keeping the infant from being exposed to waterborne contaminants. In developing countries, many water supplies are contaminated with bacteria and chemicals. Using this water to mix formula increases the exposure of the baby to these pathogens and toxins. Breastfed babies do not have to worry about being exposed to this type of contamination.

Another advantage of breastfeeding is that infants are unlikely to gain too much weight. **Childhood obesity** is a major concern in the United States. Since mothers are unable to measure how much breast milk their baby consumes, they are less likely to encourage overfeeding. Research suggests that breastfed babies have a lower risk of developing type 2 diabetes. Other research suggests that the rate of other chronic diseases such as **asthma**, **celiac disease**, inflammatory bowel disease, and various **allergies** appear to be lower in breastfed babies than in babies fed formula. Premature babies especially appear to benefit from reduced chronic disease as a result of breastfeeding.

Breastfeeding also provides benefits to the nursing mother. To start with, breastfeeding is more economical than buying formula, even taking into account the extra food—about 500 calories daily—that the mother needs to eat when she is nursing. Since breastfed babies on average get sick less than formula-fed babies, the family is also likely to save money on doctor visits, medicine, and time off from work to care for a sick child.

The mother's health also benefits from breastfeeding. Nursing mothers tend to lose the weight they put on during pregnancy faster than mothers who do not nurse. The hormones that are released in the mother's body when her infant nurses also help her uterus contract and become more nearly the size it was before pregnancy. Mothers who nurse their babies also seem to be less likely to develop breast, ovarian, or uterine **cancer** early in life. Finally, breastfeeding offers psychological benefits to the mother as she bonds with her baby and may reduce the chance of postpartum depression.

DISADVANTAGES OF BREASTFEEDING Although breast milk is the best food for an infant, breastfeeding does cause some disadvantages to the mother. Initially babies breastfeed about every two to three hours. Some women find it exhausting to be available to the baby so frequently. Later, when the infant is older, the mother may need to pump breast milk for her child to eat while she is away or at work. Fathers sometimes feel shut out during the early weeks of breastfeeding because of the close bond between mother and child. In addition, women who are breastfeeding must watch their diet carefully. Some foods or substances, such as **caffeine**, can pass into breast milk and cause the baby to be restless and irritable. Finally, some women simply find the idea of breastfeeding messy and distasteful, and resent the fact that they need to be "on tap" much of the time. For women who cannot or do not want to breastfeed, infant formula provides an adequate alternative.

Formula feeding

Although infant formula is not as perfect a food as breast milk for infants (it is harder for them to digest and is not a chemical replica of human milk), formula does provide all the nutrients a baby needs to grow up healthy. The United States Food and Drug Administration (FDA) regulates infant formula under the Federal Food, Drug, and Cosmetic Act (FFDCA). The FDA sets the minimum amounts of 29 nutrients that must be present in infant formula and sets maximum amounts for 9 other nutrients. Some of these nutrients include Vitamins A, D, E, and K, and calcium. Some formulas contain iron, while others do not.

Substances used in infant formulas must be foods on the approved Generally Recognized as Safe (GRAS) list. Facilities for manufacturing infant formula are regularly inspected by the FDA and the manufacturer must keep process and distribution records for each batch of formula. Every container of formula must show an expiration or use by date. The FDA must be informed of any changes made to the formula.

Infant formulas are either cow's milk based or soy based. Infants who show signs of lactose-intolerance (colicky, restless, gassy, spitting up) usually do well on soy-based formula. Formula comes in three styles:

- Ready-to-feed. This is the easiest type of formula to use. It can be poured straight from the can into a bottle. It is also the most expensive form of formula.
- Concentrated liquid. This needs to be mixed with an equal portion of water. Concentrated liquid is less expensive than ready-to-feed.
- Powder. This needs to be mixed with water. Advantages are that it is the least expensive formula and that it keeps longer than the liquid varieties. The main disadvantage is that it requires accurate measuring of powder and water.

Reasons to formula feed

Not every woman wants or is able to breastfeed. Aside from personal preference, here are some reasons why some women should formula feed.

- They are adoptive parents.
- They have HIV, active tuberculosis, or hepatitis C. These diseases can be passed on to their infants through breast milk.
- They use street drugs or abuse prescription medicines. Many drugs pass into breast milk and can permanently damage a baby's health.
- They are taking chemotherapy drugs, certain mood stabilizers, migraine headache medications or other drugs that pass into breast milk and whose effect on the infant is negative or unknown.
- They have alcoholism or are binge drinkers. The alcohol they drink will be present in breast milk.
- They have difficult to control diabetes and may have increased difficulty controlling their blood sugar level if they choose to breastfeed.
- They are going to be separated from their baby for significant periods.

- They have had breast surgery that interferes with milk production.
- They are emotionally repelled by the idea of breast-feeding.
- A few babies are born with a genetic inborn error in metabolism that prevents them from digesting any mammalian milk. These babies must be fed soy-based formula in order to survive.

Pros and cons of formula feeding

Formula feeding has some definite advantages. Anyone, not just the mother, can feed the infant. This gives the mother more flexibility in her schedule and allows the father or other relatives to enjoy a special closeness with the baby that comes with feeding. Also, the mother does not need to be concerned about how her diet affects her baby and she does not need to worry about breast milk leakage. In addition, since formula is digested more slowly than breast milk, feedings are less frequent. Some women feel uncomfortable nursing in front of other people or find it difficult to locate places to nurse in private. Formula feeding eliminates this problem.

There are also disadvantages to formula feeding. Aside from the fact that formula is not an exact duplicate of breast milk and is harder to digest, it also costs more and requires more advance preparation. Bottles need to be washed, and the water used to mix formula, at least in the early months, needs to be boiled or be special bottle water suitable for infants. The Academy of General Dentistry warns that some public water supplies are fluoridated at levels too high for infants, and that fluorodosis of the primary (baby) teeth may result. Fluorodosis is a cosmetic problem. It causes brown spots on the teeth, but does not weaken them in any way. Finally, formula must be refrigerated once it is mixed or a can is opened. It can only be kept about 2 days in the refrigerator so is there is more likely to be waste. Likewise, when traveling, bottles need to be refrigerated. Although most babies do not mind cold formula, many parents like to heat their child's bottle to body temperature, another inconvenience when traveling.

Transitioning to solid foods

When an infant is between four and six months old, most pediatricians recommend introducing the infant to solid food. By this age, infants begin to have the muscle coordination to swallow runny solids. If there is a family history of **food allergies**, some pediatricians recommend waiting until 6 months or older to start solid food.

Normally solid feeding begins with a small amount of iron-fortified rice or other single-grain cereal mixed into a slurry the consistency of thin gravy with formula or breast milk. The infant is then offered a small amount of cereal on a small spoon. It may take many attempts before the infant is happy with the new food. After runny cereal is accepted, a thicker cereal can be offered. When the child eats this with ease, parents can begin feeding one new pureed food every week. Commercial baby food is available in jars or frozen. Baby food can also be made at home using a blender or food processor. Portions can be frozen in an ice cube tray and thawed as needed.

About the same time babies begin eating solid food, they are ready to take small sips of apple, grape, or pear juice (but not citrus juices) from a cup. Juice should not be served in a bottle. By the end of the first year, infants can eat a variety of ground or chopped soft foods that the rest of the family eats.

Foods that should not be fed to infants

Some foods are not appropriate for children during their first year. These include:

- homemade formula. The nutrient requirements for infants are very specific and even a small excesses or deficits of a particular nutrient can permanently harm the child's development.
- cow's milk. Plain cow's milk should not be offered before 6 months, after this it can be introduced in small amounts as part of weaning foods but should not be offerd as the main drink before age 1. The cow's milk in formula has been altered to make it acceptable for infants.
- honey. Honey can contains spores of the bacterium *Clostritium botulinum.* This bacterium causes a serious, potentially fatal disease called infant botulism. Older children and adults are not affected. *C. botulinum.* can also be found in maple syrup, corn syrup, and undercooked foods.
- well cooked eggs can be offered between 6–9 months (later if any family history of atopy), fish (can be offered from 6–9 months, shellfish, peanuts, and peanut butter. These often trigger an allergic reaction during the first year.
- orange, grapefruit, or other citrus juices. These often cause a painful diaper rash during the first year.
- home prepared spinach, collard greens, turnips, or beets. These may contain high levels of harmful nitrates from the soil. Jarred versions of these foods are okay.
- raisins, whole grapes, hot dog rounds, hard candy, popcorn, raw carrots, nuts, and stringy meat. These and similar foods can cause choking, a major cause of accidental death in infants and toddlers.

Precautions

Mothers with certain health conditions such as those mentioned above should not breastfeed. Women with chronic diseases should discuss this with their healthcare provider.

Mothers using certain drugs should not breastfeed.

Parents using concentrated liquid and powdered formulas must measure and mix formula accurately. Inaccurate measuring can harm the infant's growth and development. Water used in mixing formula must be free of pathogens, contaminants, and excessive levels of fluoride.

Interactions

Street drugs, many prescription and over-the-counter drugs, and alcohol pass into breast milk and have the potential to permanently harm an infant's growth and development. Before taking any drugs, a pregnant or breastfeeding woman should consult her healthcare provider. Caffeine also passes into breast milk. Some women find that even moderate amounts of coffee or caffeinated sodas cause their infant to become restless and irritable, while others find little effect. Breastfeeding women should monitor their caffeine intake and try to keep it to a minimum.

Complications

Many women have trouble getting the newborn to latch on and begin breastfeeding. This can usually be overcome with the help of a **lactation** consultant or pediatric nurse. Breastfeeding can cause the mother to develop sore, infected nipples. This is usually a temporary condition that should not be a reason to stop breastfeeding.

Complications from bottle feeding tend to be related to the infant's difficulty in digesting formula. Some infants become gassy and colicky and may fuss, cry for long periods, and spit up cow's milk-based formula. A switch to soy-based formula on the advice of a healthcare professional usually relieves this problem. Other complications of formula feeding are generally related to improper mixing of formula.

Parental concerns

Breastfeeding parents often are concerned about whether their baby is getting enough milk, since there is no way to directly measure how much milk a baby consumes when nursing. Newborns should have a minimum of 6–8 wet diapers and four bowel movements during the first two weeks of life. As the child grows, these numbers will gradually decrease. In addition, a woman's breasts should feel hard and full (sometimes even painful) before nursing and softer after nursing. Newborns nurse every 2–3 hours but they should seem satisfied after nursing. The most definite sign that the baby is getting enough food is that he or she is gaining weight.

Infants grow in irregular spurts. They may eat hungrily for a few days and then eat little few days later. Parents often worry about this but it is a normal occurrence.

The transition to solid food is often a slow process. Infants eat very small amounts and often must be exposed to a new food multiple times before they will eat it willingly. Since childhood obesity is a major problem in the United States, parents and caregivers should avoid encouraging the infant to overeat.

Resources

BOOKS

Berggren, Kirsten. *Weaning Without Working: A Working Mother's Guide to Breastfeeding.* Amarillo, TX: Hale Pub., 2006.

Bhatia, Jatinder, ed. *Perinatal Nutrition: Optimizing Infant Health and Development.* New York: Marcel Dekker, 2005.

Curtis, Glade B. and Judith Schuler. *Your Pregnancy Quick Guide: Feeding Your Baby In The First Year.* Cambridge, MA: Da Capo Life Long, 2004.

Mohrbacher, Nancy and Kathleen Kendall-Tackett. *Breastfeeding Made Simple: Seven Natural Laws for Nursing Mothers.* Oakland, CA: New Harbinger Publications, 2005.

Moran, Victoria H. and Fiona Dykes, eds. *Maternal and Infant Nutrition and Nurture: Controversies and Challenges.* London: Quay, 2006.

Samour, Patricia Q. and Kathy K. Helm, eds. *Handbook of Pediatric Nutrition.* Sudbury, MA: Jones and Bartlett, 2005.

Torgus, Judy and Gwen Gotsch, eds. *The Womanly Art of Breastfeeding,* 7th ed. rev. Schaumburg, IL: La Leche League International, 2004.

PERIODICALS

American Academy of Pediatrics. "Breastfeeding and the Use of Human Milk (Policy Statement)." *Pediatrics* 115 no.2 (February 2005): 496-506, http://aappolicy.aappublications.org/cgi/content/full/pediatrics; 115/2/496.

OTHER

International Food Information Council. "Questions and Answers About the Nutritional Content of Processed Baby Food." October 13, 2009. [Accessed December 8, 2010], http://www.foodinsight.org/Resources/Detail.aspx?topic=-Questions_and_Answers_About_the_Nutritional_Content_of_Processed_Baby_Food_.

International Food Information Council. "Starting Solids: Nutrition Guide for Infants and Children 6 to 18 Months of Age." January 2005. [Accessed December 8, 2010], http://ific.org/publications/brocuhres/solidsbroch.cfm.

Mayo Clinic Staff. "Introducing Solid Foods: What You Need to Know." MayoClinic.com, June 26, 2010. [Accessed December 8, 2010], http://www.mayoclinic.com/health/healthy-baby/PR00029.

Nemours Foundation "Breastfeeding vs. Formula Feeding." Kid's Health, July 2005. [Accessed December 8, 2010], http://www.kidshealth.org/parent/food/infants/breast_bottle_feeding.html.

United States Department of Agriculture, Food and Nutrition Information Center. "Infant Nutrition and Feeding Resource List." October 2009. [Accessed December 8, 2010], http://www.nal.usda.gov/fnic/pubs/bibs/gen/infnut.html.

United States Department of Agriculture, Food and Nutrition Information Service. "WIC at a Glance." March 8, 2010. [Accessed December 8, 2010], http://www.fns.usda.gov/wic/aboutwic/wicataglance.htm.

United States Department of Health and Human Services, Office of Women' Health. "HHS Blueprint for Action on Breastfeeding." August 1, 2010. [Accessed December 8, 2010], http://www.womenshealth.gov/breastfeeding/government-programs/hhs-blueprints-and-policy-statements/.

United States Food and Drug Administration (FDA). "Frequently Asked About FDA's Regulation of Infant Formula." March 1, 2006. [Accessed December 8, 2010], http://www.fda.gov/Food/GuidanceComplianceRegulatoryInformation/GuidanceDocuments/InfantFormula/ucm056524.htm.

ORGANIZATIONS

American Academy of Pediatrics (AAP), 141 Northwest Point Boulevard, Elk Grove Village IL, 60007, (847) 434-4000, http://www.aap.org.

American Dietetic Association, 120 S. Riverside Plaza, Suite 2000, Chicago IL, 60606, (800) 877-1600, http://www.eatright.org.

International Food Information Council, 1100 Connecticut Avenue, NW Suite 430, Washington DC, 20036, (202) 296-6540, (202) 296-6547, http://www.ific.org.

La Leche League InterNational, 1400 N. Meacham Road, Schaumburg IL, 60168-4079, (847) 519-7730, (847) 592-7570 (TTY), (847) 519-0035, http://www.lalecheleague.org/.

United States Department of Agriculture, 1400 Independence Avenue SW, Room 1180, Washington DC, 20250, http://www.usda.gov/wps/portal/usdahome.

United States Food and Drug Administration (FDA), Center for Food Safety and Applied Nutrition, Office of Nutritional Products, Labeling, and Dietary Supplements, 5100 Paint Branch Parkway, College Park MD, 20740, (301) 436-2639, http://www.cfsan.fda.gov/~dms/onplds.html.

Tish Davidson, A.M.

Infant screening *see* **Newborn screening**

Infectious disease

Definition

Infectious disease—also called communicable disease—is any illness caused by an infective agent—a germ, microbe, or parasite. Infective agents include bacteria, viruses, fungi, parasitic protozoa, and worms.

Demographics

Virtually all children contract infectious disease, especially during infancy and early childhood. Respiratory and gastrointestinal infections are the most common causes of illness in children. Respiratory infections affect as many as 32% of all infants. Up to 26% of infants contract gastrointestinal infections.

Worldwide, more children and adults die from infectious disease than any other single cause. The vast majority of these deaths occur in poorer counties with limited access to prevention, medical care, and drugs. In 2008, infectious disease killed 5,970,000 children under the age of five, accounting for 68% of all deaths in that age group: an estimated 18% died of **pneumonia**, 15% of **diarrhea**, and eight percent of **malaria**. According to the World Health Organization (WHO), more than 800,000 children under five die every year from **pneumococcal pneumonia** and **meningitis**. Children under age two are at particular risk for serious pneumococcal infections. Children with HIV/AIDS are 20–40 more likely than others to contract pneumococcal infections. Pneumococcal meningitis is disabling or fatal in 40–70% of affected children.

Among American children, the frequency and severity of infectious disease has declined dramatically in recent decades, primarily due to the development of vaccines for common childhood infections. The United States is one of the few places in the world where **polio** has been completely eradicated. Childhood pneumococcal infections caused by vaccine-targeted bacterial strains have been almost completely eliminated.

Description

When an infective agent enters the body and begins to multiply, the immune system responds with various defensive mechanisms that protect against most infectious disease. However when an infective agent temporarily evades or overwhelms the immune system and begins to damage tissues, signs and symptoms of disease develop.

The most common infectious diseases are contagious—they spread via direct transfer of an infective agent from one person to another. Shaking hands, kissing, or coughing or sneezing on someone can directly transmit contagious diseases such as colds, flu, or **tuberculosis** (TB). Some infective agents, including cold viruses, can be contracted by indirect contact with a contaminated surface such as a faucet, doorknob, or computer keyboard. International airplane travel is responsible for the spread of contagious diseases around the world. Infant diarrhea caused by rotavirus or the protozoan *Giardia lamblia* often spreads among babies and young children through the accidental transferring of feces from hand to mouth after diaper changes. Some infectious diseases can be passed from a mother to her unborn child across the placenta or during birth.

Other infectious diseases can be transmitted from animals or animal waste to humans. Dog and cat saliva may contain more than 100 different types of infective agents. *Pasteurella* bacteria are the most common microbes transmitted via pet **bites**. These bacteria can cause serious—sometimes fatal—infectious diseases such as meningitis, an inflammation of the lining of the brain and spinal cord. **Toxoplasmosis** is a bacterial infection that is transmitted via cat feces. Pet reptiles, such as turtles, snakes, and iguanas, can transmit *Salmonella* bacteria. Wild animals can directly or indirectly transmit a wide variety of infectious disease.

Some infectious diseases are transferred between human hosts by insect vectors:

- Mosquitoes transfer the protozoan that causes malaria, as well as West Nile virus, dengue fever, and viral encephalitis.
- Body lice can transmit typhus.
- Fleas can transmit typhus and transfer plague bacteria from rodents to humans.
- Deer ticks—which are actually more closely related to crabs than to insects—can transfer the bacterium that causes Lyme disease from mice to humans.
- Ticks can also transmit the bacterium that cause Rocky Mountain spotted fever and tularemia and the protozoan that causes babesiosis.

Some infectious diseases are spread from a single source to many people through contaminated food or water. For example, the bacterium ***Escherichia coli*** (*E. coli*) can be transmitted via unwashed fruit or vegetables or undercooked meat.

Some infectious diseases have recently emerged, re-emerged, or become much more widespread and dangerous by acquiring drug resistance. Examples include:

- methicillin-resistant *Staphylococcus aureus* (MRSA) bacteria
- multi- and extensively drug-resistant TB bacteria
- 2009 H1N1 influenza virus
- H5N1 avian influenza virus
- West Nile virus
- Ebola virus
- Marburg virus
- Nipah virus
- SARS virus
- dengue virus
- polio virus
- malaria parasite

Risk factors

Risk factors for respiratory or gastrointestinal infectious diseases in babies include:

- premature birth
- low birth weight
- low socioeconomic status
- multiple siblings
- daycare
- parental smoking

Children with weakened immune systems are at increased risk for infectious disease. Infection can occur if a child:

- has HIV/AIDS
- has an autoimmune disease
- is taking steroids or anti-rejection drugs for a transplanted organ
- is being treated for cancer

In 2010, scientists reported the discovery of mutations that increase susceptibility to infectious disease. The mutations are in a gene called CISH that encodes a protein that regulates the immune system's response to infectious disease. A child who inherits one of these mutations from a parent has an 18% increased risk for infectious disease. Inheriting four or more of the mutations increases the risk to 81%.

Causes and symptoms

Although most bacteria are not harmful—and some types are essential for proper functioning of the human body—some bacteria produce toxins that cause infectious disease. *Streptococcus* can cause infections ranging from relatively mild ear infections to **strep throat** to potentially fatal pneumococcal pneumonia, meningitis, and **sepsis** or blood poisoning. Children can be especially vulnerable to bacteria that cause:

- diphtheria
- pertussis or whooping cough

- tetanus
- urinary tract infections

Viruses cause many childhood diseases including:

- common colds
- influenzas
- diarrhea from rotaviruses
- measles
- mumps
- rubella (German measles)
- chicken pox
- polio
- hepatitis
- human papillomavirus (HPV)
- herpes
- HIV/AIDS

Fungi cause various infectious diseases including:

- thrush, a mouth and throat infection in infants caused by *Candida albicans*
- skin conditions, such as ringworm and athlete's foot
- pneumonia caused by *Pneumocystis carinii*

Protozoan parasites cause infectious diseases such as malaria, **giardiasis**, and toxoplasmosis. Helminths are larger parasites—such as tapeworms and roundworms—that can infect the intestinal tract, lungs, liver, skin, or brain.

Symptoms of infectious disease vary with the type of infection. However many infectious diseases have symptoms that include:

- fever and chills
- loss of appetite
- muscle aches
- fatigue

Diagnosis

Examination

A medical history and physical exam—including the child's breathing pattern and respiratory rate, body temperature, and other symptoms—may be sufficient for diagnosing an infectious disease. Sometimes an infectious organism in a blood or urine sample can be seen under a microscope.

Tests

Blood, urine, throat swabs, or other bodily secretions may be cultured in a laboratory to identify the infective agent. Diagnosis of some infectious diseases requires a **lumbar puncture** or spinal tap to obtain a sample of cerebrospinal fluid.

KEY TERMS

Bacteria—Single-celled microorganisms that live in soil, water, organic matter, plants, and animals, and are associated with a number of infectious diseases.

Fungi—A kingdom of saprophytic and parasitic spore-producing organisms that include mushrooms and yeast.

Helminths—Parasitic worms, such as tapeworms or liver flukes, that can live in the human body.

Immunization—Treatment, usually by vaccination, to produce immunity to a specific infective agent.

Meningitis—An infection or inflammation of membranes surrounding the brain and spinal cord.

Pneumococcal—Infection by the bacterium *Streptococcus pneumoniae*) that causes acute pneumonia.

Pneumonia—Inflammation of the lungs, usually caused by infection with a bacterium, virus, or fungus.

Protozoa—Single-celled microorganisms of the Kingdom Protista, some of which can cause infectious disease in humans.

Vaccine—A preparation of live, weakened, or killed microorganisms that is administered to produce or increase immunity to specific diseases.

Procedures

Diagnostic procedures may include:

- a chest x ray to diagnose pneumonia
- computerized tomography (CT) scans or magnetic resonance imaging (MRI)
- a biopsy—the removal of a tiny amount of tissue from an infected area, such as the lung for diagnosing fungal pneumonia

Treatment

Traditional

Treatment depends on the type of infectious disease. Some diseases resolve on their own without any treatment other than possibly relieving symptoms.

Drugs

- Bacterial infections are treated with antibiotics.
- A very few antiviral drugs, such as acyclovir, are available for treating viral infections such as flu and herpes.

- Various drugs may be used to treat hepatitis B and C.
- HIV/AIDS is treated with a combination of drugs known as highly active antiretroviral therapy (HAART).
- Fungal infections of the skin and nails may be treated with over-the-counter or prescription medications applied directly to the affected area.
- Oral antifungal medications are used to treat systemic fungal infections, such as histoplasmosis, or severe infections of the mouth and throat in children with weakened immune systems.
- Only a very few anti-parasitic drugs are available and some of these are either very toxic or are becoming less effective with the spread of drug-resistant parasites.

Alternative

A wide variety of alternative therapies are used to treat infectious disease, although bacterial infections usually require **antibiotics**. Yogurt containing healthy gut bacteria can ease gastrointestinal symptoms and has been shown to reduce the incidence of some common infections in children.

Home remedies

Many mild infectious diseases respond well to home remedies. Bed rest and drinking plenty of fluids are the most common remedies.

Prognosis

Prognosis varies greatly depending on the type of infectious disease. Some, such as the **common cold**, usually resolve quickly without medical treatment, and most infectious diseases have only minor complications. However some—such as pneumonia or meningitis—can be life-threatening. Even some common and usually mild infectious diseases—such as **measles**, **mumps**, chicken pox, or seasonal flu—can be dangerous or life-threatening in very young children.

Prevention

Many common infectious diseases are preventable with good hygiene and vaccines. The best protection is frequent and thorough hand washing:

- before, during, and after handling food
- before eating
- after using the toilet
- after changing diapers
- after touching animals or their toys, leashes, or waste
- after touching trash, cleaning rags, drains, or soil
- after contact with body fluids, including blood, vomit, saliva, or nasal secretions
- before cleaning a wound, administering medicine, or inserting contact lenses
- more often, if someone in the home is ill

Hands should be washed by:

- wetting with water and applying soap
- rubbing them together vigorously to lather and scrub all surfaces for 20 seconds
- rinsing well under running water
- drying with a paper towel or air dryer
- turning off the faucet with a paper towel
- using alcohol-based disposable hand wipes or sanitizers if soap and water are not available

Other practices for preventing infectious disease include:

- breastfeeding, which helps protect infants from respiratory and gastrointestinal infections
- avoiding touching one's eyes, nose, and mouth
- covering one's mouth and nose when coughing or sneezing
- rinsing fresh fruit and vegetables under running water and scrubbing firm-skinned produce with a vegetable brush
- keeping meat, poultry, seafood, and eggs separated from other foods at all times
- refrigerating foods promptly at a constant temperature of 40°F (4°C) or below, with enough room for cold air to circulate freely
- freezing foods at 0°F (–18°C) or below
- using separate cutting boards for produce and meat, poultry, seafood, or eggs
- washing cutting boards, dishes, utensils, and counter tops with hot, soapy water between preparation of each food item
- never reusing marinades from raw foods without boiling first
- thoroughly cooking all foods, especially meat, at the correct temperature
- cleaning with disposable paper towels or sanitizing wipes, cloth towels that are washed in hot water, or sponges that are washed in the dishwasher or microwaved daily for 30 seconds
- cleaning and disinfecting all bathroom surfaces, especially when someone in the home has an infectious disease

- avoiding sharing personal items, including toothbrushes, combs, drinking glasses, and eating utensils
- keeping children home when they are sick
- not flying when ill
- practicing safer sex or abstaining from sex entirely to avoid sexually transmitted infections that can be passed to unborn children

Precautions against contracting infectious disease from animals include:

- adopting pets from an animal shelter or purchasing from a reputable store or breeder
- obtaining routine care and immunizations for your pet from a veterinarian
- obeying leash laws
- cleaning litter boxes daily, except when a person is pregnant
- keeping children away from pet waste
- keeping sandboxes covered
- washing one's hands thoroughly after contact with animals
- keeping wild animals away from the house
- using insect repellent and routinely checking for ticks and removing them immediately by applying gentle, steady pressure with tweezers

Children should be immunized as follows:

- at birth or as soon as possible: hepatitis B (HBV)
- at 1–4 months: HBV
- at 2 months: diphtheria, tetanus, and acellular pertussis (DTaP); haemophilus influenza type b (Hib); inactivated poliovirus (IPV); pneumococcal conjugate (PCV); rotavirus (RV)
- 4 months: DTaP; Hib; IPV; PCV; RV
- 6 months: DTaP; Hib; PCV; RV
- 6 months and annually: seasonal flu
- 6–18 months: HBV; IPV
- 12–15 months: varicella (chicken pox, Var); Hib; PCV; measles, mumps, and rubella (MMR)
- 12–23 months: hepatitis A (HepA)
- 15–18 months: DTaP
- 4–6 years: IPV; Var; DTaP; MMR
- 11–12 years: DTaP booster; meningitis (MCV)
- girls at 11–12 years: human papillomavirus (HPV) to prevent genital warts and cervical cancer
- additional immunizations for foreign travel

Resources

BOOKS

Finn, Adam, and Andrew J. Pollard, editors. *Hot Topics in Infection and Immunity in Children IV.* New York: Springer, 2008.

Shah, Samir S., editor. *Pediatric Practice: Infectious Diseases.* New York: McGraw-Hill Medical, 2009.

Shannon, Joyce Brennfleck. *Contagious Diseases Sourcebook: Basic Consumer Information About Disease Spread from Person to Person,* 2nd ed. Detroit: Omnigraphics, 2010.

PERIODICALS

Black, Robert E., et al. "Global, Regional, and National Causes of Child Mortality in 2008: A Systematic Analysis." *Lancet* 375 (9730) (June 5-11, 2010): 1969-87.

Khor, Chiea C., et al. "CISH and Susceptibility to Infectious Diseases." *New England Journal of Medicine* 362 (22) (June 3, 2010): 2092.

Rockoff, Jonathan D. "More Parents Seek Vaccine Exemption." *Wall Street Journal* (July 6, 2010): A19.

"Science and Technology: Mens Sana in Corpore Sano; Disease and Intelligence." *Economist* 396 (8689) (July 3, 2010): 75.

OTHER

"Breast Milk Reduces Infections in Babies." HealthDay. June 21, 2010. [Accessed September 26, 2010], http://www.nlm.nih.gov/medlineplus/news/fullstory_100207.html.

"Childhood Diseases: What Parents Should Know." MedlinePlus. Spring 2008. [Accessed September 26, 2010], http://www.nlm.nih.gov/medlineplus/magazine/issues/pdf/spring2008.pdf.

"Infectious Diseases." MedlinePlus. June 30, 2010. [Accessed September 26, 2010], http://www.nlm.nih.gov/medlineplus/infectiousdiseases.html.

Mayo Clinic Staff. "Germs: Understand and Protect Against Bacteria, Viruses and Infection." MayoClinic.com. April 30, 2009. [Accessed September 26, 2010], http://www.mayoclinic.com/health/germs/ID00002/METHOD=-print.

Mayo Clinic Staff. "Infectious Diseases." MayoClinic.com. July 21, 2009. [Accessed September 26, 2010], http://www.mayoclinic.com/health/infectious–diseases/DS01145.

"An Ounce of Prevention Keeps the Germs Away: Seven Keys to a Safer Healthier Home." Centers for Disease Control and Prevention. [Accessed September 26, 2010], http://www.cdc.gov/ounceofprevention/docs/oop_brochure_eng.pdf.

"Understanding Microbes in Sickness and in Health." National Institute of Allergy and Infectious Diseases. September 2009. [September 26, 2010], http://www.niaid.nih.gov/topics/microbes/documents/microbesbook.pdf.

ORGANIZATIONS

National Foundation for Infectious Diseases (NFID), 4733 Bethesda Ave., Suite 750, Bethesda MD, 20814, (301)

656-0003, (301) 907-0878, info@nfid.org, http://www.nfid.org.

National Institute of Allergy and Infectious Diseases, Office of Communications and Public Liaison (NIAID), 6610 Rockledge Dr., Bethesda MD, 20892–66123, (866) 284-4107, http://www3.niaid.nih.gov.

U.S. Centers for Disease Control and Prevention (CDC), 1600 Clifton Rd., Atlanta GA, 30333, (800) CDC-INFO (232-4636), cdcinfo@cdc.gov, http://www.cdc.gov.

Margaret Alic, PhD

Infectious mononucleosis

Definition

Infectious mononucleosis is a contagious illness caused by the Epstein-Barr virus that can affect the liver, lymph nodes, and oral cavity. While mononucleosis is not usually a serious disease, its primary symptoms of fatigue and lack of energy can linger for several months.

Description

Infectious mononucleosis, frequently called "mono" or the "kissing disease," is caused by the Epstein-Barr virus (EBV) found in saliva and mucus. The virus affects a type of white blood cell called the B-lymphocyte producing characteristic atypical lymphocytes that may be useful in the diagnosis of the disease.

While anyone, even young children, can develop mononucleosis, it occurs most often in young adults between the ages of 15 and 35 and is especially common in teenagers. The mononucleosis infection rate among college students who have not previously been exposed to EBV has been estimated to be about 15%. In younger children, the illness may not be recognized.

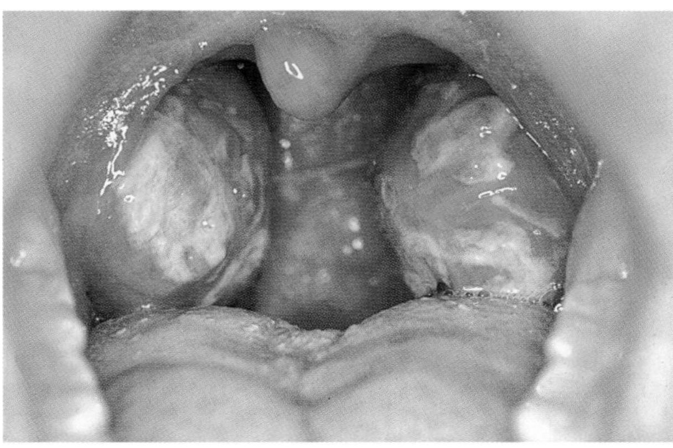

Sore throat and swollen tonsils caused by infectious mononucleosis, frequently called mono or the kissing disease. *(Dr. P. Marazzi/Science Photo Library/Photo Researchers, Inc.)*

The disease typically runs its course in four to six weeks in people with normally functioning immune systems. People with weakened or suppressed immune systems, such as **AIDS** patients or those who have had organ transplants, are particularly vulnerable to the potentially serious complications of infectious mononucleosis.

Causes and symptoms

The EBV that causes mononucleosis is related to a group of herpes viruses, including those that cause **cold sores**, chickenpox, and shingles. Most people are exposed to EBV at some point during their lives. Mononucleosis is most commonly spread by contact with virus-infected saliva through coughing, sneezing, kissing, or sharing drinking glasses or eating utensils.

In addition to general weakness and fatigue, symptoms of mononucleosis may include any or all of the following:

- Sore throat and/or swollen tonsils
- Fever and chills
- Nausea and vomiting, or decreased appetite
- Swollen lymph nodes in the neck and armpits
- Headaches or joint pain
- Enlarged spleen
- Jaundice
- Skin rash.

Complications that can occur with mononucleosis include a temporarily enlarged spleen or inflamed liver. In rare instances, the spleen may rupture, producing sharp **pain** on the left side of the abdomen, a symptom that warrants immediate medical attention. Additional symptoms of a ruptured spleen include light headedness, rapidly beating heart, and difficulty breathing. Other rare, but potentially life-threatening complications may involve the heart or brain. The infection may also cause significant destruction of the body's red blood cells or platelets.

Symptoms do not usually appear until four to seven weeks after exposure to EBV. An infected person can be contagious during this incubation time period and for as many as five months after the disappearance of symptoms. Also, the virus will be excreted in the saliva intermittently for the rest of their lives, although the individual will experience no symptoms. Contrary to popular belief, the EBV is not highly contagious. As a result, individuals living in a household or college dormitory with someone who has mononucleosis have

KEY TERMS

Antibody—A specific protein produced by the immune system in response to a specific foreign protein or particle called an antigen.

Herpes viruses—A group of viruses that can cause cold sores, shingles, chicken pox, and congenital abnormalities. The Epstein-Barr virus which causes mononucleosis belongs to this group of viruses.

Reye's syndrome—A very serious, rare disease, most common in children, which involves an upper respiratory tract infection followed by brain and liver damage.

a very small risk of being infected unless they have direct contact with the person's saliva.

Diagnosis

If symptoms associated with a cold persist longer than two weeks, mononucleosis is a possibility; however, a variety of other conditions can produce similar symptoms. If mononucleosis is suspected, a physician will typically conduct a physical examination, including a "Monospot" antibody blood test that can indicate the presence of proteins or antibodies produced in response to infection with the EBV. These antibodies may not be detectable, however, until the second or third weeks of the illness. Occasionally, when this test is inconclusive, other blood tests may be conducted.

Treatment

The most effective treatment for infectious mononucleosis is rest and a gradual return to regular activities. Individuals with mild cases may not require bed rest but should limit their activities. Any strenuous activity, athletic endeavors, or heavy lifting should be avoided until the symptoms completely subside, since excessive activity may cause the spleen to rupture.

The **sore throat** and **dehydration** that usually accompany mononucleosis may be relieved by drinking water and fruit juices. Gargling salt water or taking throat lozenges may also relieve discomfort. In addition, taking over-the-counter medications, such as **acetaminophen** or ibuprofen, may relieve symptoms, but aspirin should be avoided because mononucleosis has been associated with **Reye's syndrome**, a serious illness aggravated by aspirin.

While **antibiotics** do not affect EBV, the sore throat accompanying mononucleosis can be complicated by a streptococcal infection, which can be treated with antibiotics. Cortisone anti-inflammatory medications are also occasionally prescribed for the treatment of severely swollen tonsils or throat tissues.

Prognosis

While the severity and length of illness varies, most people diagnosed with mononucleosis will be able to return to their normal daily routines within two to three weeks, particularly if they rest during this time period. It may take two to three months before a person's usual energy levels return. One of the most common problems in treating mononucleosis, particularly in teenagers, is that people return to their usual activities too quickly and then experience a relapse of symptoms. Once the disease has completely run its course, the person cannot be re-infected.

Prevention

Although there is no way to avoid becoming infected with EBV, paying general attention to good hygiene and avoiding sharing beverage glasses or having close contact with people who have mononucleosis or cold symptoms can help prevent infection.

Resources

OTHER

"Communicable Disease Fact Sheet." New York State Department of Health. November 2006. [Accessed December 8, 2010], http://www.nyhealth.gov/diseases/communicable/mononucleosis/fact_sheet.htm.

"Mononucleosis: A Tiresome Disease." *Mayo Clinic Online*. [Accessed December 8, 2010], http://www.mayoclinic.com/health/mononucleosis/DS00352.

ORGANIZATIONS

National Institute of Allergy and Infectious Disease 31 Center Drive MSC 2520, Building 31, Room 7A-50, Bethesda MD, 20892-2520, (301) 496-5717, (800) 877-8339 (TTY), http://www.niaid.nih.gov/default.htm.

Susan J. Montgomery

Influenza

Definition

Usually referred to as the flu or grippe, influenza is a highly infectious respiratory disease. The disease is caused by certain strains of the influenza virus. When the virus is inhaled, it attacks cells in the upper respiratory tract, causing typical flu symptoms such as fatigue, **fever** and chills, a hacking **cough**, and body aches. Influenza victims are also susceptible to potentially life-threatening

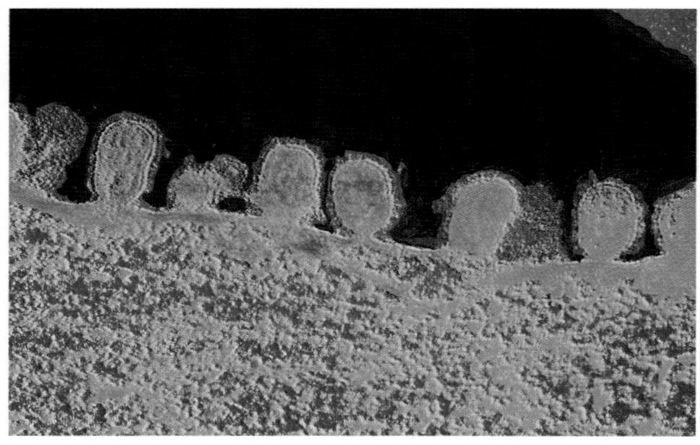

A transmission electron micrograph (TEM) of influenza viruses budding from the surface of an infected cell. *(SPL/ Photo Researchers, Inc.)*

secondary infections. Although the stomach or intestinal "flu" is commonly blamed for stomach upsets and **diarrhea**, the influenza virus rarely causes gastrointestinal symptoms. Such symptoms are most likely due to other organisms such as rotavirus, *Salmonella*, *Shigella*, or *Escherichia coli*.

Description

The flu is considerably more debilitating than the **common cold**. Influenza outbreaks occur suddenly and infection spreads rapidly. The annual **death** toll attributable to influenza and its complications averages 20,000 in the United States alone. In the 1918–1919 Spanish flu pandemic, the death toll reached a staggering 20–40 million worldwide. Approximately 500,000 of these fatalities occurred in America.

Influenza outbreaks occur on a regular basis. The most serious outbreaks are pandemics, which affect millions of people worldwide and last for several months. The 1918–1919 influenza outbreak serves as the primary example of an influenza pandemic. Pandemics also occurred in 1957 and 1968 with the Asian flu and Hong Kong flu, respectively. The Asian flu was responsible for 70,000 deaths in the United States, while the Hong Kong flu killed 34,000.

Epidemics are widespread regional outbreaks that occur every two to three years and affect 5–10% of the population. The Russian flu in the winter of 1977 is an example of an epidemic. A regional epidemic is shorter lived than a pandemic, lasting only several weeks. Finally, there are smaller outbreaks each winter that are confined to specific locales.

The earliest existing descriptions of influenza were written nearly 2500 years ago by the ancient Greek physician Hippocrates. Historically, influenza was ascribed to a number of different agents, including "bad air" and several different bacteria. In fact, its name comes from the Italian word for "influence" because people in 18th century Europe thought that the disease was caused by the influence of bad weather. It was not until 1933 that the causative agent was identified\as a virus.

There are three types of influenza viruses, identified as A, B, and C. Influenza A can infect a range of animal species, including humans, pigs, horses, and birds, but only humans are infected by types B and C. Influenza A is responsible for most flu cases, while infection with types B and C virus are less common and cause a milder illness.

In the United States, 90% of all deaths from influenza occur among persons older than 65. Flu-related deaths have increased substantially in the United States since the 1970s, largely because of the aging of the American population. In addition, elderly persons are vulnerable because they are often reluctant to be vaccinated against flu.

A new concern regarding influenza is the possibility that hostile groups or governments could use the virus as an agent of bioterrorism. A report published in early 2003 noted that Type A influenza virus has a high potential for use as such an agent because of the virulence of the Type A strain that broke out in Hong Kong in 1997 and the development of laboratory methods for generating large quantities of the virus. The report recommended the stockpiling of present **antiviral drugs** and speeding up the development of new ones.

Causes and symptoms

Approximately one to four days after infection with the influenza virus, the victim is hit with an array of symptoms. "Hit" is an appropriate term because symptoms are sudden, harsh, and unmistakable. Typical influenza symptoms include the abrupt onset of a **headache**, dry cough, and chills, rapidly followed by overall achiness and a fever that may run as high as 104°F (40°C). As the fever subsides, nasal congestion and a **sore throat** become noticeable. Flu victims feel extremely tired and weak and may not return to their normal energy levels for several days or even a couple of weeks.

Influenza complications usually arise from bacterial infections of the lower respiratory tract. Signs of a secondary respiratory infection often appear just as the victim seems to be recovering. These signs include high fever, intense chills, chest pains associated with breathing, and a productive cough with thick yellowish green sputum. If these symptoms appear, medical treatment is necessary. Other secondary infections, such as sinus or ear infections, may also require medical intervention.

Heart and lung problems, and other chronic diseases, can be aggravated by influenza, which is a particular concern with elderly patients.

With children and teenagers, it is advisable to be alert for symptoms of **Reye's syndrome**, a rare, but serious complication. Symptoms of Reye's syndrome are nausea and **vomiting**, and more seriously, neurological problems such as confusion or delirium. The syndrome has been associated with the use of aspirin to relieve flu symptoms.

Diagnosis

Although there are specific tests to identify the flu virus strain from respiratory samples, doctors typically rely on a set of symptoms and the presence of influenza in the community for diagnosis. Specific tests are useful to determine the type of flu in the community but they do little for individual treatment. Doctors may administer tests, such as throat cultures, to identify secondary infections.

Since 1999, however, seven rapid diagnostic tests for flu have become commercially available. These tests appear to be especially useful in diagnosing flu in children, allowing doctors to make more accurate treatment decisions in less time.

Treatment

Essentially, a bout of influenza must be allowed to run its course. Symptoms can be relieved with bed rest and by keeping well hydrated. A steam vaporizer may make breathing easier, and **pain** relievers will take care of the aches and pain. Food may not seem very appetizing but an effort should be made to consume nourishing food. Recovery should not be pushed too rapidly. Returning to normal activities too quickly invites a possible relapse or complications.

Drugs

Since influenza is a viral infection, **antibiotics** are useless in treating it. However, antibiotics are frequently used to treat secondary infections.

Over-the-counter medications are used to treat flu symptoms but it is not necessary to purchase a medication marketed specifically for flu symptoms. Any medication that is designed to relieve symptoms, such as pain and coughing, will provide some relief. Medications containing alcohol, however, should be avoided because of the dehydrating effects of alcohol. The best medicine for symptoms is simply an analgesic, such as aspirin, **acetaminophen**, or naproxen. Without a doctor's approval, aspirin is generally not recommended for people under 18 owing to its association with Reye's syndrome, a rare aspirin-associated complication seen in children recovering from the flu. To be on the safe side, children should receive acetaminophen or ibuprofen to treat their symptoms.

There are four antiviral drugs marketed for treating influenza. To be effective, treatment should begin no later than two days after symptoms appear. Antivirals may be useful in treating patients who have weakened immune systems or who are at risk for developing serious complications. They include amantadine (Symmetrel, Symadine) and rimantadine (Flumandine), which work against Type A influenza, and zanamavir (Relenza) and oseltamavir phosphate (Tamiflu), which work against both Types A and B influenza. Amantadine and rimantadine can cause side effects such as nervousness, **anxiety**, lightheadedness, and nausea. Severe side effects include seizures, delirium, and hallucination, but are rare and are nearly always limited to people who have kidney problems, seizure disorders, or psychiatric disorders. The new drugs zanamavir and oseltamavir phosphate have few side effects but can cause **dizziness**, jitters, and insomnia.

Alternative treatments

There are several alternative treatments that may help in fighting off the virus and recovering from the flu, in addition to easing flu symptoms.

- Acupuncture and acupressure. Both are said to stimulate natural resistance, relieve nasal congestion and headaches, fight fever, and calm coughs, depending on the acupuncture and acupressure points used.
- Aromatherapy. Aromatherapists recommend gargling daily with one drop each of the essential oils of tea tree (*Melaleuca* spp.) and lemon mixed in a glass of warm water. If already suffering from the flu, two drops of tea tree oil in a hot bath may help ease the symptoms. Essential oils of eucalyptus (*Eucalyptus globulus*) or peppermint (*Mentha piperita*) added to a steam vaporizer may help clear chest and nasal congestion.
- Herbal remedies. Herbal remedies can be used stimulate the immune system (echinacea), as antivirals (*Hydrastis canadensis*) goldenseal and garlic (*Allium sativum*), or directed at whatever symptoms arise as a result of the flu. For example, an infusion of boneset (*Eupatroium perfoliatum*) may counteract aches and fever, and yarrow (*Achillea millefolium*) or elderflower tinctures may combat chills.
- Homeopathy. To prevent flu, a homeopathic remedy called *Oscillococcinum* may be taken at the first sign of flu symptoms and repeated for a day or two. Although oscillococcinum is a popular flu remedy in Europe, however, a research study published in 2003 found it to be ineffective. Other homeopathic remedies recommended

vary according to the specific flu symptoms present. *Gelsemium* (*Gelsemium sempervirens*) is recommended to combat weakness accompanied by chills, a headache, and nasal congestion. *Bryonia* (*Bryonia alba*) may be used to treat muscle aches, headaches, and a dry cough. For restlessness, chills, hoarseness, and achy joints, poison ivy (*Rhus toxicodendron*) is recommended. Finally, for achiness and a dry cough or chills, *Eupatorium perfoliatum* is suggested.

- Hydrotherapy. A bath to induce a fever will speed recovery from the flu by creating an environment in the body where the flu virus cannot survive. The patient should take a bath as hot as he/she can tolerate and remain in the bath for 20–30 minutes. While in the bath, the patient drinks a cup of yarrow or elderflower tea to induce sweating. During the bath, a cold cloth is held on the forehead or at the nape of the neck to keep the temperature down in the brain. The patient is assisted when getting out of the bath (he/she may feel weak or dizzy) and then gets into bed and covers up with layers of blankets to induce more sweating.
- Traditional Chinese medicine (TCM). Practitioners of TCM recommend mixtures of herbs to prevent flu as well as to relieve symptoms once a person has fallen ill. There are several different recipes for these remedies but most contain ginger and Japanese honeysuckle in addition to other ingredients.
- Vitamins. For adults, 2–3 grams of vitamin C daily may help prevent the flu. Increasing the dose to 5–7 grams per day during the flu can felp fight the infection. (The dose should be reduced if diarrhea develops.)

Prognosis

Following proper treatment guidelines, healthy people under the age of 65 usually suffer no long-term consequences associated with flu infection. The elderly and the chronically ill are at greater risk for secondary infection and other complications but they can also enjoy a complete recovery.

Most people recover fully from an influenza infection but it should not be viewed complacently. Influenza is a serious disease and approximately 1 in 1,000 cases proves fatal.

Prevention

The Centers for Disease Control and Prevention recommend that people get an influenza vaccine injection each year before flu season starts. In the United States, flu season typically runs from late December to early March. Vaccines should be received two to six weeks prior to the onset of flu season to allow the body enough time to establish immunity. Adults only need one dose of the yearly vaccine but children under nine years of age who have not previously been immunized should receive two doses with a month between each dose.

Each season's flu vaccine contains three virus strains that are the most likely to be encountered in the coming flu season. When there is a good match between the anticipated flu strains and the strains used in the vaccine, the vaccine is 70–90% effective in people under 65. Because immune response diminishes somewhat with age, people over 65 may not receive the same level of protection from the vaccine; even if they do contract the flu, the vaccine diminishes the severity and helps prevent complications.

The virus strains used to make the vaccine are inactivated and will not cause the flu. In the past, flu symptoms were associated with vaccine preparations that were not as highly purified as modern vaccines, not to the virus itself. In 1976, there was a slightly increased risk of developing Guillain-Barré syndrome, a very rare disorder, associated with the swine flu vaccine. This association occurred only with the 1976 swine flu vaccine preparation and has never recurred.

Serious side effects with modern vaccines are extremely unusual. Some people experience a slight soreness at the point of injection, which resolves within a day or two. People who have never been exposed to influenza, particularly children, may experience one to two days of a slight fever, tiredness, and muscle aches. These symptoms start within 6–12 hours after the **vaccination**.

It should be noted that certain people should not receive an influenza vaccine. Infants six months and younger have immature immune systems and will not benefit from the vaccine. Since the vaccines are prepared using hen eggs, people who have severe **allergies** to eggs or other vaccine components should not receive the influenza vaccine. As an alternative, they may receive a course of amantadine or rimantadine, which are also used as a protective measure against influenza. Other people who might receive these drugs are those that have been immunized after the flu season has started or who are immunocompromised, such as people with advanced HIV disease. Amantadine and rimantadine are 70–90% effective in preventing influenza.

There are two types of influenza vaccines: the flu shot and the flu mist. The flu shot consists of inactivated (killed) influenza viruses and is given by injection into the muscle. With the flu mist, the live, attenuated (weakened) influenza vaccine (LAIV) is sprayed into the nostrils but this type of vaccination is not recommended for persons over the age of 49. Both injectable and mist vaccine typically contain three influenza viruses, two of

KEY TERMS

Bioterrorism—The intentional use of disease-causing microbes or other biologic agents to intimidate or terrorize a civilian population for political or military reasons. Type A influenza virus could be used as an agent of bioterrorism.

Common cold—A mild illness caused by upper respiratory viruses. Usual symptoms include nasal congestion, coughing, sneezing, throat irritation, and a low-grade fever.

Epidemic—A widespread regional disease outbreak.

Guillain-Barré syndrome—Also called acute idiopathic polyneuritis, this condition is a neurologic syndrome that can cause numbness in the limbs and muscle weakness following certain viral infections.

Pandemic—A worldwide outbreak of an infection, afflicting millions of victims.

type A virus and one of type B virus. The strain of viruses included in the vaccine change yearly based on international surveillance data of influenza cases and estimations by scientists on what types and strains of viruses will be prevalent in the coming influenza season. When the strains included in the vaccine are well matched to the strains present in the community, the vaccine usually can protect seven to nine out of ten vaccinated persons. However, in elderly people, the vaccine may not work as well in preventing influenza, but will result in decrease in severity of symptoms and in the risk of health complications.

In April 2009, the United States Department of Health and Human Services declared a public health emergency regarding human cases of H1N1 influenza A, more commonly called swine flu. Swine flu was of special concern because for several reasons. Experts believed that the virus was a new strain of influenza with a genetic composition different from the familiar viruses that cause seasonal influenza. Because it was radically different, individuals were especially susceptible to developing serious illness. In addition, the virus often caused more intense symptoms in young, healthy people than in the elderly or the very young who are the greatest target of seasonal flu. Because the decision had already been made about which strains of seasonal flu were to be included in the vaccine for the next flu season and manufacture had already begun, a special push was made to make a separate vaccine against the swine flu. Thus, in the winter of 2009 through the 2010 flu season, people were advised to get two separate flu shots, one against seasonal flu and one against the new H1N1 influenza A.

Certain groups are strongly advised to be vaccinated because they are at increased risk for influenza-related complications:

- All people 65 years and older
- Residents of nursing homes and chronic-care facilities, regardless of age
- Adults and children who have chronic heart or lung problems, such as asthma
- Adults and children who have chronic metabolic diseases, such as diabetes and renal dysfunction, as well as severe anemia or inherited hemoglobin disorders
- Children and teenagers who are on long-term aspirin therapy
- Women who will be in their second or third trimester during flu season or women who are nursing
- Anyone who is immunocompromised, including HIV-infected persons, cancer patients, organ transplant recipients, and patients receiving steroids, chemotherapy, or radiation therapy
- Anyone in contact with the above groups, such as teachers, care givers, health-care personnel, and family members
- Travelers to foreign countries.

A person need not be in one of the at-risk categories listed above, however, to receive a flu vaccination. Anyone who wants to forego the discomfort and inconvenience of an influenza attack may receive the vaccine.

Resources

BOOKS

Beers, Mark H., MD, and Robert Berkow, MD, editors. "Respiratory Viral Diseases: Influenza." In *The Merck Manual of Diagnosis and Therapy.* 18th ed., Whitehouse Station, NJ: Merck Research Laboratories, 2006.

Pelletier, Kenneth R., MD. *The Best Alternative Medicine*, Part II. "CAM Therapies for Specific Conditions: Colds/Flu." New York: Simon & Schuster, 2002.

PERIODICALS

Elkins, Rita. "Combat Colds and Flu." *Let's Live.* 68 (January 2000): 81+.

Jonas, W. B., T. J. Kaptchuk, and K. Linde. "A Critical Overview of Homeopathy." *Annals of Internal Medicine* 138 (March 4, 2003): 393-399.

Krug, R. M. "The Potential Use of Influenza Virus as an Agent for Bioterrorism." *Antiviral Research* 57 (January 2003): 147-150.

Oxford, J. S., S. Bossuyt, S. Balasingam, et al. "Treatment of Epidemic and Pandemic Influenza with Neuraminidase and M2 Proton Channel Inhibitors." *Clinical Microbiology and Infection* 9 (January 2003): 1-14.

Roth, Y., J. S. Chapnik, and P. Cole. "Feasibility of Aerosol Vaccination in Humans." *Annals of Otology, Rhinology, and Laryngology* 112 (March 2003): 264-270.

Shortridge, K. F., J. S. Peiris, and Y. Guan. "The Next Influenza Pandemic: Lessons from Hong Kong." *Journal of Applied Microbiology* 94, Supplement (2003): 70S-79S.

Storch, G. A. "Rapid Diagnostic Tests for Influenza." *Current Opinion in Pediatrics* 15 (February 2003): 77-84.

Thompson, W. W., D. K. Shay, E. Weintraub, et al. "Mortality Associated with Influenza and Respiratory Syncytial Virus in the United States." *Journal of the American Medical Association* 289 (January 8, 2003): 179-186.

OTHER

"Flu (Influenza): 2009 H1N1, Seasonal, Avian (Bird), Pandemic." National Institute of Allergy and Infectious Diseases. December 6, 2010, [Accessed December 8, 2010]http://www.niaid.nih.gov/topics/Flu/Pages/default.aspx.

"About the Flu." United States Department of Health and Human Services. [Accessed December 8, 2010], http://www.flu.gov/individualfamily/about/index.html.

ORGANIZATIONS

Centers for Disease Control and Prevention (CDC), 1600 Clifton Road, Atlanta GA, 30333, (404) 498-1515, (800) 311-3435, http://www.cdc.gov.

National Institute of Allergy and Infectious Disease, 31 Center Drive MSC 2520, Building 31, Room 7A-50, Bethesda MD, 20892-2520 (301) 496-5717, (800) 877-8339 (TTY), http://www.niaid.nih.gov/default.htm.

Julia Barrett
Rebecca J. Frey, PhD

Influenza vaccination

Definition

An **influenza vaccination** is a vaccination that is used to protect individuals against the viruses that cause influenza, which is also called the flu.

Purpose

Influenza vaccination helps to protect people against getting influenza. Protection is imperfect because the viruses that cause influenza are constantly changing (mutating). Influenza vaccines are updated every year to reflect the current stains of flu that are most expected to be most prevalent and re-vaccination is recommended every year.

Description

Every year in the United States, about 226,000 people are hospitalized and 36,000 die of influenza-related complications, most often bacterial **pneumonia**, **dehydration**, or a worsening of chronic medical conditions, such as congestive heart failure, **asthma**, or diabetes. 90% of the deaths occur in individuals 65 years and older. During influenza epidemics, hospitalization rates for older people increase 2–5 times compared to other seasons of the year and more than half of the hospitalizations are people 65 and older.

An influenza vaccination is the best way to be protected from contracting influenza. Older Hispanic and African-American adults are much less likely to be vaccinated against influenza than their white counterparts. The rate of vaccination of senior citizens as of 2005 was 65% in the U.S. African-Americans 65 years and older lag behind whites by about 21% in getting annual vaccinations, while Hispanic Americans 65 years and older lag behind whites by 19%. In large urban areas with high levels of unvaccinated persons, there is a potential for outbreaks of influenza; thus improving overall immunization coverage rates is essential. Studies have also shown that elderly people who choose to be vaccinated are generally in better health than those who fail to get the vaccine so influenza control strategies should be developed to target those who are not being vaccinated. The United States Center for Disease Control (CDC) has set a target date of 2010 to increase influenza vaccinations to 90% among all adults aged 65 years and older with an emphasis on vaccinating minority groups. In the U.S. the influenza vaccination is provided at no cost to all senior citizens covered by Medicare.

There are two types of influenza vaccines: the flu shot and the flu mist. The flu shot consists of inactivated (killed) influenza viruses and is given by injection into the muscle. With the flu mist, the live attenuated (weakened) influenza vaccine (LAIV) is sprayed into the nostrils but this type of vaccination is not recommended for persons over the age of 49. Both injectable and mist vaccine typically contain three influenza viruses: two of type A virus and one of type B virus. The strain of viruses included in the vaccine change yearly based on international surveillance data of influenza cases and estimations by scientists on what types and strains of viruses will be prevalent in the coming influenza season. When the strains included in the vaccine are well matched to the strains present in the community, the vaccine usually can protect 7–9 out of 10 vaccinated persons. However, in elderly people, the vaccine may not work as well in preventing influenza, but will result in decrease in severity of symptoms and in the risk of health complications.

In April 2009, the United States Department of Health and Human Services declared a public health emergency regarding human cases of H1N1 influenza A, more commonly called swine flu. Swine flu was of special concern for several reasons. Experts believed that the virus was a new strain of influenza with a genetic composition different from the familiar viruses that cause seasonal influenza. Because it was radically different, individuals were especially susceptible to developing serious illness. In addition, the virus often caused more intense symptoms in young, healthy people than in the elderly or the very young who are the greatest target of seasonal flu. Because the decision had already been made about which strains of seasonal flu were to be included in the vaccine for the next flu season and manufacturing had already begun, a special push was made to make a separate vaccine against the swine flu. Thus, in the winter of 2009 through the 2010 flu season, people were advised to get two separate flu shots, one against seasonal flu and one against the new H1N1 influenza A.

Vaccinations against influenza are especially important for those who are not in good health. The vaccination is recommended for persons who have trouble swallowing or breathing, are receiving long term steroid therapy, or who have had heart attacks, heart disease, lung diseases such as asthma, emphysema, or chronic **bronchitis**, diabetes, HIV, blood disorders, such as sickle cell **anemia** or other hemoglobinopathies, kidney or liver disease, or weakened immune systems. Individuals with such conditions are at an increased risk of developing serious influenza-related complications. Those who are at a high risk of complications and who have not received their influenza vaccination the preceding fall or winter should be vaccinated before travel to the tropics, travel with tourist groups, or travel to the Southern Hemisphere between April and September.

KEY TERMS

Guillain-Barre Syndrome—A disorder characterized by progressive symmetrical paralysis and loss of reflexes, usually beginning in the legs. The paralysis characteristically involves more than one limb (most commonly the legs), is progressive, and usually proceeds from the end of an extremity toward the torso. Guillain-Barre usually occurs after a respiratory infection, and it is apparently caused by a misdirected immune response that results in the direct destruction of the myelin sheath surrounding the peripheral nerves or of the axon of the nerve itself.

Influenza—Commonly known as flu; an infectious disease of birds and mammals caused by viruses of the family Orthomyxoviridae (the influenza viruses); common symptoms of the disease are the chills, then fever, sore throat, muscle pains, severe headache, coughing, weakness and general feelings of illness.

Vaccination—Injection of a killed or weakened microbe in order to stimulate the immune system against the microbe, thereby preventing disease. Vaccinations, or immunizations, work by stimulating the immune system, the natural disease-fighting system of the body. The healthy immune system is able to recognize invading bacteria and viruses and produce substances (antibodies) to destroy or disable them. Vaccinations prepare the immune system to ward off a disease. To immunize against viral diseases, the virus used in the vaccine has been weakened or killed.

Recommended dosage

As of 2010, the United States centers for Disease Control and Prevention (CDC) recommended that the following groups be vaccinated against seasonal influenza.

- children between the ages of 6 months and 19 years
- pregnant women
- all individuals age 50 or older
- people with certain chronic medical problems
- health care workers
- people caring for or living with children under age 5
- people caring for or living with someone at high risk for complications from influenza
- healthy individuals of any age who wish to reduce their chances of getting the flu, especially those living in group situations such as dormitories or military barracks

All persons 50 years of age and older should receive one dose intramuscularly of the inactivated seasonal influenza vaccine every year. Individuals ages 2–49 may be given flu mist rather than an injection. Ideally vaccination should occur during the period from September to mid-November but a vaccination received later may still be beneficial. Influenza can occur any time from November through May in the northern hemisphere, with cases usually peaking occurring in January or February. The influenza vaccine can safely be given with other vaccines, including the pneumococcal vaccine.

As of the 2009–2010 influenza season, additional vaccination against H1N1 swine flu was recommended for everyone with first responders, health care workers, and other high-risk individuals given priority.

Precautions

People who should not be vaccinated against influenza without first contacting a physician for advice include:

- those who have a severe allergy to chicken eggs
- those who have had a severe reaction to an influenza vaccination previously
- those who previously developed Guillain-Barre Syndrome (a very rare condition that results in weakness and paralysis of muscles of the body) within six weeks of getting an influenza vaccination

In addition, a person who has a moderate or severe illness with a **fever** should wait to get vaccinated until their symptoms decrease.

It takes up to two weeks to develop protection after the shot with the protection from the vaccination lasting up to one year.

Side effects

Although the risk of the influenza vaccine causing serious harm or is small, and is much less than the health risks from contracting influenza, the vaccine, as with any medicine, can cause problems such as severe allergic reactions. Because the viruses in the vaccine have been killed, no one can get influenza from the vaccine. Mild problems that can occur soon after the vaccination is given and lasting 1 to 2 days include:

- soreness, redness, or swelling where the shot was given
- low grade fever
- aches
- chills
- general feelings of ill health
- runny nose (flu mist only)
- wheezing (flu mist only)
- sore throat (flu mist only)

More severe problems that can be associated with the influenza vaccine are life-threatening allergic reactions. These will occur within a few minutes to a few hours after the shot. A person should stay in the clinic where the shot was given for 15 minutes in case an immediate reaction occurs. Such reactions could include **hives**, difficulty breathing, or swelling of the throat, tongue, or lips. If a severe reaction occurs after the person leaves the clinic, the affected person should immediately be taken to an emergency health care facility. The chance of such an adverse reaction occurring is estimated at less than one in a million people. Any adverse reaction should be reported to the U.S. Department of Heath and Human Services through the Vaccine Adverse Event Reporting Service. If a person has had a serious reaction to a vaccine, a federal program, the National Vaccine Injury Compensation Program, is available to help pay for the care of the person harmed or injured by the shot.

Interactions

Influenza vaccines are not known to interact with any drugs or foods.

Resources

OTHER

"Influenza Vaccine." Medline Plus. October 3, 2010. [Accessed December 8, 2010], http://www.nlm.nih.gov/medlineplus/ency/article/002025.htm.

"Flu Vaccine (Influenza Immunization)." MedicineNet.com. November 2, 2009. [Accessed December 8, 2010], http://www.medicinenet.com/flu_vaccination/article.htm.

"Vaccines." United States Centers for Disease Control and Prevention (CDC). March 30, 2010. [Accessed December 8, 2010], http://www.cdc.gov/vaccines.

ORGANIZATIONS

United States Centers for Disease Control and Prevention (CDC), 1600 Clifton Road, Atlanta GA, 30333, (404) 639-3534, 800-CDC-INFO (800-232-4636), TTY: (888) 232-6348, inquiry@cdc.gov, http://www.cdc.gov.

World Health Organization, Avenue Appia 20, 1211 Geneva 27 Switzerland, +22 41 791 21 11, +22 41 791 31 11, info@who.int, http://www.who.int.

Judith L. Sims
Tish Davidson, AM

Inhalants and related disorders

Definition

Inhalants are chemicals that are inhaled through the nose or mouth for a quick "high." They include a broad range of chemicals found in hundreds of different readily available products. Inhalant intoxication, abuse, and dependence are classified as substance use disorders.

Demographics

Inhalants are one of the few substance abuse disorders that more often affect younger children. Because inhalants are inexpensive and readily available,

Percentage of high school students who used inhalants,* by sex, race/ethnicity, and grade, 2009

	Female %	Male %	Total %
Race/ethnicity			
White†	12.8	10.4	**11.5**
Black†	9.4	7.1	**8.2**
Hispanic	15.3	12.8	**14.0**
Grade			
9	16.7	9.7	**13.0**
10	13.1	12.0	**12.5**
11	11.5	11.6	**11.5**
12	9.3	8.9	**9.1**
Total %	**12.9**	**10.6**	**11.7**

*Sniffed glue, breathed the contents of aerosol spray cans, or inhaled any paints or sprays to get high one or more times during their life
†Non-Hispanic

SOURCE: Centers for Disease Control and Prevention. Youth Risk Behavior Surveillance—United States, 2009. Surveillance Summaries, June 4, 2010. *MMWR* 2010;59(No. SS-5).

(Table by PreMediaGlobal. Reproduced by permission of Gale, a part of Cengage Learning.)

they are often used by children aged 6–16, as well as by people with little money. In 2008, two million Americans aged 12 and over abused inhalants. It has been estimated that 10–20% of youths aged 12–17 have tried inhalants and about 6% of Americans tried inhalants prior to the fourth grade. The peak period for inhalant use appears to be the 7th through 9th grades. However inhalant use among American teens may be on the decline.

Among adults and children younger than 12, inhalant use is more common among males than females. However there are no gender differences in inhalant use in teens between the ages of 12 and 17.

The use of inhalants and inhalant dependence are common among those who do not have access to other drugs or are otherwise isolated, such as prison inmates. As with other substance use disorders, people who have greater access to inhalants are more likely to develop dependence. This group includes workers in industrial settings.

Description

Inhalants include volatile solvents—liquids that vaporize at room temperature—and aerosols—sprays that contain both solvents and propellants. Examples of inhalants include:

- glue
- gasoline
- paint thinner
- hairspray
- lighter fluid
- spray paint
- nail polish remover
- correction fluid
- rubber cement
- felt-tip marker fluids
- vegetable sprays
- certain cleaners

Inhalants are generally used by breathing in the vapors directly from the container ("sniffing"), by inhaling fumes from substances placed in a bag ("bagging"), or by inhaling from a cloth soaked in the substance ("huffing"). Inhalants take effect very quickly because they enter the bloodstream directly from the lungs. The "high" from inhalants is usually brief so they are often used repeatedly over several hours. This pattern of use can be particularly dangerous, leading to unconsciousness or even **death**.

The American Psychiatric Association's *Diagnostic and Statistical Manual of Mental Disorders*, fourth edition, text revision (*DSM-IV-TR*) does not include use of anesthetic gases (such as nitrous oxide, chloroform, and ether) or nitrites (such as amyl and butyl nitrites) as inhalant-related disorders because they have slightly different intoxication properties. Rather, use of these substances is classified with other substance-related disorders. However the symptoms are very similar to those of inhalants and related disorders.

Although only a small proportion of inhalant use meets the diagnostic criteria for abuse or dependence, all use of chemical inhalants constitutes abuse since they are not being used for their intended purposes. Unlike all other substance dependencies, inhalants and related disorders may not result in clinically significant withdrawal syndromes. Instead inhalants are sometimes considered to be "gateway" drugs because inhalant use often precedes the use of other substances such as alcohol, **marijuana**, or cocaine.

Risk factors

Factors associated with inhalant disorders include poverty, a history of childhood abuse, poor grades, and dropping out of school. However the latter two factors may be a result of inhalant use rather than a cause. Inhalants are often used in group settings and are highly subject to peer influence.

Causes and symptoms

The symptoms of inhalant intoxication differ slightly depending on the type of inhalant, the amount used, and other factors. In general, intoxication from an inhalant usually occurs within 5 minutes and lasts for 5–30 minutes. Inhalants typically depress the central nervous system, with effects similar to those of alcohol, and produce euphoria, excitement, **dizziness**, and slurred speech. Inhalant intoxication can cause a feeling of floating or a sense of power.

An overdose of inhalant can result in coma or death. The most serious medical risk of inhalant use is "sudden sniffing death." Inhalants, especially repeated use in a single, prolonged session, can cause a rapid and irregular heartbeat or severe breathing difficulties, followed by heart failure and death. Sudden sniffing death can occur within minutes. Inhalant use also can cause permanent damage to the brain, lungs, kidneys, muscles, and heart. In addition to damage from the vapors themselves, many inhalants contain dangerously high levels of copper, zinc, and heavy metals.

The *DSM-IV-TR* requires the following criteria for a diagnosis of inhalant intoxication:

- Use: There was recent intentional inhalant use.
- Personality changes: There are significant behavioral or psychological changes during or shortly after inhaling. These might include provoking a fight, assault, using poor judgment, apathy, or impaired functioning at work or school or in a social situation.
- Inhalant-specific intoxication syndrome: Two or more of the following symptoms occur during or shortly after inhalant use or exposure: dizziness; involuntary side-to-side eye movements (nystagmus); loss of coordination; slurred speech; unsteady gait (difficulty walking); lethargy (fatigue); slowed reflexes; psychomotor retardation (moving slowly); tremor (shaking); generalized muscle weakness; blurred or double vision; stupor or coma; euphoria.

Inhalant abuse is defined as significant negative consequences from the recurrent use of inhalants without physical dependence on the substance. Abusers typically use inhalants less frequently than those with inhalant dependence but nevertheless suffer negative consequences. For example inhalant abuse may contribute to poor grades or school **truancy**. According to the *DSM-IV-TR*, to meet the diagnostic criteria for inhalant abuse, one or more of the following symptoms must occur and cause significant impairment or distress within a 12-month period:

- Interference with role fulfillment: Inhalant use frequently interferes with obligations at work, home, or school. Users may be unable to perform chores or pay attention at school.
- Danger to self: The user repeatedly uses inhalants in physically hazardous situations such as while driving a car.
- Legal problems: The user has recurrent legal problems related to inhalant use, such as assault arrests.
- Social problems: The user continues to use inhalants despite repeated interpersonal or relationship problems caused by or worsened by his/her use. For example the affected person may have arguments related to inhalant use.

Inhalant dependence or **addiction** is a syndrome in which inhalant use continues despite significant problems caused by or worsened by the use. The problems may involve employment, **family** relationships, and/or physical impairments such as kidney or liver damage. Users may find it difficult to stop using inhalants despite these problems. Heavy users of inhalants may develop a tolerance to the substance that suggests physical dependence. Dependent users may inhale daily or several times per week. The solitary use of inhalants is associated with heavy, prolonged use and may indicate dependency. To meet the diagnostic criteria for inhalant dependence the *DSM-IV-TR* requires that three or more of the following symptoms occur and cause significant impairment or distress within a 12-month period:

- Tolerance: The user has developed tolerance to the inhalant, as indicated by the same amount having less effect over time or by the need to use increasingly higher amounts to achieve the same effect. After a period of regular inhalant use, users often find that they require at least 50% more than the original amount to achieve the same effect.
- Loss of control: The user repeatedly uses a larger amount of inhalant than planned or uses over a longer period of time than planned; for example using inhalants on school days after initially limiting their use to weekends.
- Inability to stop using: The user has either unsuccessfully attempted to cut down or stop using inhalants or has a persistent desire to stop.
- Time: The user spends large amounts of time obtaining inhalants, using them, being under their influence, and recovering from their effects. Although inhalants may be readily available for very little money, they may be used repeatedly for hours every day.
- Interference with activities: The user either abandons or reduces the amount of time devoted to recreational and social activities and/or occupational activities

KEY TERMS

Aerosols—Sprays that contain propellants and solvents, including many household products.

Delusion—A persistent false belief held in the face of strong contradictory evidence.

Euphoria—An exaggerated state of psychological and physical well-being.

Hallucinations—False sensory perceptions; hearing sounds or seeing people or objects that are not there. Hallucinations can also affect the senses of smell, touch, and taste.

Tolerance—The body's adjustment to a drug so that it takes more and more to produce the same physiological or psychological effects.

Volatile solvents—Liquids that vaporize at room temperature, including a variety of industrial and household products and art and office-supply solvents.

because of inhalant use. Inhalant use may replace sports, time with friends, or work.

- Harm to self: Inhalant use continues despite physical problems, such as liver or heart damage, or psychological problems, such as depression or memory loss, that are caused by or worsened by the inhalant use.

Diagnosis

Users rarely seek diagnosis and treatment for inhalant abuse or dependence on their own. A child or adolescent may be brought to a doctor by a parent or other relative who is concerned about personality changes, a chemical odor on the child's breath, or other signs of inhalant abuse. The parent may have discovered empty containers of the inhaled substance. Sometimes inhalant use by a child or adolescent is diagnosed in a hospital emergency room after an overdose or accidental injury.

Examination

Inhalant use is sometimes diagnosed by the existence of:

- auditory, visual, or tactile hallucinations
- other perceptual disturbances, such as illusions
- delusions, such as a belief that one can fly

Inhalant disorder may be difficult to diagnose, since intoxication from alcohol, sedatives, hypnotics (medications to induce **sleep**), or anxiolytics (tranquilizers) can resemble inhalant intoxication. The use of other substances is not uncommon among inhalant abusers and those with inhalant dependency often have other **substance abuse** disorders as well. In the latter case inhalant use is usually secondary to other substance use since inhalants are only occasionally the primary drug of choice.

Tests

Although inhalants can be detected in blood or urine samples, laboratory tests may not always confirm a diagnosis of inhalant disorder since the substances do not remain in the body for very long.

Treatment

Traditional

Inhalant intoxication is often treated in a hospital emergency room because of serious psychological or medical consequences. The latter may include **headache**, nausea, **vomiting**, severe breathing difficulties, heart failure, or injuries sustained while under the influence of inhalants, such as falls or auto accidents. Life-threatening **burns** are common since many inhalants are highly flammable. Users may also require emergency treatment for suffocation from inhaling from a plastic bag placed over the head or from **choking** on inhaled vomit.

Treatment of inhalant and related disorders usually takes a long period and involves:

- family support
- different social networks if the individual uses inhalants with friends
- new coping skills
- increased self-esteem

Prognosis

The course of inhalant use, abuse, and dependence differs somewhat depending on the user's age. Younger children who regularly abuse inhalants, especially after school and on weekends—and even children who are dependent on inhalants—often stop on their own as they get older. They may avoid substance use altogether or move on to other substances. Adults suffering from inhalant abuse or dependence may continue to use regularly for years. Alternatively they may binge frequently—using inhalants much more often for shorter periods of time. This pattern of use can also continue for years. Chronic inhalant users are difficult to treat because they often have other serious personal and social problems, have difficulty avoiding inhalants, and frequently relapse.

Prevention

Comprehensive prevention programs that involve families, schools, communities, and media such as television can be effective in reducing substance abuse. The focus of such programs is the avoidance of any initial contact with abused substances. This is the most effective method for preventing inhalant and related disorders.

Parents and teachers can help prevent inhalant abuse by educating children about the negative effects of inhalants and by recognizing signs of inhalant use including:

1. chemical odors on a child's breath or clothes
2. slurred speech
3. drunken or disoriented behavior
4. nausea or lack of appetite
5. inattentiveness
6. poor coordination

Resources

BOOKS

American Psychiatric Association. *Diagnostic and Statistical Manual of Mental Disorders,* 4th ed., text rev. Washington, DC: American Psychiatric Association, 2000.

Flynn, Noa. *Inhalants and Solvents: Sniffing Disaster.* Philadelphia: Mason Crest, 2008.

Kuhn, Cynthia, et al. *Buzzed: The Straight Facts About the Most Used and Abused Drugs from Alcohol to Ecstasy,* 3rd ed. New York: W. W. Norton, 2008.

McCage, Crystal. *Inhalants.* San Diego, CA: ReferencePoint Press, 2008.

Robinson, Matthew. *Inhalant Abuse.* New York: Rosen Central, 2008.

PERIODICALS

Magid, Jennifer. "HUFFING: A Deadly High." *Current Health 1* 33, no. 3 (November 2009): 20-22.

Perron, Brian E., and Matthew O. Howard. "Adolescent Inhaler Use, Abuse and Dependence." *Addiction* 104, no. 7 (July 2009): 1185.

OTHER

Howard, Matthew O. "Epidemiology of Inhalant Use in the United States." American Psychological Association. October 5, 2009. [Accessed December 8, 2010], http://www.apa.org/about/gr/science/spin/2009/10/epidemiology.pdf.

"Inhalants." *unitalicize*, http://www.nlm.nih.gov/medlineplus/inhalants.html.

"Trends in Adolescent Inhalant Use: 2002 to 2007." *The National Survey on Drug Use and Health Report.* March 16, 2009. [Accessed December 8, 2010], http://oas.samhsa.gov/2k9/inhalantTrends/inhalantTrends.htm.

"NIDA InfoFacts: Inhalants." *unitalicize.* March 2009. [Accessed December 8, 2010], http://www.drugabuse.gov/infofacts/inhalants.html.

"Inhalants." *Drugabuse.gov.* [Accessed December 8, 2010], http://www.inhalants.drugabuse.gov/.

ORGANIZATIONS

American Psychological Association, 750 First Street, NE, Washington DC, 20002-4242, (202) 336-5500, (800) 374-2721, http://www.apa.org.

National Clearinghouse for Alcohol and Drug Information, P.O. Box 2345, Rockville MD, 20847-2345, (877) SAMHSA7, (240) 221-4292, http://ncadi.samhsa.gov/default.aspx.

National Institute on Drug Abuse, 6001 Executive Boulevard, Room 5213, Bethesda MD, 20892-9561, (301) 443-1124, information@nida.nih.gov, http://www.drugabuse.gov/NIDAHome.html.

Substance Abuse & Mental Health Services Administration (SAMHSA) Health Information Network (SHIN), PO Box 2345, Rockville MD, 20847-2345, (877) SAMHSA-7 (726-4727), (240) 221-4292, SHIN@samhsa.hhs.gov, http://www.samhsa.gov/shin.

Jennifer Hahn, PhD
Margaret Alic, PhD

Inner ear infection ***see* Labyrinthitis**

Insect bites ***see* Bites and stings**

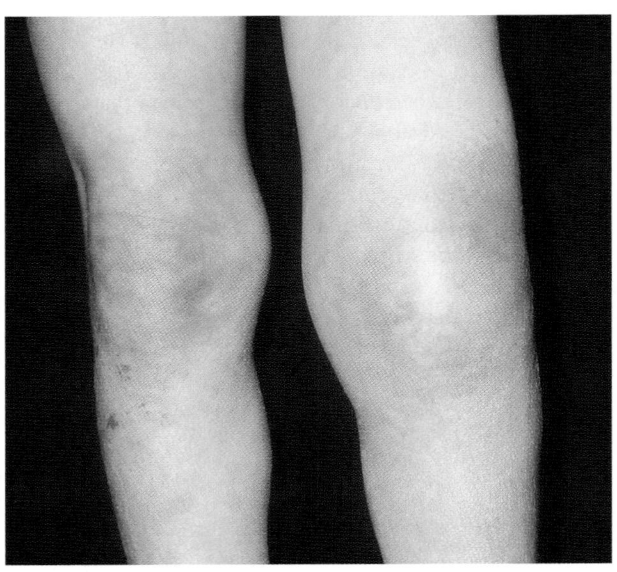

Swelling in the patient's left knee from an allergic reaction to a wasp sting. *(Dr. P. Marazzi/Photo Researchers, Inc.)*

Insect sting allergy

Definition

An insect sting allergy is an allergic reaction on the part of a human or other animal to the venom of a stinging insect (bees, wasps, hornets, some ants) or the anticoagulant injected by a biting insect (mosquitoes, ticks). The reaction may be local or systemic.

Demographics

It is estimated that over 2 million Americans are allergic to stinging insects. Another figure given is that 5%–10% of the general population is allergic to stinging insects. Up to 1 million emergency room visits occur annually because of insect **stings**. In 2007, the last year for which data are available, the American Association of Poison Control Centers reported 42,620 cases of exposures to insects in the United States. Slightly more than 200 of these were listed as resulting in moderate or major reactions.

About 40 Americans die each year as a result of insect sting-induced **anaphylaxis**, although some studies give estimates of 50–100 deaths each year. It is possible that this number may be markedly underestimated. Bee, wasp, and insect stings cause more deaths in the United States than any other kind of injection of venom. Most of these deaths, however, occur in adults between 35 and 45 years of age. About 1 out of 100 children has a systemic allergic reaction to the sting of an insect. 50% of deaths from insect stings occur within 30 minutes of the sting, and **death** can occur in as little as 10 minutes.

The majority of insect stings in the United States are from wasps, hornets, bees, yellow jackets, and fire ants. The class of insects capable of injecting venom into a person is called Hymenoptera. With the exception of fire ants, all of these insects are found throughout the United States. Fire ants are found primarily in the southeastern region of the country but have also been noted in some Western states. In recent years, doctors in the United States and Canada have noted an increase in health problems in frequent travelers that result from exposure to exotic insects in Africa and South America.

Description

Many people experience insect stings or **bites** every year. For most of them, these stings cause only mild **pain** and discomfort lasting for a few hours. Symptoms might include swelling, **itching**, and redness at the sting site. Some individuals, however, are allergic to insect stings. When they are stung by an insect to which they are allergic, their bodies produce an antibody called immunoglobulin E (IgE). IgE reacts with the insect venom and triggers the release of various chemicals, including histamine, which causes the allergic reaction. Stings may be life-threatening for a small number of such persons. These severe allergic reactions may develop quickly and can involve several body organs. This type of reaction is called anaphylaxis and can be fatal.

Insect venom is made up of proteins and other substances that usually cause only itching, pain, and swelling in those who are stung. This local reaction is usually confined to the site of the sting. Sometimes the redness and swelling may extend from the sting site and cover a larger area of the body. These large local non-allergic reactions can persist for days. Occasionally the site may become infected, which requires antibiotic treatment. Although most local reactions are not serious, if they are near the face or neck, swelling can block the airway and cause serious problems.

Although mosquitoes are biting rather than stinging insects, some people can develop allergic reactions to mosquito bites known as skeeter syndrome. The syndrome is characterized by inflammation and **fever**.

Some people are allergic to insect venom and may develop more serious reactions if they are stung. It is important to note that allergic reactions to stings normally do not occur after the initial sting. A reaction may take place after two or more stings that have happened over an extended period of time. Therefore, it is essential to be aware of the possibility for allergic symptoms in people in any age group even if they have been stung previously and had no reaction.

Risk factors

Risk factors for insect bites or stings include:

- A job that requires being outdoors, particularly in warm weather.
- Frequent travel abroad.
- Hiking or travel within or to wilderness areas.
- Homelessness.
- Recent hurricane or storm. Stinging insects may be displaced or their nests or hives destroyed by bad weather, and may seek shelter indoors or in other locations where they are not usually found.

The most significant risk factor for an allergic reaction to insect **bites and stings** is a personal history of an allergy like hay fever, or a past allergic reaction (even a minor one) to an insect sting.

In late 2009, a group of European researchers reported that older age, male sex, and a high baseline concentration of tryptase (an enzyme associated with allergic response) in the blood increase an allergic person's risk of a severe anaphylactic reaction to bee or wasp venom.

Causes and symptoms

Causes

Allergic reactions to insect stings result from an overreaction of a person's **immune system** to the venom injected by the insect. After the first sting, the person's body produces an allergic substance called immunoglobulin E (IgE) antibody, which reacts with the insect venom. If the person is stung again by the same type of insect or by one from a similar species, the insect venom will interact with the IgE antibody produced in response to the previous sting. This reaction in turn triggers the release of histamine and several other chemicals that cause allergic symptoms.

Symptoms

The sting of an insect may cause only a local response, in which pain, redness, itching, and swelling are confined to the site of the sting. This type of reaction is considered normal. The normal reaction to fire ant stings is different. Clear blisters usually form within several hours then become cloudy within 24 hours. The reaction usually presents in a ring or cluster, since a fire ant pivots and repeatedly stings. Also, fire ants travel in groups and a person may receive multiple stings from many ants.

Larger allergic reactions often affect almost the entire arm, leg, foot, hand, or other part of the body in the area of the sting. Swelling occurs and may last as long as 7 to 10 days. The affected person may also experience a low-grade fever, fatigue, and nausea.

Some people experience a more severe allergic reaction. For a small percentage of these individuals, insect stings may be life threatening. Severe allergic reactions can involve multiple body organs and may progress rapidly. This reaction is called anaphylaxis. Anaphylaxis is considered a medical emergency and may be fatal. The symptoms of anaphylaxis include the following:

- wheezing
- difficulty breathing
- hives and itching over large areas of the body
- swelling of the tongue or throat
- dizziness, fainting, rapid heartbeat, chest pain
- nausea, vomiting, or diarrhea

KEY TERMS

Allergen—Any non-parasitic antigen capable of triggering an IgE hypersensitivity reaction in susceptible individuals.

Allergy shots—Injections given by an allergy specialist to desensitize an allergic person to a known allergen. Also known as immunotherapy treatment.

Anaphylaxis—Also called anaphylactic shock; a severe allergic reaction characterized by airway constriction, tissue swelling, headache, nausea, and lowered blood pressure.

Histamine—A chemical that triggers the inflammatory response to an allergen.

Immunoglobulin E (IgE)—A type of antibody found only in mammals that is involved in allergic responses to insect venom and other allergens.

Radioallergosorbent (RAST) test—A type of blood test used to evaluate a patient for allergic reactions if the skin prick test is inconclusive or if the patient has a skin condition that would interfere with a skin prick test.

Skeeter syndrome—An informal term for a severe reaction to mosquito bites, characterized by fever and a rash or large area of swelling at the site of the bite.

- headache
- metallic taste in mouth
- feeling of impending doom

In severe cases, a rapid fall in blood pressure may result in shock and loss of consciousness. This systemic reaction is less common in children than in adults. The progression of these symptoms may take only a few minutes. In rare cases, **coagulation disorders** have been reported to result from anaphylactic reactions to wasp venom.

Diagnosis

For the majority of insect stings, home care is all that is necessary. However, in many cases medical attention is warranted. If any of the following occur, people should seek professional assistance at once:

- Symptoms progress beyond the site of the sting.
- Swelling becomes extensive and painful.
- The sting is located on the head or neck area.
- The affected person has had severe reactions to insect stings in the past.

- There is evidence of infection, such as increased pain, redness, warmth, and swelling at the sting site.

If a person who has been stung develops **hives**, has difficulty breathing or swallowing, swelling of the lips or face, fainting, or **dizziness**, he or she should be transported to an emergency department immediately.

Examination

An allergy to insect stings is determined by the doctor who takes a thorough history from the patient or the parents, in the case of a child. The history will usually show that the individual has been stung previously. The doctor will also note the presence of the various symptoms common to insect sting allergic reactions during the office examination. In some cases the doctor may be able to identify the insect that caused the sting(s) by examining the location, number, and pattern of the stings or bites. The patient may also be referred to an allergist to determine specific sensitivities.

Tests

The most common tests used by allergists to evaluate a patient for hypersensitivity to insect venom are skin prick tests and radioallergosorbent (RAST) blood tests. In the skin prick test, a small amount of purified insect venom is pricked with a needle into the skin of the arm or upper back. If the patient is allergic to the insect venom, he or she will develop a hive at the site of the test. The skin prick test is usually considered the most accurate test.

If the allergist thinks that the patient is allergic to insect venom even though the skin prick test is negative, a RAST test may be ordered. In the RAST test, a sample of the patient's blood is sent to a medical laboratory. In the lab, a small quantity of the suspected allergen (in this case, insect venom) is added to an insoluble substance. The patient's blood is then added. If it contains IgE antibodies to the allergen, the antibodies will bind to the allergen. Radioactive anti-IgE antibody is then added to the insoluble material in those locations where IgE antibodies are bound to the allergen. The amount of radioactivity will indicate the level of IgE antibodies in the patient's blood, hence the level of his or her sensitivity to the allergen.

Treatment

Traditional

If a person has been stung by an insect that has left its stinger, it should be removed by flicking the fingers at it. Avoid squeezing the venom sac, as this maneuver can force more venom into the skin. If fire ants have stung the person, they should be carefully brushed off to prevent repeated stings.

Drugs

Any symptoms that progress beyond the local area of the sting require immediate attention. Allergic reactions to insect stings are considered medical emergencies and are treated by medications. The physician will treat the child with epinephrine (adrenaline), which is usually given as an injection into the arm. An antihistamine such as diphenhydramine is usually given by mouth or injection to diminish the histamine reaction. Such gluococorticoids as prednisone or methylprednisolone are often given to decrease any swelling and to suppress the immune response. The physician may write prescriptions for both **antihistamines** and **steroids** to take after the child leaves the hospital.

After a person has experienced a severe allergic reaction and received emergency treatment, the doctor may write a prescription for a self-injecting epinephrine device called an EpiPen. This device should be carried by the individual at all times especially when out of reach of medical care, such as on an airplane or in the woods. Sometimes epinephrine is not enough, however, and other treatment may be needed. Whenever people with a known severe insect sting allergy are stung, they should receive prompt medical attention, even if they have received an epinephrine injection.

Immunotherapy

Allergy shots for insect stings, also known as venom immunotherapy, can be an effective treatment for children who experience a severe reaction to insect stings. Any child who has had a significant reaction to an insect sting should be evaluated by an allergy specialist. Not all children who have had a reaction will get allergy shots but many should. Experts once believed that most children outgrow insect sting **allergies** and that allergy shots were not needed. They now know, however, that about one child in five will remain allergic into adulthood. Because of this pattern, it is recommended that immunotherapy should be used for the approximately 40% of children who experience moderate to severe systemic reactions to insect stings.

Venom immunotherapy is a highly effective **vaccination** program that actually prevents future sting reactions in most patients who receive them. The person is initially tested to determine his or her individual sensitivities. The treatment normally involves twice weekly injections of venom in dosages that are gradually increased over about 10–20 weeks. At this point, a maintenance dosage is administered about every one to two months. Allergy shots given in childhood can protect a person for 10–20 years.

Home remedies

Home treatment is normally all that is needed for minor skin reactions to insect stings. The affected arm or leg should be elevated and an ice pack applied to the area to reduce swelling and pain. Over-the-counter products can also be used to decrease the pain and itching. These include the following:

- products with a numbing effect, including topical anesthetics like benzocaine and phenol
- hydrocortisone products, which may decrease inflammation and swelling
- skin protectants, such as calamine lotion and zinc oxide, which have astringent, cooling, and antibacterial effects
- diphenhydramine, an antihistamine, which will help to control itching, and will counter some of the substances produced as part of the reaction
- ibuprofen or acetaminophen for pain relief
- a paste made with baking soda and water and applied to the affected area

It is important to keep the area of the sting clean. The site should be gently cleansed with mild soap and water. Avoid breaking any blisters, as breaks in the skin can increase the chances of a secondary infection.

Prognosis

Prompt treatment of insect stings normally prevents immediate complications but a delay in the treatment of a severe allergic reaction can result in rapid deterioration and even death. The long-term prognosis is usually good with the rare exception of possible local infections. If a person develops anaphylaxis after an insect sting, they are at increased risk of developing anaphylaxis if stung again.

Prevention

The best way to avoid an allergic reaction from an insect sting is to avoid getting stung in the first place. One way to do this is to be able to identify the most common stinging insects and where they live:

- Honeybees have fuzzy rounded bodies with dark brown coloring and yellow markings. After stinging, the honeybee normally leaves its barbed stinger in its victim and then the bee dies. Honeybees are usually not aggressive and will sting only if provoked. However, the so-called killer bees, or Africanized honeybees, are far more aggressive and may sting in swarms. Wild honeybees live in honeycombs or colonies in cavities of buildings or in hollow trees. Africanized honeybees may nest in old tires or holes in the ground, in house frames, or between fence posts.
- Yellow jackets are black with yellow markings. Their nests have a papier-maché appearance and are usually located underground. They can also be found in woodpiles, in the walls of frame buildings, or in masonry cracks.
- Paper wasps have slender elongated bodies and are black, red, or brown with yellow markings. Their nests are also made of a paper-like substance that opens downward in a circular comb of cells. Their nests are often located behind shutters, in shrubs or woodpiles, or under eaves.
- Hornets are the largest wasps and can grow to more than 2 inches (1 centimeter) in length. They prefer dark sheltered locations like hollow tree trunks. Unlike bees, hornets can sting multiple times.
- Fire ants are reddish brown to black stinging insects. They build nests of dirt in the ground that may be quite tall. Fire ants attack with little warning.

A variety of precautionary measures will decrease the chances of getting stung:

- Avoid walking barefoot on lawns; wear closed-toe shoes. The majority of honeybee stings occur on the bottom of the foot when someone steps on the bee.
- Hire a professional exterminator to destroy nests and hives around the home.
- The smell of food attracts insects so be careful when eating, drinking, or cooking outdoors. Keep food covered.
- Remain calm and quiet if flying insects are noted and move away slowly. Do not attempt to swat them.
- Avoid using highly scented perfumes, colognes, or hair sprays.
- Avoid wearing brightly colored clothing.
- Do not wear loose fitting garments that can trap insects between the material and skin.
- Keep the areas around trash containers clean and at some distance away from where children are playing.
- Before traveling abroad, consult the Centers for Disease Control and Prevention (CDC) for travelers' advisories about exotic stinging insects, particularly if the destination country is in Africa or South America.

In the case of children, parents should be aware of the potential risks of insect stings and should teach their children to take measures to avoid being stung. If their child does get stung, parents need to begin treatment immediately and watch the child closely for any signs of allergic reaction. If these do occur, parents should transport their child immediately to a hospital emergency department.

Resources

BOOKS

Backer, Howard D., et al. *Wilderness First Aid: Emergency Care for Remote Locations*, 3rd ed. Sudbury, MA: Jones and Bartlett Publishers, 2008.

Grammer, Leslie C., and Paul A. Greenberger, editors. *Patterson's Allergic Diseases*, 7th ed. Baltimore, MD: Wolters Kluwer Health/Lippincott Williams and Wilkins, 2009.

PERIODICALS

Demain, J.G., et al. "Anaphylaxis and Insect Allergy." *Current Opinion in Allergy and Clinical Immunology* 10 (August 2010): 318-22.

Diaz, H. "Recognition, Management, and Prevention of Hymenopteran Stings and Allergic Reactions in Travelers." *Journal of Travel Medicine* 16 (September-October 2009): 357-64.

Hamilton, R. G. "Diagnosis and Treatment of Allergy to Hymenoptera Venoms." *Current Opinion in Allergy and Clinical Immunology* 10 (August 2010): 323-29.

Heddie, R.J., and S.G. Brown. "Venom Immunotherapy: Worth the Time and Trouble!" *Clinical and Experimental Allergy* 39 (June 2009): 774-76.

Lombardini, C., et al. "'Heparinization' and Hyperfibrinogenolysis by Wasp Sting." *American Journal of Emergency Medicine* 27 (November 2009): 1176.

Pollyea, D.A., et al. "When Yellow Jackets Attack: Recurrent and Severe Anaphylactic Reactions to Insect Bites and Stings." *American Journal of Hematology* 84 (December 2009): 843-46.

Rueff, F., et al. "Predictors of Severe Systemic Anaphylactic Reactions in Patients with Hymenoptera Venom Allergy: Importance of Baseline Serum Tryptase—A Study of the European Academy of Allergology and Clinical Immunology Interest Group on Insect Venom Hypersensitivity." *Journal of Allergy and Clinical Immunology* 124 (November 2009): 1047-54.

OTHER

American Academy of Allergy, Asthma, and Immunology (AAAAI). "Tips to Remember: Stinging Insect Allergy." [Accessed September 21, 2010], http://www.aaaai.org/patients/publicedmat/tips/stinginginsect.stm.

"Insect Bites." eMedicine. [Accessed December 8, 2010], http://www.emedicinehealth.com/insect_bites/article_em.htm.

"Insect Sting Allergy." Aukland Allergy Clinic. [Accessed December 8, 2010], http://www.allergyclinic.co.nz/guides/20.html.

Kemp, Stephen F., and G. William Palmer. "Anaphylaxis." eMedicine. April 29, 2009. [Accessed September 21, 2010], http://emedicine.medscape.com/article/135065–overview.

Mayo Clinic. "Bee Stings." [Accessed September 21, 2010], http://www.mayoclinic.com/health/bee–stings/DS01067.

ORGANIZATIONS

American Academy of Allergy, Asthma, and Immunology (AAAAI), 555 East Wells St., Suite 1100, Milwaukee WI, 53202, (414) 272-6071, info@aaaai.org

American College of Emergency Physicians (ACEP), 1125 Executive Circle, Irving TX, 75038-2522, (972) 550-0911, (800) 798-1822, (972) 580-2816, http://www.acep.org/.

Centers for Disease Control and Prevention (CDC), 1600 Clifton Rd., Atlanta GA, 30333, (800) 232-4636, cdcinfo@cdc.gov, http://www.cdc.gov.

National Institute of Allergy and Infectious Diseases (NIAID), 6610 Rockledge Dr., MSC 6612, Bethesda MD, 20892-6612, (301) 496-5717, (866) 284-4107, (301) 402-3573, http://www3.niaid.nih.gov.

Deanna M. Swartout–Corbeil, RN
Rebecca J. Frey, PhD

Insomnia **see Sleep disorders**

Insulin shock **see Hypoglycemia**

Intelligence

Definition

A term referring to a variety of mental capabilities, including the ability to reason, plan, solve problems, think abstractly, comprehend complex ideas, learn quickly, and learn from experience.

Description

Throughout the 19th- and 20th centuries scientists debated the nature of human intelligence, including its heritability and whether (and to what extent) it exists or is measurable. There are almost as many definitions of intelligence as there are researchers in the field. David Wechsler, a psychologist who helped design one of the most commonly used tests of intelligence, defined it as "the aggregate or global capacity of the individual to act purposefully, to think rationally, and to deal effectively with his environment" John Kotter defined it as "a keen mind," which in his opinion included strong analytical ability, good judgment, and the capacity to think strategically and multidimensionally. Cyril Burt defined it as "innate cognitive ability," while Howard Gardner emphasizes skill in problem-solving as a hallmark of intelligence. The 1994 publication of Richard J. Herrnstein and Charles Murray's volume *The Bell Curve* brought these debates to the forefront of public attention by discussing links between social class, race, and

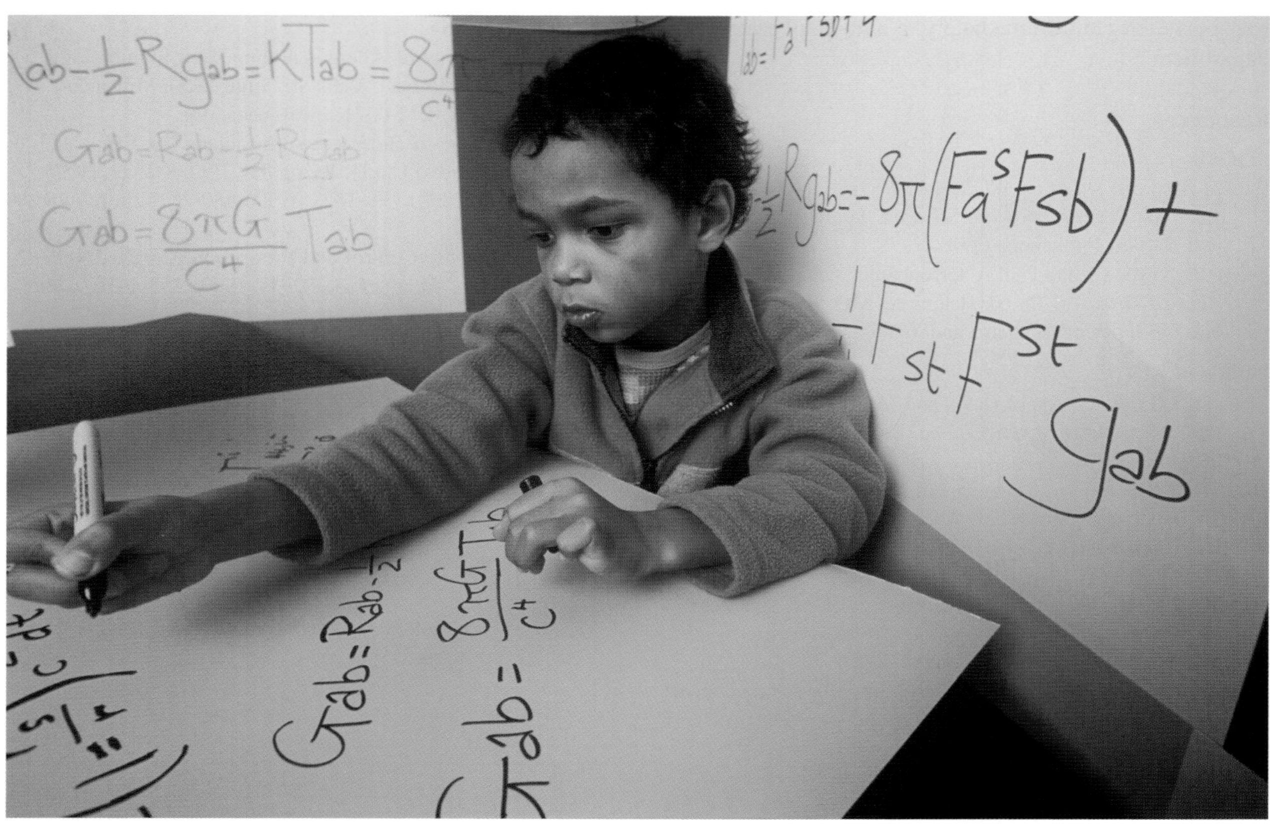

Young child completing physics equations. *(David Hay Jones/Photo Researchers, Inc.)*

IQ scores, despite the fact that many have questioned the validity of IQ tests as a measurement of intelligence or a predictor of achievement and success.

Although the **assessment** of mental abilities through standardized testing has had many detractors, especially over the past 30 years, the notion that intellect is a measurable entity—also called the psychometric approach—lies at the heart of much modern theorizing about the nature of intelligence. A rudimentary forerunner to 20th-century intelligence testing was developed in the 1860s by Charles Darwin's younger half-cousin, Sir Francis Galton. Galton was inspired by the social implications of *On the Origin of Species* and set out to prove that intelligence was inherited using quantitative studies of prominent individuals and their families. Galton is thus regarded as the founder of psychometrics, which can be defined as the branch of psychology that measures intelligence as well as other abilities and personality traits.

Galton's work was followed in 1905 by that of the French psychologist Alfred Binet, who introduced the concept of mental age, which match eschronological age in children of average ability. Mental age would be higher than chronological age in bright children and lower in those of lesser ability. Binet's test was introduced to the United States in a modified form in 1916 long with the concept of the **intelligence quotient** or IQ. IQ represents a person's mental age divided by chronological age and multiplied by 100.

In the meantime, one of the central concepts of the psychometric approach to intelligence had been introduced in England in 1904 by Charles Spearman; he noted that people who perform well on one type of intelligence test tend to do well on others also. Spearman gave a name to the general mental ability that carried over from one type of cognitive testing to another—*g* for general intelligence—and ultimately decided that *g* consists mainly of the ability to infer relationships based on one's experiences. Although the concept of *g* has the disadvantage of being based solely on a particular statistical analysis rather than direct observation, it has remained an important concept psychometric research. Perhaps the best-known contemporary researcher of the *g* factor is Arthur Jensen, whose 1998 book on the subject sparked a firestorm of controversy because he suggested that differences in *g* between whites and African Americans are biological rather than cultural. Jensen's work has been defended by such other psychologists as Hans J. Eysenck, Christopher F. Chabris, and Linda S. Gottfredson.

In order to understand why the findings of such psychometricians as Jensen are controversial, we must return briefly to Sir Francis Galton who introduced the concept of eugenics in 1883. Eugenics refers to the belief that society should direct or control the process of human mating in order to improve the intelligence of the human race. Galton carried out a statistical study of the number of children born in English families of high achievement and noted that such families had relatively few children because the adults tended to marry late. Galton proposed that the British government should encourage eugenic marriages by supplying incentives for early marriage among the gifted. Although Galton himself did not favor what has since come to be called social engineering, some intellectuals who were influenced by his writings (including H. G. Wells and George Bernard Shaw) thought that the state should compel gifted people to marry and forbid the less able to have children. Some even advocated forced sterilization of the "unfit." In the 1930s, Nazi Germany practiced euthanasia of the mentally retarded. Thus eugenics has come to be associated with human-rights violations and coercive government policies. Although Jensen, Eysenck, and other researchers in the field of cognitive differences have never advocated anything remotely resembling the practices carried out by Hitler's regime, they have been accused of racism nonetheless. The media have been particularly sensationalistic in this regard. In 1994, for example, ABC broadcasted a show about *The Bell Curve* in which news anchor Peter Jennings followed photographs of Murray, Herrnstein, and Jensen with footage of Nazi concentration camps.

The other factor involved in opposition to psychometric research is the fact that above-average intelligence is necessary to enter college and education is the chief avenue to well-paying and prestigious jobs in the early 2000s. Technological change has gradually reduced the number of jobs that can be done by persons of below-average intelligence. This development in turn has led to concern that intelligence research will be used as a social gatekeeper; that is, IQ scores and similar data about individuals' intelligence will be misused to give some test-takers unfair advantages and to unfairly stigmatize others.

Psychometrics is still considered by many to be a valid scientific area of inquiry but it has been challenged by researchers who approach intelligence in different ways. Instead of studying the structure of intelligence (i.e., what it is) some scientists have focused on the processes involved (how it works). A leader in this information-processing approach is Robert Sternberg, whose triarchic theory of intelligence not only addresses internal thought processes but also explores how an individual uses them to solve problems within his or her environment. The first part of Sternberg's theory, like psychometric theories, is concerned with the internal components of intelligence, although its emphasis is on process rather than structure. It analyzes the processes involved in interpreting sensory stimuli, storing and retrieving information in short- and long-term memory, solving problems, and acquiring new skills. The second part of the triarchic theory addresses the interaction between mental processes and experience, centering on the fact that, while a new experience requires complex mental responses, as it becomes increasingly familiar, the required response gradually becomes routine and automatic. In the third part of his theory, Sternberg analyzes the way that people use their intelligence to survive in the "real world" by either adapting to their environments, modifying them, or abandoning them in favor of new ones.

Another approach is Howard Gardner's theory of multiple intelligences, which replaces the general intelligence factor (*g*) with seven different types of intelligence: linguistic; logical-mathematical; spatial; interpersonal (ability to deal with other people); intrapersonal (insight into oneself); musical; and bodily-kinaesthetic (athletic ability). According to Gardner, each of these areas of competence includes a separate set of problem-solving skills that can be mobilized by various symbolic systems. Every person has all the different types of intelligence, although some may be developed far more fully than others. The most dramatic example of this uneven development is found in autistic savants, children who suffer from autistic spectrum disorders but who nonetheless have exceptional abilities in a few highly specialized areas, usually involving arithmetical calculations.

Gardner regards his theory as radical in its rejection of *g* and in its reliance on psychometric premises. He claims that Spearman's *g* (a purported general intelligence factor enabling people to perform fairly consistently on different types of mental tests) is an artificial construct made possible by the fact that standard IQ tests assess only the first three of the seven types of intelligence, ignoring the others. He also argues that IQ tests can predict school performance only because formal education emphasizes those abilities measured by the tests, rather than truly assessing all aspects of human intelligence. In recent years, Gardner's theory has become popular among educators and a number of schools have instituted programs based on his ideas.

Another focus for recent studies of intelligence has been the evolutionary development of the brain. Scientists with this research orientation are interested in the ways that human mental capacities developed over hundreds of thousands of years or more in response to changing problem-solving challenges in the environment. From this perspective, the *g* factor of the psychometricians could be viewed as a specialized ability that has evolved in response to humankind's expanded exposure to tests of all kinds rather than an innate ability that enables us to deal with them. An evolutionary perspective on the phenomenon of similar performance in a variety of cognitive tests might also take into account the selective pairing of cognitively matched couples that has resulted from the modern freedom to marry for love, producing children whose abilities are more and more likely to be uniformly high or low across a series of different cognitive tasks.

Other areas of research that have been stimulated by the evolutionary theory of human intelligence include animal cognition and artificial intelligence. Animal cognition research seeks to answer such questions as whether animals can think, whether they have rudimentary languages, how they solve problems, and whether they are capable of such emotions as empathy and love. Psychologists who specialize in animal cognition also study the similarities and differences between the cognitive capacities of different animal species (for example, dogs vs. cats) and the similarities and differences between animal and human cognition.

Artificial intelligence refers to a branch of computer science and engineering that deals with intelligent behavior, learning, and reasoning ability in machines. Researchers in this field are interested in developing machines to perform real-life tasks that require intelligence, such as speech and handwriting recognition, game strategy, and case-based reasoning. Some of these scientists have developed robots that can perform jobs that are dangerous to humans if they lose their concentration, such as welding and other tasks in car assembly. In Japan, over 500,000 robots are already in use in various manufacturing processes.

Resources

BOOKS

The Intelligence Controversy. New York: Wiley, 1981.

Eysenck, H. J. *The IQ Argument: Race, Intelligence, and Education.* New York: Library Press, 1971.

Fraser, Steven. *The Bell Curve Wars: Race, Intelligence, and the Future of America.* New York: Basic Books, 1995.

Gardner, Howard. *Frames of Mind: The Theory of Multiple Intelligences.* New York: Basic Books, 1983.

Goleman, Daniel. *Emotional Intelligence.* New York: Bantam, 1995.

Gottfredson, Linda S. "Suppressing Intelligence Research: Hurting Those We Intend to Help." In R. H. Wright and N. A. Cummings, eds. *Destructive Trends in Mental Health: The Well-Intentioned Path to Harm.* New York: Taylor and Francis, 2005.

Herrnstein, Richard J., and Charles Murray. *The Bell Curve: Intelligence and Class Structure in American Life.* New York: Free Press, 1994.

Jensen, Arthur R. *The "g" Factor.* Westport, CT: Praeger, 1998.

Kline, Paul. *Intelligence: The Psychometric View.* London: Routledge, 1991.

Sternberg, R. J. *Beyond IQ: A Triarchic Theory of Human Intelligence.* Cambridge, UK: Cambridge University Press, 1985.

PERIODICALS

Chabris, Christopher F., and Critics. "Does IQ Matter?" *Commentary* 106 (November 1998): 13-23.

Chabris, Christopher F. "IQ Since 'The Bell Curve.'" *Commentary* 106 (August 1998): 33-40. Available online at, *http://www.wjh.harvard.edu/~cfc/Chabris1998a.html.*

OTHER

American Psychological Association Task Force. "Intelligence: Knowns and Unknowns." *American Psychologist* 51 (1996). Available online at, http://www.lrainc.com/swtaboo/taboos/apa_01.html

Gardner, Howard. "Multiple Intelligences after Twenty Years." Paper presented to the American Educational Research Association, Chicago, Illinois, April 21, 2003.

ORGANIZATIONS

American Educational Research Association (AERA) 1230 Seventeenth Street, NW., Washington DC, 20036, (202) 223-9485, http://www.aera.net.

American Psychological Association (APA), 750 First St. NE, Washington DC, 20002-4242 (202 336-5700, http://www.apa.org.

Intelligence quotient (IQ)

A measurement of **intelligence** based on standardized test scores.

Although intelligence quotient (IQ) tests are still widely used in the United States, there has been increasing doubt voiced about their ability to measure the mental capacities that determine success in life. IQ testing has also been criticized for being biased with regard to race and gender. In modern times, the first scientist to test mental ability was Alfred Binet, a French psychologist who devised an intelligence test for children in 1905, based on the notion that intelligence can be expressed in terms of age. Binet created the concept of "mental age," according to which the test performance of a child of average intelligence would match his or her age, while a gifted child's performance would be on par with that of an older child and a slow learner's abilities would be equal to those of a younger child. Binet's test was introduced to the United States in a modified form in 1916 by Lewis M. Terman, a professor at Stanford University. The scoring system of the new test, devised by the German psychologist William Stern, consisted of dividing a child's mental age by his or her chronological age and multiplying the quotient by 100 to arrive at an "intelligence quotient," which would equal 100 in a person of average ability.

The Wechsler Intelligence Scales, developed in 1949 by David Wechsler, chief psychologist at Bellevue Psychiatric Hospital in New York, addressed an issue that still provokes criticism of IQ tests today: the fact that there are different types of intelligence. The Wechsler scales replaced the single mental-age score with a verbal scale and a performance scale for nonverbal skills to address each test taker's individual combination of strengths and weaknesses. The Stanford-Binet and Wechsler tests (in updated versions) remain the most widely administered IQ tests in the United States. Average performance at each age level is still assigned a score of 100 but today's scores are calculated solely by comparison with the performance of others in the same age group rather than with test takers of various ages. Among the general population, scores cluster around 100 and gradually decrease in either direction in a pattern known as the normal distribution (or bell-shaped) curve.

With regard to the heritability of IQ, data from hundreds of family studies provide the primary supporting evidence that IQ is shaped more by heredity than environment. The correlation percentage of IQ tests with various human relationships is as follows:

- Test and retest of the same subject: 87 percent
- Identical twins reared in the same family: 86 percent
- Identical twins reared apart: 76 percent
- Fraternal twins reared in the same family: 55 percent
- Full biological siblings: 47 percent
- Parents and children in intact families: 40 percent
- Parents and children living apart: 31 percent
- Adopted children living with the adoptive family: 0 percent

At the lower end of the bell-shaped curve are those groups of people defined as mentally retarded. **Mental retardation** is known to be familial; about 25 percent is thought to be due to chromosomal abnormalities or organic brain damage. The American Psychiatric Association's *Diagnostic and Statistical Manual of Mental Disorders*, fourth edition (DSM-IV), defines and describes IQ score ranges among the mentally retarded as follows:

- Mild mental retardation (IQ 55 to 70): children are educable and require only mild support as adults.
- Moderate mental retardation (IQ 35 to 55): children require moderate supervision and care as adults.
- Severe mental retardation (IQ 20 to 40): children can be taught basic life skills.
- Profound mental retardation (IQ below 20): children require ongoing custodial care even when they are chronologically adults.

Although IQ scores are good predictors of academic achievement in elementary and secondary school, the correspondence between IQ and academic performance is less consistent at higher levels of education and many have questioned the ability of IQ tests to predict success later in life. The tests do not measure many of the qualities necessary for achievement in the world of work, such as persistence, self-confidence, motivation, and interpersonal skills, or the ability to set priorities and to allocate one's time and effort efficiently. In addition, the **creativity** and intuition responsible for great achievements in both science and the arts are not evaluated in IQ tests. For example, creativity often involves the ability to envision multiple solutions to a problem (trait educators call this divergent thinking); in contrast, IQ tests require the choice of a single answer or solution to a problem, a type of task that could penalize highly creative people. In spite of this well-known limitation of IQ tests, such companies as Microsoft use their own versions of **intelligence tests** when evaluating potential employees.

One interesting finding in recent years is that IQ appears to have a positive correlation with health and longevity as well as income and accomplishment in later life. One group of British researchers reported in 2004 that the results of IQ testing of adults in late middle age predicted the onset of Alzheimer's disease up to 11 years after the testing more accurately than the possession of a gene known to be associated with Alzheimer's. Another group in Scotland reported that childhood IQ is a significant factor among the variables that can be used to predict age at **death**; people with higher IQs live longer than those with average IQs.

The value of IQ tests has also been called into question by recent theories that define intelligence in ways that transcend the boundaries of tests chiefly designed to measure abstract reasoning and verbal comprehension. For example, Robert J. Sternberg's triarchical model addresses not only internal thought processes but also the ways in which they operate in relation to past experience and to the external environment. Howard Gardner, a psychologist at Harvard University, has posited a theory of multiple intelligences that includes seven different types of intelligence: linguistic and logical-mathematical (the types measured by IQ tests); spatial; interpersonal (ability to deal with other people); intrapersonal (insight into oneself);

musical; and bodily-kinaesthetic (athletic ability). It is interesting that the test battery administered to potential military recruits, the Armed Services Vocational Aptitude Battery, or ASVAB, revised in 2002, consists of nine sections that measure a range of mechanical as well as verbal and mathematical skills: general science; arithmetic; word knowledge; paragraph comprehension; mathematical reasoning; electronics information; auto and shop skills; mechanical comprehension; and assembling objects. Each branch of the military has its own set of standards for assigning recruits to different specialties on the basis of their ASVAB scores.

Critics have also questioned whether IQ tests are a fair or valid way of assessing intelligence in members of ethnic and cultural minorities. Early in the 20th century, IQ tests were used to screen foreign immigrants to the United States; roughly 80% of Eastern European immigrants tested during the World War I era were declared "feeble-minded," even though the tests discriminated against them in terms of language skills and cultural knowledge of the United States. The relationship between IQ and race became an inflammatory issue with the publication of the article "How Much Can We Boost IQ and Scholastic Achievement?" by the educational psychologist Arthur Jensen in *the Harvard Educational Review* in 1969. Flying in the face of prevailing belief in the effects of environmental factors on intelligence, Jensen argued that the effectiveness of the government social programs of the 1960s had been limited because the children they had been intended to help had relatively low IQs, a situation that could not be remedied by government intervention. Jensen was widely censured for his views, and standardized testing underwent a period of criticism within the educational establishment. The National Education Association called for a moratorium on testing and major school systems attempted to limit or even abandon publicly administered standardized tests. Another milestone in the public controversy over testing was the 1981 publication of Stephen Jay Gould's best-selling *The Mismeasure of Man*, which critiqued IQ tests as well as the entire concept of measurable intelligence.

Many educators still maintain that IQ tests are unfair to members of minority groups because they are based on the vocabulary, customs, and values of the mainstream, or dominant, culture. Some observers have cited cultural bias in testing to explain the fact that, on average, African-Americans and Hispanic-Americans score 12 to 15 points lower than European-Americans on IQ tests. (Asian-Americans, however, score an average of four to six points higher than European-Americans.) A new round of controversy was ignited with the 1994 publication of *The Bell Curve* by Richard Herrnstein and Charles Murray, who explored the relationship between IQ, race, and such pervasive social problems as unemployment, crime, and illegitimacy. Given the proliferation of recent theories about the nature of intelligence, many psychologists have disagreed with Herrnstein and Murray's central assumptions that intelligence is measurable by IQ tests, that it is genetically based, and that a person's IQ essentially remains unchanged over time. From a sociopolitical viewpoint, the book's critics have taken issue with *The Bell Curve*'s use of arguments about the genetic nature of intelligence to cast doubt on the power of government to remedy many of the nation's most pressing social problems. In 1995 the American Psychological Association formed a task force to examine the implications of Herrnstein and Murray's work. The report, titled "Intelligence: Knowns and Unknowns," was published in the APA's official journal in 1996.

Another explosive issue in the early 2000s is the significance of differences between men and women on IQ tests. While men and women have the same average IQ, women score higher on tests of verbal knowledge and memory while men score higher on tests of spatial aptitude and mathematical ability. Neuroimaging studies have confirmed that men and women activate different parts of the brain when performing various tests of general intelligence; as of 2006, there is a general consensus that these differences in brain design result in equivalent intellectual performance; they do not indicate that one sex is "brighter" than the other. Men's IQ scores also display a wider variance than women's; that is, there are more men than women at the upper and lower extremes of the bell-shaped curve. Although these differences refer to large groups and not to individuals, the topic is sensitive enough, particularly within college and university faculties, to generate considerable controversy. The president of Harvard University, Lawrence Summers, was forced to resign in 2006 after a year-long dispute over a lecture in which he raised the possibility that women are underrepresented at the highest levels of achievement in such fields as engineering and mathematics because of innate differences in intellectual preferences between men and women. Unfortunately, Summers was misunderstood by many as suggesting that women on average are less intelligent than men.

The U.S. government does make use of IQ testing in the selection of officer candidates in the armed forces. Results of studies of the Armed Forces Qualifying Test (AFQT) indicate that higher scores on the test correlate with more effective performance, for units as well as individual soldiers. As of 2006, 31 is the cutoff score for volunteers; those with lower scores are considered disqualified for military service. Another area in which IQ tests are of interest to the government is forensic evaluation of persons convicted of capital crimes. In 2002 the Supreme Court ruled in *Adkins v. Virginia* that the execution of the mentally retarded constitutes cruel and unusual punishment, which is prohibited by the Eighth Amendment to the Constitution. Lastly, the government uses IQ scores as a basis for deciding claims for Social Security Disability benefits.

Yet another topic for debate has arisen with the discovery that IQ scores in the world's developed countries–especially scores related to mazes and puzzles–have risen dramatically since the introduction of IQ tests early in the century. Scores in the United States have risen an average of 24 points since 1918, scores in Britain have climbed 27 points since 1942, and comparable figures have been reported throughout Western Europe, as well in Canada, Japan, Israel, Australia, and other parts of the developed world. This phenomenon–named the Flynn effect for the New Zealand researcher who first noticed it–raises important questions about intelligence testing. It has implications for the debate over the relative importance of heredity and environment in determining IQ, since experts agree that such a large difference in test scores in so short a time cannot be explained by genetic changes.

A variety of environmental factors have been cited as possible explanations for the Flynn effect, including expanded opportunities for formal education that have given children throughout the world more and earlier exposure to some types of questions they are likely to encounter on an IQ test (although IQ gains in areas such as mathematics and vocabulary, which are most directly linked to formal schooling, have been more modest than those in nonverbal areas). For children in the United States in the 1970s and 1980s, exposure to printed texts and electronic technology–from cereal boxes to video games–has been cited as an explanation for improved familiarity with the types of maze and puzzle questions that have generated the greatest changes in scores. Improved mastery of spatial relations has also been linked to **video games**. Other environmental factors mentioned in connection with the Flynn effect include better **nutrition** and changes in parenting styles.

Resources

BOOKS

American Psychiatric Association. *Diagnostic and Statistical Manual of Mental Disorders*, fourth edition, text revision. Washington, DC: American Psychiatric Association, 2000.

Eysenck, H. J. *The Intelligence Controversy*. New York: Wiley, 1981.

Fraser, Steven. *The Bell Curve Wars: Race, Intelligence, and the Future of America*. New York: Basic Books, 1995.

Herrnstein, Richard J., and Charles Murray. *The Bell Curve: Intelligence and Class Structure in American Life*. New York: Free Press, 1994.

Kline, Paul. *Intelligence: The Psychometric View*. London: Routledge, 1991.

Sternberg, R. J. *Beyond IQ: A Triarchic Theory of Human Intelligence*. Cambridge, UK: Cambridge University Press, 1985.

PERIODICALS

Cervilla, J., M. Prince, S. Joels, et al. "Premorbid Cognitive Testing Predicts the Onset of Dementia and Alzheimer's Disease Better Than and Independently of APOE Genotype." *Journal of Neurology, Neurosurgery and Psychiatry* 75 (August 2004): 1100-1106.

Dickens, W. T., and J. R. Flynn. "Heritability Estimates Versus Large Environmental Effects: The IQ Paradox Resolved." *Canadian Psychological Review* 108 (April 2001): 346-369.

Flynn, J. R. "Searching for Justice: The Discovery of IQ Gains over Time." *American Psychologist* 54 (1999): 5-20.

Haier, R. J., R. E. Jung, R. A. Yeo, et al. "The Neuroanatomy of General Intelligence: Sex Matters." *Neuroimage* 25 (March 2005): 320-327.

Neubauer, A. C., R. H. Grabner, A. Fink, and C. Neuper. "Intelligence and Neural Efficiency: Further Evidence of the Influence of Task Context and Sex on the Brain-IQ Relationship." *Brain Research/Cognitive Brain Research* 25 (September 2005): 217-225.

Whalley, Lawrence J. "Longitudinal Cohort Study of Childhood IQ and Survival up to Age 76." *British Medical Journal* 322 (April 7, 2001): 819.

OTHER

American Psychological Association Task Force. "Intelligence: Knowns and Unknowns." *American Psychologist* 51 (1996). Available online at, http://www.lrainc.com/swtaboo/taboos/apa_01.html

Gardner, Howard. "Multiple Intelligences after Twenty Years." Paper presented to the American Educational Research Association, Chicago, Illinois, April 21, 2003.

ORGANIZATIONS

American Educational Research Association (AERA) 1230 Seventeenth Street, NW., Washington DC, 20036, (202) 223-9485, http://www.aera.net.

American Psychological Association (APA), 750 First St. NE, Washington DC, 20002-4242, (202) 336-5700, http://www.apa.org.

National Institute of Mental Health (NIMH), 6001 Executive Boulevard, Room 8184, MSC 9663, Bethesda MD, 20892-9663, (301) 443-4513, (866) 615-6464, nimhinfo@nih.gov, http://www.nimh.nih.gov.

Intelligence tests

Definition

Intelligence tests are **psychological tests** that are designed to measure a variety mental functions, such as reasoning, comprehension, and judgment.

Purpose

The goal of intelligence tests is to obtain an idea of the person's intellectual potential. The tests center around a set of stimuli designed to yield a score based on the test maker's model of what makes up intelligence. Intelligence tests are often given as a part of a battery of tests.

Precautions

There are many different types of intelligence tests and they all do not measure the same abilities. Although the tests often have aspects that are related with each other, we should not expect that scores on one intelligence test, that measures a single factor, will be similar to scores on another intelligence test, that measures a variety of factors. Also, when determining whether or not to use an intelligence test, a person should make sure that the test has been adequately developed and has solid research to show its reliability and validity. Additionally, psychometric testing requires a clinically trained examiner. Therefore, the test should only be administered and interpreted by a trained professional.

A central criticism of intelligence tests is that psychologists and educators use these tests to distribute the limited resources of our society. These test results are used to provide rewards such as special classes for gifted students, admission to college, and employment. Those who do not qualify for these resources based on intelligence test scores may feel angry and as if the tests are denying them opportunities for success. Unfortunately, intelligence test scores have not only become associated with a person's ability to perform certain tasks but also with self-worth.

Many people are under the false assumption that intelligence tests measure a person's inborn or biological intelligence. Intelligence tests are based on an individual's interaction with the environment and never exclusively measure inborn intelligence. Intelligence tests have been associated with categorizing and stereotyping people. Additionally, knowledge of one's performance on an intelligence test may affect a person's aspirations and motivation to obtain goals. Intelligence tests can be culturally biased against certain minority groups.

Description

When taking an intelligence test, a person can expect to do a variety of tasks. These tasks may include having to answer questions that are asked verbally, doing mathematical problems, and doing a variety of tasks that require eye hand coordination. Some tasks may be timed and require the person to work as quickly as possible. Typically, most questions and tasks start out easy and progressively get more difficult. It is unusual for anyone to know the answer to all of the questions or be able to complete all of the tasks. If a person is unsure of an answer, guessing is usually allowed.

The four most commonly used intelligence tests are:

- Stanford-Binet Intelligence Scales
- Wechsler-Adult Intelligence Scale
- Wechsler Intelligence Scale for Children
- Wechsler Primary & Preschool Scale of Intelligence

Advantages

In general, intelligence tests measure a wide variety of human behaviors better than any other measure that has been developed. They allow professionals to have a uniform way of comparing a person's performance with that of other people who are similar in age. These tests also provide information on cultural and biological differences among people.

Intelligence tests are excellent predictors of academic achievement and provide an outline of a person's mental strengths and weaknesses. Many times the scores have revealed talents in many people, which have lead to an improvement in their educational opportunities. Teacher, parents, and psychologists are able to devise individual curriculum that matches a person's level of development and expectations.

Disadvantages

Some researchers argue that intelligence tests have serious shortcomings. For example, many intelligence tests produce a single intelligence score. This single score is often inadequate in explaining the multidimensional aspects of intelligence. Another problem with a single score is the fact that individuals with similar intelligence test scores can vary greatly in their expression of these talents. It is important to know the person's performance on the various subtests that make up the overall intelligence test score. Knowing the performance on these various scales can influence the understanding of a person's abilities and how these abilities are expressed. For example, two people have identical scores on intelligence tests. Although both people have the same test score, one person may have obtained the score because of strong verbal skills while the other may have obtained the score because of strong skills in perceiving and organizing various tasks.

Furthermore, intelligence tests only measure a sample of behaviors or situations in which intelligent behavior is revealed. For instance, some intelligence tests do not measure a person's everyday functioning, social knowledge, mechanical skills, and/or **creativity**. Along with this, the formats of many intelligence tests do not capture the complexity and immediacy of real-life situations.

Therefore, intelligence tests have been criticized for their limited ability to predict non-test or nonacademic intellectual abilities. Since intelligence test scores can be influenced by a variety of different experiences and behaviors, they should not be considered a perfect indicator of a person's intellectual potential.

Results

The person's raw scores on an intelligence test are typically converted to standard scores. The standard scores allow the examiner to compare the individual's score to other people who have taken the test. Additionally, by converting raw scores to standard scores the examiner has uniform scores and can more easily compare an individual's performance on one test with the individual's performance on another test. Depending on the intelligence test that is used, a variety of scores can be obtained. Most intelligence tests generate an overall **intelligence quotient** or **IQ**. As previously noted, it is valuable to know how a person performs on the various tasks that make up the test. This can influence the interpretation of the test and what the IQ means. The average of score for most intelligence tests is 100.

Resources

BOOKS

Kaufman, Alan, S., and Elizabeth O. Lichtenberger. *Assessing Adolescent and Adult Intelligence.* Boston: Allyn and Bacon, 2001.

Matarazzo, J. D. *Wechsler's Measurement and Appraisal of Adult Intelligence.* 5th ed. New York: Oxford University Press, 1972.

Sattler, Jerome M. and Lisa Weyandt. "Specific Learning Disabilities." In *Assessment of Children: Behavioral and Clinical Applications.* 4th ed. Written by Jerome M. Sattler. San Diego: Jerome M. Sattler, Publisher, Inc., 2002.

Sattler, Jerome M. "Issues Related to the Measurement and Change of Intelligence." In *Assessment of Children: Cognitive Applications.* 4th ed. San Diego: Jerome M. Sattler, Publisher, Inc., 2001.

Keith Beard, Psy.D.

Intermittent explosive disorder

Definition

Intermittent explosive disorder (IED) is a mental disturbance that is characterized by specific and repeated episodes of violent and aggressive behavior that may involve harm to others or destruction of property. Throwing and breaking of objects are often part of the behavior. Often the anger and violence seen in such an individual reaches a point of uncontrollable rage. Such behavior seems out of context to the situation at hand during such outburst. Common signs of IED are temper **tantrums**, domestic abuse, and road rage. IED is sometimes grouped together as an impulse–control disorder with other such behavioral disorders such as **kleptomania**, **pyromania**, and pathological gambling.

A person must meet certain specific criteria to be diagnosed with IED:

- There must be several separate episodes of failure to restrain aggressive impulses that result in serious assaults against others or property destruction.
- The degree of aggression expressed must be out of proportion to any provocation or other stressor prior to the incidents.
- The behavior cannot be accounted for by another mental disorder, substance abuse, medication side effects, or such general medical conditions as epilepsy or head injuries.

Many psychiatrists do not place intermittent explosive disorder into a separate clinical category but consider it a symptom of other psychiatric and mental disorders. In many cases individuals diagnosed with IED do in fact have a dual psychiatric diagnosis. IED is frequently associated with mood and **anxiety** disorders, **substance abuse**, **eating disorders**, and narcissistic, paranoid, and antisocial **personality disorders**.

Demographics

With regard to sex and age group, the majority of individuals diagnosed with IED in the United States are adolescent and adult males. Women do experience IED, however, and have reported it as part of **premenstrual syndrome** (PMS). IED may appear in childhood but is usually misdiagnosed as temper tantrums. Later in life, it often goes undiagnosed for years because it is a relatively rare condition.

According to researchers at the National Institutes of Health, in 2006, approximately 2.2 million persons in the United States (about 7.3% of the total population) met the criteria for IED, with a total of 11.5 to 16 million meeting the lifetime criteria for the disorder.

Description

People diagnosed with IED sometimes describe strong impulses to act aggressively prior to the specific incidents reported to the doctor and/or the police. They may experience racing thoughts or a heightened energy level during the aggressive episode, with fatigue and depression developing shortly afterward. Some report various physical sensations, including tightness in the chest, **tingling** sensations, increased energy, tremor, hearing echoes, irritability, or a feeling of pressure inside the head.

Many people diagnosed with IED appear to have general problems with anger or other impulsive behaviors between explosive episodes. Some are able to control aggressive impulses without acting on them while others act out in less destructive ways, such as screaming at someone rather than attacking them physically.

Causes and symptoms

Causes

As with other impulse-control disorders, the cause of IED has not been determined. As of 2010, researchers disagree as to whether it is learned behavior (environmental in nature), the result of biochemical or neurological abnormalities (biological in nature), or a combination of factors. Some scientists have reported abnormally low levels of serotonin, a neurotransmitter that affects mood, in the cerebrospinal fluid of some anger-prone persons, but the relationship of this finding to IED is not clear. Generally, IED patients also have higher levels of the hormone testosterone in their systems. Similarly, some individuals diagnosed with IED have a medical history that includes migraine headaches, seizures, attention-deficit hyperactivity disorder, or developmental problems of various types but it is not clear that these cause IED, as most persons with migraines, learning problems, or other neurological disorders do not develop IED.

Some psychiatrists who take a cognitive approach to mental disorders believe that IED results from rigid beliefs and a tendency to misinterpret other people's behavior in accordance with these beliefs. According to American psychologist Aaron Beck (1921–), a pioneer in the application of cognitive therapy to violence-prone individuals, most people diagnosed with IED believe that other people are basically hostile and untrustworthy, that physical force is the only way to obtain respect from others, and that life in general is a battlefield. Beck also identifies certain characteristic errors in thinking that go along with these beliefs:

- Personalizing. The person interprets others' behavior as directed specifically against him or her.
- Selective perception. The person notices only those features of situations or interactions that fit his or her negative view of the world rather than taking in all available information.
- Misinterpreting the motives of others. The person tends to see neutral or even friendly behavior as either malicious or manipulative.
- Denial. The person blames others for provoking his or her violence while denying or minimizing his or her own role in the fight or other outburst.

Symptoms

The symptoms that can precede episodes of IED, or can accompany the disorder, include:

- Rage
- Increased energy
- Tingling
- Tremors
- Palpitations
- Irritability
- Headache or feeling of pressure in the head
- Tightness in the chest

Risks

People with increased risk of having intermittent explosive disorder may have these other characteristics:

- Substance abuse (more likely to have abused drugs or alcohol)
- Age (younger people are more prone to IED)
- Gender (men are more likely than women to have IED)
- Other mental health problems (people with other mental illnesses, such as anxiety attacks or depression, are more likely to also have IED)
- Previous physical abuse (people previously abused physically as children are at higher risk of IED)

Diagnosis

The diagnosis of IED is basically a diagnosis of exclusion, which means that the doctor will eliminate such other possibilities as neurological disorders, mood or substance abuse disorders, anxiety syndromes, and personality disorders before deciding that the patient meets the DSM-IV criteria for IED. In addition to taking a history and performing a physical examination to rule out general medical conditions, the doctor may administer one or more psychiatric inventories or screeners to determine whether the person meets the criteria for other mental disorders.

In some cases the doctor may order imaging studies or refer the person to a neurologist to rule out brain tumors, traumatic injuries of the nervous system, **epilepsy**, or similar physical conditions.

Patients diagnosed with IED are also usually diagnosed with at least one other disorder, such as personality disorders, substance abuse, or neurological disorders.

Along with these other evaluations, the doctor will also investigate the personal and professional history of the patient. People with IED often have problems in school, keeping a job, and interpersonal relationships (including **divorce**), along with numerous automobile accidents and law enforcement crimes.

Treatment

Emergency room treatment

A person brought to a hospital emergency room by family members, police, or other emergency personnel after an explosive episode will be evaluated by a psychiatrist to see whether he or she can safely be released after any necessary medical treatment. If the patient appears to be a danger to him/herself or others, the person may be involuntarily committed for further treatment. In terms of legal issues, a doctor is required by law to notify the specific individuals as well as the police if the patient threatens to harm particular persons. In most states, the doctor is also required by law to report suspected abuse of children, the elderly, or other vulnerable family members.

The doctor will perform a thorough medical examination to determine whether the explosive outburst was related to substance abuse, withdrawal from drugs, head trauma, delirium, or other physical conditions. If the patient becomes assaultive inside the hospital, he or she may be placed in restraints or given a tranquilizer (usually either lorazepam [Ativan] or diazepam [Valium]), usually by injection. In addition to the physical examination, the doctor will obtain as detailed a history as possible from the family members or others who accompanied the patient.

Medications

Medications that have been shown to be beneficial in treating IED in nonemergency situations include lithium, carbamazepine (Tegretol), propranolol (Inderal), and such selective serotonin reuptake inhibitors as fluoxetine (Prozac) and sertraline (Zoloft). Adolescents diagnosed with IED have been reported to respond well to clozapine (Clozaril), a drug normally used to treat **schizophrenia** and other psychotic disorders.

KEY TERMS

Cognitive therapy—A form of short-term psychotherapy that focuses on changing people's patterns of emotional reaction by correcting distorted patterns of thinking and perception.

Delirium—An acute but temporary disturbance of consciousness marked by confusion, difficulty paying attention, delusions, hallucinations, or restlessness. Delirium may be caused by drug intoxication, high fever related to infection, head trauma, brain tumors, kidney or liver failure, or various metabolic disturbances.

Kleptomania—A mental disorder characterized by impulsive stealing.

Neurotransmitter—Any of a group of chemicals that transmit nerve impulses across the gap (synapse) between two nerve cells.

Pyromania—A mental disorder characterized by setting fires.

Serotonin—A neurotransmitter or brain chemical that is responsible for transporting nerve impulses.

Psychotherapy

Some persons with IED benefit from cognitive therapy in addition to medications, particularly if they are concerned about the impact of their disorder on their education, employment, or interpersonal relationships. Psychoanalytic approaches are not useful in treating IED.

Prognosis

The prognosis of IED depends on several factors that include the individual's socioeconomic status, the stability of his or her family, the values of the surrounding neighborhood, and his or her motivation to change. As some patients age the disorder tends to decrease in its severity. However, in others the disorder becomes chronic.

Prevention

There is not a clear way to prevent this disorder. It is also difficult to diagnose until symptoms begin to appear. Since the causes of IED are not fully understood as of the early 2010s, preventive strategies should focus on treatment of young children (particularly boys) who may be at risk for IED before they enter **adolescence**. Teaching self-control skills at a young age is been shown helpful in controlling the disorder.

Resources

BOOKS

Aboujaoude, Elias, and Lorrin M. Koran. *Impulse Control Disorders*. New York: Cambridge University Press, 2010.

Beers, Mark H., editor. *The Merck Manual of Diagnosis and Therapy,* 18th ed., Whitehouse Station, NJ: Merck Research Laboratories, 2006.

Diagnostic and Statistical Manual of Mental Disorders, 4th ed. St. Paul, MN: Thomson/West, 2009.

Grant, Jon E. *Impulse Control Disorders: A Clinician's Guide to Understanding and Treating Behavioral Addictions.* New York: W. W. Norton, 2008.

Hollander, Eris, and Dan J. Stein, editors. *Clinical Manual of Impulse-Control Disorders.* Arlington, VA: American Psychiatric, 2006.

OTHER

"Intermittent Explosive Disorder Affects up to 16 Million Americans." National Institutes of Health. June 5, 2006. [Accessed September 5, 2010], http://www.nih.gov/n ews/pr/jun2006/nimh–05.htm.

"Intermittent Explosive Disorder." Mayo Clinic. June 10, 2010. [Accessed September 5, 2010], http://www.mayoclinic.com/health/intermittent–explosive–disorder/DS00730.

American Academy of Child and Adolescent Psychiatry, 3615 Wisconsin Ave., NW, Washington DC, 20016-3007, (202) 966-7300, (202) 966-2891, http://www.aacap.org.

American Psychiatric Association, 1000 Wilson Blvd, Suite 1825, Arlington VA, 22209, (888) 357-7924, http://www.psych.org.

National Institute of Mental Health, 6001 Executive Blvd., Room 8184, MSC 9663, Bethesda MD, 20892-9663, (866) 615-6464, http://www.nimh.nih.gov.

Janie F. Franz
Rebecca Frey, PhD

Intersex states

Definition

Intersex states are conditions where a newborn's sex organs (genitals) look unusual, making it impossible to identify the sex of the baby from its outward appearance.

Description

All developing babies start out with external sex organs that look female. If the baby is male, the internal sex organs mature and begin to produce the male hormone testosterone. If the hormones reach the tissues correctly, the external genitals that looked female change into the scrotum and penis. Sometimes, the genetic sex (as indicated by chromosomes) may not match the appearance of the external sex organs. About 1 in every 2,000 births results in a baby whose sex organs look unusual.

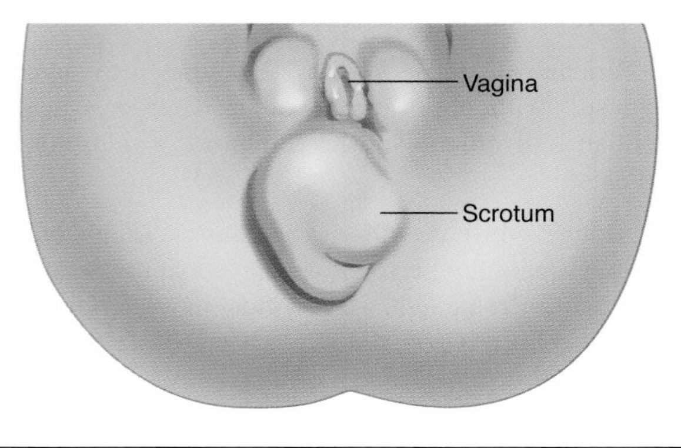

Illustration of an infant born with female and male genitalia. *(Illustration by Electronic Illustrators Group. Reproduced by permission of Gale, a part of Cengage Learning.)*

Patients with intersex states can be classified as a true hermaphrodite, a female pseudohermaphrodite, or a male pseudohermaphrodite. This is determined by examining the internal and external structures of the child.

A true hermaphrodite is born with both ovaries and testicles. They also have mixed male and female external genitals. This condition is extremely rare.

A female pseudohermaphrodite is a genetic female. However, the external sex organs have been masculinized and look like a penis. This may occur if the mother takes the hormone progesterone to prevent a miscarriage, but more often it is caused by an overproduction of certain hormones.

A male pseudohermaphrodite is a genetic male. However, the external sex organs fail to develop normally. Intersex males may have testes and a female-like vulva, or a very small penis.

Causes and symptoms

Any abnormality in chromosomes or sex hormones, or in the unborn baby's response to the hormones, can lead to an intersex state in a newborn.

Intersex states may also be caused by a condition called **congenital adrenal hyperplasia**, which occurs in about 1 out of every 5,000 newborns. This disease blocks the baby's metabolism and can cause a range of symptoms, including abnormal genitals.

KEY TERMS

Chromosomes—Spaghetti-like structures located within the nucleus (or central portion) of each cell. Chromosomes contain the genetic information necessary to direct the development and functioning of all cells and systems in the body. They pass on hereditary traits from parents to child (like eye color) and determine whether the child will be male or female.

Diagnosis

When doctors are uncertain about a newborn's sex, a specialist in infant hormonal problems is consulted as soon as possible. Ultrasound can locate a uterus behind the bladder and can determine if there is a cervix or uterine canal. Blood tests can check the levels of sex hormones in the baby's blood and chromosome analysis (called karyotyping) can determine sex. Explorative surgery or a biopsy of reproductive tissue may be necessary. Only after thorough testing can a correct diagnosis and determination of sex be made.

Treatment

Treatment of intersex states is controversial. Traditional treatment assigns sex according to test results, the potential for the child to identify with a sex, and the ease of genital surgery to make the organs look more normal. Treatment may then include reconstructive surgery followed by hormone therapy. Babies born with congenital adrenal hyperplasia can be treated with cortisone-type drugs and sometimes surgery.

Counseling should be given to the entire **family** of an intersex newborn. Families should explore all available medical and surgical options. Counseling should also be provided to the child when he or she is old enough.

Prognosis

Since the mid-1950s, doctors have typically assigned a sex to an intersex infant based on how easy reconstructive surgery would be. The **American Academy of Pediatrics** states that children with these types of genitals can be raised successfully as members of either sex and recommends surgery within the first 15 months of life.

Some people are critical of this approach, including intersex adults who were operated on as children. The remolded genitals do not function sexually and can be the source of lifelong **pain**. They suggest that surgery be delayed until the patient can make informed choices about surgery and intervention.

Resources

ORGANIZATIONS

Pacific Center For Sex And Society, University of Hawaii at Mānoa, 1960 East-West Road, Honolulu Hawaii, 96822, http://www.hawaii.edu/PCSS/index.html.

Intersex Society of North America, 979 Golf Course Drive #282, Rohnert Park CA, 94928, http://www.isna.org/.

Intersex Initiative, PO Box 40570, Portland OR, 97240, (971) 570-8698, http://intersexinitiative.org/index.html.

Carol A. Turkington

Intestinal obstructions

Definition

Intestinal obstructions, sometimes also called bowel obstructions, refers to the partial or complete mechanical or non-mechanical blockages of fluids or foods of the small or large intestine (which includes the colon, cecum, and rectum). When such obstructions occur, they can lead to reduced or blocked passage of digested materials through the intestines. They are often caused by intestinal adhesions, hernias, or tumors.

Demographics

The disorder occurs in people of all ages, genders, and ethnic backgrounds.

Description

There are two types of intestinal obstructions, mechanical and non-mechanical. Mechanical obstructions occur because the bowel (intestines) is physically blocked and its contents cannot get past the obstruction. Mechanical obstructions can occur for several reasons. Sometimes the bowel twists on itself (volvulus) or telescopes into itself (intussusception). Mechanical obstruction can also result from hernias, impacted feces, abnormal tissue growth, the presence of foreign bodies in the intestines (including gallstones), or inflammatory bowel disease (Crohn's disease). Non-mechanical obstruction, called **ileus**, occurs because the wavelike muscular contractions of the intestine (peristalsis) that ordinarily move food through the digestive tract stop.

Mechanical obstruction in infants

Infants under one year of age are most likely to have intestinal obstruction caused by meconium ileus, volvulus,

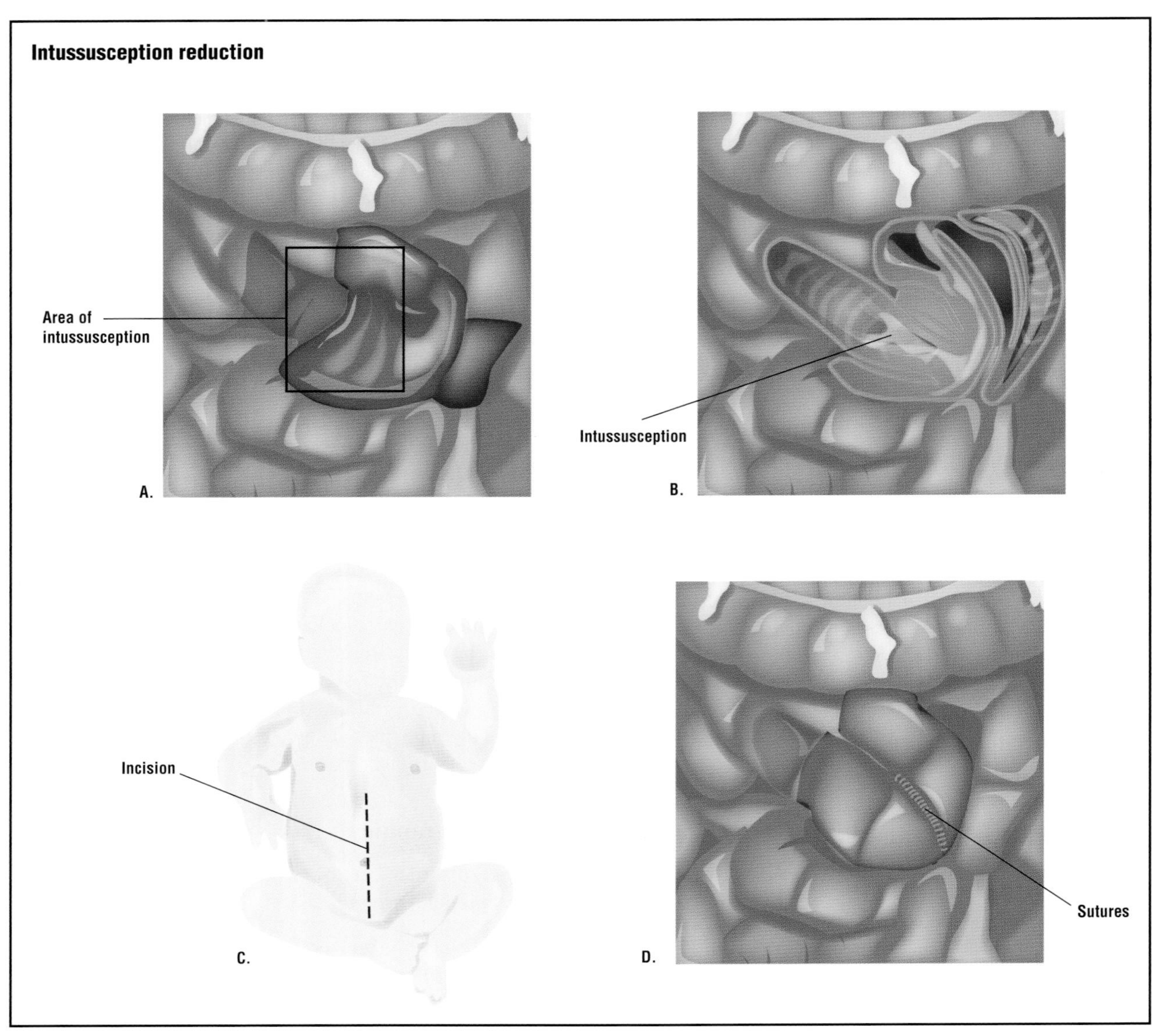

Intussusception of the bowel results in the bowel telescoping onto itself (A and B). An incision is made in the baby's abdomen to expose the bowel (C). If the surgeon cannot manipulate the bowel into a normal shape manually, the area of intussusception will be removed and remaining bowel sutured together (D). *(Illustration by PreMediaGlobal. Reproduced by permission of Gale, a part of Cengage Learning.)*

and intussusception. Meconium ileus, which is the inability to pass the first fecal excretion after **birth** (meconium), is a disorder of newborns. It is an early clue that the infant has **cystic fibrosis** but may also occur in very low birth weight (VLBW) infants. In meconium ileus, the material that is blocking the intestine is thick and stringy, rather than the collection of mucus and bile that is passed by normal infants. The abnormal meconium must be removed with an enema or through surgery.

Volvulus is the medical term for twisting of either the small or large bowel. The twisting may cut off the blood supply to the bowel, leading to tissue **death** (gangrene). This development is called a strangulating obstruction.

In intussusception, the bowel telescopes into itself like a radio antenna folding up. Intussusception is most common in children between the ages of three and nine months, although it also occurs in older children. Almost twice as many boys suffer intussusception as girls. It is, however, difficult for doctors to predict which infants will suffer from intestinal obstruction.

Mechanical obstruction in adults

Obstructions in adults are usually caused by tumors, trauma, volvulus, the presence of foreign bodies such as gallstones, or hernias, although they have also been reported in adults with cystic fibrosis. Volvulus occurs most often in elderly adults and psychiatrically disturbed patients. Intussusception in adults is usually associated with tumors in the bowel, whether benign or malignant.

More recently, gastroenterologists have described a postsurgical complication known as early postoperative small bowel obstruction, or EPSBO. Although this condition was at one time confused with postoperative ileus, it is now known to be caused by mechanical obstructions resulting from radiation therapy for **cancer** or laparoscopic surgery. Most cases can be successfully treated within 10–14 days of surgery.

Causes and symptoms

Causes

Causes of intestinal obstructions can be subdivided into two primary groups: small bowel obstruction and large bowel obstruction. Causes of small bowel obstruction include:

- adhesions (usually from abdominal surgery, but sometimes present at birth)
- hernias (protrusion of intestines through cavity that contains it)
- Crohn's disease (inflammatory disease of the intestines)
- neoplasm (abnormal growth of tissue mass)
- intussusception (layering [telescoping] of sections of intestines within other sections, children only)
- volvulus (abnormal twist in bowel)
- superior mesenteric artery syndrome (compression of part of duodenum by abdominal aorta and superior mesenteric artery)
- intestinal atresia (narrowing or absence of part of intestine)
- carcinoid (neuroendocrine tumor)
- foreign bodies (such as gall stones or swallowed objects)
- ischaemic stricture (abnormal narrowing of intestines usually at outlet from stomach)

Large bowel obstruction can be caused by the following:

- neoplasm
- hernias
- cancer
- inflammatory bowel disease (inflammation of the colon)
- diverticulitis (small pouches in digestive tract become inflamed or infected)
- colonic volvulus (twist in colon)
- fecal impaction (blocked, impacted feces in rectum)
- intestinal atresia
- endometriosis (uterine tissue found outside of uterus, in women only)

Almost all of the causes of intestinal obstructions occur in the small intestines rather than the large intestines.

Symptoms

One of the earliest signs of mechanical intestinal obstruction is abdominal **pain** or cramps that come and go in waves. Infants typically pull up their legs and cry in pain, then stop crying suddenly. They will then behave normally for as long as 15–30 minutes, only to start crying again when the next cramp begins. The cramping results from the inability of the muscular contractions of the bowel to push the digested food past the obstruction.

Vomiting is another symptom of intestinal obstruction. The speed of its onset is a clue to the location of the obstruction. Vomiting follows shortly after the pain if the obstruction is in the small intestine but it is delayed if found in the large intestine. The vomited material may be fecal in character. When the patient has a mechanical obstruction, the doctor will first hear active, high-pitched gurgling and splashing bowel sounds while listening with a stethoscope. Later these sounds decrease and then stop. If the blockage is complete, the patient will not pass any gas or feces. If the blockage is only partial, however, the patient may have **diarrhea**. Initially there is little or no **fever**.

When the material in the bowel cannot move past the obstruction, the body reabsorbs large amounts of fluid and the abdomen becomes sore to the touch and swollen. The balance of certain important chemicals (electrolytes) in the blood is upset. Persistent vomiting can cause the patient to become dehydrated. Without treatment, the patient can suffer shock and kidney failure.

Strangulation occurs when a loop of the intestine is cut off from its blood supply. Strangulation occurs in about 25% of cases of small bowel obstruction. It is a serious condition that can progress to gangrene within six hours.

Risks

The following pre-existing conditions can add to the risk of contracting intestinal obstructions:

- Crohn's disease
- abdominal or pelvic surgeries
- long-lasting constipation

- malrotation (congenital condition in which intestines do not develop normally)

If someone has advanced intestinal obstruction of one type or the other, certain symptoms will be apparent due to infection within the lining of the abdominal cavity (a condition known as peritonitis). These symptoms include:

- tenderness, pain, and swelling in abdominal area
- thirst, but low urine output
- fluid in abdomen
- vomiting and nausea
- fever and chills
- inability to pass gas or have a bowel movement

When advanced peritonitis occurs, more severe symptoms occur. They include:

- weak, rapid pulse
- either abnormally slow, shallow breathing or rapid breathing
- pale, clammy skin
- inability to pass gas or have a bowel movement
- dilated pupils in the eyes
- eyes that stare off into the distance

If such symptoms occur, the patient has most likely gone into shock, and immediate emergency care should be sought.

Diagnosis

Imaging studies

If the doctor suspects intestinal obstruction based on the physical examination and patient history, he or she will order **x rays**, a computed tomography scan (CT scan), or an ultrasound evaluation of the abdomen. In many cases the patient is given a barium enema. A suspension of barium sulfate, which is a white powder, is inserted through the rectum, and the intestinal area is photographed. Barium acts as a contrast material and allows the location of the obstruction to be visualized on film.

Laboratory tests

The first blood test of a patient with an intestinal obstruction usually gives normal results but later tests indicate electrolyte imbalances. There is no way to determine if an obstruction is simple or strangulated except by performing surgery.

Treatment

Initial assessment

All patients with suspected intestinal obstruction are hospitalized. Treatment must be rapid because strangulating obstructions can be fatal. The first step in treatment is inserting a nasogastric tube to suction out the contents of the stomach and intestines. The patient is then given intravenous fluids to prevent **dehydration** and correct electrolyte imbalances.

Nonsurgical approaches

Surgery can be avoided for some patients. In some cases of volvulus, guiding a rectal tube into the intestines will straighten the twisted bowels. In infants, a barium enema may reverse intussusception in 50–90% of the cases. An air enema is sometimes used instead of a barium enema. This treatment successfully relieves the obstruction in many infants. The children are usually hospitalized for observation for two to three days after these procedures. In patients with only partial obstruction, a barium enema may dissolve the blockage.

Surgical treatment

If these efforts fail, surgery is necessary. Strangulated obstructions require emergency surgery. The obstructed area is removed and part of the bowel is cut away. If the obstruction is caused by tumors, polyps, or scar tissue, they are removed. Hernias, if present, are repaired. **Antibiotics** are given to reduce the possibility of infection.

Alternative treatment

Alternative practitioners offer few suggestions for treatment. They focus on preventive strategies, particularly the use of high-fiber diets, to keep the bowels healthy through regular elimination.

Prognosis

The prognosis for intestinal obstructions depends on age, previous illnesses (especially lung, heart, or kidney problems), and the specific cause of the obstruction within the intestines. Generally, healthy people have good prospects. However, when intestinal obstructions are associated with cancer, the prognosis is not as favorable.

Mortality

Untreated intestinal obstructions can be fatal. Delayed diagnosis of volvulus in infants has a mortality rate of 23–33% with prompt diagnosis and treatment the mortality rate is 3–9%. The bowel either strangulates or perforates, causing massive infection. Tissues within the intestines soon die, which leads to perforation of the intestines and infection. The patient

KEY TERMS

Electrolytes—Salts and minerals that ionize in body fluids. Electrolytes control the body's fluid balance as well as performing other important functions.

Gangrene—The death of soft tissue in any part of the body when the blood supply is obstructed.

Ileus—Obstruction of the intestines caused by the absence of peristalsis.

Intussusception—The slipping or telescoping of one part of the intestine into the section next to it.

Meconium—A greenish fecal material that constitutes the first bowel movement of an infant.

Peristalsis—The waves of muscular contraction in the intestines that push the food along during the process of digestion.

Strangulated obstruction—An obstruction in which a loop of the intestine has its blood supply cut off.

Volvulus—A twisting of the intestine that causes an obstruction.

eventually goes into shock. With prompt treatment, however, most patients recover successfully without complications.

Recurrence

As many as 80% of patients whose volvulus is treated without surgery have recurrences. Recurrences in infants with intussusception are most likely to happen during the first 36 hours after the blockage has been cleared. The mortality rate for unsuccessfully treated infants is 1–2%.

Prevention

Most cases of intestinal obstruction are not preventable. Surgery to remove tumors, polyps, or gallstones helps prevent recurrences. Other medical treatments and therapies may help to reduce the risk from many forms of intestinal obstructions.

Resources

BOOKS

Beers, Mark H., et al., editors. *The Merck Manual of Diagnosis and Therapy,* 18th ed. Whitehouse Station, NJ: Merck Research Laboratories, 2006.

Feldman, Mark., et al., editors. *Sleisenger and Fordtran's Gastrointestinal and Liver Disease: Pathophysiology/Diagnosis/Management.* Philadelphia: Saunders/Elsevier, 2006.

Townsend, C. M, et al. editors. *Sabiston Textbook of Surgery: The Biological Basis of Modern Surgical Practice,* 18th ed. Philadelphia: Saunders/Elsevier, 2008.

OTHER

Heller, Jacob L. "Intestinal Obstruction." Medline Plus, U.S. National Library of Medicine and National Institutes of Health. July 23, 2008. [Accessed September 5, 2010], http://www.nlm.nih.gov/medlineplus/ency/article/000260.htm.

"Intestinal Obstruction—Overview." University of Maryland Medical Center. [Accessed September 5, 2010], http://www.umm.edu/ency/article/000260.htm.

"Intestinal Obstruction." Mayo Clinic. July 8, 2010. [Accessed September 5, 2010], http://www.mayoclinic.com/health/intestinal–obstruction/DS00823.

Tish Davidson, AM
Rebecca Frey, PhD

Intrauterine growth retardation

Definition

Intrauterine growth retardation (IUGR) occurs when the unborn baby (fetus) is at or below the 10th weight percentile for his or her gestational age (in weeks). In other words, the unborn baby is developing poorly (more slowly then normal) within the womb. After being born, these babies usually have low weights and are likely to continue having health problems later in life.

Description

There are standards or averages in weight for unborn babies according to their age in weeks. When the baby's weight is at or below the 10th percentile for his or her age, it is called intrauterine growth retardation, or fetal growth restriction. These babies are smaller than they should be for their age. How much a baby weighs at **birth** depends not only on how many weeks old it is but also the rate at which it has grown. This growth process is complex and delicate. There are three phases associated with the development of the baby. During the first phase, cells multiply in the baby's organs. This occurs from the beginning of development through the early part of the fourth month. During the second phase, cells continue to multiply and the organs grow. In the

Intrauterine growth retardation (IUGR)

Conditions associated with IUGR	
Maternal history	Alcohol use Cocaine use Smoking Malnutrition Use of prescription drugs warfarin (Coumadin, Panwarfarin) and phenytoin (Dilantin) Prior history of IUGR pregnancy Residing at altitude over 5,000 ft (1,500 m)
Medical conditions (of mother)	Chronic hypertension Preeclampsia early in gestation Diabetes mellitus Systemic lupus erythematosus Chronic kidney disease Inflammatory bowel disease Severe lung disease
Infectious diseases	Syphilis Cytomegalovirus Toxoplasmosis Rubella Hepatitis B Herpes simplex virus 1 or 2 HIV-1
Congenital disorders (of fetus)	Trisomy 21 (Down syndrome) Trisomy 18 (Edwards syndrome) Trisomy 13 (Patau syndrome) Turner's syndrome

(Table by PreMediaGlobal. Reproduced by permission of Gale, a part of Cengage Learning.)

third phase (after 32 weeks of development), growth occurs quickly and the baby may gain as much as seven ounces (200 grams) per week. If the delicate process of development and weight gain is disturbed or interrupted, the baby can suffer from restricted growth.

IUGR is usually classified as symmetrical or asymmetrical. In symmetrical IUGR, the baby's head and body are proportionately small. In asymmetrical IUGR, the baby's brain is abnormally large when compared to the liver. In a normal infant, the brain weighs about three times as much as the liver. In asymmetrical IUGR, the brain can weigh five or six times as much as the liver.

Causes and symptoms

Doctors think that the two types of IUGR may be linked to the time during development that the problem occurs. Symmetrical IUGR may occur when the unborn baby experiences a problem during early development. Asymmetrical IUGR may occur when the unborn baby experiences a problem during later development. While not true for all asymmetrical cases, doctors think that sometimes the placenta may allow the brain to get more oxygen and **nutrition** while the liver gets less.

There are many IUGR risk factors involving the mother and the unborn baby. A mother is at risk for having a growth restricted infant if she:

- Has had a previous baby who suffered from IUGR
- Has poor weight gain and lack of nutrition (malnutrition) during pregnancy
- Is socially deprived
- Uses substances (like tobacco, narcotics, alcohol, and some prescription drugs, such as anticonvulsants) that can cause abnormal development or birth defects
- Has a vascular disease (like chronic hypertension [high blood pressure], preeclampsia [hypertension during pregnancy], or heart disease)
- Has chronic kidney disease
- Has sickle cell anemia
- Has a coagulation/antibody disorder called antiphospholipid antibody syndrome that causes blood clots
- Has a serious lung disease
- Has a low total blood volume during early pregnancy
- Is pregnant with more than one baby (multiple pregnancies)

A mother that is very small in size (weight) is more likely to have a fetus that is underweight when compared to normally sized unborn babies. Such a situation is not always caused by IUGR. About one out of three babies born smaller than normal have IUGR, while the other two are born smaller usually because the mother is smaller herself.

Additionally, an unborn baby may suffer from IUGR if it has:

- Exposure to an infection, including German measles (rubella), cytomegalovirus, tuberculosis, syphilis, or toxoplasmosis
- A defect in the kidneys, abdominal wall, or in the cardiovascular system
- A chromosome defect, especially trisomy 18 (Edwards' syndrome), Down syndrome, or anencephaly (missing parts of the brain)
- A primary disorder of bone or cartilage
- A chronic lack of oxygen during development (hypoxia), such as from living at high altitudes
- Placenta or umbilical cord defects such as placenta previa (placenta too low in uterus) or placental abruption (placenta detaching from uterus)
- Developed outside of the uterus.

KEY TERMS

Preeclampsia—Hypertension (high blood pressure) during pregnancy.

Diagnosis

IUGR can be difficult to diagnose and in many cases doctors are not able to make an exact diagnosis until the baby is born. A mother who has had a growth-restricted baby is at risk of having another during a later pregnancy. Such mothers are monitored closely during pregnancy. The length in weeks of the pregnancy must be carefully determined so that the doctor will know if development and weight gain are appropriate.

Checking the mother's weight and abdomen measurements can help diagnose cases when other risk factors are not present. Measuring the girth of the abdomen is often used as a tool for diagnosing IUGR. During pregnancy, the healthcare provider will use a tape measure to record the height from the pubic bone to the top of the uterus (the uterine fundal height, in centimeters).

As the pregnancy continues and the baby grows, the uterus stretches upward in the direction of the mother's head. Between 18 and 30 weeks of gestation, the uterine fundal height equals the weeks of gestation. For example, if the mother is 26 weeks pregnant, then the fundal height should be about 26 centimeters. If the uterine fundal height is more than 2–3 centimeters below normal, then IUGR is suspected. Ultrasound is used to evaluate the growth of the baby. Usually, IUGR is diagnosed after week 32 of pregnancy. This is during the phase of rapid growth when the baby should be gaining more weight. IUGR caused by genetic factors or infection may sometimes be detected earlier.

Treatment

Treatment is not available that improves fetal growth but IUGR babies who are at or near term have the best outcome if delivered promptly. If IUGR is caused by a problem with the placenta and the baby is otherwise healthy, early diagnosis and treatment of the problem may reduce the chance of a serious outcome. Pregnant women suspected of carrying a fetus with IUGR will be monitored closely with several ultrasounds during the course of the pregnancy.

Measurements of movement, blood flow, growth, and fluid surrounding the fetus, will be carefully taken. Fetal monitoring is one test that indicates the health of a fetus. **Amniocentesis**, where a tiny amount of amniotic fluid is withdrawn from the uterus, is a way to test for chromosomal abnormalities.

A fetus that cannot tolerate the stress of natural labor may be delivered by **cesarean section** (c-section).

Prognosis

Babies who suffer from IUGR are at an increased risk for intrauterine (inside the womb) **death**, stress during vaginal delivery, abnormally high red blood cell count, low blood sugar (**hypoglycemia**), low body temperature (hypothermia), lower resistance to infection, difficulty maintaining body temperature, and abnormal development of the nervous system. These risks increase with the severity of the growth restriction. The growth that occurs after birth cannot be predicted with certainty based on the size of the baby when it is born. Infants with asymmetrical IUGR are more likely to catch up in growth after birth than are infants who suffer from prolonged symmetrical IUGR.

However, doctors cannot reliably predict an infant's future progress. Each case is unique. Some infants who have IUGR will develop normally, while others will have complications of the nervous system or intellectual problems like **learning disorders**. If IUGR is related to a disease or a genetic defect, the future of the infant is related to the severity and the nature of that disorder. Generally, most IUGR babies will attain a normal weight and height within two years of birth.

Prevention

The risk factors that can complicate pregnancies should be strictly controlled. Avoid alcohol, tobacco products, and drugs that are not part of the pregnancy. Make sure that regular prenatal care is obtained from medical professionals.

Movement of the unborn baby inside the mother is a reliable way to indicate its general health. A healthy baby moves and kicks often. Your **caregiver** may request a fetal kick count in between prenatal appointments to check on the number of kicks. A baby that has moved frequently in the past but has stopped kicking may be a sign of a problem. In such cases, call the **pediatrician** or other medical profession caring for the mother and baby.

The more nutrients that the mother takes in, means the more nutrients for the unborn baby. Eat healthy foods and always go by the amount of calories recommended by the doctor. Plenty of rest is essential. At least eight hours of **sleep** each night should be taken by the mother, and naps during the day are also helpful.

Resources

BOOKS

Bianchi, Diana W., et al. *Fetology: Diagnosis and Management of the Fetal Patient.* New York: McGraw-Hill Medical, 2010.

Cunningham, F. Gary, et al. *Williams Obstetrics,* 22nd ed. Stamford, CT: Appleton & Lange, 2005.

Kiess, Wieland, et al. *Small for Gestational Age: Causes and Consequences.* Basel, Switzerland: Karger, 2009.

Preedy, Victor R., and Ronald R. Watson, editors. *Handbook of Disease Burdens and Quality of Life Measures.* New York: Springer, 2010.

OTHER

"Intrauterine Growth Restriction." FamilyDoctor.org. April 2008. [Accessed September 21, 2010], http://familydoctor.org/online/famdocen/home/women/pregnancy/fetal/313.html.

"Intrauterine Growth Restriction (IURG)." BabyCenter L.L.C. May 2006. [Accessed September 21, 2010], http://www.babycenter.com/0_intrauterine–growth–restriction–iugr_142740 6.bc.

"Intrauterine Growth Restriction." Medline Plus, U.S. National Library of Medicine and National Institutes of Health. February 19, 2009. [Accessed September 21, 2010], http://www.nlm.nih.gov/medlineplus/ency/article/001500.htm.

Linda Jones

Intravenous rehydration

Definition

Rehydration is the process of replenishing the human body with water, or water and electrolytes, which have been previously lost through **dehydration**. This process can be performed orally or intravenously. With mild dehydration, oral rehydration is usually used. However, for more severe cases, which can cause serious and permanent injury or even **death**, intravenous rehydration is the method of choice within the medical community. For the method of intravenous (IV) rehydration, a sterile water solution containing small amounts of salt or sugar (and usually essential **minerals** and

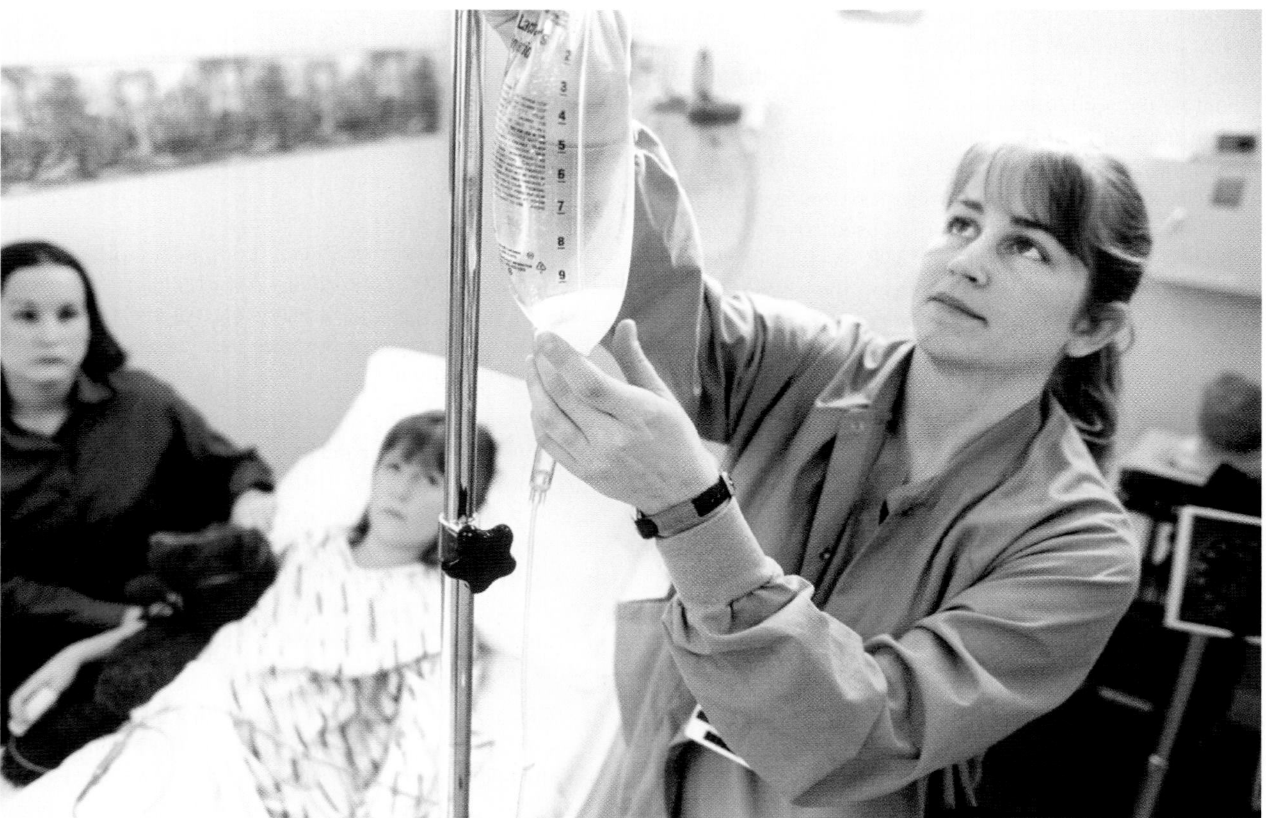

A child receiving fluids through an intravenous (IV) bag. *(© Tom Stewart/Corbis.)*

vitamins), are injected into the body through a tube attached to a needle, which is inserted into a vein.

Purpose

Fever, **vomiting**, and **diarrhea** can cause a person to become dehydrated fairly quickly. Infants and children are especially vulnerable to dehydration because of their smaller body weights, of a higher turnover of water and electrolytes, and due to their increased susceptibility to sicknesses such as those involving vomiting and diarrhea. Adult patients can become dehydrated due to an illness, surgery, or accident. Athletes, who have overexerted themselves and, thus, become dehydrated, may also require rehydration with IV fluids. An IV for rehydration can be used for several hours to several days, and is generally used if a patient cannot drink fluids.

Precautions

Patients receiving IV therapy need to be monitored to ensure that the IV solutions are providing the correct amounts of fluids and minerals needed. People with kidney and heart disease are at increased risk for **overhydration** so they must be carefully monitored when receiving IV therapy.

Demographics

Because dehydration is common throughout the human population, intravenous rehydration may be used on any persons in need of such medical treatment. Infants and children, due to their young age, are at greater risk of becoming dehydrated. Adults recovering from surgeries and those that are sick are also vulnerable for dehydration. Athletes that overexert themselves may also become dehydrated. Hot weather, accidents, and medical problems can also cause a person to become dehydrated.

Description

Basic IV solutions are sterile water with small amounts of sodium chloride (salt) or dextrose (sugar) supplied in bottles or thick plastic bags that can hang on a stand mounted next to the patient's bed. Additional minerals like potassium, phosphate magnesium, chloride, calcium, vitamins, or drugs can be added to the IV solution by injecting them into the bottle or bag with a needle.

Risks

There is a small risk of infection at the injection site. It is possible that the IV solution will not provide all of the nutrients needed, leading to a deficiency or an imbalance. If the needle becomes dislodged, it is possible that the solution may flow into tissues around the injection site rather than into the vein.

Causes and symptoms

Initial symptoms of dehydration that indicate the possible need for intravenous rehydration include:

- headache
- flushing in the face
- dry, warm skin
- muscle cramps, especially in the legs and arms
- lower than normal, and sudden decrease, in blood pressure
- dizziness or fainting when standings
- abnormal thirst or the inability to drink
- decreased urine output and unusually dark yellow-colored urine
- tiredness, weakness, sleepiness, lethargic
- irritability, confusion
- dry mouth, dry tongue with thick saliva

More serious symptoms of dehydration that indicate a more critical need for intravenous rehydration include:

- low blood pressure
- delirium
- unconsciousness/comotose
- swelling of the tongue
- no urine output
- lethargy or extreme sleepiness
- fainting
- rapid, deep breathing
- weak, fast pulse
- severe muscle contractions, especially in the arms, legs, back, and stomach
- bloated stomach
- dry eyes, sunken look to eyes
- wrinkly look to skin, a lost firmness (elasticity) to the skin

Diagnosis

Anyone who exhibits signs and symptoms of moderate to severe dehydration should be taken promptly to a emergency medical professional for appropriate care. At the medical facility, the team will observe for physical characteristics as to indicate low blood pressure, rapid heart rate, appearance of shock, poor skin features (lack of elasticity), delayed capillary refill (rate at which blood refills capillaries), and other such signs that indicate dehydration.

KEY TERMS

Intravenous—Into a vein; a needle is inserted into a vein in the back of the hand, inside the elbow, or some other location on the body. Fluids, nutrients, and drugs can be injected.

Tests that may be performed to indicate moderate to severe dehydration include: complete blood count (CBC), creatinine, blood urea nitrogen (BUN), urine specific gravity, and various blood chemistries (such as those indicating sodium, bicarbonate, and potassium).

Treatment

Moderate and severely dehydrated persons should be initially treated by emergency personnel. Take such people to an emergency room at the hospital or other such facility where immediate emergency care can be given. The person should receive intravenous rehydration with salts and fluids through the vein (intravenously) because such a method provides a fast way to introduce water and essential nutrients into the body. This is especially important in life-threatening situations.

Preparation

A doctor orders the IV solution and any additional nutrients or drugs to be added to it. The doctor also specifies the rate at which the IV will be infused. The IV solutions are prepared under the supervision of a doctor, pharmacist, or nurse, using sanitary techniques that prevent bacterial contamination. Just like a prescription, the IV is labeled clearly to show its contents and the amounts of any additives. The skin around the area where the needle is inserted is cleaned and disinfected. Once the needle is in place, it will be taped to the skin to prevent it from dislodging.

The vein usually used are those in the arm, however, those veins in the back of the hand or the median cubital vein on the inside of the elbow can also be used. Generally, any appropriate vein can be used.

Aftercare

Patients need to take fluids by mouth before an IV solution is discontinued. After the IV needle is removed, the site should be inspected for any signs of bleeding or infection.

Prognosis

People with mild to serious dehydration will usually recover when they are given intravenous rehydration promptly and effectively at the first signs of being dehydrated. However, seizures, permanent brain damage and, even, death can result to people who are not given such treatment.

Prevention

To prevent the need for intravenous rehydration, make sure the body is properly hydrated. Consume plenty of fluids on a daily basis, along with foods that are high in water content such as fruits and vegetables. When exercising or performing other strenuous activities, make sure sufficient water is consumed before, during, and after such events. If a person is overly sweating and feels overheated during hot conditions, stop all activity and rest in a shady area to lower the body temperature. Drink fluids to replace any that have been lost. However, do not consume too much water because such a condition can also cause problems.

Fluids can be lost in the body in cold weather, not only in hot weather. **Exercise** or strenuous activity in cold weather, while wearing insulated clothing, can cause sweating and, thus, lost of hydration in the body. Even conditions inside involving very low humidity can contribute to a person losing moisture within the body. In addition, locations of high altitudes, usually over 8,200 feet, or 2,500 meters, can cause a body to need more fluids.

During illnesses, such as those that include vomiting or diarrhea, make sure water or other fluids that can replenish lost electrolytes are taken promptly and regularly.

Resources

BOOKS

Kliegman, Robert, and Waldo E. Nelson. *Nelson Textbook of Pediatrics.* Philadelphia: Saunders, 2007.

Marx, John A., et al., editors. *Rosen's Emergency Medicine: Concepts and Clinical Practice.* Philadelphia: Mosby/Elsevier, 2010.

Shils, Maurice, et al., editors. *Modern Nutrition in Health and Disease.* Philadelphia: Lippincott Williams and Wilkins, 2006.

OTHER

"Dehydration." Mayo Clinic. July 25, 2009. [Accessed July 17, 2010], http://www.mayoclinic.com/health/dehydration/DS00561.

"Dehydration." Medline Plus, National Library of Medicine and National Institutes of Health. [Accessed July 17, 2010], http://www.nlm.nih.gov/medlineplus/ency/article/000982.htm.

Altha Roberts Edgren

Intussusception **see Intestinal obstructions**

Iowa tests of basic skills

Definition

The Iowa Tests of Basic Skills (ITBS) are probably the most widely administered, nationally standardized, comprehensive assessments of academic achievement for kindergarten through the eighth grade. They are group-administered traditional achievement test batteries that measure the development of the basic skills required for academic success. At least some of the school districts in all 50 states use the ITBS, with more than four million children taking the batteries every year.

Purpose

The purposes of the ITBS include:

- assessing the developmental level of each student in each tested subject area
- identifying each student's relative strengths and weaknesses within each subject area
- comparing individual student achievement with peers nationwide
- monitoring the year-to-year progress of individuals and groups of students in basic skills and major subject areas
- providing a basis for parental reports to promote home and school cooperative efforts
- providing comprehensive data about the development of basic skills and critical thinking
- providing schools with benchmark data on student performance at the start of the school year
- providing educators with diagnostic data for planning remedial instruction
- evaluating the effectiveness of instructional programs and specific curricula
- preparing students for high-stakes reading and math assessments, especially criterion-referenced state competency exams
- fulfilling some state- or locally-mandated testing requirements
- comparing progress and achievements of home-schooled, Catholic, and other private school students with public school students
- providing a basis for selecting students for charter schools, magnet schools, and other educational programs
- conducting educational research studies

The ITBS levels 5–8, for kindergarten through second grade, are designed to:

- help determine the background and skills of individual students
- estimate general developmental levels for adapting materials and instructional procedures
- identify areas for individual early interventions
- establish an achievement baseline for monitoring year-to-year progress
- provide information for administrative planning
- identify group strengths and weaknesses for planning procedural and curricular changes

In addition:

- Level 5, for kindergarten, assesses cognitive preparedness to begin an academic curriculum. It does not measure school or reading readiness.
- Level 6, usually administered in the fall or midyear of first grade, is similar in purpose and content to level 5, but has an optional reading test for students with beginning literacy skills.
- Level 7, usually administered during the spring of first grade or fall of second grade, and level 8, for midyear or spring of second grade, are designed to provide information about student progress in an expanding curriculum.

The primary purpose of the ITBS levels 9–14, for 3rd–8th grades, is to provide unique information for improving instruction, including:

- selecting learning objectives and procedures
- designing and choosing materials
- creating effective learning environments
- helping teachers determine whether individual students have the knowledge and skills to succeed in the planned program
- helping teachers adapt materials and procedures to meet individual needs
- identifying individual strengths and weaknesses to help plan goals and approaches
- monitoring yearly progress

States and school districts have varying requirements for administration of the ITBS. Some states require that all schools administer the ITBS at specific grade levels.

Description

The ten levels of the ITBS are available in three forms—A, B, and C. The ITBS is available as a complete battery, a core battery, or a survey battery.

The ITBS levels 5–8, for the primary grades, measure content and skills in separate tests. The levels 5 and 6 tests are not timed and, except for the level 6 reading test, are read aloud by the teacher. The test booklets have large picture responses and the children mark their answers in a machine-scorable booklet. Levels 7 and 8 are also orally administered, except for the vocabulary and reading tests. The tests consist of:

- a practice page of six questions in several different test areas, preceding the first test for levels 5 and 6
- a listening vocabulary test for levels 5 and 6
- a reading vocabulary test for levels 7 and 8
- word analysis to assess recognition of letters and letter-sound relationships
- a listening comprehension test
- reading comprehension tests for levels 6–8
- language tests
- math tests for levels 5 and 6
- separate math concepts, problem solving, and computation tests for levels 7 and 8
- social studies, science, and information sources tests for levels 7 and 8, with the latter being replaced by an information literacy test in 2011

The ITBS levels 9–14, for grades 3–8, include the following tests:

- general vocabulary
- a two-session reading comprehension test
- spelling
- capitalization
- punctuation
- usage and expression
- math concepts and estimation
- math problem solving and data interpretation
- math computation
- social studies
- science
- maps and diagrams
- reference materials
- word analysis and listening tests for level 9

Teachers are given exact instructions for administering the ITBS. Each timed test takes 30 minutes or less. The complete ITBS battery for grades 3–8 requires five and a half hours—five hours and ten minutes of actual testing—with another 20 minutes for the level 9 word analysis test and 25 minutes for the level 9 listening test. The complete battery should be administered in 6 or 11 sessions on 6 different days, with the order and number of sessions per day up to the school district. Test results are of the most value to teachers if testing is done in the fall, usually in early October, so that results are available in early December for instructional planning.

In some cases it is necessary to modify ITBS administration in order to obtain meaningful information about individual students. A student's individualized education program (IEP) usually guides the type of accommodation required for a particular student. Large-print and Braille versions of the ITBS are available. An enlarged answer folder or an assistant can be provided for students with physical disabilities that prevent them from marking the standard answer folder. Some students also may require extended time limits. Accommodations for English-language learners (ELLs) may include:

- extending time limits
- using a translation dictionary
- reading some parts of the test to the student, although not the reading vocabulary or reading comprehension tests
- supplying pronunciations or word meanings, when this does not interfere with the subject content or skills being tested

The ITBS includes a career guidance and counseling tool, the Interest Explorer, in which students indicate their degree of interest in described activities corresponding to 14 career areas. Level 1 is designed for the 8th grade and level 2 is designed for high school students. The Iowa Tests of Education Development (ITED) are a continuation of the ITBS for grades 9 through 12, with more complex material and advanced skill testing.

Origins

The ITBS was originally developed by E. F. Lindquist, Harry Greene, Ernest Horn, Maude McBroom, and Herbert Spitzer in 1935, as the Iowa Every Pupil Test of Basic Skills. Since then, it has been in ongoing development by the faculty and professional staff of the Iowa Testing Programs at the University of Iowa. Thus, the ITBS is one of the best-studied academic assessments.

New ITBS questions are added continuously. They are written by educators and examined for fairness and accuracy by a panel of educators. The new questions are then field tested by students in Iowa. In 2010, school districts began testing a computerized version of the ITBS.

Preparation

Before taking the ITBS, students should understand what the tests are like and why they are being given. Students should be assured that there is no reason for **anxiety** about the ITBS. Parents should also be informed

KEY TERMS

Achievement test—An exam designed to assess knowledge and proficiency in a specific subject or group of subjects.

Criterion-referenced—Test performance measurements based on a defined, independent standard, rather than relative to the performance of a population.

Grade equivalent—A position on an achievement continuum, in terms of beginning grade level and additional months; a decimal number that indicates the grade and month of a typical student who earns that score; most useful for monitoring the development of an individual student over time.

Literacy—The ability to efficiently comprehend and interpret written language and to communicate through written language.

Norm—A standard of achievement, usually derived from the average or median achievement of a large group of a particular age.

Norm-referenced test (NRT)—A test with results that are assessed based on results previously achieved by a selected sample of subjects, rather than by independent or absolute standards.

Percentile—A rank in a population that has been divided into 100 equal groups; thus, test results in the 50th percentile indicate that half of those who took the test scored higher and half scored lower.

Reading First—A federal program that helps states and school districts implement scientifically based reading programs for kindergarten through the third grade.

Standardized—A test with established norms and procedures that serve as the standard for future test results.

about the purpose and nature of the tests and what they can do to support their children. Teachers' attitudes can help make testing a positive experience and ensure accurate test results. There should be a discussion of procedures for new students, including:

- how to mark answers in the answer booklet
- how to pace oneself
- not to expect to know the answers to all questions
- how to make thoughtful guesses about answers

Each test within the ITBS begins with at least one sample question to provide practice with the content and format of the test. Teachers should not prepare students for the ITBS with practice questions or tests. Commercial ITBS preparation materials may raise test scores without improving student achievement, which leads to inaccurate results and undermines the purposes of testing.

Results

The ITBS can hand-scored, locally scored with optical scanning equipment, or centrally scored by a scoring service. Raw scores (RS) and the percent correct are the numbers of questions that students answered correctly. They have little meaning on their own. ITBS results are reported as developmental standard scores or scaled scores (SS) and national percentile ranks (NPR). SS are standard scores that correspond to the average performance of grade groups in the fall of the school year. NPRs compare a student's scores to those of a national sample of students in the same grade who were tested at the same point in the school year—fall, midyear, or spring.

Other ITBS scores that may be reported include:

- grade equivalent—a decimal number that describes a student's achievement on a continuum, in terms of grade level and months, but which is not an indication of the appropriate grade placement of that student
- primary reading profile for levels 5–9—information from all literacy-related tests to diagnosis the needs of individuals or an entire class
- core total score—the average of the reading, language, and mathematics test scores
- total composite score—the average of the reading, language, mathematics, social studies, and science test scores
- group item analysis or class item record reports—information about a specific group or classroom performance

The norms for the ITBS are from 2000 and 2005. The norms used for comparison can be national, local, for Catholic or private schools only, or for specific socioeconomic brackets. Although the ITBS is designed primarily as a norm-referenced test, it can also be interpreted by criterion-referencing, although the administrator must establish the criterion levels or performance standards to be referenced.

Performance on the ITBS correlates well with the American College Test (ACT), commonly used for college admissions. It also correlates fairly well with high school grade point averages (GPAs).

Parental concerns

The ITBS is designed as a supplement to teacher observations and ongoing classroom assessments. Skills develop at widely varying rates among children of the same age or grade. Many highly motivated and conscientious children learn more slowly than others. Proficient skill areas also vary greatly among children. Some children progress faster than others with specific methods, materials, and teaching styles. Thus, the ITBS should never be used except as one achievement measure among many.

The ITBS does not cover all of the important aspects of school curricula. However, studies have found that certain programs and curricula improve ITBS scores. These include Reading First, elementary school foreign language study, and playing bridge.

Many parents and educators believe that standardized tests, such as the ITBS, place an inordinate amount of pressure on small children, take up an inordinate amount of classroom time, and provide too little information about specific skills. Increased emphasis on standardized testing can also result in the neglect of non-tested areas of the curriculum. Finally, the ITBS can be expensive for school districts. With the increase in state-mandated tests, some schools are eliminating the ITBS. Other schools are substituting online tests that automatically adapt to a student's individual level and provide immediate results for classroom implementation.

Tests such as the ITBS also have been criticized because the results, rather than indicating the skill and knowledge levels of individual students, indicate only how each student compares with others. The test is designed such that 50% always score below the average and 50% score above.

ITBS scores are sometimes used inappropriately. These inappropriate uses include:

- evaluating early childhood programs
- screening children for readiness for school enrollment
- retaining children at a grade level
- selecting students for special remedial and talented and gifted education programs
- deciding on instructional objectives for specific grade levels
- evaluating the effectiveness of a school

Resources

BOOKS

Hoover, H. D., et al. *Iowa Tests of Basic Skills Guide to Research and Development.* Itasca, IL: Riverside, 2003.

Hoover, H. D., S. B. Dunbar, and D. A. Frisbie. *Iowa Tests of Basic Skills, Forms, A, B, and C.* Itasca, IL: Riverside, 2001.

Salkind, Neil J., and Kristin Rasmussen. *Encyclopedia of Measurement and Statistics.* Thousand Oaks, CA: SAGE, 2007.

PERIODICALS

Gutierrez, Bridget. "Get Schooled: ITBS: What's It Good For?" *Atlanta Journal-Constitution* (December 19, 2007).

OTHER

"Frequently Asked Questions about the Iowa Test of Basic Skills (ITBS)." Utah State Office of Education. [Accessed October 9, 2010], http://www.schools.utah.gov/assessment/DOCUMENTS/IOWA_FAQ.pdf.

"Iowa Test of Basic Skills (ITBS) Results." Great Schools. [Accessed October 9, 2010], http://www.greatschools.org/test/landing.page?state=IA&tid=27.

"The Iowa Tests of Basic Skills." Iowa Testing Programs. [Accessed October 9, 2010], http://www.education.uiowa.edu/itp/itbs/Default.aspx.

"Iowa Tests of Basic Skills (ITBS) Forms A, B, and C." Riverside Publishing. [Accessed October 9, 2010], http://www.riversidepublishing.com/products/itbs/index.html.

ORGANIZATIONS

Iowa Testing Programs, University of Iowa College of Education, 340 Lindquist Center S, Iowa City IA, 55242-1529, (319) 335-5408, (800) 323-9540, (Riverside Publishing), http://www.education.uiowa.edu/itp.

Margaret Alic, PhD

IQ *see* **Intelligence quotient (IQ)**

Iron deficiency anemia

Definition

Anemia is a condition, which is the result of insufficient numbers of healthy red blood cells, that can be caused by iron deficiency, folate deficiency, vitamin B_{12} deficiency, and other causes. The term iron deficiency anemia means anemia that is due to iron deficiency—that is, the insufficient dietary intake or absorption of iron in the body. Iron deficiency anemia is characterized by the production of smaller than normal red blood cells and less than the normal number of red cells in the blood. When examined under a microscope, the red blood cells also appear pale or light colored due to too little iron in the blood. For this reason, the anemia that occurs with iron deficiency is also called hypochronic microcytic anemia. Because fewer healthy red blood cells are produced (which causes less hemoglobin to be produced and, thus, less oxygen to be carried throughout the body), people with iron deficiency anemia often a lack of energy throughout their daily lives.

Demographics

Anyone has the potential for acquiring iron deficiency anemia. In the United States, approximately 20% of all women of child-bearing years, about 50% of pregnant women, and between 2 and 3% of all men of similar ages have iron deficiency anemia. Women are generally at higher risk for iron deficiency anemia because they lose iron during **menstruation**.

Description

Iron deficiency anemia is the most common type of anemia throughout the world. In the United States, iron deficiency anemia occurs to a lesser extent than in developing countries because of the higher consumption of red meat and the practice of food fortification (addition of iron to foods by manufacturers). Anemia in the United States is caused by a variety of sources, including excessive losses of iron in menstrual fluids and excessive bleeding in the gastrointestinal tract. The condition can also be produced by **lead poisoning**, often in children ingesting lead-based paints while playing. In developing countries located in tropical climates, the most common cause of iron deficiency anemia is infestation with hookworm.

Risks

The following groups have more chance of getting iron deficiency anemia than other groups: women, infants and children, and people with certain medical conditions. The following are factors that can contribute to increased risk of getting iron deficiency anemia: pregnancy (additional iron is needed for support of the fetus), heavy menstrual periods (which depletes iron in the body), low iron diet (such as vegetarian diets in which iron in allowed foods, such as vegetables, are not absorbed as well as iron in not-allowed foods, such as meat), and internal bleeding (such as from an ulcer or polyps). Donating blood and eating unhealthy foods on a regular basis are also other ways to increase one' risk of iron deficiency anemia.

Causes and symptoms

Infancy is a period of increased risk for iron deficiency. The human infant is born with a built-in supply of iron, which can be tapped during periods of drinking low-iron milk or formula. Both human milk and cow milk contain rather low levels of iron (0.5–1.0 milligrams of iron per liter [mg iron/l]). However, the iron in human milk is about 50% absorbed by the infant, while the iron of cow milk is only 10% absorbed. During the first six months of life, growth of the infant is made possible by the milk in the diet and by the infant's built-in supply. However, premature infants have a lower supply of iron and, for this reason, it is recommended that preterm infants (beginning at 2 months of age) be given oral supplements of 7 mg iron/day, as ferrous sulfate. Iron deficiency can be provoked where infants are fed formulas that are based on unfortified cow milk. For example, unfortified cow milk is given free of charge to mothers in Chile. This practice has the fortunate result of preventing general **malnutrition** but the unfortunate result of allowing the development of mild iron deficiency.

The normal rate of blood loss in the feces is 0.5–1.0 milliliter per day (mL/day). These losses can increase with colorectal **cancer**. About 60% of colorectal cancers result in further blood losses, where the extent of blood loss is 2–10 mL/day. Cancer of the colon and rectum can provoke losses of blood, resulting in iron deficiency anemia. The fecal blood test is widely used to screen for the presence of cancer of the colon or rectum. In the absence of testing, colorectal cancer may be first detected because of the resulting iron deficiency anemia.

Infection with hookworm can provoke iron deficiency and iron deficiency anemia. The hookworm is a parasitic worm. It thrives in warm climates, including in the southern United States. The hookworm enters the body through the skin, as through bare feet. The hookworm then migrates to the small intestines where it attaches itself to the villi (small sausage-shaped structures in the intestines that are used for the absorption of all nutrients). The hookworm provokes damage to the villi, which results in blood loss. They also produce anti-coagulants, which promote continued bleeding. Each worm can provoke the loss of up to 0.25 mL of blood per day.

Bleeding and blood losses through gastrointestinal tract can be provoked by colorectal cancer and hookworms, as mentioned above, but also by hemorrhoids, anal fissures, **irritable bowel syndrome**, aspirin-induced bleeding, blood clotting disorders, and diverticulosis (a condition caused by an abnormal opening from the intestine or bladder). Several genetic diseases exist, which lead to bleeding disorders, and these include **hemophilia** A, hemophilia B, and von Willebrand disease. Of these, only von Willebrand disease leads to gastrointestinal bleeding.

The symptoms of iron deficiency anemia include weakness and fatigue. These symptoms result because of the lack of function of the red blood cells, and the reduced ability of the red blood cells to carry iron to exercising muscles. Iron deficiency can also affect other tissues, including the tongue and fingernails. Prolonged iron deficiency can result in changes of the tongue; such as, it may become smooth, shiny, and reddened. This condition is called glossitis. The tongue may also become sore and inflamed. The fingernails may grow abnormally, acquiring a spoon-shaped appearance. They may also grow out brittle in texture and appearance.

The whites of the eyes may appear bluish in color. Other symptoms can include irritability, **headache**, cravings of food and other unusual substances while generally having a overall poor appetite, pale skin color, shortness of breath, irregular heartbeat, dizziness/light-headedness, cold feeling of the extremities (hands and feet), and irritability. If iron deficiency anemia is mild, however, symptoms may not appear. Symptoms begin to show up as the condition worsens.

Decreased iron intake is a contributing factor in iron deficiency and iron deficiency anemia. The iron content of cabbage, for example, is about 1.6 milligrams per kilogram (1.6 mg/kg) food, while that of spinach (33 mg/kg), lima beans (15 mg/kg), potatoes (14 mg/kg), tomatoes (3 mg/kg), apples (1.5 mg/kg), raisins (20 mg/kg), whole wheat bread (43 mg/kg), eggs (20 mg/kg), canned tuna (13 mg/kg), chicken (11 mg/kg), beef (28 mg/kg), corn oil (0.6 mg/kg), and peanut butter (6.0 mg/kg), are indicated. One can see that apples, tomatoes, and vegetable oil are relatively low in iron, while whole wheat bread, spinach, and beef are relatively high in iron. The assessment of whether a food is low or high in iron can also be made by comparing the amount of that food eaten per day with the **recommended dietary allowance (RDA)**, which is part of the Dietary Reference Intakes (DRIs), for iron. The **RDA** for iron for the adult male (19 to 50 years of age) is 8 milligram per day (mg/day), while that for the adult woman (of the same age range) is 18 mg/day. For adult males and females (51 years and older) the RDA for iron is 8 mg/day. The RDA during pregnancy is 27 mg/day. The RDA for infants of 7 to 12 months of age is 11 mg/day, for children 1 to 3 years of age it is 7 mg/day, for children 4 to 8 years it is 10 mg/day, for children 9 to 13 years it is 8 mg/day, and for children 14 to 18 years it is 11 mg/day for males and 15 mg/day for females. The RDA values are based on the assumption that the consumer eats a mixture of plant and animal foods.

The above list of iron values alone may be deceptive, since the availability of iron in fruits, vegetables, and grains is very low, while that the availability from meat is much higher. The availability of iron in plants ranges from only 1–10%, while that in meat, fish, chicken, and liver is 20–30%. The term availability means the percent of dietary iron that is absorbed via the gastrointestinal tract to the bloodstream. Non-absorbed iron is lost in the feces.

Interactions between various foods can influence the absorption of dietary iron. Vitamin C can increase the absorption of dietary iron. Orange juice is a rich source of vitamin C. Thus, if a plant food, such as rice, is consumed with orange juice, then the orange juice can enhance the absorption of the iron of the rice. Vitamin C is also added to infant formulas and the increased use of formulas fortified with both iron and vitamin C has led to a marked decline in anemia in infants and young children in the United States. In contrast, if rice is consumed with tea, certain chemicals in the tea (tannins) can reduce the absorption of the iron. Phytic acid is a chemical that naturally occurs in legumes, cereals, and nuts. Phytic acid, which can account for 1–5% of the weight of these foods, is a potent inhibitor of iron absorption. The increased availability of the iron in meat products is partly due to the fact that heme-iron is absorbed to a greater extent than free iron salts, and to a greater extent than iron in the phytic acid/iron complex. Nearly all of the iron in plants is nonheme-iron. Much of the iron in meat is nonheme-iron as well. The nonheme-iron in meat, fish, chicken and liver may be about 20% available. The heme-iron of meat may be close to 30% available. The most available source of iron is human milk (50% availability).

Diagnosis

Iron deficiency anemia in infants is defined as a hemoglobin level below 109 mg/mL of whole blood, and a hematocrit (percentage of blood volume with respect to red blood cells) of under 33%. Anemia in adult males is defined as a hemoglobin under 130 mg/mL and a hematocrit of under 39%. Anemia in adult females is defined as hemoglobin under 120 mg/mL and a hematocrit of under 35%. Anemia in pregnant women is defined as hemoglobin of under 110 mg/mL and hematocrit of under 31%.

When an abnormally high presence of blood is found in the feces during a fecal occult blood test, the physician needs to examine the gastrointestinal tract to determine the cause of bleeding. Here, the diagnosis for iron deficiency anemia includes the examination using a sigmoidoscope. The sigmoidoscope is an instrument that consists of a flexible tube that permits examination of the colon to a distance of 60 centimeters (cm). A barium enema, with an x ray, may also be used to detect abnormalities that can cause bleeding.

The diagnosis of iron deficiency anemia should include a test for oral iron absorption, where evidence suggests that oral iron supplements fail in treating anemia. The oral iron absorption test is conducted by eating 64 mg iron (325 mg ferrous sulfate) in a single dose. Blood samples are then taken after 2 hours and 4 hours. The iron content of the blood serum is then measured. The concentration of iron should rise by an increment of about 22 micromolar, where iron absorption is normal. Lesser increases in concentration mean that iron absorption is abnormal and that therapy should involve injections or infusions of iron.

Treatment

Oral iron supplements (pills) may contain various iron salts. These iron salts include ferrous sulfate, ferrous gluconate, or ferrous fumarate. These pills are most effective if they are taken with an empty stomach. Milk and antacids should not be taken with such pills. However, vitamin C, such as in orange juice, increases the absorption of iron. Injections and infusions of iron can be carried out with a preparation called iron dextran. In patients with poor iron absorption (by the gut), therapy with injection or infusion is preferable over oral supplements. Intravenous injections are often made into a vein or muscle. Treatment of iron deficiency anemia sometimes requires more than therapy with iron. Where hemorrhoids provoke iron deficiency, surgery may prove essential to prevent recurrent iron deficiency anemia. Where iron deficiency is provoked by bleeding due to aspirin treatment, aspirin should be discontinued. Where iron deficiency is provoked by hookworm infections, therapy for this parasite should be used, along with protection of the feet by wearing shoes whenever walking in hookworm-infested soil.

Prognosis

The prognosis for treating and curing iron deficiency anemia is excellent. Perhaps the main problem is failure to take iron supplements. With adequate treatments most cases of iron deficiency anemia goes away in a few weeks. In cases of pregnant women, the health care worker may recommend taking 100–200 mg of iron everyday. This dose is rather high and can lead to nausea, **diarrhea**, or abdominal **pain** in 10–20% of women taking this dose. The reason for using this high dose is to affect a rapid cure for anemia, where the anemia is detected at a mid-point during the pregnancy. The above problems of side effects and noncompliance can be avoided by taking iron doses (100–200 mg) only once a week, where supplements are initiated some time prior to conception, or continuously throughout the fertile period of life. The problem of compliance is not an issue where infusions are used, however a fraction of patients treated with iron infusions experience side effects, such as flushing, headache, nausea, **anaphylaxis**, or seizures. A number of studies have shown that iron deficiency anemia in infancy can result in reduced **intelligence**, where intelligence was measured in early childhood. It is not certain if iron supplementation of children with reduced intelligence, due to iron-deficiency anemia in infancy, has any influence in allowing a "catch-up" in intellectual development.

If left untreated, iron deficiency anemia can lead to heart problems such as irregular or rapid heartbeat (as the heart tries to pump more blood that contains less oxygen) or angina (chest pains that occur then the heart does not receive sufficient oxygenated blood). It can also cause complications during pregnancy in women and delayed mental and physical growth spurts in children.

KEY TERMS

Hematocrit—The proportion of whole blood in the body, by volume, that is composed of red blood cells.

Hemoglobin—Hemoglobin is an iron-containing protein that resides within red blood cells. Hemoglobin accounts for about 95% of the protein in the red blood cell.

Protoporphyrin IX—Protoporphyrin IX is a protein. The measurement of this protein is useful for the assessment of iron status. Hemoglobin consists of a complex of a protein plus heme. Heme consists of iron plus protoporphyrin IX. Normally, during the course of red blood cell formation, protoporphyrin IX acquires iron, to generate heme, and the heme becomes incorporated into hemoglobin. However, in iron deficiency, protophoryrin IX builds up.

Recommended Dietary Allowance (RDA)—The Recommended Dietary Allowances (RDAs) are quantities of nutrients of the diet that are required to maintain human health. RDAs are established by the Food and Nutrition Board of the National Academy of Sciences and may be revised every few years.

Prevention

In the healthy population, all of the mineral deficiencies can be prevented by the consumption of inorganic nutrients at levels defined by the RDA. Iron deficiency anemia in infants and young children can be prevented by the use of fortified foods. Liquid cow milk-based infant formulas are generally supplemented with iron (12 mg/l). The iron in liquid formulas is added as ferrous sulfate or ferrous gluconate. Commercial infant cereals are also fortified with iron, and here small particles of elemental iron are added. The levels used are about 0.5 gram iron/kg dry cereal. This amount of iron is about ten fold greater than that of the iron naturally present in the cereal. Foods that are rich in iron include, poultry, red meat (such as liver), pork, seafood, egg yolks, whole-grain breads, raisins, legumes (such as beans and peas), dark green leafy vegetables (such as spinach), nuts and seeds and dried fruits (such as apricots and raisins). Many other foods are fortified with iron (such as breakfast foods).

Parental concerns

Understanding iron metabolism and the ways to ensure that iron deficiency anemia in infants and children can be successfully treated and prevented from recurring may be concerns of parents. It is important to remember that although iron deficiency anemia is common in infants and toddlers, it is easily corrected by feeding infants mother's milk or iron-fortified formulas. In older children, the diet usually balances iron usage and replacement. In teenage years, when demands for iron increase for rapid growth and to compensate for menstruation in girls, parents will need to pay attention once again to providing adequate food sources. However, supplementation of iron should only be done with a doctor's recommendation.

Resources

BOOKS

Null, Gary, and Amy McDonald, editors. *Be a Healthy Woman!* New York: Seven Stories Press, 2009.

Rosenfeld, Gary C. and David S. Loose. *Pharmacology.* Philadelphia: Wolters Kluwer Health/Lippincott Williams and Wilkins, 2010.

Shils, Maurice, et al., editors. *Modern Nutrition in Health and Disease.* Philadelphia: Lippincott Williams and Wilkins, 2006.

OTHER

"Dietary Supplement Fact Sheet: Iron." Office of Dietary Supplements, National Institutes of Health. August 24, 2007. [Accessed July 17, 2010], http://ods.od.nih.gov/factsheets/iron.asp.

"Iron Deficiency Anemia." Mayo Clinic. March 24, 2009. [Accessed July 17, 2010], http://www.mayoclinic.com/health/iron-deficiency-anemia/DS00323.

"Iron Deficiency Anemia." Medline Plus, National Library of Medicine and National Institutes of Health. March 21, 2010. [Accessed July 17, 2010], http://www.nlm.nih.gov/medlineplus/ency/article/000584.htm.

Tom Brody, PhD

Irritable bowel syndrome

Definition

Irritable bowel syndrome (IBS) is a common intestinal condition characterized by abdominal **pain** and cramps; changes in bowel movements (**diarrhea**, **constipation**, or both); gassiness; bloating; nausea; and other symptoms. There is no cure for IBS. Much about the condition remains unknown or poorly understood; however, dietary changes, drugs, and psychological treatment are often able to eliminate or substantially reduce its symptoms.

Demographics

No one knows for sure how many Americans suffer from IBS. Surveys indicate a range of 10–20%, with perhaps as many as 30% of Americans experiencing IBS at some point in their lives. IBS normally makes its first appearance during young adulthood and in half of all cases symptoms begin before age 35. Women with IBS outnumber men by two to one for reasons that are not yet understood. IBS is responsible for more time lost from work and school than any medical problem other than the **common cold**. It accounts for more than half of all the patients seen by specialists in diseases of the digestive system (gastroenterologists). Yet only half—possibly as few as 15%—of IBS sufferers ever consult a doctor.

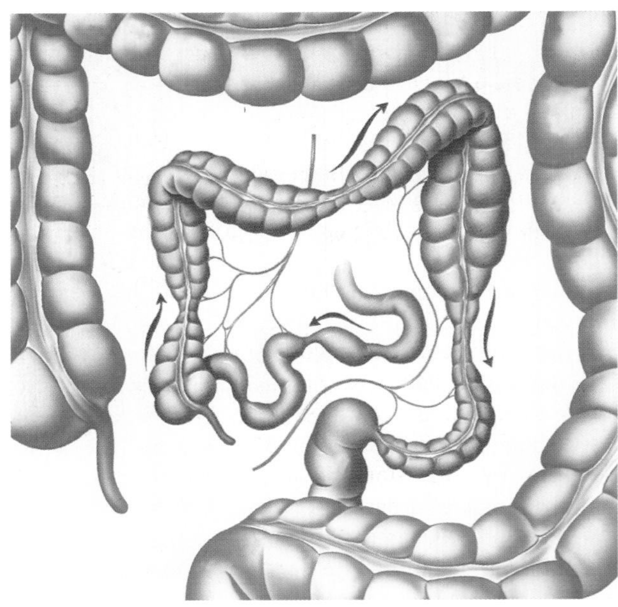

Normal and diseased (center) colons. Areas of constriction in the colon cause constipation, while areas of distention cause diarrhea. *(Custom Medical Stock Photo, Inc. Reproduced by permission.)*

Description

IBS is the name people use today for a condition that was once called colitis, mucous colitis, spastic colon, nervous colon, spastic bowel, and functional bowel disorder. Some of these names reflected the now outdated belief that IBS is a purely psychological disorder, a product of the patient's imagination. Although modern medicine recognizes that stress can trigger IBS attacks, medical specialists agree that IBS is a genuine physical disorder—or group of disorders—with specific identifiable characteristics.

Causes and symptoms

Symptoms

The symptoms of IBS tend to rise and fall in intensity rather than growing steadily worse over time. They always include abdominal pain, which may be relieved by defecation; diarrhea or constipation; or diarrhea alternating with constipation. Other symptoms—which vary from person to person—include cramps; gassiness; bloating; nausea; a powerful and uncontrollable urge to defecate (urgency); passage of a sticky fluid (mucus) during bowel movements; or the feeling after finishing a bowel movement that the bowels are still not completely empty. The accepted diagnostic criteria—known as the Rome criteria—require at least three months of continuous or recurrent symptoms before IBS can be confirmed. According to Christine B. Dalton and Douglas A. Drossman in the *American Family Physician,* an estimated 70% of IBS cases can be described as "mild;" 25% as "moderate;" and 5% as "severe." In mild cases the symptoms are slight. As a general rule, they are not present all the time and do not interfere with work and other normal activities. Moderate IBS occasionally disrupts normal activities and may cause some psychological problems. People with severe IBS often find living a normal life impossible and experience crippling psychological problems as a result. For some, the physical pain is constant and intense.

Causes

Researchers remain unsure about the cause or causes of IBS. It is called a functional disorder because it is thought to result from changes in the activity of the major part of the large intestine (the colon). After food is digested by the stomach and small intestine, the undigested material passes in liquid form into the colon, which absorbs water and salts. This process may take several days. In a healthy person the colon is quiet during most of that period except after meals, when its muscles contract in a series of wavelike movements called peristalsis. Peristalsis helps absorption by bringing the undigested material into contact with the colon wall. It also pushes undigested material that has been converted into solid or semisolid feces toward the rectum, where it remains until defecation. In IBS, however, the normal rhythm and intensity of peristalsis is disrupted. Sometimes there is too little peristalsis, which can slow the passage of undigested material through the colon and cause constipation. Sometimes there is too much, which has the opposite effect and causes diarrhea. A Johns Hopkins University study found that healthy volunteers experienced 6–8 contractions of the colon each day, compared with up to 25 contractions a day for volunteers suffering from IBS with diarrhea, and an almost complete absence of contractions among constipated IBS volunteers. In addition to differences in the number of contractions, many of the IBS volunteers experienced powerful spasmodic contractions affecting a larger-than-normal area of the colon; according to one of the investigators, it was "like having a Charlie horse in the gut."

DIET Some kinds of food and drink appear to play a key role in triggering IBS attacks. Food and drink that healthy people can ingest without any trouble may disrupt peristalsis in IBS patients, which probably explains why IBS attacks often occur shortly after meals. Chocolate, milk products, **caffeine** (in coffee, tea, colas, and other drinks), and large quantities of alcohol are some of the chief culprits. Other kinds of food have also been identified as problems, however, and the pattern of what can and cannot be tolerated is different for each person. Characteristically, IBS symptoms rarely occur at night and disrupt the patient's **sleep**.

STRESS Stress is an important factor in IBS because of the close nervous system connections between the brain and the intestines. Although researchers do not yet understand all of the links between changes in the nervous system and IBS, they point out the similarities between mild digestive upsets and IBS. Just as healthy people can feel nauseated or have an upset stomach when under stress, people with IBS react the same way but to a greater degree. Finally, IBS symptoms sometimes intensify during **menstruation**, which suggests that female reproductive hormones are another trigger.

Diagnosis

Diagnosing IBS is a fairly complex task because the disorder does not produce changes that can be identified during a physical examination or by laboratory tests. When IBS is suspected, the doctor (who can be either a family doctor or a specialist) needs to determine whether the patient's symptoms satisfy the Rome criteria. The doctor must rule out other conditions that resemble IBS, such as Crohn's disease and ulcerative colitis. These disorders are ruled out by questioning the patient about his or her physical and mental health (the medical history), performing a physical examination, and ordering laboratory tests. Normally the patient is asked to provide a stool sample that can be tested for blood and intestinal parasites. In some cases **x rays** or an internal examination of the colon using a flexible instrument inserted through the anus (a sigmoidoscope or colonoscope) is necessary. The doctor also may ask the patient to try a lactose-free diet for two or three weeks to see whether **lactose intolerance** is causing the symptoms.

Treatment

Dietary changes, sometimes supplemented by drugs or psychotherapy, are considered the key to successful treatment. The following approach, offered by Dalton and Drossman, is typical of the advice found in the medical literature on IBS. The authors tie their approach to the severity of the patient's symptoms:

Mild symptoms

Dalton and Drossman recommend a low-fat, high-fiber diet. Problem-causing substances such as lactose, caffeine, beans, cabbage, cucumbers, broccoli, fatty foods, alcohol, and medications should be identified and avoided. Bran or 15–25 grams a day of an over-the-counter psyllium laxative (Metamucil or Fiberall) may also help both constipation and diarrhea. The patient can still have milk or milk products if lactose intolerance is not a problem. People with irregular bowel habits—particularly constipated patients—may be helped by establishing set times for meals and bathroom visits.

Moderate symptoms

The advice given by Dalton and Drossman in mild cases applies here as well. They also suggest that patients keep a diary of symptoms for two or three weeks, covering daily activities including meals, and emotional responses to events. The doctor can then review the diary with the patient to identify possible problem areas.

Although a high-fiber diet remains the standard treatment for constipated patients, such **laxatives** as lactulose (Chronulac) or sorbitol may be prescribed. Loperamide (Imodium) and cholestyramine (Questran) are suggested for diarrhea. Abdominal pain after meals can be reduced by taking antispasmodic drugs such as hyoscyamine (Anaspaz, Cystospaz, or Levsin) or dicyclomine (Bemote, Bentyl, or Di-Spaz) before eating.

Dalton and Drossman also suggest psychological counseling or **behavioral therapy** for some patients to reduce **anxiety** and to learn to cope with the pain and other symptoms of IBS. Relaxation therapy, hypnosis, biofeedback, and **cognitive-behavioral therapy** are examples of behavioral therapy.

Severe symptoms

When IBS produces constant pain that interferes with everyday life, **antidepressants** can help by blocking pain transmission from the nervous system. Dalton and Drossman also underscore the importance of an ongoing and supportive doctor-patient relationship.

Alternative treatment

Alternative and mainstream approaches to IBS treatment overlap to a certain extent. Like mainstream doctors, alternative practitioners advise a high-fiber diet to reduce digestive system irritation. They also suggest avoiding alcohol, caffeine, and fatty, gassy, or spicy foods. Recommended stress management techniques include **yoga**, meditation, hypnosis, biofeedback, and reflexology. Reflexology is a technique of foot massage that is thought to relieve diarrhea, constipation, and other IBS symptoms.

Alternative medicine also emphasizes such herbal remedies as ginger (*Zingiber officinale*), buckthorn (*Rhamnus purshiana*), and enteric-coated peppermint oil. Enteric coating prevents digestion until the peppermint oil reaches the small intestine, thus avoiding

KEY TERMS

Anus—The opening at the lower end of the rectum.

Crohn's disease—A disease characterized by inflammation of the intestines. Its early symptoms may resemble those of IBS.

Defecation—Passage of feces through the anus.

Feces—Undigested food and other waste that is eliminated through the anus. Feces are also called fecal matter or stools.

Lactose—A sugar found in milk and milk products. Some people are lactose intolerant, meaning they have trouble digesting lactose. Lactose intolerance can produce symptoms resembling those of IBS.

Peristalsis—The periodic waves of muscular contractions that move food through the intestines during the process of digestion.

Ulcerative colitis—A disease that inflames and causes breaks (ulcers) in the colon and rectum, which are parts of the large intestine.

irritation of the upper part of the digestive tract. Chamomile (*Matricaria recutita*), valerian (*Valeriana officinalis*), rosemary (*Rosemarinus officinalis*), lemon balm (*Melissa officinalis*), and other herbs are recommended for their antispasmodic properties. The list of alternative treatments for IBS is in fact quite long. It includes aromatherapy, homeopathy, hydrotherapy, juice therapy, acupuncture, chiropractic, osteopathy, naturopathic medicine, and Chinese traditional herbal medicine.

Prognosis

IBS is not a life-threatening condition. It does not cause intestinal bleeding or inflammation, nor does it cause other bowel diseases or **cancer**. Although IBS can last a lifetime, in up to 30% of cases the symptoms eventually disappear and symptoms decrease significantly with treatment in about 60%. Even if the symptoms cannot be eliminated, with appropriate treatment they can usually be brought under control to the point where IBS becomes merely an occasional inconvenience. Treatment requires a long-term commitment, however; six months or more may be needed before the patient notices substantial improvement.

Prevention

Because the cause of IBS is not understood, there are no definitive ways to prevent it. However, some of the following may generally improve digestion:

- Drink sufficient water, about 8 glasses per day
- Follow a high-fiber diet
- Avoid foods that make you feel uncomfortable. For some people, these include highly acidic or spicy foods, caffeinated beverages, and alcohol.
- Physical activity can help improve digestion
- Learn to avoid and cope with stress in your life
- Eating many small meals a day is preferable to eating fewer very larfge meals
- Be aware of medications that you may take that could cause constipation, or irritate your stomach

Nutritional concerns

To help prevent or decrease the child's symptoms, parents can:

- help the child identify and avoid problematic foods
- work with a registered dietitian to facilitate specific dietary changes
- incorporate changes in the child's diet gradually so his or her body has time to adjust
- establish set times for meals; not allowing the child to skip a meal
- encourage the child to drink at least eight 8-ounce glasses of water per day
- serve small portions during meals
- teach the child to eat slowly, to avoid swallowing too much air that can produce excess gas
- try offering smaller, more frequent meals
- keep a regular schedule for bathroom visits

Parental concerns

Parents should reinforce with the child that IBS is not a life-threatening condition and that dietary changes and stress reduction can help reduce symptoms. Remind the child that six months or more may be needed before he or she notices substantial improvement in symptoms.

Resources

BOOKS

Berkowitz, Jonathan M. *A Victim No More: Overcoming Irritable Bowel Syndrome: Safe, Effective Therapies for Relief From Bowel Complaints.* North Bergen, NJ: Basic Health Publications, 2003.

Dean, Carolyn and L. Christine Wheeler. *IBS for Dummies.* Hoboken, NJ: Wiley Pub., 2006.

Feldman, M, et al. *Sleisenger & Fordtran's Gastrointestinal and Liver Disease.* 8th ed. St. Louis: Mosby, 2005.

Nicol, Rosemary. *Irritable Bowel Syndrome: A Natural Approach.* Berkeley, CA: Ulysses Press, 2007

Peikin, Steven R. *Gastrointestinal Health: The Proven Nutritional Program to Prevent, Cure, or Alleviate Irritable Bowel Syndrome (IBS), Ulcers, Gas, Constipation, Heartburn, and Many Other Digestive Disorders.* rev ed. New York, NY: Perennial Currents, 2004.

Talley, Nicholas J. *Conquering Irritable Bowel Syndrome: A Guide to Liberating Those Suffering with Chronic Stomach or Bowel Problems.* Hamilton, Ontario: BC Decker, 2006.

OTHER

Lehrer, Jenifer K. and Gary R Lichtenstein. "Irritable Bowel Syndrome." eMedicine.com. August 9, 2009. [Accessed December 9, 2010], http://emedicine.medscape.com/article/180389-overview.

International Foundation for Functional Gastrointestinal Disorders "Frequently Asked Questions." October 5, 2009. [Accessed December 9, 2010], http://www.iffgd.org/site/about-iffgd/.

Lichtenstein, Gary R. and Jenifer K. Leher. "Irritable Bowel Syndrome." eMedicineHealth.com, October 26, 2005. [Accessed December 9, 2010], http://www.emedicine-health.com/irritable_bowel_syndrome/article_em.htm.

Mayo Clinic Staff. "Irritable Bowel Syndrome." MayoClinic.com, July 29, 2009. [Accessed December 9, 2010], http://www.mayoclinic.com/health/irritable-bowel-syndrome/DS00106.

American Academy of Family Physicians. "Irritable Bowel Syndrome: Tips on Controlling Your Symptoms." Familydoctor.org. October 10, 2010. [Accessed December 9, 2010], http://familydoctor.org/online/famdocen/home/common/digestive/disorders/112.printerview.html.

National Digestive Diseases Information Clearinghouse (NDDIC). "Irritable Bowel Syndrome." February 2006. [Accessed December 9, 2010], http://digestive.niddk.nih.gov/ddiseases/pubs/ibs.

ORGANIZATIONS

American College of Gastroenterology, P.O. Box 342260, Bethesda MD, 20827-2260, (301) 263-9000, http://www.acg.gi.org.

American Gastroenterological Association, 4930 Del Ray Avenue, Bethesda MD, 20814, (301) 654-2055, (301) 654-5920, http://www.gastro.org.

IBS Self Help and Support Group, 1440 Whalley Avenue, New Haven CT, 06515, http://www.ibsgroup.org.

International Foundation for Functional Gastrointestinal Disorders, P. O. Box 170864, Milwaukee WI, 53217, (888) 964-2001, (414) 964-7176, http://www.iffgd.org.

National Digestive Diseases Information Clearinghouse (NDDIC), 2 Information Way, Bethesda MD, 20892-3570, (800) 891-5389, (703) 738-4929, http://digestive.niddk.nih.gov.

Howard Baker

Itching

Definition

Itching is an intense, distracting irritation or tickling sensation that may be felt all over the skin's surface, or confined to just one area. The medical term for itching is pruritus.

Description

Itching instinctively leads most people to scratch the affected area. Different people can tolerate different amounts of itching and anyone's threshold of tolerance can be changed due to stress, emotions, and other factors. In general, itching is more severe if the skin is warm and if there are few distractions. This is why people tend to notice itching more at night.

Causes and symptoms

The biology underlying itching is not fully understood. It is believed that itching results from the interactions of several different chemical messengers. Although itching and **pain** sensations were at one time thought to be sent along the same nerve pathways, researchers reported the discovery in 2003 of itch-specific nerve pathways. Nerve endings that are specifically sensitive to itching have been named pruriceptors.

Research into itching has been helped by the recent invention of a mechanical device called the Matcher, which electrically stimulates the patient's left hand. When the intensity of the stimulation equals the intensity of itching that the patient is experiencing elsewhere in the body, the patient stops the stimulation and the device automatically records the measurement. The Matcher was found to be sensitive to immediate changes in the patient's perception of itching as well as reliable in its measurements.

Stress and emotional upset can make itching worse, no matter what the underlying cause. If emotional problems are the primary reason for the itch, the condition is known as psychogenic itching. Some people become convinced that their itch is caused by a parasite; this conviction is often linked to burning sensations in the tongue, and may be caused by a major psychiatric disorder.

Generalized itching

Itching that occurs all over the body may indicate a medical condition such as **diabetes mellitus**, liver disease, kidney failure, **jaundice**, thyroid disorders (and rarely, **cancer**). Blood disorders such as leukemia, and lymphatic conditions such as Hodgkin's disease may sometimes cause itching as well.

Some people may develop an itch without a rash when they take certain drugs (such as aspirin, codeine, cocaine); others may develop an itchy red "drug rash" or **hives** because of an allergy to a specific drug. Some medications given to cancer patients may also cause itching.

Itching also may be caused when any of the family of hookworm larvae penetrate the skin. This includes swimmer's itch and creeping eruption caused by cat or dog hookworm, and ground itch caused by the "true" hookworm.

Many skin conditions cause an itchy rash. These include:

- Atopic dermatitis
- Chickenpox
- Contact dermatitis
- Dermatitis herpetiformis (occasionally)
- Eczema
- Fungus infections (such as athlete's foot)

- Hives (urticaria)
- Insect bites
- Lice
- Lichen planus
- Neurodermatitis (lichen simplex chronicus)
- Psoriasis (occasionally)
- Scabies.

On the other hand, itching all over the body can be caused by something as simple as bathing too often, which removes the skin's natural oils and may make the skin too dry and scaly.

Localized itching

Specific itchy areas may occur if a person comes in contact with soap, detergents, and wool or other rough-textured, scratchy material. Adults who have hemorrhoids, anal fissure, or persistent **diarrhea** may notice itching around the anus (called "pruritus ani"). In children, itching in this area is most likely due to worms.

Intense itching in the external genitalia in women ("pruritus vulvae") may be due to **candidiasis**, hormonal changes, or the use of certain spermicides or vaginal suppositories, ointments, or deodorants.

It is also common for older people to suffer from dry, itchy skin (especially on the back) for no obvious reason. Younger people also may notice dry, itchy skin in cold weather. Itching is also a common complaint during pregnancy.

Diagnosis

Itching is a symptom that is quite obvious to its victim. Someone who itches all over should seek medical care. Because itching can be caused by such a wide variety of triggers, a complete physical exam and medical history will help diagnose the underlying problem. A variety of blood and stool tests may help determine the underlying cause.

Treatment

Antihistamines such as diphenhydramine (Benadryl) can help relieve itching caused by hives, but will not affect itching from other causes. Most antihistamines also make people sleepy, which can help patients **sleep** who would otherwise be awake from the itch.

Specific treatment of itching depends on the underlying condition that causes it. In general, itchy skin should be treated very gently. While scratching may temporarily ease the itch, in the long run scratching just makes it worse. In addition, scratching can lead to an endless cycle of itch-scratch-more itching.

To avoid the urge to scratch, a person can apply a cooling or soothing lotion or cold compress when the urge to scratch occurs. Soaps are often irritating to the skin, and can make an itch worse; they should be avoided or used only when necessary.

Creams or ointments containing cortisone may help control the itch from insect **bites**, **contact dermatitis** or **eczema**. Cortisone cream should not be applied to the face unless a doctor prescribes it.

Probably the most common cause of itching is dry skin. There are a number of simple things a person can do to ease the annoying itch:

- Do not wear tight clothes
- Avoid synthetic fabrics
- Do not take long baths
- Wash the area in lukewarm water with a little baking soda
- For generalized itching, take a lukewarm shower
- Try a lukewarm oatmeal (or Aveeno) bath for generalized itching
- Apply bath oil or lotion (without added colors or scents) right after bathing.

Itching may also be treated with whole-body medications. In addition to antihistamines, some of these systemic treatments include:

- tricyclic antidepressants
- sedatives or tranquilizers
- such selective serotonin reputake inhibitors as paroxetine (Paxil) and sertraline (Zoloft)
- binding agents (such as cholestyramine which relieves itching associated with kidney or liver disease).
- aspirin
- cimetidine

People who itch as a result of mental problems or stress should seek help from a mental health expert.

Alternative and complementary therapies

A well-balanced diet that includes carbohydrates, fats, **minerals**, proteins, **vitamins**, and liquids will help to maintain skin health. Capsules that contain eicosapentaenoic acid, which is obtained from herring, mackerel, or salmon, may help to reduce itching. Vitamin A plays an important role in skin health. Vitamin E (capsules or ointment) may reduce itching. Patients should check with their treating physician before using supplements.

KEY TERMS

Atopic dermatitis—An intensely itchy inflammation often found on the face of people prone to allergies. In infants and early childhood, it is called infantile eczema.

Creeping eruption—Itchy irregular, wandering red lines on the foot made by burrowing larvae of the hookworm family and some roundworms.

Dermatitis herpetiformis—A chronic very itchy skin disease with groups of red lesions that leave spots behind when they heal. It is sometimes associated with cancer of an internal organ.

Eczema—A superficial type of inflammation of the skin that may be very itchy and weeping in the early stages; later, the affected skin becomes crusted, scaly, and thick. There is no known cause.

Hodgkin's disease—A type of cancer characterized by a slowly-enlarging lymph tissue; symptoms include generalized itching.

Lichen planus—A noncancerous, chronic itchy skin disease that causes small, flat purple plaques on wrists, forearm, ankles.

Neurodermatitis—An itchy skin disease (also called lichen simplex chronicus) found in nervous, anxious people.

Pruriceptors—Nerve endings specialized to perceive itching sensations.

Pruritus—The medical term for itching.

Psoriasis—A common, chronic skin disorder that causes red patches anywhere on the body. Occasionally, the lesions may itch.

Scabies—A contagious parasitic skin disease characterized by intense itching.

Swimmer's itch—An allergic skin inflammation caused by a sensitivity to flatworms that die under the skin, causing an itchy rash.

Homeopathy has been reported to be effective in treating systemic itching associated with hemodialysis.

Baths containing oil with milk or oatmeal are effective at relieving localized itching. Evening primrose oil may soothe itching and may be as effective as corticosteroids. Calendula cream may relieve short-term itching. Other herbal treatments that have been recently reported to relieve itching include sangre de drago, a preparation made with sap from a South American tree; and a mixture of honey, olive oil, and beeswax.

Distraction, **music therapy**, relaxation techniques, and visualization may be useful in relieving itching. Ultraviolet light therapy may relieve itching associated with conditions of the skin, kidneys, blood, and gallbladder. There are some reports of the use of acupuncture and transcutaneous electrical nerve stimulators (TENS) to relieve itching.

Prognosis

Most cases of itching go away when the underlying cause is treated successfully.

Prevention

There are certain things people can do to avoid itchy skin. Patients who tend toward itchy skin should:

- Avoid a daily bath
- Use only lukewarm water when bathing
- Use only gentle soap
- Pat dry, not rub dry, after bathing, leaving a bit of water on the skin
- Apply a moisture-holding ointment or cream after the bath
- Use a humidifier in the home.

Patients who are allergic to certain substances, medications, and so on can avoid the resulting itch if they avoid contact with the allergen. Avoiding insect bites, bee **stings**, **poison ivy** and so on can prevent the resulting itch. Treating sensitive skin carefully, avoiding overdrying of the skin, and protecting against diseases that cause itchy **rashes** are all good ways to avoid itching.

Resources

BOOKS

Beers, Mark H., MD, and Robert Berkow, MD, editors. "Pruritus." In *The Merck Manual of Diagnosis and Therapy.* 18th ed., Whitehouse Station, NJ: Merck Research Laboratories, 2006.

PERIODICALS

Al-Waili, N. S. "Topical Application of Natural Honey, Beeswax and Olive Oil Mixture for Atopic Dermatitis or Psoriasis: Partially Controlled, Single-Blinded Study." *Complementary Therapies in Medicine* 11 (December 2003): 226-234.

Browning, J., B. Combes, and M. J. Mayo. "Long-Term Efficacy of Sertraline as a Treatment for Cholestatic Pruritus in Patients with Primary Biliary Cirrhosis." *American Journal of Gastroenterology* 98 (December 2003): 2736-2741.

Cavalcanti, A. M., L. M. Rocha, R. Carillo Jr., et al. "Effects of Homeopathic Treatment on Pruritus of Haemodialysis

Patients: A Randomised Placebo-Controlled Double-Blind Trial." *Homeopathy* 92 (October 2003): 177-181.

Ikoma, A., R. Rukwied, S. Stander, et al. "Neurophysiology of Pruritus: Interaction of Itch and Pain." *Archives of Dermatology* 139 (November 2003): 1475-1478.

Jones, K. "Review of Sangre de Drago (*Croton lechleri*)—A South American Tree Sap in the Treatment of Diarrhea, Inflammation, Insect Bites, Viral Infections, and Wounds: Traditional Uses to Clinical Research." *Journal of Alternative and Complementary Medicine* 9 (December 2003): 877-896.

Ochoa, J. G. "Pruritus, a Rare but Troublesome Adverse Reaction of Topiramate." *Seizure* 12 (October 2003): 516-518.

Stener-Victorin, E., T. Lundeberg, J. Kowalski, et al. "Perceptual Matching for Assessment of Itch; Reliability and Responsiveness Analyzed by a Rank-Invariant Statistical Method." *Journal of Investigative Dermatology* 121 (December 2003): 1301-1305.

Zylicz, Z., M. Krajnik, A. A. Sorge, and M. Costantini. "Paroxetine in the Treatment of Severe Non-Dermatological Pruritus: A Randomized, Controlled Trial." *Journal of Pain and Symptom Management* 26 (December 2003): 1105-1112.

Carol A. Turkington
Rebecca J. Frey, PhD

J

Japanese encephalitis

Definition

Japanese **encephalitis** is an infection of the brain caused by a virus. The virus is transmitted to humans by mosquitoes.

Demographics

Many of these areas are in Asia, including Japan, Korea, China, India, Thailand, Indonesia, Malaysia, Vietnam, Taiwan, and the Philippines. Areas where the disease-causing arbovirus is always present are referred to as being endemic for the disease. In such areas, blood tests will reveal that more than 70% of all adults have been infected at some point with the arbovirus.

Because the virus that causes Japanese encephalitis is carried by mosquitoes, the number of people infected increases during those seasons when mosquitoes are abundant. This tends to be in the warmest, rainiest months. In addition to humans, wild birds and pigs are susceptible to infection with this arbovirus. Because the specific type of mosquito carrying the Japanese encephalitis arbovirus frequently breeds in rice paddies, the disease is considered to be primarily a rural problem.

About 45,000 cases of Japanese encephalitis are reported each year; however, the disease is thought to be seriously underreported. The disease is about 1.5 times more common in men than in women, possibly because men are likely to spend more time outdoors in areas where the disease is endemic. Cases in the United States are exceedingly rare (less than 1 case per year) and usually occur in military personnel or other Americans who have returned home after living in affected areas.

Description

The virus that causes Japanese encephalitis is called an arbovirus, which is an arthropod-borne virus. Mosquitoes are a type of arthropod. Mosquitoes in a number of regions carry this virus. The virus is passed to humans when the mosquitoes bite them. The disease cannot be passed directly from human to human, nor can it be passed directly from animals infected with the virus to human. Not all infections cause severe symptoms; in many cases the only symptoms are a **fever** and **headache**. In areas where the virus is common, most people become infected by the time they are young adults.

Causes and symptoms

The virus is transferred to a human when an infected mosquito sucks that person's blood. Once in the body, the virus travels to various glands where it multiplies. The virus can then enter the bloodstream. Ultimately, the virus settles in the brain, where it causes serious problems.

The time from becoming infected to starting to show symptoms (incubation period) usually is 5–15 days. Serious cases of Japanese encephalitis begin abruptly with fever, severe headache, nausea, and **vomiting**. As the tissue covering the brain and spinal cord (the meninges) becomes infected and swollen, the patient will develop a stiff and painful neck. By day two or three, the patient begins to suffer the effects of swelling in the brain. These effects include:

- problems with balance and coordination
- paralysis of some muscle groups
- tremors
- seizures
- lapses in consciousness
- a stiff, mask-like appearance of the face.

The patient becomes dehydrated and loses weight. If the patient survives the illness, the fever will decrease by about day seven and the symptoms will begin to improve by about day 14. Other patients will continue to have extremely high fevers and their symptoms will get worse.

KEY TERMS

Encephalitis—A swelling of the brain, potentially causing serious brain damage.

Endemic—Naturally and consistently present in a certain geographical region.

In these cases, coma and then **death** occur in 7–14 days. Many patients who recover have permanent disabilities due to brain damage.

Diagnosis

Most diagnostic techniques for Japanese encephalitis do not yield results very quickly. The diagnosis is made primarily on the basis of the patient's symptoms and the knowledge of the kinds of illnesses endemic to a particular geographic region.

Tests

Immunofluorescence tests, where special viral markers react with human antibodies that have been tagged with a fluorescent chemical, are used to verify the disease. However, these results tend to be unavailable until week two of the infection. Other tests involve comparing the presence and quantity of particular antibodies in the blood or spinal fluid during week one with those present during week two of the illness.

Treatment

There are no treatments available to stop or slow the progression of Japanese encephalitis. Only the symptoms of each patient can be treated. Fluids are given to decrease **dehydration** and medications are given to decrease fever and **pain**. Medications are available to attempt to decrease brain swelling. Patients in a coma may require mechanical assistance with breathing.

Prognosis

While the majority of people infected with arbovirus never become seriously sick, those who develop Japanese encephalitis become very ill. Death ranges can range from 30–60%. A variety of long-term problems may haunt those who recover from the illness. These problems include:

- movement difficulties where the arms, legs, or body jerks or writhes involuntarily
- shaking
- paralysis
- inability to control emotions
- loss of mental abilities
- mental disturbances, including schizophrenia (that may affect as many as 75% of Japanese encephalitis survivors)

Young children are most likely to have serious, long-term problems after an infection.

Prevention

Two different vaccines are available for immunization against Japanese encephalitis. A three-dose vaccine is available for Japanese encephalitis and is commonly given to young children in areas where the disease is endemic. A two-dose vaccine can be give to people age 17 and older. Both vaccines are given over the period of a 28–30 days and should be completed at least 7–10 days before entering an area where the Japanese encephalitis virus is common.

The vaccine is not 100% effective, thus controlling the mosquito population with insecticides is an essential preventive measure. Visitors to regions with high rates of Japanese encephalitis should take precautions (like using mosquito repellents such as DEET and sleeping under a bed net) to avoid contact with mosquitoes.

Resources

OTHER

Jani, Asim A. and Alexander J. Kallin. Japanese Encephalitis. eMedicine.com. May 6, 2009, http://emedicine.medscape.com/article/233802-overview.

Japanese Encephalitis. United States Centers for Disease Control and Prevention. March 12, 2010, http://www.cdc.gov/ncidod/dvbid/jencephalitis/.

Japanese Encephalitis vaccine. MedlinePlus. March 22, 2010, http://www.nlm.nih.gov/medlineplus/druginfo/meds/a607019.html.

The Yellow Book. Chapter 2—The Pre-Travel Consultation: Travel-related Vaccine Preventable Diseases. United States Centers for Disease Control and Prevention. January 25, 2010 (and frequently updated), http://wwwnc.cdc.gov/travel/yellowbook/2010/chapter-2/japanese-encephalitis.aspx.

ORGANIZATIONS

United States Centers for Disease Control and Prevention (CDC), 1600 Clifton Road, Atlanta GA, 30333, (404) 639-3534, 800-CDC-INFO (800-232-4636). TTY: (888) 232-6348, inquiry@cdc.gov, http://www.cdc.gov.

World Health Organization, Avenue Appia 20, 1211 Geneva 27 Switzerland, +22 41 791 21 11, +22 41 791 31 11, info@who.int, http://www.who.int.

Rosalyn Carson-DeWitt, MD
Tish Davidson, AM

Jaundice

Definition

Jaundice is a condition in which the skin and whites of the eyes turn yellowish from increased levels of a waste product called bilirubin. Although jaundice is common in newborn infants, at any time after the first few weeks of life it can be a symptom of a serious underlying condition. Jaundice is sometimes called hyperbilirubinemia or icterus from the Greek word for the condition.

Demographics

Newborn jaundice affects more than half of all full-term newborns and 80% of premature newborns within the first few days of life, although only about 10% of newborns require treatment. Jaundice is often more severe in Asian and Native American infants. **Biliary atresia**, a congenital defect in the bile ducts that can cause severe hyperbilirubinemia in otherwise healthy infants, occurs in about one in every 15,000 live births and girls are slightly more at risk than boys.

Description

Bilirubin is a yellow pigment that is formed from the breakdown of hemoglobin—the oxygen-carrying protein in red blood cells (RBCs). RBCs normally are removed from the blood and broken down in the spleen and other parts of the body after about 120 days in circulation. About 1% of RBCs are normally broken down and replaced each day. Bilirubin is carried to the liver where it is attached or conjugated to another molecule and added to bile. Conjugated bilirubin is known as direct or soluble bilirubin and unconjugated bilirubin is known as indirect or insoluble bilirubin.

Bile that is formed in the liver passes into the network of hepatic bile ducts, which join to form a single tube. One branch of this tube carries bile to the gallbladder where it is stored and concentrated. When food enters the stomach, the gallbladder is stimulated to release bile to the intestines through the common bile duct. Before the common bile duct reaches the intestines, it is joined by a duct from the pancreas. Bile and pancreatic juice enter the intestine through a valve called the ampulla of Vater. After entering the intestine, bile and pancreatic secretions assist in digestion and bile is excreted in the stool. However if bilirubin accumulates in the blood rather than being excreted, it discolors tissues, turning the skin and whites of the eyes yellow.

Risk factors

Risk factors for newborn jaundice include:

- Asian or Native American parentage
- a parent or sibling who had high bilirubin levels at birth
- maternal diabetes
- premature birth
- induced labor
- birth at a high altitude
- bruising during birth
- excessive weight loss during the first few days after birth

Causes and symptoms

Although jaundice is always caused by a buildup of bilirubin in the blood and tissues, there are many different causes for this buildup. The causes can be divided into three categories based on where they occur in the bilirubin cycle: before, in, or after the liver—pre-hepatic, hepatic, or post-hepatic.

The pre-hepatic cause of jaundice is hemolysis—the **death** of RBCs at a faster-than-normal rate, which releases hemoglobin and causes bilirubin to accumulate. The many causes of hemolysis include:

- Malaria. The malaria parasite develops inside RBCs and destroys them when it matures. Bilirubin can enter the urine in sufficient quantities to cause "blackwater fever," which is often lethal.
- Certain drugs. Hemolysis is a rare but sudden side effect of some antibiotics, anti tuberculosis medications, drugs that regulate heartbeat, and levodopa for treating Parkinson's disease.
- Certain drugs in combination with an inherited deficiency in the enzyme glucose-6-phosphate dehydrogenase (G6PD). G6PD deficiency affects more than 200 million people worldwide. Some of the drugs listed above, as well as certain others, especially vitamins C and K and anti-malarial medications such as quinine, can cause hemolysis in people with G6PD deficiency.
- Poisons. Snake and spider venoms, certain bacterial toxins, copper, and some organic industrial chemicals cause hemolysis by directly attacking RBC membranes.
- Artificial heart valves. The inflexible moving parts of artificial heart valves damage RBCs.
- Hereditary RBC disorders. Sickle cell disease that results in abnormal hemoglobin, spherocytosis, weakens the outer membrane of RBCs, and various other

inherited defects that affect the internal chemistry of RBCs can all cause hemolysis.

- Enlargement of the spleen. The spleen filters the blood and destroys old RBCs. If it becomes enlarged, healthy RBCs also are filtered out resulting in hemolysis. A wide variety of conditions can cause enlargement of the spleen.
- Diseases of the small blood vessels. As the RBCs move through diseased capillaries they can be damaged by rough surfaces on the inside of vessel walls.
- Immune reactions. The immune system can produce antibodies that destroy RBCs.
- Blood transfusions. Hemolysis can result from a transfusion with an incompatible blood type.
- Kidney failure and other serious diseases. Several diseases cause defective blood coagulation that destroys RBCs.
- Erythroblastosis fetalis. This results from too many immature RBCs (erythroblasts) in a newborn, usually because of a blood factor incompatibility between the mother and infant that causes maternal antibodies to destroy the newborn's RBCs.

Newborn jaundice results from both pre-hepatic and hepatic sources of excess bilirubin. At **birth** the newborn immediately begins converting from fetal to adult-type hemoglobin. The removal of the fetal hemoglobin can overload the immature liver for a week or two after birth, resulting in excess bilirubin and jaundice. Bilirubin gives a newborn's stools their yellow color. Jaundice usually appears first on the face, on the third or fourth day after birth, and progresses downward to the chest, abdomen, legs, and feet. If newborn feeding is delayed for any reason, such as illness, a digestive tract problem, or low fluid intake due to inefficient **breastfeeding**, the infant produces fewer stools, which can result in critically high blood levels of bilirubin and severe jaundice.

Jaundice at birth or within the first 24 hours can be a sign of abnormal jaundice, which can be very dangerous, particularly in preterm or unhealthy newborns. **Erythroblastosis fetalis** is the most common cause of abnormal newborn jaundice.

Other causes of hepatic jaundice include a variety of liver diseases in which the damaged organ cannot to keep up with bilirubin processing. These hepatic causes of jaundice include:

- starvation
- circulating (systemic) infections
- certain medications
- hepatitis
- cirrhosis
- hereditary defects in liver chemistry, including Gilbert's syndrome and Crigler-Najjar syndrome

Obstructive jaundices are post-hepatic forms caused by failure of soluble bilirubin to reach the intestines after leaving the liver. The most common cause of obstructive jaundice is gallstones in the ducts of the biliary system. Other causes of obstructive jaundice include:

- birth defects such as biliary atresia or infections that damage the bile ducts
- drugs
- cancers
- physical injury
- certain drugs—and rarely, pregnancy—that simply cause the bile in the ducts to stop flowing

Jaundice has no symptoms other than discoloration of the skin and eyes and is usually harmless, although the underlying condition may cause other symptoms and complications. However if unconjugated bilirubin reaches the newborn brain, it can cause permanent damage. Prolonged jaundice can also upset the balance of chemicals in the bile and cause the formation of stones.

Diagnosis

Examination

Jaundice is usually evident from the yellowish tint of the eyes and complexion. All newborns are examined under good light for signs of jaundice. The physician will feel (palpate) the liver and spleen to check for enlargement and evaluate any abdominal **pain**. The location and severity of abdominal pain and the presence or absence of **fever** help distinguish between hepatic and obstructive jaundice.

Tests

Blood tests measure the levels of total and/or conjugated bilirubin in the blood. Total bilirubin in the blood serum is normally between 0.3 milligrams (mg) per deciliter (dl) and 1.9 mg/dl. Conjugated or direct bilirubin is normally 0–0.3 mg/dl. Jaundice occurs when the total bilirubin level rises to 3 mg/dl or higher. It may be necessary to repeatedly measure bilirubin levels in jaundiced newborns because of the danger of insoluble bilirubin reaching the brain. An instrument called a bilirubinometer can be held against the infant's skin to assess the level of jaundice, eliminating the need for blood tests.

Additional tests may include:

- blood cell counts to detect anemia
- tests for blood-clotting function

KEY TERMS

Ampulla of Vater—The widened portion of the duct through which bile and pancreatic juices enter the intestine. Ampulla is a Latin word for a bottle with a narrow neck that opens into a wide body.

Anemia—A deficiency in hemoglobin, red blood cells, or total blood volume.

Bile—A liquid secreted by the liver and passed through ducts to the small intestine where it aids in the digestion and absorption of fats.

Biliary atresia—The underdevelopment or absence of bile ducts.

Biliary system/bile ducts—The gall bladder and the system of tubes that carries bile from the liver into the intestine.

Bilirubin—A reddish-yellow pigment that is a breakdown product of hemoglobin and is excreted by the liver into the bile.

Cirrhosis—Disruption of liver function due to damage from chronic progressive disease.

Crigler-Najjar syndrome—A moderate to severe form of hereditary jaundice.

Erythroblastosis fetalis—A disorder of newborn infants marked by a high level of immature red blood cells (erythroblasts).

Gilbert's syndrome—A mild hereditary form of jaundice.

Glucose-6-phosphate dehydrogenase (G6PD) deficiency—A hereditary disorder that, in combination with certain medications, can lead to episodes of hemolytic anemia.

Hemoglobin—The red substance in blood cells that carries oxygen.

Hemolysis—The destruction or breakdown of red blood cells.

Hepatic—Referring to the liver.

Hepatitis—Inflammation of the liver or the disease or condition causing liver inflammation.

Hyperbilirubinemia—An excess of bilirubin in the blood.

Icterus—Jaundice.

Microangiopathic—Pertaining to disorders of the small blood vessels.

Pancreas—The organ beneath the stomach that produces digestive juices, insulin, and other hormones.

Sickle cell disease—A hereditary defect in hemoglobin that changes the shape of red blood cells.

Splenectomy—Surgical removal of the spleen.

- tests for excess destruction of RBCs
- blood tests to assess liver function
- urine and stool samples to check for signs of bacterial or viral infection

Procedures

Various procedures may be used to diagnose a disorder underlying jaundice:

- Sometimes a bone marrow biopsy is necessary to diagnose blood-formation disorders.
- Ultrasound or a nuclear scan may be used to evaluate the spleen.
- A liver biopsy may be necessary to diagnose liver disease. A thin needle is used to remove a tiny core of liver tissue, which is sent to the laboratory for microscopic examination.
- Computed tomography (CT) or magnetic resonance imaging (MRI) scans are very useful for imaging certain conditions such as cancers in and around the liver or gallstones in the common bile duct.
- Various imaging techniques can be used to diagnose diseases of the biliary system. X rays for obtaining functional as well as anatomical information are taken one day after swallowing a contrast agent that is secreted into the bile. Alternatively contrast dye can be injected directly into the bile ducts, through a thin needle pushed into the liver or through a scope that is passed through the stomach to inject the dye into the ampulla of Vater.

Treatment

Traditional

Jaundice itself is treated only in newborns with dangerously high bilirubin levels. In the past it was necessary to exchange most of the infant's blood. Now the newborn can be fitted with eye protection and placed under a high-intensity, cool, blue-fluorescent light. The light is absorbed by the bilirubin and converts it into a harmless form than can be excreted in the bile and urine. Other phototherapy methods—such as a fiber optic bilirubin blanket—incorporate the light into a blanket so that the child can be breastfed during treatment or treated at home. Frequent feedings lead to more frequent stools, which reduces the reabsorption of bilirubin from the intestines into the blood. The infant also may be given additional fluids, possibly intravenously, to help remove bilirubin.

Obstructive jaundice frequently requires surgery. Surgery for biliary atresia must be performed within the first few weeks of life to prevent fatal liver damage. A common technique is to stitch an open piece of intestine over a bare patch of liver. Tiny bile ducts in that part of the liver will begin to discharge their bile into the intestine and pressure from the obstructed ducts elsewhere will release in that direction. As the bile flow increases, the ducts grow to accommodate it until all of the bile is redirected through the open pathways.

There are a variety of treatments for other conditions underlying jaundice:

- Any medications that are causing hemolysis or arresting the flow of bile are stopped immediately.
- Hemolytic diseases are treated, if at all, with medications and blood transfusions, except in the case of an enlarged spleen. Surgical removal of the spleen (splenectomy) can sometimes cure hemolytic anemia.
- Although there are no specific cures for most liver diseases, the liver can recover from even severe damage and regenerate from only a small remnant of original tissue.

Prognosis

Prognosis depends on the condition underlying the jaundice. Normal newborn jaundice is not harmful and disappears after one–two weeks. In cases of severe newborn jaundice, phototherapy usually returns bilirubin levels to normal within a few days. Infants with a duct obstruction within the liver itself usually require a liver transplant by the age of two.

Prevention

Prevention of jaundice involves preventing the underlying condition:

- Malaria in tropical or subtropical countries can often be prevented by precautions such as bed nets treated with insecticides or mosquito repellants and prophylactic drugs such as mefloquine.
- Hemolytic side effects from medications can be minimized with early detection and immediate cessation of the drug.
- G6PD-deficiency hemolysis can be prevented by testing patients before administering the causative drugs.
- Erythroblastosis fetalis can be prevented by treating an Rh-negative mother with a gamma-globulin solution called RhoGAM if there is a possibility that she is developing antibodies against her baby's blood.

The **American Academy of Pediatrics** recommendations for identifying and managing **neonatal jaundice** include:

- assessing all newborns for risk of severe jaundice, including measuring bilirubin levels before hospital discharge
- a follow-up visit within 3–5 days after birth when bilirubin levels are likely to peak
- breastfeeding a newborn at least 8–12 times per day, since effective breastfeeding significantly reduces the risk of hyperbilirubinemia

Resources

BOOKS

Sargent, Suzanne. *Liver Diseases: An Essential Guide for Nurses and Health Care Professionals.* Ames, IA: Wiley-Blackwell, 2009.

Valman, H. B., and Roslyn Thomas. *ABC of the First Year,* 6th ed. Hoboken, NJ: Wiley-Blackwell, 2009.

PERIODICALS

Charles, Katie. "Yellow Alert for Parents" *New York Daily News* (February 18, 2009): 27.

Jacobi, Tillmann. "Jaundice in an Adult." *GP* (March 27, 2009): 35.

Moerschel, Sarah K., Lauren B. Cianciaruso, and Lloyd R. Tracy. "A Practical Approach to Neonatal Jaundice." *American Family Physician* 77, no. 9 (May 1, 2008): 1255–1262.

OTHER

American Association for Clinical Chemistry. "Bilirubin." *Lab Tests Online*, http://www.labtestsonline.org/understanding/analytes/bilirubin/test.html.

American Association for Clinical Chemistry. "Jaundice." *Lab Tests Online*, http://www.labtestsonline.org/understanding/conditions/jaundice.html.

"Jaundice." *freeMD*, http://www.freemd.com/jaundice/visit-virtual-doctor.htm.

"Jaundice." *MedlinePlus*, http://www.nlm.nih.gov/medlineplus/jaundice.html.

Questions and Answers: Jaundice and Your Newborn. American Academy of Pediatrics, http://www.aap.org/family/jaundicefaq.htm.

ORGANIZATIONS

American Academy of Pediatrics, 141 Northwest Point Blvd., Elk Grove Village IL, 60007-1098, (874) 434-4000, (874) 434-8000, kidsdocs@aap.org, http://www.aap.org.

American Liver Foundation, 75 Maiden Lane, Suite 603, New York NY, 10038, (212) 668-1000, (212) 483-8179, http://www.liverfoundation.org.

National Institute of Diabetes and Digestive and Kidney Diseases, Building 31, Room 9A06, 31 Center Drive, MSC 2560, Bethesda MD, 20892-2560, (301) 496-3583, http://www2.niddk.nih.gov.

J. Ricker Polsdorfer, MD
Teresa G. Odle
Margaret Alic, PhD

Jaundice test ***see* Bilirubin test**

Jock itch ***see* Ringworm**

Juvenile arthritis

Definition

Juvenile arthritis (JA) is not a single disorder but a group of arthritides (plural of arthritis) that affect children and teenagers below the age of 16. JA has been known by various names since 1970, including juvenile rheumatoid arthritis (JRA), juvenile idiopathic arthritis (JIA), and juvenile chronic arthritis (JCA). All the conditions included under the general term of JA strike children under age 16, and all have immune-mediated joint inflammation as their major manifestation. The International League of Associations for Rheumatology (ILAR) has tried to bridge these differences with a unifying set of criteria to define juvenile arthritis.

Demographics

According to the American College of Rheumatology (ACR), as of 2010 about one child in every 1,000 in the United States develops some form of JA. Doctors estimate that around 300,000 children in the United States have been diagnosed with JIA. Native Americans in both Canada and the United States have somewhat higher rates of JA than members of other racial and ethnic groups. Internationally, Norway and Australia have the highest rates of JA, while Africa and individuals of African ancestry appear to have lower than average rates. The reason for these differences is not yet known.

Description

The skeletal system of the body is made up of different types of the strong, fibrous tissue known as connective tissue. Bone, cartilage, ligaments, and tendons are all forms of connective tissue that have different compositions, and thus different characteristics.

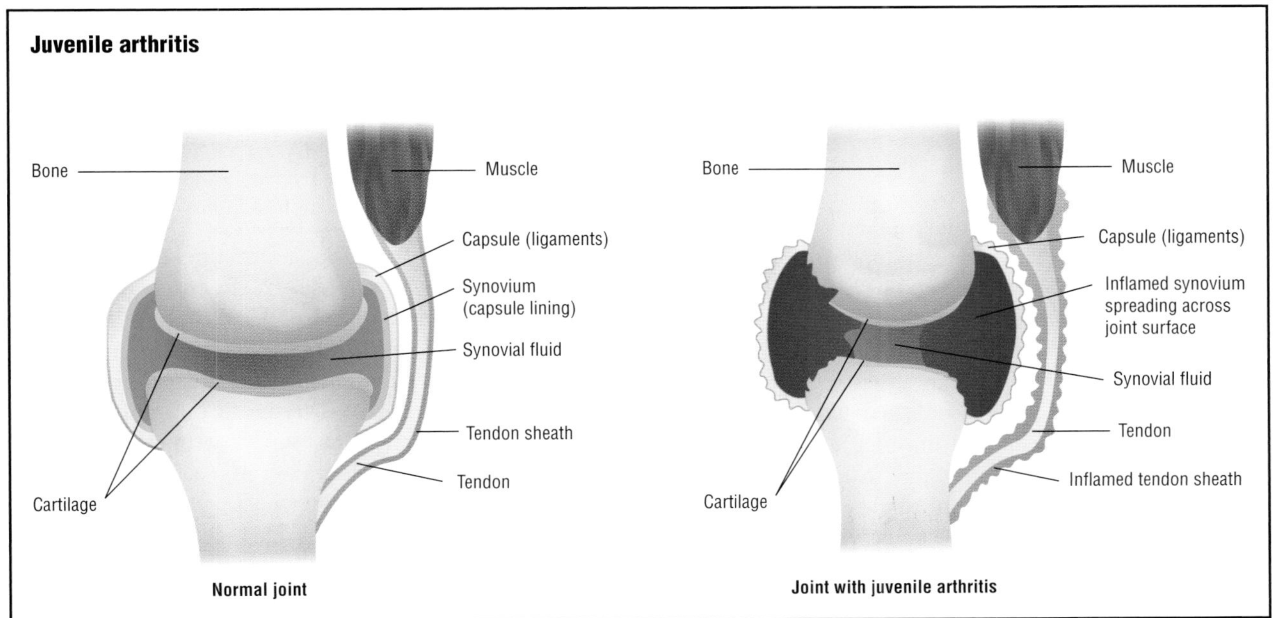

Normal knee joint (left) and one affected by juvenile arthritis, which shows damaged cartilage and inflammation of the synovial fluid and tendon sheath. *(Illustration by PreMediaGlobal. Reproduced by permission of Gale, a part of Cengage Learning.)*

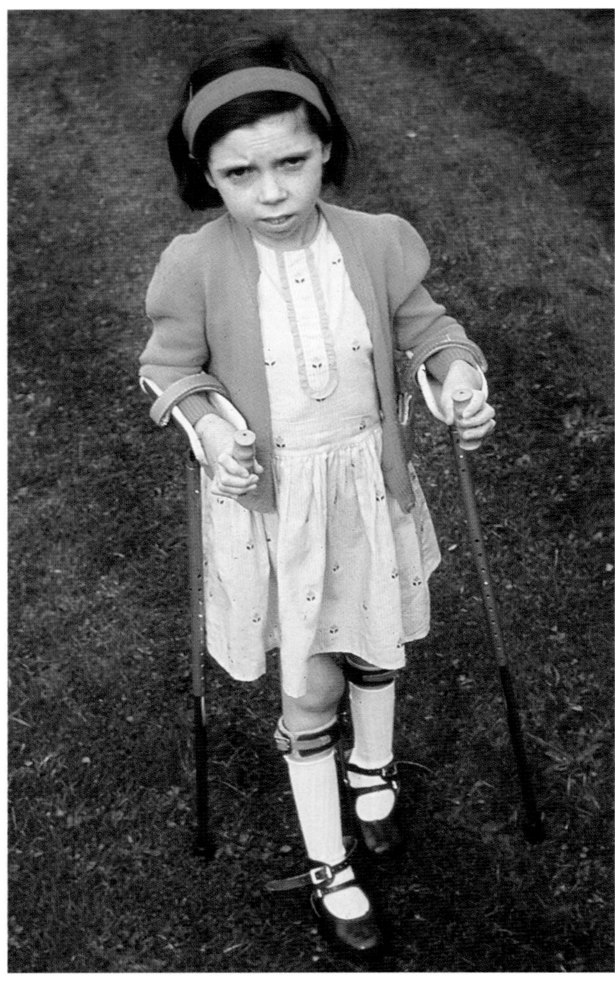

A young girl with juvenile arthritis uses braces to help rest painful joints and prevent deformities. *(John Moss/Photo Researchers, Inc.)*

The joints are structures that hold two or more bones together. Some joints (synovial joints) allow for movement between the bones being joined (called articulating bones). The simplest model of a synovial joint involves two bones, separated by a slight gap called the joint cavity. The ends of each articular bone are covered by a layer of cartilage. A tough tissue called the articular capsule surrounds both articular bones and the joint cavity. The articular capsule has two components: the fibrous membrane on the outside, and the synovial membrane (or synovium) on the inside. The fibrous membrane may include tough bands of fibrous tissue called ligaments that are responsible for providing support to the joints. The synovial membrane has special cells and many capillaries (tiny blood vessels). This membrane produces a supply of synovial fluid that fills the joint cavity, lubricates it, and helps the articular bones move smoothly about the joint.

In JA, the synovial membrane becomes intensely inflamed. Usually thin and delicate, the synovium becomes thick and stiff, with numerous infoldings on its surface. The membrane becomes invaded by white blood cells, which produce a variety of destructive chemicals. The cartilage along the articular surfaces of the bones may be attacked and destroyed, and the bone, articular capsule, and ligaments may begin to be worn away. These processes severely interfere with movement in the joint.

JA specifically refers to chronic arthritic conditions that affect a child under the age of 16 years and last for a minimum of three to six months. JA is often characterized by a waxing and waning course, with flares separated by periods during which no symptoms are noted (remission). Some of the medical literature refers to JA as juvenile rheumatoid arthritis, although most types of JA differ significantly from the adult disease called rheumatoid arthritis, in terms of symptoms, progression, and prognosis.

Risk factors

The two major risk factors for JA are sex and race. Most forms of JA are more common in girls than in boys (the major exception being eye disorders), and more common in Caucasian and Native American children than in children of other races.

Causes and symptoms

Causes

A number of different causes have been sought to explain the onset of JA. There seems to be some genetic link, because the tendency to develop JA sometimes runs in a particular **family**, and because certain genetic markers are more frequently found in patients with JA and other related diseases. Genes that have been linked to increased susceptibility to JA as of 2010 include the *IL2RA/CD25* gene and the *VTCN1* gene.

Many researchers have looked for some infectious cause for JA, but no clear connection to a particular organism has ever been made. JA is considered by some to be an autoimmune disorder. **Autoimmune disorders** occur when the body's **immune system** mistakenly identifies the body's own tissue as foreign and goes about attacking those tissues as if trying to rid the body of an invader (such as a bacteria, virus, or fungi). While an autoimmune mechanism is strongly suspected, certain markers of such a mechanism (such as rheumatoid factor, often present in adults with such disorders) are rarely present in children with JA.

Symptoms

Joint symptoms of arthritis may include stiffness, **pain**, redness and warmth of the joint, and swelling.

Bone in the area of an affected joint may grow too quickly, or too slowly, resulting in limbs that are of different lengths. When the child tries to avoid moving a painful joint, the muscle may begin to shorten from disuse. This is called a contracture.

Symptoms of JA depend on the particular subtype. According to criteria published by the American College of Rheumatology (ACR) in 1973 and modified in 1977, JRA is classified by the symptoms that appear within the first six months of the disorder:

- Pauciarticular JA: This is the most common and the least severe type of JA, affecting about 40–60% of all JA patients. This type affects fewer than four joints, usually the knee, ankle, wrist, and/or elbow. Other more general (systemic) symptoms are usually absent, and the child's growth usually remains normal. Very few children (less than 15%) with pauciarticular JA end up with deformed joints. Some children with this form of JA experience painless swelling of the joint. Some children with JA have a serious inflammation of structures within the eye, which if left undiagnosed and untreated could lead to blindness. This condition is known as uveitis, and affects about 20% of children diagnosed with JRA. While many children have cycles of flares and remissions, in some children the disease completely and permanently resolves within a few years of diagnosis.
- Polyarticular JA: About 40% of all cases of JA are of this type. More girls than boys are diagnosed with this form of JA. This type is most common in children up to age three or after the age of 10. Polyarticular JA affects five or more joints simultaneously. It usually affects the small joints of both hands and both feet, although other large joints may be affected as well. Some patients with arthritis in their knees experience a different rate of growth in each leg. Ultimately, one leg will grow longer than the other. About half of all patients with polyarticular JA have arthritis of the spine and/or hip. Some patients with polyarticular JA have other symptoms of a systemic illness, including anemia (low red blood cell count), decreased growth rate, low appetite, low-grade fever, and a slight rash. The disease is most severe in those children who are diagnosed in early adolescence. Some of these children test positive for a marker present in other autoimmune disorders, called rheumatoid factor (RF). RF is found in adults who have rheumatoid arthritis. Children who are positive for RF tend to have a more severe course, with a disabling form of arthritis that destroys and deforms the joints. This type of arthritis is thought to be the adult form of rheumatoid arthritis occurring at a very early age.
- Systemic-onset JA: Sometimes called Still disease (after a physician who originally described it), this is a type of JA that occurs in about 10–20% of all patients with JA. Boys and girls are equally affected, and diagnosis is usually made between the ages of 5–10 years. The initial symptoms are not usually related to the joints. Instead, these children have high fevers; a rash; decreased appetite and weight loss; severe joint and muscle pain; swollen lymph nodes, spleen, and liver; and serious anemia. Some children experience other complications, including inflammation of the sac containing the heart (pericarditis); inflammation of the tissue lining the chest cavity and lungs (pleuritis); and inflammation of the heart muscle (myocarditis). The eye inflammation often seen in pauciarticular JA is uncommon in systemic onset JA. Symptoms of actual arthritis begin later in the course of systemic onset JA, and they often involve the wrists and ankles. Many of these children continue to have periodic flares of fever and systemic symptoms throughout childhood. Some children will go on to develop a polyarticular type of JA.
- Enthesis-related arthritis (sometimes called spondyloarthropathy): This type of JA most commonly affects boys older than eight years of age. The arthritis occurs in the knees and ankles, moving over time to include the hips and lower spine. Inflammation of the eye may occur occasionally, but usually resolves without permanent damage.
- Psoriatic JA: This type of arthritis usually shows up in fewer than four joints, but spreads to include multiple joints (appearing similar to polyarticular JA). Hips, back, fingers, and toes are frequently affected. A skin condition called psoriasis accompanies this type of arthritis. Children often have pits or ridges in their fingernails. The arthritis usually progresses to become a serious, disabling problem.

There is some disagreement among specialists about the classification of JRA. Some prefer the EULAR classification, introduced in 1977, to the ACR system. More recently the International League of Associations for Rheumatology (ILAR) has identified a unifying set of criteria to define juvenile arthritis. As of 2010, inconsistencies in naming the specific types of juvenile arthritis and their criteria for diagnosis continue to exist.

Diagnosis

The diagnosis of JA is not always obvious and may be delayed because some children do not complain of pain, and swelling of the joints may not be obvious.

Diagnosis of JA is usually made on the basis of the child's collection of symptoms together with elimination of other possible causes of the symptoms. Disorders to be ruled out include lupus, **Lyme disease**, certain bone disorders, infections, and childhood **cancer**. The

KEY TERMS

Articular bones—Two or more bones connected with each other via a joint.

Biologics—A class of drugs produced by means of biological processes involving recombinant DNA technology.

Congenital—Present at birth.

Contracture—Shortening of a muscle or joint due to a disease condition or injury.

Flare—A recurrence or worsening of the symptoms of JA.

Idiopathic—Of unknown cause or spontaneous origin. JRA is sometimes called juvenile idiopathic arthritis or JIA because its causes are still not fully known.

Joint—A structure that holds two or more bones together.

Rheumatology—The branch of medicine that specializes in the diagnosis and treatment of disorders affecting the muscles and joints.

Synovial joint—A particular type of joint that allows for movement in the articular bones.

Synovial membrane—The membrane that lines the inside of the articular capsule of a joint and produces a lubricating fluid called synovial fluid.

Uveitis—Inflammation of the pigmented vascular covering of the eye, which includes the choroid, iris, and ciliary body. Uveitis is a common complication of JRA.

diagnosis will usually involve a referral from the child's **pediatrician** to a rheumatologist, a physician specializing in disorders of the muscles and joints).

Examination

Symptoms of JA that the doctor can observe or measure during an office physical include:

- limping
- fever
- difficulty in moving or using an arm or leg
- swollen joint(s)
- skin rash on the chest, arms, or legs that comes and goes with fever
- swollen lymph nodes
- enlarged liver and spleen
- red eyes
- pain when a bright light is shone in the eye.

Tests

There is no blood test as of 2010 that can be used to diagnose JA, and other laboratory tests often show normal results. A blood test may be useful in ruling out certain infections as a cause of the child's symptoms. Some nonspecific indicators of inflammation may be elevated, including white blood cell count, erythrocyte sedimentation rate, and a marker called C-reactive protein. As with any chronic disease, **anemia** may be present. Children with an extraordinarily early onset of the adult type of rheumatoid arthritis will have a positive test for rheumatoid factor.

Imaging studies (most often **x rays**) may be taken to rule out broken or fractured bones, congenital defects in the joints, tumors, or some types of infectious disease. X-ray studies may also be done to monitor the development of the child's bones. **Magnetic resonance imaging** (MRI) and ultrasound are used increasingly as of 2010 to detect damage caused by JA in order to prevent further damage to the child's joints.

Procedures

In some cases the doctor may tap a swollen joint by inserting a small hollow needle into the joint to withdraw some of the fluid. This fluid can be analyzed to help determine the cause of the arthritis. In addition, withdrawing fluid may ease the discomfort in the joint.

Treatment

Traditional

Mainstream treatment of JA involves the use of appropriate medications together with physical and **occupational therapy** as needed. Some children with JA may eventually need surgery, including joint replacement, and others may require psychological counseling to cope with depression or anger related to their symptoms. The goal of therapy is to control symptoms, maintain functioning of the child's joints, and prevent damage to the joints.

Drugs

Treating JA involves efforts to decrease the amount of inflammation in order to preserve movement. Medications that can be used for this include such nonsteroidal anti-inflammatory agents (NSAIDs) as ibuprofen (Motrin, Ibuprin), naproxen (Aleve, Naprelan, Naprosyn), diclofenac (Voltaren, Cataflam), and Tolmetin (Tolectin). Oral steroid medications are effective but have many serious side effects with long-term use. Injections of **steroids** into an affected joint can be helpful. Steroid eye drops are used to treat eye inflammation. Occasionally, splints are used to rest painful joints and to try to prevent or improve deformities.

Children who do not respond to treatment with NSAIDs may be given disease-modifying antirheumatic drugs or DMARDs. DMARDs include such medications as hydroxychloroquine (Plaquenil), sulfasalazine (Azulfidine), and methotrexate (Rheumatrex). More recent agents used to treat JA include biologics, which are drugs produced using recombinant DNA technology. Biologics used to treat JA include etanercept (Embrel), infliximab (Remicade), adalimumab (Humira), and abatacept (Orencia). Biologics work by blocking high levels of proteins that cause inflammation in the body.

Alternative

Juice therapy has been suggested as an alternative treatment for arthritis. It works to detoxify the body, helping to reduce JA symptoms. Some recommended fruits and vegetables to include in the juice are carrots, celery, cabbage, potatoes, cherries, lemons, beets, cucumbers, radishes, and garlic. Tomatoes and other vegetables in the nightshade family (potatoes, eggplant, red and green peppers) are discouraged.

As an adjunct therapy, aromatherapy preparations use cypress, fennel, and lemon. Massage oils include rosemary, benzoin, chamomile, camphor, juniper, and lavender. Other types of therapy that have been used include acupuncture, acupressure, and bodywork.

Nutritional supplements that may be beneficial include large amounts of antioxidants (**vitamins** C, A, E, zinc, selenium, and flavenoids), as well as B vitamins and a full complement of **minerals** (including boron, copper, manganese). Other nutrients that assist in detoxifying the body, including methionine, cysteine, and other amino acids, may also be helpful. A number of autoimmune disorders, including JA, seem to have a relationship to **food allergies**. Identification and elimination of reactive foods may result in a decrease in JA symptoms. Constitutional homeopathy can work to quiet the symptoms of JA and bring about balance to the whole person. None of these alternative treatments, however, have been proven effective in clinical trials that meet the standards of conventional Western medicine.

Prognosis

The prognosis for pauciarticular JA is quite good, as is the prognosis for spondyloarthropathy. Polyarticular JA carries a somewhat worse prognosis; children who have many joints involved, or who have a positive rheumatoid factor are more likely to have chronic pain, disability, and problems with school attendance. Systemic onset JA has a variable prognosis, depending on the organ systems affected, and the progression to polyarticular JA. JRA is rarely life-threatening; however, about 1–5% of all JA patients die of such complications as infection, inflammation of the heart, or kidney disease. In addition, depression and other psychological problems are common in children with JA, particularly when they enter their teen years. Many children benefit from support groups and special summer camp programs for children with JA.

Prevention

Because so little is known about the causes of JA, there are no recommendations as of 2010 for preventing its development.

Resources

BOOKS

Huff, Charlotte. *Raising a Child with Arthritis*. 2nd ed. Atlanta, GA: Arthritis Foundation, 2008.

Rouba, Kelly. *Juvenile Arthritis: The Ultimate Teen Guide*. Lanham, MD: Scarecrow Press, 2009.

Szer, Ilona S., et al., eds. *Arthritis in Children and Adolescents: Juvenile Idiopathic Arthritis*. New York: Oxford University Press, 2006.

PERIODICALS

Angeles-Han, S., and S. Prahalad. "The Genetics of Juvenile Idiopathic Arthritis: What Is New in 2010?" *Current Rheumatology Reports* 12 (April 2010): 87–93.

Damasio, M.B., et al. "Synovial and Inflammatory Diseases in Childhood: Role of New Imaging Modalities in the Assessment of Patients with Juvenile Idiopathic Arthritis." *Pediatric Radiology* 40 (June 2010): 985–98.

Haber, L., et al. "Clinical Manifestations and Treatment of the Pediatric Rheumatoid Patient." *Clinics in Podiatric Medicine and Surgery* 27 (April 2010): 219–33.

Kalinina Ayuso, V., et al. "Male Gender as a Risk Factor for Complications in Uveitis Associated with Juvenile Idiopathic Arthritis." *American Journal of Ophthalmology* 149 (June 2010): 994–99.

Oen, K., et al. "Early Outcomes and Improvement of Patients with Juvenile Idiopathic Arthritis Enrolled in a Canadian Multicenter Inception Cohort." *Arthritis Care and Research* 62 (April 2010): 527–36.

Philpott, J.F., et al. "Physical Activity Recommendations for Children with Specific Chronic Health Conditions: Juvenile Idiopathic Arthritis, Hemophilia, Asthma, and Cystic Fibrosis." *Clinical Journal of Sport Medicine* 20 (May 2010): 167–72.

Shin, S.T., et al. "Nutritional Status and Clinical Characteristics in Children With Juvenile Rheumatoid Arthritis." *Journal of Microbiology, Immunology, and Infection* 43 (April 2010): 93–98.

OTHER

Abramson, Leslie. "Arthritis in Children." American College of Rheumatology (ACR). June 2008, http://www.rheumatology.org/practice/clinical/patients/diseases_and_conditions/juvenilearthritis.asp (accessed September 25, 2010).

Borigini, Mark James. "Juvenile Rheumatoid Arthritis." *MedlinePlus*. May 31, 2009, http://www.nlm.nih.gov/medlineplus/ency/article/000451.htm (accessed September 25, 2010).

"Juvenile Arthritis Fact Sheet." JA Alliance, http://www.arthritis.org/ja-fact-sheet.php (accessed September 25, 2010).

"Juvenile Rheumatoid Arthritis." *MayoClinic*. October 16, 2009, http://www.mayoclinic.com/health/juvenile-rheumatoid-arthritis/DS00018 (accessed September 25, 2010).

Rabinovich, C. Egla. "Juvenile Rheumatoid Arthritis." *eMedicine*. June 1, 2010, http://emedicine.medscape.com/article/1007276-overview (accessed September 25, 2010).

ORGANIZATIONS

American College of Rheumatology (ACR), 2200 Lake Boulevard NE, Atlanta GA, 30319, (404) 633-3777, (404) 633-1870, acr@rheumatology.org, http://www.rheumatology.org.

Arthritis Foundation, PO Box 7669, Atlanta GA, 30357-0669, (800) 283-7800, http://www.arthritis.org.

European League against Rheumatism (EULAR), Seestrasse 240, ZürichSwitzerland, CH 8802 Kächberg, +41 44 716 30 30, +41 44 716 30 39, http://www.eular.org.

International League of Associations for Rheumatology (ILAR), ndavidai@rheumatology.org, http://www.ilar.org.

National Institute of Arthritis and Musculoskeletal and Skin Diseases (NIAMS), 1 AMS Circle, Bethesda MD, 20892-3675, (301) 495-4484, (877) 22-NIAMS, (301) 718-6366, NIAMSinfo@mail.nih.gov, http://www.niams.nih.gov.

Rosalyn Carson-DeWitt, MD
Rebecca J. Frey, PhD
Tish Davidson, AM

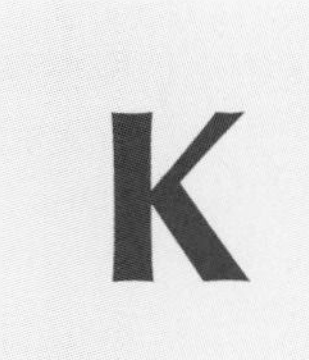

Kaufman assessment battery for children

Definition

The Kaufman Assessment Battery for Children (K-ABC) is a standardized test that assesses **intelligence** and achievement in children aged two years, six months to 12 years, 6 months. The edition published in 1983 by Kaufman and Kaufman was revised in 2002 to expand its age range (to cover children ages three to eighteen) and enhance its usefulness. In addition, new subtests were added and existing subtests updated.

Purpose

The K-ABC was developed to evaluate preschoolers, minority groups, and children with learning disabilities. It is used to provide educational planning and placement, neurological **assessment**, and research. The assessment is to be administered in a school or clinical setting and is intended for use with English speaking, bilingual, or nonverbal children. There is also a Spanish edition that is to be used with children whose primary language is Spanish.

Precautions

The K-ABC is especially useful in providing information about nonverbal intellectual abilities. However, it has been criticized for not focusing on measures of verbal intelligence in the Mental Processing Composite score that measures intelligence. Additionally, the separation of intelligence and achievement scores has been questioned by researchers who claim the two terms are misleading. For example, many subtests in the achievement composite are in fact measures of intelligence rather than achievement (knowledge acquired through school and/or home environment). The K-ABC should be used with caution as the primary instrument for identifying the intellectual abilities of children.

Administration and interpretation of results (as with all psychometric testing) requires a competent examiner who is trained in psychology and individual intellectual assessment—preferably a psychologist.

Description

Administration of the K-ABC takes between 35 and 85 minutes. The older the child, the longer the test generally takes to administer. It is comprised of four global test scores that include:

- sequential processing scales
- simultaneous processing scales
- achievement scales
- mental processing composite

There is an additional nonverbal scale that allows applicable subtests to be administered through gestures to hearing impaired, speech/language impaired, or children who do not speak English.

The test consists of 16 subtests—10 mental processing subtests and six achievement subtests. Not all subtests are administered to each age group, and only three subtests are administered to all age groups. Children ages two years, 6 months are given seven subtests, and the number of subtests given increase with the child's age. For any one child, a maximum of 13 subtests are administered. Children from age seven years to 12 years, 6 months are given 13 subtests.

The sequential processing scale primarily measures short-term memory and consists of subtests that measure problem-solving skills where the emphasis is on following a sequence or order. The child solves tasks by arranging items in serial or sequential order including reproducing hand taps on a table, recalling numbers that were presented. It also contains a subtest that measures a child's ability to recall objects in correct order as presented by the examiner.

The simultaneous processing scale examines problem-solving skills that involve several processes at once. The seven subtests comprising this scale are facial recognition, identification of objects or scenes in a partially completed picture, reproduction of a presented design by using rubber triangles, selecting a picture that completes or is similar to another picture, memory for location of pictures presented on a page, and arrangement of pictures in meaningful order.

The achievement scales measures achievement and focuses on applied skills and facts that were learned through the school or home environment. The subtests are expressive vocabulary; ability to name fictional characters, famous persons, and well known places; mathematical skills; ability to solve riddle; reading and decoding skills; and reading and comprehension skills.

The sequential and simultaneous processing scales are combined to comprise the mental processing composite. This composite measures intelligence on the K-ABC and concentrates on the child's ability to solve unfamiliar problems simultaneously and sequentially. The simultaneous processing scales have a greater impact on the mental processing composite score than do the sequential processing scales. The mental processing composite score is considered the global estimate of a child's level of intellectual functioning.

Results

The K-ABC is a standardized test, which means that a large sample of children in the two years, six months to 12 years, six months age range was administered the exam as a means of developing test norms. Children in the sample were representative of the population of the United States based on age, gender, race or ethnic group, geographic region, community size, parental education, educational placement (normal versus special classes), etc. From this sample, norms were established.

Based on these norms, the global scales on the K-ABC each have a mean or average score of 100 and a standard deviation of 15. For this test, as with most measures of intelligence, a score of 100 is in the normal or average range. The standard deviation indicates how far above or below the norm a child's score is. For example, a score of 85 is one standard deviation below the norm score of 100.

Test scores provide an estimate of the level at which a child is functioning based on a combination of many different subtests or measures of skills. A trained psychologist is needed to evaluate and interpret the results, determine strengths and weaknesses, and make overall recommendations based on the findings and behavioral observations.

Resources

BOOKS

Sattler, Jerome. *Assessment of Children.* 3rd Edition. San Diego, CA: Jerome Sattler, Publisher Inc. 1992.

PERIODICALS

Cahan, S. and A. Noyman. "The Kaufman Ability Battery for Children Mental Processing Scale: A Valid Measure of 'Pure' Intelligence?" *Educational and Psychological Measurement* 61, no. 5 (2001): 827-840.

ORGANIZATIONS

American Psychological Association, 750 First St., NE, Washington DC, 20002-4242, (202) 336-5500, www.apa.org.

National Association of School Psychologists, 4340 East West Highway, Suite 402, Bethesda MD, 20814, (301) 657-0270, http://www.nasponline.com.

Jenifer P. Marom, Ph.D.

Kawasaki syndrome

Definition

Kawasaki syndrome is a potentially fatal inflammatory disease that affects several organ systems in the body, including the heart, circulatory system, mucous membranes, skin, and **immune system**. It occurs primarily in

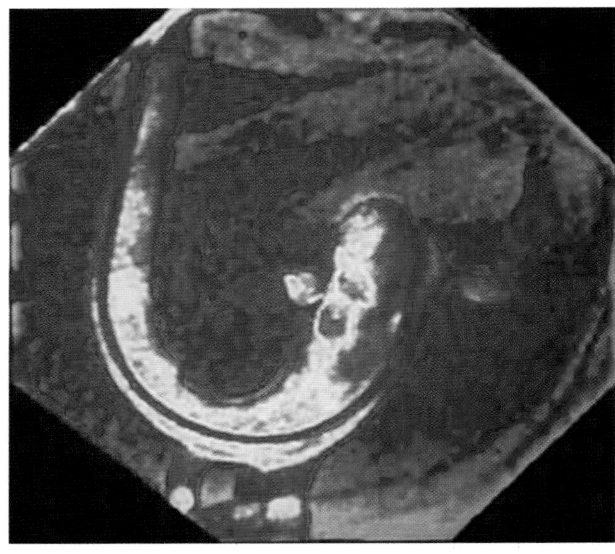

An angiogram showing abnormal coronary arteries in a child suffering from Kawasaki syndrome. The coronary arteries bulge into balloon shapes, called aneurysms, along their lengths. *(Mehau Kulyk/SPL/Photo Researchers, Inc.)*

infants and children but has also been identified in adults as old as 34 years. Its cause is unknown.

Description

Kawasaki syndrome, also called mucocutaneous lymph node syndrome (MLNS), is an inflammatory disorder with potentially fatal complications affecting the heart and its larger arteries. Nearly twice as many males are affected as females. Although persons of Asian descent are affected more frequently than either black or white individuals, there does not appear to be a distinctive geographic pattern of occurrence. Eighty percent of cases involve children under the age of four. Although the disease usually appears in individuals, it sometimes affects several members of the same family and occasionally occurs in small epidemics.

Causes and symptoms

The specific cause of Kawasaki syndrome is unknown, although the disease resembles infectious illnesses in many ways. It has been suggested that Kawasaki syndrome represents an allergic reaction or other unusual response to certain types of infections. Some researchers think that the syndrome may be caused by the interaction of an immune cell, called the T cell, with certain poisons (toxins) secreted by bacteria.

Kawasaki syndrome has an abrupt onset, with **fever** as high as 104°F (40°C) and a rash that spreads over the patient's chest and genital area. The fever is followed by a characteristic peeling of the skin beginning at the fingertips and toenails. In addition to the body rash, the patient's lips become very red, with the tongue developing a "strawberry" appearance. The palms, soles, and mucous membranes that line the eyelids and cover the exposed portion of the eyeball (conjuntivae) become purplish-red and swollen. The lymph nodes in the patient's neck may also become swollen. These symptoms may last from two weeks to three months, with relapses in some patients.

In addition to the major symptoms, about 30% of patients develop joint pains or arthritis, usually in the large joints of the body. Others develop **pneumonia**, **diarrhea**, dry or cracked lips, **jaundice**, or an inflammation of the membranes covering the brain and spinal cord (**meningitis**). A few patients develop symptoms of inflammation in the liver (hepatitis), gallbladder, lungs, or tonsils.

About 20% of patients with Kawasaki syndrome develop complications of the cardiovascular system. These complications include inflammation of the heart tissue (myocarditis), disturbances in heartbeat rhythm (arrhythmias), and areas of blood vessel dilation (aneurysms) in the coronary arteries. Other patients may develop inflammation of an artery (arteritis) in their arms or legs. Complications of the heart or arteries begin to develop around the tenth day after the illness begins, when the fever and rash begin to subside. A few patients may develop gangrene, or the **death** of soft tissue, in their hands and feet. The specific causes of these complications are not yet known.

Diagnosis

Because Kawasaki syndrome is primarily a disease of infants and young children, the disease is most likely to be diagnosed by a **pediatrician**. The physician will first consider the possible involvement of other diseases that cause fever and skin **rashes**, including **scarlet fever**, **measles**, **Rocky Mountain spotted fever**, **toxoplasmosis** (a disease carried by cats), juvenile rheumatoid arthritis, and a blistering and inflammation of the skin caused by reactions to certain medications (Stevens-Johnson syndrome).

Once other diseases have been ruled out, the patient's symptoms will be compared with a set of diagnostic criteria. The patient must have a fever lasting five days or longer that does not respond to **antibiotics**, together with four of the following five symptoms:

- inflammation of the conjunctivae of both eyes with no discharge
- changes in the mucous membranes of the mouth and throat such as "strawberry" tongue; cracked lips; or swollen throat tissues
- changes in the hands or feet such as swelling caused by excess fluid in the tissues; peeling of the skin; or abnormal redness of the skin
- skin eruption or rash associated with fever (exanthem) on the patient's trunk
- swelling of the lymph nodes in the neck to a size greater than 0.6 in (1.5 cm)

Since the cause of Kawasaki syndrome is unknown, there are no laboratory tests that can confirm the diagnosis. The following test results, however, are associated with the disease:

- blood tests show a high white blood cell count, high platelet count, a high level of protein in the blood serum, and mild anemia
- chest x ray may show enlargement of the heart (cardiomegaly)
- urine may show the presence of pus or an abnormally high level of protein
- an electrocardiogram may show changes in the heartbeat rhythm

KEY TERMS

Aneurysm—Dilation of an artery caused by thinning and weakening of the vessel wall.

Arrythmia—Abnormal heart rhythm.

Arteritis—Inflammation of an artery.

Cardiomegaly—An enlarged heart.

Conjunctivae—The mucous membranes that cover the exposed area of the eyeball and line the inner surface of the eyelids.

Exanthem—A skin eruption associated with a disease, usually one accompanied by fever as in Kawasaki syndrome.

Gangrene—The death of soft tissue in a part of the body, usually caused by obstructed circulation.

Hepatitis—Inflammation of the liver.

Meningitis—Inflammation of the membranes, called the meninges, covering the brain and spinal cord.

Mucocutaneous lymph node syndrome (MLNS)—Mucocutaneous lymph node syndrome, another name for Kawasaki syndrome. The name comes from the key symptoms of the disease, which involve the mucous membranes of the mouth and throat, the skin, and the lymph nodes.

Myocarditis—Inflammation of the heart muscle.

Stevens-Johnson syndrome—A severe inflammatory skin eruption that occurs as a result of an allergic reaction or respiratory infection.

T cell—A type of white blood cell that develops in the thymus gland and helps to regulate the immune system's response to infections or malignancy.

In addition to these tests, it is important to take a series of echocardiograms during the course of the illness because 20% of Kawasaki patients will develop coronary aneurysms or arteritis that will not appear during the first examination.

Treatment

Kawasaki syndrome is usually treated with a combination of aspirin, to control the patient's fever and skin inflammation, and high doses of intravenous immune globulin to reduce the possibility of coronary artery complications. Some patients with heart complications may be treated with drugs that reduce blood clotting or may receive corrective surgery.

Follow-up care includes two to three months of monitoring with chest **x rays**, electrocardiography, and echocardiography. Treatment with aspirin is often continued for several months.

Prognosis

Most patients with Kawasaki syndrome will recover completely, but about 1–2% will die as a result of blood clots forming in the coronary arteries or as a result of a heart attack. Deaths are sudden and unpredictable. Almost 95% of fatalities occur within six months of infection, but some have been reported as long as 10 years afterward. Long-term follow-up of patients with aneurysms indicates that about half show some healing of the aneurysm. The remaining half has a high risk of heart complications in later life.

Resources

BOOKS

Shandera, Wayne X., and Maria E. Carlini. "Infectious Diseases: Viral & Rickettsial." In *Current Medical Diagnosis and Treatment, 1998*, edited by Stephen McPhee, et al., 37th ed. Stamford: Appleton & Lange, 1997.

Rebecca J. Frey, PhD

Kidney development and function

Definition

Kidney development involves the formation and maturation of the kidneys from conception to adulthood. Kidney function involves the removal of metabolic wastes, regulation of urine production, and regulation of blood pressure required to keep the body in balance.

Description

The kidneys are a pair bean-shaped, fist-sized organs located below the rib cage on either side of the back. In adults they filter the about 200 quarts (190 L) of blood every day to remove waste products that result from the normal metabolism of tissues in the body. These wastes circulate in the blood. It they are not removed, they build up and damage the body. The kidneys play a role in controlling the amount of urine produced and participate in the control of blood pressure. They are also involved in regulating the effects of vitamin D on the body and in stimulating bone marrow to create new red blood cells. When the kidneys do not function properly, a person can become very ill; when they fail to function at all, a person will die without dialysis or a kidney transplant.

Kidney development

The kidneys, along with the ureters, bladder, and urethra, make up the urinary system. During embryonic development, the urinary system goes through a three-stage process resulting in a mature kidney. The first stage involves the formation of the pronephros. This begins early in the fourth week after conception when the cells of the future kidney come together in the neck region of the embryo. These cells do not form a functional kidney. This is a brief stage lasting less than a week.

The second stage is the formation of the mesonephros. It begins near the end of the fourth week and produces a large, temporary kidney that produces urine that is released into the amniotic fluid. The final stage involves the formation of the metanephros or mature kidney. The mature kidney forms from a part of the mesonephros (the rest degenerates). Metanephros formation begins at about five weeks after conception. During the next four weeks, the kidneys will develop, move, and rotate until they reach their final position in the abdomen just below the level of the waist. By week 9 the embryo has a functional kidney that produces urine. The urine is released into the amniotic fluid until **birth**. During pregnancy, however, the mother's placenta and kidneys filter out most of the fetal waste products.

At birth, a full-term infant's kidneys weigh about 0.5 ounce (14 g) each. After delivery, the infant's kidneys take over filtering waste products from the blood. Most infants urinate for the first time within 24 hours of birth and between 8 and 20 times or more a day after that. Infants' urine generally ranges from clear to pale yellow in color, although foods, **vitamins**, and even urate (one of the salts contained in the urine) may cause it to change color. The urine of infants under age two has practically no odor. As children age, the urine becomes more concentrated and its odor becomes stronger. Infants and toddlers cannot control urination until the sphincter muscles and the nerves at the base of the bladder are sufficiently developed. This does not occur until at least the age of two. Most children learn to control their bladders during the daytime by the age of three. However, **enuresis** (**bedwetting**) may occur in a healthy child (especially one who is a sound sleeper) until the age of five or six.

Kidney structure and function

The mature kidney consists of two layers of tissue encased in tough connective tissue. The outer layer is the called cortex and the inner layer is called the medulla.

Within the cortex and extending partially into the medulla are about one million tiny filtering units called nephrons. Blood enters the kidney by way of the renal artery at the rate of about 1.5 quarts (1.4 L) per minute. Once in the kidney, it passes through a series of tiny blood vessels called capillaries. Each capillary forms a tangled know called a glomerulus that is closely associated with a single nephron. Waste removal and urine formation then occurs as follows:

- The capillaries forming the glomeruli are separated by only a thin layer of cells from a part of the nephron known as Bowman's capsule. The glomerular capillaries are "leaky" so that blood pressure forces water, sodium ions (salt), potassium ions, amino acids (small proteins), and glucose (sugar) out of the capillaries and into Bowman's capsule. Red blood cells, white blood cells, and large plasma proteins are too big to leave the capillaries.
- The material in Bowman's capsule, called renal filtrate, begins to move along the part of the nephron called the proximal tubule. In the proximal tubule, sodium ions, glucose and about two-thirds of the water in the renal filtrate are reabsorbed into the blood
- The remaining renal filtrate moves on to the part of the nephron called the distal tubule. Here, most of the remaining water is reabsorbed. The amount of water returned to the blood is controlled by the concentration of antidiuretic hormone (ADH) circulating in the blood. The higher the concentration of ADH, the more water is reabsorbed from the distal tubule. The lower the level of ADH, the more water is removed from the body as urine.
- In the distal tubule, certain drugs and hydrogen ions also are secreted into the renal filtrate. The concentration of hydrogen ions in the blood is important because it regulates the acidity of the blood. The blood must remain within a very narrow, stable range of acidity (about pH 7.4) for a person to remain healthy.
- The material that remains in the distal tubules is urine. It enters collecting ducts, which eventually lead to ureters that carry the urine to the bladder where it is stored until it is released into the urethra and exits the body. The urine of a healthy person is about 95% water and 5% waste.

In addition to filtering and cleansing the blood, the kidneys also release three regulatory chemicalsmdash; erythropoietin, renin, and calcitriol—that affect other functions in the body. Erythropoietin stimulates the bone marrow to produce new red blood cells. Renin helps regulate blood pressure, and calcitriol is an active form of vitamin D and is important in maintaining bones and the level of calcium in the body. Any defect in kidney function can have far-reaching effects on other systems in the body.

Common problems

Kidney disease (also called renal disease) is a general term for any damage that reduces the functions of the kidney. Please see the topic urological disorders for a discussion of specific kidney disorders and the tests done to diagnose them. In general, there are three types of common kidney problems.

- Congenital abnormalities are problems in the structure or function of the kidney that are present at birth. Most often they originate during the seventh to ninth week after conception when the kidneys are moving into their permanent position. Congenital abnormalities can range from undetected conditions that cause no symptoms to potentially fatal abnormalities.
- Acute kidney disorders are abrupt and serious disruptions in the function of the kidney. These can be caused by infection, severe blood loss, or trauma to the kidney, as from a motor vehicle accident or sports injury. Kidney stones, caused by mineral deposits in the kidney and ureter, also can cause a painful an acute kidney disorder. Individuals who receive prompt and appropriate medical treatment often recover from acute kidney disorders.
- Chronic kidney disorders are slow to develop, have few symptoms until they are well advanced, and have no cure. Gradually the kidney loses the ability to cleanse the blood and the individual becomes progressively more ill. The only way to maintain health when the kidney fails is through regular dialysis sessions (usually three times a week) or a kidney transplant. Chronic kidney disorders occur mainly in older individuals. Hypertension (high blood pressure) and poorly controlled diabetes are the two main causes of chronic kidney failure. Long-term use of certain drugs (e.g., aspirin, acetaminophen) and exposure to environmental toxins also can contribute to chronic kidney disorders.

Parental concerns

Most parental concerns center on congenital kidney abnormalities. Some children are born with only one kidney (renal agenesis), a condition that poses no health threat as long as the remaining kidney stays healthy. Other children are born with an ectopic, or misplaced, kidney. The kidney often functions normally, although it may cause a malformation of the ureter, obstructing the flow of urine. This usually can be promptly corrected with surgery. In other cases, A two kidneys may be joined, forming a U-shaped structure (horseshoe kidney) that lies lower than the normal position. The joint kidney may or may not act as a single organ. Kidneys may also be underdeveloped (hypoplastic) or develop abnormally (dysplastic), conditions that are not necessarily debilitating if they affect only one kidney. With two hypoplastic kidneys, however, renal failure eventually occurs.

Although people can live normal, healthy lives with a single kidney, parents who have a child with only one healthy kidney may wish to wish to restrict their child's participation in contact **sports** such as football, ice hockey, and rugby or sports such as horseback riding where serious abdominal injury can occur.

KEY TERMS

Electrolyte—Salts and minerals that ionize in body fluids. The major human electrolytes are sodium (Na+), potassium (K+), calcium (Ca 2+), magnesium (Mg2+), chloride (Cl-), phosphate (HPO4 2-), bicarbonate (HCO3-), and sulfate (SO4 2-). Electrolytes control the fluid balance of the body and are important in muscle contraction, energy generation, and almost all major biochemical reactions in the body.

Glomerulus—Derived from a Greek word meaning filter. The glomerulus is a knot of blood vessels that have the job of filtering the blood.

Metabolism—All the physical and chemical changes that occur in cells to allow growth and maintain body functions. These include processes that break down substances to yield energy and processes that build up other substances necessary for life.

Ureter—A tube that carries urine from the kidney to the bladder.

Urethra—The tube that carries urine from the bladder to outside the body.

Resources

BOOKS

Field, Michael J., Carol A. Pollock, and David C. Harris. *The Renal System,* 2nd ed. New York: Churchill Livingstone, 2010.

Townsend, Raymond R. and Debbie L. Cohen. *100 Questions & Answers About Kidney Disease and Hypertension* Sudbury, MA: Jones and Bartlett Publishers, 2009.

OTHER

How Your Kidneys Work. National Kidney Foundation. Undated [accessed September 8, 2010], http://www.kidney.org/kidneydisease/howkidneyswrk.cfm.

The Kidneys and How They Work. National Kidney and Urologic Diseases Clearinghouse. February 2009 [accessed September 8, 2010], http://kidney.niddk.nih.gov/Kudiseases/pubs/yourkidneys.

ORGANIZATIONS

American Board of Urology, 6000 Peter Jefferson Parkway, Suite 150, Charlottesville VA, 22911, (434) 979-0059, (434) 979-0266, http://www.abu.org.

March of Dimes Foundation, 1275 Mamaroneck Avenue, White Plains NY, 10605, (914)997-4488, askus@marchofdimes.com, http://www.marchofdimes.com.

National Kidney Foundation, Inc., 30 East 33rd Street, New York NY, 10016, (212) 889-2210, (800) 622-9010, (212) 689-9261, http://www.kidney.org.

National Kidney and Urologic Disease Information Clearinghouse, 3 Information Way, Bethesda MD, 20892-3580, (800) 891-5390 TTY: (866) 569-1162, (703) 738-4929, nkudic@info.kidney.niddk.nih.gov, http://kidney.niddk.nih.gov.

Tish Davidson, AM

Kleptomania

Definition

Kleptomania is an irresistible urge to steal items of trivial value. The name of the disorder comes from two Greek words meaning "to steal" and "morbid impulse."

Demographics

Kleptomania is a relatively uncommon impulse control disorder; the incidence in the general population is estimated to be 0.6%. Kleptomania can begin at any age, although its onset is typically associated with **puberty**, and is reported to be more common among females. The average age of patients in Canada and the United States diagnosed with the disorder as of 2010 is 35, and the average duration of the disorder is 16 years. Some patients report that the disorder began as early as age 5; however, women usually do not enter treatment for the disorder until their 30s, and men typically are in their 50s when they enter treatment.

Description

Persons with kleptomania experience a recurring and irresistible urge to steal. They do not, however, steal for the value of the item, for its use, or because they cannot afford the purchase. Stolen items are often thrown or given away, returned, or hidden. Kleptomania is distinguished from deliberate theft or shoplifting, in which the individual is motivated by a desire to acquire the item, to seek revenge, or to fulfill a dare from peers. Shoplifting is more common than kleptomania; it is estimated that less than 5% of individuals who shoplift exhibit symptoms of kleptomania.

The most recent (2000) edition of the *Diagnostic and Statistical Manual of Mental Disorders-IV, Text Revision* (also known as the *DSM-IV-TR*) classifies kleptomania as a disorder of impulse control and groups it together with such other behavioral disorders as pathological gambling, **trichotillomania** (hair-pulling), and **pyromania** (fire setting). The tenth edition (2007) of the International Classification of Diseases (ICD-10) classifies kleptomania as a "habit and impulse disorder." Some psychiatrists maintain that kleptomania is related to **obsessive-compulsive disorder** (OCD) and should therefore be considered an obsessive-compulsive spectrum disorder. One problem with this identification, however, is that studies of persons with kleptomania do not show a high rate of comorbidity with OCD (about 6.5%, according to one study), and conversely, persons diagnosed with OCD have low rates of co-occurring kleptomania (2.2–5.9%).

Risk factors

The only known risk factors for kleptomania as of 2010 are **substance abuse**; a diagnosis of paranoid, schizoid, or borderline personality disorder; and a family history of kleptomania, **mood disorders**, or substance abuse. There are a few isolated cases reported of kleptomania being triggered by traumatic brain injury or exposure to high levels of carbon monoxide.

Causes and symptoms

The cause of kleptomania is not known as of 2010. No genes have as yet been identified with susceptibility to the disorder. One theory holds that kleptomania may be linked to abnormally low levels of serotonin, a neurotransmitter that helps to regulate mood. Another theory maintains that kleptomania is related to various substance and behavioral addictions.

The symptoms of kleptomania are outlined in the *DSM-IV* diagnostic criteria described below.

Diagnosis

The diagnosis of kleptomania is based on the patient's history and the diagnostic criteria of the disorder as given in *DSM-IV*:

- The patient recurrently fails to resist impulses to steal objects that are not needed for personal use or monetary value.

KEY TERMS

Comorbidity—The presence of one or more additional diseases or disorders in a patient diagnosed with a primary disorder.

Mental status examination (MSE)—A structured way of observing a patient's state of mind in the course of an office interview that takes into account such factors as mood, insight, judgment, ability to reason, as well as general appearance and tone of voice.

Neurotransmitter—Any of several chemicals secreted in the brain that serve to transmit nerve impulses from one neuron to another.

- The patient feels a rising sense of tension immediately before stealing the item.
- The patient experiences gratification, relief, or pleasure at the time of the theft.
- The patient is not experiencing delusions or hallucinations, and is not stealing as an act of revenge or anger.
- The stealing is not better accounted for by a conduct disorder, a manic episode, or antisocial personality disorder.

Examination

The doctor may administer a mental status examination (MSE) to rule out the possibility that the patient is suffering from delusions, hallucinations, thought disorders, or drug or alcohol intoxication at the time of the interview.

Tests

There are no laboratory or imaging tests as of 2010 that can be used to diagnose kleptomania.

Treatment

It is important for persons with kleptomania to obtain a definite diagnosis and seek treatment as soon as possible. One reason is that the sense of shame associated with impulsive **stealing** can lead to such other mental disorders as depression, **eating disorders**, compulsive shopping or gambling, and substance abuse. Another important reason is that kleptomania is one of the **impulse control disorders** that can lead to arrest and involvement with the criminal justice system.

There is no standard course of treatment for kleptomania as of 2010. Some doctors recommend a combination of psychotherapy, medication, and support groups. The most common form of psychotherapy used in patients with kleptomania is **cognitive-behavioral therapy** or CBT. CBT works by teaching patients to identify destructive and unhealthy thoughts and behaviors and replace them with healthy ones. CBT techniques that can be applied to patients with kleptomania include aversion therapy, in which the patient is taught to perform a mildly uncomfortable action (like breath-holding or digging a fingernail into the palm) when confronted with the urge to steal; and covert sensitization, in which the patient is asked to imagine negative consequences for the stealing, such as being arrested or losing a job.

Some patients with kleptomania are apparently helped by Twelve-Step programs, even when there is not one in their area dealing specifically with kleptomania. Alcoholics Anonymous, Gamblers Anonymous, and similar programs can be helpful in tackling the addictive dimension of kleptomania.

Drugs

Several different types of drugs have been tried as therapy for patients with kleptomania. They include the selective serotonin reuptake inhibitors (Prozac, Paxil); benzodiazepines (tranquilizers, including Xanax and Klonopin); antiseizure drugs (Depakene, Topamax); lithium and other mood stabilizers; and naltrexone (Revia), an **addiction** medication that appears to reduce the urges associated with addictive behaviors like stealing.

The drawbacks of medication therapy for kleptomania include the fact that almost all these drugs have side effects; some, like the benzodiazepines, are habit-forming; and some interact with alcohol or other prescription medications. In addition, there are relatively few studies of the effectiveness of drug therapy in treating kleptomania. As of 2010, there is only one clinical trial of drug therapy for kleptomania under way—a study of memantine, a drug currently used to treat Alzheimer's disease.

Prognosis

Kleptomania is generally considered a difficult disorder to treat, in part because there is no standard therapy, as described above. Relapses are common and the disorder can last for years.

Prevention

There are no known ways to prevent kleptomania as of 2010 because the causes of the disorder are not yet understood.

Resources

BOOKS

Aboujaoude, Elias, and Lorrin M. Koran. *Impulse Control Disorders*. New York: Cambridge University Press, 2010.

Abramowitz, Jonathan S., Dean McKay, and Steven Taylor, eds. *Clinical Handbook of Obsessive-Compulsive Disorder and Related Problems*. Baltimore, MD: Johns Hopkins University Press, 2008.

Adamec, Christine. *Impulse Control Disorders*. New York: Chelsea House, 2008.

American Psychiatric Association. *Diagnostic and Statistical Manual of Mental Disorders*. 4th ed., Text rev. Washington, D.C.: American Psychiatric Association, 2000.

PERIODICALS

Bohne, A. "Impulse-control Disorders in College Students." *Psychiatry Research* 176 (March 30, 2010): 91–92.

Bonfanti, A.B., and E.M. Gatto. "Kleptomania, An Unusual Impulsive Control Disorder in Parkinson's Disease?" *Parkinsonism and Related Disorders* 16 (June 2010): 358–59.

Dick, D.M., et al. "Understanding the Construct of Impulsivity and Its Relationship to Alcohol Use Disorders." *Addiction Biology* 15 (April 2010): 217–26.

Wetterneck, C.T., et al. "Current Issues in the Treatment of OC-Spectrum Conditions." *Bulletin of the Menninger Clinic* 74 (Spring 2010): 141–66.

OTHER

Mayo Clinic. *Kleptomania*, October 30, 2009, http://www.mayoclinic.com/ [accessed December 2010].

Menaster, Michael. "Psychiatric Illness Associated with Criminality." *eMedicine*, May 18, 2010, http://emedicine.medscape.com/article/294626-overview [accessed December 2010].

ORGANIZATIONS

American Psychiatric Association, 1000 Wilson Boulevard, Suite 1825, Arlington VA, 22209-3901, (703) 907-7300, apa@psych.org, http://www.psych.org/.

National Alliance on Mental Illness (NAMI), 2107 Wilson Blvd., Suite 300, Arlington VA, 22201-3042, (703) 524-7600, Hotline: (800) 950-NAMI (6264), (703) 524-9094, http://www.nami.org/Hometemplate.cfm.

National Institute of Mental Health (NIMH), 6001 Executive Boulevard, Room 8184, MSC 9663, Bethesda MD, 20892-9663, (301) 443-4513, (866) 615-6464, (301) 443-4279, nimhinfo@nih.gov, http://www.nimh.nih.gov/index.shtml.

Rebecca J. Frey, PhD

Klinefelter syndrome

Definition

Klinefelter syndrome is a chromosomal disorder that affects only males. People with this condition are born with at least one extra X chromosome. The syndrome was first identified and described in 1942 by Harry Fitch Klinefelter, Jr., an American physician.

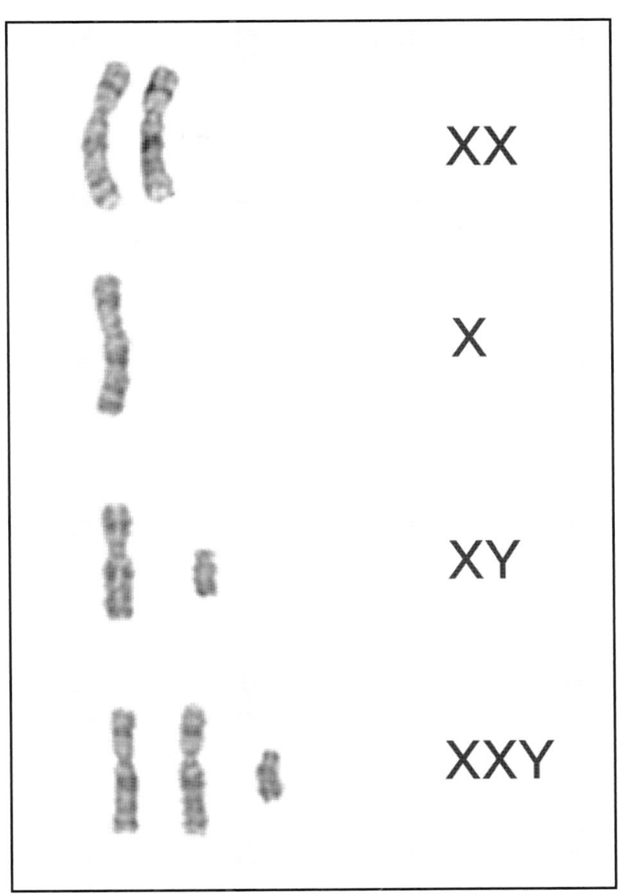

Sex chromosomes showing different phenotypes: XX, normal female; X, female with Turner syndrome; XY, normal male; and XXY, male with Klinefelter. *(Illustration by Argosy, Inc. Reproduced by permission of Gale, a part of Cengage Learning.)*

Description

Klinefelter syndrome is a condition in which one or more extra X chromosomes are present in a male. Boys with this condition appear normal at **birth**. They enter **puberty** normally, but by mid puberty have low levels of testosterone causing small testicles and the inability to make sperm. Affected males may also have learning disabilities and behavior problems such as **shyness** and immaturity, and an increased risk for certain other health problems.

Klinefelter syndrome is one of the most common chromosomal abnormalities. About 1 in every 500–800 males is born with this disorder; approximately 3,000 affected boys are born each year in the United States.

About 3% of the infertile male population have Klinefelter syndrome. The condition appears to affect all racial and ethnic groups equally.

Causes and symptoms

Chromosomes are found in the cells in the body. Chromosomes contain genes, structures that tell the body how to grow and develop. Chromosomes are responsible for passing on hereditary traits from parents to child. Chromosomes also determine whether the child will be male or female. Normally, a person has a total of 46 chromosomes in each cell, two of which are responsible for determining that individual's sex. These two sex chromosomes are called X and Y. The combination of these two types of chromosomes determines the sex of a child. Females have two X chromosomes (the XX combination); males have one X and one Y chromosome (the XY combination).

In Klinefelter syndrome, a problem very early in development results in an abnormal number of chromosomes. About 60% of embryos with Klinefelter syndrome do not survive the fetal period. Most commonly, a male with Klinefelter syndrome will be born with 47 chromosomes in each cell, rather than the normal number of 46. The extra chromosome is an X chromosome. This means that rather than having the normal XY combination, the male has an XXY combination. Because people with Klinefelter syndrome have a Y chromosome, they are all male.

Approximately 1/3 of all males with Klinefelter syndrome have other chromosomal abnormalities involving an extra X chromosome. Mosaic Klinefelter syndrome occurs when some of the cells in the body have an extra X chromosome and the others have normal male chromosomes. These males can have the same or milder symptoms than non-mosaic Klinefelter syndrome. Males with more than one additional extra X chromosome, such as 48,XXXY, are usually more severely affected than males with 47,XXY.

Klinefelter syndrome is not considered an inherited condition. The risk of Klinefelter syndrome reoccurring in another pregnancy is not increased above the general population risk.

The symptoms of Klinefelter syndrome are variable and not every affected person will have all of the features of the condition. Males with Klinefelter syndrome appear normal at birth and have normal male genitalia. From childhood, males with Klinefelter syndrome are taller than average with long limbs. Approximately 20–50% have a mild intention tremor, an uncontrolled shaking. Many males with Klinefelter syndrome have poor upper body strength and can be clumsy. Klinefelter syndrome does not cause **homosexuality**. Approximately 1/3 of males with Klinefelter syndrome have gynecomastia or breast growth, some requiring breast reduction surgery.

Most boys enter puberty normally, though some can be delayed. The Leydig cells in the testicles usually produce testosterone. With Klinefelter syndrome, the Leydig cells fail to work properly causing the testosterone production to slow. By mid-puberty, testosterone production is decreased to approximately half of normal. This can lead to decreased facial and pubic hair growth. The decreased testosterone also causes an increase in two other hormones, follicle stimulating hormone (FSH) and luteinizing hormone (LH). Normally, FSH and LH help the immature sperm cells grow and develop. In Klinefelter syndrome, there are few or no sperm cells. The increased amount of FSH and LH causes hyalinization and fibrosis, the growth of excess fibrous tissue, in the seminiferous tubules, where the sperm are normally located. As a result, the testicles appear smaller and firmer than normal. With rare exception, men with Klinefelter syndrome are infertile because they can not make sperm.

While it was once believed that all boys with Klinefelter syndrome are mentally retarded, doctors now know that the disorder can exist without retardation. However, children with Klinefelter syndrome frequently have difficulty with language, including learning to speak, read, and write. Approximately 50% of males with Klinefelter syndrome are dyslexic.

Some people with Klinefelter syndrome have difficulty with social skills and tend to be more shy, anxious, or immature than their peers. They can also have poor judgment and do not handle stressful situations well. As a result, they often do not feel comfortable in large social gatherings. Some people with Klinefelter syndrome can also have **anxiety**, nervousness and/or depression.

The greater the number of X chromosomes present, the greater the disability; each extra X chromosome lowers the child's **IQ** by about 15 points. Boys with several extra X chromosomes have distinctive facial features, more severe retardation, deformities of bony structures, and even more disordered development of male features.

Diagnosis

Diagnosis of Klinefelter syndrome is made by examining chromosomes for evidence of more than one X chromosome present in a male. This can be done in pregnancy with prenatal testing such as a chorionic villus sampling or **amniocentesis**. Chorionic villus sampling is a procedure done early in pregnancy (approximately 10–12 weeks) to obtain a small sample of the placenta for testing. An amniocentesis is done further along in pregnancy (from approximately 16–18 weeks) to obtain a sample of fluid surrounding the baby for testing. Both procedures have a risk of miscarriage. Usually these procedures are done for a reason other than diagnosing Klinefelter syndrome. For example, a prenatal diagnostic procedure may be done on an older woman to determine if her baby has **Down syndrome**. If the diagnosis of Klinefelter syndrome is suspected in a young boy or adult male, chromosome testing can also be on a small blood or skin sample after birth.

Many men with Klinefelter syndrome go through life without being diagnosed. The two most common complaints leading to diagnosis of the condition are gynecomastia and infertility.

Treatment

Children with Klinefelter syndrome may benefit from **speech therapy** for speech problems or other educational interventions for learning disabilities. Testosterone injections started around the time of puberty may help to produce more normal development including more muscle mass, hair growth and increased sex drive. Testosterone supplementation will not increase testicular size, decrease breast growth or correct infertility. Psychiatric consultation may be helpful when the boy reaches **adolescence**.

Some doctors recommend mastectomy as a surgical treatment for gynecomastia, on the grounds that the enlarged breasts are often socially stressful for affected males and significantly increase their risk of breast **cancer**.

Prognosis

While many men with Klinefelter syndrome go on to live normal lives, nearly 100% of these men will be sterile (unable to produce a child). However, a few men with Klinefelter syndrome have been reported who have fathered a child through the use of assisted fertility services.

Males with Klinefelter syndrome have an increased risk of several systemic conditions, including **epilepsy**, osteoporosis, such **autoimmune disorders** as lupus and arthritis, diabetes, and breast and **germ cell tumors**. One Danish study reported in 2004 that men with Klinefelter's syndrome have a slightly shortened life span, dying about 2.1 years earlier than men without the syndrome.

KEY TERMS

Chromosome—A microscopic thread-like structure found within each cell of the body and consists of a complex of proteins and DNA. Humans have 46 chromosomes arranged into 23 pairs. Changes in either the total number of chromosomes or their shape and size (structure) may lead to physical or mental abnormalities.

Gonadotrophin—Hormones that stimulate the ovary and testicles.

Gynecomastia—Excessive growth of breast tissue in males.

Leydig cells—Cells that make up the endocrine tissue of the testis and produce testosterone. They are named for Franz von Leydig (1821–1908), the German professor of anatomy who first identified them.

Testosterone—Hormone produced in the testicles that is involved in male secondary sex characteristics.

Resources

BOOKS

Beers, Mark H., MD, and Robert Berkow, MD., editors. "Chromosomal Abnormalities." In *The Merck Manual of Diagnosis and Therapy*. 18th ed., Whitehouse Station, NJ: Merck Research Laboratories, 2006.

Beers, Mark H., MD, and Robert Berkow, MD., editors. "Infertility." In *The Merck Manual of Diagnosis and Therapy*. 18th ed., Whitehouse Station, NJ: Merck Research Laboratories, 2006.

Probasco, Teri, and Gretchen A. Gibbs. *Klinefelter Syndrome*. Richmond, IN: Prinit Press, 1999.

PERIODICALS

Bojesen, A., S. Juul, N. Birkebaek, and C. H. Gravholt. "Increased Mortality in Klinefelter Syndrome." *Journal of Clinical Endocrinology and Metabolism* 89 (August 2004): 3830–3834.

Chen, Harold, MD. "Klinefelter Syndrome." *eMedicine* December 17, 2004. http://emedicine.com/ped/topic1252.htm.

Diamond, M., and L. A. Watson. "Androgen Insensitivity Syndrome and Klinefelter's Syndrome: Sex and Gender Considerations." *Child and Adolescent Psychiatric Clinics of North America* 13 (July 2004): 623–640.

Grosso, S., M. A. Farnetani, R. M. Di Bartolo, et al. "Electroencephalographic and Epileptic Patterns in X Chromosome Anomalies." *Journal of Clinical Neurophysiology* 21 (July-August 2004): 249–253.

Lanfranco, F., A. Kamischke, M. Zitzmann, and E. Nieschlag. "Klinefelter's Syndrome." *Lancet* 364 (July 17, 2004): 273–283.

Tyler, C., and J. C. Edman. "Down Syndrome, Turner Syndrome, and Klinefelter Syndrome: Primary Care throughout the Life Span." *Primary Care* 31 (September 2004): 627–648.

OTHER

Klinefelter Syndrome Support Group Home Page, http://klinefeltersyndrome.org/index.html.

ORGANIZATIONS

Klinefelter's Organization, PO Box 60, OrpingtonUK, BR68ZQ, http://hometown.aol.com/KSCUK/index.htm.

Klinefelter Syndrome and Associates, Inc, PO Box 119, Roseville CA, 95678-0119, (916) 773-2999, (916) 773-1449 (888) 999-9428, ksinfo@genetic.org, http://www.genetic.org/ks.

National Organization for Rare Disorders (NORD), 55 Kenosia Avenue, PO Box 1968, Danbury CT, 06813-1968, (203) 744-0100, (800) 999-6673, http://www.rarediseases.org.

Carin Lea Beltz, MS
Rebecca J. Frey, PhD

Knee injuries

Definition

The knee joint consists of bone, ligaments, cartilage, and fluid. It moves with the help of surrounding muscles and tendons. When any of these structures is degraded, the knee can become injured. According to the Mayo Clinic, nearly one out of three Americans older than 45 years of age have some type of knee **pain**. Whether it is a minor or major problem, it usually involves a certain amount of pain and a degree of difficulty in walking.

The five most common knee problems are arthritis, tendonitis, **bruises**, cartilage tears, and damaged ligaments, with arthritis being the most common problem of the bones of the knee. The ligaments and tendons of the knee can also become injured. Damage to the anterior cruciate ligament (ACL) is a common problem of knee ligaments and tendons. Knee injuries can be caused by accidents, impacts and other such traumas, sudden or awkward movements (misalignments), and gradual wear and tear of the knee joint (degeneration).

Most injuries of the knee are minor and are usually treated at home with rest and ice packs. Serious injuries necessitate treatments by physicians and rehabilitation experts. Often, various types of surgeries are needed to correct the worst knee injuries such as a ruptured ligament or tendon.

Demographics

Because the knee joint is both vulnerable and used extensively in many activities, it is prone to injuries in all peoples young and old. The American Academy of Orthopaedic Surgeons (AAOS) estimates that approximately nine million American adults are diagnosed with knee osteoarthritis each year. Osteoarthritis of the knee is deterioration (degradation) of the knee joint. Over half of all people with knee osteoarthritis were over the age of 65 years. The AAOS states that knee osteoarthritis is a leading cause of disability in the United States. In some **sports** including football, skiing, gymnastics, and racket sports, injury rates to avid practitioners can be nearly 50%, and knee injuries are the most common reason patients visit orthopedic doctors. An estimated one in five runners gets a knee injury at some point in their lives. The majority of knee injuries, however, are minor and do not require intensive treatment.

Description

The knee, the largest joint in the body, connects the thighbone (femur) to the lower leg (tibia). It is a complex and efficient joint consisting of ligaments, cartilage, and the bone of the kneecap (patella). All of these parts can be injured. Inside the knee joint is synovial fluid that protects and lubricates the parts, which may increase as the result of an injury, causing swelling. The bursa are sacs in the knee that contain synovial fluid and provide cushioning and lubrication.

Four ligaments comprise the knee joint. The medial collateral ligament (MCL) runs along the inside of the knee, while the lateral collateral ligament (LCL) is on the outside of the knee. The cruciate ligaments cross inside the knee. The anterior cruciate ligament (ACL) is deep inside the knee and limits rotation of the joint. The posterior cruciate ligament (PCL) is also inside the knee and limits the backward movement of the joint. Ligaments in the knee can be partially or completely torn, depending on the extent of the injury.

The minisci cartilage are two thin, oval-shaped tissues that act as cushions between the ends of the leg bones. The medial miniscus is the cartilage closest to the other leg while the lateral miniscus is nearer the outside of the knee. Injuries to the minisci include tears from injuries and impact and degenerative wearing away of the structure. The minisci can be partially or completely torn during injury.

The bones around the knee, including the kneecap, can be broken, fractured, or chipped. The patellar tendon connects the kneecap to the shinbone, while the quadriceps tendon connects the quadriceps muscle to the patella. The patellar tendon can be torn or can develop injury and pain from degeneration. It can also be fully dislocated or partially dislocated (called subluxation). The tendons in the knee may develop pain and inflammation known as tendonitis.

The bones of the knee joint are covered with tissue known as articular cartilage. This cartilage can be injured or fractured, and can also develop a degenerative condition called chondromalacia. Osteoarthritis is the condition associated with the wearing down of this cartilage.

There are many risks that increase one's chance of having a knee injury. These risks include:

- Excessive weight, being obese, because of the additional weight being carried in part by the knees.
- Sports and activities that are considered high risk for knee injuries, such as basketball, racquetball, downhill skiing, and tennis.
- Overuse, repeated activities can lead to fatigue in the muscles around the joints and contribute to tissue damage.
- Neuromuscular abnormalities, such as different lengths for legs and misaligned knees, can increase the likelihood of knee injuries.
- Muscle inflexibility and weakness provides less support for the knee and adds to more stress placed upon the knees.
- Previous injuries to the knee make is more likely that future knee injuries will occur.
- Gender increases the likelihood of certain types of knee problems; that is, males are more likely to have some knee problems (such as a dislocated kneecap), while females are more likely to have others (such as Osgood-Schlatter disease).
- Age increases the likelihood of more knee problems.

Causes and symptoms

Knee injuries are commonly caused by the following: impact (such as from an accident, landing after a fall, and a blow from an object), repeated stress/overuse, sudden motion (excessive turning, pivoting, or stopping), rapidly growing bones, and age-related degeneration.

There are many specific causes of knee injuries. Arthritis may develop from an autoimmune disorder, known as rheumatoid arthritis, or may be caused by the gradual wear and tear of the joint, known as osteoarthritis. Symptoms of arthritis in the knee include pain ranging from dull aches to severe pain, and may be accompanied by swelling and range of movement loss. Arthritic symptoms may tend to be worst in the morning and decrease throughout the day as the knee is used. Arthritis can be caused by lupus, **Lyme disease**, and other infections.

Hyperextended knee can occur when the knee is extended beyond its normal range. When this happens the knee bends back on itself, which usually causes minor damage, along with pain and swelling. However, hyperextended knee can also cause a partial or complete tear in a ligament, which produces more problems. Then the patella, the bone that covers the front of the knee, is dislodged from its normal position, so a dislocated kneecap can occur. The kneecap will look obviously out of place, and it can even be moved from side to side with ease. Symptoms of a hyperextended knee include swelling, intense pain, problems straightening the knee, and difficulty walking.

Cartilage injuries may include chondromalacia, with symptoms including dull pain at any time and more intense pain while climbing stairs. Damage to the minisci cartilage often occurs from sudden twists, forceful plants, and awkward movements. (The meniscus is a C-shaped piece of cartilage that curves inside of the knee joint.) A torn cartilage may make a popping sound, and may be accompanied by mild to severe pain, particularly while straightening the leg. Swelling, stiffening, and loss of movement are also symptoms of cartilage tears, as are clicking sounds and friction in the knee during movement. A knee suffering from a cartilage injury may become completely immobile.

Ligament injuries, which produces immediate pain when it occurs, may cause dull or severe pain, swelling, loss of the range of movement of the joint, and loss of the stability and strength of the knee. Ligament injuries typically occur from strong blows and forces applied to the knee. Injuries to the MCL are the most common, often caused by impact to the side of the knee joint. Of the cruciate ligaments, the PCL is less commonly injured than the ACL. Typically, forceful blows to the knee, such as during car accidents, injure the PCL, while the ACL can be injured by impacts and by sudden twists. Torn ligaments may be accompanied by a popping sound indicating the rupture, and may not always cause pain, so that some of them go unnoticed. Torn ligaments may weaken the knee and cause buckling or folding under weight.

Tendon injuries range from tendonitis to torn tendons. Symptoms of tendonitis include pain that worsens when movement occurs such as running or climbing, irritation, inflammation, inability to completely extend or straighten the knee, and swelling (especially in the front of the knee or just below the kneecap), while ruptured tendons can cause more intense pain, swelling, and loss of movement.

Osgood-Shlatter disease is a condition common in young boys and girls who play running and jumping sports. Symptoms include swelling, tenderness of the tibial tuberosity located below the kneecap, and inflammation of the patellar tendon and pain in the front of the knee during and after strenuous activity.

Iliotibial band syndrome is common in running and other repetitive sports, characterized by a sharp, burning pain at the outer side of the knee caused by stress on the band of tendons there. Sometimes this condition causes a snapping sensation when the knee is straightened. Long-distance runners are especially susceptible to illiotibial band syndrome. The pain usually goes away when at rest after running but returns when climbing occurs. Swelling usually does not occur with this problem and normal range of motion within the knee is usually present.

Bursitis is a problem caused by inflammation in the bursa, or the small fluid sacs that cushion the outside of the knee joint. Symptoms of bursitis include redness, swelling, constant pain, stiffness or aching while walking, and added pain when climbing. Infection may also occur within the bursae, which can cause **fever**, and additional pain and swelling.

Diagnosis

Depending on the severity of the condition, family physicians or orthopedic physicians who specialize in the knee joint may be consulted. A complete physical examination will be performed, along with a comprehensive review of past medical records. If arthritis is suspected, a rheumatologist may be consulted. The diagnostic process includes taking a complete patient history with details of the pain and the circumstances of the injury. During a physical exam, the doctor will specifically include several manual techniques of moving the knee joint and legs in various positions to help determine the type of injury. An experienced practitioner can often make an accurate diagnosis of injuries by performing a sequence of manual diagnostic tests.

Laboratory tests may be ordered to further or clarify the diagnosis. **X rays** can show damage to the bones as well as the narrowing of the knee space that may imply cartilage problems. For more in-depth diagnosis, a computerized axial tomographic (**CAT**) scan is an x-ray technique that can provide three-dimensional views of the bones in the knee. A **magnetic resonance imaging** (MRI) scan gives a computerized portrait of the interior of the knee, and may show damage to the ligaments and cartilage. Arthroscopy is a form of minor surgery in which a tiny camera is inserted into the knee, giving a very accurate view of the joint. Radionuclide scanning (bone scans) use radioactive material injected into the bloodstream to monitor the blood flow in particular areas. If infection or rheumatoid arthritis is suspected, a physician may order blood tests for diagnosis. Biopsies, in which pieces of tissue are laboratory tested, may also be used for diagnosis.

Treatment

When a person suspects a knee injury, the first treatment recommended by the Mayo Clinic is a process called P.R.I.C.E., that stands for protection, rest, ice, compression, and elevation. First, the person should "protect" the knee from further motion by using a wrap that immobilizes the knee and/or crutches or braces if necessary. Then, cease the activity that caused the injury and immediately "rest" and immobilize the joint. "Ice" may be applied to reduce pain and swelling, and "compression", such as wraps and braces, may be used to immobilize the knee. "Elevating" the leg is also helpful in reducing swelling and aiding circulation. Immediate care will prevent the worsening of the injury.

Generally, pain relievers such as nonsteroidal anti-inflammatory drugs (NSAIDs) can be used. They include aspirin, ibuprofen (such as Advil), and naproxen (such as Aleve). Physical therapy may also be necessary so that the knee regains is normal movement.

Treatment options for knee injuries can range from rest and light activity, to physical therapy, to surgery. Most knee injuries are treated with proper rest, **exercise**, and strengthening programs recommended by physicians. For injuries that require surgery or deeper diagnosis, arthroscopy is the least invasive technique and involves a short recovery time. Arthroscopy is commonly used to repair cartilage and partially torn ligaments. For severe knee injuries, reconstructive surgery or open knee surgery may be required. Full knee replacements may also be performed for severely damaged knees. After surgery, physical therapy programs for rehabilitation are recommended. Treatment for osteoarthritis includes over-the-counter painkillers, exercise, and weight reduction. For rheumatoid arthritis, more powerful prescription medications, such as **steroids** and stronger painkillers, and intensive physical therapy may be ordered. Knee injuries associated with infection may require **antibiotics**.

Alternative treatment

Alternative therapies for knee injuries focus on supporting the body's ability to heal itself. Various therapies may include bodywork and postural adjustments such as chiropractic and Rolfing work, in addition

KEY TERMS

Lupus—Chronic inflammatory disease caused by immune system disorder.

Lyme disease—Bacterial infection spread by ticks.

Orthopedist—Physician specializing in the diagnosis and treatment of problems involving the skeletal system.

Rheumatologist—Physician specializing in the diagnosis and treatment of arthritis and related conditions.

to physical therapy and gentle exercise routines. Herbal remedies and nutritional supplements may be used to aid the healing process and reduce symptoms. Acupuncture may be used for pain relief, and **yoga** is a low-impact exercise routine that increases flexibility, good alignment, and strength.

Prevention

The best prevention for knee injuries is being aware of activities that carry high risks for knee injuries and acting carefully. The knees can be strengthened by evenly building the muscles in the quadriceps and hamstrings. Increasing flexibility in the body through stretching can also help reduce injuries. Properly fitting shoes and other sports equipment are essential for preventing injury as well. Finally, before engaging in activities that stress the knee, a thorough and gradual warm-up routine, including aerobic activity and stretching, will lessen the chances of knee injury.

General lifestyle habits are also recommended to reduce the risk for knee injuries. These include maintaining a health height-to-weight ratio (commonly called the body mass index); exercising on a regular basis (to keep the knees and the surrounding materials strong and flexible); warming up before exercising and cooling down after exercising; not over exercising the knees if they are hurting; and using protective devices when involved in high-risk sports (such as knee pads in basketball). It is also important to wear a seat belt and harness while driving because kneecap injuries are common when automobiles crash into other cars and objects along the road.

Resources

BOOKS

Miller, Mark D., Jennifer A. Hart, and John M. MacKnight, editors. *Essential Orthopaedics.* Philadelphia: Saunders/Elsevier, 2010.

Noyes, Frank R., and Sue D. Barber-Westin, editors. *Noyes' Knee Disorders: Surgery, Rehabilitation, Clinical Outcomes.* Philadelphia: Saunders/Elsevier, 2010.

Starkey, Chad, Sara D. Brown, and Jeffrey L. Ryan. *Examination of Orthopedic and Athletic Injuries.* Philadelphia: F. A. Davis, 2010.

OTHER

"Knee and Leg." American Academy of Orthopaedic Surgeons, http://orthoinfo.aaos.org/menus/leg.cfm (accessed September 6, 2010).

"Knee Injuries and Disorders." Medline Plus, National Library of Medicine and National Institutes of Health. (March 1, 2010), http://www.nlm.nih.gov/medlineplus/kneeinjuries anddisorders.html (accessed September 6, 2010).

"Knee Osteoarthritis Statistics." American Academy of Orthopaedic Surgeons. (October 2009), http://orthoinfo.aaos.org/topic.cfm?topic=A00399 (accessed September 6, 2010).

"Knee Pain." Mayo Clinic. (September 9, 2008), http://www.mayoclinic.com/health/knee-pain/DS00555 (accessed September 6, 2010).

"Save Your Knees." American Academy of Orthopaedic Surgeons, http://www.saveyourknees.org (accessed September 6, 2010).

ORGANIZATIONS

American Academy of Orthopaedic Surgeons, 6300 North River Rd., Rosemont IL, 60018-4262, (847) 823-7186, (800) 824-BONE (2663), (847) 823-8125, http://www.aaos.org/.

National Athletic Trainers' Association, 2952 Stemmons Fwy., Suite 200, Dallas TX, 75247, (214) 637-6282, (214) 637-2206, http://www.nata.org.

American Physical Therapy Association, 1111 North Fairfax St., Alexandria VA, 22314–1488, (703) 684-APTA (2782), (800) 999-2782, (703) 684-7343, http://www.apta.org.

Douglas Dupler

Kohlberg's theory of moral reasoning

Definition

Theory featuring six stages of **moral development** advanced by American psychologist Lawrence Kohlberg.

Description

Lawrence Kohlberg (1927–1987), an American psychologist, pioneered the study of moral development in the late 1950s. Kohlberg's theory of moral reasoning involved six stages through which each person passes in order, without skipping a stage or reversing their order.

His theory states that not all people progress through all six stages.

In the 1950s, science as a whole held to the positivist belief that scientific study should be free of moral values, maintaining instead a purely "objective," value-free stance. Western psychology at that time was dominated by behaviorists who focused on behavior rather than reasoning or will. In 1958, Lawrence Kohlberg published a study that broke with both the positivists and behaviorists by presenting a theory of moral development (bringing together science and moral values) based on cognitive reasoning rather than behavior. Kohlberg's theory initiated an entirely new field of study in Western science that gained momentum in the 1960s and 1970s and continues to inspire new research today.

Kohlberg's theory of moral development expands upon Jean Piaget's work in the 1930s concerning cognitive reasoning. Piaget proposed three *phases* of **cognitive development** through which people pass in a loose order. In contrast, Kohlberg posited six *stages* (in three levels, with two stages each) of moral development, based on cognitive reasoning, through which each person passes in unvarying and irreversible order. According to Kohlberg, every person begins at Stage 1 moral reasoning and develops progressively to Stage 2, then Stage 3, etc. Not everyone makes it through all six stages; in fact, people who use Stage 5 or 6 moral reasoning are quite rare. Kohlberg claimed that his stages of moral development are universal, applying equally to all human beings across cultural divisions.

In brief, Kohlberg's theory of moral development presents three levels: the preconventional, conventional, and postconventional. Each level contains two stages. Stages 1 and 2 in the preconventional level involve an "egocentric point of view" and a "concrete individualistic perspective" in which the person makes choices based on the idea of punishment. In stage 1 the knowledge that a person would be punished for a certain action is used as evidence of that action's wrongness. In stage 2 different viewpoints are recognized as being possible, and the punishment is just something to be avoided. In Stages 3 and 4 of the conventional level, persons make choices from a "member-of-society" perspective, considering the good of others, the maintenance of positive relations, and the rules of society. In stage 3 the motivations behind actions are considered of primary importance, and positive motivations are often what define good behavior. In stage 4 the person is concerned more with upholding the law for the good of society than of the good of individual people. Persons in the final stages of the postconventional level, Stages 5 and 6, reason from a "prior-to-society" perspective in which abstract ideals take precedence over particular societal laws. A stage 5 person spends more time thinking about what a society should be like, and what laws make a society a good one, than just the idea that all laws should be upheld. In stage 6 a person would believe that there is such a thing as universal justice that can be more important than anything and applies to all people equally.

To measure the level at which persons are operating morally, Kohlberg developed a highly refined interview process in which hypothetical situations are presented that involve a moral dilemma. The person's answers to questions surrounding that dilemma determine the stage at which he or she is reasoning. One of the best-known examples of hypothetical moral dilemmas presented in Kohlberg's interview is that of an impoverished man who needs a certain medicine for his wife who is ill: is the man justified in **stealing** the medicine from the pharmacy when he does not have enough money to pay for it? Why or why not? The details of the hypothetical situation can then be altered slightly to bring out the nuances of a person's moral reasoning (e.g., does it depend on how ill the wife is, how poor the husband is, whether it is a small, family-owned corner drugstore or a large, nationwide chain, etc.).

Kohlberg also developed a method of moral education based on an expanded form of the interview process. He believed that participation in moral discussions spurs growth in moral reasoning. The "just community" approach to education that Kohlberg helped create has three basic aims: 1) to encourage moral development through discussions of moral issues; 2) to develop a culture of moral norms through community-building and the democratic establishment of rules; and 3) to create a context where students and teachers can *act* on their moral decisions. Just Community programs were put into effect in a number of public schools, with a fair amount of success (see Power, Higgins, and Kohlberg 1989).

However, there have been many criticisms of Kohlberg's theory of moral development and his methods. Some critics claim that the use of hypothetical situations skews the results because it measures abstract rather than concrete reasoning. When children (and some adults) are presented with situations out of their immediate experience, they turn to rules they have learned from external authorities for answers, rather than to their own internal voice. Therefore, young children base their answers on rules of "right" and "wrong" they have learned from parents and teachers (Stages 1 and 2 according to Kohlberg's theory). If young children are presented with situations familiar to them, on the other hand, they often show care and concern for others, basing their moral choices on the desire to share the good and maintain harmonious relations, placing them in Stage 3 or 4 (which Kohlberg claimed was not possible at their age).

Kohlberg's emphasis on abstract reasoning also creates confusing results in which habitual juvenile delinquents can score at a higher stage of moral development than well-behaved children. Because behaviors are not considered and reasoning is determined through hypothetical situations, children who behave in immoral ways may be able to answer hypothetical moral dilemmas in a more advanced fashion than better-behaved children who think less abstractly. Early criticisms of Kohlberg's lack of attention to behaviors led Kohlberg to add an emphasis on moral action to his Just Community educational program. For those who are looking for concrete help in developing moral values in children, however, Kohlberg's theory is still of little practical use.

Another strong criticism of Kohlberg's theory is that it devalues the morality of care and community. Carol Gilligan was the first to attack this aspect of Kohlberg's theory, relating it to gender differences between men and women (all of Kohlberg's original subjects were male, as was Kohlberg himself). Although Gilligan's critique has weaknesses of its own, her assessment of Kohlberg's theory as incomplete has many supporters, though others relate the absence of communitarian morality to class rather than gender differences.

Kohlberg, as a member of the educated, elite, white, male, Western culture, viewed individual autonomy and justice as the premier moral values. He even went so far as to equate morality with justice (ignoring other moral values such as courage, self-control, empathy, etc.). Members of the working and rural classes, however, tend to have a more communitarian approach to life, viewing the common good as the highest value, promoting care and harmonious relationships over individual justice. (Women, having been relegated to "lower class" status for centuries, may have developed a more communitarian approach to life for that reason, rather than simply because they are female.) Non-Western and tribal societies also frequently see the community as more important than the individual.

According to Kohlberg's upper-class Western view of moral reasoning, communitarian morality is doomed to rest forever at a lower stage of development (Stages 3 and 4). This view disregards the possibility that communitarian morality may be as advanced as individualistic morality, if not more so. It also places Western culture at the top of the scale, with little room for cross-cultural inclusion. Although Kohlberg insisted that his theory was culturally inclusive, he found little empirical evidence to back this up. In all of his interviews, only a few people showed Stage 5 reasoning, and nearly all were well-educated Westerners. Stage 6 reasoning was never substantiated conclusively in interviews; Kohlberg created it more as an "ideal" and pointed to examples such as Gandhi and the Reverend Martin Luther King Jr. to support its existence. After a tremendous amount of criticism over the fact that Stage 6 was purely hypothetical, Kohlberg removed it from the empirical stages but retained it as a "theoretical construct in the realm of philosophical speculation." Despite equally heavy criticism, Kohlberg refused to remove Stage 5 from his system.

With all its possible flaws, however, Kohlberg's theory of moral development was the first of its kind and remains the springboard for subsequent research into moral reasoning. Critiques of Kohlberg's theory have led, and continue to lead, to more expansive and inclusive understandings of the development of moral reasoning. Kohlberg's Just Community program also yielded significant results and led to the ongoing creation of other similar alternative education programs.

Resources

BOOKS

Kohlberg, Lawrence. *Child Psychology and Childhood Education: A Cognitive-Developmental View.* New York: Longman, 1987.

Kohlberg, Lawrence. *Essays on Moral Development, I: The Philosophy of Moral Development: Moral Stages and the Idea of Justice.* San Francisco: Harper & Row, 1981.

Kohlberg, Lawrence. *Essays on Moral Development, II: The Psychology of Moral Development.* San Francisco: Harper & Row, 1984.

Elliot, Deni. *Ethics in the First Person: A Guide to Teaching and Learning Practical Ethics.* Lanham, MD: Rowman & Littlefield Publishers, 2007.

Killen, Melanie and Judith G. Smetana. *Handbook of Moral Development.* Mahwah, NJ: Lawrence Erlbaum Associates, 2006.

Lapsley, Daniel K. and Darcia Narvaez. *Moral Development, Self, and Identity.* Mahwah, NJ: Lawrence Erlbaum Associates, 2004.

Moore, Diane. *Parenting the Heart of Your Child.* Minneapolis, MN: Bethany House Publishers, 2005.

Pass, Susan. *Parallel Paths to Constructivism: Jean Piaget and Lev Vygotsky.* Greenwich: CT, 2004.

Dianne K. Daeg de Mott

Kohs block design test

Description

The Kohs Block Design Test is a cognitive test for children or adults with a mental age between 3 and 19. It was designed by Samuel C. Kohs (1890–1984), a sociologist, in 1923. The test is mainly used to assess the intelligence of persons with language or hearing handicaps but also given to disadvantaged and non-English-speaking children. The child is shown 17 cards with a variety of colored designs and asked to reproduce them using a set of 16 colored cubes. The administrator's instructions can be given in pantomime, which is why the test can be given to deaf children or those with little command of English. The Kohs test, which requires about 40 minutes to complete, is regarded as a more accurate measure of intelligence than the Binet and other verbal tests because the results are less likely to be influenced by school training. Performance **assessment** is based not just on the accuracy of the **drawings** but also on the examiner's observation of the child's behavior during the test, including such factors as attention level, self-criticism, and adaptive behavior (such as self-help, communication, and social skills). The Kohs Block Design Test is sometimes included in a battery of such other tests as the Merrill-Palmer and Arthur Performance scales.

Since the mid-1980's two versions of the Kohs test have been designed for persons with visual impairments and upper limb disabilities respectively. The Ohwaki-Kohs Tactile Block Design Test for the Blind, which is sometimes called the Adapted Kohs Block Design Test, is considered to have the same reliability as a measure of intelligence as the original version. In 1997, a group of Japanese rehabilitation specialists designed a software program for use by persons whose impairments of arm, hand, or finger function make it difficult for them to lift, move, and reposition the cubes used in the Kohs test. The software program displays all six surfaces of each block, which allows the test subject to "rotate" the block on the computer screen and select one of the six surfaces.

Resources

BOOKS

McCullough, Virginia. *Testing and Your Child: What You Should Know About 150 of the Most Common Medical, Educational, and Psychological Tests.* New York: Plume, 1992.

Walsh, W. Bruce, and Nancy E. Betz. *Tests and Assessment.*, 4th ed. Upper Saddle River, NJ: Prentice Hall, 2001.

PERIODICALS

Brand, H. J., M. J. Pieterse, and M. Frost. "Reliability and Validity of the Ohwaki-Kohs Tactile Block Design Test for the Blind." *Psychological Reports* 58 (April 1986): 375–380.

Reid, Juliet M. V. "Testing Nonverbal Intelligence of Working-Age Visually Impaired Adults: Evaluation of the Adapted Kohs Block Design Test." *Journal of Visual Impairment and Blindness* 96 (August 2002): 585–595.

ORGANIZATIONS

Stoelting Company [publisher of the Kohs test] , 620 Wheat Lane, Wood Dale IL, 60191, (630) 860-9700, http://www.stoeltingco.com.

Kwashiorkor *see* Protein-energy malnutrition